CHILDHOOD LANGUAGE DISORDERS IN CONTEXT: INFANCY THROUGH ADOLESCENCE

SECOND EDITION

NICKOLA WOLF NELSON
WESTERN MICHIGAN UNIVERSITY

ALLYN AND BACON
Boston   London   Toronto   Sydney   Tokyo   Singapore

To my parents,
Betty Anderson Wolf
and the memory of Lawrence Winton Wolf,
who provided the context for developing roots and wings,

And to my grandmothers,
Marjorie Waggoner Anderson,
who showed that education is where you find it,
and the memory of
Pauline Keimig Wolf,
who first made me think I could write

Executive Editor: Stephen D. Dragin
Editorial Assistant: Elizabeth McGuire
Editorial-Production Administrator: Joe Sweeney
Editorial-Production Service: Walsh & Associates, Inc.
Composition Buyer: Linda Cox
Manufacturing Buyer: Megan Cochran

Copyright © 1998, 1993 by Allyn & Bacon
A Viacom Company
160 Gould Street
Needham Heights, MA 02194

Internet: www.abacon.com
America Online: keyword: College Online

Library of Congress Cataloging-in-Publication Data
Nelson, Nickola.
      Childhood language disorders in context : infancy through
adolescence / Nickola Wolf Nelson. — 2nd ed.
            p.   cm.
      Includes bibliographical references.
      ISBN 0-205-19787-6
      1. Language disorders in children.   2. Language disorders in
adolescence.   I. Title.
RJ496.L35N46   1998
618.92'855—dc21   97-32508
                                                                              CIP

Printed in the United States of America
10 9 8 7 6 5 4 3 2   02 01 00 99

Photo Credits
pp. 5, 23, 40, 94, 151, 182, 231, 288, 344, 385, 427, 491, John Cosby.

CONTENTS

This book is for children with language disorders. Although the immediate audience comprises graduate students and upper-level undergraduate students preparing to serve children with language disorders, ultimately the book is for the children themselves.

As a textbook it will be more accessible to students who have some background in linguistics and in normal and disordered language acquisition. Although the book is introductory in breadth, it covers many issues with relative depth. I am a speech–language pathologist, and I have used the book primarily with classes of graduate students in speech–language pathology. I have also taught courses that included graduate students in special education, and I have included some background material with those students in mind (particularly Chapter 2 and parenthetical explanations of terminology). I hope that the book will be useful to practicing professionals and to parents as well. My experiences with them have certainly helped me write it.

THE CENTRAL FOCUS

The book's central focus is the development of language and communication. It is not about a particular kind of child; it is about all kinds of children at all ability levels and ages from infancy through adolescence. The common factor is their difficulty in learning to communicate with language. That is not to say that the conditions that put children at risk for normal language learning are not important. I believe that they are, and the reader will find an etiological thread regarding theories about causes throughout the book. However, the book's ultimate purpose—and the primary reason for considering the nature of language disorders—is to find ways to facilitate language learning when it does not proceed naturally. In fulfilling this purpose, the book focuses on communicative meanings, forms, and interactions that arise in the course of normal development from infancy through adolescence. It focuses secondarily on the causative conditions likely to limit that development.

PART ONE: TAKING A BROAD VIEW OF LANGUAGE-LEARNING SYSTEMS

A variety of pathways may be taken to facilitate positive change in language-learning systems. Viewed comprehensively, a language-learning system includes not only the developing skills, knowledge, and biological systems that children bring to the task, but also the contexts and communicative partners that contribute to the acquisition process.

Part One addresses these issues from varied perspectives. Chapter 1 sets the stage by presenting the conceptual framework for the book. It introduces the theme that *problems are not just within children, and neither are the solutions.* Readers are urged to ask insightful questions not only about children's language abilities and impairments, but also about the communicative needs and opportunities that arise in the important contexts of children's lives.

Chapter 2 provides background information about language, speech, and communication. Multidisciplinary perspectives are introduced, and language, speech, and communication are defined. I emphasize the strong links among the three systems but also present evidence for their relative separability and argue for considering each during language assessment and intervention. Nonlinguistic and paralinguistic communication are also reviewed, as are the five systems of language—phonology, morphology, syntax, semantics, and pragmatics. Issues on bilingualism and dialect difference are introduced.

Because issues related to bilingualism and dialect difference cannot be isolated from broader issues of language learning and education, neither are they isolated in a single chapter of this book. Although most examples illustrate the acquisition of standard American English, this bit of ethnocentricity is countered by equal emphasis on the need for multicultural sensitivity. To exhibit multicultural sensitivity, language specialists must appreciate the richness of cultural variation, be familiar with language systems other than standard English, and recognize the need for modified language assessment and intervention strategies for children from varied language-learning communities. Guidance on such issues is provided throughout the book.

Chapter 3 introduces six theoretical perspectives that explain language acquisition alternatively by emphasizing biological maturation, linguistic rule induction, behaviorism, information processing, cognitivism, and social interaction. Whether it is clearly recognized, one or more theoretical perspectives always guide language assessment and intervention practices. Even when a professional does not custom design a program but "buys" a ready-made approach, that professional is assuming that the theoretical basis of the "store-bought" approach is consistent with the child's needs. This may be the case. The position taken here, however, is that professionals must make choices that are deliberate and individualized in the context of collaborative interactions with others who know the child well and that are not based on chance, dogma, or prepackaged decision making.

Chapter 4 provides an overview of causes, categories, and contributing factors, including a discussion of the value of categorization. Causative conditions associated with language disorders are presented under three main headings: (1) central processing factors, (2) peripheral sensory and motor system factors, and (3) environmental and emotional system factors. Central processing categories include specific language disability, mental retardation, autism, attention-deficit hyperactivity disorder, and acquired brain injury. Peripheral sensory and motor system categories include hearing impairment, visual impairment, and physical impairment. Environmental and emotional system categories include neglect and abuse and behavioral and emotional development problems. Mixed factors are also considered. Within each category, I present the available evidence for subtypes and for differentiating language disorder from delay, referring to the six theories introduced in Chapter 3. Diagnostic features associated with categorical conditions are summarized in boxes. Chapter 4 concludes with a section on prevention.

Chapter 5 addresses the relationship between public policy and service delivery. As a result of federal mandates, individuals employed in school settings and other public agencies bear a major responsibility for language intervention with children. The text therefore emphasizes information about Public Laws 94–142, 99–457, 101–476, and 105–17, now known collectively as the Individuals with Disabilities Education Act (IDEA). Chapter 5 also provides general information about service delivery settings, people, and scheduling.

Chapter 6 concludes Part One with an overview of issues related directly to language assessment and intervention. The chapter begins with a flowchart outlining decisions from the point a problem is suspected until a child or adolescent no longer needs special services. Assessment and intervention are not viewed as separate, but as highly integrated processes. The remaining sections of the chapter extend discussions related to the assessment issues of team process—diagnosing disorder, determining eligibility for service, establishing prognosis, and outlining parameters of impairment, functional limitation, and disability. The sections on intervention address processes for selecting goal areas and gathering baseline data, designing and implementing intervention plans, monitoring progress, using exit criteria, and judging program accountability.

PART TWO: BALANCING AGES AND DEVELOPMENTAL STAGES

Part Two is organized developmentally into three pairs of chapters addressing assessment and intervention during early, middle, and later stages of development. Chapter 13 addresses assessment and intervention for individuals with severe communication impairments. Historically, a developmental focus too often has meant that professionals have attempted to measure a child's current level of functioning relative to quantitative norms for variables such as vocabulary size and mean length of utterance. Based on such standards, programs have been devised and implemented, often in separate, specialized settings, to teach children discrete language structures that normally developing children would learn at about the same stage. Aspects of this approach are still pertinent, but the narrowness of its focus has been recognized, and it is now being replaced by more comprehensive approaches and a broader perspective of "normal." Newer strategies are based on greater collaboration among family members and multidisciplinary professionals, a view of the language learner as a whole person, and recognition of the rights and needs of children to participate in activities with their same-age, normal-learning peers.

Although individual differences are emphasized, general descriptions of normal development nevertheless remain helpful templates for guiding selection of intervention targets, strategies, and contexts when language development is impaired. Part Two therefore provides perspectives from normal development as the dominant but not the only focus. Chapters 7 and 8 examine expectations for the early developmental stages, which include infancy through toddlerhood; Chapters 9 and 10 address the middle developmental stages, which include preschool through early elementary years starting with three-word utterances and going through grade three; and Chapters 11 and 12 address the later developmental stages, which include middle elementary through later adolescent years. Chapters 7, 9, and 11 are organized with parallel structure addressing two issues: (1) the identification of children needing intervention and (2) the commonly used tools and strategies for measuring the needs and abilities for each stage. Chapters 8, 10, and 12 address methods and targets of intervention for individuals at those stages of development. Objectives and outcome statements are provided for major goal areas. Chapter 13 addresses the needs of children, adolescents, and young adults who are at middle or later stages chronologically, but at earlier stages developmentally. It also addresses the needs of individuals with severe speech impairments whose cognitive and linguistic skills are commensurate with their chronological ages. In this way, a balance between consideration of ages and developmental stages is maintained.

Throughout the book, "facts," theories, issues, and clinical experience are combined to help current and future professionals contemplate the relationships between their own organized thoughts (theories) and actions (interventions) regarding language disorders in children. I believe that such a combination is the one most likely to generate positive and productive change in the lives of children with language disorders and their families. That is the ultimate goal of this book.

SPECIAL FEATURES

A few special features have been included to make the text more readable and applicable. Sprinkled throughout are individuals' personal reflections relevant to service provision to children with language disorders. These encourage readers to think about the body of knowledge related to language disorders in children as dynamic, shaped by the people who have studied it. The personal reflections also introduce meaningful statements from workers in related fields—parents, teachers, and children. In addition, I use case examples liberally to integrate theory and basic information with application. Some illustrate a major point and are more fully developed. Others illustrate minor points and are less fully developed.

Finally, pedagogical tools are provided to help readers organize their approach to the text, to raise issues for discussion, and to provide guidance to further resources. These include outlines of main topics and guiding questions at the beginning of sections within chapters. In addition to traditional tables and figures, boxes and appendices summarize key points and present data for organizing assessment and intervention. Each chapter ends with a summary and with review points and questions. Activities for extended thinking are also suggested. Chapter appendices provide bibliographies of formal tests for early, middle, and later stages to augment the discussions of informal assessment techniques highlighted in the chapters. The appendices to Chapter 13 summarize developmental information in the four domains—cognitive underpinnings, receptive language, expressive language, and social interaction and play. They can be used to assist in making placement and programming decisions for children with severe disabilities. Appendices for Chapter 9 present the scoring criteria for Developmental Sentence Scoring (Lee, 1974) and Black English Sentence Scoring (Nelson & Hyter, 1990a, 1990b). Course instructors should also request the accompanying instructor's manual, which includes practice exercises for these procedures.

Nothing is sacred about reading the chapters of this book in order. Although there is some logic to this order and some cross-referencing of information, alternative approaches are equally appropriate. Readers who are already familiar with aspects of language, speech, and communication may wish to skim Chapter 2. Readers seeking information on a specific developmental stage may start with Chapter 7, 9, or 11. Readers less concerned about public policy may skip Chapter 5 or save it until last.

ACKNOWLEDGMENTS

Completing this second edition brings a flood of feelings almost as intense as with the first. Relief is again high among them, as well as a sense of connectedness with the individuals who responded so positively to the first edition and gave me encouragement for writing the second.

Steve Dragin is the editor at Allyn and Bacon who has prodded and fostered its completion. Kathy Whittier was a wonderful chief copyeditor and indexer for Walsh & Associates, Inc. I am also still indebted to the reviewers for the first edition—Lynn S. Bliss, Wayne State University; Cheryl D. Gunter, Iowa State University; Mareile Koenig, West Chester University; Marilyn A. Nippold, University of Oregon; Kenneth G. Shipley, California State University–Fresno; and Carol Stoel-Gammon, University of Washington—who read outlines and early drafts, wrote words of criticism, praise, and encouragement, and saved me from a few embarrassing mistakes. I also appreciate the input of the reviewers for the second edition: Mona R. Griffer, Nova Southeastern University; Celeste Roseberry-McKibbin, California State University-Fresno; and Debra Reichert Hoge, Southern Illinois University at Edwardsville.

Another part of the cast is the set of colleagues and close friends known to me but who are too broad a group to name in full. They listened to me gripe and wax enthusiastic; shared their libraries, references, and prepublication copies of their work; took my phone calls at all hours; stimulated my thinking; and made me look at old ideas in new ways. You will recognize some of them from the impact they had on the ideas represented in this book. I have tried to give them scholarly credit, but I also want them to feel my personal appreciation for making this project a lot more fun. I particularly appreciate those who provided specific suggestions for improving the second edition, including (alphabetically) David Beukelman, Bonnie Brinton, Kay Butler, Kathy Coufal, David Ertmer, Martin Fujiki, Diane German, Barbara Hoskins, Alan Kamhi, Mabel Rice, Rosalind Scudder, Elaine Silliman, Sandra Tattershall, and Steve Warren. In addition, I paid close attention to the anonymous reviews gathered by my former editor, Anne Castel Davis.

A third set of active participants is the group of my own graduate students and other anonymous students who have provided critical feedback. They continue to be sitting with me as the primary audience when I write.

A number of former students made significant contributions to the book content and to my understandings of childhood language disorders as well. Their names appear with their contributions throughout the book. Not fully acknowledged are the equally important contributions of graduate student trainees for Project Collaborate (Grant No. HO2910245) and Project Connect (Grant No. HO29B40183), the two personnel preparation projects in which we have experimented with new ideas and learned from the perspectives of our clients. Two graduate assistants have played major roles in preparing the manuscript for the second edition. Rachel Hauser served as copymeister and did original work updating the chapter appendices on formal tests. She also went through the entire manuscript *twice* performing reference checks, earning her the title of reference-meister as well. Nicole McDonnell carefully proofread early drafts of chapters, checked the references, and made savvy suggestions for edits and additions. With Shannon Kersten, Nicole McDonnell assumed major responsibility for updating the instructor's manual, which was prepared for the first edition by Kelly Wenzler. Carrie McCarter-Barnes and Sue Eberstein pitched in in the final stages of manuscript preparation and transmission. They all have my most heartfelt appreciation.

In this second edition, as in the first, I acknowledge and try to be true to the legacy of Charles Van Riper, who sadly, no longer lives down his lane, but continues to inspire me to remember that I am writing about people for people, including those "in the trenches." Finally, I acknowledge those who are closest to me in the writing process, my family and my Western Michigan University and local colleagues—Mick Hanley, in his role of understanding department chair; Michael Clark, as personnel preparation grant project co-director; also Jan Bedrosian and Adelia Van Meter, as fellow travelers in the world of language intervention and research; as well as colleagues from across campus, Constance Weaver and Kathryn Kinnucan-Welsch, who keep me attuned to general education issues; and special education colleagues, Christine Bahr, project co-director for research on Linking Text Processing Tools to Student Needs (Grant No. H180G20005) and Barbara Harris and Patricia Williams, who have worked closely on our collaborative summer program activities. Adelia particularly, thank you. I appreciate the support of the U.S. Department of Education for the aforementioned federal projects too. The contents of the book, however, do not reflect the policy or views of the department, and no official endorsement should be inferred.

Between the first and second editions, my three children, David, Nicky, and Clayton, became adults and left home, but they still have been aware of just what chapter Mom was working on. It has been a lot more quiet writing this edition, except for the wonderful little voices of four-year-old Jessica and two-year-old Justin. I can't say they make writing any easier, but they do make life more interesting—as does Larry. Thanks for doing the cooking.

PART ONE

Viewing Childhood Language Disorders from Varied Perspectives

Part I lays the foundation for understanding the needs of children with language disorders. The dominant perspective is developmental, in preparation for the second part of the book, which is organized into chapters covering early, middle, and later stages of language learning, as well as severe communication impairment. The developmental perspective, however, is only one of several that can be used when working with children with language disorders.

Other perspectives considered in Part I relate to general concerns that extend across developmental ages and stages. Chapter 1 builds a basic framework for working with children with language disorders and their families and teachers. It introduces the importance of asking questions and presents a framework of questions to address the needs of these children. The traditional question about *impairment,* "What is wrong with the way this person processes language?" should be supplemented by questions about *functional limitations* (formerly called *disability*), "What does this person need to do to succeed in this particular context?" and *disability* (formerly called *handicap*), "What opportunities does the person have to participate in desired contexts?" (Beukelman & Mirenda, 1992).

The focus on contextually based need is important for exceeding the limitations of strictly developmental approaches for assessment and treatment. This focus is part of treating these children as members of whole systems, rather than fragmenting them into a collection of separable parts. The "fragmentation fallacy" (Damico, 1988) is one of several potential problems that language specialists should avoid. Others, also suggested by Damico and considered in Chapter 1, are therapist bias, acquiescence, lack of follow-up, and negative effects of bureaucratic policies and procedures.

Strategies for avoiding these mistakes are suggested, using **system theory** as a general framework and tools borrowed from several other disciplines. **Ecological thinking,** borrowed from biology, is critical for understanding the contextual nature of change and the interactive influences at all levels of environmental and biological systems. **Phenomenology,** borrowed from philosophy, is critical for understanding the relativity of truth and the influence of observational perspectives and tools on how truth is perceived by different observers of the same event or person. **Collaborative consultation** and **cooperative goal setting,** borrowed from educational theorists and group managers, are critical tools for creating change within larger systems. **Ethnographic methodology,** borrowed from anthropologists, is critical for understanding a culture, whether an ethnic group or an elementary school

1

classroom, through the eyes of its participants. These tools provide a framework for considering the information about childhood language disorders in the rest of the book.

Chapter 2 addresses questions about multidisciplinary perspectives on language, speech, and communication. The strong linkages among them are stressed, but evidence of some degree of isolation of each is presented as well. This chapter suggests that professionals should be clear about the relative impairment and retention of speech, language, and communication variables when working with children with language disorders. Chapter 2 reviews basic organizational principles about language rule systems and nonlinguistic and paralinguistic communicative features. The reviews summarize key aspects of systems that children must learn to become competent communicators; later chapters consider evidence about what can go wrong with those systems. Because not all children learn the same language, speech, and communication systems, issues of dialect and language differences are also considered here. Summaries of key features follow in the areas of phonology, morphology, syntax, semantics, and pragmatics, plus traditional methods for measuring knowledge of linguistic rule systems. Here, the key distinction is between naturalistic methods that assess **intrinsic knowledge** of linguistic rules, by inferring regularities based on observable evidence such as spontaneous language samples, and controlled methods that assess **metalinguistic knowledge,** by asking individuals to reflect on and to talk about language. Chapter 2 also provides an overview of sociolinguistic contributions related to the importance of context, reasons for communicating, and cultural variation in discourse interactions.

Chapter 3 explores varied developmental perspectives in preparation for considering multiple aspects of assessment and intervention services for children with language disorders. Contributions from six theoretical perspectives (and limitations) are considered: (1) **biological maturation,** (2) **linguistic rule induction,** (3) **behaviorism,** (4) **information processing,** (5) **cognitivism,** and (6) **social interaction.**

Chapter 4 explores categorical views of childhood language disorders. This is a touchy area because there are advantages and disadvantages to applying labels to problems. Labels can stereotype children and can seem to reduce the need for individualization. Labels do not always accurately predict an individual child's language abilities and needs, and care must be taken so that labels do not function as blinders. On the other hand, knowledge of labels, and the causative conditions they represent, can open doors to past learning about those conditions and can even reduce the likelihood of repeating previous mistakes.

The categorical system used in Chapter 4 is divided into three major sections: (1) central factors, (2) peripheral factors, and (3) environmental–emotional factors. The first grouping includes **specific language disability** (including conditions labeled as specific language impairment, learning disabilities and dyslexia), **mental retardation, attention-deficit hyperactive disorder,** and **acquired brain injury.** The second grouping includes **hearing, visual,** and **physical impairments.** The third grouping includes **child neglect and abuse** and **behavioral–emotional impairment.** Mixed factors are also considered.

Chapter 5 addresses questions about public policy and service delivery. The public policy sections are based on laws and regulations in the United States related to service provision in schools. The service-delivery system is divided into federal, state, intermediate, and local levels. I recognize that readers from other countries and nonschool settings must learn about different public policy systems that apply to them; perhaps the public policy portion of this chapter will provide a framework for doing so, even if it does not apply directly to everyone's needs. The second part of Chapter 5 is a more generic discussion of service-delivery variables and it is divided into three major sections: (1) setting, (2) people, and (3) scheduling. Preferences of children and their parents regarding service-delivery decisions are also considered.

The final chapter in Part I, Chapter 6, overviews factors related to assessment and intervention. It starts with a decision-making flowchart (Figure 6.1) that characterizes the major stages in providing services to children and a sequence of questions asked from the time concern is voiced until the child appears no longer to need special services. The remainder of the chapter describes procedures to implement assessment and intervention as integrated processes. Assessment topics include using team process and assessment activities to diagnose disorder, to determine eligibility for service, and to establish prognosis. Intervention topics include selecting goal areas and gathering baseline data, designing and implementing an intervention plan, monitoring progress during intervention, using exit criteria to determine when to quit, and judging program accountability.

Part I sets the stage for Part II, which considers early, middle, and later stage language disorders, as well as the unique needs of individuals with severe language impairments. The questions and information in Part I are intended to assist readers to develop rich perspectives for looking at developmental needs in Part II. Both parts are designed to encourage an appreciation of the guiding principle of this book: *Problems are not just within children—and neither are their solutions.*

1

A Framework

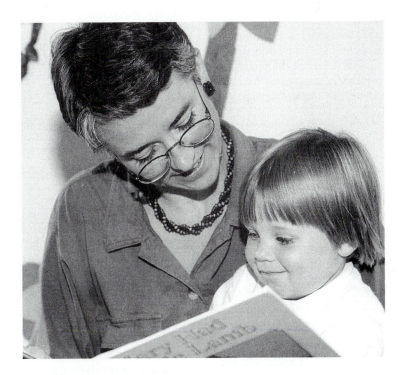

THE IMPORTANCE OF ASKING QUESTIONS

THE PURPOSE OF LANGUAGE INTERVENTION

THE FOREST AND THE TREES PROBLEM (AND HOW TO AVOID IT)

BALANCING AGES AND DEVELOPMENTAL STAGES

STRATEGIES FOR CHANGING SYSTEMS

5

THE IMPORTANCE OF ASKING QUESTIONS

This is a book about childhood language disorders. It is designed to help readers: (1) understand the conditions and symptoms associated with disordered language development, (2) appreciate how language disorders affect the lives of infants, children, adolescents, and their families, and (3) develop assessment, intervention, and collaboration skills for assisting children and their families and teachers to improve those lives. Collaboration relies more on asking good questions than having all the answers.

Questions Reduce Information Anxiety

Wurman's (1989) words, "My expertise has always been my ignorance" (p. 53) (see Personal Reflection 1.1), suggest a strategy for managing complex information. This is sage advice in this era of information explosion, when computers and the information highway keep us busy reading, transmitting, and storing all kinds of information. The best human recourse, in such an overwhelming world, is not to try to act as data banks for mountains of facts, but as framers of relevant questions for organizing knowledge and facilitating further learning.

Questions Guide Scientists, Teachers, and Clinicians

Asking good questions is a key both to science and to clinical practice. Information can be found in books, and research assistants can be hired to gather data, but scientists only make truly new discoveries when they ask questions that lead to new insights. The same is true of good clinicians and teachers. Good questions permit

PERSONAL REFLECTION 1.1 _____

"My expertise has always been my ignorance, my admission and acceptance of not knowing. My work comes from questions, not from answers" (p. 53).

"By giving yourself permission not to know, you can overcome the fear that your ignorance will be discovered. The inquisitiveness essential to learning thrives on transcending this fear" (p. 54).

Richard Saul Wurman (1989), author of the book *Information Anxiety.*

selection of appropriate procedures, tools, and contexts for assessment and intervention. Rather than thinking of education or treatment as what *they* do, such professionals focus on child-centered questions such as: "What is important for the children to know? How will I help them learn it? Are they getting it? What parts are still confusing to them? Does it matter? In what contexts does it matter?" Effective teachers and clinicians view themselves not as transferring information or "getting through" a set of material, but as helping individuals develop new knowledge, skills, and strategies (see Personal Reflection 1.2).

Questions Scaffold Language Acquisition and Intervention Across the Age Span

Intervention involves facilitating others to ask good questions as well. With strategic questions and cues, the language interventionist builds a **scaffold,** much as a painter or bricklayer does, to help students see new relationships, to expect that even complex language should make sense, and to reach higher levels of competence. The concept of **scaffolding** comes from the literature on language acquisition in infancy and early childhood (Bruner, 1975, 1977; Cazden, 1983) where language is largely embedded in the meaningful contexts of personal, familiar events. Parents scaffold their infants' and toddlers' understanding by drawing their attention to key features and patterns in "joint referencing" interactions (Bruner, 1975, 1978). That is, parents find the focus of their children's attention and use language and gestures to segment the experiences into meaningful elements within their children's range of understanding, helping them to understand more and to say more than they could independently:

PARENT: Oh, did you get an owie?
CHILD: Door.
PARENT: Did that door hit your toe?
CHILD: Door unh toe.

PERSONAL REFLECTION 1.2 _____

"Teaching is not telling. Being told is not being taught."

David Johnson (1989), who with his brother, Roger, has been a primary contributor to the development of cooperative learning strategies (e.g., D. W. Johnson & Johnson, 1975).

Questions Guide Metacognitive, Strategic Thinking for Older Children and Adolescents

Adults who work with school-age children adapt the techniques of scaffolding within the context of individualized instruction (Cazden, 1983; Wood, Bruner, & Ross, 1976; Wood, Wood, & Middleton, 1978). In the school-age years, most children, including those with language disorders, have already cracked the basic linguistic code, but need to develop their language for new and more sophisticated purposes (Nippold, 1988b).

School-age children and adolescents become independent when they begin to ask themselves guiding questions. The independent older child or adolescent has internalized such questions as: "What am I supposed to do here? Does this make sense? What does this mean? How does this work? Am I doing this right? Can I do this better? How is this organized? What happens next?"

Questioning and self-talk foster metacognition. **Metacognition** is a conscious awareness of the thinking process (discussed further in Chapter 12). It allows students to acquire deliberate **strategies** for guiding their own attention and learning processes.

STUDENT (**reading a story she's been writing**): *She saw her. She went with her friends.*

INSTRUCTOR: I like what you added to your story. I'm just a little confused about who this "she" is? (pointing to pronoun with unclear referent)

STUDENT: That's Sheila, and that's Nadia. I guess I better put their names in my story.

INSTRUCTOR: Great idea.

Instructors can help build scaffolds, but should avoid making students dependent on them. Dismantling metacognitive scaffolds involves teaching such self-questioning as "Is my story clear?" When we work with school-age students in our university clinic, we talk directly about the "question transplant operation," which involves moving the questions from our brains to theirs ("kind of like 'Frankenstein,' " I tell them, "but not quite"). Then we encourage them to use their own **thinking language,** also called **self-talk** or **think alouds.**

Questions Underlie Early Sensemaking

The ability to direct one's own attention with questions is clearly important to school-age children and adolescents attempting to compete academically. But what about young children or individuals with severe disabilities who

PERSONAL REFLECTION 1.3 _____

"Attention is perhaps best conceptualized as questions being asked by the brain, and our perceptions are what the brain decides must be the answers."

Frank Smith (1975, p. 28).

have difficulty grasping concepts of cognitive self-control or forming linguistically oriented questions? For them as well, it is helpful to think of **attention** as "questions asked by the brain" (in the words of psycholinguist Frank Smith in Personal Reflection 1.3).

Consider the infant just beginning to make sense of the world. When a baby begins to pay attention to sounds, such as someone entering the house, it is as if the baby is thinking, "What is that? Isn't that something pleasant? Is that my daddy? Is that my mommy?" In the early phases of learning, such attention-directing "questions" are not linguistic, but they may become so as the scaffolding parent or day-care worker asks, "Ooh, who's coming? Is that mommy?" Sensemaking by young children depends on recognition of familiar events guided by the internalized questions of natural curiosity. The act of weaving them into organized cognitive perceptions occurs when scaffolding is provided by supportive adults.

This alternative view of attention helps clinicians understand why the old therapy technique of prompting children to "look at me" (for tangible reinforcement) was never enough. The mere *appearance* of attention might orient children to a stimulus, but it is not the same as the focused attention that children demonstrate when they *want* to see something to make sense of the world.

THE PURPOSE OF LANGUAGE INTERVENTION

Perhaps most important is the question of purpose— "What am I trying to accomplish here?" It should never be far from the language interventionist's mind. Although the ultimate purpose of language intervention may be to facilitate normal functioning, that is not always possible. Some children have severely impaired biological and neurological systems that will never support the development of normal language functioning.

The statement of purpose in Box 1.1 represents an attempt to focus on both change and relevance within the three communicative contexts—**social, educational,** and **vocational** (or avocational). Change is central to the

Box 1.1 _____

The Purpose of Language Intervention

To bring about change in the communicative systems of individuals, and in the important communicative contexts of their lives, that are relevant to their needs for

- Social appropriateness, acceptance, and closeness
- Formal and informal learning
- Gainful occupation (whether paid or unpaid)

_____

process and should be measured in systematic ways relevant to the person's needs. The questions directing the therapeutic process then shift from "What am I going to do today with this person?" to "What needs to change if life is to improve for this person?" The process is also tempered by the question, "What can be changed?"

In addition, it is important to keep in mind the communicative contexts in which change is needed.

THE FOREST AND THE TREES PROBLEM (AND HOW TO AVOID IT)

This keeps clinicians from losing sight of the forest for the trees. That is, clinicians can easily become so absorbed in "fixing" isolated language and speech behaviors that they lose sight of the whole picture. This is the danger when using a traditional approach to analyze a person's linguistic skills and then to design intervention activities for missing or delayed skills. Beukelman and Mirenda (1988, 1992) called this assessment approach the **communication processes model** and contrasted it with two other models, a **communication needs model** and a **communication opportunities model.** Avoiding the forest and the trees problem requires all three of these models. Each asks a different critical question and each is uniquely related to reducing a different level of concern: **impairment, functional limitation,** or **disability.** (see Box 1.2).

Communication Processes Model— Reducing Impairment

In the communication processes model (Beukelman & Mirenda, 1988), the primary question is "What is wrong *within* the individual?" This model is designed to ask questions about impairment.

Impairment, as currently defined by the community of international disability specialists (Pope & Tarlov, 1991), is the *loss or abnormality of mental, emotional, physiological, or anatomical structure or function* (see Box 1.2). The communication processes model focuses on reducing impairment. Essentially, the questions asked when implementing the communication processes model are, "What is wrong here?" and "Can it be fixed?"

Related questions that should be asked when using a communication processes model is, "What is right with this individual?" "What strengths does this person have that can help the intervention work?"

The communication processes model is the one most frequently used in providing traditional intervention services. It is an approach in which an individual's language skills are analyzed as relatively separate components— usually, **phonology, morphology, syntax, semantics,** and **pragmatics,** often with controlled standardized tests. The problem with such an approach is that, rather than simply controlling contextual variables, an entirely new context is introduced that is unlike any natural context (see Personal Reflection 1.4).

When they recognize the importance of context, language specialists may be more likely to see impaired communicative processes as the outcomes of interactions between internal systems and external contextual expectations. Children may appear more or less impaired depending on the nature of a particular task and the current environmental support. The key question of this approach then becomes, "What is wrong (and right) with this child's communicative processes in these varied contexts?" (see Personal Reflection 1.5)

A modified version of the communication processes model might avoid the problem of splintering language processes artificially and studying them in isolated contexts, but alone, it is not enough. It misses a perspective provided by the communication needs model.

Personal Reflection 1.4 _____

"As theorists and researchers, we tend to behave as if context were the enemy of understanding rather than the resource for understanding which it is in our everyday lives."

Elliot G. Mishler (1979, p. 2), Harvard Medical School.

_____

Box 1.2 _____

Two Frameworks for Organizing Concepts about Disability
(Based on Pope & Tarlov, 1991)

THE WORLD HEALTH ORGANIZATION'S (WHO) INTERNATIONAL CLASSIFICATION OF IMPAIRMENTS, DISABILITIES, AND HANDICAPS (ICIDH)

The first system was proposed by members of the WHO (see Frey, 1984; Wood, 1980) as a trial supplement to the International Classification of Diseases. It includes four basic concepts: **disease, impairment, disability,** and **handicap.** Several European countries (e.g., France, the Netherlands) use it extensively.

- Disease   Abnormal process at the level of cells and tissue that interferes with normal physiological and developmental processes and structures

- Impairment   Loss or abnormality of psychological, physiological, or anatomical structure or function

- Disability   Reduced ability to meet daily living needs; varies with context and stage of life

- Handicap   Social disadvantage that results from impairment or disability; its extent depends on impairment, disability, and the attitudes and biases of others in contact with the individual

THE FUNCTIONAL LIMITATION (ALSO CALLED NAGI'S) FRAMEWORK

The second model avoids the word "handicap," which has assumed negative connotations in the United States. This model, proposed by Nagi and the Institute of Medicine (Pope & Tarlov, 1991), includes the four levels, **pathology, impairment, functional limitation,** and **disability.** In this model the first three components are viewed as stages of a "disabling process," which may or may not result in full disability, depending on the interventions that are provided to restore function and to prevent the onset of secondary impairments and functional and social limitations.

- Pathology   Interruption or interference of normal bodily processes or structures.

  Level: Cells and tissues

Example: Congenitally absent corpus callosum makes it difficult for a child to coordinate and integrate sensory and linguistic input

- Impairment   Loss or abnormality of mental, emotional, physiological, or anatomical structure or function

  Level: Organs and organ systems (including "mental" systems, such as language)

Example: Impaired ability to acquire language appears as simplified syntax and inconsistent use of language rules, such as plural and past tense endings

- Functional Limitation   Restriction or lack of ability (resulting from impairment) to perform an action or activity in a manner considered normal

  Level: Organism (child)—in the context of performing a particular action or activity

Example: A child has difficulty convincing kindergarten friends to play a certain way because of inadequate language skills

An adolescent is unable to integrate listening, reading, and writing well enough to take notes in social studies class

- Disability   Limitation in performing socially defined activities and roles expected of individuals within a social and physical environment

  Level: Society—task performance within a social and cultural context

Example: A child is not scheduled to go to the library with age peers because of being defined as a nonreader.

PERSONAL REFLECTION 1.5 _____

"A child is not a computer that either 'knows' or 'does not know.' A child is a bumpy, blippy, excitable, fatiguable, distractible, active, friendly, mulish, semi-cooperative bundle of biology. Some factors help a moving child pull together coherent address to a problem; others hinder that pulling together and tend to make a child 'not know.'"

Sheldon H. White (1980, p. 43), psychologist at Harvard.

Communication Needs Model—Reducing Functional Limitation

In the communication needs model the focus shifts from what is wrong (or right) within the person—in terms of knowledge, skills, and sensory and motor processes—to what the person *needs* to do to function successfully in important life contexts (Beukelman & Mirenda, 1988, 1992). This model is designed to ask questions about **functional limitation.**

Functional limitation, as currently defined by the community of international disability specialists (Pope & Tarlov, 1991), is the inability to perform a particular activity in a particular context and to meet daily living needs—it varies in different contexts and life stages. For example, a person who has dyslexia and cannot read but who functions normally in other ways might only have functional limitations and be at risk for disability in societies where literacy is valued highly.

Because functional limitation is defined by the contexts in which an individual needs a particular skill or ability, it is amenable to intervention either by (1) modifying the expectations of the context, or (2) providing access to the important activity through compensation. Compensations allow a person to accomplish what needs to be done but only by using specialized tools and strategies. For example, a nonspeaking person who needs to communicate orally might use a communication board or computerized augmentative communication device. A person who has a severe spelling problem might use an electronic spelling device.

Choices must be made wisely about when to modify contexts and when to provide compensatory devices and techniques to reduce functional limitations. Before placing individuals in isolated "special" contexts, interven-

tion teams ask increasingly about the future as well as the present. In the short term, what skills does this person need to participate in classrooms? In the long term, what skills will lead to independent adulthood? The price is high if special classrooms in segregated settings are engineered to make students feel successful, but the students appear more limited when they face the greater demands of the "real world." That is the dilemma faced by the mother whose priorities for her child were illustrated by her frustrated comment, "We'll buy him Velcro!" (see Personal Reflection 1.6).

The dilemma of the mother in Personal Reflection 1.6 indicates that questions about what a child with a language disorder needs should be formed with two parts:

1. The first part should ask about need, and
2. The second part should consist of an if-clause, stating the contexts important to the child.

For example, teams of individuals, including parents, and students themselves, if appropriate, might ask questions such as "What does this student need *if* he is going to become an independent young adult?" or "What does this student need *if* she is going to function in a regular classroom?"

A related dilemma is whether to label a disability. Thomas Mautner (1984) (see Personal Reflection 1.7) was relieved when, at the age of 32, he was finally identi-

PERSONAL REFLECTION 1.6 _____

"We'll buy him Velcro!"

Ann Barnes, mother of a child with cerebral palsy, commenting during an exchange with school district personnel about the Individualized Educational Program (IEP) objectives for her son. The school personnel, following a strictly developmental model, told this mother that her son was not close to being ready to work on reading in his special classroom, because dressing came earlier in the developmental sequence, and he could not yet even zip his pants. The boy's mother surveyed the relative merits of what her son needed to do to compete in school, and decided that pants zipping was less necessary (and perhaps impossible, given his motor impairments) than reading, despite its developmental precedence. As a result, she pronounced that his dressing impairment could be minimized through an adaptive device, but that if he did not learn to read, he would be permanently disabled in an area for which he could not easily compensate. (Courtesy of Barbara Hoskins)

PERSONAL REFLECTION 1.7 _____

"I spent four years in the private school doing the minimum amount of work I could get away with, going to summer school, and excelling in sports. During my high school years, friction between my parents and me increased. There were ugly scenes at grade time, and I was constantly told by teachers, administrators, and my parents that my grades would improve if I would stop being so lazy and begin to apply myself. I graduated with a C minus average (a gift) and was mysteriously accepted by a college. I did not want to go to college, and I certainly did not have the academic background or the maturity. However, my parents insisted that I attend college; there was no other choice. My college experience lasted one semester—I flunked out" (pp. 304–305).

"Being constantly told, 'You are lazy . . . you don't apply yourself . . . if you would only try harder' creates long-term damaging results. It is very difficult to try hard or to apply yourself when you believe you cannot do the work because nothing will 'sink in.' If you are told these things often enough, eventually you will believe what you hear and give up" (p. 310).

Thomas S. Mautner (1984), mechanical engineer, talking about what it was like as an adolescent to have dyslexia when everybody knew that he was not doing his work, but nobody knew why.

_____

fied as having dyslexia (see Chapter 4 for a description of the symptoms of dyslexia). Based on Mautner's experience, questions arise: Is it better to provide special services in special contexts or to keep children in regular classrooms? Would Mautner's struggle have been less if his learning disability had been recognized earlier in his life? Mautner considered himself disabled without being labeled "disabled." In hindsight, he viewed his condition as having been worse for lack of special recognition of the nature of his difficulties.

Another perspective on being labeled as having a learning disability was provided by 13-year-old Anna (Reid & Button, 1995). In Personal Reflection 1.8, Anna expresses the ambivalence of wanting to be viewed like her peers, but needing her teachers to understand her functional limitations.

Communication Opportunities Model—Reducing Disability and Increasing Participation

In the communication opportunities model (Beukelman & Mirenda, 1988, 1992), the focus shifts again. This model considers opportunities individuals have to participate in the important contexts of their lives. It is designed to ask questions about disability as social limitation.

Disability, as currently defined by the community of international disability specialists (Pope & Tarlov, 1991), involves limitation in performing socially defined activities and roles expected within a social and cultural context—it varies with the attitudes and biases of others in contact with the individual.

PERSONAL REFLECTION 1.8 _____

When asked how teachers treated her, Anna said:

"Well, some teachers know that I'm special ed. They treat me, 'You're just like a regular student still.' And it's like, 'Yes.' And I get along with it. And sometimes they forget that that I'm special ed. And they think that I can do this. But, I can't do this. I just can't do it."

Anna, was a 13-year-old adolescent who was labeled as having language disabilities as the age of 5 (Reid & Button, 1995). Reid and Button reported that Anna's mother:

"recounted to us that at the time Anna was diagnosed, she and her husband were told 'not to bother' saving for a college education for Anna, because she would never have the requisite academic ability. They were instead advised to take their savings and 'go on a vacation.'" (p. 604)

Implementation of the participation model is consistent with the philosophical stance, taken throughout this book, that *problems are not just within children—and neither are the solutions.* Questions should be asked regularly about whether intervention contexts provide sufficient opportunity for children to practice communicative skills and abilities needed to participate in the broader social, educational, and vocational contexts of their lives. A philosophy underlying this approach is that if intervention can be provided in the real world, rather than separate from it, individuals with visible handicaps may be less isolated from the rest of society throughout their lives (see Personal Reflection 1.9).

Contributions of the communication opportunities model to decision making might be viewed on two levels—conservative and radical. Advocates of the conservative version seek to increase participation opportunities through a continuum of experiences, some of which might occur in a special education setting. Advocates of the more radical version seek out (and even demand) opportunities for children with severe disabilities to be **included** full time in contexts with persons who are not disabled (Fuchs & Fuchs, 1994, analyze both positions).

Debate centers around interpretation of the federal requirement that all children with disabilities must be educated in the least restrictive environment (LRE) (see Chapter 5 for further discussion of policies). The Education for All Handicapped Children Act (EHA; PL 94–142) was originally passed in 1975. Reflecting changes in labels and definitions, the act is now known as the Individuals with Disabilities Education Act (IDEA). The definition of LRE for a particular child continues to be left to the Individualized Education Planning Committee formed for that child.

In many states and communities, the LRE was traditionally interpreted to mean that children with severe disabilities should have access to specialized facilities and professionals (e.g., physical therapists, occupational therapists, speech–language pathologists, and special educators). The result of such an interpretation, however, was often that children with severe disabilities were educated in isolated classrooms and buildings, sometimes after long bus rides from their homes. Advocates for **full inclusion** of all children with disabilities in the schools and classrooms within their home communities have pointed out that segregated contexts do not provide opportunities for children with or without disabilities to interact with each other (Knoll & Meyer, 1987; Ruben, 1988) (see Personal Reflection 1.10). This perpetuates long-standing biases and attitudes that increase social penalties and lead to full disability.

Advocates for change note that individuals with disabilities have the right to be integrated within the mainstream, emphasizing the similarity to civil rights movements of the past (Markus, 1988) (see Personal Reflection 1.11). When applied to decision making about

---

PERSONAL REFLECTION 1.9 _____

"Life is not a dress rehearsal!"

Sarah Blackstone (1989, p. 1), speech–language pathologist and editor of *Augmentative Communication News*, commenting on the questionable advisability of designing segregated programs for persons with severe disabilities on the assumption that such programs will somehow help those individuals become more "ready" to enter integrated settings later.

PERSONAL REFLECTION 1.10 _____

"You used to see those kids in the mall or something, and you'd shy away. . . .Now you just go up and talk to 'em without worrying about it."

Tom Luick, high school sophomore in Ankeny, Iowa. Luick was quoted in an article by Ruben (1988, p. 121) about how mothers convinced their school district to keep their children in the community instead of busing them to Des Moines. As a result, Tom Luick and his friends participated with Dan Piper, an 18-year-old with Down syndrome, to form a group called the "Greasers." The group backed up Piper as he mimed John Travolta in a rendition of "Greased Lightnin' " for a school lip-sync program. At the end of the year, Piper's junior high school yearbook was full of such inscriptions as:

"To a narly dude, homeroom and anywhere else."

"Your [*sic*] a real cool person. I've really enjoyed you."

"Keep on jammin' with the football team!!" [Piper had served as manager.]

" '93 rules." (Ruben, 1988, p. 120)

Although not at all unusual as yearbook inscriptions go, these particular in were highly special for Dan. In earlier years, when visiting his brothers' school, Dan had said repeatedly, "This be my school" (Ruben, 1988, p. 120). His mother reported that he only wanted to be a "Hawk." Finally, he was one.

PERSONAL REFLECTION *1.11* _____

"For years . . . we have maintained a public policy of protectionism toward people with disabilities. We have created monoliths of isolated care in institutions and in segregated education settings. It is that isolation and segregation that has become the basis of the discrimination faced by many disabled people today. Separate is not equal. It wasn't for blacks; it isn't for the disabled."

Lowell Weicker, former U.S. Senator, making the connection between full inclusion and other civil rights movements explicit when testifying in support of the Americans with Disabilities Act (quoted by Blackstone, 1989, p. 17).

special services for children, **inclusion** refers to a process whereby children with special needs interact with normally learning children in an ordinary school structure that represents an educational whole (Flynn, 1990). Attempts to include children with severe disabilities into regular education settings represent a dramatic shift away from a philosophy of "change the child" to "adapt the mainstream" (W. Stainback, Stainback, Courtnage, & Jaben, 1985).

An important function of the current advocacy movement is to shake some old stereotypes about special education contexts for children with special needs. It should lead intervention teams away from the strategy of testing and labeling children and then placing them in service-delivery models, classrooms, and even school buildings simply by matching labels.

Beware of Missing the Trees for the Forest

Improved service delivery, however, is not a foregone conclusion. If instituted as a blanket policy, full inclusion models have the same potential as any other to overlook the needs of individual children. The American Speech-Language-Hearing Association (1996, Spring) passed a policy statement that affirms the value of **inclusive practices** but acknowledges the need for a continuum of service delivery models. Some parents and professionals worry that the movement may simply represent a swing of the pendulum to former times when the needs of their children for individualized programming were not recognized and they were left to fail in regular classrooms.

The potential problem of missing the forest for the trees is based on the premise that holistic needs of

language-impaired children will not be met if intervention and education practices become bogged down in piecemeal definitions and activities. When all children are treated alike, it is also possible to lose sight of the trees for the forest. That sometimes happens when administrators of large programs become so involved with looking at program costs that they lose sight of individual children.

Examining Past Mistakes and Learning from Them

Thus far in this chapter, I have suggested that problems of missing the whole or missing the parts can be avoided by asking questions to illuminate communication processes, needs, and opportunities. Another strategy is to learn from mistakes (Damico, 1988) (see Box 1.3).

What went wrong in Debbie's case? Damico (1988) identified five factors that contributed to the failure (additional factors are identified relative to the perspectives discussed in this chapter): (1) the fragmentation fallacy, (2) therapist bias, (3) acquiescence, (4) lack of follow-up, and (5) bureaucratic policies and procedures.

The Fragmentation Fallacy. As described by Damico (1988), the fragmentation fallacy arises out of discrete-point approaches to assessment in which phonology, morphology, syntax, semantics, and pragmatics are viewed as discrete "modules" that can be evaluated and treated separately. This approach results in fragmentation because it "breaks the elements of language apart and tries to test them separately with little or no attention to the way those elements interact in a larger context of communication" (Damico, 1988, p. 56). Modular views can be contrasted with molar views of language as a system that can be understood only in the contexts of real communicative interactions, not contrived tasks. In Debbie's case Damico later recognized the need to ask comprehensive questions about the skills she would need in the social and educational contexts of school.

Therapist Bias. The problem Damico (1988) identified as therapist bias is tied to theories of cognitive dissonance. According to such theories, therapists internalize a view of each client and tend to filter and reinterpret evidence contrary to that view to eliminate dissonance with it. Therapist bias can have two effects (Nisbett & Wilson,

Box 1.3 _____

Damico's Example of Failed Language Intervention

Debbie was first seen by Damico during her first-grade year for a language problem that her teacher described as "lack of correct pronouns and the omission of words during conversation" (p. 52). Damico described Debbie as a sociable child of well-educated, involved parents. She made frequent eye contact with the examiner and was curious and readily engaged in the assessment tasks. Her scores on most standardized measures, however, were below her chronological age level. In addition, Debbie's spontaneous language sample included an error rate higher than 40% for some grammatical forms, including pronoun case substitutions (e.g., *her* for *she*), omitted auxiliary verbs (e.g., "The dog running"), irregular plurals (e.g., *womens* for *women*), and past-tense markers (e.g., *comed* for *came*). Further analysis of the language sample showed 34 instances of "semantic confusion" in which Debbie used excessive generic terms (e.g., *stuff* and *thing*) or misused deictic terms when referring to concepts of space (e.g., *here* versus *there*), time (e.g., *to-morrow* versus *today*), or person (*I* versus *you*).

For the remainder of her first-grade year, Debbie participated in a traditional language-intervention program that was designed to target her grammatical form problems and did not address semantic confusions. At the end of the period, although Debbie's grammatical errors had not disappeared entirely, her error rate involving grammatical forms in spontaneous language sampling had dropped significantly, while her mean length of utterance remained at 5.0. These findings were taken as evidence that she was in a phase of spontaneous carryover. Therefore, a decision was made to dismiss her from therapy. After the first 3 months of the following school year, Debbie transferred to another school.

Damico did not see Debbie again until seven years later, when he was asked to evaluate a seventh-grade student who was exhibiting a severe communication disorder. When Debbie entered the evaluation room, Damico did not immediately recognize her: "While she still presented an attractive appearance, she was less friendly and somewhat introverted. Upon identification, however, the significance of the situation was realized. A student dismissed from language management as 'normalized' several years ago still manifested language difficulties. Indeed, she exhibited more severe problems" (p. 54).

Debbie was now reading four grades below grade level and was unable to perform tasks expected of most seventh graders. She claimed to have only three friends (two of whom were in special education programs) and was described by others as being shy, quiet, and having poor social skills. At this point, formal testing showed Debbie to have severe difficulty in recognizing and expressing semantic attributes and in being pragmatically appropriate. Analysis of grammatical form showed Debbie still to be capable of producing fairly long and complex sentences with few grammatical errors (with a mean length of utterance of 8.4 morphemes). However, Debbie had many problems using pragmatic rules to participate in interactive discourse. Problems included difficulty judging the amount of information to provide to a listener, giving appropriate answers to questions, maintaining conversational topics, and producing an unusual number of linguistic nonfluency and revision errors, both with her peers as well as with the clinician. Based on these findings, Debbie was described as a "severely [language] disordered individual with concomitant academic and social problems" (p. 56).

Note. From "The Lack of Efficacy in Language Therapy: A Case Study" by J. Damico, 1988, *Language, Speech, and Hearing Services in Schools,* 19, pp. 51–66. Copyright 1988 by American Speech-Language-Hearing Association. Adapted by permission.

_____

1977): (1) based on the **halo effect,** the therapist sees results of therapy as more positive than they actually are; (2) based on the **Rosenthal effect,** the therapist introduces subtle, and often unconscious, positive bias into the collection, analysis, and interpretation of data.

Acquiescence.   By acquiescence, Damico (1988) meant "the tendency to agree or assent to the impressions or opinions of others without dispute" (p. 59). Professional uncertainty or a desire to build a personal or working relationship with others contributes to acquiescence.

The potential of acquiescence has some interesting implications related to cooperative goal setting and collaborative consultation strategies, described later in this chapter. When a teacher, speech–language pathologist, and parent all collaborate in the setting of goals, no one must acquiesce, because all have worked together to establish mutually defined goals.

Lack of Follow-up.   The need for follow-up after children have been "dismissed" from therapy has rarely been discussed in the literature (Damico, 1988). Perhaps the evolution of school services from primary focus on speech to include language is partially responsible (L. Miller, 1989). Although not invariably, some speech impairments involving articulation, stuttering, and voice problems may actually be "corrected." The strategy that seems to have been adopted—by analogy—for children with language disorders is to work with them until their language skills reach normal limits according to some standardized test and then to dismiss them from therapy as corrected. This, essentially, is what Damico (1988) did with Debbie.

Such a strategy can have negative life effects, however, if the skills measured by assessment tasks are not the same as those required in real life. In Debbie's case, although she developed sufficient skills to produce well-formed sentences of adequate length, she did not have the skills she needed to meet the communicative demands of real educational and social contexts. Debbie's symptoms of early language disability began to shift as she grew older. Unless follow-up services are provided in the form of classroom observations and interviews, problems that are barely noticeable in some contexts may evolve into highly significant disabilities in others (see Personal Reflection 1.12).

PERSONAL REFLECTION 1.12 _____

"Language deficits which begin early in life . . . may persist into young adulthood and emerge again and again in later life. They tend to come out when new circumstances—perhaps a new line of study, a new job, or a promotion—place different and unexpected demands upon language processing and use in speaking or writing."

Elisabeth H. Wiig and *Eleanor Messing Semel* (1980, p. 20).

Bureaucratic Policies and Procedures.   Damico's (1988) explanation of bureaucratic policies and procedures fits the analogy in which one misses the trees for the forest. In the system responsible for meeting Debbie's needs, professionals carried 45 to 90 children on their caseloads. Children were "taken and molded to fit the service plan rather than the reverse" (p. 61).

Perhaps a different set of accountability criteria would have averted the problems with Debbie's case. Rules should be written and implemented consistent with goals to reduce impairment, meet needs, and increase opportunities.

BALANCING AGES AND DEVELOPMENTAL STAGES

Children have different language assessment and intervention needs at different points in their development. That is, the same child will need different services (or no services) at varied developmental points. Although some age-based needs stem from individual differences, some can also be predicted according to developmental stages. The second half of this book is organized into three sections based on three stages of normal development: **early, middle,** and **later.**

Early Stages

In the early stages of language development—birth to 3 years—children develop the building blocks of speech, language, and communication. The birth cry, cooing, and babbling demonstrate the preparation and natural unfolding of physiological, perceptual, and sensorimotor aspects of **speech** production. First words and early word combinations show that infants and toddlers are acquiring the building blocks of **language.** The early exhibition of a desire to establish social **communication** is the hallmark of the early stages.

Middle Stages

In the middle stages of language development—preschool through early elementary years—children work at figuring out the rules of language. Language learning problems at this stage often reflect children's impaired abilities to figure out the linguistic rules of language content and form. This is also when they acquire many socially defined rules of language use.

Later Stages

In the later stages of language development—later elementary years through adolescence—most children with language impairments know *something* about most of the rules of language. The problems of preadolescents and adolescents center around selecting information from their knowledge base and implementing it to solve integrative language problems, rather than in learning basic linguistic and communicative rules.

When Developmental Stage and Chronological Age Do Not Match

Many language specialists assume a developmental focus in treating childhood language disorders. That is, they assess a child's development across relevant communicative domains, find the area that is most delayed but relevant to the child's needs, and foster a more normalized development within that area using the child's relative strengths to support the process. For children with large mismatches between their chronological age and developmental stage (in one or more areas), however, a strictly developmental approach may be inappropriate.

For example, a 13-year-old student with profound cognitive and multiple other impairments functioning at a presymbolic level would be assessed as functioning at an early stage of language acquisition and would be viewed primarily in the context of what is known about infant and toddler development. When a 13-year-old is functioning at a 13-month-old level, it does, after all, make sense to start at that child's level when planning intervention. Such a unidimensional approach, however, misses the other two facets of comprehensive programming discussed throughout this book—contextual needs and opportunities.

The questions "What abilities does this child need to participate in the important contexts of his or her life?" and "What communication opportunities should the environment provide?" cannot be answered by focusing on a single developmental dimension. The child's language system may have remained at a 1-year-old level, but his or her body and social interaction needs may not. Even the child's language and speech behaviors may not

be accurately characterized by describing them as similar to those of a 1-year-old. The normally developing 1-year-old changes rapidly. Every day brings new exploration and shifts of experience and ability. The 13-year-old with profound impairments may have behavioral routines that are much more closely tied to particular contexts and people.

Questions of need and opportunity are equally important for the 8-year-old with language skills at a 6-year-old level as they are for the profoundly impaired individual. No one wants to put children in situations where they are sure to fail. Yet, removing children from contexts with their peers to ensure success on a short-term basis may, in the long-run, ensure failure in adulthood. Interventions should focus on whole systems to avoid this problem.

STRATEGIES FOR CHANGING SYSTEMS

System Theory

Effective programming for infants, children, and adolescents with language disorders is complex. Problems of too narrow a focus may be avoided by viewing language as one aspect of a much larger system.

System theory offers a theoretical framework for conceptualizing complex nonlinear problems. System theory was developed in the 1920s by German biologist Ludwig von Bertalanffy (1968) to avoid mechanistic explanations for biological phenomena. The principles of system theory have been applied therapeutically in a wide variety of work, including disturbed families (Minuchin, 1985), adults with aphasia as a result of stroke (Norlin, 1986), and children with language disorders (L. Miller, 1978; N. W. Nelson, 1986). Six basic principles have been discussed:

1. Any system is an organized whole, and elements within the system are necessarily interdependent (Minuchin, 1985). When describing ecosystems, Capra (1982) commented that "what is preserved in a wilderness area is not individual trees or organisms but the complex web of relationships between them" (pp. 266–267). This principle is also illustrated by Damico's (1988) "fragmentation fallacy" discussion about systems whose properties are lost when one attempts to reduce them to smaller units. It suggests that childhood language disorders can only be understood within a network of complex external and internal relationships.

2. Causative patterns in a system are circular rather than linear (Minuchin, 1985). The principle of complex causality is illustrated by research on the communicative interaction patterns of parents with their language-delayed children. When children have language impairments, parents tend to be more directive, ask more questions, and do more correcting (e.g., Conti-Ramsden & Friel-Patti, 1983; Cross, 1984; Lasky & Klopp, 1982; Leonard, 1987). Given these results, it might be tempting to suggest that the slower language development of such children is caused at least partially by their parents' interaction styles. The causative system theory principle, however, suggests that parents' interaction styles may also be partially caused by the reduced communicative capabilities of their children (Cross, 1984; Leonard, 1987).

3. Systems have homeostatic features that maintain the stability of their patterns. This principle of homeostasis represents the tendency of biological systems, family systems, and classroom systems to remain stable (Minuchin, 1985). Without it, change would occur randomly, and chaos would result. Yet homeostatic forces tend to maintain systems in maladaptive as well as adaptive states. For example, children who have never raised their hands to speak in class may find it difficult even after they have the basic skills to do so. It just does not "feel" right to them, and no one expects them to talk in class. For such a student, carryover will come only when the homeostatic pattern is altered.

4. Evolution and change are inherent in open systems (Minuchin, 1985). The principle of morphogenesis balances the principle of homeostasis. The openness of systems means that they will inevitably change. The question is whether the change will be positive or negative. The purpose of language intervention is to influence change within systems to be positive. For example, to change classroom patterns about asking questions, participants might agree that talking is a valuable goal. Then, it may be possible to modify the classroom system so that the teacher gives the child more opportunity to participate, the language interventionist helps the child acquire new language skill for participating, and the child commits to risk participating.

5. Complex systems are composed of subsystems (Minuchin, 1985). This fifth principle provides a balance to the first. Although systems are wholes that cannot be reduced without losing some of their essence, they do nevertheless have subsystem components. The ability to analyze complex systems into smaller units allows the language specialist to examine various dimensions of a problem sequentially to understand how subcomponents work together simultaneously (which is the point of the exercise described in Box 1.4). Choosing the size of the units to address is an important part of the decision-making process. Language specialists must learn to shift their focus from whole systems to subsystem components and back again. Important subsystems for children with language disorders include

Box 1.4

Steps for Maintaining Balanced Focus on Client Needs

1. Focus on one small aspect of a particular language problem.
2. Think about possible immediate causes and effects of the problem and their implications.
3. Shift to a medium level of focus, perhaps thinking about other aspects of the problem and effects within a particular family or a classroom context.
4. Use your cognitive "wide-angle lens" to imagine how the problem might interact with needs the child has (or will have) to communicate in the broader contexts of life and to imagine circumstances in which it might be less of a problem. Try to keep multiple factors all in focus at the same time.
5. Switch back and forth between thinking about a subpart of the problem and the whole system in which the problem appears in various forms.

their internal linguistic, psycholinguistic, neurolinguistic, sensorimotor, emotional, and cognitive subsystems; their external family, classroom, peer, ethnic, and other social subsystems; and the physical environments in which they participate.

6. The subsystems within a larger system are separated by boundaries, and interactions across boundaries are governed by implicit rules and patterns (Minuchin, 1985). This final principle about subsystem boundaries also applies to multiple levels of the intervention process. For example, an intervention team will be effective with a teenage mother who feels estranged from the values and methods of the team only if the team acknowledges the existence of the boundaries and works with the mother to design an intervention plan that is ecologically valid. Similarly, a language specialist will be effective consulting with a classroom teacher only if the classroom is acknowledged as the teacher's domain.

Patterns are interactive. Systems are whole. Subcomponents, however, can be viewed separately within the context of the whole. Patterns tend to perpetuate themselves. Change is inevitable. These are the essential principles of system theory that can be used to make a difference in the lives of children with language disorders.

Ecological Thinking—A Biological Perspective

Ecological viewpoints, borrowed from biologists, represent attention to environmental systems. They emphasize balance between living beings and their environments and recognize disrupting effects of aberrations on ecosystems. Because children with language disorders may be more or less disabled depending on context, ecological implications are important. Capra (1982), writing about physical and social systems (not language disorders), described the distinction between rational and ecological approaches as a distinction between linear and nonlinear thinking. Nonlinear (ecological) thinking requires "awareness of the essential interrelatedness and interdependence of all phenomena" (p. 265). Capra noted that "ecosystems sustain themselves in a dynamic balance based on cycles and fluctuations, which are nonlinear processes" (p. 41). These he viewed as conflicting with linear, mechanistic enterprises (see also Personal Reflection 1.13).

PERSONAL REFLECTION 1.13

"We live today in a globally interconnected world, in which biological, psychological, social, and environmental phenomena are all interdependent. To describe this world appropriately we need an ecological perspective which the Cartesian world does not offer." "Reductionism and holism, analysis and synthesis, are complementary approaches that, used in proper balance, help us obtain a deeper knowledge of life."

Fritjof Capra (1982, pp. 16, 267–268) in his book *The Turning Point.*

To be effective, language specialists must envision systems holistically (in collaboration with others), while using specialized knowledge to analyze system subparts and modify interactions among them. This requires a sort of inner switching between rational thinking about linear relationships and holistic thinking about interactions.

Phenomenology—A Philosophical Perspective

When childhood language disorders disrupt systems, the philosophy of phenomenology may help. **Phenomenology** is the philosophical perspective that phenomena are influenced by the methods used to observe them. It counters the notion that any phenomenon (e.g., a child, a classroom, a school system) has an identifiable, objective essence that can be discovered if all of the contributing variables are stripped away. Rather, the theory holds that any phenomenon contains multiple, equally valid truths, and its essence can only be understood by considering multiple perspectives (Mishler, 1979). This allows professionals and families to move away from the need to determine what is "right" and "wrong" regarding a particular child's needs and to consider that multiple perspectives may be "right."

For example, John was a first-grade student with a language-learning disability who had trouble handling the communicative demands of the regular curriculum. John's teacher felt that he should be moved to a self-contained classroom in another building. John's mother felt that John belonged in his home school and that his problems did not warrant moving him. What was the true picture of John's abilities and needs?

The contribution of phenomenology to this dilemma was to accept that each participant had a valid perspective of John's problem. In John's case, participants included not only his parents and regular classroom teacher but also the school psychologist, two special education teachers (one who worked with him in the morning and one in the afternoon), his building principal, and the district's special education administrator. The varied perspectives of each of these participants had developed through observation of different aspects of the problem. Each was "true." My students and I also had developed a perspective from our formal tests and informal observations and interviews. To act as effective consultants in this complex system, we had to recognize that the varied perspectives were all valid.

Accepting viewpoints as valid does not mean accepting them as unchangeable. If "truth" about a phenomenon is a natural outcome of the attitudes, tools, and contexts used to observe it, then views of phenomena can be altered by helping observers modify their observational approaches. For example, one math teacher expressed disgust with a language-impaired child who never asked a question during class but missed all of the questions on a quiz. The teacher wondered why the student did not ask for help if he did not know what to do. As we looked together for clues to the student's understanding in the pattern of errors on the quiz, the teacher began to ask different questions. Instead of focusing on the lack of "trying," this teacher began to focus on the lack of knowledge of a particular kind. His view of the "truth" about this student shifted from one of lack of trying to lack of knowing. The teacher also began to recognize that perhaps the student did not ask questions because he did not know when he did not understand and would rather fail than ask a stupid question. Based on this modified perspective, the teacher devised a plan to meet with the student each day to make sure that he understood. In this case, an "unreachable" student became "teachable," not because of an inherent change in the child, but because of a shift in the nature of the interaction between the student and the teacher.

Collaborative Consultation and Cooperative Goal Setting

A variety of service-delivery models may be used in the language intervention process (see Chapter 5). Regard-less of which is chosen, **collaborative consultation** is a problem-solving strategy that applies across situations, service-delivery settings, and types of disability. Collaborative consultation is

> *an interactive process that enables teams of people with diverse expertise to generate creative solutions to mutually defined problems. The outcome is enhanced, altered, and produces solutions that are different from those that the individual team members would produce independently. (Idol, Paolucci-Whitcomb, & Nevin, 1986, p. 1)*

This mutual definition of problems relates directly to the previous discussion about the importance of asking questions. When collaborating participants begin with more questions than answers, they avoid confrontational approaches to problem solving.

Increasingly, I have learned the power of entering problem-solving situations in a collaborative mode. This is what happened when my student and I observed John in his regular and special education classrooms after his mother asked us to consult about his placement needs. When we left the observations, our thank-you notes included the message that the next step would be to set up some **joint problem solving.** The school staff called the next week to arrange the meeting. At the meeting, all three of John's teachers and his speech–language clinician explained John's interactions with them and the problems they had observed. His teachers realized, for example, that John had two spelling lists to learn in a week (one for regular classroom and another for his special education classroom), while his normally developing classmates had only one. Based on such realizations, John's teachers began to coordinate their curricular demands and to design deliberate program interfaces. For example, his speech–language clinician decided to use some regular classroom materials to teach him how to follow directions, because his first-grade teacher identified that as a major problem. The catalyst for this problem solving was a set of questions such as, "What does John have to do to be successful in your class? What seems to give him the most trouble?" By formulating mutual questions, the group abandoned confrontational goal setting for mutual goal setting. Rather than arguing over where John should be placed, they began to decide how best to meet his educational needs and eventually decided to keep John where he was.

Another key concept in the definition of collaborative consultation is the emphasis on **diverse expertise.** Individual problems are best understood and solved when approached through multiple perspectives. Collaboration can result in an intervention system that is more than the sum of its parts. That is what is meant by producing creative solutions "that are different from those that the individual team members would produce independently" (Idol, Paolucci-Whitcomb, & Nevin, 1986, p. 1).

As John's case exemplifies, collaborative consultation works best when it involves **cooperative goal setting.** Cooperative goal setting has been contrasted with two other kinds of goal setting (D. W. Johnson & Johnson, 1975):

1. Competitive goal setting. Competitive goal setting involves "negative interdependence" (D. W. Johnson & Johnson, 1975) among the participants. It is typical of games that have an "I win/You lose" quality. In competitive goal setting, members perceive that they can obtain their goals if, and only if, other members fail to obtain theirs. In John's case, the participants had become locked into a competitive goal-setting mode. John's first-grade teacher wanted him to move out of her classroom, his mother wanted him to stay, and his two special education teachers seemed ambivalent. As mentioned, part of the intervention process for John involved backing away from premature placement goals to focus instead on what he needed to do each day in school.

2. Individualistic goal setting. Individualistic goal setting involves "no interdependence" (D. W. Johnson & Johnson, 1975) among participants. It occurs when actions of one team member are unrelated to those of others. Individualistic goal setting is typical of some multidisciplinary assessment teams when members do not have time or opportunity to interact with each other. Report writing in such cases may be of the variety, "I'll do mine, and you do yours, and we'll staple them together and call it a team report."

3. Cooperative goal setting. Cooperative goal setting involves "positive interdependence" (D. W. Johnson & Johnson, 1975) among participants. It occurs when members of a team perceive that they can obtain their goals if, and only if, other team members also obtain theirs. The essence of using cooperative goal setting to escape from competitive goal-setting contexts is for participants to find a level where they can agree on goals for a particular child and to work from there.

Ethnographic Methodology— An Anthropological Perspective

For cooperative goal setting to work, participants must start with rich concepts of systems. Techniques may be borrowed from anthropologists for studying children as part of the "cultural systems" of their families, classrooms, and peer groups.

To learn about a culture through the eyes of its participants, anthropologists use ethnographic techniques of informant interview, case history, case study, and participant observation. Using field notes, they map and chart patterns that appear and recur, define events the way participants do, and identify unspoken rules of behavior. When a cultural description is developed, ethnographers validate it by checking it with the participants. In the process, they become participants themselves. They do not judge what occurs as good or bad; they simply describe what is occurring. In the traditional anthropological sense, the process of ethnography is one of

> studying a "whole" culture. The product of an ethnography is a definition of what the culture under study is, what being a member of that culture means, and how the culture under study differs from other cultures. In carrying out an ethnography, the anthropologist generally spends an extended period of time in the field in order to develop a description of the whole culture under study. (Green & Wallat, 1981, p. xii)

To already overextended language specialists, the thought of spending "an extended period of time in the field" is prohibitive; many barely have time to conduct traditional assessment and intervention activities. The process of studying must be streamlined. If intervention were to begin only after all the pertinent information were gathered, it would never begin.

Intervention starts as soon as the language specialist first begins to participate in the child's system (see Personal Reflection 1.14). The techniques of ethnography are useful for obtaining multidimensional perspectives of the system. In the process of information gathering and learning about a problematic situation, the system begins to change.

This smaller version of the holistic process has been described as "microethnography" by Green and Wallat (1981). They defined microethnographies as producing "descriptions of what it means to participate in various social situations that occur within the whole culture" (p. xii). The key to success when using this level of analysis, noted Green and Wallat, is to lay out carefully

"When pediatric interns asked me when the counseling began, I always told them, 'As soon as you ask the first question about history.' "

Sylvia O. Richardson, M. D., speech–language pathologist, pediatrician, and former President of the American Speech-Language-Hearing Association and the Orton Dyslexia Society, commenting in a private discussion about what was most important about intervention with children.

_____

which part of the culture will be studied and define what size units are "whole." F. Erickson (1977) commented:

> *It is in this sense that ethnographic work is "holistic," not because of the size of the social unit, but because the units of analysis are considered analytically as wholes, whether that whole be a community, a school system . . . or the beginning of one lesson in a single classroom. (p. 59)*

For the language interventionist, units of analysis are events and contexts that are relevant to the child's needs and opportunities as defined by the important players in the child's life. It is not necessary to define everything relevant to a child's needs; it is only necessary to define something relevant to the child's needs and to begin to work there.

SUMMARY _____

The theme of this chapter has been the need for change and for good questions to guide the process of change. Change is needed not only in the language and communication skills of children with disorders but in the systems designed to serve them. Old methods guided by limited theories may not be adequate for meeting the needs of children with language disorders. To those who have a history of serving children with language disorders in traditional ways, the need for change may be seen as either a threat or an opportunity.

To facilitate the process of change when dealing with childhood language disorders, a philosophical framework has been developed in this chapter on the central idea that problems are not just within children. Rather, problems arise in interactions between children and contexts when children's skills are inadequate to meet specific contextual demands.

Assessment and intervention should go beyond fixing isolated impairments. The traditional communica-

tion processes model should be expanded to include communication needs and opportunities models as well (Beukelman & Mirenda, 1988).

The forest and the trees analogy was used to describe a clinical process in which the whole is lost by looking too closely at details. It is affected adversely by fragmentation, professional bias, acquiescence, lack of follow-up, and bureaucratic policies and procedures (Damico, 1988). A system theory framework, guided by ecological, phenomenological, and ethnographic theories and methods could be used to avoid such problems. As communities begin to address questions of early intervention, family involvement, and integration of people with disabilities, techniques of collaborative consultation will be essential.

Change in children enhanced by innovations in systems—those are the goals that occupy language interventionists heading into the twenty-first century. Those goals undergird the remainder of this book as questions are addressed about language and related processing systems, about what children need to do in varied contexts, and about the opportunities provided in collaboration with parents and teachers to encourage growth and development of children's language and communicative skills from infancy through adolescence.

REVIEW TOPICS _____

- Information anxiety
- Scaffolding
- Attention and perception (Smith's views)
- Metacognition
- Self-talk
- Impairment, functional limitation, disability
- Least Restrictive Environment (LRE)
- Individuals with Disabilities Education Act (IDEA)
- Assessment using communication processes, needs, and participation models
- Fragmentation fallacy, therapist bias (halo and Rosenthal effects), acquiescence, lack of follow-up, bureaucratic policies and procedures
- Ecology, system theory, ethnography, microethnography, phenomenology
- Collaborative consultation
- Competitive, individualistic, and cooperative goal setting
- Negative interdependence, no interdependence, positive interdependence

REVIEW QUESTIONS

1. What does it imply to say, "My expertise is my ignorance"?
2. How do scientists, teachers, and clinicians use questions to guide their thinking?
3. How do children, from infancy through their school-age years, use questions (or questioning attitudes) to guide their thinking?
4. What is **scaffolding?** How does it differ in early and later childhood?
5. What three domains should be included when thinking about the **purpose of language intervention?**
6. What are the two versions of the **forest and the trees** (part-whole) problem? What is an example of each?
7. What is the definition of **impairment** and what assessment model and questions are designed to identify it?
8. What is the definition of **functional limitation** and what assessment model and questions are designed to identify it?
9. What is the definition of **disability** and what assessment model and questions are designed to identify it?
10. What are the five problems that Damico (1988) related to his case study of Debbie?
11. What are the six principles of **system theory?**
12. What are the three modes of **goal setting?** Which is associated with **collaborative consultation?**

ACTIVITIES FOR EXTENDED THINKING

1. Think about one or more children with language disorders in your own experience. Perform the exercise in Box 1.4 using primarily the communication processes model. If possible, interview the people who are part of the child's family and educational systems to get information from communication needs and opportunity (participation) perspectives. Go through the steps of Box 1.4 again. This time use the information from the communication needs and participation model questions. How does this influence your thinking? What would be the best language targets for the child? What parts of the child's broader life systems should be targeted for change?

2. Think of some collaborative interactions of your own (might be clinical or practicum experiences, group academic projects, or projects outside of school or university). Can you find an example of each of the three goal-setting modes in your own experience? If so, what were the mutual problems that allowed you and your cooperative team members to work collaboratively? What factors caused you to work independently in the individualistic model, and how could they be modified? What were the opposing views that led to negative interdependence in your competitive example? Try to imagine you and your team members in this example setting aside the win/lose decision and defining a mutual problem at another level where you *could* work toward a common goal.

2

Language, Speech, and Communication

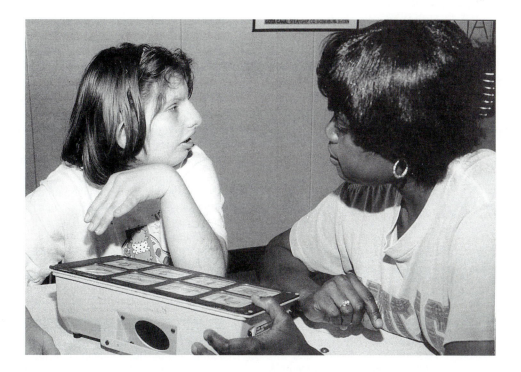

MULTIDISCIPLINARY PERSPECTIVES

THE LINKING (AND UNLINKING) OF
LANGUAGE, SPEECH, AND
COMMUNICATION

LANGUAGE AND COMMUNICATION AS
SOCIAL INTERACTION EVENTS

LANGUAGE AND COMMUNICATION AS
NEUROPSYCHOLOGICAL EVENTS

23

MULTIDISCIPLINARY PERSPECTIVES

Many disciplines study the development of language and its disorders, and a number have goals for improving the language skills of individuals with disorders (see Box 2.1). In this chapter, first the linking (and unlink-

ing) of language, speech, and communication are considered. Then two separate looks are taken at the use of language in real-life contexts. The first is an outside-in perspective. It relates to language and communication as social interaction events. This section includes a

Box 2.1

Disciplines That Contribute to Understanding Language Developments and Disorders

DISCIPLINE	STUDY OF:	GOAL AND FOCUS
Communication sciences and disorders/ Speech–language pathology	Human communication and its disorders and how to assess and treat them	Describe the acquisition, use, and disorders of human communication as well as methods for assessing and treating individuals with disorders of communication, including oral and written language.
General education	How to educate children and adults with typical development and learning	Describe methods for educating children and adults, including helping them become literate, and increasingly, with the goal of including individuals who do not learn typically as well as those who do.
Linguistics	Implicit knowledge that humans use to understand and produce utterances in their native languages	Describe the rules of inner grammar (not textbook grammar) that allow a person to "know" a language.
Neurolinguistics	Language and brain	Describe the representation of language in the brain, often by studying people who have lost aspects of language ability through specific insults to the brain.
Neuropsychology Cognitive psychology	Human learning and information-processing and disorders	Describe mechanisms of the brain that underlie typical and disordered information processing and learning as well as methods for assessing and treating learning and processing disorders, including disorders of language.
Psycholinguistics	Language and mind	Describe the interrelationships between the structures and processes underlying the ability to acquire, speak, and understand language.
Sociolinguistics	How humans use language in social settings	Describe the unconscious nonlinguistic and linguistic rules that people in a culture use to interact appropriately in particular social contexts.
Special education	How to educate children and adults with conditions that lead to atypical development and learning	Describe methods for educating individuals with learning systems that do not respond to general education approaches without additional help, including individuals with oral and written language problems associated with learning disabilities, mental retardation, autism, and other developmental and acquired disabilities.

consideration of cultural, linguistic, and dialectal differences and their relations to assessing and treating language disorders. The second is an inside-out perspective. It relates language and communication as neuropsychological events. The normal neuropsychological model is what I call a "pinball wizardry" model of integrated language use. It is the goal. It is a model of what individuals do when they use language effectively and efficiently for a variety of communicative purposes. The clinician who has a thorough understanding of this model has a built-in guide for the intervention process.

THE LINKING (AND UNLINKING) OF LANGUAGE, SPEECH, AND COMMUNICATION

In this book, language is the primary system of focus, but the language system is linked closely with related systems of speech and communication. Although the three systems overlap and intersect, it is possible, either in normal or disordered development, for speech and communication to be relatively more advanced or delayed than language. This leads to some intriguing questions about the brain, behavior, and social contexts.

For example, a college student who is profoundly deaf and communicates primarily through sign language or written language has both language and com-munication, but limited speech. A child with autism who produces speech sounds but combines them in strings of jargon or as echolalia has speech-like behavior but demonstrates low levels of language and communication. A baby who squeals and babbles to show delight has aspects both of speech and of communication but not language. An adolescent with motor impairments who communicates with computerized speech has both language and communication—but has speech only with compensation.

One of the first questions to guide assessment and intervention for children with language disorders is about relative strengths and needs across the areas of language, speech, and communication. The following sections examine the interrelatedness, but separability, of these three systems.

Language

Although most adults have an intrinsic sense of what language is, language is slippery to define. The definition proposed by the Committee on Language of the American Speech-Language-Hearing Association (Box 2.2) was written to guide public policy regarding language assessment and intervention activities. Its perspective therefore is broad, with a heavy sociolinguistic influence.

Box 2.2 _____

Definition of Language Proposed by the Committee on Language, American Speech-Language-Hearing Association (1983)

"Language is a complex and dynamic system of conventional symbols that is used in various modes for thought and communication. Contemporary views of human language hold that:

- language evolves within specific historical, social and cultural contexts;
- language, as rule governed behaviors, is described by at least five parameters—phonologic, morphologic, syntactic, semantic, and pragmatic;
- language learning and use are determined by the interaction of biological, cognitive, psychosocial, and environmental factors;
- effective use of language for communication requires a broad understanding of human interaction including such associated factors as nonverbal cues, motivation, and sociocultural roles."

Note: From "A Definition of Language" by Committee on Language, American Speech-Language-Hearing Association, 1983, *ASHA, 25*(6), p. 44. Copyright 1983 by ASHA. Reprinted by permission.

Bare-bones definitions of language (e.g., Bloom, 1988; Owens, 1992) usually include several key elements. *Language is a socially shared code that uses a conventional system of arbitrary symbols to represent ideas about the world that are meaningful to others who know the same code.* What are the key elements of this definition? Language is a **code** in the respect that it is not a direct representation of the world, as a drawing or a photograph might be. It is a **socially shared** code in the respect that, to qualify as a language, a group of people must know the same code and use the same **conventions** or **rules** to generate and to understand the symbols of the language. Language uses **arbitrary symbols** in the respect that words and their components and combinations generally bear no physical resemblance to the concepts they represent (except for some onomatopoetic words, e.g., *buzz* or *click,* and some iconic symbols in sign languages, e.g., two hands formed as wings to represent *butterfly*).

The association of arbitrary symbols and abstract meaning is particularly difficult for some children with language disorders. For some, the problem seems to be confined primarily to attaching meaning to bound morphemes, such as plural and possessive endings. These are tied closely to the form of language. For others, the problem extends to content vocabulary. Children with autism have particular difficulty in acquiring language symbols that represent conventional meanings. These children are more likely to use words and phrases idiosyncratically, as "giant words" in association with a particular situation (see Box 2.3 for an example).

When used to communicate, language provides a meaningful way of representing ideas about the world to others who speak the same language. Ideas, not things, are encoded into words. Words represent speakers' and listeners' concepts about what words mean. Because speakers and listeners share similar life experiences, they have similar concepts about the world. Because they share words and rules for combining words, they can communicate with each other. Finally, because people share language, they can develop new concepts about the world through language alone.

A variety of systems may be used for subcategorizing language. Two distinct but compatible taxonomies are used frequently by speech–language pathologists and other language specialists. The traditional set includes the five linguistic categories (1) **phonology,** (2) **morphology,** (3) **syntax,** (4) **semantics,** and (5) **pragmatics.**

Box 2.3

An Example of Unconventional Language Use

A teacher of autistic children described being present when a student of hers first learned a phrase as a "giant word" for a particular emotional situation. It started when Robbie, while visiting the home of a classmate, was attracted to play in the cat litter box. The classmate's father, quite upset, yelled, "Get the hell out of there!" Robbie's teacher reported that, thereafter, whenever he was particularly upset, and especially when he was trying to control himself from engaging in forbidden activity, Robbie repeated the phrase with the original intonation. Such language can be described as delayed echolalia that serves a self-directive function (Prizant & Rydell, 1984), but for Robbie, it also seemed to be a giant word that was evoked by a certain kind of situation much as a proper name goes with a certain person or place.

These categories are useful for guiding detailed assessment and intervention activities with children. The other set of categories (L. Bloom & Lahey, 1978; Lahey, 1988) consists of: (1) **form,** (2) **content,** and (3) **use.** Because there are fewer of them, and because the terms are more easily understood by the general public, the categories form, content, and use are particularly helpful when discussing language deficits with teachers and parents.

Speech and Other Modalities

Speech is made up of arbitrary bits of information that are combined in conventional ways to convey meaning. Speech is one modality through which language can be expressed. As Slobin (1979) pointed out, an important distinction between speech and language is that speech has a corresponding verb form, whereas language does not. People *speak,* but we do not say that they *language.* Speech is behavior. It can be recorded with audio or videotape as it is produced. Language is a body of knowledge. It is represented in the brains of people who know that language, but it cannot be observed directly. To be assessed, language must be observed as behavior produced by users of the language. Speech is one modality for doing so.

Speech is the oral modality used both for **speaking** and **listening.** Other modalities include **written lan-**

guage and conventionalized systems of gesture, or **sign language,** which can also be used either expressively or receptively. Language can also be used to support **thinking,** and is sometimes called "private speech" (Vygotsky, 1962). Speech, however, holds a special place in the development and use of language. Individuals in all cultures learn to speak and understand speech if their auditory, motor, and central nervous systems are intact and if they receive a minimal amount of exposure to it. On the other hand, written language is generally learned in the context of formal schooling. Not all cultures have developed systems of literacy for communicating through writing, but all cultures have developed equally complex spoken language systems.

Language can be learned without speech. Some deaf individuals learn sign language as their first language. When language is learned without speech, however, some other modality must serve as a substitute behavioral system to represent the knowledge system of language, and special circumstances influence the language-learning process. Studies of deaf children of deaf parents have shown that the acquisition of American Sign Language (ASL) by these children is comparable to the acquisition of spoken English by normal-hearing children (Bellugi & Klima, 1982; Collins-Ahlgren, 1975; Meier, 1991; Newport & Ashbrook, 1977). In fact, both hearing and deaf children of deaf parents start signing in their infancy and move through typical language acquisition stages of babbling in sign and using incompletely formed "baby signs" to communicate early words and phrases (Pettito & Marentette, 1991). However, ASL was not developed to be spoken or written; it evolved as an alternative to oral communication for use by deaf individuals. That can be a problem when people who have learned to communicate using ASL attempt to learn to read and write standard English, although this is a controversial topic among the Deaf community (Golan, 1996).

Other factors can make it difficult to learn to speak, although the ability to understand speech is relatively intact. For example, individuals who have severe motor control problems but normal cognitive abilities may find it impossible to produce speech, but their lack of speaking ability may interfere minimally with their comprehension of spoken language. Such people may need to use augmentative and alternative communication (AAC) devices such as computers with synthesized speech to talk and to write. When using AAC devices to write, the individual's expressive language weaknesses may become evident. The written language of non-speaking individuals often demonstrates omission of bound morphemes and function words and problems with complex syntactic structures (Kelford-Smith, Thurston, Light, Parnes, & O'Keefe, 1989). Legitimate needs to conserve time and physical effort make it desirable to omit these elements in face-to-face communication. It is difficult to determine whether written language problems of AAC users are tied directly to such expressive language practices, indirectly to reduced educational opportunity, or to some combination of factors (Koppenhaver, Coleman, Kalman, & Yoder, 1991; Koppenhaver & Yoder, 1988).

Uses of language for listening, speaking, reading, writing—and thinking—are closely intertwined, but their separability must be considered as well. This is particularly true when developmental and acquired disorders of language, speech, reading, or writing affect some modalities more than others.

Communication

Communication is defined as the sharing of needs, experiences, ideas, thoughts, and feelings with other persons (Wood, 1976). It can occur through a variety of modalities. It is possible to communicate without using speech or language. For example, humans use nonlinguistic systems when they communicate how to move a huge airplane into its bay (with large arm movements and standard gestures). Babies engage in fairly sophisticated communication exchanges with their caregivers before they can control their speech systems sufficiently to produce intelligible words or their language systems sufficiently to use linguistically formulated utterances (e.g., Bateson, 1971; Bullowa, 1979; Trevarthen, 1974).

Nonverbal communication behaviors can be produced in isolation or in conjunction with messages being transmitted via speech or writing. Two kinds of communicative features that intersect with speech and language processing in unique ways are termed **nonlinguistic** and **paralinguistic.**

Nonlinguistic Communication. Nonlinguistic features may communicate information alone or in conjunction with linguistically encoded messages. Examples are gestures, body posture, facial expression, eye contact, head and body movement, and physical distance or proxemics (Owens, 1992). Box 2.4 summarizes proxemic expectations and Box 2.5 summarizes kinesic factors in typical Western culture communicative interactions.

Nonlinguistic features are particularly evident when two people engage in face-to-face communication. For example, mothers and neonates communicate with intensity during the first few moments after birth. Nonlinguistic features also influence written language communication events. The choice of writing utensil, stationery, text format, and punctuation style all commu-

nicate something about the formality of a note or letter. Students with language-learning disabilities risk social disvalue when they fail to master nonlinguistic rules for communicating via social notes. Similarly, readers who are insensitive to nonlinguistic context may have difficulty comprehending broader meanings when they read.

Some forms of nonverbal communication, such as smiles and angry faces, are universal and appear to be part of human genetic makeup. Others communicate different meanings depending on the culture in which they were learned. For example, some African American and Native American children learn in their home cultures to drop their eyes as a sign of respect while listening to adults.

Knowledge about proxemic and kinesic factors involved in nonlinguistic communication also can facilitate team building and intervention planning. For example, I have watched student clinicians distance themselves from collaborative planning efforts by pulling their chairs away from the group meeting or by holding a clipboard between themselves and their colleagues or clients. Simply changing such physical characteristics of the communication context can set the stage for further collaboration. Similarly, clinicians can

---

Box 2.4 _____

Proxemic Communication Expectations in Western Cultures
(adapted from Higginbotham & Yoder, 1982)

Public	12 feet or more (to a visible limit)
Social-consultive	4 to 12 feet
Personal	18 inches to 4 feet
Intimate	direct contact to 18 inches

Box 2.5 _____

Nonlinguistic Features of the Kinesic Communication System
(adapted from Higginbotham & Yoder, 1982)

- **Emblems:** Convey meaning, modify associated linguistic message.
  Examples: "yes/no"headshake, hitchhiking gesture, finger pointing, middle finger gesture.

- **Illustrators and other body motion:** Modify or clarify linguistic message; indicate level of interpersonal involvement and attention; mark phonetic, syntactic, and semantic boundaries.
  Examples: Gestures, such as those tracing the outlines of a referent; other fine and gross body movements using eyes, fingers, facial expressions, head, limbs, or trunk, often in temporal synchrony with speech rhythms.

- **Regulators:** Initiate and terminate conversations, regulate turn taking, provide listener and speaker feedback, maintain or direct attention of communicative partner.
  Examples: Head movements, gaze direction and shifts, arm movements, hand tension and gesticulation, postural shifts, facial displays.

- **Adaptors:** Indicate psychological anxiety, discomfort, or emotional arousal.
  Examples: Body or object-focused movements, such as biting fingernails, picking nose, touching face, cracking knuckles, tapping foot, rotating ring, twirling pencil.

encourage small groups of students to talk to each other rather than the adult facilitator by moving to the outside of the group and prompting the students to direct their gaze, comments, and questions to each other.

Paralinguistic Communication. Paralinguistic features are related to speech because they are produced with the vocal tract, but they differ from speech because they are not produced as articulated speech sounds or words. Speech-production elements such as vowels, consonants, and syllables are considered to be the **segments** of a language. Paralinguistic devices, on the other hand, extend across the individual segments of speech that form a message. Hence, they are called **suprasegmental** devices. Rather than resulting in the production of articulated sounds and words, suprasegmental devices modify the more extensive envelopes of utterances. They provide the melody of speech that is known as its **prosody** (See Personal Reflection 2.1). Prosody is sometimes defined as the "residue" that is "left after one has studied the vowel/consonant/syllabic system of sounds" (Crystal, 1979, p. 33). Traditionally, the term has referred primarily to variation in such features as pitch, loudness, speed, and rhythm (including pauses) when speaking. Such features are related to the production of linguistic meaning, but whether they are truly linguistic is subject to debate. To Crystal (1979), such

PERSONAL REFLECTION 2.1 _____

"If you haven't got the melody, you can't decipher the words."

Sylvia O. Richardson, M.D. (personal communication, September 21, 1989), speech-language-hearing pathologist, pediatrician, and former President of the American Speech-Language-Hearing Association and the Orton Dyslexia Society, commenting on the diagnostic significance of aberrant prosody among babies, which Richardson believes indicates a risk for lack of sensitivity to the paralinguistic features of human speech, a negative prognostic indicator for learning language easily.

Richardson relates this to the difficulty she experienced herself when attempting to learn Portuguese as an adult in South America. Although she had learned Italian easily (her family was Italian and she had heard it spoken at home) and the two languages had seemed similar on the surface, they had different rhythms. She said: "They were doing the Samba; I was doing the foxtrot."

features are linguistic; to others, they are paralinguistic. Box 2.6 contains an outline of types of devices used to produce prosodic variation in linguistic messages.

At the discourse level, paralinguistic features can be used to convey such indirect shades of emotionally toned meaning as sarcasm, teasing, mocking, or parody. In such cases, the paralinguistic aspects extend beyond single words or sentences to influence an entire piece of

Box 2.6 _____

Prosodic Devices
(based on Crystal, 1975, 1979)

1. **Intonation.** The linguistic use of pitch is one of the several prosodic characteristics of speech that is integrated with others to produce a totality that expounds meaning.
2. **Pitch direction and range.** Directional tones may rise, fall, stay level, or do some combination of these things within a given phonological unit such as a syllable. As a system of contrast, tones may also vary in their range. For example, a falling pitch may occur within a relatively high, middle, or low range, and the range itself may be relatively wide or narrow. This results in syllable tone that may be characterized by linguists as high-falling-wide, low-rising-narrow, and so on.
3. **Tone-units.** When features of pitch direction and range are organized into prosodic configurations along with features of rhythm and pause, they are known as **tone units, primary contours,** or **sense groups.** Slant lines are used by linguists to mark off tone-unit boundaries, which generally correspond to grammatical clauses but expound meaning beyond the accompanying linguistic meanings. For example:

   If you want/I'll come along/

4. **Syllable prominence.** Prominent, or *tonic,* syllables are produced primarily using pitch movement, but extra loudness, duration, and pause may also be used to heighten the contrast. Tonic syllables may be indicated with capital letters when spoken utterances are coded for prosodic features. Two contrasting views of syllable prominence are (a) that it acts mainly as a syntactic feature to disambiguate sentences and (b) that it acts mainly as a semantic feature to signal new information in context.

coherent discourse. When describing first-, third-, and fourth-grade children's arguments in an article titled "You Fruithead," Brenneis and Lein (1977) noted how suprasegmental stylistic conventions can mark a speech event as an argument, "Even without hearing the words, most listeners can tell what sort of speech event is occurring by noticing such gross stylistic variables as pitch, volume, and speed" (p. 53).

Prosodic emphasis can also enhance semantic comprehension among listeners. Bean, Folkins, and Cooper (1989) found that listeners could answer multiple-choice questions better when words associated with correct answers had been emphasized in passages read aloud to the subjects. Leonard (1973) also found that prosodic stress on key words could influence the recall of verbal material.

Conversely, AAC system users sometimes find that the invariant synthetic speech of their communication devices results in miscommunication. It is difficult to program paralinguistic features with such devices. Proficient AAC users and their communicative partners use natural voicing, laughter, and nonlinguistic gestures, such as twinkling eyes and extra body movement, to signal when they have made a joke or twisted literal meaning. Message interpretation aids can also be programmed into AAC systems to assist listeners to know, for example, "that was a joke."

LANGUAGE AND COMMUNICATION AS SOCIAL INTERACTION EVENTS

Discourse Events and Contextual Variations— An Outside-In Look

Communication does not "happen" within an individual. Communication happens when a listener or a reader understands the language that a speaker or a writer has produced (Hoskins, 1990). In other words, it takes two (at least) for language to be communicative. Of course, people can "talk" to themselves either overtly or subliminally, but talking to oneself relates more closely to cognitive processing than to communicative social interaction. Most talking and writing occurs in social contexts that involve not only the influence of immediately present environmental and cultural variables, but the past histories and future expectations of the participants as well.

The term **sociolinguistics** has been used "both to refer to differences in the linguistic structures of socially

defined groups, and to those rules of speech that incorporate contextual features rather than purely linguistic or referential choices" (Ervin-Tripp & Mitchell-Kernan, 1977, p. 3). The central themes of the sociolinguistic perspective (as compared with the traditional linguistic perspective) were outlined by Ervin-Tripp and Mitchell-Kernan to include five points: (1) Natural conversations, rather than contrived tasks, are used to learn about the nature of language and communication. (2) Discourse structures, rather than sentences, are treated as the highest level. (3) Social context, beyond the linguistic structure of sentences, is recognized as influencing how language is interpreted. (4) Variability is viewed as a systematic component of linguistic rules, including those of phonology and grammar, and it appears to be related not only to linguistic context but also to social features such as sex, age, and setting. (5) Language functions are viewed as diverse, rather than merely representational, in that functions are related to cultural and developmental expectations.

The Importance of Context.   The sociolinguistic perspective plays a critical role in making decisions for children with language disorders. The questions introduced in Chapter 1 about language needs and opportunities require a sociolinguistic perspective. The variability many children with language disorders show can be understood best against a backdrop of different kinds of speech events. Because contexts vary, the ethnomethodological tools of sociolinguistics are important to language specialists as they conduct language assessment and intervention activities, both within and across cultures.

Variation with Context.   A major element in contextual sensitivity is being able to make predictions based on prior experiences with human communication as a medium and with particular communicative partners as individuals. Expectations partially relate to implications that must be inferred. Such inferences are called **implicature** (Grice, 1975). They are based on the four **conversational maxims** that the philosopher Paul Grice (1975) outlined: (1) the maxim of **quantity**—Provide no more or less information than is needed; (2) the maxim of **quality**—Be truthful and only say what you know to be true; (3) the maxim of **relation**—Only say things that are relevant; (4) the maxim of **manner**—Be organized and avoid vagueness, wordiness, or ambiguity.

When a person with a communication problem seems strange to talk with, but you are not sure why, consider whether the individual might be violating one or more of Grice's conversational maxims. Damico (1985/1991) suggested a discourse analysis procedure for doing so.

Reasons for Communicating.   Whether working with an infant in the context of family or a school-age child in the context of the regular or special education classroom, professionals should help assess whether the child has sufficient reasons for communicating. If not, the intervention process could encourage increased authentic reasons for communicating (see Personal Reflection 2.2). Part of the intervention process is to work with the people in the child's living and learning environments to facilitate the child's opportunities and reasons for communicating.

Cultural and Linguistic Differences

Playing the Discourse Game by Different Rules.   The sociolinguistic perspective encourages practitioners to appreciate the language development of children in ways that are relevant to the children's own cultures. Iglesias (1989) noted that the important shift from a time when there was "study after study comparing how the performance of minority children is inferior to that of White children" (p. 75) to a time when cultural sensitivity is more the norm. Personal Reflection 2.3 illustrates a situation when cultural mismatch could have led a clinician astray.

For language specialists to provide culturally fair and nonbiased language assessment and intervention services, it may not be possible to start with a full understanding of the differing expectations of every language and culture, but it is always possible to start with

PERSONAL REFLECTION 2.2 _____

"Unless bludgeoned into an unthinking form of rote learning or forced to play the game of attempting to guess what the teacher wants to hear, children are active learners, attempting to construe what is new in terms of what they already know."

Gordon Wells (1986, p. 101).

PERSONAL REFLECTION 2.3 _____

"*The researcher's perspective.* One of the boys was particularly intriguing even from the beginning of taping. His language seemed advanced for his age, and he talked frequently. His tapes had more entries per minute than any other child's tapes. From my perspective he was a very bright and very verbal little boy. As time went on I became curious as to why he seemed to talk more than the others. I asked an Inuk teacher for her reactions to this child.

"*The Inuk teacher's perspective.* The teacher listened to my description of how much he talked and then said:

> Do you think he might have a learning problem? Some of these children who don't have such high intelligence have trouble stopping themselves. They don't know when to stop talking.

I was amazed by her response. It was as if my perspective had been stood on its head."

Martha Borgmann Crago (1990, p. 80), in an article based on her doctoral thesis at McGill University. Crago used ethnographic techniques to analyze cultural differences in such discourse exchanges as question asking and answering.

an attitude of recognition that some of the rules may be different. Professionals can then seek opportunities to learn about another culture by using published sources, cultural informants, and participant observation within the culture itself. Ethnographic techniques, including strategies of participant observation and interviewing, can be helpful as long as professionals remember that their own cultural backgrounds and expectations affect the interview (Westby, 1990). The phenomenological perspective that was introduced in Chapter 1 can facilitate this process.

Bilingualism.   Language specialists and language textbooks in the United States often seem to approach issues concerning language disorders in children as if all children were learning standard English. The evolving demographics of North America, however, are not at all consistent with that assumption. It is projected that, by the turn of the century, at least one third of the school-age population in the United States will be either black, Hispanic, Asian, or Native American (Bouvier & Gardner, 1986). As Taylor (1995) commented:

The demographic issue cannot be overemphasized. According to the 1990 census, for example, people of color (African Americans, Hispanics, Asian Americans, Native Americans, Aleuts, Eskimos, Pacific Islanders, and others) comprised almost 28% of the American population. Moreover, they comprised more than 35% of the school-age children and were a majority of the population in most of America's urban centers. If current birth rates and immigration patterns continue, they will comprise a majority of the American population by the middle of the 21st century. This is true already in the state of California, and will become so in Texas by the turn of the century. More importantly, these rapidly growing populations will continue to comprise a substantial portion of the pool of individuals seeking services from professionals in the rehabilitation and educational fields. (p. x)

Although membership in a minority group provides some hint about cultural and linguistic differences, primary language is by no means isomorphic (i.e., exactly matched) with cultural heritage (Taylor & Payne, 1983). L. Cole (1989) summarized the heterogeneity of linguistic minority populations and commented on the problems that result when trying to use or develop norm-referenced measures for providing speech and language intervention services to members of such populations:

Linguistic minority populations cannot be categorized into the same four groups as have racial/ethnic minorities. The vast majority of Hispanics in this country are Mexican, Puerto Rican, Cuban, Central American, or South American, each representing varying dialects of Spanish. Asian language populations rank among the five largest linguistic minority groups, including about two million speakers of Chinese, Philippine languages, Japanese, Korean, Vietnamese, Cambodian, and Laotian. About 250 different languages are spoken by American Indians, some of which are spoken by only a few. Others, such as Cherokee, Dinneh, and Teton Sioux are spoken by many thousands. (p. 70)

Thus, language interventionists need to bear in mind that variation is possible even within a language and that such variation should be explained as language difference rather than language disorder.

Dialect Differences.   Not all children who acquire language systems other than standard English acquire completely different linguistic systems. Some acquire dialectal variations of English. A **dialect** is defined by linguists as "any aspect of variation which differentiates

groups of speakers" (Wolfram, 1979, p. 1). Such variation is systematic and patterned, and it is always governed by regular rules. Everyone who speaks a language speaks a dialect of it. The development and maintenance of dialects is affected by multiple factors, not just linguistic ones. "Dialects develop when speakers of a common language are separated from each other, either by geographical or social distance" (Fasold & Wolfram, 1970, p. 42).

The boundaries that differentiate dialects and languages are not always clear because language evolves in concert with a variety of social and geopolitical influences. Many of the features of the dialect called Black English Vernacular (BEV) (also called *Ebonics*) can be traced to features of West African languages via Caribbean Creole languages, which developed through processes of pidginization during the years of slave trading (Dillard, 1972; O. Taylor, 1972). As a result, BEV exhibits features not shared by other dialects of English. In fact, Bickerton (1983) noted that "the grammatical structures of creole languages are more similar to one another than they are to the structures of any other language" (p. 121). The controversy over whether Ebonics is a separate language was a topic of extensive national discussion in the United States in 1997. Children who come from homes where languages other than English are spoken, but who interact with speakers of a variety of English dialects, also may show mixed influences in the dialects they speak.

Problems related to language dialect occur because of mismatch between the linguistic expectations of the context and the dialect of a person who must communicate in that context (see Personal Reflection 2.4). Some of the problems associated with using a different dialect relate more to the differential prestige with which individuals hold various dialects than to any risk of actual miscommunication. When the rules of a dialect, however, diverge sufficiently from the linguistic rules used in a particular context, communication may be misunderstood in either direction. For example, a teacher who speaks only standard English may have difficulty understanding the communicative attempts of a speaker who uses BEV, just as that student may not always understand the teacher's exact meaning.

Discriminatory educational practices may be deeply intertwined with language differences. For example, the "ability" tracking that goes on in many of America's schools may actually be based in a profound way on language. Cleary (1988) suggested that social class distinc-

"My English is terrible. My English to me I understand what I am saying; to other people, they don't understand. I just don't wanna speak; don't know what words to use. My English crashes into Spanish. It mixed together. If I ever try to speak Spanish, Spanish people would say, 'Are you Spanish?' I say, 'Yes.' They say, 'You don't talk like you're Spanish; you don't know how to speak well.' My mother is always telling me I should be ashamed. I don't feel like I'm Spanish; I don't feel like anything. I just feel . . . like a plant."

Carlos, a pseudonym given to a high school student, described by Cleary (1988, p. 62). Carlos was born into a large family in a large city to a Puerto Rican mother, who spoke Spanish, with 11 brothers and sisters, who taught him what he called "street talk," a dialect of English that showed both Spanish language and Black English Vernacular influence.

---

tions are perpetuated by a practice that relegates "basic" writers to "work at the word/exercise level, thus preventing them from becoming fluent in written expression, from getting any joy in the process, or in practicing abstract thought" (p. 63). Cleary also reported that, although children whose language is influenced by completely different systems such as Spanish might seem to be at the greatest risk, actually children who use "working class English" and BEV are also affected because teachers are likely to see them as problems of poor "grammar" and ignorance rather than use of dialect.

Such problems highlight the influence of attitude toward low-prestige dialects. Linguists have been pointing out that all language systems are equally sophisticated and rule based since the late 1960s (Baratz, 1969; Labov, 1966, 1969; Taylor, Stroud, Moore, Hurst, & Williams, 1969). U.S. District Court Judge Charles W. Joiner, in the well-known "Ann Arbor case" (*Martin Luther King Junior Elementary School Children et al. v. Ann Arbor School District Board,* 1979), ruled that a school system must appreciate a child's dialect within the context of the community and must use knowledge of dialectal difference in the educational process. Furthermore, the judge ruled that children must not be found to have language disorders when they are developing normally within their own linguistic communities. However, old attitudes die hard. Smitherman (1985) commented that, across time, "research on language attitudes consistently

indicates that teachers believe Black English speaking youngsters are non-verbal and possess limited vocabulary. They are slow learners or ineducable. Their language is unsystematic and needs constant corrections and improvement" (p. 50).

Difficult questions arise for language disorders specialists when they attempt to differentiate language disorder from language difference. Professionals may either "undercompensate" for language difference—and run the risk of identifying children as disabled when they are merely using language skills different from those tapped by most testing methods—or they may "overcompensate" for language difference and assume that any child from a sociolinguistic community that differs from the mainstream must not have a language disorder (Terrell & Terrell, 1983). Both practices are discriminatory and must be avoided.

LANGUAGE AND COMMUNICATION AS NEUROPSYCHOLOGICAL EVENTS

Differentiating Competence and Performance—An Inside-Out Look

The five rule systems of language (phonology, morphology, syntax, semantics, pragmatics) are part of the intrinsic knowledge possessed by users of a language. That knowledge cannot be measured directly. **Intrinsic** linguistic knowledge differs from **explicit** or **metalinguistic** knowledge in that it can only be inferred by observing the output of a system.

A common method used by psycholinguists and by speech–language pathologists for assessing intrinsic knowledge of language rules is to gather samples of oral or written language using audio- and videotape recordings. Intrinsic language knowledge may also be assessed by devising special tasks. For example, a child's intrinsic knowledge of semantic or syntactic rules might be assessed by asking him or her to judge whether it is acceptable for a puppet to say particular sentences in certain ways. By contrast, explicit knowledge of language rules is demonstrated when a child tells the rule for forming passive sentences or plurals.

Language judgment tasks are not explicit, but they are **metalinguistic.** Metalinguistic tasks require individuals to treat language as an object of focus in its own right, in which it becomes "opaque," rather than the "transparent" tool that it usually is as a medium of communication.

Metalinguistic tasks involve conscious focus on language, on using language to talk about language, and on thinking about language on more than one level at once.

Any task that is metalinguistic introduces an extra variable into the process of assessing children's knowledge of linguistic rules. If a child fails to demonstrate knowledge of language rules when metalinguistic strategies are used, language specialists must consider the possibility that it may be failure to understand the task rather than lack of intrinsic knowledge of the rules under question. A continuum of assessment tasks is shown in Figure 2.1. Notice in this figure that there is

---

LANGUAGE PERFORMANCE

Explicit Knowledge Tasks

State the rule: "What is the rule for forming plurals?"

Intuition Tasks

Paraphrasing: "What's another way to say _____?"
           "Does _____ mean the same as _____?"

Linguistic "My puppet is learning to talk. You have to help. Is it
judgment: OK to say, 'Boy the spilled the milk'?"

Contrived Demonstrated Tasks

Closure: e.g., The Wug Test (Berko, 1958)

           "This is a wug.
           Now there is another one.
           There are two of them.
           There are two _____.

Comprehension: "Here are my toy animals.
           "Show me 'The giraffe kicked the zebra.'
           Show me 'The giraffe was kicked by the zebra.' "

Modeling: (with puppet)

           Adult: "I can see."
           Puppet: "I can't see."
           Adult: "I will come."
           Puppet: "I won't come."

   Now you make my puppet talk.

           Adult: "I can run."
           Puppet: [child talks]

Spontaneous Samples

Adult-initiated and controlled samples
           (e.g., using story retelling, specific questioning, indirect
           modeling, tasks contrived to elicit certain verb tenses)

Child-initiated and controlled samples
           (e.g., using play scenarios with little or no adult
           questioning; peer-to-peer samples)

Continuum of Metalinguistic Demands

Continuum of Naturalness

FIGURE 2.1   Continuum of tasks for using language performance to assess knowledge of linguistic rules.

no way to gain access directly to a person's intrinsic knowledge of the rules.

Chomsky differentiated between nonobservable intrinsic linguistic knowledge and the observable extrinsic evidence of that knowledge as competence and performance. Chomsky (1965, 1968) defined **language competence** as the idealized internalized grammar that allows native speakers of a language to judge sentences as being grammatical, ungrammatical, or ambiguous, and to generate all and only the sentences of the language. He accounted for the observation that native speakers of a language sometimes produce agrammatical sentences or fail to analyze perfectly grammatical ones by saying that these represent errors of **performance.** Performance errors might include such things as lapses of memory or attention and malfunctions of the psychological mechanisms underlying speech.

If performance errors are typical of normal speakers in everyday situations, how can language disorders specialists hope to identify children who are not learning and using language normally? The answer to that question often lies in four kinds of judgments that will be considered further in Chapter 6: (1) judgments of **degree** (children with language disorders may be observed to make more performance errors than their peers in similar contexts); (2) judgments of **kind** (children with language disorders may be observed to make different kinds of performance errors than their peers in similar contexts); (3) judgments **relative to some standard** (children with language disorders may be observed to make more and different performance errors than a standardized sample of their peers did in a highly controlled context); and (4) judgments relative to **assessment of need and opportunity** (children with language disorders may be observed and described as not having all of the language skills they need to take advantage of the opportunities that are, or could be, available to them).

A Pinball Wizardry Model

Thus far in this chapter, language has been viewed as a set of five systems that people need to know to communicate effectively. People use the five linguistic systems, phonology, morphology, syntax, semantics, and pragmatics, to communicate in five modalities—or, with sign language, seven. The modalities are (1) listening [or (2) reading sign language], (3) speaking [or (4) producing sign language], (5) reading, (6) writing,

and (7) thinking. Language users support their linguistic communications with additional paralinguistic (e.g., intonation and syllable stress) and nonlinguistic (e.g., gestural or picture) cues to communicate meanings. You may be surprised to find thinking as a mode of communication. Thinking is indeed possible without language. In at least some forms of thinking, however, people use language to manipulate ideas internally to communicate with themselves and to remember.

How does this happen? How does a mature language user pull together all of these abstract rule systems to produce and understand messages? It is the highly complex apparatus of the human brain that makes it all possible (see Figure 2.2). Although the workings of the brain are far from completely understood, neurolinguists, neuropsychologists, and speech–language pathologists have fairly strong evidence about some neuropsychological operations that relate to language.

The clinician or teacher who wants to help a child develop a neuropsychological system that can manage mature language processing needs an internalized model of what that entails. The pinball wizardry model is intended for that purpose. It is built on evidence of how the human brain works when approaching language-related tasks, but I take a few liberties of interpretation. Take a look at Figure 2.3. Compare it with Figure 2.2, showing Wernicke's and Broca's areas in the left hemisphere connected with the arcuate fasciculus. Current research shows that many brain resources are brought to bear in communicating. Not only the left hemisphere, but the right as well, connected with the corpus callosum (Springer & Deutsch, 1985). Some subcortical structures play important roles too, along with the many white matter projection pathways that connect cortical, subcortical, and peripheral structures (Aram, Ekelman, & Gillespie, 1989).

The metaphor of a pinball machine is offered as a clinical model of all that goes on when language is being processed. As you study Figure 2.3, think about the various parts of the brain lighting up when needed to handle a particular language-related task. If you have seen computer-generated color photographs of the output of brain imaging, picture those. Different areas of the brain light up when different activities take place, both simultaneously and in sequence. You might also picture the small arrows illustrating connections among the components as the running lights associated with holiday decorations. Try not to get too hung up on which part of the

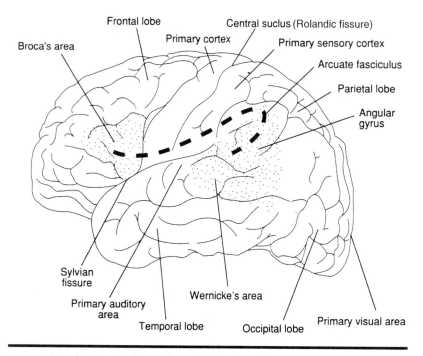

FIGURE 2.2   Left hemisphere of an adult brain showing the major lobes and primary sensory and motor cortical areas. The arcuate fasciculus, a subcortical white matter tract, is shown connecting Wernicke's and Broca's areas.

model represents which part of the brain. I have built the model as if you were looking down on a brain, with largely left hemisphere functions on the left, and largely right hemisphere functions on the right. The top of the model correlates loosely with prefrontal parts of the cortex. The bottom of the model correlates loosely with the brain stem and end organs of audition and vision (receptively) and speaking and writing (expressively). It is through these that information passes in and out as it is transformed from physical (sound or light waves) to physiological (tympanic membrane movements or coordinated oral motor activity) to neurological (cranial and peripheral nerves) data, and back again.

The pinball wizardry model represents competent mature language processing as four different but interrelated and synergistic systems, all of which relate to the central purpose of constructing meaning and making sense (represented at the center of the model):

1. Six sets of knowledge structures are represented by boxes in the model, but they are not localized so sepa-

rately in a real brain. They are separated in the model to help clinicians and teachers tease out which kinds of cues are being attended to, which rule systems are being brought on line, and which rule systems support adequate processing (production or comprehension). The six knowledge structures include three linguistic systems (graphophonemic, semantic, and syntactic) that are traditionally associated with strong left hemisphere control and three additional systems (world knowledge, pragmatic, and discourse) that are known to benefit from strong right hemisphere contributions.

2. Peripheral processing skills for interacting with the environment and getting information in and out are represented by the large bidirectional arrow at the bottom of the figure. It represents the connections between internal aspects of visual, auditory, oral-motor and grapho-motor processing and the two external boxes that represent linguistic and nonlinguistic tasks and contexts. Much of what happens inside the brain is influenced by contexts outside the brain. This is the basic

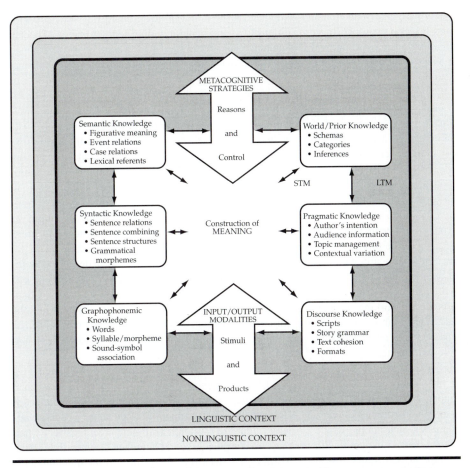

FIGURE 2.3   Pinball wizardry model representing integrated language processing.
© 1996 N. W. Nelson.

belief behind analyzing children's language-related difficulties with reference to specific contexts. It also underlies the expectation that intervention (i.e., adjustments in the context for fostering normal development) can make a difference.

3. Central processing skills are represented by small black bidirectional arrows connecting the knowledge structures with each other. Information-processing skills perform such functions as holding information in short-term memory, analyzing it, encoding it, associating it, storing it in long-term memory, and retrieving it when appropriate. The neurological bases for such functions are not fully understood, but they probably depend on a combination of parallel (simultaneous) and serial (se-

quential) neural activity at multiple levels of the brain. These appear to include serial aspects of signal recognition, which are influenced by interactions between the clarity of incoming information and the integrity of the system (bottom-up aspects) as well as by simultaneous aspects of message construction the language user brings to bear by predicting from past experience and focusing on making sense (top-down aspects).

4. Conscious metacognitive strategies for guiding attention and for directing and organizing all of the other processes and making them work efficiently are represented by a large bidirectional arrow at the top of the model. This arrow represents the interaction of internal and external forces on the executive functions of reason and control. These seem to draw particularly on frontal lobe contributions in the brain, but also on some lower cortical and subcortical contributions related to emotional state, resources for guiding and maintaining attention, and social aspects of interactions with communication partners that support the construction of meaning.

This model is complex because human information-processing systems are complex, but it will pay off if you take time to learn it. That is because it will help you juggle the many variables that influence how well a child learns and uses language in the midst of clinical or educational activities. Whether your work is with an infant, toddler, child, or adolescent, with either a developmental or acquired language disorder, you will need an internal model to guide your assessments and interventions. By envisioning the parts of the model as you assess the youngster or interact therapeutically with him or her, you can ask yourself, which parts of the model does this child seem to have mastered at an expected level of wizardry? Which parts are not working so well? Which seem underdeveloped? Which can I get to light up by focusing the child on missed cues and opportunities so the system can begin to work better?

This model will reappear in Chapter 11, so I encourage you to spend some time with it now, perhaps even sketching it from memory. Do remember (from system theory in Chapter 1) that the model represents a holistic system comprising smaller subsystems, which have boundaries and which interact synergistically with each other. These make the whole greater than the sum of its parts. It is also an abstract model because it represents many processes that can only be inferred on the basis of data from normal development, modern neuroimaging techniques, and behaviors of people with localized brain lesions. Finally, remember that it is not an exhaustive model because the subpoints within each of the six knowledge modules are only representative of the kinds of rules a person must be able to know in order to be a competent language user.

SUMMARY

Chapter 2 addressed the question of what children must learn to acquire language normally, viewed from the perspectives of multiple disciplines: linguistics, psycho-

linguistics, neuropsychology, neurolinguistics, sociolinguistics, and general and special education. Speech, language, and communication are linked as intertwined but somewhat separable systems. The relatively normal language learning of many individuals with deafness or severe physical disability illustrates this relative separability. The written language-learning deficits these individuals often experience, however, suggest links between language and speech that require further exploration and attention in assessment and intervention. Elements of paralinguistic and nonlinguistic communication also may be linked with speech and language in varied ways. All children eventually must develop competence with five different rule systems of language: phonology, morphology, syntax, semantics, and pragmatics.

Language and communication were described as social interaction events. Social interaction theory is one of six language acquisition theories discussed in Chapter 3. Here the importance of context, different reasons for communicating, and sociolinguistic variation across cultures were discussed as critical factors when language is learned in a social context.

Many factors influence the nature of the language a child learns. Some children are exposed to more than one language (bilingualism) or more than one dialect of English. It is important to recognize the special challenges that face children with language disorders when they are learning a second language or when they speak a different dialect. It is also critical to separate language disorder from language difference.

When assessing intrinsic knowledge of language rule systems, the specialist must still consider how the nature of the task may influence what a child appears to know. For example, tasks that involve metalinguistic awareness add a level of processing demand that may obscure a child's intrinsic knowledge of the rule systems of language.

Language and communication were also described as neuropsychological events from the inside-out. Finally, a pinball wizardry model was used to represent what goes on inside a human brain during language-processing events. The model is proposed as having clinical value that can guide the questions a clinician or teacher asks during language assessment and intervention.

REVIEW TOPICS _____

- Disciplines that consider language development and disorders (speech–language pathology, general education, special education, linguistics, neurolinguistics, neuropsychology, cognitive, psychology, psycholinguistics, sociolinguistics)
- Connections (and possible disconnections) among speech, language, and communication
- Five rule systems of language (phonology, morphology, syntax, semantics, pragmatics)—alternatively called language content, form, and use
- Nonlinguistic communication features
- Paralinguistic communication features
- Cultural difference, bilingualism, dialectal difference, nonbiased assessment
- Differentiating competence and performance, metalinguistic demands of assessment tasks
- Pinball wizardry as a neuropsychological model for clinical use

REVIEW QUESTIONS _____

1. What are some developmental conditions in which links among speech, language, and communication vary? For example, consider a person who is a member of Deaf culture, a child with severe physical disabilities but typical cognition, a person with autism whose speech is difficult to interpret. What other examples could you suggest?
2. List different disciplines that contribute to understanding language development and disorders. Describe their varied contributions.
3. What circumstances would lead you to use the 5 subcategories of language? When would you choose to use the 3 category system?
4. What dangers need to be avoided when assessing individuals from different cultures or linguistic groups than those represented by the examiner or test?

5. Can you sketch the components of the pinball wizardry model or visualize it in order to use it clinically?

ACTIVITIES FOR EXTENDED THINKING _____

1. Pair up with one or two partners. Have Partner 1 communicate to Partner 2 what he or she did last night using no speech or language (Partner 3 should observe and take notes about modalities and systems used). Have Partner 2 communicate a similar message to Partner 3 using language but no speech (Partner 1 should observe and take notes this time).

2. Set up communicative partnerships again. This time, take turns relaying personal narratives to each other while consciously violating each of Grice's four conversational maxims. That is, tell something interesting that happened to you, but violate the Quantity Rule first by giving too much, then too little information. Then violate the Quality Rule by adding details that you have no way to substantiate and convey them as facts. Third, violate the Relation Rule by adding irrelevant comments. Finally, violate the Manner Rule by telling the story in disorganized fashion. You might also mix these up to see if the partner can detect which rule you are trying to violate.

3. Use the pinball wizardry model to discuss the components a child would need to bring into play for communication events typical of different ages and developmental stages. Examples might be a toddler looking at a book with a parent; preschoolers doing pretend play about going to the doctor; a first grader learning to read; a third grader writing a story; a high school student reading and answering questions about a social studies textbook. In each case, consider which rule systems and other components would be particularly important, and how they would be brought into play.

Language Acquisition Theories: Contributions to Language Assessment and Intervention

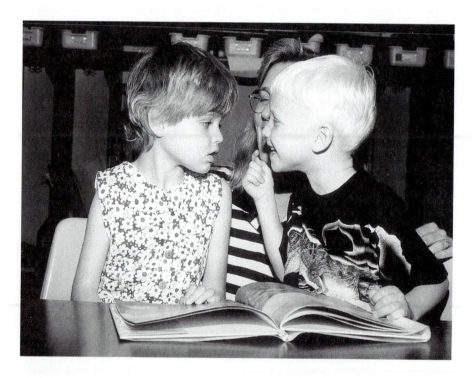

SIX THEORIES OF LANGUAGE ACQUISITION AND INTERVENTION

This chapter includes a review of six theories of normal language acquisition and their contributions to language assessment and intervention choices. The six theories alternatively emphasize: (1) biological maturation, (2) linguistic rule induction, (3) behaviorism, (4) information processing, (5) cognitivism, and (6) social interactionism.

Of these, only linguistic rule induction and behaviorism have been proposed as comprehensive theories of necessary and sufficient conditions for language learning. The others relate to factors that are *necessary* for language acquisition to proceed normally rather than describing factors that are *sufficient* for explaining it. Theories of this type are often considered to be interactionist because they acknowledge the presence of multiple essential factors but do not claim that any single factor can explain the process of language acquisition completely.

In the six major sections below, each theory is discussed with its principal explanations, its contributions to language assessment and intervention, and its limitations. Finally, an argument is made for clinicians working with children with language disorders to draw on eclectic resources to guide their practices.

BIOLOGICAL MATURATION THEORY

Theories that tie normal language acquisition to biological maturation are related to observations of the universality of language acquisition by human beings (Box 3.1). Because a system so complex as language is learned with such rapidity and at such a young age, its learning must be made possible by innate mechanisms. Such theories are called **nativist.** They contrast with **empiricist** theories, which emphasize the role of learning and influences of the environment on language acquisition (e.g., Bohannon & Warren-Leubecker, 1989; Cairns, 1996). Basically, this is the traditional nature versus nurture debate, but with the admission by each side that some (although limited) contribution comes from the other. That is, empiricists claim that biological maturation plays a generalist role that is not unique to language, and nativists (including bio-maturationists) claim that the human brain is specially designed to learn language, but accept that the environment plays a role as well. As Cairns (1996) expressed this **interactionist** form of nativism in the view of contemporary psycho-

---

Box 3.1 _____

Primary Assumptions of Biological Maturation Theories of Language Development

1. Some macrostructures of the brain are more critical than others for language learning (e.g., the left hemisphere, parts of the temporal and frontal lobes, the arcuate fasciculus, and some subcortical structures).
2. Microstructure factors—including brain cell organization, branching and spines on dendrites, myelination of axons, and axodendritic synapses—contribute to language acquisition and other developmental advances (but in ways as yet unknown).
3. Although scientists who study biological maturation of the language system adopt nativist views of language acquisition, they recognize both genetic and environmental factors as influencing human brain development and, by consequence, language acquisition.

---

linguists, "We now see the phenomenon of human language and its acquisition as a special case of the close linkage between nature and nurture" (p. ix) (see also Personal Reflection 3.1).

Neuroscientists who study brain maturation and growth (e.g., Lenneberg, 1967) are linked theoretically to linguists who view language as a distinctly human "instinct" (e.g., Chomsky, 1965, 1976; Pinker, 1994; Sapir, 1949). Both point out that talking is like other biologically determined activities, such as walking, in that it has a regular sequence of development shared by all members of a species. Both hypothesize the existence of structures and systems of the brain that specifically support language. The difference is that linguists focus

---

PERSONAL REFLECTION 3.1 _____

"What is really meant by the claim that human language is innate is that it is biologically based. Human infants are specially prepared by virtue of being human to acquire a language with the unique features of human language." (p. 11)

Helen Smith Cairns (1996), professor of communication arts and sciences at Queens College of the City University of New York.

on the rules and mechanisms for acquiring language (see linguistic theory discussion later in chapter); whereas neuroscientists focus directly on mechanisms of the brain itself. Explanations of language development as a biologically based phenomenon also explain language disorder as involving pathology at the level of cells and tissues within the organism. If brain development abnormalities can be detected, perhaps they can be corrected, compensated for, or prevented from occurring in other children. Explanations of language development as a biologically based phenomenon rest on evidence of several types: (1) cerebral asymmetries and critical periods, (2) brain weight changes during normal development, (3) neuronal growth patterns, (4) macro-organizational evidence, and (5) genetic evidence.

Explanations

Cerebral Asymmetries and Critical Periods. Cerebral asymmetry in the developing human brain implies biological predisposition to learn language. Concepts of cerebral dominance have been debated ever since Broca first claimed in 1865 that "although the left hemisphere was 'innately' pre-eminent in language skills, its dominance could be strengthened, modified or reversed by experience or injury during certain critical periods" (cited in Marshall, 1979, p. 446). The traditional wisdom about such periods suggested that:

1. The two cerebral hemispheres are equally capable at birth of supporting the acquisition of language.
2. They remain equipotential in this sense for approximately two years.
3. Then, a slow process of specialization begins, with complete lateralization reported to be complete by puberty, or in the opinion of some, by age 5 years.

This traditional view, however, has been contradicted by evidence from several sources:

First, strong evidence now indicates that right–left brain asymmetries are present at birth (Galaburda, Corsiglia, Rosen, & Sherman, 1987; Geschwind & Levitsky, 1968; Wada, 1977; Wada, Clark, & Hamm, 1975) and even before—as early as 31 weeks of gestation (Chi, Dooling, & Gilles, 1977). Furthermore, asymmetries are greatest in areas that are known to be critical for normal language functioning in adults. For example, the Sylvian

fissure is longer and the planum temporale is larger on the left than on the right in the majority of fetal and newborn brains (see Figure 3.1). The degree of asymmetry, however, seems to grow as brains mature. It is greater in adults than in infants (Wada et al., 1975), suggesting at least some role of maturational factors. As Marshall (1979) put it, "To assert that the left hemisphere is 'innately pre-eminent' as a neurological substrate for language still leaves open the possibility that the young brain is more 'plastic' than the mature brain" (p. 448).

Second, evidence has accumulated that infants as young as 3 months of age, and even as young as 3 weeks, can make highly sophisticated perceptual discriminations in the speech mode and that this processing is lateralized to the left hemisphere (Eimas, 1975; Kuhl, 1992). Studies provide strong evidence that cerebral dominance for phoneme perception is innate (Marshall, 1979), but this is not the same as saying that language is lateralized at 3 months (Wada, 1977).

Along with the evidence of structural and functional cerebral asymmetry at birth, evidence still exists that the brain has critical periods in which it is more plastic than others. Babies are better at 6 months than at 10 months at distinguishing fine phonetic differences in multiple languages (Werker & Lalonde, 1988). Second languages are much easier to learn without accent before puberty than after (Seliger, Krashen, & Ladefoged, 1975). The occasional child who is not exposed to language before puberty has difficulty acquiring the morphological and syntactic rules of language. An unfortunate example is the child called Genie (Curtiss, 1977; Curtiss, Fromkin, Krashen, Rigler, & Rigler, 1974). Although apparently normal biologically, Genie was kept from hearing speech until she was 13 years old by her abusive father who isolated her to a room and provided only physical care. After being discovered, Genie eventually learned some words and word order, but never mastered the rules of syntax and morphology. Evidence of critical periods of brain plasticity also comes from research that shows that damage to the left hemisphere is much less likely to result in permanent aphasia if it occurs before puberty than in adulthood (Aram, Ekelman, & Gillespie, 1989; Foss & Hakes, 1978).

Brain Weight Changes during Normal Development. The human brain increases in size and weight in a series of spurts. The most rapid period of brain growth is in the first two years of life, when the brain more than

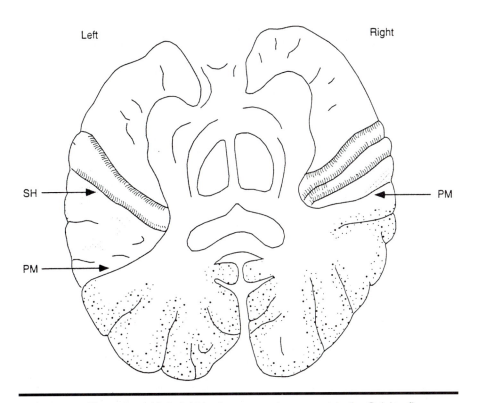

Left   Right

SH ———→   ←——— PM

PM ———→

FIGURE 3.1   Illustration of left-right brain asymmetry present in the Sylvian fissure and planum temporale (top surface of the temporal lobe) of the majority of newborns at birth. Typical left-right differences are shown. The posterior margin (PM) of the planum temporale (top surface of the temporal lobe) slopes back more sharply on the left than on the right, and the anterior margin of the sulcus of Heschl (SH) slopes forward more sharply on the left.

Note: From "Human Brain: Left–Right Asymmetries in Temporal Speech Region" by N. Geschwind and W. Levitsky, 1968, *Science, 161,* pp. 186–187. Copyright 1968 by the AAAS. Reprinted by permission.

triples its weight (Love & Webb, 1986). The timing of brain weight gains correlates closely with the appearance of new behavioral competencies (Epstein, 1974, 1978). In particular, the first four stages of brain growth coincide with the four main stages of cognitive development outlined by Piaget (1969).

Neuronal Growth Patterns.   Increased brain weight may result from several neural network factors, including increased elongations and branching of axons (long cellular processes that transmit signals away from neuronal cell bodies) and dendrites (shorter cellular process

with numerous branches that transmit signals toward neuronal cell bodies) (D. L. Maxwell, 1984). This process has been described as an explosion of neural connectors in the left hemisphere of the child's cortex during the first two years of life (Foss & Hakes, 1978).

Myelination is the process by which the long axon projections of neurons undergo "anatomical and chemical changes as they are wrapped progressively in several alternating layers of lipids and proteins" (D. L. Maxwell, 1984, p. 45). Myelination is a prime correlate of speech and language development (Love & Webb, 1986; D. L. Maxwell, 1984).

Macro-Organizational Evidence. Evidence from adults who have lesions in specific areas of the brain due to stroke suggests amazing consistency in the manner in which language is organized in adult brains. Such organizational consistency surely does not occur by accident. Similarities between the developmental language learning problems of children and the symptoms of adult aphasia (e.g., Aram & Nation, 1975) do not necessarily imply that the mechanisms of impairment are similar, however. Scientists looking for biological differences in the brains of children with developmental language disorders have found that, unlike acquired lesions, they generally are not gross enough to be detectable through standard brain scanning methods. For example, when Hier and Rosenberger (1980) examined the computerized tomography (CT) brain scans of children with developmental language disorders, only 2 of the 30 had detectable focal lesions of the temporal lobe. Nevertheless, 19 of them (63%) had a family history of language disorder, suggesting the possibility of at least some biological mechanism at work.

Other intriguing possibilities for understanding the biological bases of developmental language disorders come from brain asymmetry studies. When Hier, Le-May, and Rosenberger (1978) conducted CT brain scans on 24 children diagnosed with dyslexia, they found reversed asymmetry in the linguistically important parieto-occipital region among 42%. An additional 25% showed symmetrical hemisphere relationships, compared with the expectation that the left planum temporale is larger than the right in 66% of normal brains (Geschwind & Levitsky, 1968). Hynd, Marshall, and Gonzalez (1991) summarized this and eight other studies using either CT or magnetic resonance imaging (MRI) techniques. They concluded that the studies showed significantly less expected left–right asymmetry among individuals with severe reading disability or dyslexia.

Galaburda (1989) later reported on the autopsies of eight brains of individuals with dyslexia. All showed symmetry (rather than the expected asymmetry) in the planum temporale, but in addition, all of the six males and one female showed abnormalities in the organization of neural networks of the perisylvian region, especially in their left hemispheres. Galaburda also noted abnormal cortical cell layering (see Figure 3.2) in some and scarring in others, which could be related to injury

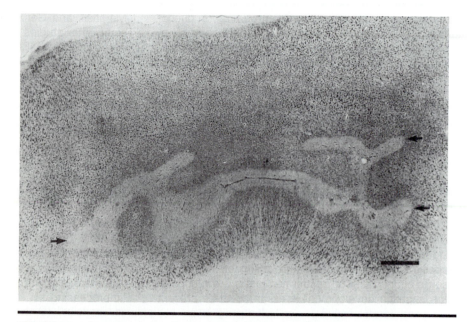

FIGURE 3.2   Arrows point to distorted lamination of cerebral cortex in the brain of an individual with dyslexia (courtesy of Albert M. Galaburda).

dated to the end of pregnancy through the end of the second year.

Genetic Evidence. The biological basis of language is also supported by evidence from genetic studies of children with specific language impairment (SLI). For example, Tomblin (1989) reported that family members of second graders with SLI demonstrated substantially increased odds for language impairments. Similarly, Tallal, Ross, and Curtiss (1989) found that children with specific language impairment had significantly higher rates of affected close relatives. Other genetic studies show strong patterns of inheritance, with some whole families affected (Gopnik, 1990; Samples & Lane, 1985).

Roles of Nature and Nurture in Brain Development Revisited. The body of evidence leads to the conclusion that it is no longer appropriate to dichotomize nature and nurture influences on brain maturation. The equipment that a language learner is born with interacts with the experiences the language learner has.

Contributions

Language specialists sometimes make assumptions about the child's brain activity as they assess and assist a child to learn language. They may use a neuropsychological model, such as the pinball wizardry model presented in Chapter 2, to guide their assessment observations. They may also use such a model to provide scaffolding designed to encourage children to make new linguistic and nonlinguistic connections.

Biological Maturation Theory and Assessment. Tests of central auditory processing based on neuropsychological theory are designed to identify such brain-related disturbances as lack of hemisphere dominance of language; inability to localize sounds; difficulty separating, synthesizing, or integrating sounds presented to the two ears; or difficulty separating a foreground message from a background noise. Keith (1981) provided a rationale for such testing by noting that language learning problems may result from "situations where the neurological structure is inadequate for processing a complex acoustic signal in an imperfect listening environment" (p. 63). He designed his Screening Test for Auditory Processing Disorders (SCAN; Keith, 1986) to look for such difficulties.

In a variation on the central auditory processing theme, Tallal (1988) and her colleagues (Tallal & Piercy, 1978; Tallal & Stark, 1976) found that many children with specific language-learning impairments are unable to detect differences between such syllables as [ba] and [da] when the phonemes are presented in normal rapid succession, but they can discriminate them when the acoustic formant transitions from consonants to vowels are extended artificially (Tallal & Piercy, 1975). Tallal and her colleagues (1996) used this finding to support their claim that the basic deficit underlying specific language impairment is neurological weakness for processing rapidly changing sensory inputs, and not a primary linguistic or cognitive system deficit.

One assessment question based on biological maturation is whether to refer children for pediatric neurological evaluation when language disorder appears to be the primary concern. Every child should have access to good general health care of all types—auditory, visual, and dental. Whether a specific neurological evaluation is warranted is generally a decision made by the entire health team and the family. Neurological referral is critical when a child loses previously acquired language abilities or when a child has seizures. Medical assessment is not called for when language disorder is suspected but no evidence of immediate neurologic pathology is present. A magnetic resonance scan, for example, can cost about $1,000, and its contribution to clinical decision making is limited in the absence of suspected treatable pathological processes.

Biological Maturation Theory and Intervention. If central nervous system dysfunction at the macro- or microstructural (cellular) level causes language learning difficulty, and if assessment can be designed to isolate the source of the problem, it might be possible to design treatment approaches that encourage the development of critical brain structures and connections that have not developed or have been injured. A number of intervention approaches have, in fact, been developed based on this theory (see Boxes 3.2 and 3.3). As Carrow-Woolfolk (1988) described it, intervention based on neuropsychological theory "is directed to improving the function of that part of the brain that is damaged or developmentally immature and/or encouraging other parts of the brain to 'take over' the function of the disordered part" (p. 66).

Box 3.2 _____

First Example of Language Intervention Based on Biological Maturation and Neuropsychological Theory

We (Sturm & Nelson, 1989) found a neuropsychological perspective helpful in providing assessment and intervention for Sarah, a child with postleukemia encephalopathy whose description and magnetic resonance image appear in Chapter 4. Sarah's MRI scan showed massive reduction in white matter across wide areas, with damage particularly concentrated in posterior temporoparietal cortical and subcortical regions. Her clinical symptoms included significantly reduced language comprehension abilities, with better language expression abilities, particularly when she was allowed to initiate topics. Sarah also demonstrated immediate echolalia fairly regularly, particularly echoing direct questions rather than answering them.

We interpreted the echolalia as a processing aid that might help Sarah move linguistic input from her relatively more impaired auditory comprehension system to her relatively more intact language production system and thus did not try to discourage it. We did, however, try to reduce the numbers of direct questions asked of her at first, and we made a concentrated effort to provide meaningful contexts in which Sarah might do most of the initiating or use modeled comments to stay on topic. For example, while looking at one of Sarah's favorite books, instead of saying, "What will the bunny do next, Sarah?" the clinician would say, "I wonder what that bunny is going to do." Gradually, we were able to reintroduce direct questions, and Sarah began to be able to answer them. The echolalia reduced in frequency as her other productive language abilities increased.

Box 3.3 _____

Second Example of Language Intervention Based on Biological Maturation and Neuropsychological Theory

In the "Fast ForWord" approach, children engage in "aerobics for the brain" three hours a day, five days a week by playing a computer game with a circus theme or "Old MacDonald's Flying Farm" for 20 sessions or more. They wear earphones and listen to sound pairs, pressing buttons to indicate which of 2 CV (e.g., [ba] versus [da]) or VCV (e.g., [aba] versus [ada] or CVC (e.g., "pat" versus "pack") syllable pairs they hear first. The computer game provides feedback. For example, in the farm game, the object is to catch a flying cow. Children listen to a series of syllables, such as "pat, pat, pat, pack." If they release the computer mouse button quickly enough when the syllable changes, the cow goes into the barn. After three successful responses, the computer program systematically reduces the temporal intervals in the stimuli until the children can make finer and finer judgments. This process was explained in news media accounts as "rewiring their brains." Tallal (1997, p. 12) described the approach, now called Fast ForWord, as a "series of seven computerized exercises that hierarchically train important components of auditory processing, memory, phonological analysis, and grammar."

[This description is based on scientific reports by Tallal et al., 1996, and Merzenich et al., 1996, as well as news accounts in the popular media by Kotulak, 1996, and Nash, 1996. The Web site is *http://www.scientificlearning.com*.]

The pinball wizardry model introduced in Chapter 2 and discussed in Chapter 12 is one such approach. Although it is only loosely tied to hypotheses and evidence on the representation of language in the brain, it can guide the clinician about cueing strategies to use within the context of curriculum-based language intervention (N. W. Nelson, 1994).

Tallal and Merzenich and their colleagues (Merzenich et al., 1996; Tallal et al., 1996) designed a more specific neuropsychological intervention based on their claim that a primary temporal processing deficit is at the root of specific language-learning impairment (LLI). They also based their approach on evidence from animal studies that practice can change neural structures. Box 3.3 contains a description of the computer programs the research team designed to provide intensive daily practice in making temporally based phonological decisions. The results of one study (Merzenich et al., 1996) showed children with LLI to improve markedly in their abilities to recognize brief and fast sequences of nonspeech and speech stimuli after the treatment. The results of a related study (Tallal et al., 1996) showed that children with LLI could improve speech discrimination and comprehension (as measured by several other tests) with four weeks of listening exercises.

A considerable body of evidence now also shows that children with specific language impairment, who often have difficulty learning to read, demonstrate deficits of **phonological awareness.** Phonological awareness deficits can be identified with tasks that have children manipulate sounds in words and syllable, such as in rhyming tasks or sound segmentation and deletion (also called "elision") tasks (e.g., "cowboy" without the "cow" is _____ [boy]; "thread" without the [th] is _____ [red]) (Blachman, 1994; Kamhi & Catts, 1989). In neuropsychological models, relating sounds and symbols and manipulating them seems to involve multiple left hemisphere contributions, probably with parietal lobe integration of processed information about the auditory, visual, motoric (articulatory), and linguistic characteristics of sounds and their symbols. Interventions aimed at improving phonological awareness include rhyming and other sound-based manipulations of words, syllables, and phonemes, and relating them to print (Blachman, 1994; van Kleeck, 1994a).

On a broader scale, biological maturation theories have implications for comprehensive treatment of children with all kinds of conditions. Many conditions associated with frank impairments of biological systems justify transdisciplinary intervention strategies to address those peripheral impairments. When hearing impairment exists, for example, a combination of services should be provided early and consistently to ensure that: (1) the biological hearing mechanism is the best that it can be, (2) compensatory technology, in the form of personal hearing aids and other amplification devices are provided, and (3) the child learns to use the hearing system. Similarly, children with craniofacial anomalies such as cleft palate justify early attention and ongoing follow-up by transdisciplinary teams, including attention to language development.

Limitations

A primary limitation is that the central nervous system is basically inaccessible to direct treatment. Medical-surgical techniques may be used to treat conductive hearing loss, and cochlear implants may be used to stimulate the auditory nerve. Drugs may be prescribed for seizure disorders and attention-deficit hyperactivity disorder (ADHD). Such treatments, however, are designed more to provide a system accessible to learning than to modify any part of the language learning system directly. For the most part, the central nervous system is modifiable only indirectly, through learning processes, and any of the other theoretical models contributes more to understanding how to foster learning than does the biological maturation model.

Another limitation is that assessment tasks designed to tap particular kinds of brain functioning are only guesses about what might be happening in the brain. As U. Kirk (1983) pointed out, most neuropsychological models of brain functioning are limited in their ability to explain "the consistency and variability that characterize the developing system, the matured system, and the system that is recovering from damage" (p. 23). Many tasks for assessing neuropsychological processing were developed for adults with known lesions. The child's developing brain may not be organized in the same way. Additionally, there is no way to clearly isolate the functioning of one part of the brain from contributions of other parts.

Nowhere is this problem more evident than in the assessment of central auditory processing skills. Tasks designed to measure selective auditory attention, short-term memory, auditory sequencing, and dichotic listening cannot prevent an intact language system, or even a disordered one, from playing a role in the outcome. Rees (1973, 1981) pointed out that causal relationships are not clear. It is as likely that language problems "cause" auditory processing problems as vice versa.

LINGUISTIC THEORY

Linguistic theories of language acquisition propose that language develops because of an innate language acquisition device (LAD). The LAD is a biologically based system that needs only to be triggered by evidence in the environment (see Personal Reflection 3.2). Thus, theories of biological maturation and linguistic rule induction are not separate theories but alternate sides of the same coin. Biological maturation not only is related to confirmation of the linguistic induction theory, however, but to other theories as well.

Chomsky proposed the innate LAD, but he left the actual functioning of the LAD largely a mystery. In his more recent work, Chomsky's (1981) focus shifted slightly from the abstract structure of language to the constraints associated with "learnability." He did this by developing his concept of an innate Universal Grammar (UG), which is compatible with the existing and possible grammars of the world.

Explanations

Child as Miniature Linguist.   A major element of linguistic theories is that a child learning language is very much like a small linguist working in the field (McNeill, 1970). When presented with a finite number of examples, the child must use the limited and imperfect linguistic evidence to induce the general rules of an idealized grammar (see major assumptions of linguistic rule-induction in Box 3.4). Linguistic theorists argue that, because this process is accomplished with such relative ease at a time when children seem unable to

PERSONAL REFLECTION 3.2 _____

"There are very deep and restrictive principles that determine the nature of human language and are rooted in the specific character of the human mind."

Noam Chomsky, in his book *Language and Mind* (1968).

Box 3.4 _____

Primary Assumptions of Linguistic Theories of Language Acquisition

1. The end product of language learning is an internalized formal **grammar,** which is a finite set of rules, shared by all of the speakers of a language, that can generate an infinite variety of possible sentences.
2. The majority of the rules of formal grammar are learned very early (before age 5 years), with similar patterns of development observed across languages and cultures, indicating that the environment must play a relatively minor role in the process and, therefore, that human genetics must play a major role.
3. Only indirect links can be observed between the language input the child hears and the language output the child produces; furthermore, direct teaching efforts as correction are rarely observed.
4. Yet children learn with little or no formal training to do such things as to understand ambiguous sentences (those with the same surface structure but different deep structures) and to understand and produce paraphrases (those that have different surface structure but the same deep structure).

---

use sophisticated inductive reasoning for other purposes, some aspects of the grammar must be preprogrammed. McNeill (1970) held that children come equipped with such innate linguistic universals as concepts of sentences, grammatical classes, and some aspects of phonology.

Constraints on Language Learning.   More recently, linguistic theorists (Slobin, 1979; Wells, 1986) have proposed that children function with a special set of "operating principles." These lead children to do such things as (1) pay attention to the ends of words (thus allowing children to acquire inflectional morphemes); (2) recognize that linguistic elements encode relationships between words (thus allowing children to recognize basic differences between classes of words such as *things* and *acts* and ways they relate in sentences); (3) analyze the utterances they hear into smaller units (thus allowing children to comprehend and construct unique sentences by selecting and rearranging pieces);

and (4) prefer to work with principles of maximum generalizability (thus allowing children to induce the rules but also leading them to produce such "errors" of overgeneralization as *foots* and *goed*).

Other constraints are viewed as inherent characteristics of innate Universal Grammar (UG) itself. That is, "there are *constraints* on the rules that form sentences, and many of them are the same for all human languages" (Cairns, 1996, p. 9, italics in original). These are the **principles** that limit language variation. Linguists also hypothesize that UG comprises a set of **parameters.** Parameters do vary and can be set differently for different languages. For example, one parameter is the presence of subjects in sentences. English is a language that requires subjects to be present for a sentence to be grammatical. This parameter leads speakers of English to include meaningless expletives when a sentence needs a subject, as in the standard English, "It's raining," and "There are five of us," or the Vernacular Black English, "Here goes the book" (comparable to the standard English, "This is the book"). Many other languages (e.g., Spanish, Italian, and Chinese) do not require subjects if the speaker and hearer both know who the subject is.

Looking at UG as a set of principles and parameters that act as constraints helps one to understand what is considered innate by linguists. To say that "Each child is born 'knowing' UG . . . is, of course, a metaphor. What we actually mean is that the child's developing brain will construct only those representations allowed by the constraints on human language" (Cairns, 1996, p. 18). It is constraints that linguists see as making the rapid acquisition of language possible. Crain's (1991/ 1994) explanation was that, "From the standpoint of acquisition, constraints reduce the number and kind of hypotheses children can entertain in response to their linguistic experience" (p. 368).

Relationships between "Input" and "Intake." An abstract representation of the LAD appears in Figure 3.3. This representation acknowledges the central role of the LAD in working toward a final grammar for the child's adult native language, but it also notes the need for language **input,** which can be used by the child because the child is capable of active and selective language feature **intake.** These reciprocal aspects of input and intake may be particularly important for understanding disordered language development. For example, Leonard and his colleagues (Leonard, 1989; Leonard, Bortolini, Caselli, McGregor, & Sabbadini, 1992) proposed that children with specific language impairment may possess an intact UG but have a problem converting linguistic input into intake and using it to construct adult grammar.

Some linguists hold that at each stage of the process of working toward adult grammar, the child constructs an **intermediate grammar,** which is consistent with the constraints of UG, but with all of the parameters of the child's own language not yet set. Pinker (1984) called the theory that all intermediate grammars conform to UG **continuity theory.** Alternative views of how a child's grammar differs from adult grammar in its interim states have been proposed by other psycholinguists. Some claim that it is always related to adult

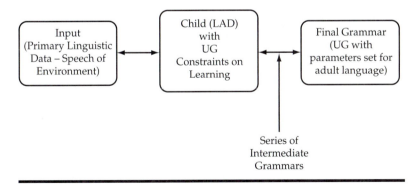

FIGURE 3.3 How the language acquisition device (LAD) is supposed to work (based on Cairns, 1996; Crain, 1991/1994).

grammar, developing in stages as a primitive subset of that grammar (Gleitman & Wanner, 1982; Wexler, 1982). Others argue that children go through stages in which their internalized grammar differs qualitatively from that of adults (Bloom, 1970; Bowerman, 1982, Pinker, 1987).

Bootstrapping as a Mechanism of Acquisition.   Part of linguistic theory is that young children must have some means of relating language to the events of the world that it represents. They also must be able to identify the relevant units of the language they hear without explicit help from adults. For example, how does the child identify three separate words in the sentence, "The birdie ate," in order to detect the agent and action? The speech stream could just as well be segmented, "*theber deeate* or *thebirdie* ate" (Bedore & Leonard, 1995, p. 67, italics in original).

The explanations for these two concerns, mapping language onto meanings and knowing how to segment language into meaningful units, are often tied to bootstrapping. Three kinds of bootstrapping mechanisms have been proposed: semantic, prosodic, and syntactic.

The essence of **semantic bootstrapping** (Pinker, 1984) is that a child first figures out subjects, verbs, and objects of sentences by relating them to events in the environment. According to this hypothesis, the acquisition of units within phrases and sentences like "The birdie ate," is facilitated by the fact that the child hears the sentence while watching bird behavior and interacting with an adult who provides the linguistic evidence to match the event. This explanation seems plausible, particularly as a boost to learning the meaning of concrete nouns and verbs with observable actions, but it contributes less to explaining the acquisition of function words and content words with abstract meanings.

Prosodic bootstrapping (Gleitman, Gleitman, Landau, & Wanner, 1988) depends on the fact that adult speech to young children is more fluent and melodic than to older children and adults. This feature appears to make the input more accessible. That is:

> *it appears that the speech children hear contains a number of prosodic cues to the most relevant units of the language. These cues do not label the units for the child, nor inform the child of the relationships that hold among the units. However, they provide a means for the child to separate one unit from another, thus making his or her job*

> *of discovering specific linguistic function of each unit more manageable. (Bedore & Leonard, 1995, p. 67)*

Syntactic bootstrapping seems necessary to help the child learn abstract meanings of words like verbs. For example, it is unlikely that semantic bootstrapping would be sufficient to help a child learn the meaning of a verb whose meaning conflicts with the action of the moment in the accompanying event. Consider the toddler who is opening the door to a toy garage at the same time the adult says, "Are you getting ready to drive away" (Bedore & Leonard, 1995, p. 69). The acquisition of meaning and syntactic possibilities of a phrase such as *getting ready* is more likely facilitated by hearing the verb phrase in multiple syntactic frames, each of which contributes to narrowing its meaning and syntactic functions, as in "Are we *getting ready* to go to Grandma's," and "We are now *getting ready* to go to bed."

Support for linguistic acquisition theory.   Several forms of evidence are cited consistently in support of linguistic theories of language acquisition (e.g., Crain, 1991/1994; Pinker, 1994). Key arguments relate to (1) the poverty of the stimulus, (2) universality, (3) early emergence, and (4) separability of language from intelligence.

The **poverty of the stimulus argument** (Crain, 1991/1994; Pinker, 1990, 1994) is that the LAD must be innate because there is no way that the child receives enough language input to explain the richness of the language the child develops. The constraints that allow a child to narrow infinite possible linguistic combinations to those allowable by UG, and to further set the parameters of his or her own language, do not come from adults. Adults hardly ever provide negative evidence about utterances that are ungrammatical, and when they do, the feedback is inconsistent (Pinker, 1990). Therefore, the child is left with the task of constructing the grammar only from positive evidence, and with evidence that is limited at that. Thus, a major component of the process must be preset by the UG that is within the child's LAD.

The **universality argument** is that the most basic constraints of UG show up in all of the world's languages. Any principle that appears universally "is a prime candidate for consideration an an innate linguistic property" (Crain, 1991/1994, p. 369). The phrase is one example. Another is that "Many languages, widely scattered over the globe, have auxiliaries, and like English, many languages move the auxiliary to the front of the sentence to form questions and other constructions, always in a structure-dependent way" (Pinker, 1994, p. 43).

The **early emergence argument** is that children across the world develop complex grammars rapidly and without formal instruction at a time when their other problem solving abilities are still limited. Therefore, something like the LAD must be innate.

The **separability of language from intelligence argument** is that language development must emerge from a specific linguistic module within the brain because there are instances of individuals whose cognitive skills appear normal, but whose language is specifically impaired, as well as individuals whose language appears normal, but whose cognitive skills are impaired. Pinker (1994) used the genetic evidence of the "K family" studied by Gopnik (1990; Gopnik & Crago, 1991) as an example of the former, and reports of individuals with Williams syndrome or spina bifida as examples of the latter. Williams syndrome is a genetic syndrome associated with a defective gene on chromosome 11 that affects calcium regulation and interferes with the development of the brain, skull, and internal organs. Children with this syndrome have an elfin or pixie-like appearance due to their unusual skull formation. The important feature here is that despite having intelligence that tests in the moderately to severely retarded range, individuals with Williams syndrome can engage in conversation that sounds fluent and grammatical, even using an extensive vocabulary (Bellugi, Bihrle, Jernigan, Trauner, & Doherty, 1991). Similarly, some children born with spina bifida who test in the severely retarded range (although others test within normal limits) can carry on a fluent form of conversational speech, sometimes called "cocktail party chatter" (Cromer, 1991; Curtiss, 1989).

Contributions

When based primarily on linguistic theory, the overriding goal of language assessment is to represent a child's underlying grammar or knowledge of the rules of language. The primary goal of intervention is to develop that grammar further. This is done by setting up conditions to lead children to induce rules they have not acquired naturally.

Linguistic Theory and Assessment. Linguistic approaches to language assessment focus on observable aspects of language performance as a way to infer what children know about the rules of language (i.e., children's nonobservable language competence). Children are seen as active participants in language acquisition, not as imperfect little adults whose primary developmental efforts are directed toward making fewer and fewer errors. Spontaneous samples of linguistic behavior are particularly important assessment tools because the things children say and do during language acquisition are thought to permit glimpses of their hidden generative hypotheses about language. Assessments based on linguistic theory tend to involve speaking more than other communication modes because oral language acquisition is considered primary to written language development, and because language expression is easier to observe than language comprehension.

When linguistic theory guides language assessment, the primary outcome is a profile of linguistic rules the child does and does not use. Particularly, following the introduction of Chomsky's linguistic theory (1957, 1965), assessment efforts focused on language form rules in spontaneous language and on structured language elicitation tasks. Then, "If the child missed a certain language structure on a test, that structure was listed as a goal of intervention. If the child responded correctly to a given language structure, the clinician assumed that the child 'knew' that structure, and it was not a target for intervention" (Launer & Lahey, 1981, p. 16).

Linguistic Theory and Intervention. Early efforts to apply Chomsky's theory to language intervention included the admonition for clinicians to view "language as a linguistic structure having phonemic, semantic, syntactic, and morphological features" (Lee, 1966, p. 311). In operation, however, the focus tended to be more on form than meaning. Pragmatics was not yet a part of the picture.

The application of linguistic theory to language assessment and intervention began to change as developmental psycholinguistics contributed to its evolution. A particularly important influence was Bloom's (1970) focus on the need for a rich semantic-grammatic interpretation of children's early two-word utterances. Bloom also emphasized that context was an essential part of determining meaning. These two contributions foreshadowed the blending of linguistic, cognitive, and sociolinguistic elements into the content–form–use model of language development and disorders that Bloom and Lahey introduced in their influential text in 1978 (see Figure 3.4). Even earlier, Bloom (1967) had pointed out that clinical techniques based on unidimensional aspects of linguistic theory, such as those analyzing the form of utterances in spontaneous language samples without considering their communicativeness, were limited and even distorted by their lack of contextual information.

Contemporary linguistic theory, with its emphasis on UG and learnability of principles and parameters, is just beginning to influence clinical decision making. It has been used to explain specific language impairment (SLI) as a condition in which children have a "young" grammar for an extended period of time. For example, Rice, Wexler, and Cleave (1995) found SLI children to show a cluster of problems with finite marking of verbs for number and tense (third person singular -s or past tense -ed or inflected forms of the auxiliaries, *be* and *do*)

when other aspects of grammar (longer MLU and inclusion of plural and possessive morphemes) were more advanced. They called this an Extended Optional Infinitive (EOI) stage because children with SLI seem to treat all verbs as non-finite. Infinitival (non-finite) forms do not have to be inflected. Compare the inflected finite forms in "She *walks,*" "She *is walking,*" or "She *walked,*" with the uninflected nonfinite "She liked *to walk,*" and "She made him *walk.*" Sentences of the type, "She walk," are commonly produced by children with SLI in place of any of the finite forms. Questioning the presence of clusters of grammatical immaturities can guide clinical assessment.

Two components of linguistic theory that are particularly relevant to language intervention are the **input-intake** relationship and **bootstrapping.** The bootstrapping of linguistic theory differs fundamentally from the "scaffolding" of social interaction theory in the degree of independence from social interaction partners. One pulls oneself up by the bootstraps, whereas scaffolding is essentially a phenomenon of social interaction between a more mature mentor and less mature learner. Cairns (1996) noted the distinction between normal and disordered development:

> *It is unnecessary to improve on nature; a normal linguistic environment will provide normally developing children with the information they need. For people dealing with children with language disorders, however, knowledge about input speech is highly practical. If a child is not developing language normally, the entire therapeutic enterprise is about providing input to facilitate language development. (p. 28)*

How should such input be modified? Triggering the LAD of a child with a language impairment to turn language **input** into language **intake** may require enhancing natural cues to make them more salient. All three forms of bootstrapping—semantic, prosodic, and syntactic—might be fostered deliberately by the clinician. The staging of language intervention activities within meaningful communicative events seems to be the best approach to facilitate semantic bootstrapping. That is, the adult can talk about what the child is doing or attending to. This approach is reminiscent of the traditional Van Riper suggestion of using parallel talk to provide "a running commentary on what the client is doing, perceiving, or probably feeling" (Van Riper & Erickson, 1996, p. 195). Bedore and Leonard

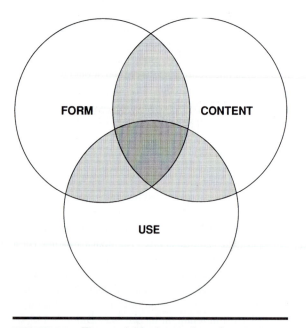

FIGURE 3.4   The model for interaction of content, form, and use in language.

Note: Reprinted with the permission of Macmillan Publishing Company from *Language Disorders and Language Development* (p. 22) by Margaret Lahey. Copyright © 1988 by Macmillan Publishing Company.

(1995) offered some additional suggestions for facilitating prosodic and syntactic bootstrapping (see Box 3.5).

Limitations

Probably the greatest limitation of linguistic theory for directing language assessment and intervention practices is its relatively narrow focus on learning the syntactic rules for forming single sentences. Rules related to pragmatics and to producing and understanding connected discourse are conspicuously missing. Linguistic theory seems best suited to explaining syntactic and phonological processes, which appear to unfold with relatively scant need for support from environmental factors. "Other aspects of language, however, such as semantic and pragmatic domains, may well exploit more general human information-processing mechanisms and are less strictly or exclusively tied to a 'language organ' "(Gardner, 1983, p. 81).

Box 3.5 _____

Example of Language Intervention Based on Linguistic Theory
(Bedore & Leonard, 1995)

TECHNIQUES BASED ON PROSODIC BOOTSTRAPPING

Research indicates that it is easier for children to pick out important content words from prosodic contexts that include both strong and weak syllables. Therefore, rather than using such telegraphic phrases as "eat cookie," or "push car," linguistic theorists recommend simple, but complete phrases:

> *He's eating the cookie* or *She pushed the car*

Words and morphemes also have longer durations and are easier for children to take in at the ends of sentences. Clinicians, therefore, modify their linguistic input so that targeted elements appear at the ends of sentences. Targeted elements include function words, such as the copula forms of *be,* the auxiliary forms of *be,* the "dummy" auxiliary *do* (see Chapter 8 for an explanation of the auxiliary construction rule), and modals such as *can* and *will,* as well as inflectional morphemes, such as plurals and possessives:

> *Now where is Letizia? Oh, there she is.* [copula]
>
> *Do you like dogs? I do.* [dummy *do*]
>
> *Can Tim count to ten? I can.* [modal *can*]
>
> *This is Paula's. It's Paula's coat.* [possessive inflectional morpheme]
>
> *I know what Bob wants. He wants a cookie.* [third person singular inflectional morpheme]

TECHNIQUES BASED ON SYNTACTIC BOOTSTRAPPING

Syntactic bootstrapping involves placing a targeted structure, such as a verb form, in a series of syntactic frames designed to help children infer aspects of the verb's meaning and its syntactic privileges:

> *Let's look at the pictures in the book* (*look is* transitive [i.e., takes an object])
>
> *Let's look at the pictures* (but it does not need a third component [e.g., like *put* does])
>
> *Let's look at what she's doing* (it can take an event as complement [not just person or place])
>
> *Look!* (it can be used as an imperative and is an active verb of perception)

Unlike theoreticians, clinicians cannot afford to ignore some aspects of language development to focus exclusively on others. Presentation of multiple exemplars of a particular syntactic formation rule (e.g., *is* + [Verb]*ing*) in single isolated sentences presented to correspond to a stack of pictures fails to consider the child's comprehensive needs (e.g., Gray & Ryan, 1973). Damico's (1988) case study of Debbie, which appears in Chapter 1, illustrates the limitations of this "fragmentation fallacy."

A second limitation associated with narrow clinical applications of linguistic theory is the potential to focus on a single stage of linguistic development, the preschool years, which I identify as the **middle stage of language acquisition.** It is only one of three important stages. Most professionals now recognize that although the majority of syntactic and morphological rule acquisition activity occurs during the years 3 through 7, some extremely important communicative events precede that period. Prelinguistic events occurring during the **early stage,** the communicative interactions of infancy, are now viewed to establish a foundation for language acquisition. The **later stage** of language acquisition is also now recognized for its significant developments, particularly in metalinguistics, abstract language use, and sophisticated discourse strategies. The linguistic-induction strategies that seem so important for supporting certain aspects of language acquisition in a particular stage may not be so important for supporting other aspects in other stages.

BEHAVIORAL THEORY

The general assumptions of behavioral theories of language development are outlined in Box 3.6. Behavioral explanations focus on the learning process rather than the linguistic system. The primary proponent of behavioral theories of language acquisition has been B. F. Skinner (1957). Skinner's book *Verbal Behavior* was published in the same year as Chomsky's (1957) first major book *Syntactic Structures*. The polarity of concepts advocated by these two theorists in the areas of function versus structure, performance versus competence, and nurture versus nature contributed to interesting debates in the scientific community (see Personal Reflection 3.3).

Box 3.6 _____

Primary Assumptions of Behavioral Theories of Language Development

1. Language acquisition can be explained by focusing on the observable and measurable aspects of language behavior.
2. Explanations of language acquisition should not rely on mentalistic constructs such as intentions or implicit knowledge of grammatical rules.
3. Rather, language acquisition is related to observable environmental conditions (stimuli) that co-occur with specific verbal behaviors (responses).
4. The term **verbal behavior** is preferred over **language** because the structural aspects of linguistics are irrelevant to the language-learning process; language as a skill does not differ essentially from any other behavior. Language is something people do, not something that they know.
5. The units of focus in the acquisition of verbal behavior should not be words or sentences but "functional units."

Personal Reflection 3.3 _____

"These were the mental and physiological theories I opposed. But I did not oppose them because they appealed to unobservables. Private events had to be taken into account in any successful analysis of human behavior, but they were mediators or by-products, not initiators of behaviors."

B. F. Skinner (1983, p. 279), writing in his autobiography, *A Matter of Consequences.*

Explanations

The mechanisms behaviorists propose for language acquisition are the same **stimulus–response–reinforcement** links used to explain other types of learning. The processes of **classical conditioning** are used to explain associations between arbitrary verbal stimuli and internal responses, such as for learning word meanings (Staats, 1971). The processes of **operant conditioning** are used to explain selective reinforcement and shaping of key verbal behaviors in a series of successive approximations. As explained by B. F. Skinner (1957), "Any response which vaguely resembles the standard behavior of the community is reinforced. When these begin to appear frequently, a closer approximation is insisted upon. In this manner very complex verbal forms may be reached" (p. 29). Behaviorists also propose that **imitation** plays a major role in language learning. The next section briefly addresses how behaviorists explain the acquisition of such language behaviors as phonological characteristics, words, sentences, and communicative functions.

Behavioral Explanations for Phonological Learning. Behaviorists explain phonological development as a product of operant conditioning. Elements of modeling and imitation also play a role. Behaviorist theory suggests that parents provide models to demonstrate for their children the important phonological characteristics of their native language. Then they selectively reinforce the child's attempts to imitate those characteristics. As parents reinforce attempts that come closest to those of their native language through attention, soothing, feeding, and handling, the frequency of appearance of desired phonological characteristics is shaped. Meanwhile, phonological characteristics that are not distinctive in the child's native language are ignored, and they eventually become extinguished because of lack of reinforcement.

Behavioral Explanations for Word Learning. Both operant and classical conditioning are used to explain word learning. When operant shaping principles shape phonological characteristics, they also contribute to the development of words. Phonological productions that sound like words (such as vocal play productions of *mamama* and *dadada*) are responded to with enthusiasm by parents.

Behaviorists cite classical learning principles to explain how children build associations between words and the things they represent. For example, the child may have a previously conditioned internal response to the environmental stimuli associated with going "bye-bye." When the parent labels this event, the child begins to associate the new "conditioned stimulus" (word + gesture) with the existing internal response. In similar ways, other conditioned stimuli (words) are associated with the event, with each other, and with other mediat-

ing stimuli. This process is sometimes called **stimulus clustering.** When the child learns to respond "bye-bye" under slightly different stimulus conditions (e.g., when someone else leaves or at bedtime), the process is called **stimulus generalization.** Stimulus generalization is necessary to explain how children learn that the word *dog* is associated with furry, four-legged creatures that can look widely different from one another.

Behavioral Explanations for Learning Sentences. The development of early two-word combinations and later sentences is explained as successive associative learning. Children learn to associate one word with the next in a left-to-right response chain. Meanwhile, they learn to associate the word chain with events in the environment. This is where the idea of functional units comes in. To explain how children can produce and understand unique sentences, behaviorists claim that what children learn is a set of increasingly larger functional units and how to combine them. For example, children might learn to treat prepositional phrases as a functional unit (or grammatical frame). Then, to create or understand novel utterances, they need only insert previously learned lexical items into the slots of the grammatical frame that they have already learned.

Behavioral Explanations for Communicative Function Learning. Behaviorists do not rely exclusively on explicit reinforcement from parents to explain the learning that takes place. Reinforcement patterns are more complicated than that. B. F. Skinner (1957) differentiated between several kinds of verbal responses, depending on their effect and other control factors. An **autoclitic** is the type of verbal behavior just described, in which speakers fill slots in grammatical frames (e.g., as subject–verb–object chains). It is a speaker response that is controlled by other verbal behaviors of that speaker. A **mand** is a verbal behavior, such as a demand, command, or request (e.g., "I want to see you") that specifies its reinforcer. In a sense, it is controlled by the reinforcer it specifies. An **echoic** verbal behavior is an imitative one. According to behaviorist theory, imitation allows a child to develop conditioned responses that can be elicited by environmental stimuli without the intervening model. An **intraverbal behavior** has no one-to-one correspondence to the stimuli that immediately evoke it. It is thought to be stimulated (and controlled) by previously learned associations from within the speaker's own system. For example, social rituals and spontaneous comments in conversational small talk fall into this category. A **tact** is a verbal behavior that relates to elements of the nonlinguistic context that speakers discuss. When speakers learn to name items in their environment, they are learning to treat those items as discriminative stimuli that elicit tact responses.

The Importance of Environmental Factors—Nature and Nurture Revisited.   To summarize, the major difference between linguistic and behavioral theories is the emphasis of behaviorists on nurture over nature. That is, behaviorists accord more importance to what occurs outside the child than inside. Behaviorists avoid talking about events that are not directly observable. They do not think it necessary to hypothesize that what children are learning is a set of linguistic rules. They argue instead that discussion of verbal behavior is enough.

Contributions

Behaviorism offers a well-developed technology for designing language intervention. This characteristic prompted Fey (1986) to note that, "Since the early 1960s, operant theory, or behaviorism, probably has had a greater impact on intervention practices than any other theory" (p. 3).

One of the most basic tenets of behaviorism is that nothing is hidden or mysterious. Everything that needs to be known can be observed by analyzing the effects of antecedent and consequent events on behavior. In addition, the stimulus–response–reinforcement paradigm offers a ready-made plan to modify a person's behavior.

Behavioral Theory and Assessment.   The tools of behaviorism include elements of both analysis and control. According to B. F. Skinner's (1957) view of radical behaviorism, language is treated either as a response to a presenting stimulus (a **tact**) or as an operant (a **mand**), which is either strengthened or weakened by subsequent reinforcement. The analysis techniques of behaviorism are used to define observable and measurable behavioral targets. Hidden, central processes, such as those representing mental states or motivational elements are considered to be beyond the purview of the observer and not critical to the outcome of interactions.

The basic tenets of a behavioral perspective on language assessment and intervention were outlined by Craig (1983):

(1) all behavior, including language, can be observed, described, and characterized in peripheral terms without involving the mind or central behavior; (2) complex behaviors are the sum of a set of simple behaviors; and (3) learning is the relationship between time and response strength. (pp. 103–104)

The view of complex behaviors as the sum of a set of simple behaviors invites the breakdown of language into steps that can be mastered one at a time. In behaviorism, the assessment process not only involves analysis of current levels of functioning, it also involves the use of task analysis procedures to outline learning goals. Under this theoretical umbrella, when deciding what to teach next, developmental level may be considered less important than task simplicity, and functionality may be viewed as more important than linguistic sophistication. In contrast with traditional linguistic or cognitive approaches, behaviorists give little weight to developmental prerequisites (e.g., Guess, Sailor, & Baer, 1974). Early examples of behavioral programs especially "placed no 'entrance requirements' on the learner" (L. McCormick, 1990a, p. 188).

One tool of assessment that behaviorists employ is called an **A-B-C assessment.** The acronym stands for Antecedent-Behavior-Consequence. It can be implemented with varying degrees of structure. Its purpose is to "establish hypothesized relations between naturally occurring environmental antecedents and consequences" (Cooper & Harding, 1993, p. 46). One strategy is to divide a piece of paper into three columns, each with one of the three headings. Usually the inventory starts with an entry in the "Behavior" column, arising from a need to figure out why a particular behavior, often an undesirable one, is interfering with communication or serving as an aberrant form of communication (see Box 3.7). The objective of the assessment is to identify antecedent stimuli or consequences that may be inadvertently triggering or reinforcing the undesirable behavior so they may be targeted in intervention.

Behavioral Theory and Intervention.   In behavior modification approaches, context is engineered. Environmental influences are considered paramount in determining whether a certain desired behavior will be

Box 3.7

Example of A-B-C Assessment Based on Behavioral Theory

My students and I were working with a fifth-grade girl with autism and severe communication impairment. Her Individualized Education Plan was designed to "include" her in a general education classroom with her typically learning fifth-grade classmates. She exhibited a behavior, however, that interfered with implementing the plan. It was the occasional emission of a high-pitched, extremely loud and piercing squeal. The noise effectively stopped the learning and teaching process for everyone and typically got her removed from the classroom. Even with systematic use of the A-B-C assessment procedure, her educational team was never able to identify a clear pattern of antecedent events (e.g., too much pressure, not enough attention) that seemed to trigger the behavior. The squeal seemed more a response to an internal state than to predictable environmental stimuli. The student's educational team did have to use the removal consequence consistently to protect the learning environment for the other students. They were able to conclude from the assessment, however, that removal was not acting as an inadvertent reinforcer for the squealing, as the squealing did not increase in frequency over time. In fact, it decreased in frequency as the student's learning and communicative repertoire increased, which allowed the student to participate in class discussions. In spite of improvements, the squealing never disappeared entirely, even into the student's high school years.

emitted, and once produced, whether it will occur again in the future. Thus, the behaviorist may write highly structured programs specifying all critical dimensions for sequences of interactions (e.g., Costello, 1977; Gray & Ryan, 1973; Sloane & MacAulay, 1968).

The technology of behaviorism involves control of antecedent and consequent events to shape responses and sometimes to encourage children to initiate behaviors. A variety of strategies can be used, some of which may also be employed in programs based on theories other than behaviorism with slight modifications of procedure and terminology:

Attention training involves an initial intervention objective in which a child is trained to "look at me," or

to "look at this," to receive a reinforcer just before the presentation of a new target stimulus (Kent, 1974).

Modeling involves presentation of a demonstrative model essentially indicating, "Here's how it's done."

Imitation training is the other side of modeling. It is the behavior produced by the child rather than by the trainer (McCormick, 1990b, p. 218). Imitation may be taught directly if the child has difficulty reproducing the behavior of another. This is usually done in a series of steps:

1. In a period of mutual imitations, the trainer imitates a behavior produced spontaneously by the child.
2. The trainer models behaviors the child has produced earlier in the same session.
3. The trainer models behaviors the child has produced in the past.
4. The trainer models a modified behavior close to one in the child's repertoire with the hope that the child will be able to imitate the modification (using reinforcers at every step to strengthen the child's attempts at responding).
5. Gradually, the child is able to imitate completely novel behaviors.

Reinforcement strategies all serve to strengthen the behavior they follow, but not all reinforcers are positive: **Positive reinforcers** are positive events whose presence increases the probability that a response will recur. For example, the act of requesting desired objects (called **manding** by behaviorists) may be reinforced with the objects requested. **Negative reinforcers** are aversive events whose removal increases the probability that a response will recur. For example, a child with tantrums may be placed in a "time-out" booth until the tantrum subsides, at which point the child is removed from the booth. Negative reinforcers are sometimes also viewed as "escape factors" that work to sustain undesirable behavior. Carr, Newsom, and Binkhoff (1980) described two children for whom aggressive behavior seemed to be negatively reinforced (i.e., increased in frequency) because it resulted in their being removed from undesired work situations whenever it occurred. Donnellan, Mirenda, Mesaros, and Fassbender (1984) recommended that caregivers infer from this type of behavior the communicative message, "Leave me alone! I don't want to do this!" (p. 202).

Varied reinforcement schedules are used in different stages of behavioral training. Reinforcement schedules of 100% (i.e., a positive reinforcer presented after every desired behavior) are often used initially, but frequency of reinforcement may be gradually reduced as new behaviors are stabilized. Eventually, only intermittent reinforcement, or only naturally reinforcing environmental consequences, are used to maintain the behavior. Planners generally try to avoid removing reinforcement entirely or too abruptly, for fear that a newly acquired behavior will be extinguished entirely but they try to avoid a situation in which a desired response can only be maintained with artificial reinforcers.

Punishment strategies are used to reduce an undesirable behavior. Like reinforcement, punishment is defined by its effect on behavior. Any consequence that reduces the frequency of a preceding behavior is considered to be punishing for a particular individual.

For example, echolalia may be defined as undesirable by behaviorists, who would shout, "Don't echo!" as a punishing consequence. However, as Duchan (1984) has pointed out, such a theoretical stance fails to recognize the potential communicative value of the echolalia, and punishment may suppress more than echolalia.

Parents and professionals debate whether other **aversives** should ever be used to punish behaviors of individuals with severe disabilities. Some parents and professionals feel that strong aversive punishments, such as those involving administration of electric shock or water or vinegar squirted in the face, are justified when needed to reduce self-injurious behaviors such as hand biting or head banging. Others feel that extreme use of aversive measures, such as physical restraint or ongoing isolation, is never justified. This position is summarized in Box 3.8 in a *Resolution on Abusive Treatment and Neglect* passed in 1988 by the Board of Directors of the Autism Society of America.

Prompting and **cuing** are used to highlight the salient features of a stimulus. The terms **prompt** and **cue** may be used interchangeably (McCormick, 1990b), but some prefer to reserve the term **prompt** to refer to direct efforts to guide a person into making a particular response (e.g., by guiding a person's hand or touching him on the elbow to initiate a response). **Putting through** and **hand-over-hand** prompts are used to physically assist motor responses.

Fading is used when cues and prompts are successful by reducing their intensity or frequency and reinforcing the child for the desired behavior. The idea is to remove prompts entirely, so that natural stimuli alone

---

Box 3.8

Autism Society of America: Excerpt from Resolution on Abusive Treatment and Neglect

The Society calls for a cessation of treatment and/or intervention that results in any of the following:

1. Obvious signs of physical pain experienced by the individual;
2. Potential or actual physical side effects, including tissue damage, physical illness, emotional stress, or death;
3. Dehumanization of an individual with autism by the use of procedures that are normally unacceptable for non-handicapped persons in all environments;
4. Ambivalence of discomfort by family, staff, and/or caregivers regarding the necessity of such extreme strategies or their involvement in such intervention; and
5. Revulsion or distress felt by handicapped and non-handicapped peers and community members who cannot reconcile extreme procedures with acceptable human conduct.

Note. "Resolution on Abusive Treatment and Neglect" by the Autism Society of America, July 16, 1988, *The Advocate,* 20(3), p. 17. Reprinted courtesy of the Autism Society of America.

---

result in the desired response; then, behaviorists say the response is under **stimulus control.**

Shaping is a basic strategy of operant conditioning. It involves selective reinforcement of responses increasingly close to the target. For example, behaviorists might advise the parent of a nonverbal child to respond "Oh, you want some cereal" first, when the child merely looks at a cabinet where a favorite cereal is kept; next, only when the child uses a whole-hand reach as well as a look; after that, only when the child points; then, only when the child points and vocalizes at the same time; and finally, only when the child produces increasingly close approximations of words and then phrases.

Discrimination training is a basic behavioral training technique. It involves differential reinforcement of particular responses to particular stimuli. For example, when a word is spoken, a child might be expected to discriminate it from others and to select the particular object or picture the word represents. In another session, the child might be expected to discriminate an object on the basis of its function, for example, "What do you use to fix your hair?" or "What do you use to sweep the floor?"

Chaining is used to build complex behaviors from simpler ones. It is particularly useful when sequence is important (e.g., washing hands independently). Either backward chaining or forward chaining approaches may be used. Both approaches take advantage of selective limits on short-term memory. Backward chaining takes advantage of the "recency effect," which represents the finding that the last item of a sequence is usually the easiest to remember. Using backward chaining, a speech–language pathologist might teach a child to produce a multisyllabic word like hamburger by asking the child to imitate each of the following syllabic combinations in sequence:

> -ger
>
> -burger
>
> hamburger

Forward chaining takes advantage of the primacy effect of short-term memory (STM) and starts by modeling early elements in a chain, adding on later elements as success is experienced.

Generalization is the goal of a behavior training program. Stimulus generalization occurs when the child learns to use a new label, such as *hat,* to go with many types of headgear, some of which the child has never seen before, as well as with a picture of a particular kind of hat. The technical explanation is that varied stimuli begin to take on controlling properties for that same response. Response generalization occurs when the conditioning of a particular response results in increased probability of other responses similar to the original. This happens when varied responses are in the same response class. An example is when a child learns to use plural morphemes in response to a set of pictures of duplicate items and then asks for "two pretzels" at snacktime.

Repeated trials are used to strengthen new responses.

Discrete trials are also typical of behavioral programs. Three formats (Mulligan, Guess, Holvoet, & Brown, 1980) are: (1) **massed trials,** with no other responses or spontaneous comments permitted; (2) **spaced trials,** grouped in clusters but with a rest period between;

and (3) **distributed trials,** interspersed with other activities, in which relevant responses are permitted and even encouraged.

Direct teaching is the term used to describe behaviorist intervention approaches. They are characterized by: (1) task analysis of targeted skills into discrete parts, (2) adult-directed choices of carefully specified content, (3) specific prompts and reinforcement, (4) rapid massed trial instruction, and (5) frequent test-questions to assess learning (Warren & Yoder, 1994).

The "Lovaas approach" (Lovaas, 1981; Lovaas, Schaeffer, & Simmons, 1965) is one of the most well known, but controversial, behavioral approaches. Lovaas has worked with children with autism and other developmental disabilities since the 1960s at the University of California at Los Angeles. Many parents of children with Pervasive Developmental Disorders (PDD), including autism, seek Lovaas therapy because of a study (Lovaas, 1987) that showed autistic children younger than 3 years gain apparently normal intellectual and educational functioning after intensive 40-hour-per-week treatment. This approach, like other behaviorist approaches for autism (Maurice, 1996), is highly structured. For example, the Lovaas (1981) training sequence for hugging goes as follows:

Step 1: Say, "Hug me," and prompt (e.g., physically move) the child so that his cheek makes momentary contact with yours. Reward him with food the moment his cheek makes contact.

Step 2: Gradually fade the prompt while keeping the instruction ("Hug me") loud and clear.

Step 3: Gradually withhold the reward contingent on longer and longer hugs. Move in slow steps from a 1-second hug to one lasting 5 to 10 seconds. At the same time, require a more complete hug such as placing his arms around your neck, squeezing harder, etc. Prompt these additional behaviors if necessary.

Step 4: Generalize this learning to many environments and many persons. Gradually thin the reward schedule so that you get more and more hugs for less and less reward. (p. 50)

The DISTAR Language Program I (Engleman & Osborn, 1976) is another example of a language instructional program, but one used with a wide range of children in general education as well as special education classrooms. DISTAR uses all of the direct teaching techniques, as in the sequence for teaching *tall* and *short:*

Listen. Is this bottle tall? [touch]
No.
Say the whole thing. [touch]
This bottle is not tall.
Is this bottle short? [touch]
Yes.
Say the whole thing. [touch]
This bottle is short.
[Repeat until all children's responses are firm.] (p. 58)

Personally, I confess that I do not like this approach. My own intervention bias is toward social-interaction approaches that are natural, meaningful—and fun. Cole and Dale (1986), however, compared DISTAR with a social-interactionist approach by implementing each with a randomly assigned group of preschoolers with delayed language. Both groups improved significantly and substantially on syntactic and semantic measures, and no posttest differences were found between them.

Yoder, Kaiser, and Alpert (1991) compared another direct approach, the Communication Training Program (Waryas & Stremel-Campbell, 1983) with a Milieu Teaching Program (see Box 3.9), which is also based on behaviorist theory, but with an eclectic theoretical flavor (Warren & Yoder, 1994). In this research, Yoder and his colleagues found that children benefited differentially from the two approaches, depending on their incoming characteristics. That is, lower functioning preschoolers benefited more from the Milieu method, and higher functioning preschoolers (who also had developmental disabilities) benefited more from the Communication Training Program. In particular, direct instruction was less effective than milieu teaching for teaching early vocabulary or facilitating the development of pragmatic skills.

Limitations

Few contemporary language specialists take behavioral explanations of normal language acquisition seriously.

Associative learning and selective reinforcement paradigms may explain some aspects of sound and word learning, but behavioral theory is woefully inadequate for explaining the rapidity and complexity of normal acquisition of grammatical knowledge in early childhood. Nevertheless, the question remains for *clinicians* whether behavioral principles, either in pure or modified forms, should guide language intervention decisions when language acquisition does not proceed normally. Perhaps children with specific language impairment have different learning needs. For example, Connell (1987) found young children with SLI to generalize a novel morpheme more extensively following imitation teaching; whereas their peers without SLI generalized more extensively after learning the morpheme through a more naturalistic modeling approach.

Direct instruction is widely criticized by cognitivists and social interactionists for being so adult-directed that language learners are not actively engaged in the language acquisition enterprise. This distinction is sometimes characterized as a dichotomy between *instruction* and *construction* (although Warren & Yoder, 1994, consider it a false dichotomy), or between teaching *skills* and encouraging the acquisition of *knowledge*. When adults engineer the teaching choices so completely, children are more likely to *imitate* utterances for artificial reinforcement than to *generate* them for authentic communicative purposes. A danger then exists that learning may only occur on the surface and may only appear in the highly structured teaching context. In our clinic at Western Michigan University, we have worked with a number of children with specific learning and reading disabilities whose prior direct reading instruction with a DISTAR approach had taught them to focus on sound to the exclusion of meaning, to expect words to rhyme but not to fit into meaningful sentences, and to sound out words letter-by-letter rather than to use knowledge about language and stories to predict what might fit.

Another limitation of behaviorist approaches to language assessment and intervention stems from the lack of a rich model of the structure of language. Repeated trials with the same stimulus can turn meaningful language meaningless. For example, if you were to sit in front of a set of objects and be asked repeatedly, "Is this a brush?," you might begin to wonder after a while. Even after reaching criterion on this task the child may have no concept of what a brush can be used for or how to request one. The crux of this problem is that lan-

Box 3.9 _____

Examples of Milieu Prompting Episodes Using the Mand-Model and Incidental Teaching Procedures

MAND-MODEL

Example 1	*Example 2*
Context: Child is scooping beans with a ladle and pouring them into a pot.	Context: Trainer gives each child a turn to blow bubbles.
TRAINER: "What are you doing?" (target probe question) CHILD: No response TRAINER: "Tell me." (mand) CHILD: "Beans" TRAINER: "Say, pour beans." (model) CHILD: "Pour beans." TRAINER: "That's right, you're pouring beans into the pot." (verbal acknowledgment + expansion)	TRAINER: (holds the wand up to the child's mouth) "What do you want to do?" (target probe question) CHILD: "Bubbles" TRAINER: "*Blow* bubbles" (model) CHILD: "Blow bubbles" TRAINER: "OK, you want to blow bubbles. Here you go." (verbal acknowledgment + expansion + activity participation)

INCIDENTAL TEACHING

Example 1	*Example 2*
Context: Making pudding activity. Trainer gives peer a turn at stirring the pudding as the subject looks on.	Context: Trainer and subject are washing dishes together in a parallel fashion.
CHILD: "Me!" (Child initiates) and reaches for ladle. TRAINER: "Stir pudding" (model) CHILD: "Stir pudding" TRAINER: "All right. You stir the pudding, too." (verbal acknowledgment + expansion + activity participation)	CHILD: "Wash" (Child initiates with an action-verb, partial target response) TRAINER: "Wash what?" (elaborative question) CHILD: "Wash" (incorrect response) TRAINER: "Wash *what*?" (elaborative question) CHILD: "Wash cups" TRAINER: "That's right. We're washing cups." (verbal acknowledgment + expansion)

Note: From "An Experimental Analysis of Milieu Language Intervention. Teaching the Action–Object Form" by S. Warren and L. Bambara, 1989, *Journal of Speech and Hearing Disorders,* 54, p. 461. Copyright 1989 by American Speech-Language-Hearing Association. Reprinted by permission.

---

guage seems to be too complex a system for some children to master on their own, but breaking it down into manageable pieces does not make it simpler so much as different.

Many children taught with behaviorist methods find it difficult to generalize newly learned behaviors to complex real-life situations. Some behaviorists have attempted to address this problem by focusing on the functionality of language and other behaviors (McCormick & Schiefelbusch, 1990). **Functional re-**

sponses are natural and necessary in children's everyday interactions. They produce immediate, specific, and potentially naturally reinforcing consequences (Guess, Sailor, & Baer, 1978). For example, when a child learns to imitate bringing a cup to the mouth to get juice or pointing to a cookie to get a bite of it the reinforcers are received as natural consequences of the child's actions.

Another problem is that behavioral analysis tends to result in focus on pieces of behavior rather than interactions among people (e.g., Duchan, 1995b). The principles of behaviorism generally have been demonstrated in the laboratory and in small-scale experiments. Progress is measured in terms of specific pieces of behavior targeted for intervention and not in terms of broader situational outcomes. Studies that have attempted to assess generalization from training contexts to natural environments (e.g., Hughes & Carpenter, 1983; Warren & Rogers-Warren, 1983) or to teach it directly (e.g., Stokes & Baer, 1977) have shown poor or mixed results. Broad scale efficacy of strict behavioral-oriented approaches across multiple aspects of children's lives is difficult to demonstrate.

Additionally, by denying the relevance (or even existence) of internal processes and emotional states such as interest and motivation, reductionistic behavioral programs fail to take advantage of the rich opportunities afforded by the more active learning paradigms based on linguistic, cognitive, or social-interaction theories. For example, classic behaviorism treats echolalia as a behavior to be extinguished rather than as communicative, perhaps representing inner states such as frustration or discomfort. By responding to a child's behavior, rather than asking questions about the child's need, important learning and participation opportunities may be missed.

Overcoming Past Limitations through Communicative Analysis.   More recent behavioral approaches analyze possible communicative functions of aberrant behavior and design intervention approaches in which such behaviors might be treated as communicative (Donnellan et al., 1984; Reichle & Wacker, 1993a). Modified behavioral approaches are also designed to reduce the passivity that frequently results when children are taught exclusively in stimulus–response–reinforcement modes. Such children tend to become **prompt-dependent** and thus never learn to recognize the assertive and communicative possibilities of language use. (Behaviorists explain this as too much reinforcement of tact behaviors and not enough of mands.) Mirenda and Santogrossi (1985) developed a "prompt-free" approach for starting over with an 8½-year-old nonspeaking girl. Amy only pointed to pictures on her communication board when an adult or peer asked "What do you want?" or "Show me what you want." In the revised program, only one symbol was available, and Amy was only reinforced when she spontaneously touched it (a picture of a can of pop). First, this occurred accidentally, and then, intentionally.

Overcoming Past Limitations through Milieu Teaching.   Others have overcome limitations of behaviorism by using naturally occurring learning contexts rather than highly structured ones; keeping interaction events whole rather than breaking them down into component parts; using topics initiated by children, not by adults; using naturally occurring, not contrived, reinforcers; and using dispersed, not massed, trials. These approaches have been called **milieu** or **incidental teaching.** The principles of incidental teaching were first reported by Hart and Risley (1968) and have since been expanded (Hart & Risley, 1975, 1986; Hart & Rogers-Warren, 1978; Kaiser & Warren, 1988; S. F. Warren & Kaiser, 1986; S. F. Warren & Rogers-Warren, 1985).

According to Warren and Yoder (1994), milieu teaching subsumes modeling, mand-model, time delay, and incidental teaching procedures (see Box 3.9 for examples of mand-model and incidental teaching discourse). These behaviorist strategies are described as follows:

1. **Modeling.** Models of desired responses are presented in environmentally appropriate contexts.
2. **Mand-model.** When children show interest in a particular item or activity, they are directly prompted (e.g., "Tell me what you want to do") and may even be prompted to "Give me a whole sentence." If further modeling is needed, it is provided, and when a satisfactory response is obtained, it is reinforced with the desired object or activity.
3. **Time delay.** This technique is used to avoid prompt dependence. Rather than prompting, the adult arranges the environment to elicit the child's interest. When the child looks at the object and then the adult, the adult seeks to establish and maintain eye contact. If the child does not speak, the adult may model a response twice (with adequate time between models), and then, if the child still does not speak, the object or activity is provided nevertheless.
4. **Incidental teaching as a specific procedure.** Each episode starts with an initiation by the child. Adults attend to the child's interest and help the child to make more elaborate requests or comments through modeling and reinforcement within the natural contexts of the events.

Although incidental teaching approaches use natural learning contexts, they are not particularly naturalistic (Duchan, 1995a). Kirchner (1991) commented that "milieu teaching may be the most 'naturalistic' of the behaviorally derived approaches, but can hardly be considered pragmatic" (p. 83). On the other hand, Warren and Yoder (1994) argued that:

> *Milieu teaching represents a truly eclectic approach to intervention. By basing teaching on the child's attentional lead (as constructivist approaches do), the child plays a significant role in determining the topic and pace of learning. But by allowing adults to elicit target production, direct teaching attempts are also built in as a critical source of input and deliberate scaffold for children's conversational participation (as behavioral approaches do). (p. 252)*

INFORMATION PROCESSING THEORY

Explanations

Like behavioral theories, information processing theories focus on how language is learned rather than the rules presumed to underlie it (see Box 3.10). Contrasting with behavioral theories, information processing theories (in several versions) emphasize the role of internal information processing mechanisms in language acquisition and use.

Information processing theory in the older version proposes a set of **serial information processes** that act on incoming perceptual input from auditory (speech) or visual (print) sources to analyze it, comprehend it, formulate a response, and transform it back into physical form. Carrow-Woolfolk (1988) noted that this "single-path serial model of cognitive processing (sensation → perception → cognition → memory) has been in existence since the time of Aristotle" (p. 10).

A second, newer version is based on computer modeling of the language acquisition process. It proposes a **parallel distributed processing** (PDP) or **connectionist** model in which incoming information is distributed to several processing nodes simultaneously. PDP models are designed to overcome limitations of linguistic theory by providing a working model for the mysterious LAD. Johnson-Laird (1983) noted that a working model would "not require any decisions to be made on the basis of intuition or any other such 'magical' ingredient" (p. 6) (see Personal Reflection 3.4).

In this section, several aspects of information processing theory are considered: bottom-up processing, top-down processing, interactive processing, attention, working memory, and central auditory processing. Then

---

Box 3.10 _____

Primary Assumptions of Information Processing Theories of Language Development

1. The information processing system encodes stimuli from the environment, interprets them, stores the results in memory, and allows retrieval of information previously stored.
2. Language acquisition depends on empiricist principles in that experience with linguistic evidence from the environment causes changes within processing mechanisms.
3. Rather than starting with innate patterns of (probably neural) connections, all original connections are equal; through experience, some connections become strengthened by repeated activations, whereas others (primitive patterns) are weakened (owing to lack of empirical evidence to activate them) until they disappear.
4. Newer models claim that the patterns of information processing that account for language learning are parallel rather than serial.
5. The order of acquisition of language forms is cued by the functions (e.g., requesting, identifying location) of the forms. Forms that appear more frequently and that regularly serve the same function (even if they are less frequent) are learned first.

PERSONAL REFLECTION 3.4 _____

"To understand a phenomenon is to have a working model of it, albeit a model that may contain simulated components."

Phillip N. Johnson-Laird (1983, p. 4), writing in his book, *Mental Models.*

---

computer models and connectionist (also called **competition**) theories are discussed.

Bottom-up Processing. The sequence of processes involved in language interactions usually includes a list of processes that allow an individual to: (1) sense information, (2) attend to it, (3) separate it from environmental noise, (4) perceive it, (5) hold it in working memory, (6) recognize it, (7) make sense of it, (8) compare it with prior experience, (9) formulate new information,

(10) make adjustments in long-term memory, and (11) produce expressions that can be received by others. Serial models have been proposed for listening and speaking and for reading and writing. The emphasis is on perception of auditory input in the first, and visual input in the second. Bottom-up information processing models share an emphasis on accurate reception and preliminary perceptual processing of sensory input before it can be processed at higher levels of meaning. The arrows in the sequence, "sensation → perception → cognition → memory," suggest this unidirectional view.

Myklebust (1954, 1957) popularized bottom-up processing models for auditory-oral language. He pointed to the language learning problems of individuals with severe hearing loss as evidence that accurate reception and perception of peripheral auditory information are critical to language learning. Linguists, such as Bellugi and Klima (1982) and Pettito (1992/1994), countered arguments about the essential nature of auditory processing to language learning by showing that deaf infants of parents who use American Sign Language acquire language in much the same way as hearing infants whose parents use spoken language. They argued that this supports the linguistic theory of a more general LAD rather than modality-specific information processing theories.

Serial models for reading typically emphasize the sensory role the eyes play as visual end-organs for scanning texts. Perceptual processes follow, which include relating print to sound, after which input is processed for meaning and higher order thinking (Singer & Ruddell, 1985). Both auditory and visual bottom-up models are considered **data-driven.** They emphasize **decoding** as preliminary to sensemaking and the importance of signal clarity and accurate perception for successful processing. Bottom-up processing models also suggest that language processing moves from **part-to-whole.**

Top-down Processing.   As the name suggests, top-down processing models emphasize the influences of higher order thinking processes over lower order perceptual ones. Such models explain human beings making sense of their world as going from **whole-to-part** (Norris & Hoffman, 1993). In fact, they may be better classified as **cognitivist** models. In other words, listeners or readers start with cognitive schemas constructed through experience, and they use these internalized models of reality to make predictions about the meaning of sensory input in particular contexts. Their expec-

tations that sensory input will make sense causes them to listen selectively to auditory input or to see selectively when reading.

Frank Smith (1973, 1975) is one of the major proponents of this cognitivist/information processing view. To explain the developmental mystery about how young children can detect the boundaries between words within the slippery stream of speech, Smith pointed out that meaning tells what the words are rather than words telling meaning.

A second major proponent of top-down theory is Ken Goodman (1986). Along with colleagues, including his wife Yetta Goodman, Goodman has been one of the leaders of the whole language movement in education. Describing how oral and written language acquisition are similar, he wrote:

> *Language is actually learned from whole to part. We first use whole utterances in familiar situations. Then later we see and develop parts, and begin to experiment with their relationship to each other and the meaning of the whole. The whole is always more than the sum of the parts and the value of any part can only be learned within the whole utterance in a real speech event. (p. 19)*

Although language development specialists could point to flaws in this argument, citing early production of one-word utterances by toddlers, first words generally do express "holophrastic" meanings. Evidence that mature language users employ some top-down strategies becomes apparent when a glitch occurs while listening or reading. This happens when a predicted meaning turns out not to match the perceptual data after all. When meaning construction gets too far ahead of input and listeners or readers get off track, they have to regroup and focus attention back to the perceptual data to get going again.

Interactive Processing.   The preceding example also forms part of the evidence for interactive processing models, which combine bottom-up and top-down components (Butler, 1984a). Such models suggest that either without the other is insufficient. Duchan (1983) contrasted older views of serial processing using the metaphor of an elevator (see Personal Reflection 3.5). She noted that:

> *typical language processing models have deficiencies because they incorrectly assume that listeners begin by hearing the signal and then, in a step-like manner, continue through and passively process until an interpretation is*

made. Instead, perhaps even before the signal is introduced, there is an active higher order processing going on which selects the relevant signals and processes their contents in parallel fashion. The listener uses both signal and higher order knowledge in the effort to make sense of what is going on and to fulfill particular needs. (p. 89)

Interactive theories of information processing are characterized by four features: (1) Higher level processes are viewed as exerting influence on lower ones; (2) multiple processes are viewed as operating in parallel, as modeled by computer simulations of human information processing; (3) language learners are viewed as active participants; (4) the importance of linguistic and nonlinguistic context as well as the clarity of the informational signal itself.

An example is Rumelhart and McClelland's (1981) interactive model of written language processing. According to this model, a reader is viewed as a person who comes to a text with a set of expectations about the kinds of visual input likely to be encountered. Such expectations are based on prior knowledge of the structure of letters, words, phrases, sentences, and larger pieces of discourse as well as aspects of the nonlinguistic context. Reading is viewed as a series of hypothesis testing moves that are used to construct meanings. During this process, visual information from the page is used to strengthen some hypotheses, to weaken others, and to formulate new predictions. Comprehension is defined as the state reached when the accumulated evidence most strongly supports one hypothesis.

Attention. Language learners do not give equal weight to all the sensory stimuli that bathe them at any point in time. Try the exercise in Box 3.11 to appreciate the active role attention plays in tuning our systems to process certain sources of information (the signal) and to ignore others (the noise). In other words, humans have choices about how to allocate their attention. At-

PERSONAL REFLECTION 3.5 _____

"A prevailing idea then was that processing language was something like sending a linguistic package up and down a freight elevator in a multilevel, rectilinear building." (p. 83)

Judith Felson Duchan (1983).

Box 3.11 _____

Exercise in Tuning in to the Senses

As you read this text, pause for a moment and pay attention to each of your senses.

1. If you listen, you can become aware of the noise that surrounds you; think about its characteristics and the probable sources for each of the sounds you hear.
2. Look around you, or stay focused on the page and see all that you could take in if you wanted to, even then.
3. Feel the things that you are touching, such as the chair you are sitting on, the feel of the book under your fingertips, the feel of your clothes on your body.
4. If you attend to your sense of smell, can you notice anything?
5. Are you aware of any kinesthetic sensations from movements you are making? How about your tongue? Is it completely still? Are you chewing gum?
6. Now refocus your attention on the meaning of this exercise and these words. Think about the role of attention in screening out information not critical to the purpose of the moment (noise) as well as the role of attention in screening in information that might have meaning (signal). This is sometimes called **figure-ground** perception. Perception of meaningful signals against a background of noise depends on a combination of internal filtering ability and external signal-to-noise ratio.

tention appears, as Smith (1975) suggested, to be questions asked by the brain, such as: "What is that?" "Is it important?" "Is it safe to ignore?" "Does it make sense?" "Should I pay attention to it?"

Attention allocation depends on at least two things: (1) the information available, and (2) the amount of resources (processing capability) that can be allocated to the task (Snyder & Downey, 1983). A task that lacks sufficient information for the processor to complete it is **data limited,** and a processor who lacks sufficient skill to carry out a task is said to be **resource limited.** The more existing resources a processor has, the more the person is able to rely on top-down processing to fill in data that may be missing from the signal. When prior knowledge is weak, processors become increasingly dependent on signal clarity. For example, it is much easier to listen to a lecture over a public address system that is full of static when the topic is familiar and the content interesting.

Working Memory.   In order to be able to analyze language input, listeners need to hold it in memory while making sense of it. Then the actual words can be forgotten while the meaning is retained for participating in ongoing communication events. This temporary storage is called **working memory** or **short-term memory.**

Normal language users become aware of the value of working memory and ability to **reauditorize** a partially processed speech signal when they say, "What?" then "Oh, yeah," to a communication partner before the partner has a chance to repeat the message. What happens in such cases? It is as if a little tape loop replays the partially processed auditory signal through the system, possibly involving the arcuate fasciculus, which connects Wernicke's and Broca's areas in the left hemisphere and makes it possible to repeat what others say. Meanwhile, other resources are brought online to fill in the missing data and figure out what has been said. The system that can do this must constitute a fine-tuned interaction between data-driven signal decoding and knowledge-driven narrowing of options. That is, based on prior experience with language and what people are likely to say in certain circumstances, listeners seem to narrow the options about what might have been heard and test them against limited sensory input data. It is because listeners can hold input in short-term memory that they are able to do this.

The concept of a **limited capacity processor** is used to explain variations in **short-term memory** as they relate to attentional demands of particular tasks. Lahey and Bloom (1994) explained how STM fits within the broader concept of **working memory.** In working memory:

> *A part of the system is allocated to storage and a part to processing. Working memory, therefore, contrasts with the typical view of short-term memory as a limited capacity storage-only mechanism; working memory is an information processing system with limits on both storage and processing capacity. (p. 361)*

Working memory models incorporate modality-specific storage components. Baddeley (1986) called the auditory storage mechanism the **articulatory loop** and the visual storage mechanism the **visual-spatial scratch pad.** These two storage systems have a limited capacity and can only be used for storage. The other part of working memory is the processor component, called the **central executor.** It has greater flexibility and can be used either for storage (when the capacity of the usual storage system is full) or for processing.

Lahey and Bloom (1994) described how contextual variations in processing demands can influence the allocation of resources within a limited capacity processor. Initial learning requires considerable allocation of resources from the central executor. Once an operation becomes automatic, it requires less allocation of direct attention to processing. A return to greater executor involvement may be needed, however, when demands increase from perceptual-motor, linguistic, or social-emotional factors. "For example, when listeners try to understand someone with an unfamiliar accent or dialect or to understand someone in a noisy environment, they use more processing resources than when listening to familiar speech in a quiet room" (p. 362).

Toddlers learning language show the effects of working memory when they repeat selective parts of what others say to them. When an adult says, "Let's go downstairs now and see what Grandpa is doing," a two-year-old might repeat, "Downstairs, see Grandpa." This example illustrates two marvelous traits of normal language acquisition: (1) The child has been able to hold relatively complex input in memory long enough to act on it (the storage component); and (2) the child has acted on it (the central executor component). This marvelous language learning machine demonstrates not only the effects of short-term memory, but also that memory is more than rote.

Experiments that measure short-term memory typically use lists of unrelated words in sequence (often the names of digits) rather than words related linguistically in sentences. The reason is to test the simple ability to remember without help from the sensemaking language processing mechanism, which facilitates STM and confounds the experiment. It is impossible, however, to separate memory tests from language knowledge systems entirely. To appreciate this, ask a friend to test your ability to remember sequences of the names of digits in English. Then have the friend test your ability to remember digit sequences from a language you know marginally. You should be able to repeat more number words from the language you know well.

George Miller's (1956) famous guideline for holding unrelated chunks of information in STM is 7, plus or minus 2. Miller's main point was that humans can exceed the limits of their bottom-up information processing systems, but only if they code them some way by using higher order processes to construct meaningful chunks. Miller emphasized that adult limits are related to seven **chunks,** not seven bits, of information (Bruner, 1990).

Short-term memory for unrelated words is subject to the **recency effect** and the **primacy effect.** That is, the easiest items to remember are the last heard (recency effect) and the first heard (primacy effect). Words in the middle are the hardest to remember. This is not what happened in the toddler language example, though. The toddler had to linguistically process the original message to pull out the words that conveyed the essence of the meaning. The child was clearly treating this as more than a memory task.

Language specialists know that STM is somehow associated with normal language acquisition, because reduction in STM is often associated with impaired language development (Gathercole & Baddeley, 1995; Gillam, Cowan, & Day, 1995). What is not known is precisely how the two processes are related. It may be that STM deficits reflect language acquisition problems rather than causing them (Rees, 1973, 1981). Gathercole and Baddeley (1990), for example, found limitations in phonological storage capabilities, rather than impairments of auditory perceptual processes, to explain why children with specific language impairments have exaggerated difficulty repeating nonwords (Kamhi & Catts, 1986; Kamhi, Catts, Mauer, Apel, & Gentry, 1988). Gillam and colleagues concluded, "Although we do not yet know exactly how certain constraints on memory processes affect language development and use, we do know that language learning involves both conceptually driven (top-down) and data-driven (bottom-up) memory processes" (p. 401).

Central Auditory Processing.   Others have suggested that the memory deficits of children with specific language impairment constitute a more generalized temporal processing impairment. The research conducted by Tallal and her colleagues pointed to a generalized sequential processing deficit for detecting and remembering both auditory and visual stimuli produced in rapid sequence (Tallal, 1980; Tallal & Piercy, 1978; Tallal & Stark, 1976). Tallal (1996) noted that intervention studies with children with LLIs (Merzenich et al., 1996; Tallal et al., 1996) linked improvements in the speed of discrimination decisions with improvements in other re-

ceptive speech and language abilities. Based on these results, she suggested "that the symptomatology of children with LLI may mainly reflect bottom-up processing constraints rather than a defect in language competence, per se" (p. 6).

The temporal auditory processing research involves responses to rapid transitions that mirror natural speech. Other techniques involve physiological and behavioral measurements that detect neural activity while auditory signals move from the cochlea through the brain stem on their way to the auditory cortex and association areas (American Speech-Language-Hearing Association, 1996; Keith, 1977, 1981; Lasky & Katz, 1983).

Transformations from acoustic to sensory to symbolic information take place within this system, but it is not clear where the dividing line exists between CAP and language processing, if there is one. The cause and effect relationship is also unclear. At least one study of children with specific language impairment failed to show any difference in their brain stem responses to acoustic tone shifts compared with children developing language normally (Tomblin, Abbas, Records, & Brenneman, 1995). Can a defect in the CAP mechanism cause a child to have difficulty acquiring language, or does less efficient operation of the CAP mechanism merely reflect a language system that is not working properly?

Computer Models and Competition Theory.   Information processing theories presume the existence of biological processing mechanisms, but ties between information processing and biological maturation theories are not as close as one might suppose. As Johnson-Laird (1983) pointed out, "the mind can be studied independently from the brain" (p. 9). Computer models of linguistic rule learning provide a primary means for doing so.

Computer simulations of normal language acquisition are designed to take in linguistic input of the sort children hear, "learn" the rules that govern it, and generate new linguistic forms consistent with those rules. Systems that can accomplish such a feat are based on **parallel distributive processing** models. In these computer models, as input comes in, it is distributed to several decision-making activation nodes simultaneously, where it is compared with stored data. A critical feature is that the nodes are linked or connected much as the neural cells in a human brain are. In fact, such models are sometimes called **connectionist.** Gradually, over time and with increasing environmental exposure to additional language input, the system figures out the patterns in the input. With each new input, adjustments occur in the relative strength of connections among the association nodes and output nodes (this is the learning process), so that some connective patterns are strengthened and others are weakened. While going through this process, the computer makes developmental errors like children do, but eventually reaches a level at which it can produce output that has never occurred in the input. Thus, it can be said to have "learned" the pattern.

PDP computer simulations are not yet like little futuristic robots, who can run around learning all the complexities of language the way real children do, but they are able to figure out specific rule systems when provided with relatively limited (although deliberately planned) input the way real children do. In their pioneering research, Rumelhart and McClelland (1986/1994) demonstrated regular and irregular verb learning. Like normally developing children, the system started by using each

verb correctly, then went through a stage of overregularization (producing output like "wented") and finally produced both regular and irregular forms correctly (see Figure 3.5 for a representation of how the model works).

Bates and MacWhinney (1987; MacWhinney, 1987) applied connectionist theory to explanations of children's language acquisition in their **competition model** (I know this is a lot of labels for related ideas—**PDP, connectionist,** and now **competition models** are all in the same family). According to the competition model, when children begin the language-learning process, the only thing that is innate is a powerful PDP mechanism. Children's systems are subject to no other innate biases or constraints, as linguists presume in the LAD. At first, all phonetic patterns, words, and syntactic forms *compete* equally to represent a particular meaning or communicative function. As children gain repeated experience with language exemplars in their environment, some activation patterns are strengthened (among the nodes in the PDP system) while others are weakened. Over the course of develop-

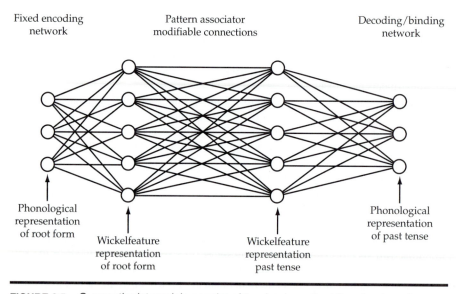

Fixed encoding network

Pattern associator modifiable connections

Decoding/binding network

Phonological representation of root form

Wickelfeature representation of root form

Wickelfeature representation past tense

Phonological representation of past tense

FIGURE 3.5   Connectionist models consist of two basic parts: (1) a simple pattern associator network, "which learns the relationships between the base form and the past-tense form," and (2) a decoding network that "converts a featural representation of the past-tense form into a phonological representation. All learning occurs in the pattern associator." (Rumelhart & McClelland, 1986/1994, p. 428)

Note. From *On Learning the Past Tenses of English Verbs* (p. 428) by D. E. Rumelhart & J. L. McClelland, 1994. Cambridge, MA: The MIT Press. Copyright 1986 by The MIT Press. Reprinted by permission.

ment, the patterns that most closely match the evidence win the competition and are used for communicating.

By avoiding reliance on a mysterious and unique LAD to explain language acquisition, information processing theory shifts the emphasis from a set of specialized linguistically tuned "operating principles" (proposed by linguistic theory) to a set of generalized cognitive "mechanisms." Such mechanisms can serve the developing child in a variety of ways and are influenced by the type of input received and the functions the child needs to perform. For example, mechanisms are affected by the frequency of stimulus input, perceptability, memory load, and semantic transparency (Bates & MacWhinney, 1987) and by goals for the communication exchange.

Bates, Bretherton, and Snyder (1988) argued that it is possible to accept that children are creative language learners who are predisposed to learn language (among other things), and that there is a biological basis for the process, without accepting that what is biological is necessarily universal or that what is universal is necessarily biological. Rather, "Individual differences in language development can be brought about by the differential strength and/or differential timing of two or more underlying mechanisms responsible for language acquisition and language processing" (p. 7).

Contributions

Information processing theory is sometimes viewed as a subcomponent of general cognitive processing theory, but cognitive theory and information processing theory are separated here because they have different implications for clinical decision making. As considered in an upcoming section, cognitive theory emphasizes the construction of schemas as primary to language use, and the development of thought as preceding and encouraging the development of language. In contrast, assessment and intervention based on information processing theory emphasize the input, output, perceptual, memory, and motor processing elements of language learning and use.

Information Processing Theory and Assessment. Myklebust (1954, 1957) applied his bottom-up model of information processing to discussions of auditory disorders and to the differential diagnosis of language and learning disorders. With Doris Johnson, Myklebust introduced the idea of learning style into the literature on assessment and intervention for learning disabilities. The Johnson and Myklebust (1967) text, *Learning Dis-*

abilities: Educational Principles and Practices, encouraged clinical identification of primarily auditory or primarily visual strengths and/or deficits in children with language learning problems. Specific processing skills were separated into "perceptual skills," such as attention and figure-ground discrimination, and "language skills," such as verbal memory, sequencing, integration, and formulation. At the same time, the popular Illinois Test of Psycholinguistic Ability (ITPA; Kirk, McCarthy, & Kirk, 1968) included subtests that were designed to look for "primarily auditory" or "primarily visual" patterns of learning.

Central auditory processing assessments (e.g., Keith, 1981, 1986; Lasky & Katz, 1983; Willeford & Burleigh, 1985) are based on information processing models. All children with suspected language deficits should have at least an audiometric screening of their peripheral hearing. CAP models suggest that it is also important to consider the possible presence of impaired central auditory processes. Table 3.1 is an outline of central auditory

TABLE 3.1 An outline of measures of central auditory processing (American Speech-Language-Hearing Association, 1990)

BEHAVIORAL MEASURES	PHYSIOLOGICAL MEASURES
A. Monotic (same signal to one or both ears)	A. Acoustic reflexes
1. Filtered speech	B. Auditory evoked potentials
2. Time-altered speech	
3. Pattern recognitions	
4. Ipsilateral competing signals	
B. Dichotic (competing signals exactly simultaneous to both ears)	
1. Digits	
2. Syllables	
3. Words and sentences	
C. Binaural (different signals to the two ears)	
1. Binaural fusion	
2. Selective listening and rapidly alternating speech	
3. Masking level differences	

processing assessment measures (American Speech-Language-Hearing Association, 1990). Research supports the value of auditory perceptual measurements for diagnosing disorder. For example, performance on a set of fine-grained auditory discrimination tasks was enough to classify 80% of a group of 6- to 7-year-olds, and 65% of a group of 8- to 11-year-olds, as either having language learning problems or progressing normally in school (Elliott, Hammer, & Scholl, 1989). Tallal and her colleagues (Merzenich et al., 1996; Tallal et al., 1996) recommended CAP assessment to identify children requiring abnormally long transitions to discriminate speech sounds.

Most assessments of information processes focus on language input, but some children with language impairments have deficits in word retrieval (Denckla & Rudel, 1976a, 1976b; German, 1979, 1994). Children with reading and spelling deficits often have slow (latent) or inaccurate word retrieval processes (Denckla, Rudel, & Broman, 1981; Snyder & Downey, 1995; Wolf & Segal, 1992). McGregor and Leonard (1995) used a parallel-access information processing model to describe how multiple related entries might be connected to each other through nodes that associate "category membership (e.g., cat and dog), functional properties, (e.g., knife and scissors), and physical characteristics (e.g., fire and sun)" (pp. 85–86) as well as phonological lexical information related to input and output. Successful word retrieval requires accurate phonetic representation, efficient short-term storage of this representation, and efficient semantic organization of lexical items in associated networks (Lahey, 1988). Tests of word retrieval (e.g., German, 1989, 1990, 1991) are designed to identify patterns of retrieval deficits, such as: (1) fast but inaccurate, (2) slow and inaccurate, and (3) slow but accurate (German, 1993).

Other output processing deficits operate more clearly at the phonological level. As noted previously, children with developmental language and reading disorders often show exaggerated difficulty producing multisyllabic words in imitation (Kamhi & Catts, 1986; Kamhi et al., 1988). Such problems probably relate to phonological representation difficulties rather than simple short-term memory deficits or motor planning deficits. Some children with language impairments do, however, exhibit co-occurring impairments of articulatory planning and motor execution processes that are diagnosed as **developmental apraxia of speech** (DAS). DAS is "a disorder of motor control of speech production, not attributable to other problems of muscular control" (Hall, Jordan, & Robin, 1993, p. 8). Other motor output prob-

lems affect writing, such as the inability to perform rapid alternating finger movements or to copy words and designs even when accurate perception can be shown (Duffy & Geschwind, 1985). Comprehensive assessments of children's needs must consider the functioning of a variety of input and output systems and analyze the information processing demands of tasks. Lahey and Bloom (1994) also suggested systematically varying perceptual-motor and social demands of assessment tasks to identify which factors might be "competing for resources in working memory for a particular child" (p. 369).

Information Processing Theory and Intervention. Information processing theory differs from linguistic theory by positing a set of processes that are not particularly unique to language (as the LAD is), but operate horizontally across multiple areas of cognitive functioning. If the linguistic model is more accurate, language intervention programs should target such elements as grammatical rules and lexical relationships. If the information processing model is more accurate, language intervention programs should target such processes as speech perception and comprehension, short-term memory, word retrieval, and other output organizational skills, depending on a student's individual profile.

Widespread use of the ITPA (Kirk, McCarthy, & Kirk, 1968) in the 1970s for planning intervention was grounded in information processing theory. This "psycholinguistic" approach to language intervention often involved direct translation of ITPA tasks into therapy tasks. This meant practicing language expressions of the sort, "It's a cup, it's pink, it's plastic, you drink out of it," which were not particularly useful for everyday interactions. Clinicians also drilled some children in remembering sequences of numbers, based on observations that their STM for digits was abnormally short.

As clinicians began to notice the limitations of specific skills approaches to language intervention and teaching to the test, top-down theories became more prominent, coinciding with the whole language movement in general education. The problem with extreme versions of whole language approaches to early reading instruction, however, is that children with limited phonological awareness tend to have difficulty figuring out the code without more explicit help. All children's brains do not seem to be equally prepared to infer the relationships between sounds and symbols by experiencing meaningful texts. Some need an adult to help them see the patterns and remember them. Research with children with specific language impairment has, in fact, shown repeatedly that such children have difficulty in the area of phonological awareness (e.g., Blachman, 1994; Kamhi & Catts, 1989).

Noting this, a number of intervention approaches have been designed to help children develop phonological awareness. Such approaches tend to rely heavily on meta-linguistic sound discrimination and segmentation tasks (Lindamood & Lindamood, 1969; Sawyer, Dougherty, Shelly, & Spaanenburg, 1985). Blachman (1994) described a procedure reported by the Russian psychologist, D. B. Elkonin, which has become known as the "Elkonin boxes" approach. Marie Clay (1979) [pronounced '*maa ree*], from New Zealand, adapted the Elkonin boxes procedure for her work with early elementary students who were struggling with reading (Clay's approach is known in North America as "Reading Recovery"). Using the slow speech and visual-motor aids of this procedure, 5- and 6-year olds can learn to segment the phonemes in words accurately (Blachman, 1994; Griffith & Olson, 1992) (see Figure 3.6).

Interventions aimed at improving temporal sequential processing abilities directly, such as the computer programs of Tallal and Merzenich (Merzenich et al., 1996; Tallal et al., 1996), are based on information processing theory also. They are built on the premise that perceptual processing deficits involving speech sound detection and sequencing can result in broader language deficits involving higher order skills. The theory suggests that helping a child to overcome deficits in perceptual processing capabilities will make it possible for the child to acquire other aspects of language normally also (see Box 3.3 earlier in this chapter).

Treatments designed to address other central auditory processing deficits often emphasize improving the loudness and clarity of input, rather than improving the processing mechanism per se. Such interventions might involve enhancing the signal input to make it easier to process with a system that is less than optimal. For example, a student might use a personal FM system with mild gain to improve the signal-to-noise ratio in his classroom, with the teacher wearing a microphone to transmit the signal to the student's headset. Alternatively, the output from the teacher's microphone might be fed to multiple speakers around the room, thus enhancing listening conditions for entire classrooms (e.g., American Speech-Language-Hearing Association, 1991, 1994, 1996; Crandell, Smaldino, & Flexer, 1995).

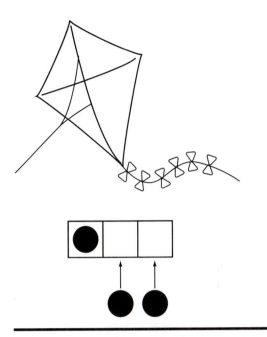

FIGURE 3.6   Example of intervention program to teach phonological sequencing consistent with an information processing model (illustrated by Griffith & Olsen, 1992). The teacher slowly articulates the word while pushing counters into the boxes, sound by sound. The child is encouraged to join in the process, perhaps by articulating the word while the teacher moves the counters and later by moving the counters herself. Gradually the responsibility should be transferred to the child. The task can be made more complex by removing the matrix and having only the counters available. Later the picture can be removed. Eventually the child should be able to count the number of sounds in a word and be able to answer questions about the order of the sounds in words, for example, What is the first sound you hear in *kite?* What sound do you hear after /ī/ in *kite?* (pp. 521–522)

Note. From "Phonemic awareness helps beginning readers break the code" by Priscilla L. Griffith & Mary W. Olson, 1992, *The Reading Teacher*, 45, 516–523. Reprinted by permission.

Treatment for word retrieval deficits takes two primary forms depending on the clinician's assumptions about levels of processing—**storage** elaboration and **retrieval** activities. If one assumes that semantic network elaborations are inadequate, intervention may focus on helping clients create more elaborate associative networks for storing related words. If one assumes that the deficit centers around retrieval processes per se, intervention may target retrieval activities to build strategies for word finding within naming or discourse activities. However, "it is unlikely that naming drills in which words are neither elaborated nor practiced in connected discourse will improve word finding beyond confrontation naming tasks" (McGregor & Leonard, 1995, p. 101). Individual children may also demonstrate different patterns of difficulty. When probing shows that children have extensive knowledge of words they have difficulty retrieving, retrieval strategies should be a major focus of intervention; if not, word comprehension should be a primary target (German, 1992, 1993).

Limitations

Treatments based on improving auditory perceptual processes have something of a "fixing the garden hose" appeal. They suggest that "plugging the leak" at the most peripheral point will make it possible for accurate information to get to the centers that are prepared to process it. If improvement in such basic CAP mechanisms as rapid sequence perception (illustrated in Box 3.3) can also improve higher level language skills without targeting them directly, a causative link might be inferred. Such interventions seem to have particular relevance to the early development of reading decoding skills, or to performing academic tasks in the elementary grades, but their relevance to primary language development and to the ability to read for meaning is less clear. To prove causation, researchers will have to show that improvement in perceptual processing thresholds leads directly to improvement in broader language skills measured by tasks that are different from tasks used in the intervention process. Tallal's (1996) expanded description of the tasks reported in preliminary intervention studies (Tallal et al., 1996) suggests that the training in the research studies included listening exercises using a "Simon Says" game. Such a game is similar to the tasks of the Token Test for Children, which was used to provide evidence of treatment efficacy. It is not clear yet whether school-age children with language deficits that cross oral and written language modalities can make comprehensive language gains through intensive listening exercises alone (Rice, 1997).

Another limitation of traditional information processing approaches is that areas identified through assessment do not necessarily make the best targets of intervention; nor should deficit areas necessarily be avoided. Assessment approaches based both on the ITPA and on Johnson and Myklebust (1967) were designed to identify learning processes that worked better in some modalities than others. When patterns of strength and weakness were identified, clinicians were advised to circumvent deficit areas rather than attack them directly. Based on this view, if a child with weak auditory sequential processing skills was having trouble with a phonics approach in the initial stages of learning to read, the recommended intervention might avoid phonics and emphasize a more visually based whole word "sight" approach. The limitation of this reasoning is that a reader and speller ultimately needs knowledge of sound-symbol relationships to decode and spell new words. Areas of strength can certainly be called on to support areas of weakness, and relationships between bottom-up and top-down processing skills may change over time, but my own belief is that most interventions should be designed to help the child make connections that will bring multiple processing systems (bottom-up and top-down) into balance with each other.

In Chapter 1, I encouraged adoption of assessment and intervention procedures that went beyond an inventory of communication processes and included questions about meeting communication needs in real-life contexts. A primary limitation of CAP approaches and other specific skills approaches is excessive focus on a laundry list of discrete processes that can obscure the real-life academic and social interaction problems that most seriously limit a child's participation opportunities. When a school-age child, parent, and teacher all express concern about the child's difficulty in learning to read, intervention should target reading in as intact a form as possible and with a balanced view of interactive bottom-up and top-down influences.

Knowing that a child scores poorly on tests of CAP may help the child's family and teachers know that the school problems are more than a matter of not trying hard enough and less than a matter of broad cognitive deficit. It does not, however, particularly help the intervention team to know what to do. For that, one must ask which communicative needs are not being met. It is the communicative events identified through such a process that make the best intervention targets.

Thankfully, gone are the times when clinicians worked on short-term memory by drilling students on sequences of digits. Along with other "psycholinguistic approaches" to language intervention based on the ITPA, therapy targeting specific changes that could not be observed in broader language contexts were largely discredited (Hammill & Larsen, 1974), and "specific skills" orientations have been replaced by approaches that target comprehensive systems of language content, form, and use (e.g., Bloom & Lahey, 1978).

Interactive processing models (Butler, 1981, 1984a) also overcome the limitations of exclusively bottom-up or top-down approaches. Such models encourage clinicians to consider the influence of varied contexts (acoustic as well as linguistic) on children's abilities to process complex auditory-linguistic signals (Lasky & Cox, 1983; Nelson, 1985, 1986). In such cases, the influence of top-down processing models can be seen in efforts to teach children to use higher order knowledge to compensate for limitations in signal-processing capabilities. At the same time, the influence of bottom-up models can be seen in efforts to make signals clear enough, loud enough, slow enough, and simple enough that children will have a chance of making sense of them.

Aspects of such interventions may extend to measuring the acoustic characteristics of key learning environments, such as classrooms of hearing impaired and language-learning impaired children. If needed, sound treatment might be applied to floors, walls, and ceilings, and amplification might be provided to make classrooms more acoustically conducive to learning (American Speech-Language-Hearing Association, 1991, 1994, 1996; Hart, 1983; Ross, 1978). Metacognitive strategy training efforts also play a role in helping children develop the cognitive questions for guiding attention and other lower level processes.

COGNITIVE THEORY

Explanations

Cognitive theorists emphasize the sequence and rate of cognitive development as influencing the sequence and rate of language development. The essence of cognitive theory (see Box 3.12) is that development can be explained across domains by postulating a general set of cognitive structures and processes, among which lan-

---

Box 3.12 _____

Primary Assumptions of Cognitive Theories of Language Development

1. Language is not innate in and of itself, but cognitive precursors are.
2. Language is neither innate nor learned but emerges as a result of the child's constructivist activity.
3. Language is only one of several symbolizing abilities for representing and manipulating mental concepts about the world, all of which result from cognitive maturation, triggered by states of disequilibrium between current cognitive structures and new evidence from the environment.
4. A child's cognitive capacities differ qualitatively as well as quantitatively from those of adults.
5. Yet, a constant across all stages of development is that adaptation processes are used either to assimilate new information into existing schemas, or, if they do not seem to fit, to accommodate the schemas by extending and combining them into new ones that are more complex.

---

guage holds no particularly special position. A primary proponent of this viewpoint was Jean Piaget.

Piaget.   The classic cognitive development theorist, Jean Piaget (1896 to 1980), was a Swiss scientist who profoundly influenced current understanding of normal cognitive development. Piaget (1926, 1952, 1969) used the **adaptation** processes of **assimilation** and **accommodation** to explain cognitive developments in the stages outlined in Box 3.13 (see Personal Reflection 3.6). He described the motivating force behind evolution of thought as **disequilibrium** between what children encounter in the world and what they already have organized in their minds.

Neo-Piagetians.   Neo-Piagetians have questioned two of Piaget's original assertions: (1) that children's devel-

---

PERSONAL REFLECTION 3.6 _____

"The idea is an organism, is born, and dies."

Jean Piaget (1977; quoted by T. Brown, 1985, p. vii).

Box 3.13 _____

Qualitative Differences in Thought during Piaget's (1926, 1952, 1969) Three Stages of Cognitive Development (pp. 68–69)

Sensorimotor Stage (birth to 18 months or 2 years):

Piaget subdivided the sensorimotor period into six substages, through which children gain increasing control over their environment by learning to differentiate and coordinate schemes (schemata) for acting on it:

- Substage i (birth to 1 month). Children rely on reflexive actions but demonstrate the beginnings of adaptive intelligence.
- Substage ii (1 to 4 months). Children demonstrate primary circular reactions, in which they demonstrate the ability to repeat a successful cycle of action, such as thumb sucking, for its own sake (with no apparent attempts to use them to an end).
- Substage iii (4 to 8 months). Children demonstrate secondary circular reactions, in which they may try out all of their existing schemes in a new situation but will repeat an activity that works especially well with the apparent aim of maintaining the effect (e.g., shaking a toy that rattles). In this substage they can also imitate an action if the behavior is already in their repertoire.
- Substage iv (8 to 12 months). Children exhibit coordination of secondary schemas as a means to solving new problems, as, for example, grasping strings and shaking them to dislodge entangled toys. In this substage they also begin to demonstrate the ability to imitate behaviors not in their repertoire, to demonstrate intention to communicate, and to demonstrate concepts of object permanence by looking actively for an object that has disappeared from view.
- Substage v (12 to 18 months). Children exhibit tertiary circular reactions in which they actively experiment to achieve new and interesting results, and they can imitate behaviors that differ markedly from those in their repertoire.
- Substage vi (18 to 24 months). Children begin the transition to representational thought in which they are able to invent new means through mental combinations and to engage in deferred imitation; they use symbols for representing objects and people not currently present, both in the acquisition of words (e.g., using the word *bird* to represent a thing that flies and sings and has wings and feathers), and in symbolic play (e.g., using a building block to represent anything from a hairbrush to a can of food).

Representational Stage:

Children further differentiate and coordinate their representational schemes within two major substages:

A. Preoperational Thought (18 months or 2 years to 7 years):

As in the sensorimotor period, children start with undifferentiated and uncoordinated schemes, but they acquire more mature schemes in a step-by-step fashion:

- At first the child's words are undifferentiated (e.g., Piaget's daughter Jacqueline used the sound "choo-choo" to indicate a train passing by her window but also to indicate any other vehicle, any other sound from the window, or anything that appeared suddenly).
- Gradually, words are used in a way that shows a differentiation between the child's actions and internal concepts, such that words can be used to *re-present* events from the past.

- At about the age of 4½ years, children enter an intuitive period, when they still cannot make comparisons mentally but must build them up one at a time in action. However, in this period children begin a transition to the period of operational thought.
- Thought still tends to be centered on one attribute at a time; it is also considered to be pre-logical in that it is irreversible (i.e., children at this stage have difficulty imagining that the amount of clay is the same when rolled into a snake as when it was formed in a ball), and it remains egocentric (i.e., they have difficulty considering any perspective other than their own).

B. Concrete Operations (7 to 11 years):

- Children develop thinking characterized by conservation, decentration, and reversibility (e.g., now they can perform the conservation task related to judging changes in mass of a ball of clay because they can mentally reverse the rolling action that changed the shape from ball to snake, and they can avoid centering on only the characteristic of shape but can hold mass in mind at the same time).
- They can now group objects and words into categorical and seriational categories without considering them in individual pairs and without overt action.
- Preadolescents can demonstrate logical thought but continue to demonstrate some difficulty in moving beyond intuitive explanations for world phenomena.

Formal Operations Stage (more than 11 years):

- Children begin to be able to form classes and series mentally by internalizing earlier physical actions, or "operations."
- Development proceeds through a series of subdevelopments (as in prior stages) until children have acquired a set of abstract intercoordinated schemes for understanding laws regulating the behavior of objects in the external world, and they can apply the operations to solving complex problems with several parts.
- Children demonstrate mental hypothesis testing, abstract and flexible thought, and complex reasoning using language.

---

opment is controlled by the emergence of general logical structures, and (2) that the transition from one stage to the next is produced by the process of equilibration (Case, 1985). Generalized logical structures have been questioned because some tasks that appear to share the same logical structure are passed at widely different ages. For example, conservation of number may be passed at 5 or 6, conservation of liquid volume at 7 or 8, and conservation of mass not until 9 or 10. All of these conservation tasks involve starting with two amounts that look the same, and that the child says are the same: beads that match 1:1 for **number,** equal amounts of liquid in same size beakers for **volume,** equal sized balls of clay for **mass.** As the child watches, the examiner next spreads out one set of beads, pours one beaker of liquid into another that is taller and thinner, or rolls one ball of clay into a long snake, then asks, "Now, do you have more, do I have more, or do we both have the same?" Only the child who can mentally reverse the action can pass this task. Although these tasks all seem to require the mental operation of reversibility, the differing ages of acquisition cast doubt that a single logical structure is involved.

Other abilities, such as imitation, also appear much earlier than Piaget originally suggested. Some infants imitate slow tongue protrusion in the first few days of life, although Piaget notes it as emerging at about 8 to 12 months. Meanwhile, correlations across developmental tasks have been found to be low or insignificant. Finally, it has been difficult to define the abstract concept of logical structure.

The other problem raised by neo-Piagetians is the assertion that new stage developments occur entirely through equilibration. Piaget viewed the young child as a young scientist who constructs ever more powerful theories of the world through the application of logico-mathematical tools of gradually increasing power. In this view, the source of change comes from within the child and is impossible to hurry. In fact, Piaget (1964) commented that "Every time we teach a child something, we prevent him from discovering it on his own." However, the assertion that the initiation of change must be prompted by disequilibrium within the child runs into trouble in view of experimental results that have shown that children who were not even on the verge of acquiring conservation could be brought to complete mastery with training (Lefebvre & Pinard, 1972).

Other recent theorists have questioned whether the stage Piaget (1926, 1952, 1969) termed **formal thought** is actually reached by all normally functioning adults. Some have proposed adding stages of postformal thought (Kamhi & Lee, 1988). Postformal stages might include the ability to combine formal operations into higher-order structures or systems. They might also include metasystematic reasoning for organizing general systems into supersystems. Kamhi and Lee (1988) summarized the evidence regarding later stage thought:

> Although questions have been raised about the universal characteristics of formal operational thought and the age at which youngsters reach this stage, most developmental psychologists would agree that adolescents reason differently than preadolescents. (p. 137)

Contextual variables can influence the appearance of later-stage cognitive competence. Nearly all adults are capable of formal thought, but many exhibit it only on problems that interest them and fall in their area of expertise. For example, an auto mechanic who troubleshoots an engine problem with formal hypothetical reasoning may rely on more concrete reasoning about other problems. The message for clinicians is that they should probe multiple contexts when adolescents and adults do not seem to be reasoning at the formal level. They should not accept that formal thought is impossible just because it is not exhibited on traditional assessment tasks (Kamhi & Lee, 1988).

Sensemaking through Play, Schemas, Scripts, and Narratives. Most cognitive theorists have had relatively little to say about language acquisition as a special case because they do not consider it to be a special case. As Owens (1988) noted, "There is no Piagetian model of language development" (p. 135). Pure cognitive theorists consider language acquisition to be only one of many cognitive developments taking place as the child constructs a sense of himself or herself in the world.

Pursuing this line of reasoning, a number of researchers have attempted, with varying degrees of success, to tie advances in language development to advances in Piagetian stages of cognition. Correlations have been found, for example, between the acquisition of linguistic concepts and symbolic play with objects, imitations of gestures and sounds, and aspects of problem solving through tool use. "Disappearance" words, such as *allgone,* are highly correlated with object permanence, but other first words are not. Noticing that people serve as agents for events in the world also seems to relate to first word productions (Bates, 1976; Bates, Benigni, Bretherton, Camaioni, & Volterra, 1979; Bates & Snyder, 1985; Corrigan, 1978).

Other cognitive psychologists, such as Katherine Nelson (1985, 1986) and Jerome Bruner (1990), do see language acquisition as unique, but related to general cognitive advances and the sensemaking that occurs through play and other socially situated routine events. Such theorists have related early language abilities to children's efforts to make sense of the world's events, the social interactions that influence them, and the stories that document them. Describing this melding of cognitive and social-interaction influences, K. Nelson (1985) noted that:

> When children learn to talk they enter into a system of shared meanings. The words that they learn to use have the power to evoke in others a conceptual representation that, ideally, matches the one they intend to express. (p. 3)

Nelson saw the process of language acquisition as one in which the "individual develops a meaning system from experience with social meanings reflecting an understanding of cultural meaning" (p. 12).

This view of cognitive constructivism takes cognitive theory beyond perceptually based, and even conceptually based, problem-solving schemes underlying Piaget's developmental stage observations. It also links cognitive development directly to language development without making either entirely dependent on the other (see Personal Reflection 3.7). Finally, it places both cognitive and language development within a sociocultural context.

Bruner (1990) contrasted constructivist cognitive theory with behavioral and information processing approaches. Describing the "cognitive revolution," he com-

PERSONAL REFLECTION 3.7 _____

"Children learn language because they are predisposed to do so. How they set about the task is largely determined by the way they are: seekers after meaning who try to find the underlying principles that will account for the patterns that they recognize in their experiences."

Gordon Wells (1986, p. 43), British psycholinguist (now at the Ontario Institute for Studies in Education), in his book, *The Meaning Makers: Children Learning Language and Using Language to Learn.*

mented that "we were not out to 'reform' behaviorism, but to replace it" (p. 3). Initial focus on the construction of meaning and the development of mind, however, was soon influenced by a shift toward information processing theory. "Very early on," Bruner commented, "emphasis began shifting from 'meaning' to 'information,' from the *construction* of meaning to the *processing* of information" (p. 4, italics in original). Arguing against the shift, Bruner credited culture as the source of higher order cognitive tools that humans use to overcome the biological limits of their information processing systems.

Bruner (1990), who is usually viewed as a primary proponent of social interaction theory, also emphasized the importance of goal-oriented behavior in the construction of meaning. In particular, he saw narratives as the primary tool for seeking meaning in the context of human experience and making sense of how things work. Bruner (1990) described narrative as "one of the most ubiquitous and powerful discourse forms in human communication"; he also noted that it appears in "social interaction before it achieves linguistic expression" (p. 77). Bruner described effective narrative structure as including four crucial constituents:

> It requires, first, a means for emphasizing human action or "agentivity"—action directed toward goals controlled by agents. It requires, secondly, that a sequential order be established and maintained—that events and states be "linearized" in a standard way. Narrative, thirdly, also requires a sensitivity to what is canonical and what violates canonicality in human interaction. Finally, narrative requires something approximating a narrator's perspective: it cannot, in the jargon of narratology, be "voiceless." (p. 77)

As evidence for the central role of narrative in cognitive-linguistic development, Bruner (1990) used the bedtime soliloquies of Emily between her eighteenth month and third year, which are described in *Narratives from the Crib* (edited by Katherine Nelson, 1989). By herself in her crib, Emily seems to construct both meaning and language, using one to pull the other along, with temporal links (e.g., *and then*) appearing as Emily needs them to order the events of the day, and causal links (e.g., *because*) appearing based on an interest in the reasons *why* people do things (See Personal Reflection 3.8). The basic force underlying all such developments seems to be a constructivist push to make sense of the world's events. As Bruner put it:

> The engine of all this linguistic effort is not so much a push toward logical coherence, though that is not absent. It is, rather, a need to "get the story right": who did what to whom where, was it the "real" and steady thing or a rogue happening, and how do I feel about it. Her language aided but did not compel her to talk or think in this way. (p. 92)

Nelson (1985) explained the process by which children relate social events and physical objects in their developing knowledge systems as storage within "scriptlike event-representations" (p. 18). She described relationships among **categories, schemas,** and **scripts. Categorical structures** group elements on the basis of similar properties, such as "food" and "furniture." Categorical structures crosscut with **schemas** that bring together elements based on contextual relationships in time or space, such as "kitchen" and "making dinner." The kitchen schema, for example, organizes a spatial scene that includes a set of objects appropriate to activities that take place there. A **script,** which is a subset of a schema, is "an ordered set of events in temporal se-

PERSONAL REFLECTION 3.8 _____

" . . . now sleeping time
now not sleeping time
Emmy make it bedtime
not sleeping time."

Emily, a child who, at the age of 23 months, 6 days, was using her crib monologue discourse (this piece is from Gerhardt, 1989, p. 225) in more than one way—to construct her world, to construct her language, and to construct herself (K. Nelson, 1989).

PERSONAL REFLECTION 3.9 _____

"Early pretend play is a type of intellectual activity that is both analogous to language and distinct from it. It is symbolic and an important tool for early reasoning, but it doesn't seem to be mediated by inner verbalization, and it certainly doesn't require auditory processing."

Judith R. Johnston (1991, pp. 300–301).

---

quence representing a familiar activity, such as making dinner" (p. 18). Scripts develop through children's participation in events and relate to the emergence of pretend play (see Personal Reflection 3.9). Similar to Bruner's narratives, Nelson (1986) described events as being organized around goals, involving "people in purposeful activities, and acting on objects and interacting with each other to achieve some result" (p. 11).

Cognitive Theory and Specific Language Impairment. A different approach to discerning the relationship between language acquisition and general cognitive development has been to look for the separability or inseparability of thought and language within the population of children with specific language impairments. By definition, children with specific language impairment score significantly higher on measures of nonverbal cognitive development than on measures of language development. Speech–language pathologists Judith Johnston (1991) and Alan Kamhi (1996) have looked closely at the evidence from studies of the "nonverbal" cognitive abilities of children with language disorders, including their own research and that of others, and have reached slightly different conclusions about its meaning.

Johnston (1991) questioned whether "specific" language impairments are all that specific. Considering her clinical experiences with children with specific language impairment, she reasoned that, "if language was both the product and the tool of human cognition, it seemed unlikely that these children could have serious difficulty learning language and be otherwise intellectually normal" (p. 299). Johnston concluded from her review of the "research on the cognitive abilities of language-disordered children" that it:

presents a convincing picture of substantial impairment. At many ages, across visual, auditory, and tactile stim-

uli, across many domains of knowledge, in symbolic and nonsymbolic activities, in tasks with little to no explicit verbal demand, language-disordered children perform below age expectations. (p. 300)

Kamhi's (1996) conclusion was slightly softer but similar. His assessment of the research was that "SLI children do not have domain-specific cognitive deficiencies, nor do they have deficits in fundamental reasoning" (p. 105), but they do show deficiencies in a range of cognitive skill areas compared with their normal learning peers. For example, studies show that children with SLI: (1) exhibit deficient symbolic, adaptive, and integrative play skills, (2) have difficulty generating, maintaining, and interpreting mental images, (3) show deficiencies in hierarchical planning, and (4) have difficulty solving certain complex reasoning problems. However, other studies show that children with SLI: (1) can solve mental imagery problems when multiple or alternative strategies can be used, (2) can use age-appropriate reasoning processes involving analogical thinking and hypothesis testing to solve problems, and (3) are adept at solving problems that require visual-spatial pattern analysis.

Reconciling Nativism and Constructivism. Psycholinguist Annette Karmiloff-Smith (1993) has been a primary proponent of the position that linguistic theory and cognitive theory can be reconciled. She noted that:

For as long as Piaget's constructivist description of the human infant held (i.e., an assimilation/accommodation organism with no constraints from built-in knowledge), then it followed that the human mind, acquiring basic knowledge via interaction with the environment, might turn out to be cognitively flexible and creative. However, in the last decade or so, exciting new paradigms for infancy research have challenged our view of the architecture of the human mind, which is now considered to be endowed from the outset with some domain-specific predispositions. (p. 563)

Many psycholinguists who accept the nativist linguistic viewpoint believe that it precludes any acceptance of constructivism, but Karmiloff-Smith (1993) argued that nativism and constructivism are not necessarily incompatible. In her view, some aspects of Piaget's developmental stage model can be questioned, but his constructivist view of biology and knowledge, as well as his "vision of the cognizer as a very active participant in his or her own ontogenesis—are still a viable way to think about how development occurs" (p. 564).

Contributions

Cognitive theories influence assessment and intervention by claiming that sequence and rate of language development are at least partially determined by sequence and rate of cognitive development. This leads to a heavy dependence on developmental scales to assess language and to decide what knowledge and skills to target as part of intervention. Earlier acquired behaviors may also be seen as prerequisites for later ones, and cognitive advances may be seen as prerequisites for linguistic ones.

Cognitive Theory and Assessment.   In a developmental approach, assessment is aimed at identifying a child's current level of functioning in multiple cognitive domains so that intervention can start at the child's current level of functioning. According to such a model, cognitive developments guide developments in other domains and are prerequisite to them. Based on the outcome of assessment and looking at the next step on developmental scales, intervention is then implemented by arranging environmental experiences to encourage children to expand their schemas about how the world works through their experiences with it. Items on developmental scales may even be translated rather directly into intervention objectives. The charts attached to Chapter 13 can be used in this way. Other examples are Westby's (1988) Symbolic Play Scale, for ages birth through 5 years (see Chapters 7 and 9), and Linder's (1990) Transdisciplinary Play-Based Assessment (TPBA), which is "both an assessment and intervention process" (p. 4). The TPBA provides a structure for observing (1) cognitive, (2) social-emotional, (3) communication/language, and (4) sensorimotor development in the context of play.

Cognitive theory also influences assessment practices when "cognitive referencing" is used as a criterion to decide who qualifies to receive special services. Policy issues related to assessment and diagnosis are considered further in Chapters 5 and 6. Here, consider what it means from a theoretical perspective to use cognitive referencing as a diagnostic criterion.

First, what is cognitive referencing? It is the practice of using separate measures to assess language and non-

verbal intelligence, then requiring a discrepancy of more than one standard deviation (sometimes 1.5 SD) between standard scores on the two measures for a child to be diagnosed as having a "specific" language impairment or learning disability. Even if a child is significantly delayed in language development relative to his or her chronological age peers, if no discrepancy can be documented, the child does not qualify for services. The person's language level, if commensurate, is presumed simply to be where it "ought to be," given the person's level of cognitive ability. The reasoning goes that such an individual is simply a slow learner (if his or her IQ is in the 70 to 90 range) or mentally retarded (if his or her IQ is 69 or less). Can a child have a true language impairment in co-occurrence with frank cognitive impairment or with IQ scores in the "dull normal" range? I think so, but many policies imply otherwise. This question has strong practical clinical implications. My own view is that it is wrong to use policies based on cognitive-linguistic discrepancy criteria to decide who gets access to language intervention services.

Policies requiring cognitive discrepancies are based on the weak form of a cognitive hypothesis. It is one of three hypotheses about relationships between cognition and language that Miller (1981) summarized:

1. *Strong form cognitive hypothesis.* Cognitive development is both necessary and sufficient for language to develop. This hypothesis would predict that no discrepancy would ever be found between language and cognition. Children with specific language impairment, who show a discrepancy in test scores by definition, provide counterevidence for this position.

2. *Weak form cognitive hypothesis.* Cognitive development is necessary, but not sufficient, for language to develop. This hypothesis forms the basis for cognitive referencing policies. It suggests that a child who shows commensurate levels of cognitive development and language development would be unlikely to benefit from language intervention service because language development is simply where the child's cognitive development predicts it would be.

3. *Correlational cognitive/language hypothesis.* Cognitive development and language development are independent, but interactive. Either can lead the other at a particular point in time for an individual child, and advances in one domain may assist a child to make advances in the other domain.

Cognitive Theory and Intervention.   The general goal of programs influenced by cognitive theory is to foster advances through developmental stages. Unlike behavioral theory, cognitive theory acknowledges a rich and active set of inner processes. This leads to a rich view of developmental "errors," not simply as mistakes to be corrected, but as evidence about the theories and schemas a child is constructing to make sense of language and other phenomena. Clinicians then use such evidence to fine-tune intervention efforts.

Cognitive theory underlies constructivist approaches to general and special education. "Constructivism is a philosophy about teaching and learning rather than a specific teaching method or approach" (Harris & Graham, 1996a, p. 135). Within such a view, "children are seen as inherently active, self-regulating learners who construct knowledge in developmentally appropriate ways within a social context" (p. 135). A good example of a constructivist approach is a whole language approach to language arts (e.g., Goodman, 1986) or to language intervention (e.g., Norris & Hoffman, 1993). Whole language teachers facilitate and assist students in the context of authentic learning experiences to construct knowledge. They eschew workbooks and direct instruction; they particularly reject teaching discrete skills in linear sequence; and they avoid labeling children who have special education needs. Box 3.14 shows how Vivian Paley (1990) encourages constructivist learning in the case of Jason, who is a different learner. Paley is kindergarten teacher who has written several books about how young children construct their knowledge systems through play and stories.

Cognitive theory, in its emphasis on self-directed learning, also contributes to the development of intervention approaches that are designed to teach older children and adolescents to adopt metacognitive strategies. **Metacognition** is thinking about thinking. Similar to metalinguistic behavior, metacognitive behavior involves a conscious awareness of processes that have primary functions that are ordinarily transparent. The training of **strategies** is particularly important for students with language-learning disabilities in upper elementary and secondary grades because they seem to have difficulty acquiring such strategies on their own.

Box 3.14 _____

A Cognitive-Constructivist Approach
(Paley, 1990)

Paley describes how the other kindergarten children respond to Jason's unusual behavior:

> They keep track of Jason's private spectacle while I worry about that which does not take place. He plays alone; he tells stories to himself; he seems unaware of our habits and customs. Ask him a question and he says his helicopter is broken. Suggest an activity and he rushes away to fix his helicopter, sometimes knocking over a building in his path. (p. 29)

In a transcript of a later class session, Paley shows how Jason's language provides clues to his world constructs:

> "It's silly," Jason says.
>
> "What's silly?" I ask.
>
> "This thing's eating draw."
>
> "What does eating draw mean, Jason?"
>
> "It means eating draw."
>
> Petey looks at Jason's paper. "He drawed on there and that's eating it," he explains. "Mine isn't because I don't use the white."
>
> Now I see what Jason means. White on white is hard to see. The white paper eats the white crayon. The paper "eats draw." (p. 42)

I am bombarded by such evidence of the distance between the children's world and mine. To me, Jason seems different from the others, but it is clear that I am the one who is different, not Jason. His thinking mirrors that of his classmates; their images creep into his play and his talk, and it is their solutions that cause him, from time to time, to stop whirling his blades in order to listen. (p. 43)

Examples of strategy training approaches are discussed more thoroughly in Chapter 12. Briefly, they involve teaching students to adopt conscious strategies of problem solving, with the aim of teaching them to direct their own learning (Buttrill, Niizawa, Biemer, Takakashi, & Hearn, 1989; Deshler, Alley, & Carlson, 1980; Lloyd, 1980; Schumaker, Deshler, Alley, & Warner, 1983; Torgesen, 1982).

Limitations

Although perspectives from normal cognitive development add to the framework for language assessment and intervention, they also have some limitations. Especially, strictly developmental approaches may restrict children to environments and activities consistent with their developmental ages rather than their chronological ages. Recall the child with physical impairments, mentioned in Chapter 1, who was not taught to read because he could not yet zip his pants.

Cognitive theory explains normal development when it unfolds spontaneously. It does not offer a strong technology for encouraging development that does not. From a strict Piagetian (1964) viewpoint, developmental advances occur only when a state of disequilibrium occurs within children. However, as Case (1985) pointed out, others have questioned this limited view and have shown that it is possible to design teaching strategies that can help children advance from one stage to the next. Pascual-Leone's (1984) solution was to combine Piagetian theory with aspects of behaviorism and information processing theories to explain how both intrinsic and extrinsic factors could help children activate new schemas through interaction of the four factors: (1) cues from the internalized scheme itself, (2) field effects that might make particular features of stimuli stand out for attention, (3) logical cues on structural relationships, and (4) mental power or attention. Case's (1985) addition of executive control structures is also consistent with strategy training approaches that are based on elements of cognitivist theory.

Rice (1983) commented that few training studies based on cognitivist theory have been reported. Those that have fail to support the idea that prior cognitive understandings are a prerequisite for training (Rice, 1980) or that training certain cognitive structures will necessarily facilitate the emergence of communicative behaviors (Steckol & Leonard, 1981). Rice (1983) summarized that "the cognition hypotheses have not fulfilled their early promise, but they have spawned a range of explanations that contribute helpful perspectives" (p. 355). For example, she identified an ongoing clinical danger as stemming from the lack of recognition of what she called the **mapping problem.** That is, although children may not enter the therapeutic interaction with a fully developed nonlinguistic concept of such things as cup-like objects, clinicians may assume

that they do and that all that is needed is teaching the child to associate the label *cup* with that notion. A cognitive perspective can help one avoid this problem.

Harris and Graham (1996a) also questioned whether a purely constructivist approach is sufficient to meet the special learning needs for some children. A concern is that "constructivism may lure some teachers into believing that individual differences are neither real nor problematic and that difficulties will resolve themselves in due developmental time" (p. 136). Harris and Graham argued for a more integrated individualized approach, which would include explicit, focused, and possibly even isolated instruction, to the extent needed by particular children.

SOCIAL INTERACTION THEORY

Explanations

Social interaction theories emphasize communicative purpose over language structure and the importance of context (see Personal Reflection 3.10). This is because the rules of social communication differ from those of linguistic structure (see Box 3.15). Rather than being static representations, social interactions vary with the situations in which they occur. They involve situated uses that are "glued to their contextual backgrounds" (Dore, 1986, p. 7). Dore provided as an example of this, when the meaning of *mine* changes in the context of the preschool playroom, where objects are temporarily possessed for play purposes (e.g., *my sponge*) rather than being owned outright as they are at home (e.g., *my room*).

Dore (1986) further contrasted linguistic and cognitive theories with social interaction (pragmatic) ones:

Structural and cognitive accounts of language typically assume that development is controlled from within the individual (whether by cognitive processes or substantive

---

PERSONAL REFLECTION 3.10 _____

"If you concentrate on communicating, everything else will follow."

Roger Brown, Harvard psycholinguist in the Introduction to *Talking to Children,* edited by Catherine Snow and Charles Ferguson (1977b, p. 26).

Box 3.15

Primary Assumptions of Social Interaction Theories of Language Development

1. Language develops, not because of any innate linguistic competence or because of strict reinforcement principles, but because human beings are motivated to interact socially and to develop concepts of self and others.
2. The important elements of development are not abstract linguistic or cognitive structures or concrete verbal behaviors, but rather they are the phenomena of intentional and symbolic acts of speech, their conversational functions, their consequences for participants, and their context-creating power and context-dependent properties (Dore, 1986).
3. Language acquisition occurs in the context of dyadic, dynamic interactions, which are motivated by the child's drive to develop a concept of self and to interact with others socially (not isolated efforts to construct a grammar, or passive processes controlled by external reinforcers).
4. Parents (and other conversational partners) contribute significantly to the language acquisition process by adjusting their linguistic input to be compatible with the child's developing linguistic and communicative abilities and by supplying a scaffold (i.e., supportive communicative structure) to allow the child to communicate despite primitive abilities (Bruner, 1978).

---

constraints) and focus on the construction and elaboration of mental products. But pragmatic approaches should begin by postulating that development proceeds from intersubjectively sustained activity to the child's cognitive-linguistic control and should focus on the emergence of self-awareness and the child's personal powers in social interactions. (p. 5)

Joint Action Routines and Scaffolding. Bruner (1968) thought that it was possible to isolate a special kind of symbolic communication learning in infancy by involving communicative eye-gaze, smiling, and vocalizing patterns, which could be distinguished from language. He called the "limited subspecies of symbolic learning involved in social interaction . . . *code learning*" (p. 56). Bruner noted the importance of the parental

role in establishing this code early in infancy. Parents respond to their child's initiative (e.g., crying) by converting some feature of the spontaneous behavior into a signal. That is, parents expect their infants to be communicative. In turn, infants learn to expect their initiations to elicit a response.

In addition, caregivers systematically assist children to differentiate between objects within events using a process Bruner (1974–1975) called **joint reference.** This involves elaborate **joint action routines** (JARs) whose development begins in early infancy with intensive eye contact between caregiver and child, followed by behaviors in which the caregiver calls to the child, points, names objects, and comments on them, thus guiding both the content and form of language input.

As development continues, caregivers modify their speech so that it is comprehensible at the assumed level of the child, but systematically advances in complexity (Snow, 1977a; Snow & Ferguson, 1977). Teachers also modify their linguistic input systematically during the elementary school years, apparently to match the developing language skills of their students (Cazden, 1988; Cuda & Nelson, 1976; Nelson, 1984; Sturm, 1990).

This process by which adults mediate experiences to assist young children to be more competent than they could be by themselves is called **scaffolding** (Bruner, 1975, 1977; Cazden, 1983). Whether it occurs early or later in development, the essence of scaffolding is that a more mature and experienced member of a culture provides systematic support to a less mature individual who is still learning to function within it.

Vygotsky and the Zone of Proximal Development (ZPD). Scaffolding techniques are probably as old as human communication, but it was the Russian psychologist Vygotsky who, in the early part of the twentieth century, promoted the idea that individual development has social origins. Vygotsky lived from 1896 to 1934, and although he died prematurely of tuberculosis at the age of 38, his ideas about child development and the relationships of thought and language continue to exert a major influence on modern educational practices. In 1962, an English translation of Vygotsky's work *Thought and Language* (originally published in Russian in 1934) was published. Vygotsky argued that early in its development, language is primarily a tool for social interaction. As development progresses, however, language becomes a medium through which children control their private interactions with the environment by talking aloud during play and verbalizing intended actions. Language eventually becomes a way of structuring actions, directing thought, and creating a concept of self.

Vygotsky (1962, 1978) thought that this transformation occurred through a process of cultural mediation. He saw cultural mediation (similar to what others have called scaffolding) as a process of assisting learners to move from elementary to higher levels of mental functioning. In Vygotsky's view, elementary mental functions are characterized by their individual origins, control by the natural environment, absence of conscious realization, and lack of mediation by psychological tools. Higher mental functions are characterized by their social origins and nature, voluntary control by the learner, conscious realization of mental processes, and independent mediation using psychological tools (Wertsch, 1985, 1991).

Vygotsky (1934/1962) commented that "with assistance, every child can do more than he can by himself—though only within the limits set by the state of his development" (p. 103). He called the range of these limits, which vary from child to child and context to context, the **zone of proximal development (ZPD).** The ZPD is the difference between what a child can accomplish independently and what that child can do with the assistance of an intentioned adult (Vygotsky, 1978).

Wertsch (1985) summarized three interrelated assumptions underlying the Vygotskian concept of ZPD: (1) what children can accomplish now is different from their potential for further learning; (2) what they can achieve alone is different from what they can achieve with the help of a knowledgeable adult or peer; and (3) a more knowledgeable person can deliberately transfer control to a less knowledgeable person through a process of mediated learning. The essence of the Vygotskian viewpoint is that "social interaction is essential for development, not only as a source of stimulation and feedback, but as the very means by which individual psychological functioning comes to be" (Schneider & Watkins, 1996, p. 157).

Social Interaction and Development of the Concept of Self. Cooper and Anderson-Inman (1988) noted that the usual interpretation of socialization is that par-

ents and other adults are the teachers or transmitters of culture and that children are the learners. Cooper and Anderson-Inman added that "This view of socialization is not erroneous, but it is somewhat incomplete. Socialization is actually an interactive process" (p. 225).

Social interaction theories depend in part on an assumption that human beings have an innate motivation to communicate (see Personal Reflection 3.11). Bruner (1968) noted that newborns seek out human faces and respond to them.

Dore (1986) used concepts of feeling-form-function-frame analyses to describe the nature of the complex social communicative interactions. Dore posited feelings between participants as motivating the particular forms, which are chosen to put into effect various intentional and sequential functions, which are relative to the contextual frames in which they occur. In describing this "house-that-Jack-built" view of the transition to language, Dore emphasized its basis in feelings and the "primacy of relationship" (p. 16). A primary example is an infant–mother pair. As Dore expressed it, "It is the infant's mother who thus endows his behavior with meaning" (1986, p. 17).

Social Interaction, Theory of Mind, and Autism. Bruner (1990), in his book, *Acts of Meaning,* related the social underpinnings of meaningfulness to the human tendency to practice "folk psychology." Folk psychology is the drive to figure out how humans act and what their feelings and motivations are (Humphrey, 1984). In fact, the human faculty to be amateur psychologists is thought by some to be the core cognitive ability, with a biological basis, which underlies all human communication, storytelling, and sensemaking (Astington, 1994). It is because humans can imagine the goals,

PERSONAL REFLECTION 3.11 _____

"Although reinforcement may explain food searching in rats, it has failed to explain the average human child's search for communicative competence."

John Neil Bohannon III, Butler University, and *Amye Warren-Leubecker,* University of Tennessee at Chattanooga, writing about theoretical approaches to language acquisition (1989, p. 209).

beliefs, and motivations of other human beings that they can develop and use language normally. The cognitive ability that permits such inferences is called the "theory of mind" (Baron-Cohen, 1995; Hobson, 1993). It is thought to be supported by several innate mechanisms.

> *The thesis is that infants are biologically "prewired" to relate to people in ways that are special to people, and that it is through the experience of reciprocal, affectively patterned interpersonal contact that a young child comes to apprehend and eventually to conceptualise the nature of persons with mental life. (Hobson, 1993, p. 194)*

The term, "theory of mind," was coined by Premack and Woodruff (1978) who commented, "In saying that an individual has a theory of mind, we mean that the individual imputes mental states to himself and to others" (p. 515). Baron-Cohen (1995) described the biological basis and normal development of four key "mindreading" mechanisms for: (1) detecting intentionality, (2) detecting eye direction, (3) interpreting shared attention, and (4) developing a theory of mind. These developments are summarized in Box 3.16.

Support for the theory of mind as a key to normal cognitive, communicative, and social development comes from observation of individuals with autism. Hobson (1993) described how children with autism differ from children developing normally:

> *They are markedly delayed in developing creative symbolic play, an ability that normally flowers around the middle of a normal child's second year of life. When representational play does emerge, it is often stereotyped and relatively impoverished in content. Their language is usually delayed to a degree that is out of keeping with their non-verbal cognitive capacities such as visuospatial (jigsaw) pattern recognition. Their social use of language is especially unusual, in that they often fail to adjust what they say to the context in which they say it, and are insensitive to the interests, needs, and knowledge of their listeners. Their thinking is often "concrete" and inflexible, unattuned to contextual subtleties, insensitive to metaphor, and often awkward and one-track in style. (p. 4)*

As Hobson (1993) suggested, the ability to imagine and relate to the thinking of other people seems to be separate from other, more general cognitive abilities, particularly perceptual ones, such as visuospatial pattern recognition. Autism involves specific impairment of the faculty Baron-Cohen (1995) called mindreading, while sparing more general cognitive and information processing abilities. In contrast, Williams syndrome selectively spares social-interaction mechanisms while impairing more general cognitive abilities. As noted in the section on linguistic theory, Williams syndrome is a genetic condition involving metabolism of calcium, "which results in a pattern of poor cognitive skills against a backdrop of excellent language, face-processing, and mindreading skills" (Baron-Cohen, 1995, p. 96). Individuals with Williams syndrome can produce and comprehend complex sentences, participate appropriately in social conversations, and generate narrative structures, but "they are significantly retarded, with an IQ of about 50, and are incompetent at ordinary tasks like tying their shoes, finding their way, retrieving items from a cupboard, telling right from left, adding two numbers, drawing a bicycle, and suppressing their natural tendency to hug strangers" (Pinker, 1994, p. 52). Their unique combination of abilities and disabilities also supports the relative separability of social interaction and linguistic mechanisms from more general cognitive mechanisms.

Contributions

Social interaction theories offer a system for blending the content and procedures of other theoretical approaches into a unified intervention approach. Biological maturation theories emphasize anatomical structure without offering much regarding target content or procedures. Linguistic theories focus on content and say little about procedures. Behaviorist theories offer a well-developed set of procedures but with relatively undefined content. Information processing theories focus on a content that is not really content and offer procedures that can support other intervention efforts but do not stand well on their own. Cognitivist theories cross wide expanses of content and offer primarily developmental expectations as procedural guidelines.

Two of the major contributions of social interaction theory are its focus on **function,** suggesting that children learn to talk and to practice their communication skills when they have a reason to do so, and **context,** suggesting that form–content language structures are determined not only by communicative function but by contextual factors.

Box 3.16 _____

Social-Interaction Views of the Predisposition to Know Oneself in Relation to Others—Developmental Phases and the Theory of Mind

PHASE 1. (0 TO 9 MONTHS)
Primary intersubjectivity

Infants seem innately endowed with mechanisms for reading mental states in behavior, detecting intentionality, and interpreting signals from eyes. The Intentionality Detector (ID) is activated when perceptual input from visual, tactile, and auditory sources identifies potential agents with goals and desires. Anything that moves with self-propelled motion or makes nonrandom sounds might be an agent. The Eye-Direction Detector (EDD) works only through vision. Infants stare longer at eyes than at other parts of the face. At least by 6 months, infants can detect whether eyes are looking directly at them or somewhere else. Researchers know this because the infants look two to three times longer at a face looking directly at them. This function allows the infant to attribute a perceptual state to another organism, inferring that "Mommy sees me."

PHASE 2. (9 TO 18 MONTHS)
Triadic representation with shared attention

The infant uses early dyadic representations and visual distinction between eye gaze directed toward self or other objects to build understanding of triadic relationships. Triadic representations involve an agent, self, and an object (which might be another agent). This Shared-Attention Mechanism (SAM) activates when the infant joins with another participant to share focus on a third object or agent. Gaze monitoring is seen in some infants from around 9 months and is observed universally by 14 months. When gaze monitoring, an infant turns to look where another person is looking,

then shows gaze alternation, checking back and forth a few times to make sure he or she is looking at the same thing. At around the same time, infants begin to use protodeclarative pointing with an outstretched index finger and the alternating gaze to check whether attention is shared.

PHASE 3. (18 TO 48 MONTHS)
Evidence of emerging theory of mind

The Theory-of-Mind Mechanism is a system of inferring the full range of mental states (pretending, thinking, knowing, believing, imagining, dreaming, guessing, and deceiving) and for theorizing about how mental states and actions are related.

(18 TO 24 MONTHS)

Toddlers begin to pretend and recognize the pretending of others, signaling a qualitative change in their play.

(36 TO 48 MONTHS)

Children show evidence of understanding such states as "knowing" and that seeing leads to knowing. They also come to understand that some beliefs are true and others are false. Thus, they can appreciate the deception at the heart of "Snow White" and other fairy tales and grow in their ability to deceive others.

Note: The term "primary intersubjectivity" is attributed to Trevarthen (1979); the naming of the "Theory-of-Mind Mechanism" is attributed to Leslie (1994); otherwise, the phases are those summarized by Baron-Cohen (1995).

Social Interaction Theory and Assessment. Recognizing the limitations of earlier form-based linguistic approaches, Lucas (1980) recommended looking at children with language disorders as potentially having a disruption in one of four areas, which she defined based on speech-act theory. The potential areas of difficulty were in:

(1) developing the rules; (2) establishing a desire or motivational cause for having an intent to linguistically express; (3) having a need to communicate to a hearer; and/or (4) being capable of participating in the active process. (p. 45)

Assessment tied to social interaction theory can be designed to uncover which of these sources of difficulty might be active for a particular child. It is difficult to imagine a formal test that could accomplish such a feat without an insightful clinician to interpret not just the test scores, but also how the individual approached the task, compensated for difficulties, and dealt with frustration. Even then, the testing procedure would offer little insight into the person's motivation or ability to create and understand novel messages and to function differently depending on the communicative demands of a particular situation. To understand contextually based variations in ability and disability, requires informal, ecologically valid approaches to assessment.

You may recognize that the framework developed in Chapter 1 is closely aligned with such a social interactionist viewpoint. The statement that "problems are not just within children, and neither are the solutions," serves as a reminder to myself, my students, and now you, that intervention is only relevant if it improves an individual's ability to meet the communicative demands of significant life contexts. By starting with a series of interviews about zones of significance for a particular individual, a clinician can focus the assessment process on those contexts. For example, when a preschool teacher expresses concern that a child with a language impairment is not getting invited to play in the block or doll corner, a clinician using this approach would assess the context first in order to understand the social and language skills of other children in this situation; and then, observe what the target child currently does while attempting to participate, gathering descriptive data and quantifying any pieces that might help capture the essence of the situation. Examples of baseline quantification efforts might be to count the number of times an aggressive child grabs another child's toy within a 10-minute observation, or to document the low frequency with which a passive child attempts to initiate interaction with another child within a 10-minute sample. Although these elements index only some of the characteristics of highly complex communication events, they set the stage for what to target in the intervention process.

Zones of significance are not to be confused with ZPDs, but they are related. By interviewing important participants in a problem (children, parents, teachers), a clinician can identify which contexts and materials should be drawn into the assessment process. Once assessment begins, a social interactionist goal is to learn about a child's zone of proximal development within a particular zone of significance. Recall Vygotsky's (1978) description of the ZPD from earlier in this section as the difference between what a child can do independently and what the child can do with the mediational support of a more competent, intentioned adult to address a particular problem. An important part of this concept is that "a child does not *have* a ZPD—it is not a feature of the child. Rather a zone is created whenever children interact with more capable others in particular activities" (Schneider & Watkins, 1996, p. 160, italics in original). To choose the particular activities that are relevant for a particular child (the child's zones of significance), it is necessary to ask the participants.

Assessment aimed at outlining the parameters of a child's ZPD for a particular activity involves figuring out how much and what kinds of supports (or scaffolds) will assist *the child* to make connections, draw conclusions, and produce responses that were impossible without the support. The idea is to start with a baseline observation in a condition of no support and then gradually to offer minimal levels of support increasing them only as necessary to focus the child on components that will lead to success, but encouraging as much independence as possible; then withdrawing the supports to see what the child can now do without them within a similar problem situation. This cycle has been called the **test-intervene-retest** (or **test-teach-retest**) format (Schneider & Watkins, 1996). It is a key aspect of the process of dynamic assessment.

Dynamic assessment has been described in a number of sources (Campione & Brown, 1987; Lidz, 1991; Olswang, Bain, & Johnson, 1992; Palincsar, Brown, & Campione, 1994; Schneider & Watkins, 1996). The term originated with Feuerstein's (1979) description of the "assessment of retarded performers," in which he questioned the concept of IQ as a static entity. Feuerstein is an Israeli psychologist who developed some of his ideas working with survivors of the Holocaust. Feuerstein used a process of systematic mediation, which he and his colleagues called "instrumental enrichment," to show the malleability of intelligence and that performance on IQ tests could be modified (Feuerstein, Rand, & Rynders, 1988).

Peña, Quinn, and Iglesias (1992) described dynamic assessment procedures as a tool for diagnosing bilingual children with language impairments. They based decisions about children who were "possibly language disordered" on their ability to benefit in a short time from dynamic interaction targeting lexical learning. Children who showed significant change on a "modifiability indicator" were thought not to be at risk, whereas those children who did not benefit in a short time were considered in need of intervention.

Working with preschoolers with specific expressive language delay, Olswang and Bain and their colleagues have conducted several studies to demonstrate the value of dynamic assessment for identifying which children are most likely to need and to benefit from intervention (Bain & Olswang, 1995; Olswang & Bain, 1991; Olswang, Bain, & Johnson, 1992; Olswang, Bain, Rosendahl, Oblak, & Smith, 1986). Children who benefit quickly and with minimal assistance are considered to have potential to develop without treatment. Children who do not respond to adult cueing may not be ready for treatment. When children do not benefit, however, an alternative explanation is that the scaffolding may have been at too high a level, and that the work simply needed to be moved into the child's true ZPD (Schneider & Watkins, 1996). Children who fall in the middle are considered to be the best candidates for intervention.

Assessment strategies also have been developed to assess a child's theory of mind; this has particular implications for children with autism. The essence of such procedures is to discover whether a person can understand that someone might hold a false belief. Informal evidence of this can be uncovered when preschoolers begin to demonstrate understanding of many common fairy tales (e.g., Snow White, Little Red Riding Hood, Hansel and Gretel) that involve deception and trickery. A more clinical version of a false-belief test was adapted by British researchers Baron-Cohen, Leslie, and Frith (1985) for studying children with autism, Down syndrome, and normal development. The "Sally-Anne Test" (Baron-Cohen, 1995) involves two doll figures, a basket and a box, and a marble. As a child watches, Sally puts the marble in her basket, then exits the scene. Along comes Anne and moves the marble (unbeknownst to Sally) from the basket into the box. Then Sally returns, and the examiner asks the child where Sally will look for her marble. Children who have established a theory of mind (most normally developing 3- to 4-year-olds) will indicate the original location. If not, they will indicate where they know the marble actually is. In the study by Baron-Cohen and colleagues, both normally developing children and those with Down syndrome could perform the task, whereas only a small minority of the children with autism did so.

Social Interaction Theory and Intervention. "As language interventionists, our practice rests on at least an implicit belief that social interaction provides the context for and has the potential to effect developmental change" (Schneider & Watkins, 1996, p. 157). Within the broad realm of programs based on social interaction theory, however, variation can be found along the naturalness of the social interaction continuum. The common elements of such programs are intervention in everyday contexts and the emphasis on the importance of communicating with real partners in sincere communicative interactions that serve a real purpose.

Duchan (1995a) described the essence of intervention based on social interaction theory (see Box 3.17):

The teacher or clinician in the situated pragmatics paradigm provides the child with contextual support to help

---

Box 3.17 _____

Social Interaction Principles for Language Intervention (from Duchan, 1995a, p. 99)

1. The **goals** of language intervention programs should be prioritized, and those that have the greatest impact on the child's improved sensemaking should be given the highest priority.
2. When determining the intervention **activities,** choose those that make sense in the child's life and are sensible in the child's cultural context.
3. If there is a need to break down language, events, or discourse into component parts to facilitate learning, **divide the task** in ways that are meaningful for the child.
4. When asking **questions** to promote understandings, ask authentic questions—ones you would like to know the answers to.
5. Use **physical props** that are meaningful to the child.
6. **Respond contingently** to the child's intent, content, and form, giving priority to the intent.
7. Minimize **frame shifts** caused by correction or metalinguistic rewards (e.g., "Remember how you're supposed to say that?" "Good talking").
8. Follow the **children's lead.** Talk with them about what they may be thinking.
9. Consider the **function** as well as form as part of a child's response, and respond accordingly. (Avoid focusing solely on "right answers.")

---

the child make sense of what is going on. The prompts need to be designed in the children's zone of under-standing to aid them not only to respond appropriately, but to interpret what is happening around them. The chil-dren's actions are not seen as responses to stimuli, but as ways of conveying intents, carrying out agendas, or ac-complishing an event. So the focus is not on providing them with the proper prompts and reinforcements but on helping them accomplish their goals and on engaging them in communicative exchanges or event sequences. (pp. 134–135)

This suggests that professionals must assume a dif-ferent kind of role in the process. Muma (1978) de-scribed the old role of clinicians in traditional direct-teaching programs as being of the "jug and mug" variety. The clinician's role was to pour language into the waiting child. In programs conceptualized within a social interaction framework, however, Muma (1983) identified three quite different basic intervention com-ponents: (1) peer modeling, (2) parallel talk, and (3) par-ent participation.

Craig (1983) contrasted the role of clinicians in be-haviorist and mentalist (here called linguistic-induction) therapy models with pragmatic approaches. She noted that, "In contrast to the 'teacher' and 'facilitator' roles of the other major paradigms, within pragmatic approaches the clinician should serve as a 'trouble shooter' for the child—locating and eliminating the source of trouble in any communication flow and thereby maximizing the child's communicative potential" (p. 114).

This role requires that clinicians function in a **child-centered** mode, with the child initiating and the adult making scaffolding decisions based on the nature of the child's errors (van Kleeck & Richardson, 1986). Norris and Hoffman (1990a) pointed out that this mode is es-sentially related to a whole-language view in which nat-uralistic strategies are used that involve "a more socially oriented, child-initiated and child-controlled interaction style of treatment. . . .The child-initiated style of inter-action assumes that language is indivisible from a con-text of shared meaning and social use, and that children discover the properties of language through immersion in the communicative process" (p. 28). Arwood (1983) labeled such an approach "pragmaticism."

These models may seem aimed exclusively at the early or middle stages of language intervention (infancy through preschool years), but some have attempted to interpret contextually based language intervention for the school-age years. For example, Norris (1988, 1989) showed how small reading groups within classrooms could be used as the context for language intervention with children in early elementary grades. In the ap-proach she dubbed *communicative reading strategies* (CRS), Norris described how language intervention spe-cialists can use the reading group context in a three-step process to (1) organize some linguistic unit for the child (e.g., a sentence within the text, a phrase within a com-plete sentence, or a concept within a word, phrase, or paragraph); (2) give the child an opportunity to use lan-guage to communicate the information by reading the relevant text to the group; and (3) provide feedback to the child (e.g., in the form of an acknowledgment, re-quest for clarification, or extension of the idea) based on the information communicated to the group.

For school-age students of all ages, I described (1989b) how curriculum-based language assessment and intervention could be grounded in the various as-pects of the curriculum that children are supposed to master. The critical dimension of this and other ap-proaches is that relevant content and contexts from the child's world guide assessment and intervention. In ad-dition, the professional assumes the role of **participant** to guide the student, rather than functioning in the usual teacher role, as the student attempts to master the lan-guage of the curriculum. This is essentially the "trou-bleshooter" role described by Craig (1983), except that it is aimed at older children (see also Palinscar, Brown, & Campione, 1994).

Elements of programs based on social interaction theory have existed at least since clinicians began trying to integrate language function into intervention. In dis-cussing approaches based on the other theoretical per-spectives in this section of the chapter, I have pointed out the influence of social interaction theory in modify-ing many of them, such as the linguistic-based content–form–use model developed by Bloom and Lahey (1978; Lahey, 1988), Linder's cognitive-based TBPA model (1993), and the behaviorism-based incidental teaching model (e.g., Hart & Risley, 1968; Warren & Kaiser, 1986).

Limitations

When specialists began to interpret pragmatic issues for clinical application, they expressed a concern that clin-icians might view pragmatics simply as a fifth linguistic rule system (added to phonology, morphology, syntax, and semantics), to be inserted into the general linguistic rule-induction framework (Craig, 1983; Gallagher & Prutting, 1983). To simply add pragmatics as a new set of intervention goals, perhaps coupled with modification in carryover strategies, would not do the theory justice. As Craig emphasized, the broader perspective of pragmatics, which is tied closely to the concept that "language is acquired and used in a social context" (Bates, 1976, p. 412), does more than influence the choice of intervention targets. It leads to a paradigm shift that dramatically influences choices about language intervention procedures.

Most of the more recent practical interpretations of this theory involve rich interpretations of its broad implications. Even in such cases, however, potential limitations remain. Because approaches based on social interaction theory tend to place a priority on targets involving language use and pragmatics, potential targets involving language content–form interactions may receive less attention than they need. Not all children have the same kind of language disorder, and not all children need the same kind of intervention. Fey (1986) noted that an uncritical implementation of a "natural is better" assumption leads some clinicians to:

> *select activities that do not allow the implementation of effective procedures. Consequently, intervention sometimes provides little more than what the child would ordinarily get from the natural environment. History has demonstrated the extreme difficulty which many of these children have in extracting conventional patterns of communication from such natural contexts. For example, children who are reasonably good communicators but who have marked difficulty with language form often seem oblivious to many of the structural details of language. Since their own efforts to communicate are reasonably effective, the need to attend and master the use of language form is often not readily apparent. In my experience, a clinician can often facilitate growth in the child's vocabulary and perhaps pragmatic and cognitive skills by providing highly natural and enriching experiences. The rate of development of syntax and morphology, however, often continues to lag. (p. 65)*

Social interaction theory provides a strong rationale that combines aspects of several other perspectives with the view that children are whole people whose development is influenced by internal as well as external variables. Because social interaction theory provides a

strong philosophical basis for selecting procedures, it translates fairly well into intervention models. It is now popular for this reason among others. Like any other model, however, it should not be adopted uncritically for all children without considering their needs as individuals (Cromer, 1981).

INTEGRATING SIX THEORETICAL PERSPECTIVES

What aspects of these six theoretical approaches can we use to guide our decisions as language interventionists? Is this merely a case of six blind men each describing the elephant as a vastly different creature, depending on the areas of evidence they explored, or are there true differences in essence among these theories that go beyond the avenues of inquiry, observational methods, and data they represent? My own sense is that there is probably some of both.

To some extent, the extreme position of any of the theoretical views considered here can make it incompatible with any of the others, but return to the discussion of system theory introduced in Chapter 1. As clinicians who must deal with the complexities of real people and problems, we cannot afford the purity of focus that a strictly theoretical orientation requires (see also Kamhi, 1993). System theory allows one to conceive of the language acquisition process as an integrated whole involving contributions from subsystems that may be quite different from one another; some subsystems may appear to be internal to the child, and others external, but all are part of the same open and interactive system.

The clinician–educator needs to understand the assumptions of the varied theoretical positions and the evidence used to support them but cannot afford to become so wedded to one theoretical approach that taking a broader perspective becomes difficult. Rather, aspects of all six of these theoretical positions may be useful in facilitating the language acquisition process when it needs a boost.

In the contexts of language assessment and intervention, the best theory may be one that allows the professional to conceive of children as having a genetic heritage, a biological mechanism that predisposes them to make cognitive sense of the world, to interact socially, and to acquire linguistic rules, but that can be molded through interactions with an external environment designed to facilitate their needs. The explanations of behaviorism can be accepted as influencing the directions of development but not without reliance on some contributions from internal cognitive structures and information processing strategies that allow children to alter their future perceptions, memories, recognitions, and expressions. Children can be viewed as active contributors to their own development.

Different children also have different needs and some theoretical perspectives are better suited to meeting some needs than others. For those who accept such a premise, the problem of decision making shifts from selecting the best theory to serve all children's needs to selecting the best theory (or theories) to serve a particular child's needs (see Personal Reflection 3.12).

The stimulus–response–reinforcement elements of a behaviorist paradigm are a part of any human interaction, whether controlled by design or not. Yet, the application of this technology might be so much richer if guided by aspects of theories that view children as active information seekers. Information processing theory might also contribute ideas about how to build the attention needed for further learning. Rather than viewing attention as a set of specific behaviors to be learned, one might view it from the cognitivist perspective, as a set of "questions being asked by the brain" (Smith, 1973, p. 28). Adopting this viewpoint can also introduce metacognitive elements that can guide the intervention process toward teaching the child to use new self-questioning strategies (this is the "question transplant" idea introduced in Chapter 1). This approach might blend disparate views that define learning as the strengthening of a stimulus–response relationship (behaviorism), as "remembering what you're interested in"

PERSONAL REFLECTION 3.12 _____

"Clinicians need to understand, judge, and exploit the plurality of theories and areas of knowledge that have a direct impact on clinical service. In doing so, clinicians will ensure that there is some logic to the clinical decisions they make in serving children with speech–language disorders." (p. 59)

Alan G. Kamhi (1993), professor at Memphis State University in Tennessee.

(social interaction; Wurman, 1989, p. 137), and as "relative to something you understand" (cognitivism; Wurman, 1989, p. 167).

On the other hand, theoretical perspectives are not unimportant. Duchan (1995a) explained how differences in behaviorist and social interactionist views affect intervention:

> *Sequences of responses cast as behavioral chains in the behavioral framework are seen in the situated pragmatics framework as a set of planned actions governed by goal structures or subscripts within a larger script. So brushing one's teeth, regarded by behaviorists as a chain, becomes a meaningful activity to a situated pragmatist, with subparts that bear a logical relationship to one another. (Taking a cap off the toothpaste enables one to get the paste out.) A pragmatist who approaches a task analysis would consider the variety of meaningful relations which the performer of the task sees among the steps in the task. The job of the learner is not seen as memorizing separated steps, but rather as learning the meaningful relations of each subpart to the whole task—as a dynamic, active and creative exercise in sensemaking. (p. 135)*

My own approach is to use cues to meaningfulness to help individuals construct logical networks that can continue to guide them when they are not in the presence of the clinician. But I also know that some skills require practice. I do not see these two positions as antithetical. Similarly, Harris and Pressley (1991) warned against setting up false dichotomies between "constructed versus instructed knowledge, understanding versus rule following, and discovery versus drill and practice" (p. 393).

As a metatheory, system theory offers a framework for problem solving that allows integration of multiple theoretical perspectives. Different theoretical explanations can be viewed not as competitive alternatives but as mutual contributors to the decision-making process. Specialists can then design intervention to assess a particular situation using the tools most suitable for identifying its critical features and can use strategies matched to particular needs. Careful thought and collaborative goal setting are required.

The best way to characterize a practice that blends the most desirable aspects of multiple theories is *eclectic:*

> **eclectic,** ek•lek'tik, *a.* [Gr. *eklektikos—ek,* and *lego,* to choose.] Proceeding by the method of selection; choos-

ing what seems best from others; not original nor following any one model or leader, but choosing at will from the doctrines, works, etc., of others. (Thatcher, 1980, p. 274)

As this dictionary definition indicates, one should not confuse eclectic with disorganized or random practices. An eclectic approach involves careful, deliberate selection from among several choices. Selecting the best involves neither lack of theory nor devotion to any one theory. Rather, it involves making intentional choices that vary as purposes vary.

SUMMARY

Chapter 3 summarized six different theories of language development: biological maturation, linguistic, behavioral, information processing, cognitive, and social interaction. Some of these theories (particularly linguistic and behavioral theories) attempt more comprehensive explanations than others. All have some relevance for understanding childhood language disorders, with varied applications to language assessment and intervention as well.

REVIEW TOPICS

- Six theoretical perspectives of normal and disordered development: biological maturation, linguistic, behavioral, information processing, cognitive, social interaction (be able to describe basic beliefs, contributions to language assessment and intervention, and limitations for each)
- Nativist versus empiricist views
- Bio-maturational theory explanations: cerebral asymmetries and critical periods, brain weight changes, neuronal growth patterns (microstructural axonal myelination and dendritic arborization), macro-organizational evidence, genetic evidence
- Neuropsychological models, including the pinball wizardry model
- Central auditory processing, temporal sequencing, and the Tallal and Merzenich Fast ForWord therapy approach
- Phonological awareness and implications for language and literacy development
- Linguistic theory explanations: the Language Acquisition Device (LAD), poverty of the stimulus ar-

gument, universality argument, early emergence argument, separability of language from intelligence argument
- Universal Grammar: principles and parameters, input and intake, intermediate grammars and Continuity Theory, bootstrapping (semantic, prosodic, syntactic)
- Behavioral theory explanations: classical conditioning, operant conditioning, imitation, stimulus clustering, stimulus generalization, word learning, sentence learning, functions (autoclitic, mand, echoic, intraverbal), nature versus nurture views
- A-B-C assessment
- Behavioral training techniques: attention, modeling, imitation, reinforcement (positive, negative, punishment), prompting and cueing (putting through, hand-over-hand, fading, stimulus control), shaping, discrimination training, chaining, stimulus and response generalization, repeated trials, discrete trial learning, direct teaching
- Methods for overcoming limitations of behavioral training models: analyzing aberrant behavior as communicative, milieu (incidental) teaching approaches
- Information processing theory explanations: serial information processes (sensation, perception, cognition, memory), parallel distributed processing models (also called connectionist or competition models), bottom-up (data driven, decoding emphasis, part-to-whole) versus top-down (constructivist, comprehension emphasis, whole-to-part) versus interactive processing models, attention, working memory, short-term memory (reauditorization, recency effect, primacy effect), central auditory processing
- Examples of bottom-up intervention (e.g., training auditory perception, short-term memory, phonological awareness), top-down intervention (e.g., whole language), interactive approaches (e.g., Reading Recovery, Elkonin boxes), treatment for word retrieval deficits (storage elaboration, retrieval processes)
- Cognitive (constructivist) theory explanations: disequilibrium, adaptation processes of assimilation and accommodation (see Box 3.12), schemas, Piagetian stages (sensorimotor, representational [pre-operations, concrete operations], formal operations), sensemaking through play, schemas, scripts, and narratives

- Cognitive referencing (strong form, weak form, correlational cognitive hypotheses)
- Cognitive-constructivist approaches to intervention (Paley example of using play, scripts, and narratives to construct meaning), metacognitive approaches and strategy training
- Social interactionist theory explanations: joint action routines and scaffolding, Vygotsky and the zone of proximal development, development of the theory of mind (intention detector, eye direction detector, shared attention mechanism, theory of mind module)
- Dynamic assessment, the "Sally-Anne Test," child-centered versus adult-centered approaches, pragmaticism, communicative reading strategies, scaffolding as an intervention technique
- Eclectic models of assessment and intervention

REVIEW QUESTIONS _____

1. Which of the six theoretical perspectives explains language acquisition:
   a. as analogous to inputting data to a computer?
   b. by referring to a species-specific predisposition to learn the regularities of language?
   c. by referring to a genetically determined predisposition of certain areas of the brain (such as the larger left hemispheres of most neonates) to learn language and the importance of myelination?
   d. as a process involving selective reinforcement?
   e. by assuming that human beings have an innate motivation to want to communicate and make their intentions known?
   f. as based on the construction of general conceptual frameworks?
2. Which of the six theoretical perspectives explains language intervention:
   a. as a process of selective reinforcement of desired responses and techniques to encourage stimulus and response generalization?
   b. as a process of arranging language input to facilitate semantic, syntactic, and prosodic bootstrapping so the child can infer the rules of adult grammar?
   c. as a process in which children are involved in meaningful activities with rich opportunities to communicate for varied interactive purposes and adults scaffold them to communicate at higher

   levels of competence than they could manage independently?
   d. as a process of encouraging the brain to develop new neural pathways?
   e. as a process of developing attentional, perceptual, and short-term memory abilities so as to support further language learning?
   f. as a process of setting up general learning experiences so the child can develop more complex schemas that will support language learning?
3. When a child looks out the window and sees a bird fly to its nest and says, "Birdie flying," which theoretical position is most closely associated with each of the following explanations?
   a. The child is demonstrating the results of learning through imitative modeling and positive consequences (e.g., parental attention) for appropriate verbal comments.
   b. The child has learned about birds and flying through multiple experiences in watching them and thus is "ready" to apply language to such concepts as agents and actions.
   c. The child's parents have interacted with her, focusing joint attention on the bird and its babies, pointing out how the bird flies and talking about it with the child.
   d. The child has learned to put noun phrases with verb structures and has formulated this utterance because of an innate language learning system that is tuned to pay attention to regular verb endings like -ing.
   e. The child has learned the -ing ending because recurrent experiences with similar structures have strengthened some nodes of the language learning system over others. Thus, the appropriate words and structures have been stored and retrieved for use in talking about the immediate experience. It is also important that through habituation, the system has learned to ignore competing stimuli that are not central to the current experience.
   f. The child has developed new neural connections fostered by environmental experience.
4. Which theoretical position is most closely aligned with each of the following descriptions?
   a. Children's two-word utterances probably represent the result of applying words to concepts they have already developed.

b. Children's two-word utterances probably represent the result of successive associative learning.

c. Children's two-word utterances probably represent the result of a parallel distributive processing system at work.

d. Children's two-word utterances probably represent the development of language to perform early speech acts.

e. Children's two-word utterances probably represent the results of micro- and macro-structural developments in the brain.

f. Children's two-word utterances probably represent the child's innate ability to induce the rules of language.

5. Which of the six theoretical perspectives are each of the following contributors most closely associated: Marshall, Dore, Vygotsky, Skinner, Chomsky, Myklebust, Piaget, Pinker, Bruner?

6. What key words might provide clues in journal articles to the theoretical orientation of the authors?

**ACTIVITIES FOR
EXTENDED THINKING** _____

1. Find journal articles on language development, assessment, or intervention that represent at least three or four of the six theoretical perspectives.

2. Divide your class into six cooperative learning groups. Each group should become "experts" on one of the theoretical perspectives and prepare a study sheet and some review questions for that theory. Then recombine the class into groups of six, with one expert from each of the first groups acting as tutor to the others regarding explanations, contributions, and limitations of each theory.

4

Causes, Categories, and Characteristics

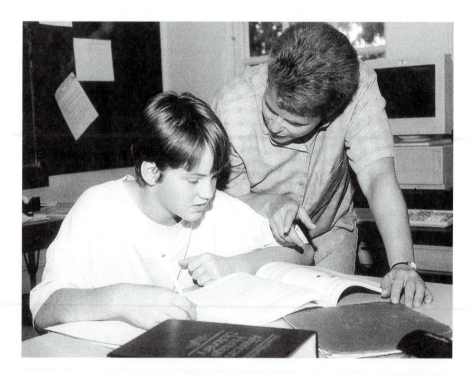

What kinds of conditions are associated with difficulty learning language? This chapter addresses the causes, categories, and characteristics of childhood language disorders. Chapter 3 included a review of factors that play complex roles in normal language acquisition. Disruptions in those factors also play complex causative roles for language disorders. As suggested by the discussion of system theory in Chapter 1, causes are not singular influences that operate at a specific time and then disappear or remain static. Rather, causative factors act as vectors that assume different levels of strength at different times. This means that a plan might be devised to strengthen the influences of positive contributing factors and reduce the influences of negative ones. Plans may also be devised to prevent language disorders on a broad scale by addressing causative factors.

A DEFINITION OF LANGUAGE DISORDERS

As noted in the preface and introduction to this book, I take a broad view of language disorders, one not restricted to "specific language impairment." A definition that encompasses the multiple elements of a broad view was offered by Bashir (1989):

> Language disorders *is a term that represents a heterogeneous group of either developmental or acquired disabilities principally characterized by deficits in comprehension, production, and/or use of language. Language disorders are chronic and may persist across the lifetime of the individual. The symptoms, manifestations, effects, and severity of the problems change over time. The changes occur as a consequence of context, content, and learning tasks. (p. 181)*

This definition recognizes the heterogeneity of language disorders, their varied symptoms, and the multiplicity of both developmental and acquired factors that can contribute to them. It acknowledges that language disorders are chronic but also changeable. Changeability partially results from developmental shifts and partially from shifts in contributing factors external to the individual (e.g., language contexts, content, and learning tasks).

On the other hand, this definition includes some elements that beg for further definition. What, in fact, *is* a "deficit in comprehension, production, and/or use of language"? That is one of the most difficult questions facing language disorder specialists. It is an integral part of the two more specific questions that practitioners (particularly those working in school settings) face

daily: (1) Who should be labeled as language impaired? (2) Who qualifies for what kind of service? In many ways, these two questions underlie and motivate the current discussion of causes, categories, and contributing factors. The discussion is extended further in Chapters 5 and 6 to more specific consideration of assessment and eligibility issues and to the provision of service. Here, it is limited to attributes of causes, categories, and contributing factors.

THE ELUSIVENESS OF CAUSE

No one fully understands the causes of childhood language disorders. Considerable information has been gathered about the conditions associated with language disorders, but clear and predictable causative patterns have yet to be demonstrated.

Even factors that appear on the surface to be related directly to language disorders have unclear causative patterns. For example, children with profound hearing impairments can be expected to have difficulty learning language through speech. Even if they learn sign language, their written language skills are generally affected. Yet, two children with highly similar hearing loss profiles may show considerably different language acquisition profiles. Similarly, an overt causative factor such as brain injury from trauma may have long-term effects on language development that are difficult to predict. Multiple factors seem to influence the direction and degree of the outcome.

TO CATEGORIZE OR NOT TO CATEGORIZE?

Any categorical approach to childhood language disorders is fraught with difficulty. A primary concern is that causative categories are not predictably related to language attributes (Bloom & Lahey, 1978). Lahey (1988) made a case for using normal development, rather than diagnostic group membership, to guide language assessment and intervention practices. The rationale is that heterogeneity within a diagnostic category and blurred distinctions across categories lead to validity and reliability problems in using categorical approaches to organize discussions of children's language disorders.

In this book, I consider a child's "membership" in a diagnostic group as only one of many factors to be considered in the decision-making process, not the determining factor. Although the organizational framework for this book is developmental, needs-based decision making is also emphasized. Readers are cautioned that any single perspective can be limiting.

Diagnostic categories can lead to trouble when *labels,* rather than individual needs, are used to determine the kinds and qualities of services a child will receive. Another problem is when a label is viewed as indistinguishable from an individual for whom it is only one of many characteristics (see Personal Reflection 4.1). This problem can be reduced by not using labels as nouns, or even as central identifying attributes. For example, instead of referring to a person as an *autistic,* or even as an *autistic person,* consider the individual a *person with autism.* Many (including me) believe such "person first" language prevents lumping individuals into categories and inappropriately limiting expectations for future growth based on preconceptions about "condition X." Establishing a prognosis is a responsibility that accompanies clinical intervention, but it should be done with an eye to avoiding stereotyping and to being realistic without limiting an individual's and a family's hopes for the future. On the other hand, a diagnosis of a language-learning disability, such as dyslexia (see Chapter 1 and Personal Reflection 4.2), can be a positive experience. It can reduce confusion and help people separate the problems they have from their basic essence.

Throughout this discussion of categories, remember that prototypes are being discussed and that space constraints limit the discussion's breadth and depth. The real world does not often offer "textbook examples." It is full of gray areas, overlaps and inexact fits. Professionals who realize that categories are inventions for the convenience of thinking and communicating about phenomena will be more likely to maintain the flexibility

PERSONAL REFLECTION 4.1 _____

"I am introducing you to my son, Joshua. Josh is 7 years old. He's diligent to the task, a unique kid, a hard worker and, yes, Josh has Down syndrome. I mention the Down syndrome last because Josh is a person first. Josh is not a 'Down's'; he's not a 'Down syndrome child'; but rather he's an individual who happens to have Down syndrome. He's not a category or a diagnosis. He is a person before he is anything else."

Thomas J. O'Neill (1987, p. xviii), President, National Down Syndrome Congress.

PERSONAL REFLECTION 4.2 _____

"The happiest day of my life occurred when I found out I was dyslexic. I believe that life is finding solutions, and the worst feeling to me is confusion." (p. 25)

Ennis Cosby, teacher (son of actor Bill Cosby and educator Camille Cosby), whose comments from a paper he had written were quoted in an article in *Time* magazine (Chua-Eoan, 1997).

needed to enter systems that include people with language disorders and contribute positively.

AN OVERVIEW OF CATEGORIES

The categories discussed in this chapter are outlined in Box 4.1. This is my own attempt to group diagnostic categories that have something in common into four groups: (1) **central processing factors,** which involve disorders of cortically supported language learning of a cognitive and/or linguistic nature; (2) **peripheral factors,** which involve disorders of sensory and/or motor systems that influence how language gets in and out of the brain (see the bottom arrow in the pinball wizardry

Box 4.1 _____

Categorical Factors Associated with Childhood Language Disorders

I. Central factors
   A. Specific language disability
   B. Mental retardation
   C. Autism
   D. Attention-deficit hyperactivity disorder
   E. Acquired brain injury
   F. Others
II. Peripheral factors
   A. Hearing impairment
   B. Visual impairment
   C. Deaf-blindness
   D. Physical impairment
III. Environmental and emotional factors
   A. Neglect and abuse
   B. Behavioral and emotional development problems
IV. Mixed factors

model introduced in Chapter 2); (3) **environmental and emotional factors,** which do not appear to be caused (at least directly) by brain organization differences (at least based on what scientists know now); and (4) **mixed factors,** which often yield severe disabilities involving cognitive, sensory, and motor systems, as well as language. Categorical discussions are organized into sections on diagnosis, subtypes, and characteristics to consider when making decisions about assessment and intervention.

CENTRAL PROCESSING FACTORS

Specific Language Impairment and Learning Disabilities

Diagnosing Specific Language Impairment and Learning Disabilities. A general definition for "specific language impairment" is that children with the diagnosis "exhibit significant limitations in language functioning that cannot be attributed to deficits in hearing, oral structure and function, or general intelligence" (Leonard, 1987, p. 1). This definition emphasizes specificity; it assumes that a relatively isolated impairment can affect language development specifically, while leaving general cognitive development and other peripheral sensory and motor functions relatively unaffected (Watkins, 1994).

Although most professionals recognize a condition known by the label **specific language impairment** (SLI) (and by other labels considered later), attempts to establish operational diagnostic criteria for the category commonly encounter two problems. These are, first, problems associated with identifying a common set of reliable symptoms that appear repeatedly in different children (inclusionary characteristics) and second, problems associated with isolating language from other cognitive, perceptual, and social functions (exclusionary characteristics).

Because the diagnosis of SLI depends on exclusion of other categorical conditions, it becomes problematic to diagnose when children have characteristics of SLI, but mixed either with other problems or with conditions of cultural diversity. Either of these circumstances may make it particularly difficult to identify the problem with standardized measures.

Inclusionary characteristics for SLI are "significant delays in the development of semantic, syntactic, phonological, and/or pragmatic abilities" (Fey, Long, &

Cleave, 1994, p. 161). As Watkins (1994) noted, however, "we have yet to establish a widely accepted profile of linguistic behavior associated with the disorder" (p. 1). Exclusionary characteristics are "the relative absence of frank neurological damage, emotional disorder, or hearing loss. Another criterion that is part of virtually every definition of specific language impairment is performance IQ of no more than 1 standard deviation below the mean (i.e., performance IQs of 85 or above)" (Fey, Long, & Cleave, 1994, p. 161).

This **cognitive referencing criterion** (also called **MA referencing** or a **discrepancy criterion**) is also part of most definitions of **learning disabilities,** including the "definition of learning disabilities provided by Public Law 94–142, which clearly requires the use of an IQ score to identify children as disabled" (Francis et al., 1996, p. 132), which specifies:

> *A severe discrepancy between achievement and intellectual ability in one or more of the following areas: (1) oral expression; (2) listening comprehension; (3) written expression; (4) basic reading skill; (5) reading comprehension; (6) mathematics calculation; or (7) mathematic reasoning. The child may not be identified as having a specific learning disability if the discrepancy between ability and achievement is primarily the results of: (1) a visual learning or motor handicap; (2) mental retardation; (3) emotional disturbance; or (4) environment, cultural, or economic disadvantage. (USOE, 1977, p. 1082)*

Discrepancy criteria are found in 31 of 50 state policies for identifying language impairment (Casby, 1992b) and in 34 of 50 state policies for identifying learning disabilities (Frankenberger & Fronzaglio, 1991). But this ubiquity does not mean that such criteria are appropriate for clinical purposes. It is one thing to find a subgroup of children with like characteristics for research purposes who demonstrate a clear discrepancy; it is quite another to say that only children who show a discrepancy need specialized interventions to succeed in school.

As considered in Chapters 3 and 6, intelligence testing for children with language disorders is fraught with difficulty. Often, when intelligence tests are administered to children with disabilities, their performance across tasks is uneven (a condition sometimes called **psychometric scatter**). As Rapin and Allen (1983) have pointed out, in intelligence testing, "The IQ is the summary score derived from performance on a psychological test battery that samples a broad range of behaviors." For children with disabilities, however, "A summary score represents neither their areas of real deficit nor their strengths" (p. 162). Although typically, children with SLIs tend to do better on "nonverbal" tests of intelligence than those designed to tap verbal abilities, when a verbal strategy can facilitate problem solving on supposedly nonverbal tests or subtests, children with SLI may also score lower on those tests because of their language deficits.

For those engaged in clinical or educational practice, Rapin and Allen (1983) commented that it is unusual to see many children with "pure" syndromes. Instead, they argued that a diagnosis of specific developmental language disorder is justified when children exhibited linguistic skills that "are much more severely deficient than their other cognitive skills and are out of proportion to their IQ" (p. 163).

What to Call Specific Language-Learning Disabilities?

Perhaps no other categorical condition has been given so many names over the years as **specific language impairment** and **learning disabilities** (LD). These two conditions, at least in my experience, overlap significantly, if not completely. The reasons for this are also many.

First, some of the names reflect theories about underlying causes prevalent at a particular point in the history of concern about the disorders. For example, the terms **minimal brain damage, minimal brain dysfunction** (U.S. Department of Health, Education, & Welfare, 1969), and **congenital aphasia** (S. F. Brown, 1959) were prevalent in earlier attempts to describe children who appear to have a specific neurological deficit that makes it difficult for them to learn language. Such diagnoses, however, were based only on "soft signs" (including language development difficulty) in the absence of hard neurological evidence. Gradually, those terms have been replaced by labels such as **learning disability,** which makes fewer assumptions about cause, or by labels such as **developmental language disability** or **developmental language disorder,** which are designed to specify a condition for which no clear cause exists but that is apparently congenital.

Second, some terminological differences reflect the varied perspectives of professional disciplines concerned with the diagnosis and remediation of relatively isolated language disorders. For example, whereas physicians might use terms such as **minimal brain dysfunction** and **dyslexia** to describe a child with such problems;

speech–language pathologists use terms such as **specific language impairment** and **language-learning disability;** special educators use terms such as **learning disability;** and reading specialists use terms such as **reading disability.**

Trends in the medical profession, however, are shifting. The *Diagnostic and Statistical Manual of Mental Disorders, Fourth Edition*—(DSM-IV™), published by the American Psychiatric Association (1994), now uses terms based more on observable symptomatology than on assumptions about cause that cannot be proven. The DSM-IV separates **learning disorders** (formerly called "Academic Skills Disorders") from **communication disorders** and recognizes subtypes within each. Learning disorders include **reading disorder, mathematics disorder,** and **disorder of written expression.** The diagnostic criteria for each of these learning disorders specify that, as measured "on individually administered, standardized tests" (p. 46), achievement is "substantially below that expected for age, schooling, and level of intelligence," and "If a sensory deficit is present, the learning difficulties must be in excess of those usually associated with it" (pp. 46–47).

Communication disorders defined in DSM-IV include the language categories of **expressive language disorder, mixed receptive-expressive language disorder, phonological disorder** (formerly developmental articulation disorder), **stuttering,** and **communication disorder not otherwise specified.** Exclusionary criteria for expressive and mixed receptive-expressive language disorders require that: language test scores be "substantially below those obtained from standardized measures of both nonverbal intellectual capacity and receptive language development" (p. 55); pervasive developmental disorder be ruled out; and "If mental retardation, a speech-motor or sensory deficit, or environmental deprivation is present, the language difficulties are in excess of those usually associated with these problems" (p. 55). Both also specify that the language difficulties must "interfere with academic or occupational achievement or with social communication" (p. 55). The difference between subtypes is that children with expressive language disorder also have test scores for expressive language that are substantially below those for receptive language. This is the version most like what speech–language pathologists call specific language impairment. **Phonological disorder** is defined in DSM-IV as "failure to use developmentally expected speech sounds that are appropriate for the individual's age and dialect" (p. 61).

Third, some terminological differences reflect evolution of symptoms of language disorders within the same children over time. For example, many children who might be categorized during their preschool years as having early language delay or early language disability may be recategorized during their school-age years as having **learning disabilities** (see Box 4.2) or **language-learning disabilities.**

What changes? Do children change or only labels? Recalling the discussions of Chapter 1 regarding contextually based definitions of disability, probably a little of both occurs, set in the context of changes in environmental expectations from the preschool years through adulthood. In my experience, children whose language impairments involve difficulty acquiring the phonological and morphological rules of oral language tend to be identified in the school-age years as having learning disabilities when their language problems start interfering with their academic developments, although not always. Other school-age children who have difficulty with language acquisition in its written forms, particularly with written language comprehension and

formulation beyond the level of single words, may not be identified as having learning disabilities until around the third or fourth grade. Language deficits can also underlie mathematical functioning (Crouse, 1996). Children whose language difficulties show up primarily as problems with written and mathematical symbol systems, and who have relatively better oral language abilities, may not be identified as having language impairments in addition to their learning disabilities unless a diagnostician or teacher looks below the surface. Rice (1994) emphasized changes over time in the nature of specific language impairments, but warned that "It is important to note that this is viewed as a likely language impairment in adulthood, not merely a language-turned-reading-impairment, as school-age learning disabilities can be regarded" (p. 69).

Out of concern that traditional views of learning disabilities are limited by their restriction to the school-age years, the National Joint Committee on Learning Disabilities (1985) developed a position paper on "Learning Disabilities and the Preschool Child," in which they noted that learning disabilities must be viewed as problems not only of the school years but also of preschool years and continuing into adult life:

> *Indiscriminate premature labeling of the preschool child as learning disabled is not warranted. Normal development is characterized by broad ranges of individual and group differences, as well as by variability in rates and patterns of maturation. During the preschool years, this variability is marked. For some children, marked discrepancies in abilities are temporary and are resolved during the course of development and within the context of experiential interaction. For other children, there is a persistence of marked discrepancies within and among one or more domains of function, necessitating the child's referral for systematic assessment and appropriate intervention. (p. 1)*

Catts, Hu, Larrivee, and Swank (1994) described a set of features of speech–language impairment that may be the "early manifestations of a reading disability" (p. 154). They noted that, "Unlike children with articulation impairments, children with language impairments are at high risk for reading problems" (p. 155). In particular, phonological awareness and rapid naming difficulties are closely linked with problems involving early word recognition skills; whereas semantic-syntactic language difficulties are linked more closely with problems involving reading comprehension.

Box 4.2 _____

Definition of Learning Disabilities by The National Joint Committee on Learning Disabilities (1991)

Learning disabilities is a general term that refers to a heterogeneous group of disorders manifested by significant difficulties in the acquisition and use of listening, speaking, reading, writing, reasoning, or mathematical abilities. These disorders are intrinsic to the individual, presumed to be due to central nervous system dysfunction, and may occur across the lifespan. Problems in self-regulatory behaviors, social perception, and social interaction may exist with learning disabilities but do not by themselves constitute a learning disability. Although learning disabilities may occur concomitantly with other handicapping conditions (for example, sensory impairment, mental retardation, serious emotional disturbance) or with extrinsic influences (such as cultural differences, insufficient or inappropriate instruction), they are not the result of those conditions or influences. (p. 19)

Fourth, varied terms may reflect the relatedness of a cluster of disorders that may or may not be parts of the same syndrome. In this category are labels such as **specific reading disability** and **dyslexia**, as well as the DSM-IV categories of **disorder of written expression** and **reading disorder.** Such labels tend to reflect a particular set of symptoms having to do with the acquisition of written rather than oral language.

Consider terminology related to **specific reading disability** a bit further. Perhaps no term is more confusing to the general public than **dyslexia.** This term grew out of recognition by a physician, Samuel Orton (1937), that childhood reading disability had some features in common with alexia, or "word blindness." The term **pure word blindness** was first used by the neurologist Dejerine in 1892 (E. Kaplan & Goodglass, 1981) to describe an adult stroke patient who exhibited serious disability in comprehending written material accompanied by a remarkable preservation of writing ability. To contrast with the acquired condition, Orton called the condition involving specific reading disability that he observed in children **developmental alexia.** The term **alexia** then evolved into the term **dyslexia,** partially because the reading disability is rarely expressed as complete inability to read. Although the general public tends to focus on Orton's explanation of symptoms related to letter reversals and word confusions in the diagnosis of dyslexia and to think of it as primarily a visual-based problem, Orton's followers in the International Dyslexia Association (formerly the Orton Dyslexia Society) use the terms **dyslexia** and **specific language disability** as interchangeable (see Box 4.3). Kamhi and Catts (1989), in a review of the evidence, also supported the view of dyslexia as a developmental language impairment, with difficulty focused in the area of phonological analysis skills.

Finally, different states, regions, and professional associations adopt different terminology, and their labels evolve over time. Because terminology used to label conditions that society views as handicapping can acquire pejorative connotations, it is particularly likely that such terminology will shift as perceptions of the disorders shift. This makes it important for parents and professionals to understand the terminology prevalent in a local area or professional group whenever they enter a new setting to be sure that they are communicating clearly about children.

Box 4.3 _____

Characteristics of Dyslexia
(Summarized from Slingerland, 1981)

1. Average or above average intelligence
2. Reversals, transpositions, and omissions in reading, spelling, and/or speech
3. Difficulty learning to read, as shown by one or more of the following:
   a. Insertion of small words in reading
   b. Silent reading slow when compared to intelligence
   c. Oral reading hesitant
   d. Poor word recall and decoding skills
   e. Reading comprehension lost during struggle to recognize words
4. Difficulty recalling images for individual letters and letter sequences readily, smoothly, and accurately
5. Features sometimes observed include:
   a. Spelling difficulty
   b. Meager writing vocabulary
   c. Awkward or slow writing
   d. Hesitancy in talking, with poor word retrieval
   e. Difficulty expressing self, talking a lot but not getting to the point
   f. Particular difficulty recalling names of acquaintances or places
   g. Poor left-to-right orientation
6. Tendency to "run in families," but can occur in isolated cases
7. Language difficulties appear in spite of adequate educational opportunities

---

Subtypes of Specific Language Impairment. Although definitions and discussions of specific language impairment and learning disabilities generally recognize their heterogeneity, few attempts have been made to differentiate subtypes. This is particularly true in the area of specific oral language impairment. More attempts have been made to differentiate subtypes of children who have specific written language problems.

Oral Language Impairment Subtypes. One of the first studies to differentiate subtypes based on language symptoms rather than presumed cause was conducted by Aram and Nation (1975). They identified six different patterns of deficit among 47 children with developmental language disorders who were between the ages of 3 and 7 years. Using performance on formal language tasks of comprehension, formulation, and repetition (imitation), Aram and Nation divided the children into six subgroups representing (1) better ability to repeat than to comprehend or formulate language; (2) generalized expressive deficiency involving formulation and repetition; (3) relatively uniform deficiency for all three kinds of language tasks; (4) specific phonological deficiency affecting comprehension, formulation, and repetition; (5) comprehension deficiency with equal or better ability to formulate language or to repeat it; and (6) specific formulation and repetition deficiency.

Rapin and Allen (1983) compiled longitudinal and cross-sectional evidence (based on such sources as neurological tests, language and cognitive tests, and direct observation) from approximately 100 children who had been referred for a pediatric neurological consultation with the chief complaint of delayed or deviant speech. From the evidence, the researchers differentiated several developmental language disorder syndromes, which they grouped into four major subtypes: (1) predominant expressive disorder (with three subgroups) (2) verbal auditory agnosia, (3) autism, and (4) a semantic-pragmatic group with some characteristics in common with autism but lacking the interpersonal deficits of autism.

Within the **predominant expressive disorder** group described by Rapin and Allen (1983) the most prevalent of the three subgroups is the **phonologic-syntactic syndrome.** It is diagnosed when children are difficult to understand, use few function words, demonstrate limited noun and verb inflection (omitting such endings as plurals and *-ing*), and rarely combine syntactic relations within a single sentence. Some, but not all, show additional signs of neurological dysfunction, particularly oromotor dysfunction. These include signs of mild dysarthria (drooling and a history of difficulty in sucking, chewing, and swallowing) and signs of oromotor apraxia (difficulty in imitating precise movements of the tongue, lips, and jaw). A second subgroup in the expressive category is **severe expressive syndrome with good comprehension** (Rapin & Allen, 1983). These children are completely mute or virtually unintelligible, with productions limited to poorly articulated two-word utterances at most, but with strikingly good language comprehension.

The third expressive subgroup is **syntactic-pragmatic syndrome** (Rapin & Allen, 1983). Children in this rare subgroup include those with grossly impaired syntax, severely limited pragmatic use of language, and impaired comprehension. They can name pictures and objects and give and follow simple commands but cannot formulate or respond to *wh-* (e.g, *what, where,* and *who*) questions. This is the only syndrome that Rapin and Allen described where syntax is affected but phonology is normal or near normal.

The second major subtype syndrome of **verbal auditory agnosia** that Rapin and Allen (1983) described might be better classified with cases of acquired childhood language disorders in this text. It is comparable to the syndrome of pure word deafness, auditory agnosia, or central deafness in adults, and its cause is thought by some to be related to encephalitic disease processes (others disagree; see Cole et al., 1988) that involve the superior temporal lobes bilaterally. Some children with this rare condition, however, appear to have had it from birth and do not have a history of marked onset; others demonstrate a period of fairly normal vocabulary and language development before the language disorder becomes apparent but with no clear causative incident. A central symptom of this disorder is severe difficulty interpreting auditory input in the presence of relatively normal peripheral hearing and audiograms. When it appears early, children with verbal auditory agnosia learn language as if they were deaf, being almost totally unable to benefit from auditory input. Thus, they have extreme difficulty acquiring spoken language. Like some children with autism, these children may remain nonspeaking, but they can be differentiated from children with autism because of their more normal responses to gestural and facial expressions and tone of voice, their more normal eye contact, and the absence of unusual autistic behaviors, such as insistence on sameness. Academically, children with verbal auditory agnosia generally do better in math than in language-intensive course work, and they may benefit from a total communication approach to language acquisition. Because of their phonological imagery problems, they are likely to have difficulty learning to read as well as to talk.

The fourth subtype Rapin and Allen (1983) described (leaving autism for a later discussion) is **semantic-pragmatic syndrome without autism.** The phrase *without autism* is necessary because this condition demonstrates some similarity to autism. Both types of children tend to share a difficulty in the pragmatic skills of considering the prior knowledge and information needs of their audience and in comprehending language spoken to them. Rather than grasping the full intent of questions, for example, they may focus on single words or short phrases and pursue tangentially related topics of their own. Sometimes this conversational pattern involves overuse of canned phrases that give it a semantically empty "cocktail party" flavor. "Cocktail party conversation" has been described particularly for children who have a history of hydrocephalus, which may impair subcortical white matter while leaving the primary peri-Sylvian cortical language areas relatively intact. However, Rapin and Allen (1983) also describe the occurrence of this syndrome in two brothers for whom a genetically determined developmental (rather than acquired neurological) cause seemed the best explanation.

Children demonstrating semantic-pragmatic syndrome without autism, like those with autism, are sometimes echolalic (repeating phrases spoken to them in part or exactly, immediately or later), particularly in their younger years, and they may show pronoun confusions. They may also be **hyperlexic** (precocious in learning to read but often reading without comprehension). They differ from children with autism primarily in their interest and ability in making and maintaining social contacts in spite of difficulties engaging in social conversation. Because teachers do not expect to find children whose verbal expression skills exceed their verbal comprehension abilities, and because school success depends to such a great extent on language comprehension (both written and spoken), these children tend to have great difficulty succeeding in school and may develop behavioral disorders.

A different approach to subtyping children with developmental language disorders based on their oral conversations was taken by Fey (1986), who devised four categories for grouping preschool-age children based on clinical experience and a theoretical view of conversational interaction (Figure 9.3). By rating children's relative assertiveness and responsiveness, Fey described four groups: (1) **active conversationalists** are communicative children high in both assertiveness and responsiveness, although they might have relatively severe impairments of language form (comparable to Rapin and Allen's, 1983, phonologic-syntactic subgroup); (2) **passive conversationalists** are low in assertiveness but adequately responsive, rarely adding information to a topic, even though they attempt to an-

swer questions (without a clear parallel in Rapin and Allen's system, although children showing severe expressive syndrome with good comprehension might be somewhat similar); (3) **inactive communicators** are children low in both assertiveness and responsiveness (comparable to Rapin and Allen's syntactic-pragmatic subgroup); (4) **verbal noncommunicators** are children high in assertiveness but low in accommodating the needs of their conversational partners (comparable to Rapin and Allen's subgroup, semantic-pragmatic syndrome without autism).

Written Language Impairment Subtypes. When children with language disorders enter schools, new sets of concerns arise. Often, difficulty in learning to read becomes the symptom of focus. Reading-impaired children without overt language disorders and language-impaired children who also exhibit reading disorders share a set of common features (Kamhi, Catts, Mauer, Apel, & Gentry, 1988). Children in these two groups perform similarly to each other on measures of phonological, lexical, syntactical, and spatial processing and differently from normal learners, suggesting common substrata for language and reading disorders.

Attempts to classify subtypes of developmental reading disorders have been numerous (e.g., A. J. Harris, 1983; Satz & Morris, 1981). Some have been based largely on clinical experience. An early example is D. W. Johnson and Myklebust's (1967) division of children with learning disabilities into the two broad subtypes of primarily auditory-based problems (difficulty remembering and sequencing auditory symbols) and primarily visual-based problems (confusion of letters and words that look similar). Others have used sophisticated empirical and statistical analysis procedures. A. J. Harris (1983) summarized these studies as suggesting three major subtypes: (1) The most common pattern is "general deficiency in language skills (coupled with normal visual and visual-motor skills) and a lower Verbal IQ than Performance IQ" (p. 53). (2) The second pattern involves "difficulty with visual perception and visual-motor tasks, coupled with relatively normal language abilities and a Verbal IQ higher than Performance IQ" (p. 53). (3) The third pattern, which has been called an "unexpected" subtype (Satz & Morris, 1981), is observed among children "whose cognitive abilities fail to show any significant deficits that could account for the reading failure" (A. J. Harris, 1983, p. 53), but whose environmental, economic, cultural, and linguistic conditions often vary widely from the mainstream. In some "disabled reader" populations, this subtype has been observed to account for 70% of the group (Denckla, 1972). Such readers probably do not have a true disability. A. J. Harris (1983) also identified a fourth subtype: children with normal verbal comprehension and vocabulary but a deficiency in verbal fluency.

One problem with subtyping studies is that they typically use single-word reading and writing tasks. Many have not even used sentence-comprehension tasks, let alone paragraph or text-comprehension tasks (A. J. Harris, 1983). Therefore, the clinically recognized category of readers who demonstrate a pattern of good word recognition with poor comprehension may have been overlooked in early subtyping studies because of experimental design problems.

Stanovich (1985) commented on four classes of cognitive processes often suggested as causes of reading failure: (1) early visual processes, (2) phonological and naming processes, (3) the use of context to facilitate word recognition, and (4) memory and comprehension strategies. His analysis of research supported the conclusion that word-decoding based on phonological abilities (rather than visual processes) accounts for a large proportion of the variance in reading ability at all levels. Stanovich commented that less-skilled readers are not characterized by a general inability to use context to facilitate word recognition. However, problems with comprehension may result from slow and inaccurate decoding of words, which tends to make the context useless.

In a later paper, Stanovich (1988) reiterated evidence supporting the position that the core disability among children with true developmental dyslexia is a **phonological decoding deficit.** He emphasized that global processes such as "general linguistic awareness, comprehension, strategic functioning, rule learning, active/inactive learning, and generalized metacognitive functioning are the wrong places to look for the key to reading disability" (p. 157). When children do have reading disabilities tied to overall deficits, their reading problems are described better by a general developmental lag model than by a specific reading disability model. Stanovich did acknowledge evidence in support of a subgroup "who have severe problems in accessing the lexicon on a visual/orthographic basis" (p. 160), but he maintained that the size of this subgroup is extremely small when compared with the subgroup of children with phonological difficulties. Stanovich concluded that one key to fluent reading "appears to be the development of an autonomously functioning module at the word recognition level" (p. 158).

Characteristics of Specific Language Impairment. If children learning language do so because they are born with a language acquisition device (LAD) specific to the language acquisition process, they may show isolated impairments that involve only language learning and that spare developmental processes in other areas. This assumption is essential to diagnosis of specific language impairment. However, evidence that the rule-induction process for children with specific language impairments is qualitatively different from that for other children is limited. On the other hand, language group subtyping efforts suggest that individual children with specific language disabilities have different patterns of abilities within the areas of language phonology, morphology, syntax, semantics, and pragmatics. Phonology, morphology, and syntax are most frequently involved when children exhibit specific language impairments (see Box 4.4).

Current accounts of the essence of specific language impairment center on explaining the exaggerated difficulty individuals with the disorder have learning grammatical morphemes. One set of theories are based on an "underlying grammar" or "missing feature" hypothesis because they propose that certain features of the innately predisposed grammatical learning system are missing. Rice and her colleagues (Rice, 1994; Rice & Oetting, 1993; Rice & Wexler, 1996a) support this view based on their observations that children with specific language impairment have more frequent difficulty with verb inflections compared to plural inflections, suggesting that they remain in a developmental period of "extended optional infinitive" in which verbs need no inflection. Other support for this view comes from a three-generation family studied by Gopnik and Crago (1991) who experienced particular difficulty acquiring rules related to number, tense, and aspect of verbs. A competing "surface hypothesis" was described by Leonard (1994), who cited cross-linguistic data to show that children with specific language impairment have more difficulty processing and developing linguistic rules related to grammatical morphemes because of the surface characteristics of the input data. According to

Box 4.4 _____

Evidence for Different (Rather Than Merely Delayed) Language Acquisition across the Rule Systems of Language for Children with Specific Language Impairment
(Based on Leonard's (1980) Review of the Literature)

1. **Phonology.** The most common pattern is for children with language disorders to demonstrate phonological simplification patterns typical of younger children, such as stopping (*pibe* for *five*), fronting (*tootie* for *cookie*), and consonant-cluster simplification (*cool* for *school*).

   Although these patterns alone provide more evidence of delay than deviance, co-occurrence patterns differ. Phonological simplification patterns are generally noted in conjunction with one- or two-word utterances in normal development. Among children with language disorders, phonological simplification patterns occur in conjunction with a wide range of utterance lengths. Occasionally, unusual phonological patterns also appear in the speech of children with language disorders (e.g., using a bilabial nasal for liquids and glides), which clearly differ from any observed in normal development.

2. **Semantics.** Children with language disorders are slow to acquire their first words, acquire additional words more slowly than their peers, and occasionally make lexical errors that are similar to the types seen in younger normally developing children. These characteristics seem to be more typical of delay than they are of qualitative differences of developmental patterns.

3. **Syntax.** Again, most syntactic differences observed between the language of children with language disorders and their same-age peers have been quantitative rather than qualitative. When children are matched on the basis of mean length of utterance (MLU) (rather than age), the differences are further minimized. Both groups follow similar developmental orders in acquiring more complex structures, such as questions (although children with language disorders have been observed to use fewer questions even after they can form them). What appears to differentiate the groups best is the co-occurrence of later-developing and earlier-developing forms in children with specific language disorders. Children with language disorders have also been observed to be delayed in their ability to paraphrase through syntactic rearrangement (Leonard, 1980, categorized this as a pragmatic skill).

4. **Pragmatics.** Studies in which children are matched for chronological age also have tended to provide more evidence of delay than difference; i.e., children with language disorders often act more like younger children without disorders. When children are matched for MLU at the one-word level, children with language disorders tend to use more nonlinguistic means to communicate about shifting contextual elements. Children with longer utterance lengths have not always shown this difference, but they do seem to have fewer options for revising their utterances and tailoring them to listener needs. Much of the literature on differences in the pragmatic skills of school-age children with language disorders came after Leonard's 1980 article. Two of the primary differences noted by Donahue, Pearl, and Bryan (1983) for adolescents with learning disabilities were their difficulties in (1) adapting form and content to varied listeners and situations and (2) understanding the rules for participating in cooperative conversational turn taking.

this hypothesis, children have difficulty learning how to use grammatical morphemes, which are transient, unstressed, and difficult to perceive, because of processing capacity limitations but an otherwise intact language-learning mechanism.

Information Processing Factors.   Although it is an area of controversy, aspects of information processing also have been implicated to explain specific language impairment. Auditory processing of rapid acoustic events has been shown repeatedly to be more difficult for children with specific language disability than for their normal language-learning peers (Tallal & Piercy, 1973, 1975; Tallal, Stark, Kallman, & Mellits, 1981; Tallal et al., 1996). As Tallal and colleagues demonstrated in a series of studies, children with specific language disability often can perceive features of nonlinguistic acoustic signals adequately when they occur in isolation or in slowly presented sequence but not when they occur in the rapid sequences more characteristic of the acoustic patterns of speech.

No one doubts that problems of short-term auditory sequential memory (particularly for rapidly produced stimuli) are associated with developmental language disorders. The controversy is over whether they are causally related. Some (e.g., Rees, 1973, 1981) state that these symptoms may represent a result of disordered language ability, or a concomitant feature, rather than its cause. Whether auditory processing should be targeted directly in language intervention plans is also a matter of controversy discussed in Chapter 3.

Cognitive Factors.   Some children with specific language impairment demonstrate symbolic deficits in nonlinguistic as well as linguistic areas. Leonard (1987), in reviewing this research, noted the implication "that specific language impairment may not be specific at all" (p. 23). From his summary of the research in symbolic play and mental imagery (often involving mental manipulations of geometric form), Leonard concluded that although some of these children "clearly fall below the performance level of same-age peers on symbolic play and imagery tasks, they appear to perform above the level of younger normal children with comparable language abilities" (p. 29).

Johnston (1991, 1994) also summarized data that suggest that specific language impairment is not all that specific. She noted that "the developmental relationships between cognition and language make it unlikely that a child could be seriously delayed in language acquisition and otherwise normal in intellect" (1994, p. 118).

Social Interaction and Self-Concept Factors.   Fujiki and Brinton (1994) noted that "the social functioning of children with SLI has typically been neglected in both research and clinical practice" (p. 123). Definitions of social competence generally comprise a variety of factors, including appropriateness and amount of social interaction, demonstration of specific behaviors, and judgments of proficiency by self and others. Children with language impairments have risks for difficulty across these areas.

Judgments of self-proficiency seem to grow in importance as children advance into the school-age years. Children must be willing to expend voluntary effort and to risk failure to participate actively in formalized language acquisition activities in school. In attempting to understand the necessary conditions for such motivation, Weiner (1979, 1980) proposed an attribution theory of achievement motivation. The theory suggests that as people experience relative success or failure in life, they search for causes to explain why their efforts are successful or unsuccessful. Four primary causes to which people may attribute their success (or lack thereof) are ability, effort, luck, and task difficulty. The nature of these causes varies in ways that determine subsequent affect, expectancies, and efforts of human beings in the long-term process of development. As Winograd and Niquette (1988) explained it:

> If individuals attribute their failures at some task to bad luck, which is usually classified as an external and unstable factor, then they may not expect to fail in the future. In contrast, if individuals attribute their failures to low ability, which is usually (but not always) classified as an internal and stable factor, then it is more likely that they will expect to fail in the future, and their consequent behavior (i.e., resignation, negative affect, passivity) will facilitate the realization of this dismal expectation. Subsequent failure will reinforce this attributional pattern, precipitating a cycle of failure, frustration and defeat. (p. 39)

Winograd and Niquette (1988) called on theories of self-concept to understand the **learned helplessness** they observed among children who have difficulty acquiring later-language skills (especially literacy) in school. Although such factors are unlikely candidates as original causes of specific language impairment and learning disability, they contribute to children's development over time, especially in later childhood and adolescence, and they should not be ignored.

Mental Retardation

Diagnosing Mental Retardation.   The definition of mental retardation provided by the American Association on Mental Deficiency (AAMD) has three critical elements. To be considered mentally retarded, a person must demonstrate (1) significantly subaverage general intellectual functioning, (2) concurrent deficits in adaptive behavior, and (3) manifestation of the problem during the developmental period (Grossman, 1983).

The determination of significantly subaverage general intellectual functioning is based on an IQ score of 70 or below (sometimes extended to 75 in educational settings) from an individually administered intelligence test. The phrase **deficits in adaptive behavior** refers to significant lags in general maturation or major limitations in academic learning, personal independence, and social responsibility. In earlier definitions of mental retardation, **developmental period** was defined as birth to 18 years, but in the current version, it extends to conception. The DSM-IV (American Psychiatric Association, 1994) specifies "the onset must occur before age 18 years" (p. 39).

The inclusion of adaptive behavior as a critical feature in the definition and diagnosis of mental retardation is a relatively recent phenomenon. Its inclusion is important for two reasons. First, IQ alone cannot perfectly predict general adaptation. Individuals with identical IQs may function very differently in society (Baroff, 1986). Second, IQ tests are biased against individuals from sociocultural communities differing from those of standardization samples (Mercer, 1973). When individuals demonstrate documented limitations of adaptive behavior within their own sociocultural developmental contexts, professionals may be less likely to diagnose them wrongly as mentally retarded than when IQ scores are used alone (Mercer & Lewis, 1975).

How do psychologists and social workers measure adaptive behavior, and what role might language specialists play? Because adaptive behavior expectations differ with chronological age, settings, and cultural groups, measurement is not easy. During infancy and early childhood, identification of adaptive behavior rests on general maturation and the acquisition of basic sensory and motor skills, language, self-help skills, and socialization. During childhood and early adolescence, cognitive and socialization functions replace general maturation as the primary determinants of adaptive behavior. They are measured as school learning, appropriateness of social judgment, and relationships established with peers and adults out of school as well as in. In the period of late adolescence and adulthood, adaptive behavior is represented by increasing independence and by the ability to assume varied social roles, for example, as employee, friend, spouse, and parent. Adaptation during this period also includes conforming to community expectations and participating as a citizen (Baroff, 1986). Speech–language pathologists and other language specialists may play key roles in identifying the maturation of speech and language skills and communication functions during each of these developmental periods.

Subtypes of Mental Retardation.   Four levels of retardation—mild, moderate, severe, and profound—are recognized by the AAMD (Grossman, 1983) and by the American Psychiatric Association (1994) in DSM-IV. They are based on the number of standard deviations below the mean on IQ tests (see Table 4.1). The characteristics of mental retardation associated with each of these levels may vary widely among individuals and with time of life (Chinn, Drew, & Logan, 1975).

Mild mental retardation is associated with delayed development of social and communication skills in the preschool years and with minimal retardation in sensorimotor areas, but the child with mild retardation may not be distinguished from normally developing children before starting school. Children with mild mental retardation acquire academic skills to approximately the sixth-grade level by their late teens but have difficulty learning high school subjects. They need special education, particularly at secondary school levels, and are often labeled **educable mentally retarded** (or **handicapped** or **impaired**), based on state guidelines. As adults, individuals with mild retardation are often capable of social and vocational independence but may need supervision under serious social or economic stress (Chinn et al., 1975).

Moderate mental retardation is associated with delays in learning to talk and communicate (but even-

TABLE 4.1 Levels of retardation, corresponding psychometric criteria, and proportions at that level within the population of all retarded persons as identified by the President's Committee on Mental Retardation (1978)

LEVEL OF RETARDATION	RANGE BASED ON STANDARD DEVIATION	RANGE BASED ON WECHSLER SCALE IQ	APPROXIMATE PERCENTAGE OF ALL RETARDED PERSONS
Mild	−2 to −3	55–69	89.0
Moderate	−3 to −4	40–54	6.0
Severe	−4 to −5	25–39	3.5
Profound	−5 to −6	0–24	1.5

tual ability to do so), with poor social awareness, and with fair motor development in the preschool years. Children with moderate mental retardation typically develop academic skills to approximately the fourth-grade level by their teen years, with special education. In school systems, they are included in the group labeled **educable mentally retarded** (or **handicapped** or **impaired**). As adults, individuals with moderate retardation may be able to work independently at unskilled or semiskilled occupations but often need supervision and guidance under conditions of even mild social or economic stress (Chinn et al., 1975).

Severe mental retardation is associated with poor motor development, minimal speech development, severely limited communication skills, and difficulty acquiring self-help abilities in the preschool years. During the school-age years, these individuals typically cannot learn functional academic skills, but they may learn to talk or to communicate in other ways, may learn elemental health habits, and generally profit from systematic training efforts. Hence, this subgroup is often called **trainable mentally retarded.** As adults, they may be able to contribute partially to self-support under complete supervision. They can also develop self-protection skills to a minimal useful level in a controlled environment (Chinn et al., 1975). Chapter 13 addresses the severe communication impairments often demonstrated by persons with severe and profound mental retardation.

Profound mental retardation is associated with minimal capacity for functioning in any sensorimotor or communication areas during the preschool years, with continued complete dependence on adults for care. During the school-age years, some motor development may occur, but such individuals continue to need total care and generally do not benefit from training in self-help

skills. As adults, some further motor, speech, and communication development may occur, but individuals with profound retardation are incapable of self-maintenance, and they continue to need complete care and supervision (Chinn et al., 1975).

Questions about the Nature of Intelligence. Theories of intelligence guide the understanding of the cognitive deficits of children, but they raise as many questions as they answer. Is intelligence a relatively unitary phenomenon, as Spearman (1923, 1927) suggested when he described the **g** factor as an index of general ability? Can intelligence be differentiated into **crystallized** (e.g., the capacity to answer questions based on word meanings, general knowledge, and language comprehension) and **fluid** abilities (e.g., the capacity to reason in nonverbal and visual-spatial contexts), as Cattell (1971) and Horn (1968) suggested? Is intelligence multifactorial in nature, as Guilford (1967) suggested? Is it best represented as a set of gradually unfolding processes for making sense of the world, as Piaget (1970) suggested? Is it a set of information processing abilities, as Sternberg suggested (1979, 1981)? Or are there multiple, relatively autonomous intelligences, as Gardner (1983) suggested?

Perhaps intelligence is all of these. Any might be shown to be affected in mental retardation (Baroff, 1986). As Sternberg (1981) noted, intelligence has traditionally been described as having the three cognitive components: (1) the ability to learn and to profit from experience and to acquire knowledge in doing so, (2) the ability to reason, and (3) the ability to adapt to changing conditions. Sternberg (1981) also posited a fourth motivational component—the will to succeed. Motivation is related to social interaction factors and communication as well as to intelligence.

Information processing theories have been posited to explain why individuals vary in basic cognitive abilities. The term *slowness,* which is often used to describe the development of persons with mental retardation, seems to literally characterize their processing abilities (Sternberg, 1979, 1981).

Persons with mental retardation have significant deficiencies in all information processing areas, including problems with planning, encoding, rapid processing, association, retention, and generalization (Baroff, 1986). Furthermore, problems in each of these areas might be expected to affect language and communication development as well as general cognitive development.

Language Characteristics Associated with Mental Retardation. Mental retardation is generally described as involving uniform developmental lags across multiple skill areas (only the degree of lag differentiates subgroups), but the group of individuals with mental retardation, even those functioning at the same level, is far more heterogeneous than homogeneous. Anyone who has worked with individuals with mental retardation knows that they are just that—*individuals.*

The Language and Cognitive Skills of Mental Retardation. Some question whether the development of individuals with mental retardation, both cognitive and linguistic, is different or delayed (see Box 4.5).

The evidence for differences in cognitive development, including attention, discrimination, organization of input memory, and transfer (or generalization) was reviewed by Owens (1989). He concluded that "In general, the mentally retarded population develops cognitively in a manner very similar to the nonretarded but at a slower rate" (p. 243). Kamhi (1981) matched retarded and nonretarded individuals for mental age. The groups performed similarly on most tasks, including haptic (touch) recognition, conservation, classification, number conservation, and linear order. Although the retarded children in the study performed slightly more poorly on tasks involving symbolic skills, they actually performed significantly better than their nonretarded mental-age-matched peers on the task involving matching ("mental displacement"). This suggests exaggerated difficulty with symbolic learning.

It is difficult to sort out the evidence for difference versus delay of language development associated with mental retardation because many variables can influence outcomes. As Owens (1989) pointed out, early

studies used research designs in which individuals were matched for chronological age. Of course, the results of such studies highlighted the differences in levels of development. More recently, studies have matched subjects on the basis of mental age or language ability, and, as the information summarized in Box 4.5 indicates, more similarities have been found.

Language Subtypes and Mental Retardation. One distinction often made clinically is whether the person with mental retardation is speaking or nonspeaking. Perceptions of subdivisions relating to whether a person is **nonspeaking** (sometimes called **nonvocal** or **nonverbal**) have evolved over recent years. Whereas in the past, the determination of the potential to talk would have been made before deciding that the individual was a candidate for alternative or augmentative communication (AAC), it is now recognized that AAC strategies and supportive technology (both low-tech and high-tech systems) may be useful at multiple stages and in multiple contexts during the developmental process. No longer does their selection imply that anyone has "given up" on speech development (although parents may still perceive the decision this way).

Another subdivision is based on whether a person with mental retardation is capable of symbolic or nonsymbolic communicative functioning (Siegel-Causey & Guess, 1989). To use language, a person must be able to understand that symbols such as words can be used to represent things and concepts. As noted previously, this skill may be particularly at risk among people with mental retardation. Some persons with mental retardation may never develop symbolic communication, but even "children and youth with the most handicapping conditions do indeed communicate; however, this communication is achieved in a variety of ways that are not readily observed or even acknowledged by many attending adults" (Guess, 1989, p. xi). As discussed in Chapter 13, nonsymbolic modes of communication include such behaviors as facial expressions, gestures, movements, postures, and touch.

At the other end of the continuum, some individuals with mild and moderate levels of retardation may learn to read and write. Again, not much evidence supports the existence of particular patterns of reading and writing disability among mentally retarded children. Yet, the efforts of these children to read and write do not necessarily mirror those of younger normally developing peers, nor are they necessarily commensurate with their oral

Box 4.5 _____

Evidence for Different (Rather Than Merely Delayed) Language Acquisition across the Rule Systems of Language for Children with Mental Retardation (Summarized from Literature Review by Owens, 1989)

1. **Phonology.** A higher incidence of articulation disorders is found. Children with retardation demonstrate the application of phonologic simplification processes similar to those used by younger normally developing children, such as reduplication (e.g., /baba/ for *bottle*) and assimilation (e.g., /dɔd/ or /gɔg/ for *dog*).

2. **Morphology.** The same order of development of inflectional morphology has been observed for retarded and nonretarded children. Although no studies are available, one might wonder whether children with mental retardation might have greater difficulty using rules of derivational morphology (e.g., prefixes such as *un-, de-,* and *re-* and suffixes such as *-ly, -tion,* and *-able*) to generate and comprehend derived word forms for which they know the roots.

3. **Syntax.** The order of development of sentence types is similar for retarded and nonretarded children, with a trend to start with simple declaratives, move through negatives, then interrogatives (in the order *what, where, when, why, how*), and later, negative interrogatives. Some differences also appear, however, in that children with mental retardation tend to use shorter, less complex sentences than those used by nonretarded peers matched for mental age. In particular, fewer complex structures such as subject elaborations and relative clauses appear. It has also been suggested that retarded persons have less flexible syntactic structure because they tend to rely on sentence word order (rather than grammatical rules for combining word classes) to formulate and understand sentences. They also tend to rely longer on more primitive syntactic forms.

4. **Semantics.** Word meanings tend to be more concrete and restricted for individuals with mental retardation, who have particular difficulty with nonliteral meanings. Retarded persons also use adjectives and adverbs less frequently than mental age-matched peers do.

5. **Pragmatics.** The pragmatic skills of children with mental retardation vary with their cognitive levels and life experiences (those who reside in institutions show the greatest deficits of communicative use). In the early stages of development, both mentally retarded and normally developing children use imperative and declarative gestures to communicate (imperative gestures enlist help and declarative gestures gain attention). Children with mental retardation, however, use more sophisticated gestures for imperative than for declarative functions. Some pragmatic skills, such as role taking, appear to be more related to social maturity than to cognitive maturity in both mentally retarded and normally developing children. Finally, although persons with mild-to-moderate mental retardation may be as skilled as their mental-age-matched peers at taking the perspective of conversational partners, they are less likely to assume assertive roles in conversation, and this pattern continues to be true of adults with mental retardation of multiple levels, even when speaking to children.

_____

language abilities. Children with mental retardation may also have difficulty learning to read and write because they are given limited educational opportunities. Chapter 13 includes some examples of what might be possible.

Anecdotal accounts describe issues related to helping individuals with Down syndrome acquire written language skills. For many, decoding seems to come more easily than comprehension. For example, Feuerstein, Rand, and Rynders (1988) presented descriptions of a series of children with Down syndrome provided by their parents. Jason was a 13½-year-old boy with Down syndrome whom his mother described as follows:

> In reading, Jason's decoding has always been extraordinarily good—but his comprehension of what he has read still gives him quite a bit of difficulty. He loves playing complicated word games, spelling words backwards, doing crossword puzzles, and performing scenes he has learned from musical shows. But his ability to answer "content questions" has been quite limited. (pp. 125–126)

Tami was a 10-year-old fourth-grade student with Down syndrome, whom her father described:

> Reading is her worst skill. She has great difficulty in reading a story, and telling us the main idea or episode. She often concentrates on a specific incident which may or may not be essential to the story. On the other hand, given a specific question, she can read several pages to find the answer.
>
> Her writing skills also are poor. She writes (and reads) cursive script, but the letters are still not well formed and not neatly arranged. She has much trouble with creative writing, where she is to make something up. (p. 124)

Behaviorism and Mental Retardation.   Children with mental retardation are thought to benefit less from natural environmental stimulation and reinforcement in the acquisition of language than their normally developing peers. Even in the absence of peripheral sensorimotor impairments, children with mental retardation seem to have difficulty recognizing subtle environmental cues. They need more repetitions of experience before they can internalize concepts. Therefore, behavioral approaches are often recommended for retarded children. They are designed to simplify and highlight discriminative properties of stimuli and to provide tangible reinforcers for targeted behaviors. Structured programs of reward, punishment, and ignoring are also used frequently to modify behaviors of individuals with severe and profound mental retardation (Baroff, 1986). Inability to generalize is a major problem for persons with retardation. Therefore, more recent behavior modification approaches tend to emphasize the use of natural contexts and consequences for facilitating the integration and retention of newly acquired behaviors.

Social Interaction and Self-Concept Factors.   Self-esteem can also influence the development of individuals with mental retardation. Baroff (1986) noted that self-esteem results from the contributions of three factors (1) personal intimacy, (2) success, and (3) autonomy. The dependence of people with mental retardation has been well documented, but this does not mean that it is safe to conclude that they are dependent by choice. All such factors seem to interact with their ability to learn, including their ability to learn to communicate (see Personal Reflection 4.3).

Autism and Other Pervasive Developmental Disorders

Diagnosing Autism and Other Pervasive Developmental Disorders.   A variety of definitions have been offered since Kanner first described the syndrome of autism in 1943. Kanner listed the characteristic features as (1) extreme autistic aloneness, (2) language abnormalities, (3) obsessive desire for the maintenance of sameness, (4) good cognitive potential, and (5) normal physical development. Kanner also described the children as having highly intelligent, obsessive, and cold parents but this description is no longer accepted.

The definition proposed by the Autism Society of America (see Ritvo & Freeman, 1978) includes the following characteristics:

1. Age of onset before 30 months.
2. Disturbances of developmental rates and sequences in the areas of motor, social-adaptive, and cognitive skills.
3. Disturbances of responses to sensory stimuli. This includes hyper- or hyporeactivity in audition, vision, touch, motor, smell, and taste. Self-stimulatory behavior is also included.
4. Disturbances of speech, language, cognition, and nonverbal communication, including mutism, echolalia, and failure to use abstract terms.

5. Disturbances of the capacity to appropriately relate to people, events, and objects, including lack of social behavior, affection, and appropriate play. Interruption of the idiosyncratic or perseverative use of objects will upset the child.

The definition of autism proposed by the American Psychiatric Association (1994) in the DSM-IV places it as a subdivision of the more general diagnostic classification **pervasive developmental disorder.** In some service-delivery systems, this label may be preferred for children with autism. Many parents, however, have worked hard to have autism treated as a separate disorder in state and federal regulations and to have it removed from status as an emotional disorder or even as a physical or health impairment. They may prefer to have autism and other "autism spectrum disorders" maintained as a distinctive category. The group of pervasive development (or autism spectrum) disorders is considered in the subsequent section on subtypes.

In the past, the labels **childhood psychosis** and **childhood schizophrenia** were sometimes used interchangeably with **autism** (sometimes called **early infantile autism**). Those conditions are now thought to be distinct. In DSM-IV, **childhood schizophrenia** is no longer a diagnostic category, although the onset of schizophrenia can occur in childhood. Autism has been contrasted with childhood onset schizophrenia by autism's early onset (before 3 years of age), less common family history of mental illness, normal or above average motor development, lower IQ, good physical health, no periods of remission and relapse, failure to develop complex language and social skills, and absence of delusions or hallucinations (all of which may appear differently in childhood schizophrenia) (Schreibman, 1988).

The DSM-IV criteria for diagnosing autism appear in Box 4.6. Diagnosis depends on identification of qualitative impairments in three areas: (1) social interaction (including nonverbal communication and play), (2) communication (including speech, language, and pragmatic communication variables), and (3) behaviors, interests, and activities (including stereotypic and repetitive sensory-motor patterns and preoccupations). As might be expected, language and communication specialists play an important role in the transdisciplinary diagnosis of the disorder.

Hypothesized Causes of Autism.   Theories of the cause of autism have changed dramatically over the years since Kanner (1943) attributed it to the lack of interaction with cold and unresponsive parents and Bruno Bettelheim (1967) wrote the book called *The Empty Fortress,* also blaming parents. Although many possibilities for explaining the social, cognitive, and linguistic, symptoms of autism have been explored, the exact mechanism by which it operates is still not understood. Current reviews, however, suggest that "the overwhelming evidence indicates that autism is a neurological rather than a psychogenic disability" (Schopler & Mesibov, 1986, p. 4).

Numerous attempts have been made to identify particular biological factors at work in autism. Factors investigated have included pregnancy and birth, genetics, neurology, and biochemistry. Some positive evidence of biological differences among children with autism has been found in all of these categories (Schreibman, 1988).

For example, prenatal histories of children with autism show an increased incidence of early complications but no particularly uniform patterns of influence. Family histories show increased incidence of speech delay (in approximately 25% of one sample) and of close family members with autism (between 2% and 6% have siblings with autism). Some evidence has also been found that autism is associated with "fragile-X" syndrome (in which a weakness or "break" appears in the structure of the X sex chromosome) (Schreibman, 1988).

Investigations of neurochemical factors have focused on neurotransmitters. Unusually high levels of serotonin (a neurotransmitter) have been found in the blood of children with autism at an age when it has begun to diminish in their normally developing peers. Another neurochemical possibility is that children with autism have an abundance of opioid peptides (brain chemicals generated naturally in normal development with the pleasure rush that comes from being cuddled and comforted). It is hypothesized that the preexistence of these chemicals in the brains of children with autism may make them less prone to seek affection and comfort. Treatment with an opioid-blocking agent has been shown to reduce such abnormal behaviors as self-stimulation, echolalia, and a tendency to shut out stimulation by covering eyes and ears (Schreibman, 1988).

Neurological pathology is often inferred from the appearance of such neurological "soft signs" as hypotonia (low muscle tone), poor coordination, and toe

Box 4.6 _____

Diagnostic Criteria for Autistic Disorders in DSM-IV™

A. A total of six (or more) items from (1), (2), and (3), with at least two from (1), and one each from (2) and (3):

  (1) qualitative impairment in social interaction, as manifested by at least two of the following:

    (a) marked impairment in the use of multiple nonverbal behaviors such as eye-to-eye gaze, facial expression, body postures, and gestures to regulate social interaction

    (b) failure to develop peer relationships appropriate to developmental level

    (c) a lack of spontaneous seeking to share enjoyment, interests, or achievements with other people (e.g., by a lack of showing, bringing, or pointing out objects of interest)

    (d) lack of social or emotional reciprocity

  (2) qualitative impairments in communication as manifested by at least one of the following:

    (a) delay in, or total lack of, the development of spoken language (not accompanied by an attempt to compensate through alternative modes of communication such as gesture or mime)

    (b) in individuals with adequate speech, marked impairment in the ability to initiate or sustain a conversation with others

    (c) stereotyped and repetitive use of language or idiosyncratic language

    (d) lack of varied, spontaneous make-believe play or social imitative play appropriate to developmental level

  (3) restricted repetitive and stereotyped patterns of behavior, interests, and activities, as manifested by at least one of the following:

    (a) encompassing preoccupation with one or more stereotyped and restricted patterns of interest that is abnormal either in intensity or focus

    (b) apparently inflexible adherence to specific, nonfunctional routines or rituals

    (c) stereotyped and repetitive motor mannerisms (e.g., hand or finger flapping or twisting, or complex whole-body movements)

    (d) persistent preoccupation with parts of objects

B. Delays or abnormal functioning in at least one of the following areas, with onset prior to age 3 years: (1) social interaction, (2) language as used in social communication, or (3) symbolic or imaginary play.

C. The disturbance is not better accounted for by Rett's Disorder or Childhood Disintegrative Disorder.

Note. From American Psychiatric Association: *Diagnostic and Statistical Manual of Mental Disorders (4th ed) DSM IV* (pp. 70–71). Washington, DC: American Psychiatric Association, 1994. Reprinted by permission.

---

walking. Such symptoms are reported in 40% to 100% of children with autism. Abnormal patterns of brain activity have also been identified in 65% of children with autism (as compared with only 39% of children with mental retardation) (DeMyer, 1975).

Structural abnormalities have been sought in the brains of individuals with autism but, for the most part, with limited success. However, Courchesne (1988) used magnetic resonance imaging (MRI) to examine the brains of persons with autism and found an area of the cerebellum that was significantly smaller than expected. This area of investigation may not be significant for all individuals with autism, but the evidence suggests that for some, abnormal brain development may have occurred at the end of the first trimester or during the second trimester. For others, abnormality may begin in the first or second year of life. Although the mechanism for cerebellar involvement is not fully understood, the cerebellum regulates incoming sensations, and its cellular irregularities may account for the sensory deficits so characteristic of autism, including insensitivity to pain or oversensitivity to sounds and textures (Schreibman, 1988). Rapin and Allen (1983) pointed out that the pattern of strengths and deficits of children with autism leads to suspicion of "multifocal brain dysfunction rather than the impairment of a single system, even one with widespread projections" (p. 174).

Subtypes of Autism and Other Pervasive Developmental Disorders.   The broader category is pervasive developmental disorder (PDD). In DSM-IV, the American Psychiatric Association (1994) includes five subtypes in this category: (1) autistic disorder, (2) Rett's disorder, (3) childhood disintegrative disorder, (4) Asperger's disorder, and (5) pervasive developmental disorder not otherwise specified (including atypical autism).

Subtypes of Autism.   Although autism is recognized as a disorder with a great deal of heterogeneity, subtype categories have not been clearly differentiated. One suggestion was that, for the purpose of research, the population of individuals with autism might be categorized into three main groups: (1) individuals with the classic symptoms of Kanner's (1943) syndrome, (2) those who have childhood schizophrenia with autistic features, and (3) those who have autism with neurological impairment (Coleman, 1976).

A more recent broadly accepted clinical and educational subdivision is based on the accompanying degree of cognitive impairment shown by individuals with autism. Approximately 60% of children with autism have measured IQs below 50; 20% have IQs between 50 and 70; and 20% have IQs of 70 or above (Schreibman, 1988). These subtypes combine the critical diagnostic features of autism with features of the accompanying level of retardation. The labels **low, middle,** and **high functioning** are often used in conjunction with these subdivisions.

The subclassifications described by Rapin and Allen (1983) for autism, mentioned earlier in this chapter, differentiate between autistic children on the basis of whether they are primarily **echolalic** or **mute.** Autistic children who are mute generally have a poorer overall prognosis (including for the development of language) than do children who are echolalic (DeMyer et al., 1973). Children with autism and echolalia often have variable **phonology** (more likely than not to be defective); faulty **prosody** resulting in wooden, nonmusical, robot-like speech; variable **morphology** (with particular difficulty developing normal pronoun reference); variable **word retrieval** (with particular difficulty in the absence of visual referents); variable **nonverbal intelligence;** impaired comprehension and semantic processing of **connected discourse** (as seen both in the echolalia and hyperlexia that tends to be evident in those with higher levels of measured intelligence); and impaired **pragmatic skills** (with limited ability to initiate and to participate in conversational discourse even after they become verbal).

Other PDD Subtypes.   Autism is only one of five types of pervasive developmental disorder recognized by the American Psychiatric Association (1994) in DSM-IV. The others are described subsequently.

Rett's disorder is diagnosed when a deceleration of head growth occurs between 5 and 48 months after apparently normal prenatal and perinatal development, psychomotor development, and head circumference for the first 5 months of life. It is associated with "severely impaired expressive and receptive language development with severe psychomotor retardation" (American Psychiatric Association, 1994, p. 73). When symptoms begin to appear, the infant or toddler shows poorly coordinated gait and trunk movements and loses previously acquired purposeful hand skills. They are replaced by stereotypic hand movements, such as hand wringing or hand washing. Social engagement skills are also lost, although social interaction abilities often develop later.

Childhood disintegrative disorder is diagnosed when children begin to show signs of PDD following apparently normal development for at least the first 2 years after birth. Criteria include: "Clinically significant loss of previously acquired skills (before age 10 years) in at least two of the following areas: (1) expressive or receptive language, (2) social skills or adaptive behavior, (3) bowel or bladder control, (4) play, (5) motor skills" (American Psychiatric Association, 1994, p. 75). In addition, children with the condition show qualitative impairments in at least two of the three areas associated with autism: (1) social interaction, (2) communication, and (3) behaviors, interests, and activities. This disorder is diagnosed when "The disturbance is not better accounted for by another specific Pervasive Developmental Disorder or by Schizophrenia" (p. 75).

Asperger's disorder is essentially what used to be called **high functioning autism.** The two key differences between Asperger's disorder and autistic disorder are in the areas of language and cognitive development. In the area of language, "There is no clinically significant general delay in language (e.g., single words used by age 2 years, communicative phrases used by age 3 years)" (p. 77). Likewise, in the area of cognition, "There is no clinically significant delay in cognitive development or in the development of age-appropriate self-help skills, adaptive behavior (other than in social interaction), and curiosity about the environment in childhood" (American Psychiatric Association, 1994, p. 77). Asperger's Disorder is similar to autism in two other key characteristics: (1) "qualitative impairment in social interaction," and (2) "restricted repetitive and stereotyped patterns of behavior, interests, and activities" (p. 77).

Pervasive developmental disorder not otherwise specified (PDD-NOS) is diagnosed when "there is a severe and pervasive impairment in the development of reciprocal social interaction or verbal and nonverbal communication skills, or when stereotyped behavior, interests, and activities are present, but the criteria are not met for a specific Pervasive Developmental Disorder, Schizophrenia, Schizotypal Personality Disorder, or Avoidant Personality Disorder" (American Psychiatric Association, 1994, p. 78). PDD-NOS includes "atypical autism," in which diagnostic criteria are not met due to late age of onset, or atypical or subthreshold symptomatology.

Language Characteristics Associated with Autism and Other Pervasive Developmental Disorders.   There is not much debate that children with autism develop in ways that are not only delayed but qualitatively different compared with normally developing children. Qualitative differences in social interaction and communication are central to the diagnosis of autism in the DSM-IV criteria (see Box 4.7 for an additional summary of language development characteristics). A question remains, how-

ever, whether children with autism follow patterns of language development similar to those of normally developing children. Swisher and Demetras (1985) reviewed the evidence. In the area of **syntax,** when children with autism are matched for nonverbal mental age with children who are mentally retarded, have specific language impairments, or are normally developing, the language-form abilities of children with autism are consistently lower than those of normally developing children but as advanced as those of children with mental retardation or specific language impairment. Swisher and Demetras (1985) interpreted these results as evidence that children with autism construct sentences with superficial form, not fully supported by an understanding of their deep structure or generative principles. Studies of **morphology** also show that children with autism have skills that are delayed relative to normally developing controls; however, not relative to children with mental retardation or specific language impairment, matched on nonverbal IQ measures (Swisher & Demetras, 1985).

In the area of **semantics,** surprisingly little research evidence is available to support the common contention that children with autism have difficulty using meaningful speech. Studies of word and sentence recall have shown children with autism to be impaired in their ability to use semantic cues to aid recall, but in the absence of further evidence, Swisher and Demetras (1985) suggested that the semantic problems of children with autism might be viewed as evidence of language delay rather than difference. They also suggested, however, that "It appears that autistic children can remember words better than they can connect them to a cognitive base" (p. 159).

In the area of **pragmatics,** evidence indicates that children with autism use language in ways that are not only delayed with respect to normally developing peers but also deviant. In particular, they tend to have difficulty in making appropriate matches between the content and form of the language they use and the contexts in which it is produced (Swisher & Demetras, 1985). This mismatch across domains of language (in the presence of patterns of delay within domains), Swisher and Demetras concluded, best characterizes the uniqueness of language development among children with autism.

Prizant (1983) also addressed the question of uniqueness. He reviewed modes of **gestalt** (holistic) versus **analytic** processing with reference to the communicative symptoms of autism. The literature shows that

Box 4.7 _____

Summary of Characteristics of the Development of Language, Speech, and Communication by Children with Autism

(Based on Reviews by Fay & Schuler, 1980; Schopler & Mesibov, 1985; Schreibman, 1988)

1. Failure to acquire language may be the first signal to parents that something is wrong.
2. Some may initially acquire such words as *mama* and *dada* but then suddenly (between 18 and 30 months) lose the acquired words and fail to progress further linguistically.
3. Approximately 50% never develop functional speech.
4. Those who speak use language qualitatively different from normally developing children and other children with language disorders, as demonstrated by the following:
   a. Echolalia, which may be produced beyond the period when it might appear normally. Echolalia may serve a variety of functions for individuals with autism, and it may be immediate or delayed (based on timing); communicative or noncommunicative (based on its apparent pragmatic function); or exact or mitigated (based on whether it is altered in any way to be more contextually appropriate). Echolalia may appear in the communicative development of other children with language disorders, particularly those with mental retardation.
   b. Pronominal reversals, with the child often referring to self with the pronouns, *you, he/she,* or the child's proper name.
   c. Noncommunicative and self-stimulatory speech, using the same sounds, words, or phrases repeatedly but without apparent attempts to communicate. (However, as professionals look more carefully at behaviors previously thought to be noncommunicative, their possible communicative value may become more apparent.)
   d. Dysprosodic, as characterized by unusual or inappropriate pitch, rhythm, inflection, intonation, pace, and/or articulation.
   e. Confusion of form, function, and context, as, for example, when a child with autism uses question

forms to express desires (e.g., "Do you want to go outside?") or make declarative statements (e.g., "Is Joe scared of lightning?").
   f. Impaired ability to produce and understand non-linguistic communicative behaviors, such as those involving eye gaze, gestures, proximity, and body contact.
5. Some higher functioning and older children with autism demonstrate language problems more similar to those of some other children with language disorders or to normally developing children at earlier stages.
   a. They are likely to have severe impairments of comprehension.
   b. They tend to form rigid semantic concepts and have particular difficulty with abstract words and concepts, including expressing their own emotions or imagination.
   c. They produce and comprehend language with almost total literalness, and they have particular difficulty understanding idioms, analogies, and metaphors (even though their own language may be characterized as metaphoric at times, in that phrases may bear only an indirect relationship to the things and ideas they represent).
   d. They may have great difficulty talking about anything outside of the immediate environment or events, having difficulty discussing past or future, and appearing stuck in the here-and-now.
6. They may be hyperlexic (reading early, but with limited comprehension).
7. Their writing may show evidence of free association of thought, with individual words appearing to have some connections based on the child's own experiences but with lack of semantic, syntactic, or thematic connectedness.

---

normally developing children are distributed on a continuum, with most children either being analytic or showing both analytic and gestalt characteristics (Peters, 1977). The analytic mode of processing is evident when single words serve as basic language units that can be combined as grammatical constituents using linguistic rules, when early language acquisition involves movement from two-to three-word phrases, and when growth in language production is flexible, creative, and generative. The gestalt mode of processing is evident when multiword utterances appear early and function as single units, when a child's syntactic development appears more sophisticated than it actually is, and when growth in language development involves segmentation and recombinations of unanalyzed chunks, with eventual movement into an analytic mode.

Prizant (1983) suggested that children with autism might function in two different modes during varied points in their development. For some, earlier language development demonstrates a high frequency of echolalia. As this pattern is gradually replaced by more spontaneous, analytic language, children produce some utterances in a gestalt mode, while at the same time, producing other utterances in the analytic mode. This pattern may confuse observers because the analytic utterances appear to regress to language of younger children (shorter in length and sometimes "telegraphic"), but as Prizant points out, they actually represent a positive sign of growth. They represent the child's emerging ability to generate unique sentences using the building blocks of language as separable units and combining them in flexible ways, rather than reusing the same inflexible word chunks over and over as unanalyzed wholes.

Language, Cognition, and Social Interaction in Autism. Competing theories have been proposed regarding the relative roles of linguistic and cognitive impairments in autism. Language deficit is agreed to be a central diagnostic feature of autism; it is always present. The question is whether linguistic impairment is central to the disorder or whether autism is primarily a disorder of cognitive development. Some theorists have suggested that language deficits are pivotal in autism, playing a major role in social interaction problems and other problems associated with autism (e.g., Churchill, 1972;

Hermelin & O'Connor, 1970; Rutter, 1965). However, this would not explain the differences noted among children with autism and children with specific language disorder, particularly in the manner in which they approach social interactions.

Qualitative impairment of social interaction is listed first in the DSM-IV definition of autism, but its nature is not fully understood. Current researchers note that when they reach adolescence, many individuals with autism show an increased interest in and awareness of others (see Personal Reflection 4.4). Their problems appear to be "a lack of social skills rather than a lack of social interest" (Schopler & Mesibov, 1986, p. 5).

The "islets of excellence" that are sometimes observed in children and adults with autism (e.g., the movie character Rainman's unusual ability to memorize playing cards and his interest in the telephone directory) appear to represent specific information processing skills that are out of balance with the person's other cognitive and linguistic abilities. Without referring specifically to autism, Bruner (1968) cautioned of the dangers of premature overspecificity in human development:

> Human infancy appears to be a guarantor against the achievement of precocities of development, a period in which very general rules of skill, or perceptual organization, and of interaction are learned in preparation for later, species-specific forms of human achievement in action, perception, and communication. In this sense, infancy can be conceived almost as a shield against premature specialization. (p. 9)

In spite of some unusual skills involving short-term memory, children with autism have difficulty integrating information from multiple levels of processing. Her-

---

PERSONAL REFLECTION 4.4 _____

I'm as good at a two way conversation as a pile of gramophone records
Or a parrot that is talking from a cage.
Some lasses seem in a rage when they talk to me
I don't seem to hold the keys to their thought processes. (p. 7)

David Miedzianik, a person with autism who lives in Scholes, Rotherham, England, writing about his loneliness in a poem.
    Note. From "I Hope Some Lass Will Want Me After Reading All This" by D. Miedzianik, 1990, *The Advocate* (newsletter of the Autism Society of America), *22* (1), p. 7. Copyright 1990 by D. Miedzianik. Reprinted by permission.

melin and O'Connor (1967) compared the recall skills of 12 children with autism and 12 children with mental retardation matched for receptive vocabulary and immediate memory span for digits. They found that children with autism had better recall skills than children with mental retardation, but they were less able to use meaning and sentence structure to aid recall.

Cognition Factors.   Cognitive factors are clearly implicated in the development of children with autism, even among the relatively small proportion (around 20%) who score near normal on IQ tests, and are considered essential contributing factors to language disorders in children with autism. Rutter (1983) has argued that children with autism have a general cognitive deficit that cannot be explained as secondary to their severe problems in social relationships. Impairment in developing the cognitive ability, **theory of mind,** is implicated in autism (Baron-Cohen, 1995; Hobson, 1993), as described in Chapter 3. On the other hand, not all children with autism demonstrate the same degree of cognitive impairment; those who do often show wide scattering in different areas of ability, and many children with significant mental retardation do not show symptoms of autism. Therefore, the two conditions must be relatively independent.

Contrasting Approaches to Intervention for Autism.   In designing an intervention for young children with autism, professionals and families have choices that differ widely in theoretical perspective. A major choice is between behavioral approaches (see Chapter 3), such as those proposed by Lovaas (1981, 1987) and Maurice (1996), and social interactionist approaches, such as described by Klinger and Dawson (1992) (see Chapter 13). Behavioral approaches require intensive scheduling of one-on-one training sessions for teaching discrete behaviors with multiple massed trials with a heavy reliance on imitation. For example, eye contact would be taught by saying, "Look at me," and then reinforcing with food and a social reinforcer (e.g., "Good looking!"). In a social interaction approach, eye contact is taught within the context of joint action routines in which the adult imitates the child and toys are held close to the face. A third approach has been developed on a cognitive-linguistic base. Blank, McKirdy, and Payne (1996a, 1996b, 1996c) designed a series of structured language-input intervention strategies for early language development

to help children with autism and other severe language impairments move from prelinguistic to linguistic (narrative) stages of developmental functioning.

Attention-Deficit Hyperactivity Disorder

Diagnosing Attention Deficit Hyperactivity Disorder. In the DSM-IV (American Psychiatric Association, 1994), attention-deficit hyperactivity disorder (ADHD) is categorized with disruptive behavior disorders (see Box 4.8 for a list of symptoms). The current label follows an earlier change in the 1980 edition of DSM-III, in which the terms **hyperkinesis** and **minimal brain dysfunction** were both replaced with the terminology **attention-deficit disorder with hyperactivity** (American Psychiatric Association, 1980). In turn, that terminology was replaced with the ADHD label in the DSM-III R (American Psychiatric Association, 1987).

ADHD is a behavioral syndrome marked by inattention, impulsivity, and hyperactivity. It occurs as much as nine times more frequently in boys than in girls (Sattler, 1988) and in 3 to 5% of all children, meaning that "more than 2 million of all those under the age of 18 in the United States could have the disorder" (Barkley, 1995, p. 78). But prevalence figures are difficult to obtain because definitions vary from place to place. In Great Britain, children with the symptoms of ADHD are diagnosed as having a conduct problem, and in eastern Europe they simply may be called undisciplined. Barkley noted that "It's unfortunate that such labels perpetuate the misperception of ADHD as a problem of personal character; the fact remains that ADHD is a neurologically determined disorder and is found throughout the world" (p. 79). The traits that lead to a diagnosis of ADHD represent just one end of a continuum that looks normal for most individuals, who show them in mild forms in limited situations. Typically, ADHD is diagnosed when symptoms occur more frequently and with greater magnitude than in others of the same age and sex (Barkley, 1995).

The "overactivity" of ADHD typically is observed first by parents and preschool teachers in early childhood. Hyperactivity is difficult to define objectively, particularly for preschool children, who normally exhibit wide ranges of activity levels (Campbell, 1985).

When children with ADHD reach school age and have difficulty meeting the demands of the classroom,

Box 4.8 _____

Diagnostic Criteria for Attention-Deficit/Hyperactivity Disorder in DSM-IV

A. Either (1) or (2):

(1) six (or more) of the following symptoms of **inattention** have persisted for at least 6 months to a degree that is maladaptive and inconsistent with developmental level:

Inattention

(a) often fails to give close attention to details or makes careless mistakes in schoolwork, work, or other activities

(b) often has difficulty sustaining attention in tasks or play activities

(c) often does not seem to listen when spoken to directly

(d) often does not follow through on instructions and fails to finish schoolwork, chores, or duties in the workplace (not due to oppositional behavior or failure to understand instructions)

(e) often has difficulty organizing tasks and activities

(f) often avoids, dislikes, or is reluctant to engage in tasks that require sustained mental effort, such as schoolwork or homework

(g) often loses things necessary for tasks or activities (e.g., toys, school assignments, pencils, books, or tools)

(h) is often easily distracted by extraneous stimuli

(i) is often forgetful in daily activities

(2) six (or more) of the following symptoms of **hyperactivity-impulsivity** have persisted for at least 6 months to a degree that is maladaptive and inconsistent with developmental level:

Hyperactivity

(a) often fidgets with hands or feet or squirms in seat

(b) often leaves seat in classroom or in other situations in which remaining seated is expected

(c) often runs about or climbs excessively in situations in which it is inappropriate (in adolescents or adults, may be limited to subjective feelings of restlessness)

(d) often has difficulty playing or engaging in leisure activities quietly

(e) is often "on the go" or often acts as if "driven by a motor"

(f) often talks excessively

Impulsivity

(g) often blurts out answers before questions have been completed

(h) often has difficulty awaiting turn

(i) often interrupts or intrudes on others (e.g., butts into conversations or games)

B. Some hyperactive-impulsive or inattentive symptoms that caused impairment were present before age 7 years.

C. Some impairment from the symptoms is present in two or more settings (e.g., at school [or work] and at home).

D. There must be clear evidence of clinically significant impairment in social, academic, or occupational functioning.

E. The symptoms do not occur exclusively during the course of a Pervasive Developmental Disorder, Schizophrenia, or other Psychotic Disorder and are not better accounted for by another mental disorder (e.g., Mood Disorder, Anxiety Disorder, Dissociative Disorder, or a Personality Disorder).

Note. From American Psychiatric Association: *Diagnostic and Statistical Manual of Mental Disorders (4th ed DSM IV)* (pp. 83–85). Washington, DC: American Psychiatric Association, 1994. Reprinted by permission.

_____

academic underachievement becomes common (see Personal Reflection 4.5). At this point, psychologists often look for a profile on the Wechsler Intelligence Scale for Children—Revised (WISC-R; Wechsler, 1974) in which children with ADHD earn scaled scores of 10 to 13 on most subtests but only achieve scores of 6 or 7 on the cluster of four subtests that demand the most selective attention: digit span, arithmetic, coding, and mazes (Newhoff, 1986). Parents and classroom teachers also contribute to the diagnosis by rating chil-

PERSONAL REFLECTION 4.5 _____

"For me, ADHD made every aspect of school a challenge . . . except getting into trouble. Impulsivity (a definite ADHD characteristic) allowed me to become frighteningly angry in seconds, to say things I shouldn't, and generally to do stupid things without carefully thinking about them first." (p. 55)

John Weaver describing what it feels like to have attention-deficit hyperactivity disorder in a book edited by his mother, Constance Weaver (1993, 1994b). The book promotes the advantages of whole language classrooms, with clear structure and a student-centered respect for diverse approaches to learning.

_____

dren's behavior with such instruments as Conners' Scales (Conners, 1969).

Because many classroom demands are conveyed through linguistic and nonlinguistic communication, it is important for language specialists to participate in the multidisciplinary diagnostic process for children with ADHD. Newhoff (1986, 1990) advocated involvement of speech–language pathologists in identifying the problem and in sorting out its relationship to possible language-learning disabilities. Among adolescents, the risk for increased psychiatric difficulty among children with ADHD is great (Sattler, 1988). Barkley (1995) reported that up to 45% of children with ADHD have at least one other psychiatric disorder, and many have two or more co-occurring problems involving anxiety, depression, and low self-esteem. "Between 20 and 30% of ADHD children have at least one type of LD [learning disability] in math, reading, or spelling" (p. 87). Up to 65% eventually have a diagnosis of oppositional defiant disorder, and "as many as 45% may progress to the more severe level of conduct disorder" (p. 91). Speech–language pathologists and special educators should probe for significant signs of previously unrecognized ADHD, along with hidden language-learning disabilities, when they consult regarding children with psychiatric difficulties.

One fairly well-controlled study (Rutter, Tizard, & Whitmore, 1970) looked for intercorrelations among psychiatric, learning, and neurological disorders among all of the children of a similar age on the Isle of Wight (an island off the coast of England). Rutter and his colleagues found that children who had "overt behavior

disorders" (such as ADD, hyperactivity, or oppositional disorders) had very high rates of learning problems, especially reading disorders. In fact, among children with reading disorders, 25% also had one of these overt psychiatric behavioral disorders.

In another study, Cantwell, Baker, and Mattison (1979), assessed 600 children in a community speech clinic. The researchers offered free psychiatric evaluations as part of the diagnostic process. Two thirds were boys and 60% were less than 6 years old. Cantwell and colleagues found that 50.3% of the group with communication impairments had diagnosable psychiatric disorders (compared with an estimated 10% of the general population) and that the most commonly diagnosed psychiatric problem was an "overt behavior disorder" (ADD, oppositional disorder, or conduct disorder), which was diagnosed in 26% of the 600 children with communicative disorders.

ADHD is not currently viewed as an educational diagnosis that justifies special education. However, when children with ADHD exhibit symptoms of learning disabilities or behavioral disorders, they may be placed in programs for children with those disorders (sometimes termed **emotional disorders** or **impairments**), or they may receive accommodations and services under Section 504 of the Rehabilitation Act (see Chapter 5).

Hypothesized Causes of Attention-Deficit Hyperactivity Disorder. It is inferred that biological factors underlie conditions of ADHD because children with the disorder often respond favorably to treatment with psychostimulant medication (Barkley, 1995). However, neither the exact mechanism for the symptoms of ADHD nor the effect of medication is fully understood. Based on studies of regional cerebral blood flow, the disorder is thought to be related to disruptions in transmission and metabolism along subcortical pathways that connect the midbrain to the prefrontal cortex. These areas play a role in directing attention, self-regulation, and planning (Bass, 1988). One hypothesis for the paradoxical finding that psychostimulants such as methylphenidate (Ritalin) appear to control hyperactivity is that they stimulate neurotransmitters that enable children to concentrate longer (Zametkin & Rapoport, 1987).

The use of psychostimulants to treat ADHD remains controversial. Although little evidence suggests that long-term learning or academic achievement is improved (Gittelman-Klein & Klein, 1976; Rie & Rie, 1977; Rie, Rie, & Stewart, 1976), research has consistently shown that psychostimulants can result in improved parent and teacher ratings of behavior and in enhancing performance on some laboratory measures (Abikoff & Gittelman, 1985; Gittelman-Klein et al., 1976; Rapport, Stoner, DuPaul, Birmingham, & Tucker, 1985). For children who can benefit, psychostimulants seem to normalize their biological systems so that they can participate in other kinds of interactions with less difficulty.

To explain the development of attention, Levine (1987) noted that individuals of all ages daily confront more data than they can possibly interpret, store, and apply. As a result, selection is necessary and involves a combination of both selective attention and selective inattention. As children mature, they gradually become better able to concentrate on important information and to ignore irrelevant stimuli. Levine said that children with ADHD are predisposed to poor selectivity, concentrating on inappropriate stimuli, and participating in purposeless activities.

Subtypes of Attention-Deficit Hyperactivity Disorder.
The DSM-IV (American Psychiatric Association (1994) recognizes three subtypes, based on parts of the definition shown in Box 4.8. A **combined type** is diagnosed "if both Criteria A1 and A2 are met for the past 6 months." A **predominantly inattentive type** is diagnosed "if Criterion A1 is met but Criterion A2 is not met for the past 6 months." A **predominantly hyperactive-impulsive type** is diagnosed "if Criterion A2 is met but criterion A1 is not met for the past 6 months" (p. 85).

Language Characteristics Associated with Attention Deficit Hyperactivity Disorder.   No evidence indicates that children with ADHD have linguistic deficits specific to the syndrome. On the other hand, children with language impairments are at increased risk for also having ADHD (Cantwell et al., 1979). A study by Rutter and colleagues (1970) supports the risk for interrelatedness of ADHD and written language disorders as well.

When meaningful linguistic distractors are used (e.g., someone reading a story) in studies of **selective auditory attention** children with hyperactivity and learning disabilities have more difficulty repeating stim-

ulus words than when nonlinguistic distractors (e.g., white noise) are used (Cherry & Kruger, 1983; Lasky & Tobin, 1973). It is difficult to interpret the results of these studies, however, because hyperactivity and learning disabilities may be confounded. The controlled conditions of laboratory testing using headphones may also fail to capture children's distractibility in natural settings (Dalebout, Nelson, Hletko, & Frentheway, 1991).

Most professionals currently recommend combined behavior and pharmaceutical treatment for children with ADHD (Barkley, 1995; C. Weaver, 1994b). Kendall and Braswell (1985) have described cognitive-behavioral therapy for "impulsive" children as an approach in which "The client and therapist work together to think through and behaviorally practice solutions to personal, academic, and interpersonal problems with a consideration of the affect involved" (p. 1). If positive reinforcement practices are not instituted consistently and deliberately, these children tend to experience only punitive responses and run increasing risks of depression and delinquency.

The role of language in cognitive-behavioral treatment is important. Vail (1987) noted that, to focus attention, children need a combination of arousal, a filter, language, and appropriate work. Attention is awakened through arousal, but then it must be focused with a filtering process that keeps out both external and internal distractions. Language enables children to organize thought and to focus their attention. It assists them to break down a task into manageable pieces, anticipate cause and effect, and categorize and sort ideas according to their relative importance. Vail noted that "Some children who appear to have trouble paying attention actually lack the language to structure their work" (p. 141). Discovering such deficits (if they exist) is a key goal of the diagnostic process.

Another element in determining how well children can attend, in Vail's (1987) view, is a "need for appropriate work," which supports the message that problems are not just within children. Before a child is diagnosed with ADHD, it is important that those in the child's environment experiment to see whether the child may be demonstrating the symptoms of ADHD because the schoolwork is too difficult (or too easy) for the child's level of ability. Vail cautioned, "Sometimes the label *attentional deficit* is applied to a student who is merely in over his head" (p. 141).

Acquired Brain Injury

Diagnosing Acquired Brain Injury.   Children with acquired brain injury constitute a heterogeneous group. To consider them to be members of one category is misleading. They also differ from children with developmental language disorders, supporting the need for a separate category.

The human brain is quite remarkable. It is complex enough to develop an impressive array of integrated sensory, motor, linguistic, cognitive, and social skills; yet it is fragile enough to be set back by a bump on the head, the bursting of a strategically placed blood vessel, or the invasion of a microscopic agent. A child's brain is also resilient enough to make an amazing recovery when a significant amount of tissue is irreparably damaged or even when an entire hemisphere is removed.

A language disorder associated with a focal-acquired lesion of the brain is termed **aphasia.** This term and its various subclassifications are applied primarily to language disorders in adults associated with brain lesions caused by cerebrovascular accidents (CVAs; strokes caused by blockage or hemorrhage). The label **congenital aphasia** has been used to represent developmental language disorders (Eisenson, 1968, 1972). The use of that term, however, can lead to confusion. Currently, it is applied rarely to children with congenital problems, except perhaps when a specific language impairment is unusually severe. Diagnosis of acquired brain injury is usually made on the basis of known etiology by a team of health professionals.

Because the role of biological maturation factors is so critical to children with acquired brain injuries, it is essential that language specialists be vigilant in recognizing any symptoms of childhood language disorder that have sudden onset or are progressive. Immediate medical referral and treatment are essential in such cases. It is not a time for "wait and see."

Subtypes of Acquired Brain Injury.   It is impossible to outline a common set of symptoms, yet some expectations vary with the cause: (1) focal-acquired lesions, (2) diffuse lesions associated with traumatic brain injury, (3) acquired childhood aphasia secondary to convulsive disorder, and (4) other brain injury or encephalopathy, such as following infection or treatment for childhood cancer.

Focal-Acquired Brain Injury in Children.   Several studies have shown that children who acquire focal (specific and localized) lesions of the left hemisphere during early childhood show generally good recovery and development of language (Aram & Ekelman, 1987; Aram, Ekelman, & Whitaker, 1986, 1987; Hecaen, 1976, 1983). Close examination of results, however, also shows some significant effects on language development and learning ability.

Although CVAs occur primarily in older adults, they can occur at any age. Children with congenital heart disorders are particularly at risk because embolic material may break loose and clog the middle cerebral artery, cutting off blood supply to the critical language areas of the brain. Children also may have congenital arteriovenous malformations, clusters of malformed and misconnected arteries and veins that are particularly susceptible to hemorrhaging (another form of CVA).

Aram and her research group conducted much of the carefully controlled research on the linguistic and cognitive sequelae of unilateral brain lesions in children. Aram (1988) reviewed the results of several of her own and others' studies regarding effects of unilateral brain lesions on language development (summarized in Box 4.9). Children who have recovered significantly from unilateral left-hemisphere lesions show predominantly left-hemisphere engagement during language tasks and predominantly right-hemisphere engagement during visuospatial tasks. This typically normal pattern suggests that, for children with unilateral lesions acquired early, the pattern of recovery and further development involves intra- rather than interhemispheric functional reorganization (Papanicolaou, DiScenna, Gillespie, & Aram, 1990).

Traumatic Brain Injury in Children.   "Each year approximately 1 to 2 million children and adolescents sustain central nervous system (CNS) injuries as a result of falls, motor vehicle accidents, sports injuries, assaults, or abuse" (Blosser & DePompei, 1994). The language development picture for such children is more mixed than that for children with unilateral lesions. The traditional wisdom is that the earlier brain injury occurs in a child's development, the more complete the expected recovery. Other interpretations of the evidence, however, suggest that age is only one factor in determining recovery (Ewing-Cobbs, Fletcher, & Levin, 1985). Al-

Box 4.9 _____

Features of Language and Cognition Observed
Following Unilateral Brain Injury in Children
(Based on Aram, 1988)

1. **Cognition.** Results from IQ tests are conflicting (probably because subject groups in many studies have been confounded with children with seizure disorders who have possibly been on medication). In children free from ongoing seizures, IQ scores may be expected to be well within normal limits, but tests may not be sensitive enough to predict persistent language or learning difficulties. The most common finding is distractibility, regardless of lesion site.

2. **Syntactic comprehension.** Studies have demonstrated at least subtle syntactic comprehension deficits following left hemisphere lesions but not right hemisphere lesions. More research is needed to assess comprehension of connected discourse and syntactic structures that are more complex than those assessed by token tests. The contributions of more primary cognitive abilities such as memory and attention also need to be teased out.

3. **Syntactic production.** In children, the most frequent early observation after acquired brain injury, even when the right hemisphere is affected, is mutism, followed by telegraphic production during the recovery process. Although the expressive syntax deficits of these children appear to lessen considerably with continued development, when tasks become more demanding, evidence of long-standing deficits can be found.

4. **Lexical and semantic aspects.** In rapid-naming tasks, children with left-hemisphere lesions tend to be significantly slower in response time and to make more errors when given rhyming cues than do matched control subjects. On the other hand, children with right-hemisphere lesions respond as rapidly or even more quickly than control subjects but produce more errors (suggesting a speed–accuracy trade-off).

5. **Written language development and academic success.** Although the oral language deficits of children with acquired unilateral brain lesions are generally subtle, with few children remaining clinically aphasic, children with both left- and right-hemisphere lesions typically exhibit academic difficulties in school. The reading abilities of children with focal left-hemisphere lesions may vary widely. Although most perform comparably to carefully selected controls on reading tests, a select subgroup (with a variety of lesion sites, including subcortical ones) exhibits severe reading disorders. Efforts to identify commonalities among this subgroup of children have been largely unsuccessful, except to note the presence of concomitant language and/or memory problems in the presence of generally intact nonverbal conceptual skills (Aram, Ekelman, & Gillespie, 1989). Children with both right- and left-hemisphere brain lesions are likely to show residual deficits of brain injury on attention, impulse inhibition, memory, reasoning, and perceptual speed, all of which may affect school functioning (Aram & Ekelman, 1988).

_____

though spontaneous recovery following brain injury is striking, a significant proportion of children exhibit persistent deficits of cognitive and linguistic processing (Satz & Bullard-Bates, 1981).

A summary of studies of long-term deficits in children following traumatic brain injury (TBI) (Ewing-Cobbs et al., 1985) showed more pervasive cognitive and behavioral sequelae than previously recognized.

These include general intellectual, language, memory, and psychosocial deficits, all of which can be expected to interfere both with communication and academic functioning. Accumulating evidence suggests that younger children may exhibit more severe and long-lasting cognitive sequelae following TBI than older adolescents or adults (Levin, Ewing-Cobbs, & Benton, 1984).

Levin and Eisenberg (1979) evaluated the language deficits of 64 children with closed head injury less than 6 months after injury. Their findings showed linguistic deficits in 31%. The most common symptom was dysnomia, both for objects presented visually (13% of the sample) or to the left hand for tactual identification (12%). Auditory comprehension was impaired in 11% and verbal repetition in only 4%.

Ewing-Cobbs and co-workers (1985) also studied children and adolescents with moderate-to-severe closed head injury, defined by the presence of neurologic deficit, CT scan findings, coma persisting for at least 15 minutes, or a combination of these findings. Their results showed that after post-traumatic amnesia (PTA) was resolved, continued deficits showed up in confrontation naming, object description, verbal fluency, and writing to dictation. Also younger children were more impaired than adolescents on measures of written language functioning.

Studies of written language processing by children and adolescents with TBI are difficult to interpret because risk for head injury is associated with preexisting learning and social problems. For example, when Shaffer, Bijur, Chadwick, and Rutter (1980) investigated 88 school-age children who sustained closed head injuries producing depressed skull fractures, they found that 55% had reading ages one or more years below their chronological ages, and 33% were two or more years behind, these effects were difficult to sort out from confounding predisposing variables.

Chadwick, Rutter, Brown, Shaffer, and Traub (1981) conducted a follow-up study of children injured between the ages of 5 and 14 years. They concluded that 25 of those who experienced PTA for more than 3 weeks (defined as the "severe head injury" group) showed reading difficulties attributable to the head injury. Of these children, seven were reported by their teachers either to be experiencing difficulties with their schoolwork or were placed in special schools. These authors

pointed out the need to consider the real-life effects of time pressures and contextual demands when evaluating children and adolescents with head injury. They noted that such individuals may be able to complete tasks under optimal, temporally controlled circumstances of psychometric testing but not in other settings.

Rather than attempting to identify subtypes of children with brain injury, rehabilitation teams tend to focus on stages of recovery. This is because different sets of concerns arise during different points in the recovery process.

In the early recovery period (sometimes called the **acute phase**), the primary goal is to increase the responsiveness of a child emerging from coma. Rosen and Gerring (1986) marked the **early recovery period** from the point of injury to the end of PTA when "patients are consistently oriented to place, date, and time and are able to store long term memories" (p. 25). During the early phase, treatment is aimed at sensory and sensorimotor stimulation to increase arousal and adaptive responses to the environment (Szekeres, Ylvisaker, & Holland, 1985). The **middle recovery period** involves efforts to channel recovery for confused patients by focusing on cognitive retraining and structured environmental compensations (see Personal Reflection 4.6). The **late recovery period** involves goals for increased independence, withdrawal of environmental supports, the development of functional integrative skills in more natural settings, and development of strategies to compensate for residual impairments (Szekeres et al., 1985). Rosen and Gerring (1986) described long-term recovery as a process that occurs over a period of months to years and that is continually influenced by concomitant processes of development. Blosser and DePompei

PERSONAL REFLECTION 4.6 _____

"My son is very fortunate to have girls as friends. Heidi has talked to him every day since the accident, even when he was in the coma. She introduced him to two other young ladies by telephone. Thank goodness for phones and friends." (p. 189)

These are the words of Sharon Hogan, the mother of Jason, age 14, who was severely injured when his bicycle was hit by a car. Her insights are quoted by Blosser and DePompei (1994) in their book on *Pediatric Traumatic Brain Injury*.

(1994) advocated a proactive approach across the stages of recovery of pediatric head injury, taking advantage of learning strengths and looking ahead to prepare for the next stage of transition.

Acquired Aphasia Secondary to Convulsive Disorder. Another type of language disorder that may be acquired in childhood is acquired aphasia secondary to a convulsive disorder, which is usually of idiopathic (unknown) origin. Normal development, varying in length (see Miller, Campbell, Chapman, & Weismer, 1984, for a review), is followed by either sudden or gradual onset of dramatic language problems (L. S. Jordan, 1980).

The condition was first described by Landau and Kleffner (1957) and is sometimes known as the **Landau syndrome** or **Landau-Kleffner syndrome.** It should be suspected whenever a child loses previously acquired language, before, during, or after seizures (Cooper & Ferry, 1978). In the United Kingdom, it is referred to as Worster-Drought (1971) syndrome.

This syndrome is characterized by the presence of electrographic epileptic discharges (whether or not overt seizures are evident), generally accompanied by severe language comprehension deficits, at least initially. Its prognosis is variable. Some children show dramatic recovery after a brief period of impairment, others show fluctuations of ability, and still others show severe, long-lasting language deficits (Mantovani & Landau, 1980). The degree of recovery appears to be weakly correlated to improvement of electrographic abnormalities and medical control of seizures.

Encephalitis has been suggested as a causative agent for this syndrome, but a variety of agents likely play a role (Cole et al., 1988). One girl I saw in my earlier practice first demonstrated listening and reading comprehension problems when she began to have seizures in third grade. She was also very embarrassed by her seizures, which often included vomiting. This girl was later found to have a temporal lobe tumor, stressing the critical need for thorough neurological assessment in such cases.

The most frequent language symptom for children with Landau-Kleffner syndrome is loss of comprehension, sometimes so profound that it is mistaken for deafness. This problem is better described as **central auditory agnosia,** i.e., hearing is intact but the ability to interpret meaning is lost because of damage to auditory reception and association areas in the brain. Expressive speech usually deteriorates secondary to the loss of ability to process receptive oral language. For older children, reading and writing may be relatively spared.

When symptoms of auditory agnosia are marked, sign language may offer a functional alternative communication mode for these children. In my experience, the condition is more difficult to diagnose in younger children because they have less history of normal development to contrast with the period of impairment, and the children themselves are less aware of their changed status. They also have acquired fewer words in their expressive vocabularies to contrast with the receptive language deficits, and they tend to show a more uniform language deficit across areas.

In cases of suddenly acquired aphasia, one of the most important early services that communication specialists can provide—aside from contributing to the assessment process, making referrals to neurologists, and assisting families to understand this scary thing that is happening to them—is to ensure that some form of communication is immediately available. Often, this involves encouraging families and educators to take advantage of all modes of communication (particularly low-technology techniques, e.g., gestures, pictures, and written communication materials, if appropriate). This role is critical in reducing frightening feelings of isolation and acting out these children are likely to experience with sudden onset.

Encephalopathy Secondary to Infection or Irradiation. Some children exhibit signs of brain injury resulting from agents that are less direct than CVA or trauma and that disrupt the normal biological maturation process over time, rather than precipitously. The direct effects of brain tumors and the aftereffects of encephalitis or cancer treatments fall into this category.

The symptoms may vary widely, again based on factors such as timing, extent, and location of involvement of cortical and subcortical tissue. They also vary qualitatively from those of children with more purely developmental disabilities. Children with acquired brain injuries of any type tend to retain some function and to have information processing and cognitive deficits of varying severity. For acquired brain injury, the risks for either over- or underexpectation, are great.

For example, in our clinic, we saw a child, Sarah, whose severe language and cognitive disabilities were acquired as an aftereffect of treatment for acute lymphocytic leukemia (ALL). Sarah had developed normally, if not precociously, up to the age of 3, when the ALL was identified. She was then treated with a combination of brain irradiation and chemotherapy (methotrexate in the spinal column), and two years later, the leukemia was basically "cured." Sarah's parents, however, faced a new set of worries after two more years passed when Sarah began to lose developmental skills she had already acquired. The worries became major as the condition worsened and her seizures became uncontrollable.

The most confusing part of the picture for those who worked with Sarah at school was her scattering of abilities. Her syntactic construction skills were more intact than her comprehension abilities. She also retained some earlier learned vocabulary in her self-initiated speech, even though she did not understand it. An effect of this was the appearance of refusing to cooperate in most standard assessment and teaching tasks (which are often the "I say and you do," or "I ask and you answer" variety). Because of her severe comprehension deficits, when Sarah did verbalize in these contexts, it was usually with off-task or echolalic remarks. Yet, when allowed more control of the topic, Sarah participated much more "normally" in conversation and play. Sarah's school district had a great deal of difficulty knowing how to provide appropriate services to meet Sarah's unique needs. She did not "fit" in any of the usual programs designed for children with developmental disabilities. This problem is common for children with acquired brain damage, especially when its effects are severe, as they were in Sarah's case. Her needs were eventually met best with an inclusive education model.

In some children with Landau-Kleffner syndrome, the "damage" may only be inferred from aberrant findings on electroencephalograms (EEGs). In cases like Sarah's, the effects of the irradiation treatment may show up clearly on MRI scans some time after treatment (see Figure 4.1). Childhood cancer survivors may demonstrate mild neuropsychological late effects of brain irradiation without apparent white matter effects on MRI scans (Kramer, Norman, Grant-Zawadzki, Albin, & Moore, 1988). A summary of results of research reports on children with ALL who have been treated with brain irradiation and chemotherapy shows (1) general lowering of functioning, with the effect most pronounced for nonlanguage skills; (2) encephalopathy (brain damage), intelligence deficits, and/or neuropsychological deficits occurring within months or years following cranial radiation and chemotherapy (Hutter, 1986; McCalla, 1985); (3) children receiving irradiation before 5 years of age

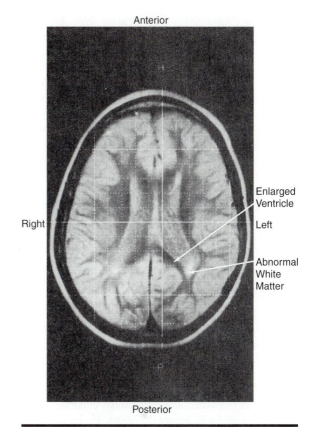

Anterior

Right

Left

Enlarged Ventricle

Abnormal White Matter

Posterior

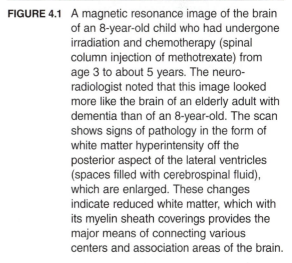

FIGURE 4.1 A magnetic resonance image of the brain of an 8-year-old child who had undergone irradiation and chemotherapy (spinal column injection of methotrexate) from age 3 to about 5 years. The neuroradiologist noted that this image looked more like the brain of an elderly adult with dementia than of an 8-year-old. The scan shows signs of pathology in the form of white matter hyperintensity off the posterior aspect of the lateral ventricles (spaces filled with cerebrospinal fluid), which are enlarged. These changes indicate reduced white matter, which with its myelin sheath coverings provides the major means of connecting various centers and association areas of the brain.

being more likely to experience cognitive difficulty (Copeland et al., 1985); and (4) children treated with chemotherapy alone showing no global or specific neuropsychological impairment (Tamaroff et al., 1982).

Language Characteristics Associated with Acquired Brain Injury. Individual variability is primary in acquired brain injury. In some cases, such as those involving left-hemisphere lesions or Landau-Kleffner syndrome, the language processing deficit may appear to be primary. Yet the linguistic processing deficits of such children may actually be secondary to auditory agnosia. In other children, such as those with TBI, specifically linguistic impairments may appear to be secondary to more general cognitive and social interaction deficits. Regardless, a comprehensive approach to assessment and intervention is needed.

The services needed by children with acquired brain injury extend beyond the area of linguistics and communication. The term **cognitive rehabilitation therapy** is commonly used when children have TBI requiring intervention (Ylvisaker, 1985). It represents the comprehensive scope of impaired abilities and the extent of rehabilitative needs.

Perhaps the most consistent characteristic of children with acquired brain injury is their wide variability as they continue to mature (N. W. Nelson & Schwentor, 1990; Rosen & Gerring, 1986; Ylvisaker, 1985). In some cases, children may be so impaired following injury that it is unrealistic to expect them to be able to compete in the social and educational contexts where they functioned well before the injury. Rosen and Gerring (1986) observed the paradoxical situation that "School is the most appropriate place for children to gain reassurance that achievement is possible again, even while being confronted with enormous new difficulties in thinking, remembering, speaking, reading or concentrating" (p. xii). Language specialists may be able to facilitate this process in ways that accentuate the positive and reduce the negative factors involved.

Other Central Factors

The central conditions considered thus far are not the only ones that can interfere with language learning. Any influence that disrupts the central nervous system can disrupt language, speech, and communication development.

Language specialists need to know about other specific conditions such as Tourette's syndrome, fragile-X syndrome, and other complexes of symptoms that may influence communicative development. Sources for information specific to communication disorders associated with these and other syndromes are Sparks (1984) and S. E. Gerber (1990).

PERIPHERAL SENSORY AND MOTOR SYSTEM FACTORS

Hearing Impairment

Diagnosing Hearing Impairment. Of impairments involving hearing, vision, and motor functioning, hearing loss is by far the most certain to be associated with difficulties in oral language acquisition. The term **hearing impairment** refers to all degrees of hearing loss, ranging from mild impairments, which may have only subtle effects on language acquisition, to profound hearing loss. Diagnosis occurs through audiological assessment by an audiologist, often teaming with an otolaryngologist who considers possible medical factors.

Subtypes of Hearing Impairment. Within the category of hearing impairment, a traditional subdivision is between **hard-of-hearing** and **deafness.** Two types of criteria are used to make this distinction: (1) the effect of the hearing loss on the ability to process linguistic information and (2) audiometric results (Northern & Downs, 1984).

An audiometric criterion for determining **deafness** is hearing loss in the better ear of 70 dB or greater hearing level (HL). HL is the average of pure-tone thresholds at 500, 1000, and 2000 Hz, the "speech frequencies." An audiometric criterion for determining **hard-of-hearing** is hearing loss in the better ear in the range of 35 to 69 dB HL (Northern & Downs, 1984). M. Ross (1977) argued that, with modern amplification methods, the physiological borderline for determining deafness should be even higher, at 95 to 100 dB HL. Boothroyd (1982) also pointed out that proper amplification can move children from one classification to another, making the audiometric distinction between deafness and hard-of-hearing questionable. Cochlear implants and tactile aids (Roeser, 1988) have also been used to help some children who previously would have been categorized as "deaf" to be aware of sounds and use them as information. Table 4.2 summarizes other terminology for categorizing degrees of hearing impairment.

Perhaps the more useful criterion for differentiating deafness is the ability to process linguistic information

TABLE 4.2 Hearing handicap as a function of average hearing threshold level of the better ear

AVERAGE THRESHOLD LEVEL AT 500–2000 HZ (ANSI)*	DESCRIPTION	COMMON CAUSES	WHAT CAN BE HEARD WITHOUT AMPLIFICATION	DEGREES OF HANDICAP (IF NOT TREATED IN FIRST YEAR OF LIFE)	PROBABLE NEEDS
0–15 dB	Normal range		All speech sounds	None	None
16–25 dB	Slight hearing loss	Serous otitis, perforation, monomeric membrane, sensorineural loss, tympano-sclerosis	Vowel sounds heard clearly, may miss unvoiced consonant sounds	Possible mild or transitory auditory dysfunction Difficulty in perceiving some speech sounds	Consideration of need for hearing aid Lip reading Auditory training Speech therapy Preferential seating Appropriate surgery
26–40 dB	Mild	Serous otitis, perforation, tympanosclerosis, monomeric membrane, sensorineural loss	Hears only some speech sounds; the louder voiced sounds	Auditory learning dysfunction Mild language retardation Mild speech problems Inattention	Hearing aid Lip reading Auditory training Speech therapy Appropriate surgery
41–65 dB	Moderate hearing loss	Chronic otitis, middle ear anomaly, sensorineural loss	Misses most speech sounds at normal conver-sational level	Speech problems Language retardation Learning dysfunction Inattention	All of the above, plus consideration of special classroom situation
66–95 dB	Severe hearing loss	Sensorineural loss or mixed loss due to sensorineural loss plus middle ear disease	Hears no speech or sound of normal conversations	Severe speech problems Language retardation Learning dysfunction Inattention	All of the above; probable assignment to special classes
96+ dB	Profound hearing loss	Sensorineural loss or mixed	Hears no speech or other sounds	Severe speech problems Language retardation Learning dysfunction Inattention	All of the above; probable assignment to special classes

*ANSI = American National Standards Institute.

Note. From *Hearing in Children* (4th ed., p. 99) by J. L. Northern and M. P. Downs, 1991, Baltimore, MD: Williams & Wilkins. Copyright 1991 by Williams. Reprinted by permission.

auditorially. Using this criterion, hard-of-hearing children are those who can develop basic communication skills through the auditory channel, whereas deaf children are those whose hearing impairments are so severe that it is impossible to process linguistic information through hearing alone, with or without amplification (Northern & Downs, 1984; Ross, 1982). To these two basic subdivisions, Ross (1982) added a third gray-area group of children who "can utilize their hearing, derive much benefit from it, and may even employ it as a primary channel in certain restricted circumstances, when they have no other choice, such as talking on the telephone on a specific topic" (p. 4). For general communication, however, this group depends primarily on vision to gather information about communicative input.

A different kind of subdivision is sometimes based on whether the hearing loss occurred **prelingually** or **postlingually.** Longitudinal research shows that, as we might expect, children who lose their hearing after they have acquired some language show superior continued development of speech and language compared with those who lose their hearing prelinguistically (Levitt, McGarr, & Geffner, 1988).

Whether a hearing loss is **unilateral** or **bilateral** can also make a difference. Although bilateral losses are, of course, most devastating, and traditionally, the hearing loss of a child's better ear is used as the best estimator of auditory functioning, unilateral hearing losses are by no means innocuous (Northern & Downs, 1984). For example, Bess (1982) found that unilateral hearing loss had a significant effect on the linguistic, educational, and auditory perceptual development of children.

Beyond the basic subdivision of hearing impairment into categories of deafness and hard-of-hearing, a separate important subtype is made up of children with mild, conductive hearing impairments associated with **otitis media with effusion** (OME). This condition may be associated with hearing losses of less than 25 dB but with air-bone gaps of 15 dB or more. Therefore, rather than using a cutoff of 25 dB HL to determine normal hearing, Northern and Downs (1984) suggested that hearing thresholds of 20, 15, or even 10 dB in the speech frequencies might be significant enough to be handicapping during the critical language-learning years for some children.

Although not all studies have shown OME to have negative effects (Brooks, 1986; Fischler, Todd, & Feldman, 1985; Roberts et al., 1986), many studies have demonstrated long-term negative effects on language

and learning, particularly when the condition occurs in the first 6 to 12 months of life and when episodes are more frequent (J. Klein, Chase, Teele, Menyuk, & Rosner, 1988; Silva, Kirkland, Simpson, Stewart, & Williams, 1982; Zinkus & Gottlieb, 1980). Adverse effects have also been reported for children in a wide variety of ethnic, socioeconomic, and racial groups. For example, G. K. Kaplan and colleagues (1973) found significant gaps in school achievement between a group of Eskimo children in Alaska whose first documented episode of OME occurred before age 2 and a control group. Disturbingly, they also found that the educational gaps tended to widen over the age range from the seven to ten years when children were followed.

In a longitudinal study in the Boston area, J. Klein and colleagues (1988) found a significant correlation between time spent with OME and lowered speech and language test scores. Gravel and Wallace (1995) followed a group of fourteen children whose first year otitis media histories were well documented. At age 6, these children had poorer academic skills, particularly involving reading, and more difficulty listening in background competition. Roberts and Medley (1995), summarizing their own research and a review of the literature, concluded that "OME may be one of many risk factors that influences a child's development" (p. 21).

Several mechanisms might account for negative effects on language and learning from OME (e.g., Dobie & Berlin, 1979; M. W. Skinner, 1978). Children with such losses might experience confusion about (1) speech-sound constancy, because of fluctuating acoustic information; (2) acoustic parameters, especially for rapid speech; (3) segmentation of linguistic boundaries, such as for plurals and tenses; (4) prosodic intonation and stress patterns that convey subtle emotional meanings; and (5) word characteristics, making it difficult to acquire new vocabulary. Significant correlations are also found between second-grade teachers' ratings of classroom attention and task orientation and the number of days of OME before 3 years of age (Roberts et al., 1986).

Language Characteristics Associated with Hearing Impairment. Patterns of development for individual children with similar hearing losses are not all alike. The summary in Box 4.10 should therefore be used with that caveat in mind. It summarizes features identified in a range of studies conducted with hearing impaired chil-

Box 4.10 _____

A Summary of Language Development Characteristics
of Hearing Impaired Children

1. **Phonology.** The phonological systems of deaf children may be so affected that intelligibility is impaired, even with familiar listeners. Phonological simplification processes used by other children with hearing impairments vary with degree of loss and generally are similar to those used by younger, normal-hearing children. They differ more in frequency than in kind. Consonant deletions are numerous, particularly in final position. The most notable differences from normal development involve impaired productions of vowels (with a tendency toward neutralization) and suprasegmental features. Problems with suprasegmental features interact with speech planning and production constraints, such as (a) reduced speech rate, which may reflect extension of consonants and vowels, slow articulatory transitions, and frequent pauses; (b) lack of coordination of breathing patterns with syntactic phrasing; (c) inappropriate use of duration to distinguish stressed and unstressed syllables. Voice and resonation qualities may also be distorted (C. Dunn & Newton, 1986).

2. **Syntax and morphology.** Developmental order of syntactic types is similar to that for normal-hearing children. Negation, conjunction, and question formation are less difficult. Relativization, complementation, the verb system, and pronominalization are most difficult. Developmental progression is dramatically delayed for most hearing impaired children, particularly those who are deaf. In some cases, deaf children may produce syntactic structures never used by normal-hearing individuals. These seem to be combinations of English grammar and attempted approximations of English grammar (Quigley, Smith, & Wilbur, 1974). Unstressed, final inflectional morphemes (such as plurals and verb endings) and some parts of speech (such as adverbs, prepositions, quantifiers, and indefinite pronouns) tend to be produced with less frequency. Delays in the acquisition of morphological and syntactic rules are noted in both receptive and expressive language, oral and written.

3. **Semantics.** Hearing impaired children encode a wide range of semantic notions using both verbal and nonverbal means from a very young age, although they tend to talk about location more frequently than normal-hearing children do (Curtiss, Prutting, & Lowell, 1979). Vocabulary production and comprehension problems include difficulty understanding and using concept words, figurative meanings of words and phrases, and multiple-meaning words. Comprehension problems also extend to connected discourse in both oral and written modalities, and they persist as children advance in age (Moeller, Osberger, & Eccarius, 1986; Robbins, 1986).

4. **Pragmatics.** Toddlers with hearing impairment employ a wide range of methods, both verbal and nonverbal (including invented gestures) to communicate their pragmatic intentions, and this ability to communicate tends to exceed their ability to encode semantic concepts linguistically (Curtiss et al., 1979). In conversational interaction, preschool deaf children may show a narrow range of complexity when they act as initiators and may be less likely to respond to partners' initiations, particularly when utterances are in the form of comments (McKirdy & Blank, 1982). Older children with hearing impairments show continued difficulty in using pragmatic rules for entering and engaging in conversations. In the rapid-moving and shifting discourse of regular classroom settings, children with hearing impairments may be particularly disadvantaged (Roeser & Downs, 1988; Wiess, 1986).

dren with varied types and degree of loss, as well as at different points along an age-level continuum.

For the most part, the characteristics in Box 4.10 are not unique to children with hearing impairments, or even to children with language disorders. Most also can be observed in normal-hearing children at some points of their development. Like the language of children with specific language impairment, the language of children with hearing impairment may be better categorized as being delayed than different, especially when considering any one system.

That was the tentative conclusion reached by Quigley, Power, and Steinkamp (1977) when they summarized research on syntactic development by 450 deaf students (ranging in age from 10 to 19 years, with 50 subjects in each age group), in comparison with 60 normal-hearing control children (20 each in 8-, 9-, and 10-year old groups). Their results showed that syntactic structures develop similarly in deaf and hearing children but at a much slower rate among deaf children.

In addition, Wilbur (1977) found that both deaf and hearing children approach the language-learning task by searching for generalities. Evidence of relatively stable, rule-based phonological development also has been found both for children with mild-to-moderate hearing losses (Oller, Jensen, & Lafayette, 1978; West & Weber, 1973) and with profound congenital deafness (Dodd, 1976).

Some have interpreted the evidence as suggesting that the order of development and strategies used are basically the same for hearing impaired and normal-hearing children; others have interpreted the evidence as suggesting that the language of deaf children differs in quality as well as quantity. Particularly, the rigidity of language used by deaf children has been cited, as well as its susceptibility to being molded by a particular language-teaching curriculum (Russell, Quigley, & Power, 1976; Simmons, 1962). To some extent, conclusions reached depend on whether comparisons are made only within systems of language or across them. Children with impaired hearing have particular difficulty acquiring features of language that carry abstract meaning, are less visible, and are produced with less prosodic stress.

Written Language Problems of Children with Hearing Impairments.   Written language is difficult for hearing impaired children to master. Geers and Moog (1989) re-

viewed the association between prelingual hearing loss and reading deficiency, which "has been abundantly documented, beginning as early as 1916" (p. 69).

Demographic studies of reading performance by hearing impaired children show that a plateau occurs at about the third-grade reading level (Schildroth & Karchmer, 1986). Most hearing impaired children reach the plateau by 15 years of age and remain there at least through age 18 (Geers & Moog, 1989). Myklebust (1964) also concluded, based on studies of read, written, and spoken language, that the syntax of deaf children of around age 17 was approximately equal to that of 7-year-old normal-hearing children. Not only that, the deaf children in Myklebust's research tended to persist in a kind of formula writing and depended on written language prompts until the age of 15 years, whereas normal-hearing children had abandoned them by age 9.

Because most studies of reading development among hearing impaired children used cross-sectional data, Geers and Moog (1989) argued that they may not adequately represent longitudinal growth for individual students. Demographic studies also are likely to miss more academically competitive students because they tend to be mainstreamed at earlier ages and may not be represented in subject groups. Therefore, Geers and Moog (1989) cautioned that "the low scores reported for older hearing impaired students may result from an increasing proportion of students with additional and more severely handicapping characteristics who remain in special education settings" (pp. 69–70). Degree of hearing loss is not necessarily the best predictor of educational success, however, because even minimal hearing loss may place students at risk for language and learning problems involving a number of psychoeducational variables (J. M. Davis, Elfenbein, Schum, & Bentler, 1986).

Geers and Moog (1989) studied 100 profoundly hearing impaired 16- and 17-year-olds enrolled in oral and mainstream high school programs and tested reading, writing, and spoken language abilities extensively. Tasks included those designed to measure both analytic "bottom-up" skills (e.g., phonics, vocabulary, and syntax) and synthetic "top-down" skills (e.g., paragraph comprehension, cloze completion, and narrative retellings). Both kinds of skills were, to the degree possible, evaluated at word, sentence, and text levels. In a multiple-regression analysis, Geers and Moog found three factors that contributed significantly to overall literacy: spoken language, hearing, and early intervention. Three other factors that were found not to contribute significantly to literacy were sign language, socioeconomic status, and mainstreaming. Test results also showed that this special subset of orally educated profoundly hearing impaired youngsters achieved reading skills commensurate with those of their normal-hearing peers (much above those traditionally reported for hearing impaired students). The authors concluded that their reading achievement was possible because they had at least average nonverbal intellectual ability, good use of residual hearing, early amplification, auditory stimulation, and oral educational management, "and—above all—oral English language ability, including vocabulary, syntax, and discourse skills" (p. 84).

Cognitive-Linguistic Factors.   Myklebust (1964) argued that loss of sensation associated with hearing impairment could impede both the development of language and the development of cognition. He based his argument on a hierarchy of processing that proceeded from lower to higher levels: sensation, perception, imagery, symbolization, and conceptualization. The loss of auditory sensation, Myklebust hypothesized, would result in an organismic shift, in which the loss of auditory sensation (and greater reliance on visual sensation) would impair auditory-linguistic symbolization, and that limitation would, in turn, impair the ability of people with hearing impairments to think abstractly.

Some disagreed with Myklebust's theory and designed studies showing few differences between the cognitive abilities of deaf and normal-hearing individuals (Furth, 1966; Vernon, 1969). For example, based on a study measuring performance on a set of Piagetian tasks, Furth concluded that deaf children's ideas about the world develop in the same sequence as those of children with normal hearing, and with only slight delay (particularly in stages of concrete and formal operations). Furth reasoned that problems demonstrated by children with hearing impairment on IQ tests represented results of communicative difficulties rather than low intelligence.

Others have suggested that the language limitations associated with hearing impairment do interfere with later stages of cognitive development, particularly for performing cognitive activities in which mental manipulation of linguistic symbols is critical (Quigley & Paul, 1984; H. S. Schlesinger & Meadow, 1972). When J. M.

Davis and colleagues (1986) measured a variety of language, intellectual, social, and academic skills, they found that performance IQ was not a good predictor of overall educational success by hearing impaired children (although it was correlated significantly to both reasoning and math scores). The best predictor of concurrent academic achievement in that study was a verbal IQ score, followed by vocabulary scores earned on the Peabody Picture Vocabulary Test—Revised (PPVT-R) (L. M. Dunn & Dunn, 1981).

Somewhat different results were found in a study of 6- to 10-year-old children who were learning a system of signed English (Watson, Sullivan, Moeller, & Jensen, 1982). In this case, nonverbal intelligence and visual memory skills were the best predictors of language performance. In fact, the average correlation of .45 between nonverbal IQ and language scores for the hearing impaired children in this study was only slightly lower than the .50 correlation reported for intelligence and measure of school achievement for normal-hearing children (Matarazzo, 1972). Watson and colleagues concluded that nonverbal intelligence is a factor in helping children acquire language (particularly a visually based system such as signed English). Studies like this contribute to growing evidence that language and cognition are closely related but not totally interdependent.

Social Interaction Factors.   Although hearing loss is generally recognized as affecting the social interactions of children with their parents, peers, and important others, the degree of hearing loss is not a particularly good predictor of problems in the psychosocial realm. This was one of the conclusions of the study by J. M. Davis and colleagues (1986) in which they assessed 45 children in a variety of areas who ranged in age from 5 to 18 years and had mild-to-moderate hearing losses. Although degree of hearing loss was not a good predictor of psychosocial difficulty, data from personality inventories administered to these youngsters did suggest that they were more likely than their normal hearing peers to show certain social interaction and self-concept problems, including aggressive tendencies and a tendency to express more physical complaints. In addition, parent observations indicated that a higher than average proportion of the hearing impaired children demonstrated significant behavior difficulties, especially school problems involving isolation and adjustment to school (see Personal Reflection 4.7)

PERSONAL REFLECTION 4.7 _____

"I don't have very many friends. Oh, people say, 'Hi, Kris, Hi Kris,' but only 'Hi Kris,' never anything–you know–go out for lunch or go out on dates or anything like that. The only friends I almost have are my teachers and my counselors."

Kris, an adolescent with hearing impairment interviewed by J. M. Davis and colleagues (1986) during their study of the effects of mild-to-moderate hearing impairments on language, educational, and psychosocial behavior in children.

Visual Impairment

Diagnosing Visual Impairment and Related Communication Problems.

Low-vision specialists, ophthalmologists, and other medical and educational professionals are typically involved in making a primary diagnosis of visual impairment. When the loss of vision is significant enough to make it difficult for a child to use visual input in the complex process of language acquisition, language specialists may be consulted, but this is not routine.

Complete loss of vision, with no light perception, is rare; rather, "the vast majority of 'blind' individuals experience and utilize some visual information, though this may be limited to sensing direct light" (Dunlea, 1989, p. 7). Measurements of vision address two primary qualities: (1) the sharpness of visual perception and (2) the integrity of the visual pathway, which is evaluated in terms of the visual field. The generally accepted legal criterion for blindness in the United States is that "central visual acuity in the better eye with best correction be no more than 20/200 Snellen" (Dunlea, 1989, p. 7). A person with this diagnosis can identify letters on the Snellen chart at 20 feet, similar to the way a person with average vision can identify them at 200 feet. Severe visual field defects, affecting the central field, the periphery, or both, are also used to classify people as legally blind. Definitions of blindness vary around the world. Dunlea noted that the World Health Organization listed 65 different definitions of blindness and visual impairment, with the result that "cross-cultural comparisons of development in blind children, as well as more epidemiological studies, are not reliable" (p. 8).

The incidence of congenital legal blindness in the United States has remained fairly constant at 14.9 per 100,000 live births since the 1950s (Dunlea, 1989). Dunlea reported that the prevalence of childhood blindness, often co-occurring with other disabilities, has increased as advances in pediatric care have allowed more children to survive. In the late 1940s and 1950s, the incidence of "congenital" blindness rose to 8 per 10,000 births because of high rates of retrolental fibroplasia (RLF). Although classified as congenital blindness, RLF actually occurs during the neonatal period when premature infants receive excessive oxygen in incubators. As a result, an opaque fibrous membrane forms over the retina, causing damage that is "severe and irreversible" (p. 8). RLF now occurs less frequently, but it continues to account for approximately 4% of congenital impairments.

When language specialists are consulted to assess the language and communication abilities of children with low vision or blindness, it is important to collaborate with low-vision specialists to adapt formal test materials so they are accessible for a particular child. Most standardized tests are inappropriate for children who are blind because of their reliance on visual stimuli. It may be possible to adapt stimuli by making them larger and adjusting lighting and placement for children with some residual vision, but standardized scoring methods cannot be used when such changes are made. It is more likely that informal language sampling techniques and observation of the child in naturalistic communicative situations will be helpful to teams concerned about a blind child's communicative development. While keeping an open mind, the language specialist may wish to focus the assessment on issues of language acquisition that are most likely to be affected by the loss of visual input.

When a child has total or near-total blindness from the earliest stages of development, three kinds of interrelated influences tend to show up in the areas of language and communication. First, a major avenue through which the child learns about the world, forms semantic concepts, and acquires **lexical knowledge** is lost (Dunlea, 1989). Katherine Nelson (1985) has pointed out that since the time of Augustine, the classic description of word learning has been that of a tutor pointing to objects while uttering their names. Although K. Nelson (1985) notes that referential–perceptual theories are not the only way, nor the most complete way, to explain the acquisition of first-word meanings, evidence has shown that children learn many new words in this way, including from photographs or other pictorial forms (Ninio, 1983; Ninio & Bruner, 1978).

Second, certain language abilities seem to be more sensitive than others to acquisition without sight. **Pro-**

noun use has been shown to be especially difficult for blind children to master (Erin, 1990; Fay, 1973; Fraiberg, 1977; House & House, 1989; Keeler, 1958). Many children with visual impairments are observed to refer to themselves by name or as "you," and, more rarely, to call others "I" or "me." Erin (1990) also found reductions in mean length of utterance and variety of sentence types. Visually impaired children also talked less about past and future events and used language less to initiate imaginative play.

The third area in which children without sight are at risk is in the area of **pragmatics.** Many of the nonverbal cues for turn taking and other aspects of conversational interaction are unavailable to children who have low vision. Limited opportunities to learn about language and communication through play and other natural interactions also may influence language learning negatively. For example, Erin (1990) hypothesized that the high frequency of questions and imperatives observed among the visually impaired children she studied could be explained by their awareness that others have more access to information from the environment. This could increase their tendency to use language to gather information and to confirm impressions about physical factors in the environment.

Other minor vision problems identified during elementary school years are not insignificant, especially because they may influence written language acquisition and the processing of academic language in school. On the other hand, when recognized, minor losses in visual acuity can be easily compensated by the fitting of glasses. Such problems are not generally associated with delays in language acquisition.

Subtypes of Visual Impairment. Children with low vision, like all children, are individuals, with highly individual sets of strengths and needs. Attempts to relate language acquisition needs to degree of visual impairment have been only partially successful.

Both age of onset and degree of loss influence the effect of visual impairment on language acquisition. Complete congenital blindness is more likely to influence language acquisition significantly than is partial blindness. Erin (1990) compared the language characteristics of four children who were **blind** (light perception or less), four who had **low vision** (legally blind but able to respond to a flashlight at 15 feet), and four who were **sighted** (none with other disabling conditions).

She found contrasts in several areas (syntactic complexity, pronoun usage, and language functions) between the two groups of visually impaired children and the sighted children. The differences were more prominent, however, in the samples of the blind children than the low-vision children.

Language Characteristics Associated with Visual Impairment. Loss of vision does not have the same devastating effect on language acquisition as loss of hearing. Because language is learned primarily through auditory–vocal modalities, vision is less critical than hearing to language acquisition. Vision, of course, plays a vital role in learning to read in the usual way, but the relative ease with which blind children learn braille when they have no concomitant cognitive impairments supports the contention that reading is far more a linguistic-communicative act than a visual one. Adaptive technology, such as talking computers and print-scanning devices, can transform printed or computer text into spoken output so that blind children can have more independent access for using language in varied modalities.

This is not to say that vision is unimportant to the process of normal language acquisition and social communicative development. The earliest form of communication between neonates and their mothers is visual. In fact, advocates of natural childbirth emphasize the importance of allowing new mothers to gaze into the eyes of their newborns as part of the bonding process. Furthermore, as considered later in the sections on child abuse and neglect, disruptions of normal patterns of gaze and eye contact tend to accompany maladaptive child-rearing patterns, perhaps in interactive patterns of cyclical cause and effect (see Personal Reflection 4.8).

If vision is so important, what is the effect of visual loss on the language acquisition process? Erin (1990) refuted the "myth of compensatory ability" (p. 181), which suggests that blind or visually impaired children must have exceptional abilities in audition and language production as automatic compensations for their losses of vision. Erin's own research results were consistent with others' in confirming risks for delay in language use in specific areas among children with visual impairments (Fraiberg, 1977, 1979; Kekelis & Anderson, 1984; Mills, 1983; D. H. Warren, 1984).

Hypotheses for explaining such pronominal problems exhibited by blind children as with the *I–you* distinction vary from psychodynamic to psycholinguistic.

PERSONAL REFLECTION 4.8 _____

"Sometimes when we have professional visitors at the project to look at films or videotapes, I steal glances at their faces when the child is seen on the screen. With sighted children it is always interesting to see the resonance of mood on the viewer's face. We smile when the baby on the film smiles; we are sober when the baby is distressed. We laugh sympathetically when the baby looks indignant at the examiner's sneakiness. We frown in concentration as the baby frowns when the toy disappears. When he drops a toy, we look below the movie screen to help him find it.

"But the blind baby on the screen does not elicit these spontaneous moods in the visitor. Typically, the visitor's face remains solemn. This is partly a reaction to blindness itself. But it is also something else. There is a large vocabulary of expressive behavior that one does not see in a blind baby at all. The absence of differentiated signs on the baby's face is mirrored in the face of the observer."

Selma Fraiberg (1979, p. 151), University of Michigan Medical School, writing about the sociolinguistic side effects when infants are unable to see.

Charney (1980) proposed that pronoun reversals can be directly explained by cognitive or linguistic deficits taking two forms: (1) either reversals are a direct by-product of echolalia and attributed to linguistic deficits, or (2) reversals and echolalia are both caused by a common cognitive deficit.

Schiff-Myers (1983) lent support to the linguistic-base hypothesis when she analyzed the pronoun reversals produced by her own normally developing daughter between 21 and 25 months and found: (1) a tendency to imitate utterances of others (possibly similar to the gestalt language acquisition style discussed in the section on autism); (2) the early production of *you* as a productive linguistic form; and (3) a tendency to use a pronoun rather than a noun for self-reference. Other attempts to explain pronoun reversal have ranged from hypotheses about blind children's need for an extended learning period to master self-representation (Erin, 1990) to more specific sensory input problems in matching the spoken *I* or *you* with the person addressed when that person cannot be seen (D. H. Warren, 1984).

House and House (1989) noted that loss of vision represents the loss of the sensory organ most uniquely

adapted for synthesis of all perceptions and the data of self. They studied children who had multiple disabilities along with blindness, had an MLU of 1.0 to 1.8, and lived in a residential setting. The researchers observed that many staff members addressed the blind children with their proper names in all activities and used the pronouns *I* and *you* infrequently. Perhaps variation in opportunity to learn pronominal reference plays a significant role in its developmental delay for some blind children.

Fraiberg (1979) noted that modifications in social interactions are to be expected when infants are without sight. She commented that, "What we miss in the blind baby, apart from the eyes that do not see, is the vocabulary of signs and signals that provides the most elementary and vital sense of discourse long before words have meaning" (p. 152). On the other hand, the usual milestones of human attachment may be observed among blind infants during the first two years of life. At this stage, they are like their sighted peers in preferences for their mothers and in differential smiling and vocalization, manual tactile seeking, embracing, and spontaneous gestures of affection and comfort seeking. From 7 to 15 months of age, blind toddlers, like sighted ones, begin to avoid and manifest stress reactions to strangers and reject them as interaction partners. During the second year, blind children's anxiety at separation and comfort at reunion provide evidence that the blind baby values the mother as an indispensable human partner.

Deaf-Blindness

Diagnosing Deaf-Blindness and Related Problems.
Children with significant loss of both their distance learning senses, hearing and vision, have particularly complex needs. As described by McInnes and Treffry (1982):

> The deaf-blind child is not a deaf child who cannot see or a blind child who cannot hear. The problem is not an additive one of deafness plus blindness. Nor is it solely one of communication or perception. It encompasses all these things and more. The deaf-blind are multisensory deprived: *they are unable to utilize their distance sense of vision and hearing to receive non-distorted information. Their problem is complex.* (p. 2)

The last sentence in this quotation may seem like a gross understatement to professionals who face the task of providing meaningful diagnostic information about the communicative abilities and needs of individuals with both hearing and visual impairments. Attempts to assess any of the three—hearing, vision, or communication—in isolation will be impeded by the complexities of their interactive effects. Although audiologists may use brain stem audiometry and other nonparticipatory assessment techniques to provide objective evidence of a child's ability to hear, and ophthalmologists may be able to provide objective evidence of a child's ability to see, understanding how the child actually uses the senses to learn and communicate may require more contextualized and dynamic assessment efforts.

Many children who are called "deaf-blind" have useful residual vision and/or hearing. "However, they must be taught to use this potential and to integrate sensory input from the damaged distance senses with past experience and input from other senses" (McInnes & Treffry, 1982, pp. 2–3). Only by observing an individual's use of varied sources of input, through extended opportunities with appropriate supports, can a diagnostic team arrive at even a semiaccurate assessment of an individual's learning potential to use various input modes and communicative systems, including fingerspelling, sign, and braille.

Before one can even begin to assess true learning potential, it is necessary to work around multiple barriers at a very basic level. I remember discovering some of the barriers through experience with a 7-year-old named Cathy, who attended our university clinic. My notes about Cathy (based on her interactions with graduate student clinician Linda Gast) are interspersed with the factors listed by McInnes and Treffry (1982, p. 2) for diagnostic and intervention teams to consider. Such teams provide better services when they recognize that persons with multisensory deprivation: (1) lack the ability to communicate with their environment in a meaningful way [for Cathy, it was necessary to use some of the strategies of a coactive movement program, described in Chapter 13, before she permitted much human contact from anyone other than her mother and was willing to use her sense of touch to explore her environment]; (2) have a distorted perception of the world [Cathy sat on her hands at the beginning of our interactions; we gently helped her pull them out and begin to explore the world]; (3) lack the ability to anticipate future events or the results of their actions [to teach cause-effect concepts, we started with familiar family routines, including a tickle game and horsey rides, then added a swinging game contingent on Cathy's "whoop," before

teaching signs for *drink, horse,* and *on,* which she used to make requests and to relate switch-activation to feeling the output of a tape recorder or hair dryer]; (4) are deprived of many of the most basic extrinsic motivations [it took a lot of exploring to find the things that Cathy enjoyed and to extend her repertoire of pleasurable events to include patting a particular ball, feeling a tape recorder playing loud rock music, and enjoying the hair dryer breeze]; (5) have medical problems that lead to serious developmental lags [we were lucky not to have these during our interactions with Cathy]; (6) are mislabeled as retarded or emotionally disturbed [we did not feel qualified to draw any conclusions about basic intelligence, we just kept trying to expand Cathy's conceptual and social-interactive boundaries]; (7) are forced to develop unique learning styles to compensate for their multiple disabilities [we tried to discover and respect Cathy's best natural modes of learning while assisting her to extend her options and communicate in ways that others could understand]; and (8) have extreme difficulty in establishing and maintaining interpersonal relationships [this was the ultimate goal; many people in Cathy's world learned to understand her requests for drink and rocking horse rides].

Subtypes of Deaf-Blindness. The category of individuals with multisensory impairment is so diverse as to make subtyping inappropriate. As Gee (1995) commented, "Persons with deaf-blindness are a highly diverse group of individuals with unique learning characteristics and a wide range of capabilities" (p. 371).

The two major causes of deaf-blindness are maternal rubella (now reduced by modern immunization efforts) and Usher's syndrome (McInnes & Treffry, 1982). **Rubella syndrome** is a congenital syndrome caused by intrauterine rubella infection that is characterized by cataracts, cardiac anomalies, deafness, and other neurological impairments. **Usher's syndrome** is "a disease transmitted genetically by an autosomal recessive gene which involves a profound congenital hearing loss and a progressive loss of vision due to retinitis pigmentosa" (p. 277). Its effects make genetic studies a priority and consideration of potential change over time a key to providing appropriate intervention services.

Language Characteristics Associated with Deaf-Blindness. Multisensory deprivation poses huge challenges to the development of communication and the formation of perceptions and concepts, but they are not insurmountable. To understand the communication possibilities for persons with deaf-blindness, it is critical to broaden the concept beyond reception and expression of oral or written language. In this broader view, "Communication can be summed up as our attempts to obtain information from and impose order upon the world around us" (McInnes & Treffry, 1982, p. 58). Box 4.11 summarizes primary communication options for individuals who are deaf-blind.

Box 4.11 _____

Types of Communication Used by Persons with Deaf-Blindness
(Summarized from a Longer Outline by McInnes & Treffry, 1982, pp. 58–61, with Additions)

UNAIDED TECHNIQUES (USED WITHOUT EXTERNAL DEVICES)

1. **Signal.** The earliest communicative interactions may involve simple body signals (e.g., to *stop* or *start* an activity), such as co-active rocking with reciprocal cues to start and stop, or even joining with the individual in self-stimulatory finger flicking before signaling *stop* through body movement.
2. **Gestures.** Conventional communicative gestures, such as waving *hi* and *bye* or shaking the head *yes* and *no,* allow individuals with deaf-blindness to establish some communicative control.
3. **Class Cues.** Class cues are used to indicate a set of coming actions so the child may begin to anticipate events. For example, a mother may use contact with a fluffy bathtowel in the living room to indicate that "It is time for your bath; let's go."
4. **Gross Signs.** Some of the conventional signs of manual communication systems will be unperceivable by individuals with deaf-blindness so it is perfectly acceptable to adapt them. To learn expressive signs, children must be manipulated through them. Efforts can begin at a gross level and be gradually shaped into finer discriminations.
5. **Fingerspelling.** Both two-hand and one-hand methods may be used, and neither method can be determined "best" for a particular child without performing individualized assessment. McInnes and Treffry reported "We have used both methods successfully with many children" (p. 59). Fingerspelling instruction may start by manipulating fingers in playful interactive finger games. Then fingers may be shaped into letters of the alphabet as name signs. The introduction of formal fingerspelling parallels early reading instruction, beginning by labeling familiar objects and actions within meaningful routines.

6. **Speech.** Vocal communication, including speech, may be a possibility for some children. McInnes and Treffry caution that children with some residual hearing and/or vision may yet find eye contact difficult, as individuals with autism do, and may have exaggerated difficulty acquiring spoken language. McInnes and Treffry emphasize that speech versus sign is not an either/or decision.
7. **Print-Braille.** Decisions to introduce a child to print and/or braille depend on multiple factors, including the child's general level of functioning, residual vision, stability of the eye condition, and ability to receive and integrate tactile information for making fine discriminations necessary to read braille.

AIDED TECHNIQUES (USED WITH HIGH OR LOW TECHNOLOGICAL SUPPORTS)

1. **Opticon.** This is an electronic device that changes print into a tactile representation. It is a tool that may assist higher functioning deaf-blind students who need braille.
2. **Teletouch.** This device enhances possibilities to communicate with sighted individuals, who type their messages into the device using a standard keyboard, so that each letter is reproduced as a raised dot braille cell.
3. **Electronic and nonelectronic communication boards and devices.** Pictures or symbols can be marked with raised braille labels or more concrete tactile identifiers and used for both receptive and expressive communication.
4. **Typing and Writing.** Individuals who can learn to type, or at least to write their names, will have expanded communicative opportunities that can be supported both with standard computers and with dedicated augmentative communication devices.

Helping children with deaf-blindness extend their academic and social interaction options may happen best in inclusive educational settings (Haring & Romer, 1995). Gee (1995) noted how the diversity among children with deaf-blindness parallels the diversity among the general student population:

> *Persons with deaf-blindness have a variety of interests, strengths, and talents. Each has a different family, different background, and different personality. When teaching, working or playing with an individual with deaf-blindness, the same bottom-line principles that are adhered to with other students, co-workers, and friends should also be followed, namely: (1) respect for the individual (and his or her choices and learning styles), (2) flexibility, and (3) cooperation. (p. 371)*

Physical Impairment and Speech Motor Control

Diagnosing Physical Impairment and Speech Motor Control Impairment.   An estimated 1,225,000 children in the United States are nonspeaking or severely speech impaired as a result of neurological, physical, or psychological disabilities (D. Yoder, 1980). For many of these children, physical impairment co-occurs with other risk factors, such as cognitive impairment or sensory loss, conditions that may themselves interfere with normal language acquisition. In cases of mixed causes, it is difficult to differentiate the influence of the motor impairment from other factors. Some children, however, exhibit a severe physical impairment, such as cerebral palsy, which greatly impedes their ability to speak but leaves their cognitive and linguistic systems relatively intact. What kinds of variations in language acquisition can be expected for such children?

Returning to the discussions about the relative separability of language, speech, and communication from Chapter 2, children can have normal potential for learning language in the presence of severe deficits of motor functioning that prevent them from acquiring intelligible speech. Limited information is available about the developmental process in such cases, however. In the past, the language development of children with severe motor impairments was rarely studied in detail because spontaneous language sampling and analysis, the usual modes of investigation, were not available. Even now, when AAC techniques are more likely to be encouraged during early language acquisition, the language expression of nonspeaking children is heavily constrained by the vocabulary and phrases that someone else has programmed into their communication devices.

Thus, it is difficult to obtain a true picture of what nonspeaking children can do with language. Language expression is confounded (Nelson, 1992a), and language comprehension tends to be overestimated (Roth & Cassatt-James, 1989). Efforts have been made to study pragmatic interaction problems (see Personal Reflection 4.9), such as passivity in conversation, but methodological problems abound in the research, and more investigation is needed in all areas of language acquisition with these children (Calculator, 1988; Light, 1988; Sutton, 1989).

Assessments of speech motor control and associated language problems are designed to differentially diagnose subtypes considered in the next section. Assessment should encompass at least four systems: (1) motor, (2) motor speech, (3) articulation/phonological, and (4) language. Assessment of the **motor system** includes examination of oral structure and function, reflexes, lingual/labial–mandibular dependency, volitional oral

---

PERSONAL REFLECTION 4.9 _____

"Recently, a language-delayed child with whom I was working vocalized and then pointed to an object in my presence. Quite confident that I understood what she wanted, I reached for the object in question, only to be stopped by her teacher who instructed both of us that she could 'point to what she wants on her communication board.' A few moments later, I was visiting with a preschool child who made a request by pointing to a pictographic symbol and was told that she needed to 'use her voice and ask for it first.' At least one result of both interactions was considerable frustration on the part of both myself and the children. The tendency to assume such narrow, 'either/or,' approaches toward communication options for children is perhaps particularly unfortunate in that it deviates so markedly from the way in which nondisabled children acquire the ability to communicate."

David R. Beukelman (1987, p. 95), University of Nebraska-Lincoln, writing about the choices made for children with communicative disorders in situations where most individuals have the opportunity to make choices for themselves.

movements (e.g., "show me how you blow"), and volitional limb movements. Assessment of the **motor speech system** includes measurement of speech diadochokinesis (rapid syllable production), and observation of basic performance in areas of prosody, fluency, nasality, voice, and maximum performance speech production tasks. Assessment of the **articulation/phonological system** includes standardized articulation tests, phonological analysis, changes with levels of complexity, and parallels with written language deficits. Assessment of the **language system** involves formal and informal measurement of comprehension and expression.

Subtypes of Physical and Speech Motor Control Impairment. Physical impairment can differ widely in degree and kind, based on such factors as varied cause and time of onset. It is beyond the scope of this chapter to consider all of the factors that can lead children to have difficulty acquiring motor control of the speech mechanism (e.g., cerebral palsy comprises several subtypes, and acquired brain injuries can result in others) or to have structural defects of the oral mechanism (e.g., burns and oral-facial anomalies). It is important, however, to differentiate the kinds of oral-motor impairment associated with symptoms of **dysarthria** from those associated with symptoms of oral-motor and **speech apraxia.**

As discussed earlier in this chapter, a subgroup of the phonologic-syntactic syndrome described by Rapin and Allen (1983) was one in which an expressive disorder seems to predominate, accompanied by additional signs of neurological oromotor dysfunction, including signs of mild **dysarthria** (demonstrated by drooling and a history of difficulty in sucking, chewing, and swallowing) or signs of **oral-motor apraxia** (demonstrated by difficulty in imitating precise movements of the tongue, lips, and jaw).

The subcategory of **developmental apraxia of speech** (Crary, 1993; Hall, Jordan, & Robin, 1993; J. C. Rosenbek & Wertz, 1972; Yoss & Darley, 1974) is controversial. It has also been called **childhood verbal apraxia** (Chappel, 1973) and **developmental verbal dyspraxia** (Aram & Nation, 1982; Crary, 1984). The controversy revolves around whether children with specific, severe expressive speech and language delay constitute a legitimate category based on deficits in motor planning that affect primarily the operation of the speech

mechanism (Crary, 1993; Hall et al., 1993), or whether the observed delays in speech production represent central problems in the phonological conceptualization of sound classes and combinations (Aram, 1984).

The primary characteristics used in diagnosing children with developmental verbal apraxia are outlined in Box 4.12. It is noteworthy that these characteristics describe speech behavior and generally fail to identify any symptoms of expressive language, except to note its significant delay relative to superior receptive language abilities. In actual practice, many children with signs of oral-motor and speech apraxia also appear to have specific language delays of probable central origin. Additionally, although dysarthria typically involves evidence of mild paresis and difficulty with such reflexive behaviors as swallowing, Rosenbek and Wertz (1972) found that 11 of 50 children with apraxia also demonstrated excessive drooling. Differential diagnosis is not a precise science. In addition, the subtypes of **dysarthria** (either as a component of cerebral palsy or as a focal problem) and **developmental apraxia of speech,** need to be differentiated from **functional articulation disorders,** and **receptive–expressive language disorders** with phonological components.

Language Characteristics Associated with Physical and Speech Motor Control Impairment. Without referring to developmental verbal apraxia (or even testing for it directly), Rescorla and Manzella (1990) reported on a group of 20 toddlers with normal cognitive ability and good receptive language at age 2 years, whom they followed until the age of 3. They identified this group of children as having specific expressive language delay (SELD). When they compared the group with 10 matched toddlers, the children with SELD continued to be significantly delayed with respect to MLU, use of obligatory morphemes, and grammatical development relative to the comparison children. Because their phonological and oral-motor skills were not reported, it is difficult to know whether any or all of these children might have exhibited signs of verbal apraxia. When individuals with physical impairments become literate, it is somewhat easier to assess their spontaneous expressive language abilities by asking them to write, particularly if they have sufficient motor control to operate a typewriter or computer keyboard (perhaps with scanning or Morse code adaptation). Of course, if they have diffi-

Box 4.12 _____

The Most Common Features in Developmental Apraxia of Speech
(Based on Summaries from Crary, 1993; Hall, Jordan, & Robin, 1993;
J. C. Rosenbek & Wertz, 1972; and Yoss & Darley, 1974)

1. **Neurological findings** of dyspraxia may be generalized, possibly including difficulty in fine motor coordination, gait, and alternating motion rates of the tongue and extremities. The condition may occur in isolation or in combination with aphasia and/or dysarthria. Oral nonverbal apraxia, often, but not always, accompanies apraxia of speech.
2. **Speech development** is delayed or deviant, with receptive abilities markedly superior to expressive ones.
3. **Repetition (imitation) tasks** may result in two- and three-feature articulation errors (e.g., /p/ for /m/ is an error in nasality, voicing, and continuancy). Groping trial-and-error behaviors may appear in the form of sound prolongations, repetitions, or silent posturing, preceding or interrupting the imitative utterances. Single-word productions on articulation tests may be surprisingly good, considering the unintelligibility of connected speech.
4. **Spontaneous speech** includes a predominance of omission errors but also evidence of other immature phonological processes (and phonetic distortions). Misarticulations include vowels as well as consonants. Errors vary with the complexity of articulatory adjustment, with more frequent errors on fricatives, affricatives, and consonant clusters, and on longer words. Metathetic errors (transpositions of sounds and syllables) and phonetic transition problems are frequent.
5. **Rate and prosody** are affected in spontaneous speaking and on diadochokinetic tasks (e.g., "puhtuhkuh"). Words and syllables are produced with slowed rate, even stress, and even spacing, perhaps in compensation for the problem.

---

culty learning to read and write, we are back to the problem of knowing whether their difficulties are related to an input/output deficit, a basic language deficit, a lack of experience (because of their motor impairments) in using formalized written language, a more isolated reading and/or writing disorder, or some other factor(s).

Some researchers have attempted to investigate the relationships of written language acquisition to frank neurological deficits. Seidel, Chadwick, and Rutter (1975) found a higher incidence of reading problems in children with perinatal brain injury than in the normally developing population. Mattis, French, and Rapin (1975) studied reading disorder subtypes by comparing the abilities of children with diagnosed neurological impairments with and without reading disabilities with those of dyslexic children (without overt neurological disorder) on several tasks. They found no difference in the types of reading disability among neurologically impaired and dyslexic children, and they also found neurologically impaired children who were good readers and showed no signs of dyslexia.

Mattis (1978) noted that many symptoms frequently associated with dyslexia (e.g., dyscoordination, dysarthria, and deficits in drawing and in puzzle and block construction) could be observed in neurologically impaired children who were good readers. If such is the case, Mattis hypothesized, then these underlying skills could not be essential to the reading process. Apparently, input/output modes used in reading and writing can vary without interfering with the central aspect of the written language processing—that is, the representation of meaning. It is recognition of the meaningfulness of orthography that is the essence of written language processing, not the manner in which stimuli and products are received or produced. It is only necessary that individuals have at least one mode of input and output available, not that they necessarily must be able to read or write in the most conventional ways (e.g., braille and AAC users).

Dorman (1987) found results that contrasted somewhat with those of Mattis (1978) regarding individuals with diagnosed neurological impairments. Dorman studied neurologically impaired students with cerebral palsy (n = 23), spina bifida (n = 9), neuromuscular impairments (n = 16), and head injury (n = 2), divided almost equally into reading disabled and nonreading disabled subgroups. Dorman found that 19 of the 23 students with cerebral palsy had symptoms of visual-spatial-perceptual disorder, whether or not they had reading impairments. When neurologically impaired individuals with visual-spatial-perceptual disorder did have reading problems, they were likely also to evidence signs of anomic language disorder, supporting the contention that language skills play a more central role in written language processing than visual-spatial-perceptual skills.

A problem for clinicians who might wish to draw on Dorman's (1987) data is that Dorman did not specify whether any of the subjects with cerebral palsy could be classified as nonspeaking. It might be assumed that they were not, because nonspeaking children would have difficulty responding to the read-aloud tasks used in Dorman's study. Many questions remain about the influence of inability to produce spoken language on written language processing. In children with specific dyslexia, phonological processing skills seem to be important (Stanovich, 1985, 1988). Therefore, one might assume that inability to speak might influence the processes of learning to read and write, and that, in such cases, phonological decoding and encoding difficulties might be expected to show up as problems in learning to read and spell.

Not much research is available on the written language processing abilities of nonspeaking individuals (Kelford-Smith et al., 1989; Koppenhaver & Yoder, 1988). Koppenhaver and Yoder summarized existing research on literacy-learning characteristics of AAC users as showing (1) delays and difficulty in learning to read and write; (2) positive relationships between number of decoding strategies and reading achievement; (3) uneven profiles of strengths and weaknesses, with some persistent difficulties even among literate individuals and adults; and (4) reports of beneficial effects from auditory feedback during instructional activities.

One study (Kelford-Smith et al., 1989) sheds some light on the acquisition of written language by individuals with severe physical impairments. Six AAC users with cerebral palsy in Toronto were given formal instruction in reading and computerized access to independent writing relatively late in childhood (at about age 10 years for all but one subject). All of the individuals were in their late adolescence to young adulthood at the time of the study. The researchers gathered and analyzed all written language output that the individuals produced using their home computers over 4 weeks. All six of the individuals had functional writing skills at the time of the study, indicating that they had made the transition from Blissymbols (a graphic symbol system) to traditional orthography "despite decreased access to normal speech upon which written language is thought to be mapped, despite the use of telegraphic output in their face-to-face interactions, and despite the fact that they were all provided with access to microcomputer systems and introduced to literacy programs relatively late in their academic careers" (p. 122). In addition to functional written language skills, however, the six individuals also demonstrated (to varying degrees) limitations in the use of morphological endings, functors, auxiliaries, and complex sentence formulation. The authors speculated that these characteristics may have been due to language-based problems among some of the subjects, performance limitations, or monitoring and editing limitations. Chapter 13 includes suggestions for increasing the literacy opportunities for individuals with severe physical impairments.

ENVIRONMENTAL AND EMOTIONAL FACTORS

Neglect and Abuse

Diagnosing Neglect and Abuse Influences. The terms **neglect** and **abuse** refer not so much to a clinical category as to a set of environmental conditions that may affect the development of infants, toddlers, and children in profound ways.

Subtypes of Neglect and Abuse. Sparks (1989a) pointed out that definitions of abuse and neglect differ, depending on whether they have been written for legal, medical, or social purposes. She commented on the inadequacy of legal definitions, which tend to focus on deliberate intent of the abuser, rather than the effect on the child. Sparks suggested the following five types:

1. **Physical abuse:** (a) shaking, beating, or burning that results in bodily injury or death; (b) physical acts that result in lasting or permanent neurological damage.
2. **Sexual abuse:** (a) nonphysical—indecent exposure, verbal attack of a sexual nature; (b) physical—genital-oral stimulation, fondling, sexual intercourse.
3. **Emotional abuse:** (a) excessive yelling, belittling, teasing–verbal attack; (b) overt rejection of the child.
4. **Physical neglect:** (a) abandonment with no arrangement made for care; (b) inadequate supervision for long periods, disregard for potential hazards in the home; (c) failure to provide adequate nutrition, clothing, personal hygiene; (d) failure to seek needed or recommended medical care.
5. **Emotional neglect:** (a) failure to provide warmth, attention, affection, normal living experience; (b) refusal of treatment or services recommended by social or educational personnel. (Sparks, 1989a, p. 124)

Of these categories, emotional neglect and abuse is probably most difficult to identify because incidents are so common. Child maltreatment occurs on a continuum. Not all occurrences are so severe that they are obvious or justify legal intervention. Yet, professionals cannot afford to ignore the possibility that emotional neglect can influence children's development. In infants, the occurrence of emotional neglect is associated with failure-to-thrive (Sparks, 1989a). Physicians diagnose this condition when a child's weight falls below the third percentile on standard growth charts without known organic cause (Barbero, 1982). Clinical criteria used to diagnose failure-to-thrive syndrome are presented in Box 4.13.

It is difficult to obtain accurate prevalence information on conditions related to neglect, but Barbero (1982) reported that 5% of pediatric admissions in his hospital met the criterion of being below the third percentile in weight and that a significant number of these met all five of the diagnostic criteria summarized in Box 4.13. The U.S. Department of Health and Human Services (1981) reported that more than 300,000 children are abused annually, and at least twice as many are neglected. Others have pointed out that, although abuse and neglect conditions co-occur about 50% of the time (Garbarino & Crouter, 1978), they are not interchangeable (Deutsch, 1983).

Language Characteristics Associated with Neglect and Abuse.   The relevant question for language specialists out of all of these discouraging statistics is

Box 4.13 _____

Clinical Criteria Used to Diagnose Failure-to-Thrive Syndrome

1. Weight below the third percentile with subsequent weight gain in the presence of normal nurturing.
2. No evidence of systemic disease or abnormality on physical examination and laboratory investigation that explained growth failure.
3. Developmental retardation with subsequent acceleration of development following appropriate stimulation and feeding.
4. Clinical signs of deprivation that decrease in a more nurturing environment.
5. Presence of significant environmental psychosocial disruption.

Note. From "Failure-to-Thrive" by G. Barbero in *Maternal Attachment and Mothering Disorders (Pediatric Round Table: 1)* (p. 3) edited by M. H. Klaus, T. Leger, and M. A. Trause, 1982, Skillman, NJ: Johnson & Johnson Baby Products Company. © 1982 by Johnson & Johnson Baby Products Company.

whether conditions of abuse and neglect have any negative effects on the development of language. The picture is cloudy because many factors confound studies associating maltreatment of children with language development (L. Fox, Long, & Langlois, 1988; McCauley & Swisher, 1987; Sparks, 1989b). Confounding variables include socioeconomic status, general cognitive delays, predisposition to language delay related to prematurity or poor prenatal care, the tendency of children at risk for communication problems to be more difficult to parent to start with, and lack of clarity in identifying varying degrees of abuse and neglect as separate or co-occurring conditions.

Several studies, however, have produced results suggesting a significant connection between maltreatment of children and developmental delay, particularly when the maltreatment extends beyond the first year of life (R. E. Allen & Wasserman, 1985; Egeland & Sroufe, 1981). It has also been suggested that patterns of abuse and neglect tend to have differing effects on different children (Augustinos, 1987). Beyond individual differences, however, the research can be summarized as showing children who have been physically abused to be more noncompliant and aggressive, whereas children who have been both physically abused and neglected to experience more problems at school, including problems of academic performance and problems of adjustment (Lamphear, 1985).

Studies of language development have shown significant correlations between maltreatment and language delay, although cause–effect relationships have been difficult to prove. For example, in an early study, L. Bloom (1975) found that children with a "high certainty" of having been physically abused showed lower expressive language scores than a group of "low-certainty" abused children, but socioeconomic status was a confounding factor. Blager and Martin (1976) and Blager (1979) also reported finding delayed speech and language development among almost all of the abused preschoolers they evaluated. By school-age level, however, the children's abilities to produce language forms seemed to have matured, but the older children continued to have difficulty with language use. In describing the communicative styles of the older children, Blager (1979) reported that they ranged from aggressive and hostile to precociously adaptive and noted that, "Regardless of the amount of talking they did, they avoided any real contact through conversation . . . keeping themselves behind a barrage of words" (p. 991).

These studies have received considerable criticism for their lack of control groups and for inadequate description of experimental procedures (McCauley & Swisher, 1987). Better controlled studies have provided additional evidence that conditions of abuse and neglect, but particularly severe neglect, are associated with language-learning difficulties (R. E. Allen & Oliver, 1982; L. Fox et al., 1988).

A few cases of neglect have been reported in the literature that are so severe that children have been almost totally isolated from the opportunity to communicate with other people, as was Genie, discussed in Chapter 3 (Curtiss, 1977; K. Davis, 1947). In such instances, both cognitive and linguistic development are impaired, and the prognosis for language development is limited even when stimulation is normalized and language intervention is provided (Curtiss, 1977; Gleitman & Gleitman, 1981). In one case, a child was discovered who was not totally isolated but who had been cared for by her deaf-mute mother (K. Davis, 1947). Despite the lack of spoken language in her environment up to the age of 6, she apparently was subsequently able to attain a normal IQ later and adequate language functions (U. Kirk, 1983).

Causative Layering and Other Complexities. Babies who exhibit failure-to-thrive often have parents who are themselves at risk. Several identified factors may play a role in disturbances of maternal attachment (Barbero, 1982) including (1) factors in the mother's past, such as childhood loss of a parent or death of prior children; (2) pregnancy events, such as protracted emotional or physical illness, or loss of key family figures; (3) perinatal events, such as birth complications, acute illness in either mother or infant, prematurity, congenital defects, diseases, and iatrogenic or institutional disruptions; and (4) current life events, such as marital strains, mental or physical illness, alcoholism or drugs, and financial crises.

Another major risk factor is adolescent pregnancy. Osofsky (1990) noted that the proportion of teen births occurring outside of marriage has risen for both blacks and whites since 1960 from 15% to 61%. Causative layering factors associated with teenage pregnancy are poverty, membership in large or single-parent families, and having a teenage mother or poorly educated parents (see Personal Reflection 4.10).

Osofsky (1990) observed that teenage mothers interacting with their dependent infants in the first year of life were likely to encourage their infants to be independent before they were ready by expecting them to hold their own bottles, to sit up early, or to scoot after toys. They also tended to use teasing behaviors toward their infants. On the more positive side, however, many infants and their teenage mothers demonstrated considerable resiliency under remarkably difficult conditions. Infant factors that seemed to contribute positively were intelli-

---

PERSONAL REFLECTION 4.10 _____

"In considering risk and protective factors for teenage mothers and infants, we must think of vulnerability and resiliency for two children—the infant and the young mother. Two immature individuals are struggling to survive, develop, and grow. We must consider protective factors for both the infants and their young mothers, and the broader family and community factors that may impact on the dyad."

Joy D. Osofsky (1990, p. 2), Louisiana State University Medical Center, New Orleans.

gence, positive temperamental characteristics, and the ability to cooperate and nurture oneself to some extent. Maternal factors that seemed to contribute positively were emotional availability and responsivity, even if they were variable, as they often are among teenage mothers.

Behavioral and Emotional Development Problems

Diagnosing Behavioral and Emotional Development Problems.   The environmental role is less clear with problems of behavioral and emotional development than with direct evidence of maltreatment. Increasingly, as investigators appreciate the intricacies of brain–behavior relationships, behavioral or emotional abnormalities are seen to involve some central processing component (Andreasen, 1984; see Personal Reflection 4.11). Indeed, as discussed earlier in this chapter, autism is no longer categorized as a "psychotic" disorder but is considered to have a likely basis in central nervous system dysfunction. In this chapter, ADHD has also been categorized as a problem of central functioning more than as a psychiatric disorder, despite its classification with Behavioral Disorders in DSM-IV (American Psychiatric Association, 1994).

What is a "psychiatric disorder"? One way to answer this question would be simply to use the subdivisions of the DSM-IV to define the domain. As Prizant and his associates (1990) pointed out, however, because of overlap with other developmental disorders (including those specifically involving speech and language), such an approach creates confusion related to differential diagnosis of communication disorders and psychiatric disorders. Perhaps better for our purposes is a working definition provided by Baker and Cantwell (1987a) of psychiatric disorder as "a disorder of behavior, emo-

PERSONAL REFLECTION 4.11 _____

"Psychiatry is moving from the study of the 'troubled mind' to the 'broken brain.' "

Nancy C. Andreasen, M.D., Ph.D., writing in the preface to her book *The Broken Brain* (1984, p. viii), which details the "biological revolution in psychiatry."

tions or relationships that is sufficiently severe and/or sufficiently prolonged, to cause disturbance in the child or disruption of his immediate environment" (p. 193).

Subtypes of Behavioral and Emotional Development Problems.   Baker and Cantwell (1987a) differentiated two major subgroups, **behavior disorders** and **emotional disorders,** on the basis of their varied behavioral symptoms. Behavior disorders include such conditions as ADHD, oppositional disorder, and conduct disorder, all of which involve overactivity and aggression, which may disturb the environment and people nearby. Emotional disorders include disorders such as anxiety disorders, phobias, and forms of depression (including dysthymic disorder), all of which are associated with internalized and/or somatic symptoms that do not directly disrupt the environment.

Language Characteristics Associated with Behavioral and Emotional Development Problems.   The most crucial question for language specialists is whether psychiatric disorders are predictably related to speech and language disorders. Perhaps the most predictable finding is that they are related. The two diagnoses occur together with an alarming frequency that tends to increase as children with language disorders get older.

Typically, epidemiological studies have examined children referred to a center specializing in diagnosis of one type of problem for co-occurrence of the other. For example, in a study of children referred to a child psychiatry inpatient facility, Gualtieri, Koriath, Van Bourgondien, and Saleeby (1983) found that 50% of the 40 children had moderate-to-severe language disorders. Prizant and co-workers (1990) reported that 67% of the children referred to their psychiatric inpatient facility failed a speech and language screening on admission.

In other studies, children were examined for psychiatric disorders when they were originally referred to community or hospital-based clinics for speech and language diagnosis. Similar proportions of co-occurrence were found. In the largest study of this type, Baker and Cantwell (1982) found that 44% of 291 children, originally referred for speech and language problems (between the ages of almost 2 years and almost 16 years), had some psychiatric disorder as defined by the DSM-

III-R. When they followed up this same group a few years later, Baker and Cantwell (1987b) found that the prevalence rate for psychiatric disorders among the original sample of children with speech and language disorders had jumped from 44% to 60%.

Subgroup analysis from the original study (Baker & Cantwell, 1982) also yielded some interesting differences in prevalence of psychiatric disorders based on whether children had pure language disorders (i.e., involving language expression, comprehension, or processing, but with normal speech), pure speech disorders, or mixed speech and language disorders. Among these three subgroups, those with "pure" language disorders were at greatest risk for also having diagnosable psychiatric problems (95% showed evidence of psychiatric problems). Those with "pure" speech disorders were at lowest risk (29%), and those with mixed speech and language problems fell in the middle (45%). These groups, however, also differed in mean chronological age, and this may have played a role in the varied prevalence rates. The pure language disorders subgroup had a mean age of 9.3 years ($SD = 3.4$) at time of referral; the pure speech disorders subgroup, 6.0 years ($SD = 2.6$); and the speech and language disorders mixed subgroup, 4.9 years ($SD = 2.3$). One implication of these results is that children with language disorders not involving speech production are less likely to be identified until they are older and, at least at that point in their lives, are more likely to have psychiatric difficulties in addition to their language problems.

Any of these studies might be said to be confounded by the fact that they involved only children whose problems were severe enough to warrant referral. Beitchman, Nair, Clegg, and Patel (1986), in Canada, used a different design in an epidemiological study of 1,655 5-year-old kindergarten children, from the general population. They identified 11% of the children as having speech and language disorders; of these, 48.7% also had a psychiatric disorder.

All of these studies placed the rate for co-occurrence of speech and language and psychiatric disorders somewhere between 40% and 67%. When considering the data, however, it is important to remember that the diagnoses included a wide range of types and severity of psychiatric disorders. Also, the diagnosis of ADD, categorized separately in this chapter, was included within the category of psychiatric disorder for these studies. In

the study by Beitchman and colleagues (1986), emotional disturbance and ADD (diagnosed using DSM-III, American Psychiatric Association, 1980, criteria) were far more prevalent in the kindergarten children diagnosed as having speech and language impairments than in those who were not. Of these, ADD was diagnosed in 30.4% of the speech and language impaired group but only in 4.5% of the control group; emotional disturbance was diagnosed in 12.8% of the speech and language-impaired group but only 1.5% of the control group. On the other hand, conduct disorder was diagnosed with similar frequency in both groups (5.5% of the speech and language-impaired group and 6.0% of the control group).

One subgroup of children with psychiatric disorder has a problem of communication as its central symptom. **Elective mutism** is a psychiatric disorder in which a child capable of talking refuses to do so, except perhaps to a small group of intimates. Its symptoms are summarized in Box 4.14. A large proportion of children who are electively mute (as many as 80%) have demonstrated long-standing personality deviations before insidious,

---

Box 4.14 _____

Symptoms of Elective Mutism
(Based on a Summary by Norman, 1983, Who Reviewed Studies by Kolvin & Fundudis, 1981, and Rosenberg & Linblad, 1978)

1. Behavioral constriction in the presence of strangers.
2. Verbal fluency documented when at home with parents or siblings (although a history of speech problems or late talking has been reported for as high as 50% of the group).
3. No evidence of reduction of key symptoms for at least one year.
4. Personality characteristics may include extreme shyness, timidity, withdrawal, anxiety and fear, and/or willfulness and a manipulative need to control.
5. History often shows at least one extremely shy parent.
6. History often shows bed wetting and bed soiling.
7. No history of disordered thought, bizarre speech patterns, or eating or sleeping disturbance.

_____

rather than abrupt, onset of the mutism (Kolvin & Fundudis, 1981; Wolff & Barlow, 1979). Higher instances of elective mutism have also been reported in cases of child abuse (Hayden, 1980), including sexual abuse.

What Is Cause and What Is Effect?   An important question regarding the relationship between psychiatric disorders and speech and language disorders is whether the relationship is causal. Prizant and co-workers (1990) summarized four hypotheses about the relationship: (1) Psychiatric disorders lead to communication disorders; (2) communication disorders lead to psychiatric disorders; (3) a third, underlying factor leads to both psychiatric and communication disorders; and (4) transactional factors between children and their environments lead to mutual influence within a longitudinal, developmental framework.

In his work on brain chemistry as a determinant of temperament, Kagan (1989) offered evidence in support of the hypothesis that a common biological factor underlies both psychiatric and communication disorders, Kagan said that the more than 150 different chemicals in our brains (e.g., the neurotransmitters norepinephrine, serotonin, and acetylcholine; peptides; endorphins and opioids; hormones), have the potential to be combined into thousands of different "broths." Although the brain is basically the same in all cases, temperamental differences are caused by the variations in the "broths" in which the brain sits and which determine the firing patterns of its varied parts.

Two of the most dramatic temperamental types Kagan (1989) studied can be recognized for their extremes. One is a group (approximately 10% to 20% of the population) of outgoing, sociable individuals, who, Kagan reported, if raised in middle-class families are generally socialized to be leaders but, if raised in neighborhoods at risk for crime, more likely become delinquents. As infants, these are the babies who appear to be relaxed and smiling when shown a mobile or played taped speech. They have a high threshold before they experience fear and anxiety, and they are willing to take risks. In the extreme, these are the children who may later show symptoms of conduct disorder. A completely different temperament is evidenced by the approximately 10% of all children who are born with tendencies to be shy (of these, Kagan said that most will overcome the problem through environmental shaping

by the time they are 8 years old). These are the infants who become easily aroused by stimulation and who respond with high tension and crying when shown a mobile or played a tape (which Kagan speculated may be due to high arousal in the limbic lobe). Children with this temperament are unlikely to take social risks. This is the group that may be more at risk for such conditions as anxiety disorders and elective mutism.

Linguistic System Factors.   The second hypothesis outlined by Prizant and co-workers (1990) is that disorders of the linguistic system may cause psychiatric disorders. This position has been argued by Baltaxe and Simmons (1988), who noted that speech and language development is a unique feature of being human and that disorders involving such critical processes can therefore be expected to have a negative impact on the developing person. The role of linguistic factors in psychiatric disorders, however, is thought to be an uncertain contributing factor.

Incidents of elective mutism have also been cited as evidence that impairments of the linguistic system may lead to the development of psychiatric disorders (Prizant et al., 1990). In one study, Wilkins (1985) found that one third of a group of 24 children with elective mutism had histories of delayed development of speech, whereas none of the matched controls had this history.

Expressive language disorders may make it difficult for some children and adolescents to express fully their ideas, feelings, fears, and needs, and eventually this lack of communication might result in the kinds of problems that justify referral to psychiatric facilities (Gualtieri et al., 1983). Prizant and co-workers (1990) concurred that such a description fits many children and adolescents:

> *These children may appear to be immature and restless, and may develop impulsive and aggressive behaviors. Other children who present with language-processing deficits may misinterpret messages and are unable to request further information or clarification, resulting in confusion and frustration. Consequently, they may demonstrate externalizing behaviors (e.g., destroying materials, physical confrontation with peers and adults), internalizing behaviors (e.g., withdrawing from interactions, self-abusive behaviors), or both. (p. 183)*

Although both experimental and clinical evidence suggest that some children and adolescents are at increased risk for psychiatric disorders based on the problems resulting from their communication impairments, if the relationship were purely causal, the proportion of communicatively impaired children with psychiatric disorders should be even higher. A related question from the other side of this coin might be, What proportion of children with early speech and language delay grow up to be psychologically healthy adults?

Although no one (to my knowledge) has yet answered that question directly, a study at the University of Iowa (Tomblin, Freese, & Records, 1990) was designed to look at outcomes following developmental language disorder in terms of language and cognitive skills, social skills, and quality of life variables. Tomblin's group gathered follow-up data on 22 adults with clear histories of developmental language disorder and compared them with a carefully matched group (with similar ages, nonverbal intelligence scores, and socioeconomic status) of 22 young adults with normal verbal and nonverbal skills. The Iowa data showed that, although language impairment continued to be evident across most language measures, the indices of life satisfaction and general affect did not differ significantly for the two groups. This suggests that at least some individuals with language and speech disorders must be able to navigate through the years of childhood and adolescence with their self-esteem fairly intact.

Behaviorist Explanations of Behavior Problems. When "behavior disorders" become so severe as to disrupt the environment, behavioral theories are often invoked to explain them and to design strategies for modifying them. Problems with this approach revolve around the fact that consequences that would be reinforcing or punishing for most children may assume twisted meanings for children with emotional or behavioral disturbances. For example, such youngsters may appear to seek out situations or punishing consequences that most children would avoid, perhaps because they have internalized messages that they are "bad" (L. Fox et al., 1988). Communication specialists, psychologists, and social workers then need to work together to analyze the highly complex sets of variables that may influence a particular behavioral system.

The subgroup of children with psychiatric disorders most likely to come to the attention of speech–language specialists is the electively mute group. As noted, a variety of explanations have been offered when children who can talk do not. No general explanation seems to work for all cases. Individual assessment is critical because knowledge of contributing factors helps to determine which intervention approaches might work best. For example, when a child who is mute has been abused, a pediatric psychotherapeutic approach is warranted (along with legal and social service system action). In most cases, however, because elective mutism is particularly disruptive to a child's ability to participate in school, transdisciplinary teams design behaviorally oriented programs for implementation in the educational setting, perhaps in conjunction with other kinds of approaches implemented elsewhere.

A strictly behaviorist approach to intervention for elective mutism might involve strategies of (1) describing the overt symptomatology without necessarily dealing with the past, (2) reciprocal inhibition, (3) desensitization, (4) shaping, (5) successive approximations, (6) reinforcement, and (7) fading. Such an approach, however, because of its superficiality, may overlook key aspects of the problem. Some advocate a more holistic approach that uses behavioral strategies (Marx & Hillix, 1979; Norman, 1983). For example, Norman implemented a combined approach with a 5-year old girl who was electively mute and in a special-needs kindergarten class. Norman employed shaping through provision of natural and secondary reinforcement contingencies, at first when the girl spoke to her sister in the protected environment of the speech room at school, then through successive approximation and desensitization procedures in a variety of rooms, with a variety of people. Later in the program, the child's initial attempts to speak in the presence of her teacher involved mouthing words or whispering. Although Norman noted that the child was always reinforced with natural consequences for talking, comments such as "Good talking!" were avoided. The focus was kept on good communication, not speech production.

It is important to avoid techniques that seek to force the child to talk, or to withhold natural reinforcers until the child does. Power struggles that result from these kinds of behavioral techniques are, in most cases, doomed to failure (Friedman, 1980). Although elective mutism tends to be frustrating to the adults in a child's environment, it helps to remember that a child who chooses not to speak may in fact be a child who, in the circumstances of the moment, cannot speak. It is not a matter of simple choice or of finding the right reinforcer. Rather, it is a matter of establishing a supportive environment in which the child can feel safe to talk and to participate.

Social Interaction Approaches to Intervention for Emotional and Behavior Problems. By definition, psychiatric disorders involve disruptions of social interactions. Psychiatric disorders considered behavioral are overt enough to disturb the environment and people nearby, whereas those that are considered emotional involve internalized symptoms that do not directly disrupt the environment (Baker & Cantwell, 1987a). Environmental factors may cause, or at least aggravate, symptoms associated with psychiatric disorders.

A role of the communicative specialist is to help normalize communicative interactions and to contribute toward aiming the system on a new course. Communication specialists and mental health workers may be most effective when they work together for assessment and intervention with young people who find themselves in psychiatric trouble using social interaction "I'm on your side" techniques.

For example, Barbara Hoskins (a specialist in speech–language pathology and learning disabilities in private practice) evaluated the language and learning abilities of a teenage boy who had tried to take his own life (personal communication, March 19, 1991). Hoskins gathered a variety of kinds of data in evaluating this boy: formal test data documenting his language and learning disabilities as well as interview and observational data. The boy went to school every day, but did nothing—no assignments, no homework, no tests. He had simply given up on himself but was still interested enough in meeting his parents' expectations to attend school. As the boy shared this information in an interview with Hoskins, he must have expected more lectures, more fix-it plans, more adult judgments. What he got instead was a person who took his perspective and tried to see the situation through his eyes. She really listened to him and then said something like, "How awful that must have been for you! I am amazed that you stayed in that situation so long. I am not sure what we are going to do, but one thing is for certain. We cannot let you go back into a situation like that one. We will put our heads together and figure out how to make some

changes. Are you willing to work with me on this one?" He agreed.

MIXED FACTORS AND CHANGES OVER TIME

Separate discussions of separate categories imply that problems of various types occur in isolation from one another, but of course, problems can co-occur in all kinds of combinations. When they do, they bring characteristics of the separate problems but with outcomes that may appear different because of complex interactions. Part of the diagnostic process is to identify the possible involvement of multiple disabilities for individual children.

Although practitioners recognize the frequency with which varied categories of impairment overlap, federal counts, and most state counts, of children with disabilities are not set up to recognize such "duplication." Children can only be counted in one category for funding purposes. Because official agencies do not make "duplicate counts," the number of children and adolescents who have speech and language impairments in conjunction with other disabling conditions is difficult to determine. It is interesting to note, however, the changes across the four age levels in patterns of occurrence of four conditions: **learning disabilities; speech-language impairments** (called **speech impairments** in the original wording of PL 94–142); **mental retardation;** and **emotional disturbance** (shown in Figure 4.2). Rather than speech and language problems disappearing, as Figure 4.2 might imply, it is more likely that they become one more component of a complex problem.

It is also important to recognize other factors that influence interpretations of the data. For example, one reason for the apparent increase in proportions of students with mental retardation in the 18 to 21 year-old "postsecondary" category is that most students with normal learning abilities graduate by around the age of 18, so this category naturally includes a higher proportion of students with mental retardation. Another factor influencing data proportions relates to students' dropping out of school before graduation. M. M. Gerber and Levine-Donnerstein (1989) reported that the proportion of the general population leaving school over the age of 16 in that same time period was less that 16%. It was less than 22% for black, Hispanic, and low-socioeconomic status young men. In contrast, the proportions of teenagers

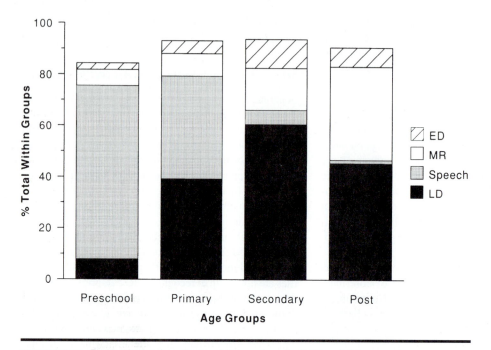

FIGURE 4.2   Proportions of students with learning disabilities (LD), speech
impairments, mental retardation (MR), and emotional disturbance (ED)
identified within four age groups.

Note. From "Educating All Children: Ten Years Later" by M. M. Gerber and D. Levine-Donnerstein,
1989, *Exceptional Children, 56,* p. 19. Copyright 1989 by The Council for Exceptional Children.
Reprinted by permission.

with disabilities dropping out during that same period was 29%. This group included 59% of the students over the age of 16 with speech impairments and almost 60% of those with emotional impairments. In contrast, only 7% of children with multiple disabilities and only 9% of students with both deafness and blindness dropped out.

PREVENTION OF CHILDHOOD
LANGUAGE DISORDERS

A discussion of causes of communicative disorders among children would be incomplete without a discussion of prevention as well. Theoreticians generally divide prevention into three types, based on the stage each attempts to address: (1) **primary prevention,** aimed at encouraging conditions to prevent problems before they start; (2) **secondary prevention,** aimed at early identification and intervention to foster conditions that will minimize long-term handicaps; and (3) **tertiary prevention,** aimed at remediating current problems and limiting further ones after they have appeared (S. E. Gerber, 1990).

Primary prevention activities attempt to ensure that children begin life with the best biological mechanisms possible. These activities include genetic counseling, avoidance of alcohol or drug consumption by mothers during pregnancy, and avoidance of other teratogens throughout life. Teratogens are environmental agents that can cause structural or functional abnormalities in a developing embryo, fetus, or child. Examples are infectious diseases, alcohol and drugs consumed by the mother, and lead in paint chips or gasoline to which the child is exposed (S. E. Gerber, 1990). Gerber has noted that the Association for Retarded Citizens—United States believes that "50 percent of mental retardation *could be prevented*" (p. xiii).

Some potential causes and contributing factors are more preventable than others. For example, a child's existing genetic and chromosomal makeup is not modifiable by current techniques. Whether it should be in the future is one of the more difficult ethical questions currently facing genetic engineers and society. Parents of a child whose language impairment is related to genetic factors should certainly have access to genetic counseling as they contemplate having additional children.

Problems stemming from substance abuse should be more preventable, but their underlying causes are also complex and not easily removed. Fetal alcohol syndrome, prenatal drug exposure, and congenital human immunodeficiency virus (HIV, the virus that causes acquired immune deficiency syndrome—AIDS), all are associated with developmental disabilities. They occur in epidemic proportions in some settings, particularly in urban centers and Native American reservations. Prevention efforts to limit causative factors like these require comprehensive social service approaches. Solutions will not be easy.

Secondary prevention, with its methods based in early identification and treatment, is the focus of Chapters 7 and 8. Secondary prevention is also an element in the treatment plans of older children and adolescents.

Tertiary prevention is a part of any attempt to intervene in a system where a problem clearly exists. Tertiary prevention efforts occur each time professionals assist in moving the process of change in a positive direction, no matter what the age of the child. It forms the primary motivation for this book.

SUMMARY

This chapter encouraged the viewpoint that not all factors that influence the course of development in children with language disorders need to be viewed as causes of the disorder. A set of categorical conditions were presented and discussed that are often associated with language disorders but not necessarily in a linear causative sense. The six theoretical perspectives introduced in Chapter 3 contribute with varying degrees of strength to

the appearance of language disorders in individual children: biological, linguistic, behavioral, information processing, cognition, and social interaction.

Also in this chapter, primary, secondary, and tertiary prevention were described. These factors can influence public policy and play a role in the modifiability of disability.

Discussions of causative factors may be fruitful, but one must also consider ways in which they may be dangerous. In particular, when parents and professionals become stuck in identifying causes that may no longer be active, they may be tempted to do so as a way of assigning blame. The statement that "Problems are not just within children, and neither are the solutions" is not intended to focus attention on determining what factors are at fault when a language-based problem is observed. Rather, it is aimed at helping those wishing to remediate the problem to look at interactions among factors internal and external to the child when designing an intervention plan. The idea is to devise a plan that can facilitate positive developmental factors, while lessening the effects of negative ones. The goals in understanding the causes of a child's difficulty in acquiring language are to reduce the child's problems with language development throughout childhood and adolescence and to reduce the probability that other children will have similar problems.

REVIEW TOPICS

- Key components of a broad definition of language disorders: heterogenous; developmental or acquired; receptive, expressive, or mixed; chronic; changeable over time; changeable relative to context, content, and learning tasks
- Four groups of causative factors, each with groups and subgroups, and information about diagnostic criteria (including cognitive referencing [also called the discrepancy criterion] and a critique of its validity; in some cases, including hypotheses about underlying causative factors), subtypes, and characteristics of language associated with the category, including discussions of evidence for different (as opposed to just delayed) language development
- Central causative factors: specific language impairment and learning disabilities, mental retardation,

autism and other pervasive developmental disorders, attention-deficit hyperactivity disorder, acquired brain injury
- Peripheral causative factors: hearing impairment, visual impairment, deaf-blindness, physical impairment and motor speech disorders
- Environmental and emotional factors: neglect and abuse (problems related to fetal alcohol syndrome [FAS] and fetal alcohol effect [FAE] are discussed in Chapter 7) and behavioral and emotional development problems
- Mixed factors, often resulting in severe communication impairments (discussed in Chapter 13)
- Prevention issues: primary, secondary, and tertiary

REVIEW QUESTIONS

1. Consider the relationships between specific language impairment and specific learning disabilities:
   a. What other labels have been applied to these and related conditions?
   b. What are some of the variables that influence children with similar profiles to be given a different label?
   c. Why is cognitive referencing a key factor in diagnosing both conditions? What factors make the practice of exclusion based on a discrepancy formula questionable (also see discussions in Chapters 3 and 6)?
   d. What inclusionary factors might be associated with specific language impairment and learning disabilities (typical characteristics involve which linguistic systems)? Why might exclusionary factors be more appropriate for research purposes than clinical and educational purposes?
   e. How great are the risks that children with specific language impairments in their preschool years will have learning disabilities and reading disorders in their school-age years?
2. What are the subtypes and differential diagnostic characteristics of:
   a. pervasive developmental disorders?
   b. mental retardation?
   c. hearing impairment?
   d. attention-deficit hyperactivity disorder?
   e. acquired brain injury?
3. What is the difference between primary, secondary, and tertiary prevention?

ACTIVITIES FOR EXTENDED THINKING

1. Some of the categories in this chapter include language impairment as a central diagnostic factor. Others have implications for affecting language development, but the diagnosis of the disorder does not depend on language factors. Provide some examples of each and discuss their distinctions.

2. In my classes, students work in pairs or groups of three. Each group selects a categorical condition in which to do additional reading and become the local "experts." Groups prepare three- to five-page handouts and duplicate sufficient copies for their classmates so that all of the students can prepare a "clinical notebook" for later quick reference. The outline for these categorical summaries is:

   PART I.
   - Definition
   - List of diagnostic characteristics
   - Discussion of associated causative factors

   PART II.
   - Appropriate assessment approaches:
        formal (suggest two measures and what particularly to look for with each)
        informal (which variables would be important to assess, given this condition?)
   - Expected variation with age
   - Expected variation with severity

   PART III.
   - Appropriate intervention methods
        Note which of the six theoretical positions addressed in Chapter 3 are most relevant for treating children who have this condition and why
        Provide detailed explanation of at least one approach
   - Note the need for any of the following:
        Augmentative and alternative communication (AAC)
        Other compensatory techniques
        Environmental modifications

   AN ANNOTATED REFERENCE LIST
        (approximately 10 sources)

5

Public Policy and Service Delivery

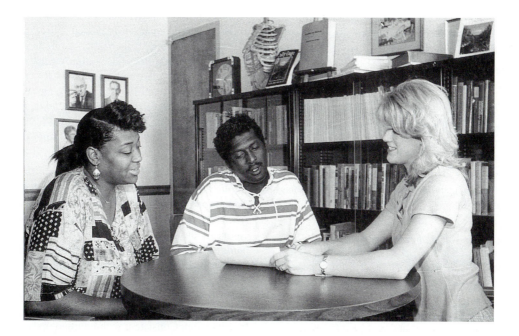

PUBLIC POLICY INFLUENCES
SERVICE DELIVERY

The systems perspective discussed in Chapter 1 can guide decisions for children with language disorders. Children function within broader systems by participating in multiple contexts that affect them and that they affect in turn. These are the recursive causative patterns of systems.

Although systems function as wholes and cannot be subdivided without losing some of their essence, they are composed of subsystems. Subsystems that exert major influences on service provision to children with language disorders operate on the levels of (1) **public policy,** including influences from federal, state, intermediate, and local levels, and (2) **service-delivery contexts,** including influences related to settings, people, and scheduling. Those two levels provide the organizational structure for this chapter.

PUBLIC POLICY INFLUENCES

Service provision to children with language disorders is constrained by public policy. This chapter begins with a consideration of public policy influences as they occur at federal, state, intermediate, and local levels.

Federal Policy

Federal policy in the United States is guided by laws passed by Congress (see Box 5.1 for a summary). Other federal influences are based on court interpretations and on position papers, newsletters, and research priorities issued by federal agencies. Such influences are considered in this section.

Section 504 of the Rehabilitation Act of 1973. Section 504 of the Rehabilitation Act of 1973 (as amended with the Rehabilitation, Comprehensive Services and Developmental Disabilities Amendments of 1978) is significant because it prohibits recipients of federal assistance from discriminating against persons on the basis of their disabilities. This piece of civil rights legislation set the stage for passage of the Education for All Handicapped Children Act in 1975.

The passage of Section 504 meant that, for the first time, children could not be excluded because of a disability from attending schools that receive federal assistance. According to the wording of the law, "No qualified handicapped person shall, on the basis of handicap, be excluded from participation in, be denied the benefits of, or otherwise be subjected to discrimination under any program or activity conducted by the agency" (28 CFR 39.130(a)).

Currently many individuals have Section 504 plans with "accommodations" to meet their special needs in schools and other agencies that receive federal support. This group includes individuals who do not qualify for special services under other programs. For example, attention-deficit hyperactivity disorder (ADHD) is not a disability addressed within the Individuals with Disabilities Education Act (IDEA), but students with ADHD can have accommodation plans under Section 504.

Public Law 94–142: The Education for All Handicapped Children Act of 1975 (Part B). The Education for All Handicapped Children Act was passed by the U.S. Congress in 1975. Often referred to as Public Law (PL) 94–142 (now known as the Individuals with Disabilities Education Act, IDEA, Part B), it is the most far-reaching piece of legislation affecting the education of children with handicaps ever passed in the United States. PL 94–142 guarantees the rights of all children in this country to a **free appropriate public education (FAPE)** in the **least restrictive environment (LRE)** (see discussion of LRE in Chapter 1). These rights are actualized by using an **Individualized Education Plan (IEP).** The rules and regulations for implementing PL 94–142 were published in the *Federal Register* on August 23, 1977. Their initial implementation was required in 1979.

Public Law 101–476: The Individuals with Disabilities Education Act of 1990 (IDEA). On October 30, 1990, when President George Bush signed into law the Education of the Handicapped Amendments of 1990, the name of the Education for All Handicapped Children Act changed to Individuals with Disabilities Education Act (IDEA) and the numbers PL 101–476 were added to the list of laws aimed at protecting the rights of all children in the United States to a free appropriate public education. Consistent with international clarification of terminology (see World Health Organization definitions of **impairment, disability,** and **handicap** in Chapter 1), the 1990 amendments changed the name of the law and specified that whenever the word *handicap* appeared in the original wording, it should be replaced with the term *disability.*

Public Law 105–17: Individuals with Disabilities Education Act Amendments of 1997 (IDEA). On June

Box 5.1

Timeline for Passage of Federal Legislation (Note That the First Number of Federal Laws Represents the Number of the Two-Year Congress That Passed It).

Years	Congress	Law
1973–75	93rd	Section 504 of the Rehabilitation Act (prohibited discrimination on the basis of disability)
1975–76	94th	PL 94–142 "The Education of All Handicapped Children Act" (Part B) (established right to Free Appropriate Public Education in Least Restrictive Environment with Individualized Education Program)
1977–78	95th	
1979–80	96th	
1981–82	97th	
1983–84	98th	
1985–86	99th	PL 99–457 "The Education of the Handicapped Act Amendments of 1986" (Part B, Preschool Grant Program; Part H, Infant and Toddler Program with IFSP, case managers)
1987–88	100th	PL 100–407 "The Technology Related Assistance for Individuals with Disabilities Act" (defined "assistive technology" to include "service" and "devices")
1989–90	101th	PL 101–476 "Education of the Handicapped Act Amendments of 1990" (renamed as Individuals with Disabilities Education Act; added autism and TBI categories; transition services)
1991–92	102nd	PL 102–119 "Individuals with Disabilities Education Act Amendments of 1991" (added assistive devices to Part H; 3- to 5-year-olds may have either IFSP or IEP; changed "case management" to "service coordination")
1993–94	103rd	
1995–96	104th	Scheduled to amend IDEA, but adjourned without reaching agreement on a bill.
1996–97	105th	PL 105–17 "Individuals with Disabilities Education Act Amendments of 1997" (reauthorized IDEA with amendments, including changing Part H to Part C)

4, 1997, President Clinton signed PL 105–17, which reauthorized IDEA. The new law preserves the rights of students with disabilities to a free and appropriate public education. Modifications include a heightened emphasis on parent involvement, revised requirements of individualized education programs in relation to the general curriculum, and a focus on collaboration between general and special educators.

Part B of IDEA. In the sections that follow, the regulations about key service delivery provisions are described with modifications in wording under PL 105–17, the "Individuals with Disabilities Education Act Amendments of 1997." Part B regulations cover procedures for service provision to school-age students with disabilities, including parent notification, comprehensive multidisciplinary evaluation and determination of disability, IEP meetings, IEP content, and periodic reevaluation.

Parent Notification. Signed, informed, parental consent is required at two points under IDEA: (1) before a preplacement evaluation and (2) "prior to conducting any reevaluation of a child with a disability, except that such informed parent consent need not be obtained if the local education agency can demonstrate that it had taken reasonable measures to obtain such consent and the child's parent has failed to respond" (Sec. 614 (c)(3)). When obtaining parental consent, school districts must provide information about parental and child rights under both IDEA and the Family Rights and Privacy Act. Those rights include parents' rights to review their children's records and to give permission before records are sent outside the district. When parents are notified, they must also be given understandable descriptions of proposed activities.

It is not easy to present so much technical information without overwhelming parents. This is true regardless of parents' backgrounds, but it is especially difficult when parents' cultural and linguistic backgrounds differ from those of school officials. To meet requirements for informing parents, districts often develop multiple-copy forms, with preprinted explanations and places for parents to sign and to check off indicating that they have been properly informed. Forms like these are designed to meet the letter of the law and to pass the inspection of state and federal officials who periodically audit districts. Districts must take care, however, that check marks in boxes do not become more important than the actual interactions with parents that lead up to them. Documentation should be used to represent important processes that have taken place; it should not become those processes.

Professionals doing assessments often have the first opportunity to develop relationships with parents. Whoever first interprets the special education process to parents should use culturally sensitive techniques. The ethnographic strategy of attempting to view the experience through the eyes of the participants can help. A face-to-face meeting is generally best for explaining the evaluation process, but if that is impossible, a telephone contact is better than a written one. The ultimate question underlying this phase of the interaction should be, "Does this parent understand what is about to happen, and the due process rights that go along with it, in his or her own terms?"

That question should be accompanied by one about the potential effects of the notification process on the family system. If you accept the premise, developed in Chapter 1, that intervention begins when the first contact with the family is made (see Personal Reflection 1.14 by Dr. Sylvia Richardson), you also ask yourself at this point, "How is this event influencing this system, and how can I enhance the chances that the influence will be positive?"

Comprehensive Evaluation. The "full and individual initial evaluation" (Sec. 614(a)(1)(A)) has two basic purposes: "(i) to determine whether a child is a child with a disability and (ii) to determine the educational needs of such child" (Sec. 614(a)(1)(B)).

Before a child is determined to have a disability, "a full and individual initial evaluation" of the child's educational needs must be conducted (Sec. 614(a)(1)(A)). The evaluation must use more than one procedure, and those procedures must be "validated for the specific purpose for which they are used" (Sec. 614(b)(3)(B)(i)). In addition, they must be "selected and administered so as not to be discriminatory on a racial or cultural basis" (Sec. 614(b)(3)(A)(i)), and they must be "provided and administered in the child's native language or other mode of communication, unless it is clearly not feasible to do so" (Sec. 614(b)(3)(A)(ii)) (see Personal Reflection 5.1).

PERSONAL REFLECTION 5.1 _____

"Since the enactment of Public Law (PL) 94–142, the Education for All Handicapped Children Act of 1975, it has been federally mandated that all test materials and procedures used for the evaluation of handicapped children be selected and administered in such a manner that they are not racially or culturally discriminatory. If this stipulation were enforced today to its fullest intent, most school systems in the United States would be in violation of the law. Eight years after PL 94–142 promised to be the salvation for all handicapped children, little has been done to improve tests and other evaluation procedures for handicapped children, especially those with communicative handicaps, to make the tests linguistically and culturally valid."

Orlando T. Taylor, Ph.D., and Kay T. Payne, Ph.D. (1983, p. 8), both of Howard University in Washington, D.C., writing in an article entitled "Culturally Valid Testing: A Proactive Approach." Their comments are still appropriate today.

Other requirements specified in the regulations passed with the 1997 Amendments to IDEA are aimed at ensuring that evaluation procedures are relevant to the child's needs. Regulations about evaluation procedures in Sec. 614(b)(2) specify that, "In conducting the evaluation, the local educational agency shall—"

(A) *use a variety of assessment tools and strategies to gather relevant functional and developmental information, including information provided by the parent, that may assist in determining whether the child is a child with a disability and the content of the child's individualized education program, including information related to enabling the child to be involved in and progress in the general curriculum or, for preschool children, to participate in appropriate activities;*

(B) *not use any single procedure as the sole criterion for determining whether a child is a child with a disability or determining an appropriate educational program for the child; and*

(C) *use technically sound instruments that may assess the relative contribution of cognitive and behavioral factors, in addition to physical or developmental factors.*

Both initial evaluation procedures and reevaluations (required once every three years) should be conducted with multiple sources of input, including a review of existing evaluation data and contributions from the child's parents and teachers. Sec. 614(c)(1) specifies that, the IEP Team "and other qualified professionals, as appropriate shall—"

(A) *review existing evaluation data on the child, including evaluations and information provided by the parents of the child, current classroom-based assessments and observations, and teacher and related services providers observation; and*

(B) *on the basis of that review, and input from the child's parents, identify what additional data, if any, are needed to determine—*

   (i) *whether the child has a particular category of disability, as described in section 602(3), or, in case of a reevaluation of a child, whether the child continues to have such a disability;*

   (ii) *the present levels of performance and educational needs of the child;*

   (iii) *whether the child needs special education and related services, or in the case of a reevaluation of a child, whether the child continues to need special education and related services; and*

   (iv) *whether any additions or modifications to the special education and related services are needed to en-*

able the child to meet the measurable annual goals set out in the individualized education program of the child and to participate, as appropriate, in the general curriculum.

Determination of Disability and Eligibility. If a child has an impairment involving language as well as speech, multiple aspects of learning are probably affected. Intact language systems are required to learn to read and write and to benefit fully from oral and written language instruction. Children whose language skills do not match the increasingly sophisticated language-processing demands of school are at serious risk for failing to learn and for developing accompanying self-esteem problems. Most children with language disorders need to be evaluated by a team of individuals who work together with the family and child to decide how best to serve the child's needs.

Deciding which children qualify to receive special services is one of the most difficult problems facing language specialists in schools. Specific rules and criteria for determining eligibility are usually established at state and local levels, as well as at federal levels. In the 1997 Amendments to IDEA, the paragraph describing "determination of eligibility" (Sec. 614(b)(4)) indicates that, "Upon completion of administration of tests and other evaluation materials—"

(A) *the determination of whether the child is a child with a disability as defined in section 602(3) shall be made by a team of qualified professionals and the parent of the child in accordance with paragraph (5); and*

(B) *a copy of the evaluation report and the documentation of determination of eligibility will be given to the parent.*

The following paragraph (Sec. 614(b)(4)) adds a "special rule for eligibility determination," which states that "In making a determination of eligibility under paragraph (4)(A), a child shall not be determined to be a child with a disability if the determinant factor for such determination is lack of instruction in reading or math or limited English proficiency."

The section that defines a child with a disability (Sec. 602(3)(A)) indicates that, "In general, the term 'child with a disability' means a child—"

   (i) *with mental retardation, hearing impairments (including deafness), speech or language impairments, visual impairments (including blindness), serious emotional disturbance (hereinafter referred to as "emotional disturbance"), orthopedic impairments,* autism, traumatic brain injury, other health impairments, or specific learning disabilities; and

(ii) who, by reason thereof, needs special education and related services.

One of the changes introduced with the Amendments of 1997, was the extension of the age period from 3 to 5 years, to an age period of "3 to 9 years," during which the term "child with disability," may "at the discretion of the State and the local education agency, include a child—"

(i) experiencing developmental delays, as defined by the State and as measured by appropriate diagnostic instruments and procedures, in one or more of the following areas: physical development, cognitive development, communication development, social or emotional development, or adaptive development; and

(ii) who, by reason thereof, needs special education and related services.

The only disability that is defined in IDEA now (and since its first appearance as PL 94–142) is specific learning disability. In the current wording of the Amendments of 1997 (Sec. 602(26)), **specific learning disability** is defined as follows:

(A) *IN GENERAL—The term "specific learning disability" means a disorder in one or more of the basic psychological processes involved in undertaking or in using language, spoken or written, which disorder shall manifest itself in imperfect ability to listen, think, speak, read, write, spell, or do mathematical calculations.*

(B) *DISORDERS INCLUDED—Such term includes such conditions as perceptual disabilities, brain injury, minimal brain dysfunction, dyslexia, and developmental aphasia.*

(C) *DISORDERS NOT INCLUDED—Such term does not include a learning problem that is primarily the result of visual, hearing, or motor disabilities, or mental retardation, or emotional disturbance, or of environmental, cultural, or economic disadvantage.*

IEP Meetings. An important vehicle of IDEA is the IEP, which is the document outlining the services to be delivered to a child. IEPs are developed at meetings so that decisions regarding the selection of a program for an individual child are not made unilaterally. After the first meeting, IEP meetings are also held at least annually (more often, if parents or school personnel request), to

review and update the child's program. Individuals who make up the IEP team include the following:

(i) *the parents of a child with a disability;*

(ii) *at least one regular education teacher of such child (if the child is, or may be, participating in the regular education environment);*

(iii) *at least one special education teacher, or where appropriate, at least one special education provider of such child;*

(iv) *a representative of the local educational agency who—*

   (I) *is qualified to provide, or supervise the provision of, specially designed instruction to meet the unique needs of children with disabilities;*

   (II) *is knowledgeable about the general curriculum; and*

   (III) *is knowledgeable about the availability of resources of the local educational agency;*

(v) *an individual who can interpret the instructional implications of evaluation results, who may be a member of the team described in clauses (ii) through (vi);*

(vi) *at the discretion of the parent or the agency, other individuals who have knowledge or special expertise regarding the child, including related services personnel as appropriate; and*

(vii) *whenever appropriate, the child with a disability. (Sec. 614(d)(1)(B))*

"Other individuals" (vi) who might attend IEP meetings may be invited either by the school district or the parents. At the first IEP meeting, it is specifically required that someone be present who can explain the evaluation results to the parents.

When you are involved in this process, it is important to remember that the familiar routine for the professionals in the IEP meeting may seem completely strange and threatening to the parents. When I was involved in many IEP meetings, I tried to interact with parents individually before the formal meetings whenever possible so that we could talk about what would happen at the meeting and the kinds of options that would be discussed. When they work well, IEP meetings offer the opportunity for cooperative goal setting and collaboration. When they do not work well, IEP meetings can be confrontational arenas of competitive goal setting at its worst.

Consider again the definition of collaborative consultation discussed in Chapter 1. It describes IEP meetings that work well, functioning as:

an interactive process that enables teams of people with diverse expertise to generate creative solutions to mutually defined problems. The outcome is enhanced, altered, and produces solutions that are different from those that the individual team members would produce independently. (Idol et al., 1986, p. 1)

Development of the IEP.   The 1997 Amendments to IDEA provide a description of the procedures to be used in developing the IEP. These procedures emphasize consideration of the child's strengths as well as needs, the child's communication needs in particular, and whether the child's needs include assistive technology devices and services. The wording in Sec. 614(d)(3) regarding development of the IEP is as follows:

(A) *IN GENERAL—In developing each child's IEP, the IEP Team, subject to subparagraph (C), shall consider—*
  (i) *the strengths of the child and the concerns of the parents for enhancing the education of their child; and*
  (ii) *the results of the initial evaluation or most recent evaluation of the child.*
(B) *CONSIDERATION OF SPECIAL FACTORS—The IEP Team shall—*
  (i) *in the case of a child whose behavior impedes his or her learning or that of others, consider, when appropriate, strategies, including positive behavioral interventions, strategies, and supports to address that behavior;*
  (ii) *in the case of a child with limited English proficiency, consider the language needs of the child as such needs related to the child's IEP;*
  (iii) *in the case of a child who is blind or visually impaired, provide for instruction in Braille and the use of Braille unless the IEP Team determines, after an evaluation of the child's reading and writing skills, needs, and appropriate reading and writing media (including an evaluation of the child's future needs for instruction in Braille or the use of Braille), that instruction in Braille or the use of Braille is not appropriate for the child;*
  (iv) *consider the communication needs of the child, and in the case of a child who is deaf or hard of hearing, consider the child's language and communication needs, opportunities for direct communications with peers and professional personnel in the child's language and communication mode, academic level, and full range of needs, including opportunities for direct instruction in the child's language and communication mode; and*

  (v) *consider whether the child requires assistive technology devices and services.*
(C) *REQUIREMENTS WITH RESPECT TO REGULAR EDUCATION TEACHER—The regular education teacher of the child, as a member of the IEP Team, shall, to the extent appropriate, participate in the development of the IEP of the child, including the determination of appropriate positive behavioral interventions and strategies and the determination of supplementary aids and services, program modifications, and support for school personnel consistent with paragraph (1)(A)(iii).*

IEP Content.   The components that must be included in a child's IEP (the acronym IEP refers to both *programs* and *plans* in the regulations for IDEA) are clearly specified in Sec. 614(a)(1)(A).

(A) *INDIVIDUALIZED EDUCATION PROGRAM—The term "individualized education program" or "IEP" means a written statement for each child with a disability that is developed, reviewed, and revised in accordance with this section and that includes—*
  (i) *a statement of the child's present levels of educational performance, including—*
    (I) *how the child's disability affects the child's involvement and progress in the general curriculum; or*
    (II) *for preschool children, as appropriate, how the disability affects the child's participation in appropriate activities;*
  (ii) *a statement of measurable annual goals, including benchmarks or short-term objectives, related to—*
    (I) *meeting the child's needs that result from the child's disability to enable the child to be involved in and progress in the general curriculum; and*
    (II) *meeting each of the child's other educational needs that result from the child's disability;*
  (iii) *a statement of the special education and related services and supplementary aids and services to be provided to the child, or on behalf of the child, and a statement of the program modifications or supports for school personnel that will be provided for the child—*
    (I) *to advance appropriately toward attaining the annual goals;*
    (II) *to be involved and progress in the general curriculum in accordance with clause (i) and to participate in extracurricular and other nonacademic activities; and*

(III) to be educated and participate with other children with disabilities and nondisabled children in the activities described in this paragraph;

(iv) an explanation of the extent, if any, to which the child will not participate with nondisabled children in the regular class and in the activities described in clause (iii);

(v)   (I) a statement of any individual modifications in the administration of State or districtwide assessments of student achievement that are needed in order for the child to participate in such assessment; and

(II) if the IEP Team determines that the child will not participate in a particular State or districtwide assessment of student achievement (or part of such an assessment), a statement of—

(aa) why that assessment is not appropriate for the child; and

(bb) how the child will be assessed;

(vi) the projected date for the beginning of the services and modifications described in clause (iii), and the anticipated frequency, location, and duration of those services and modifications;

(vii)   (I) beginning at age 14, and updated annually, a statement of the transition service needs of the child under the applicable components of the child's IEP that focuses on the child's courses of study (such as participation in advanced-placement courses or a vocational education program;

(II) beginning at age 16 (or younger, if determined appropriate by the IEP Team), a statement of needed transition services for the child, including, when appropriate, a statement of the interagency responsibilities or any needed linkages; and

(III) beginning at least one year before the child reaches the age of majority under State law, a statement that the child has been informed of his or her rights under this title, if any, that will transfer to the child on reaching the age of majority under section 615(m); and

(viii) a statement of

(I) how the child's progress toward the annual goals described in clause (ii) will be measured; and

(II) how the child's parents will be regularly informed (by such means as periodic report

cards), at least as often as parents are informed of their nondisabled children's progress, of—

(aa) their child's progress toward the annual goals described in clause (ii); and

(bb) the extent to which that progress is sufficient to enable the child to achieve the goals by the end of the year.

These requirements contribute to good professional practice in all settings. As legal requirements, however, they tend to generate preprinted paperwork monsters, with just a few blank spaces left to "individualize." Professionals and parents must try to keep IEPs concise, clear, and individualized and use them to work for children. It can be done, if the original purpose of IEP is kept forefront in mind, and if questions of the child's needs and opportunities, as well as impairments and abilities, are used to guide the deliberations that result in the written IEP.

Review and Revision of the IEP.   The 1997 Amendments to IDEA emphasize the involvement of the child's parents in the review and revision process. They point to concerns about measuring progress toward annual goals in relation to the general curriculum, which is consistent with the philosophy of this book. The wording in Sec. 614(d)(3) regarding review and revision of the IEP is as follows:

*(A) **IN GENERAL**—The local educational agency shall ensure that, subject to subparagraph (B), the IEP Team—*

(i) reviews the child's IEP periodically, but not less than annually to determine whether the annual goals for the child are being achieved; and

(ii) revises the IEP as appropriate to address—

(I) any lack of expected progress toward the annual goals and in the general curriculum, where appropriate;

(II) the results of any reevaluation conducted under this section;

(III) information about the child provided to, or by, the parents, as describe in subsection (c)(1)(B);

(IV) the child's anticipated needs; or

(V) other matters.

*(B) **REQUIREMENT WITH RESPECT TO REGULAR EDUCATION TEACHER**—The regular education teacher of the child, as a member of the IEP Team, shall, to the extent appropriate, participate in the review and revision of the IEP of the child.*

Transition Services.   Since the passage of PL 101–476, transition services have been a required part of the IEP process for students beginning no later than age 16 (and at age 14 if considered appropriate). According to Sec. 602(30), "the term 'transition services' means a coordinated set of activities for a student with a disability that—"

(A) *is designed within an outcome-oriented process, which promotes movement from school to post-school activities, including post-secondary education, vocational training, integrated employment (including supported employment), continuing and adult education, adult services, independent living, or community participation;*
(B) *is based upon the individual student's needs, taking into account the student's preferences and interests; and*
(C) *includes instruction, related services, community experiences, the development of employment and other post-school adult living objectives, and, when appropriate, acquisition of daily living skills and functional vocational evaluation.*

Transition services may seem to be primarily the responsibility of vocational education specialists, but speech–language pathologists and other language-learning specialists also should be involved in transdisciplinary efforts to plan and implement transition activities. Language and communication skills contribute to success, whether a person's transition plan is aimed primarily toward higher education or employment. Language assessment activities, for example, might include observation of functional communication demands and expectations of targeted contexts. Then intervention goals and activities should be coordinated with transition plan outlines to prepare students to meet those functional communication requirements.

Periodic Reevaluation.   Under IDEA, children must receive a comprehensive reevaluation, meeting all of the requirements of the preplacement evaluation, at least once every three years. Parents must be notified that a formal evaluation is occurring that may affect the educational placement decisions regarding their child. At the conclusion of the evaluation, the parents are invited to a meeting where the results are discussed. This meeting can be scheduled to coincide with the regularly scheduled IEP annual review.

Due Process.   Due process provisions of IDEA ensure enforcement of the rights of all children to a free ap-

propriate public education. These procedural safeguards grant parents the opportunity to examine all relevant records concerning their child, to obtain an independent evaluation if they disagree with the school district's evaluation, to receive prior notice if the school district proposes to initiate a change in the educational program, and to participate in team placement decisions. If a dispute arises regarding any of these rights, or if the parents and school district have a dispute over the child's education, either party may request an impartial due process hearing before a hearing officer, where parents can be accompanied and advised by legal counsel. Alternatively, disputes may be resolved through a mediation process if both parties agree. Mediation may not be used, however, "to deny or delay a parent's right to a due process hearing" (Sec. 614(e)(2)(A)(ii)).

The impartial officer who holds the hearing decides the outcome. Although this decision is considered final, either the parents or the school may appeal to the state department of education for review. If the "administrative remedies" of the state do not result in satisfaction, either party may initiate a lawsuit in federal or state court.

Part C of IDEA (PL 105–17): Infants and Toddlers with Disabilities.   The Education of Handicapped Amendments (PL 99–457), passed in 1986, set up the major regulations for Part H of IDEA. Part H extended the mandate for provision of special education services to children from the ages of 3 to 5 years, which had been optional in PL 94–142. In addition, Part H established a discretionary program to assist states to develop and implement early intervention services for infants and toddlers with disabilities and for their families. The 1997 Amendments to IDEA changed Part H to Part C, and introduced some other relatively minor modifications to the part of IDEA that concerns services to infants and toddlers and their families.

The involvement of families in Part H (Now Part C) represented three shifts in emphasis: (1) It involved the use of **Individualized Family Service Plans (IFSPs)** to redefine the service unit as being the family, rather than the child alone. (2) It required explicit decisions to be made about the family's service needs. (3) It mandated family representation on the decision-making team.

Another distinction is in the way that the law is handled at the level of states. Whereas implementation of Part B of IDEA is the responsibility of state public education agencies, the implementation of Part C is assigned to different designated lead agencies by governors. Governors designated education agencies as lead agencies in 21 states or territories. In the others, they designated health agencies or agencies devoted to welfare, human resources, or developmental disabilities. This is because Part C is intended to involve a "statewide, comprehensive, coordinated, multidisciplinary, interagency system to provide early intervention services for infants and toddlers with disabilities and their families" (Sec. 633), which does not supplant old ones.

Evaluation and Eligibility.   The definition of "infant or toddler with a disability" is intimately tied to the definition of "developmental delay," which is left up to states, and to the definition of "at-risk infant or toddler" as well. In the Amendments of 1997 to IDEA, these three definitions read as follows:

INFANT OR TODDLER WITH A DISABILITY—*The term "infant or toddler with a disability"—*
(A) means an individual under 3 years of age who needs early intervention services because the individual—
(i) is experiencing developmental delays, as measured by appropriate diagnostic instruments and procedures in one or more of the areas of cognitive development, physical development, communication development, social or emotional development, and adaptive development; or
(ii) has a diagnosed physical or mental condition which has a high probability of resulting in developmental delay; and
(B) may also include, at a State's discretion, at-risk infants and toddlers (Sec. 632(5)).

DEVELOPMENTAL DELAY—*The term "developmental delay," when used with respect to an individual residing in a State, has the meaning given such term by the State under section 635(a)(1) (Sec. 632(3)).*

AT-RISK INFANT OR TODDLER—*The term "at-risk infant or toddler" means an individual under 3 years of age who would be at risk of experiencing a substantial developmental delay if early intervention services were not provided to the individual (Sec. 632(1)).*

Issues related to evaluation of infants and toddlers are considered in Chapter 7.

Individualized Family Service Plan.   The IFSP is similar to the IEP but has several important distinctions. In

the regulations for Part C of IDEA, IFSPs are described as follows:

CONTENT OF PLAN—The individualized family service plan shall be in writing and contain—
(1) a statement of the infant's or toddler's present levels of physical development, cognitive development, communication development, social or emotional development, and adaptive development, based on objective criteria;
(2) a statement of the family's resources, priorities, and concerns relating to enhancing the development of the family's infant or toddler with a disability;
(3) a statement of the major outcomes expected to be achieved for the infant or toddler and the family, and the criteria, procedures, and timelines used to determine the degree to which progress toward achieving the outcomes is being made and whether modifications or revisions of the outcomes or services are necessary;
(4) a statement of specific early intervention services necessary to meet the unique needs of the infant or toddler and the family, including the frequency, intensity, and method of delivering services;
(5) a statement of the natural environments in which early intervention services shall appropriately be provided, including a justification of the extent, if any, to which the services will not be provided in a natural environment;
(6) the projected dates for initiation of services and the anticipated duration of the services;
(7) the identification of the service coordinator from the profession most immediately relevant to the infant's and toddler's or family's needs who will be responsible for the implementation of the plan and coordination with other agencies and persons; and
(8) the steps to be taken to support the transition of the toddler with a disability to preschool or other appropriate services (Sec. 636(d)).

IFSPs must be revised at least twice per year, compared with once for IEPS. Families not only must be included as active members of multidisciplinary teams, they must also be described in the IFSP. Their resources, priorities, and concerns relative to the infant or toddler with the handicap must be written down, and a service coordinator must be assigned.

This strategy is fraught with complex implications. A team of specialists, using a traditional assessment model, might approach a family, study it, analyze it, and list the family's resources, priorities, and concerns. Imagine yourself as the parent of a recently born infant with problems. How would you feel if someone decided to intervene this way? Add the consideration that you have had only a few months to become accustomed to the idea that your imagined perfect child has problems. You are likely still to be going through the stages of guilt, anger, and mourning that are part of that process (Luterman, 1979; Simons, 1987) (see Personal Reflection 5.2). Now someone comes in to analyze your family to tell you how to fix things. To a parent already dealing with issues of guilt, the most rational conclusion might be that, "Yes, I really must be the cause of my child's problems."

Now imagine a different scenario: Two caring professionals begin to get to know your family at times that are arranged jointly. You are asked to show the professionals things that you have learned about your baby. Together, you explore contexts in which your child functions differently—such as places and positions for feeding and playing, food textures, times of the day, toys, pets, and people—that seem to bring out different skills, abilities, and reactions from your baby. Gradually, joint concepts evolve so that it becomes clear that problems that may have seemed to be an inherent part of the baby actually vary with the surroundings and that the baby brings more than just problems to interactions. You become increasingly comfortable in asking the pro-

fessionals questions and learning about your baby's disability, but you appreciate that the professionals always seem to respect your role as the expert on your own baby. By the time you schedule the first IFSP meeting, you are ready to sit down together and talk about the current situation and about your hopes and expectations for the next few years. You work together to create a mutually defined statement of strengths, priorities, concerns, and needs that recognize the ecology of your own family. You are a legitimate member of the team. In which situation would you rather participate?

Other Federal-Level Influences.   Also influencing practices at the federal level are case law, federal initiatives, and federal letters of interpretation.

Outcomes of Case Law.   Laws present opportunities for varying interpretations. When litigation is used to interpret law, the implications of the outcomes of individual cases for service delivery can extend beyond the individual case. For example, in a 1989 case in New Hampshire, a U.S. District Judge ruled that 13-year-old Timothy W., who was quadriplegic and had severe disabilities, was ineligible for education services because he could not "benefit" from special education. The case (*Timothy W. v. Rochester School District,* 1989) was appealed, and three federal judges overturned the earlier ruling and reaffirmed the intention of IDEA that regardless of severity of impairment, no child is too impaired to benefit from special education. This finding is now known informally as the "no exclusion" ruling.

Practicing professionals can best remain current on case law outcomes by participating in professional associations and state and federal information networks. These groups often monitor and publish summaries of important case results in newsletters and computer bulletin board networks.

The Regular Education Initiative.   A prime example of a policy influence not based on law but on a position paper issued by a federal agency is the Regular Education Initiative (REI). It is based on a 1986 paper by Madeline Will, then Undersecretary in the U.S. Office of Special Education and Rehabilitative Services, called "Educating Students with Learning Problems: A Shared Responsibility." The essence of the REI is its proposal to "serve as many children as possible in the regular classroom by encouraging a partnership with regular

---

PERSONAL REFLECTION 5.2 _____

"I've heard this period called 'nothingness' and that's exactly how you feel. You can't move, can't think, can't do anything but feel—leaden like a rock. There's *nothing* there—but that disability."

Parent of a handicapped child speaking about the early stages of adjustment, quoted by Robin Simons (1987, p. 6), in the book *After the Tears.*

In the book, Simons introduces the task facing parents with these words: "In parenting a child with a disability you face a major choice. You can believe that your child's condition is a death blow to everything you've dreamed and worked toward until now. Or you can decide that you will continue to lead the life you'd planned—and incorporate your child into it. Parents who choose the latter course find that they do a tremendous amount of growing." (Preface written by Simons, 1987.)

education" (Will, 1986, p. 20). As originally conceived, the REI was aimed primarily at mildly handicapped students, such as students with educable mental retardation or learning disabilities (most of whom have language disorders). These children, especially those with learning disabilities, were pulled out of regular education and served in special education in record numbers in 1986.

The discussion of the REI continues through the 1990s. Byrnes (1990), a school administrator in Sudbury, Massachusetts, noted the advantages of the REI for students who had potential to keep up with the regular curriculum but expressed concerns about its appropriateness for students with more severe cognitive and behavioral control problems. Her suggestions were to "keep all options open" and to "keep opening the debate" (Byrnes, 1990, p. 348). In responding to Byrnes's comments, W. E. Davis (1990) urged participants in the debate not to see it as an either/or proposition—that is, either to keep the current special education system in place as it is currently implemented or to abandon old methods entirely and move all handicapped students into regular education settings. Both Byrnes (1990) and W. E. Davis (1990) urged a broadening of respect for diversity.

Full-Inclusion Initiatives.   Byrnes's (1990) comments illustrate the overlap between the discussion of the REI, as the original position paper was written, and discussions regarding the inclusion of all students with disabilities (no matter how severe) in regular schools and classrooms. Federal policy regarding **inclusion** is even less formally articulated than the REI position. The idea of community integration is not so much an official policy as it is a philosophy, and yet it exerts a significant influence over service provision to many children with language disorders and other disabilities.

Several ideas related to "integration" of students with disabilities were published in an article called "Community Integration: The Next Step" (Office of Special Education and Rehabilitation Services, 1989):

Over the last several years the Office of Special Education and Rehabilitation Services (OSERS) has made a major commitment to the goal of fostering greater integration of students with disabilities into the community. This commitment is based on the premise that isolation makes it harder for students with disabilities to develop appropriate interpersonal skills. The lack of such skills often creates obstacles to proper adjustment. Without the experience of living and working in community settings,

it becomes more difficult for students with disabilities to succeed in the "real world" after they leave school. (p. 1)

Terminology shifted from discussion of integration to full inclusion with the opening of the new decade. In 1992, in a report called *Winners All: A Call for Inclusive Schools,* the National Association of State Boards of Education (NASBE) extended the earlier "integration" thinking of the 1980s (Calculator & Jorgensen, 1994). The NASBE report defined inclusion as meaning that students in special education—to the maximum extent possible—would receive their in-school educational services in general education classrooms with appropriate in-class support. Included students attend their neighborhood schools in grades with their same-age peers.

Proponents of full inclusion often insist that it must be complete. Others, who support the concept of inclusionary practices, still see a role for specialized services to be provided outside of the general education classroom. The American Speech-Language-Hearing Association (ASHA, 1996), for example, recognized that "Inclusion has numerous strengths, including natural opportunities for peer interaction, and available research suggests cautious optimism regarding its effectiveness in promoting communication abilities and skills in related domains." But ASHA took the position that "the shift toward inclusion will not be optimal when implemented in absolute terms. Rather, the unique and specific needs of each child and family must always be considered" (p. 35). Box 5.2 presents the remainder of the ASHA position statement.

Interpretations of the full inclusion initiative and REI depend on policy decisions made at state, intermediate, and local levels.

Assistive Device Interpretation.   Federal level influences also appear in the form of letters of interpretation. On August 10, 1990, Judy Schrag, director of the Office of Special Education Programs in the U.S. Department of Education's Office of Special Education and Rehabilitation Services, clarified the requirements for assistive technology and services to be provided under Part B of IDEA in a letter. The essence of the interpretation was that:

if the participants on the IEP team determine that a child with handicaps requires assistive technology in order to receive FAPE, and designate such assistive technology as either special education or a related service, the child's IEP must include a specific statement of such services, in-

cluding the nature and amount of such services. 34 CFR S.300.346(c); App. C to 34 CFR Part 300 (Ques. 51).

The letter also clarified that the determination of the need for assistive technology must be made on a case-by-case basis and could be considered "special education, related services or supplementary aids and services for children with handicaps who are educated in regular classes" (Schrag, 1990).

State Policy

State education agencies bear the responsibility for implementing IDEA, Part B, in all 50 states, and they have been named as lead agencies for implementing Part C in 21 states. As specified by IDEA, states have advisory committees. They also employ staff to oversee the implementation of laws. Beyond these similarities, wide differences in public policy may exist among states.

Box 5.2 _____

Position Statement of the American Speech-Language-Hearing Association (1996) Regarding "Inclusive Practices for Children and Youth with Communication Disorders."

It is the position of the American Speech-Language-Hearing Association (ASHA) that an array of speech, language, and hearing services should be available in educational settings to support children and youths with communication disorders. The term "inclusive practices" best represents this philosophy. The inclusive-practices philosophy emphasizes serving children and youth in the least restrictive environment that meets their needs optimally. Inclusive practices consist of a range of service-delivery options that need not be mutually exclusive. They can include direct, classroom-based, community-based, and consultative intervention programming. Inclusive practices are based on a commitment to selecting and designing interventions that meet the needs of each child and family. Factors contributing to the determination of individual need include the child's age, type of disability, communication competence, language and cultural background, academic performance, social skills, family and teacher concerns, and the student's own attitudes about speech, language, and hearing services. (p. 35)

State policies generally influence service provision to children with language disorders beyond federal policies. For example, states often have guidelines for evaluating children and finding them eligible for service. They also have certification or licensure standards outlining the professional preparation needed to provide specialized services to these children. Because states are involved in funding special services, states' formulae and procedures exert major policy influences. Because states differ widely in their policies, however, readers must seek sources within their own states (or provinces) to understand the policies that affect children with language disorders there.

Intermediate Policy

Different states have different labels for the intermediate-level education agency. For example, Michigan has Intermediate School Districts; Pennsylvania has Intermediate Units; Texas, Independent School Districts; Iowa, Area Education Agencies; New York, Boards of Cooperative Educational Services (BOCES); California, cooperatives or consortiums. Not all states have policy-making bodies at this level, and not all agencies at the intermediate level perform the same functions. However, intermediate-level agencies can exert significant influence on making, implementing, and monitoring the implementation of policy. As IDEA has been implemented, a whole new set of intermediate-level agencies, including third-party payers, have been involved in making policies regarding service delivery for infants and toddlers and their families.

One contribution of intermediate-level agencies has been to provide centralized services for children with "low-incidence" conditions such as moderate-to-severe retardation, autism, and combined physical and mental impairments. These conditions are considered relatively rare and are not likely to show up frequently in any one local school district (unless it is in a large city; then city-wide school districts tend to take on many intermediate-level functions). Professionals in local districts therefore may be less familiar with the disabling conditions and their treatment. Local districts (at least small ones) also may not employ the kinds of specialized service providers (e.g., occupational therapists and physical therapists, educators of the hearing impaired, audiologists, and augmentative communication specialists) who can provide the services that such children might need. As a result, sometimes officially, sometimes simply by tradition, children are bused throughout an entire intermediate or "cooperative" district to a central location where "appropriate" services can be provided and where they are isolated from normally developing children in their own communities. The question that local planners and families now ask is whether services provided in isolation are truly more appropriate than those that might be provided at the local level.

Some of the changes that continue to evolve at the intermediate policy level in the 1990s include a shift away from the center program model of bringing children to centralized programs to an inclusion model, involving consultants with specialized expertise who go to the students in their home schools. These specialists may continue to be employed at the intermediate level but may function more as consultants. They might collaborate with regular and special education teachers and speech–language specialists in local districts rather than providing direct service themselves.

On the other hand, some children (e.g., children with hearing impairments) may benefit fully from educational experiences only when they are provided in specialized contexts (with control of variables such as room acoustics and group sizes) and by teachers who have specialized expertise in meeting their learning needs and encouraging them to develop more mature skills. Furthermore, as the sections on people variables later in this chapter attest, merely placing children side by side does not ensure that they will interact.

Local Policy

Local policy may be articulated in official documents, or it may be implemented as a part of long-standing traditions. It is impossible to outline here all of the local policy decisions that might affect services to children with language disorders. In general, local policies influence factors such as which school buildings house special programs and which rooms are used for what kinds of services.

Parents and service providers have more opportunity to influence policy locally than at any other level. For example, parents may serve on parent advisory councils, work with others in special interest groups, and run for positions on local school boards. Parents can also work cooperatively with local school officials, both spe-

cial and regular educators, to design programs that will accomplish mutually defined goals that are good for children.

Implications of Knowing About Policy and How It Is Made

Being an effective language interventionist involves participating in the process of establishing public policy. Doing so involves several strategies.

The first and most important strategy is to understand current policies and their sources. Knowledge is power when it comes to making public policy. If someone tells you that you cannot do something that you think would be good for a child with a language disorder because of policy, first try to understand the current policy that prohibits the activity. What is the actual wording of the rule? Where is it printed? Who made the rule? To answer these questions, you may ask your supervisor (in a nonthreatening manner) for a copy of the document that established the rule, or you may go to agencies at the other levels to obtain copies of important policy documents from them.

Once you believe that you understand the current policy, you can look for flexibility within it. Maybe the policy itself does not prohibit the activity, but overinterpretation does. This is where your collaborative negotiating skills are needed. Again, go to your immediate supervisor, but first be sure that your plan represents a collaborative effort with others involved in the problem-solving activity. If the problem involves a child in school, the building principal is an essential participant. So are the child's parents. At this meeting, present an organized plan to show how the desired activity is good for the child, is consistent with the current IEP or IFSP (if there is one), can be conducted so as not to violate written policy, and represents the results of collaborative planning efforts.

If current policy clearly prohibits the activity you wish to employ, you have several choices. First, you can seek to understand the rationale for the original policy and may, in the process, give up your idea. Second, you can decide that your idea, although inconsistent with prior established policy, is an innovative one, worth pursuing and good for children. In such cases, you may obtain special approval to implement your plan as an experimental or model program. Most states have provisions for these kinds of activities and may even have special sources of funding, as long as you can satisfy the appropriate groups that your idea is worthwhile and of benefit to children. Third, you can work to change the official policy.

If you elect the third choice, you will need to know not only what the current policy is, but how it was established and how it can be changed. Then you will have to set about moving through those channels. This may be a long and frustrating course, and it generally requires association with others (e.g., regional or state speech-language-hearing associations and other advocacy groups), but if the potential benefits to children with language disorders are great enough, the effort will be worth it (see O'Brien & O'Leary, 1988, for a description of a case in which they chose this course). Individuals can make a difference in public policy. It just takes patience, persistence, understanding the political process, and watching for the right place and time.

SERVICE DELIVERY

Although it is important to understand policy and how it is generated, the crucial decisions that influence children are those that are made for them as individuals. These decisions are of two broad types. One concerns daily activities of individual assessment and intervention (considered in Chapter 6 and the chapters of Part II). Another involves the broader selection of settings and people and the timing of interaction events.

Variables related to settings, people, and scheduling are combined to design service-delivery models. In this section, variables in those three areas are discussed separately to highlight their individual contributions to language intervention for children with language disorders.

As in other cases, choices should be guided by good questions. An important question underlying the selection of service-delivery variables is "How can we use intervention settings, people, and schedules to maximize the opportunities for this child to acquire the language abilities the child needs for participating in important life contexts?"

Setting Variables

When selecting service-delivery settings for individual children, it is helpful to start by considering the contexts where children would spend most of their time if they were developing normally. Such contexts serve as a baseline for determining least restrictive environments (see Personal Reflection 5.3).

Children who need assistance because of language disorders have probably experienced some degree of failure in communicating in one or more of these natural contexts. Parents and service providers may attempt to modify them. In some cases, however, specialized contexts are required to meet children's individualized language learning needs.

Language Intervention Setting Options. Options for intervention settings include home, preschool, regular classrooms, special education classrooms, small clinic-like rooms (called "pullout rooms" here), and various work and social settings (see Box 5.3 for service delivery guidelines of the American Speech-Language-Hearing Association, 1993). Traditionally, language specialists have used pullout rooms most frequently as contexts for providing language intervention services.

Pullout Rooms. The practice of using pullout rooms to provide language intervention services has evolved out of services to children with speech impairments in clinics (L. Miller, 1989). Those services traditionally have been provided in special rooms, either one-on-one or to children in small groups.

Consider first the advantages. On the basis of practicality and cost, more children can be seen in a week if

---

PERSONAL REFLECTION 5.3 _____

"Decisions about where handicapped students should be instructed have received more attention, undergone more modifications, and generated even more controversy than have decisions about how or what these students are taught. Handicapped students' educational journey has come nearly full circle. Their odyssey, which began in general education classrooms, took them first to special schools, from there to full-time special classes, and on to resource rooms with part-time placement in regular classrooms, and now they appear to be headed in the direction of full-time placement in general education classrooms."

Joseph R. Jenkins and *Amy Heinen* (1989, p. 516).

Box 5.3 _____

Service Delivery Model Options
American Speech-Language-Hearing
Association (1993).

Service delivery is a dynamic concept, and should change as the needs of the students change.

No one service delivery model need be used exclusively during treatment.

COLLABORATIVE CONSULTATIVE: The speech–language pathologist, regular and/or special education teacher(s), and parents voluntarily work together to facilitate a student's communication and learning in educational environments. It is essential that the administrator allow the speech–language pathologist and the collaborator(s) to have a regularly scheduled planning time throughout the duration of service.

CLASSROOM BASED: This model is also known as integrated services, curriculum-based, transdisciplinary, interdisciplinary, or inclusive programming. There is an emphasis on the speech–language pathologist providing direct services to students within the classroom and other natural environments. Team teaching by the speech–language pathologist and the regular and/or special education teacher(s) is frequent with this model.

PULLOUT: Services are provided to students individually and in small groups in the speech rooms. Some speech–language pathologists may prefer to provide services within the physical space of the classroom.

SELF-CONTAINED PROGRAM: The speech–language pathologist is the classroom teacher responsible for providing academic instruction and intensive speech–language remediation.

---

the children come to the specialist than if the specialist goes to the children. On a more philosophical basis, it can be argued that these children would never have been referred for special attention if they could learn language normally. Pullout rooms allow professionals to exert control over the many variables that influence whether a child can perform specific tasks such as speaking in sentences, taking conversational turns, and using new words meaningfully. For example, in small pullout rooms, auditory and visual distractions can be controlled and contexts can be structured so that chil-

dren have more turns to talk, more guidance, and more positive reinforcement for attempting to use new language skills than they do in more natural settings. Pullout rooms also allow older children with difficulties to practice new skills in environments that reduce the stress of trying to look good in front of their peers and to avoid being embarrassed by needing special help.

On the other hand, a major disadvantage of pullout settings is that, by establishing a new context, newly learned skills may not transfer to the regular contexts of the child's life, and the child may even become increasingly isolated from those contexts. Another disadvantage is that it is difficult to provide rich opportunities for developing language content and pragmatic use skills in a context that is so highly controlled.

The social interaction views of language acquisition discussed in Chapter 3 suggest that children learn to talk and to understand language because language is meaningful to them and because they need it to interact with others. It is difficult to contrive situations in pullout rooms that capture these qualities. Cognitive views suggest that children learn to talk and to interact with others because it is an integral part of learning about the world and how they relate to it. In this case as well, the context stripping that tends to accompany communication in pullout rooms can hardly be imagined to facilitate this type of language learning.

When pullout rooms are viewed solely as a context for pulling children out, taking them down the hall (or into any purely clinical area), fixing them, and putting them back, the risk is that any "fixing" will have limited relevance to children's lives (see Personal Reflection 5.4). Although pullout rooms may provide one context for intervention, they should generally be used in conjunction with attention to language use in other contexts. "Pulling-in" curricular content material may be one effective way to do this. Almost all school experiences are language rich. Individual or small group treatment in the relatively controlled context of the pullout room can provide an appropriate context for curriculum-based language intervention.

Special Classrooms in Special Buildings.   Children with severe and multiple disabilities are sometimes placed in special classrooms in special buildings. Many such "center" programs were developed during the 1970s to provide centralized services to children with low-incidence handicapping conditions in buildings specially designed to meet their needs (e.g., with ramps instead of stairs, bathrooms with access for wheelchairs, and therapeutic swimming pools). In some cases, the children served in such programs were just being returned to their home communities from state institutions, where (before Section 504 and the implementation of PL 94–142, 1977) they might have received limited or no education and special services.

In center programs, children might be bused long distances to be brought together with children with similar impairments and educational and therapy needs. Within center programs, children may be pulled out of their classrooms to receive language intervention services, or those services may be provided as part of classroom programming.

The advantage of providing services to children in center programs is that facilities can be specially designed, and specialists can be gathered together to meet the needs of children with severe disabilities and to tailor activities to their levels of functioning. These same factors, however, can be listed as disadvantages. Interpretations of children's needs have shifted. Rather than emphasizing remediation of impairments in specialized environments, the focus has shifted to encouraging socialization and education of children with severe disabilities so that they may join the rest of society.

In some cases, attempts have been made to encourage integration of peers with and without disabilities by building special facilities beside regular school education buildings. The results of such efforts in terms of peer interaction have not met expectations. For example, Mercer and Denti (1989) studied a five-year effort to integrate regular and special education students on a campus where the students were housed in separate but adjacent facilities with separate administrators. When observational data and questionnaires revealed almost total segregation after the first three years, intensive ef-

forts were undertaken to encourage integration further but without enduring effects. The authors concluded that "Physical, social, and psychological barriers created by the two-roof school erect almost insurmountable obstacles to integration. Future efforts should concentrate on building one-roof schools with a single facility and administration" (p. 30).

Special Classrooms in Regular Buildings. In some cases, children with language disorders are placed in special classrooms in regular buildings. The nature of service delivery in such classrooms depends not only on where the rooms are located but the teacher's orientation. Most teachers of special classrooms are special education teachers with credentials to teach children with disabilities such as mental retardation or learning disabilities. Many children with mental retardation and most children with learning disabilities need language intervention as well as other special education services. Such needs may be met partially within the special education classroom and partially within language intervention pullout rooms. Some children attend special education resource rooms that may function more as pullout rooms than as special classrooms, and these may be in addition to other pullout rooms where they receive speech and language intervention services (see Personal Reflection 5.5, where "Barbie" describes this situation from a student's perspective). Occasionally, speech– language pathologists serve as classroom teachers or co-teachers and assume the responsibility for teaching all or most of the curriculum to children with severe language impairments in self-contained classes (L. P. Hoffman, 1990; N. W. Nelson, 1981a). Approaches used in such classrooms are discussed in later chapters of this book.

Although children are often placed in special education classrooms based on their category of impairment, the services provided in different types of categorical rooms may not be distinguishable. In one study (Algozzine, Morsink, & Algozzine, 1989), interactions were analyzed in 40 self-contained special classes for children classified with learning disability, emotional impairment, or educable mental retardation. The results showed few differences in the teacher communication patterns, learner involvement, and instructional methods used in the three types of classes. The researchers commented that this outcome raised questions about the appropriateness of categorical grouping of students for instruction.

PERSONAL REFLECTION 5.4

"They're always trying to 'fix' Marti—as if they can't accept the fact that she's handicapped. They spend all their time working on things she *can't* do without giving her a chance to enjoy the things she *can.*"

Carol Knibbs, mother of a 14-year-old daughter who is retarded, quoted by Simons (1987, p. 48).

PERSONAL REFLECTION 5.5 _____

In this conversational sample, 11-year-old, fifth-grade *Barbie* (B) and her clinician (C), Janet Sturm (to whom I am indebted for this sample), are talking about Barbie's feelings about school. Barbie began the topic after they started talking about what is hard about school.

B: I don't know about Mrs. Y. She doesn't even let me take my books (in in) anywhere.
C: Really?
B: Yeah, (she) she's my second teacher. I have three teachers. My first one is [pause] Mrs. B. (She) she's my real teacher. Mrs. Y., she's the resource room. Mrs. M., she's my speech teacher.
C: Oh.
B: So, it's hard. You have to go, hurry, and go back, uh uh uh [motioning with her hands while she makes sound effects to represent traveling back and forth] and get [unintelligible word].
C: Like you're coming and going all the time?
B: Yeah [laughs]. Like in eighth grade.
C: Like they do in eighth grade.
B: They do nuh nuh nuh nuh nah [motioning hands as if they're going back and forth]. Say bye, hi, bye, hi.
C: Trading classrooms. See, you'll be ready for eighth grade then won't you because you're used to it?
B: But sometimes I have to, in the same room so [laughs] it's hard [laughs]. Like, ugh, you're getting dizzy and your head ache.
C: Really?
B: And sometimes I don't even eat lunch. I just pass.

Regular Classrooms.   School-age children with language disorders may spend the majority, or only limited parts, of their days in regular classrooms. What these children are expected to do in such settings may vary widely. As in the preceding discussions, whether features of regular classrooms act as advantages or disadvantages for particular children depends on complex interactions among the variables of settings, people, and scheduling.

When children can almost but not quite succeed in the regular classroom and the regular curriculum, service provision can focus on that setting, with language intervention designed to help children process the language of education. Pullout sessions may be used to implement individualized curriculum-based language intervention (N. W. Nelson, 1989b), but the child is viewed as a full member of the regular classroom. Whether the classroom itself is considered to be a language intervention context depends on the philosophy and attitudes of the entire educational team, including the building principal and, particularly, the classroom teacher. It helps when the language specialist-consultant approaches the classroom teacher with the question "How can I help you do your job?" rather than "How can you help me do mine?"

Traditionally, children have been "mainstreamed" into regular classrooms only in curricular areas where it was felt that they could be academically competitive (e.g., L. P. Hoffman, 1990). After full-inclusion policy shifts, however, children with more severe language impairments and associated disabilities may be placed in regular classrooms for all or major parts of their days, even when educators suspect that they may not be able to handle all aspects of the regular curriculum (see Personal Reflection 5.6).

Beukelman and Mirenda (1992) have written about the educational integration of students with severe disabilities and the need for augmentative communication. They distinguished three patterns of academic and social

PERSONAL REFLECTION 5.6 _____

"In order to foster change in regular education, special educators need to reduce the current emphasis on classifying, labeling, and offering 'special' programs for students who do not fit within the present regular education structure. Instead, they should put more emphasis on joining with regular educators to work for a reorganization of or modifications in the structure of regular education itself so that the needs of a wider range of students can be met within the mainstream of regular education."

William Stainback, Susan Stainback, Lee Courtnage, & Twila Jaben (1985, p. 148).

participation as (1) competitive, (2) active, or (3) involved. In this system, **competitive academic participation** is observed when students with disabilities can meet the academic standards expected of all students, at least in some areas. Some students are competitive only with compensations from specialized technology, a teacher's aide, or a reduction in the amount of work. **Active academic participation** is observed when students can participate in regular education activities and learning but cannot meet the same academic standards as peer students. **Involved academic participation** is observed when students spend time with their peers in regular academic settings but have minimal ability to compete academically at the level expected of their peers. Involvement in regular classroom settings is valued for other reasons (see Personal Reflection 5.7).

PERSONAL REFLECTION 5.7 _____

"The level of no academic participation is never acceptable or defensible, although it occurs far too often. In the level of no participation, the student is physically present in a regular classroom for a particular lesson or activity, but is passive and uninvolved for the majority of time. This may occur for a number of reasons, not the least of which is that the student does not have the AAC tools needed for participation. Even fully integrated students may be nonparticipants in one or more classroom activities, and this undesirable option requires prompt remediation."

David R. Beukelman and *Pat Mirenda* (1992, p. 209).

When mainstreaming does not work, it is generally because a child is included physically, but integrated minimally, although the child might be capable of more. This unfortunate situation tends to occur when children move in and out of regular education classrooms but are not really viewed to be part of the class. (This is what happened to Barbie, Personal Reflection 5.5.) Although the other children are reading or receiving instruction, the mainstreamed children might be completing coloring worksheets at their desks as a way of keeping them busy rather than helping them learn. Before decisions are made to remove children from regular classroom contexts, educators and language specialists might collaborate to find ways to make more of the regular curriculum accessible. Techniques for doing so are discussed in Part II.

Home and Family Contexts.   Parents are first and foremost parents. Professionals must be careful to avoid shifting that relationship by asking parents to be primarily therapists for their children (see Personal Reflection 5.8). When home and family contexts are targeted as language intervention settings, they should be used to intensify natural language experiences and interactions—experiences that cannot be provided in pullout rooms and other settings. Asking parents to turn their kitchen tables into pullout rooms may add more to parental burdens than to helping their children.

Fey (1986) reviewed the literature on homes as intervention settings for young children. He found more evidence supporting changes in parental behavior following training than evidence that parents implemented the procedures in the home. Fey reported that monitoring of changed interactions in the home has been rare,

PERSONAL REFLECTION 5.8 _____

"The speech therapist says, 'Do half an hour of therapy after dinner.' The physical therapist says, 'Do 30 minutes of therapy in your spare time.' What spare time?! I have two other kids and a husband! I finally said 'no' to all that therapy. I had to choose between being my child's extension therapist and being his mother. And I chose being his mother."

Parent of a child with multiple needs who had multiple needs herself (we all do), quoted by Simons (1987, p. 51).

but that "when such monitoring has been done, the results sometimes indicate that parents do not administer highly programmed steps as planned or trained" (p. 311). He also recommended that parents be consulted regarding their own preferences for using the home to perform primary intervention activities.

When considering home contexts, other options for using home-like settings beyond the family's home might also be considered. For example, if infants with disabilities are receiving extensive child care from someone other than their parents, such as their grandparents or day-care workers, that care setting might be considered as a possible intervention context. Here, also, the approach to be taken might be more successful if aimed at intensifying already available natural experiences rather than adding on unique therapeutic ones (see the later section on people variables).

Modern families spend much time in the car. Passing scenery offers a rich context that constantly varies but provides tangible and meaningful language interaction opportunities. For example, one child learned to produce sentences with contractible copulas (the verb *is*) and to extend her vocabulary riding in the car with her mother as part of the daily routine, playing the "There's a" game. In this activity, one person introduces the familiar game (after initial modeling) with a sentence like, "There's a barn." The other then responds with something like, "It's big," "It's old," or "It's red." The game can continue for miles in town or country, and in a home-like context where neither parent nor child could do anything else.

Social Contexts.   Social contexts can vary widely and might occur in any setting, including home, school, and work settings that are primarily social. For example, at home, language intervention might be set in social contexts involving interactions with siblings or neighborhood children. At school, it might be set in social contexts involving interactions with peers and non-teaching staff on the playground or in extracurricular activities, such as athletic events or club meetings. Other social contexts might include religious events, meals at fast-food restaurants, or shopping trips to the mall.

The advantages of social contexts are their potential for encouraging generalization of newly acquired language skills and the provision of richer contexts and content for fostering those skills than are available in most structured settings (Jenkins, Odom, & Speltz,

1989). A primary disadvantage of using social contexts as intervention settings is that the child may be embarrassed or distracted by having to meet language intervention expectations during natural social interactions. Evidence also suggests that simply placing children together in social contexts will not ensure that they will interact socially. For example, when Jenkins, Speltz, and Odom (1985) studied children with disabilities placed in integrated preschool settings with normally developing peers, they found that physical integration occurred, but social integration did not.

Varied solutions are available. Some involve consulting with others who have natural opportunities for social interactions with the child or directly facilitating social interactions between children with and without disabilities. Other solutions involve setting up role-play activities. Simulations are designed to give children practice using new language skills in more sheltered contexts with the hope of transferring them later to true social contexts. For example, Hoskins (1987) designed a program in which the language specialist (in the role of "coach") sets up conversational groups for adolescents. We practice "school skills" (e.g., handraising, passing social notes) in the Language-Based Homework Lab of our university clinic (Nelson, 1997; Nelson & Van Meter, 1996).

Vocational Contexts.   Supported employment involves the placement of workers with disabilities in the competitive marketplace but with consultants called "job coaches." Language specialists may consult with such supported employment consultants or other vocational rehabilitation specialists to analyze communicative contexts and to help adolescents and young adults develop the language and communication skills they need to succeed in vocational contexts.

People Variables

Transdisciplinary teams generally include speech–language pathologists, learning disability teachers, and other specialists, including regular educators, psychologists and health-care professionals such as occupational therapists, physical therapists, nurses, and physicians—in addition to parents and children themselves.

Provider Roles and Relationships

Language Specialist Providing Direct Service.   When language specialists provide direct service, they work with children in deliberate ways in scheduled sessions. This is the most common role assumed traditionally by language intervention specialists.

Language Specialist as Consultant. Recall the definition of collaborative consultation as

> *an interactive process that enables teams of people with diverse expertise to generate creative solutions to mutually defined problems. The outcome is enhanced, altered, and produces solutions that are different from those that the individual team members would produce independently. (Idol et al., 1986, p. 1)*

The collaborative consultation model is one in which consultation goes both ways. That is, the consultant serves as a member of a team in which all of the participants, including parents and students, are viewed as having expertise. It contrasts with expert models of consultation, which involve "an outside (the agency or profession) expert engaged in a voluntary relationship with primary interventionists (parents, teachers, care-

takers)" (Marvin, 1987, pp. 4–5) (see Personal Reflection 5.9). It is difficult to imagine the success of any intervention program for a child with a language disorder without some level of collaborative consultation by a language specialist with the other important people in the child's life.

Language Specialist as Teacher. When language specialists serve as teachers, they assume responsibility for conveying the curriculum to children whose language problems make it largely inaccessible to them under ordinary circumstances. This professional's attention necessarily extends beyond students' ability to use language for various social and academic purposes. The language specialist-teacher also assumes primary responsibility for academic development and behavior management.

Language Specialist as Co-Teacher. Language specialists sometimes co-teach with other professionals, who assume a major responsibility for teaching the reg-

---

PERSONAL REFLECTION 5.9 _____

"You listen to me politely, but you never write it down!"

Cathy Shortz, parent of a child with severe multiple impairments (SXI) in Jackson, MI.

These were the words of a frustrated parent describing her experiences with an Individualized Educational Planning (IEP) process in which her ideas about her son's needs for literacy development had not been taken seriously. This time, the message was heard. Speech–language pathologist *Mary Ann Berthiaume* asked Shortz to write down her thoughts and provide them to the team, including her son's classroom teacher, special education teacher, teaching assistants, occupational therapist, physical therapist, school psychologist, and principal.

The informal memo that Cathy Shortz wrote when the sincere invitation was issued, said:

"I'd really like to see beginning reading included in J's IEP this year. Hopefully by the end of the year he'll be able to do some sight reading—his own full name, family names—bathroom—drink—miscellaneous needs. Plus sentence structure, and how to group sentences to tell a story or have a conversation by choosing his words. I'd like to see some math. If only 1–50 and the awareness of 3 digits and up. This is a secondary desire—reading is my biggest concern.

I know this is a major request, but it's really time for academics to start showing up on his IEPs as a REAL goal. Maybe he won't be able to grasp it and at year's end it will be continued or declined, *but* either way I'd like his records to show the effort was made. Thanks for asking for my input. I'll get with you soon to work out our game plan.—C"

ular curriculum. L. Miller (1989) described three variations of the team-teaching format: (1) The language specialist teaches a portion of the regular curriculum in the regular classroom with a regular classroom teacher (e.g., Norris, 1989). (2) The language specialist shares teaching responsibilities with another specialist (usually a teacher of reading, of students with learning disabilities, or of students with behavioral disorders) (e.g., O'Brien & O'Leary, 1988). (3) The language specialist in a resource setting shares supplementary teaching responsibilities (e.g., Simon, 1977, 1987).

Mixed Models.   Children do not have to be served in unitary models, and professionals do not have to practice in only one model at a time. It is possible to mix strategies and delivery-model variables in programs individualized to meet children's needs.

Peer Roles and Relationships.   Children's peers may serve as models, assist in setting a stimulus context, or deliver natural reinforcers (L. Paul, 1985). Peers who participate in the language intervention process may or may not have disabilities themselves. They may be the same age as the target child, older, or younger. L. Paul (1985) has suggested that, when designing service-delivery options involving peers, the specialist needs to ask three essential questions: (1) Do peers provide appropriate models? (2) Do they provide sufficient opportunity for interaction? (3) Do they reinforce the child's attempts at communicating?

Peers in Social Interaction Relationships.   Numerous social advantages have been cited for integrating children with disabilities with nondisabled peers. As noted previously, however, simply placing these children together in the same classroom does not necessarily result in high-quality social interaction (Jenkins et al., 1985).

A study of the verbal productions of preschool children without disabilities in an integrated preschool showed their verbalizations to be less complex, less frequent, and less diverse when addressed to playmates with more severe handicaps than when addressed to children with mild handicaps or no handicaps, in both instructional and free-play settings (Guralnick & Paul-Brown, 1977). These findings may simply reflect the normal pragmatic abilities of children to judge the reduced comprehension abilities of their peers with disabilities. It is of concern, however, if children in integrated settings either "talk down" to their language-impaired peers unnecessarily or fail to interact with them when left to play freely.

Recognizing these tendencies, Jenkins and colleagues (1989) designed a study of both integrated and segregated preschool settings. The authors established two kinds of interactions, called **social interaction** and **child-directed play,** which differed in degree of adult direction. In the social interaction condition, teachers organized four children with heterogeneous abilities into small groups and directed the children's play in 30-minute periods by (1) suggesting play ideas, (2) modeling appropriate play behavior, and (3) prompting appropriate social interaction among the children as necessary. In the child-directed play interactions (which were modeled after those of the High/Scope Preschool Cognitive Curriculum; Hohmann, Banet, & Weikert, 1979), children were also grouped heterogeneously, but they had more freedom of choice within the activities of the 30-minute time period. The results showed a higher proportion of interactive play and higher language development in the more adult-directed social interaction conditions than in the less controlled child-directed play conditions in both settings. Children in the integrated classes also received significantly higher ratings of social competence than children in the segregated classes. Both teacher-direction and normal peer models appeared to play a role in achieving positive social interaction results for these preschoolers.

Problems facilitating quality social interactions do not lessen with age. Also, children with less obvious disabilities, such as language and learning disabilities, may have as much trouble being accepted by their peers as do those with more obvious disabilities. C. L. Fox (1989) reviewed the evidence that students with learning disabilities are socially rejected more often by their peers than students without disabilities and that mainstreaming does not automatically help such students become more accepted by their peers. Fox reported that two of techniques to influence social acceptance of children with disabilities: (1) attempts to teach specific prosocial behaviors to the children with disabilities through modeling, shaping, coaching, and cognitive problem solving and (2) attempts to influence the attitudes of children without disabilities through role playing, peer tutoring, reinforcement, enabling training, education, and sociodrama.

In a study of the second approach, C. L. Fox (1989) paired 86 low socially accepted students with learning disabilities in fourth, fifth, and sixth grades with 86 high socially accepted, same-sex, students without disabilities for 8 weeks of special activities, conducted once per week in 40-minute sessions. Student pairs were assigned randomly to one of four conditions: (1) In mutual interest groups, children were taught how to interview each other and to use information from their interviews to construct mutual interest booklets (C. L. Fox, 1980). (2) In cooperative academic task groups, children were asked to make, play, and evaluate math games. (3) In Hawthorne effect control groups (the Hawthorne effect is the potentially influencing effect of receiving experimental attention), pairs of children spent time in the room with the other groups but worked independently on the math games. (4) In control groups, pairs of children were identified but did not work cooperatively in any way and were not pulled out for special attention. The social acceptability ratings for the students in the first group rose over the 8-week period, the ratings in the second two groups did not change, and the ratings for the control group actually declined.

Eichinger (1990) also employed cooperative techniques to encourage greater social interaction between fourth- and fifth-grade regular education students and students with severe disabilities. Four pairs worked individually to complete a preassigned game or art activity, and four pairs worked cooperatively, with the same set of materials, to complete the game or art activity. The students with disabilities in the cooperative pairs expressed significantly more positive facial affect, higher cooperative play levels, and frequent vocalizations when working cooperatively. No changes were noted during free-play sessions.

The results of all of these studies suggest that, although specific social and communicative benefits can come from integrating children with disabilities with normally developing peers, benefits are unlikely without specific adult intervention. These interactions, however, have focused mostly on social outcomes. The next section discusses the use of cooperative peer interactions to influence other learning outcomes.

Peers in Cooperative Learning Relationships. Cooperative learning techniques have shown promise in regular and special education for enhancing the learning process and building a sense of community among learners (Aronson, Blaney, Stephan, Sikes, & Snapp, 1978; Augustine, Gruber, & Hanson, 1990; D. W. Johnson, Johnson, & Holubec, 1988; S. Kagan, 1990). Analysis of twelve published studies on the effects of cooperative learning on achievement by children with disabilities of varied severity, however, showed equivocal results (Tateyama-Sniezek, 1990). Only six of the studies (50%) showed cooperative learning to have positive effects on achievement. Based on this analysis, Tateyama-Sniezek reported that "the only firm conclusion is that the opportunity for students to study together does not guarantee gains in academic achievement" (p. 436).

Cooperative learning activities vary in their implementation, but in general, they involve the establishment of heterogeneous groups whose members are responsible for seeing that everyone in the group learns and understands the material. A student is not considered to have learned something until he or she has taught it to someone else (Johnson et al., 1988; Slavin, 1983).

Some cooperative learning activities are appropriate for large groups, even as large as whole classrooms. S. Kagan (1990) pointed out some of the differences between whole-class question-answer, which is the competitive structure used traditionally for large-group discussion by classroom teachers, and something he dubbed "numbered heads together." In this approach, (1) The teacher forms several groups of four students, each with heterogeneous abilities, and has the students number off within each group from 1 to 4. (2) The teacher poses a question. (3) The teacher tells the students in each small group to "put their heads together" to make sure that everyone on the team knows the answer (and how to explain it). (4) Then the teacher calls a number (1, 2, 3, or 4) to indicate that only people with that number are eligible to raise their hands to respond. The group gets credit for answers of its individual members.

Another cooperative learning technique is designed to facilitate group discussion with the three-step interview (S. Kagan, 1990) in which students (1) form pairs within their teams of four and conduct one-way interviews in pairs; (2) then reverse roles so that interviewers become interviewees; and (3) end with a roundrobin, in which each takes a turn sharing information from the interview. Kagan noted that the three-step interview is far better than the traditional discussion model "for developing language and listening skills as well as promoting equal participation" (p. 13).

Larson and McKinley (1987) noted that peers could be enlisted as tutors by using a four-step process to achieve the following: (1) gaining educators' support, (2) recruiting and selecting potential tutors, (3) training, supervising, and supporting tutors, and (4) selecting students with language disorders who could benefit from this type of approach. Murray-Seegert (1989) reported on a program in a tough inner-city high school that paired students with severe disabilities and students without disabilities in social contexts for the benefit of both.

The final word is not in. As in other areas, cooperative learning groups and peer tutors are probably good for some students, when organized in some ways, some of the time. There are no universal answers for students with language disorders.

Family Roles and Relationships.   As mentioned, home contexts can be used in a variety of ways to provide services to children with language disorders. The roles of family members in the intervention process can also vary widely, depending on sociocultural variables, the family's culture, and prior experiences of the adults in the family with health-care and educational agencies. Other influential variables are the age of the child with the language disorder, the severity of the disorder, and its association with other disabilities.

Parents have a special perspective on their children's needs at all age levels, and that perspective should be respected. Personal Reflection 5.9 is an example of a school system learning to listen better to what one parent had to say. It is a reminder to professionals of the requirements in IDEA that parents must be given the opportunity to participate as active members of the IEP team.

Fey (1986) divided parental roles into two basic types: (1) parents as aides and (2) parents as primary intervention agents. I add a third role of parents as incidental intervention agents. As you read this section, you might also extend the group of family participants that you are thinking about to include other members, such as siblings or grandparents.

Family Roles as Language Intervention Aides.   When parents act as language intervention aides, they may use the same objectives and intervention activities as in the clinical or school setting, but in the home environment (e.g., Sandler, Coren, & Thurman, 1983; Zwitman & Sonderman, 1979). Parents can also help their children transfer newly acquired language skills to more natural contexts after they have reached certain criteria in a therapeutic setting (Gray & Ryan, 1973; Hughes, 1985; Mulac & Tomlinson, 1977).

Parents and other family members also can function as aides in less formal ways. Fey (1986) noted that "We often bring family members into the clinic sessions to serve as models, to heighten the child's attention, to help the clinician to motivate and reinforce the child, to help create more naturalistic intervention contexts, and, generally, to assist the clinician in any way possible" (p. 295). In our university clinic, this is what we did with a child, "Stephen," who at the age of 3 was nonspeaking and showed many symptoms of autism. We knew that Stephen's sisters played "house" with him at home, so we brought them in to play house in a play kitchen in the language preschool area at the university clinic. As they made pretend cupcakes and played dolls, we encouraged Stephen's sisters to include him in their play. We also taped some of Stephen's favorite songs and taught his sisters the accompanying motions so that they could repeat them with him at home. When the activity was conducted in the clinic, Stephen watched his sisters closely, imitating their actions and interacting with them.

The involvement of siblings as tutors for adolescents with language disorders has also been described (Larson & McKinley, 1987). In deciding when such an approach might be appropriate, Larson and McKinley suggested that the sibling should (1) have the necessary skills and patience to work with the adolescent with the language disorder, (2) have the desire to participate, (3) be willing to be trained and supervised in carrying out assignments, (4) be willing to spend the necessary time and energy to do so, and (5) be older to maximize the potential of the interaction.

Several advantages may be realized from using family members as language intervention aides. Fey (1986) noted that such strategies can promote generalization across contexts and may allow parents to feel more involved in their children's programming. Hughes (1985) also commented that, "If parents are present during language teaching and are taught to provide stimuli (verbal or nonverbal) for eliciting the target language, then they are part of a 'common stimulus' " (p. 162), and they can also play a role in providing meaningful responses to communicative attempts.

Parents as Primary Language Intervention Agents. When parents assume primary roles as intervention agents (see Fey, 1986, and Hughes, 1985, for reviews of this literature), they become the primary providers of direct intervention. This role is generally assumed after parents are trained to set up activities, recognize appropriate language behaviors, reinforce them, and keep records documenting progress.

Positive results of studies in which parents served as primary intervention agents (summarized by Fey, 1986) have included success in reaching clinician-designated goals for the child and general improvements in the parents' adjustments. Fey cautioned, however, that most of the evidence comes from work with children with severe impairments who were learning early words and simple language structures. There is less support for parents' serving as primary intervention agents for working on more complex morphological and syntactic structures. Generalization results after parent-training programs also have not been as encouraging as might be expected.

Parents as Incidental Intervention Agents. A third level of parental interaction is as incidental intervention agent. Parents and others are taught to use naturally occurring opportunities to foster language development. They do not serve as formal teachers or as intervention aides. Rather, they watch for brief episodes, precipitated by the child (B. Hart, 1985), in which they might intervene (incidental teaching techniques are discussed further in Chapter 6). Fey (1986) categorized this role as child-oriented intervention; no specific language structures are selected as goals, and no direct teaching of specific language behaviors is attempted.

Because of its informal nature, and because of individual differences among families and children, the effectiveness of this role is especially difficult to evaluate. The evidence reviewed by Fey (1986) and Hughes (1985) suggests that simply encouraging intervention as a part of opportunities incidental to the process of daily living (rather than those that are formally planned) may not give parents sufficient information. Parents may need more direct training on how to intensity their own

language-facilitating skills and how to provide multiple language-learning opportunities.

As one approach to parental training, Ruder, Bunce, and Ruder (1984) developed a rating sheet for parents to encourage them to monitor their use of such strategies as (1) getting their child's attention before they talked, (2) talking about the here-and-now, (3) labeling objects and talking about actions, (4) pausing to give the child opportunities to talk, (5) responding meaningfully, (6) expanding the child's utterances, and (7) asking appropriate questions. Videotapes and associated training materials are sometimes used to assist parents to identify opportunities and strategies that might occur incidentally in their interactions with their children.

Hubbell (1981) characterized the goal of this kind of involvement as being "not to teach the parent to teach the child. Rather, it is to establish transactional patterns that maximize opportunity for language growth within the child" (p. 275). Hughes (1985) identified changing "parents' language and nonlanguage behaviors in such a way as to facilitate language development" as "the clinician's ultimate goal" (p. 163).

The Need for Sensitivity.   As in other areas, the "best" approach for family involvement may differ widely from one family to another, and decisions must be made individually. Fey (1986) cautioned that "clinicians must be aware of parents' sensitivities and take steps to ensure that their well-intentioned efforts to integrate parents into the intervention process reduce rather than exacerbate the parents' feelings of guilt, anxiety, and frustration" (pp. 292–293).

Scheduling Variables

To improve their language, children must have opportunities to use it. Therefore, a major concern in planning services is to maximize the time available for children to use language when talking, listening, reading, writing, and thinking. Scheduling variables are intimately tied to setting and people variables and the number of children on a caseload at any one time (see Box 5.4 for caseload sizes recommended for speech–language services in the schools by the American Speech-Language-Hearing Association, 1993). Scheduling is used to establish frequency of sessions, length of sessions, and duration of periods when special services will be provided.

Session Frequency Variables. The amount of time needed in language intervention sessions depends on the degree to which the child's other activities encourage his or her language development. Specialized intervention sessions can be less frequent when the child's language development needs are met in other contexts.

Adoption of the twice-weekly scheduling, traditional in many school and clinical settings, may be tempting. This schedule, however, may be established more because of convenience than because of a deliberate plan to meet the child's needs. Research support for selecting one schedule over another is not available. Therefore, scheduling decisions must be made by considering what will best allow professionals and family to meet the child's language development needs (while not interfering with other needs) and to provide maximum opportunities for the child to participate in desired contexts. These decisions will likely vary depending on the child's age and other factors.

If the child is an infant at risk for a language disorder, the child's parents and other caregivers play the primary role in encouraging the child's communicative development. The frequency with which a language specialist works with an infant and family to facilitate language acquisition is determined as part of the IFSP process. Generally, when children are in frequent and close contact with parents and other adults who know how to facilitate their language and communication de-velopment, language specialists do not need to be involved as frequently. When these adults have extensive needs for knowing how to interact with the child, greater time commitment from a language specialist may be required initially but may be reduced later.

Some school-age children with language disorders are mainstreamed for all or part of the day in general education classrooms and are pulled out for language intervention sessions and other special education activities. For these children, decisions about session frequency should consider not only needs for language intervention but also needs to participate in important events in other academic, social, physical, artistic, and musical contexts. It can become a scheduling nightmare, but if children with language disorders have strengths that make them successful in other activities, their opportunities to participate should be protected and not automatically considered "less important" and available as time slots for special education activities.

Other particularly negative effects of traditional scheduling on students noted by students, parents, and school staff include the following: (1) being held responsible for material presented in pullout sessions in addition to material taught in regular classes; (2) pull-out-session content irrelevant to regular education needs; (3) being held responsible for activities of the general education classroom that occur while out of the room; (4) lack of time in the regular classroom to do

---

Box 5.4.

Guidelines for Caseload Size of the American Speech-Language-Hearing Association (1993).

MAXIMUM CASELOAD SIZE = 40 EXCEPT FOR SPECIAL CIRCUMSTANCES

SPECIAL CIRCUMSTANCES THAT MAY REQUIRE CASELOAD LIMITS

Caseload of all preschool students	Caseload should not exceed 25
Self-contained classroom	Caseload should not exceed 12 students with a support person
Technologically dependent students Medically fragile students Multilingual or limited-English proficient students Homebound students	Caseload should not exceed 8 students without a support person

seatwork and receive feedback; (5) missing teacher explanations and information about how to study for tests and do assignments; and (6) receiving reduced direct instruction and teacher assistance relative to peers (G. M. Anderson & Nelson, 1988).

One way to address these needs without adding on another kind of curriculum in patchwork fashion (as described by Barbie in Personal Reflection 5.5) is to establish the language intervention schedule to include an alternative language classroom that replaces the regular language arts curriculum. This scheduling approach works particularly well at middle school, junior high, and high school levels, where children change classes hourly. Language intervention sessions then can be provided daily in a regularly scheduled hour slot for a small class of students who need assistance in gaining access to the language of instruction and in using language to organize their approach to education (e.g., G. M. Anderson & Nelson, 1988; Buttrill, Niizawa, Biemer, Takahashi, & Hearn, 1989). A similar scheduling approach was taken by Despain and Simon (1987) by using regular science, social studies, and English classes as the context for building stronger communication and study skills, but with reduced class sizes and additional consultative assistance to the teachers.

Session Length Variables. Decisions about session length are related to what can be accomplished with a particular child within various time frames and what the child might miss in other contexts at those times. When children are placed in self-contained classrooms so that the language of instruction can be tailored to fit their needs, they may attend all day every day. Preschoolers may be scheduled only for half-day periods. In one case (Mroczkowski, 1988), however, a self-contained language class was offered for kindergartners in blocks of time that included full-day classes 5 days per week.

Alternative classrooms for older students may be offered for hour-long periods (with one half hour for group instruction and one half hour for individual practice) (G. M. Anderson & Nelson, 1988). Resource room activities with specialists in learning disabilities may be scheduled for various lengths of time, and sessions with speech–language pathologists tend to be scheduled for 20 to 30 minutes in schools during school hours and for 50 to 60 minutes in clinics outside of school hours. Remember, however, that although these time periods are usual, they are not necessarily optimal. We simply do not have the evidence to know, and so many variables operate in each situation that evidence would be very difficult to obtain.

In one study (Rich & Ross, 1989), however, students' time on learning tasks was measured in various educational settings, including regular class, resource room, special class, and special school. The analysis showed significant advantages in terms of in-class learning time for the resource room over any of the more restrictive settings. In regular classrooms, students with disabilities spent approximately the same time on-task as did students without disabilities, matching earlier reported data that showed that regular elementary students spend approximately 4 hours in class, are allocated learning time of about 3 hours, and are on task about 2 hours (Denham & Lieberman, 1980).

Data also show that children spend much more of their time in regular classrooms listening than talking. Elementary students spend over one half of their day listening to teachers talk, and estimates for high school students range as high as 90% (Bellack, Kliebard, Hyman, & Smith, 1966; Griffin & Hannah, 1960).

Language specialists can consult with others to analyze the time available to children with language disorders to communicate in social and academic contexts during a schoolday. Certain children in certain contexts may be particularly at risk for having insufficient opportunities to interact. For example, Capper (1990) analyzed how three children with severe disabilities spent their time in mixed special education classrooms in rural school districts. She found some disturbing evidence about how much time the three children spent alone, with no opportunity for social or communicative interaction or instruction. As illustrated in Figure 5.1, Capper found conditions in which

> *Elizabeth was physically separated from her peers, assigned to a corner of a room that was blocked by low bookshelves and cabinets. Elizabeth and Tiffany had no learning activities with peers, but were with them primarily at recess and meals. Although Roseann spent nearly 28% of her day with classmates in group learning activities, no interaction took place. (p. 340)*

Language intervention service-delivery decisions in situations such as these should include some collaborative problem solving aimed at identifying ways to increase students' opportunities to participate (review the discussions in Chapter 1).

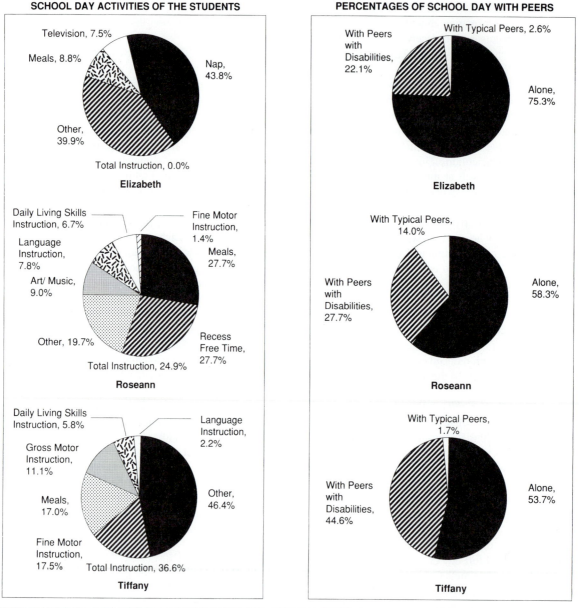

FIGURE 5.1   Relative time spent on school-day activities and with peers by three girls with severe developmental disabilities in a poor rural school district.

Note: From "Students With Low-Incidence Disabilities in Disadvantaged Rural Settings" by C. A. Capper, 1990, *Exceptional Children, 56,* p. 341. Copyright 1990 by The Council for Exceptional Children. Reprinted by permission.

Program Duration Variables.   IDEA requires that IEP content include a statement of "the projected date for the beginning of services" and the anticipated duration of the services (Sec. 614(d)(1)(A)(vi)). Similar wording is used in the statement that outlines content for IFSPs in Sec. 636(d). The difference is that a particular IEP can be in effect for a year or less before it must be revised. An IFSP must be reviewed within 6 months.

Preferences of Children and Their Parents

Children's Preferences.   Children are rarely asked whether they would prefer one type of service-delivery model over another. That is not too surprising, given children's limited experiences with different kinds of models that might give them the opportunity for comparison. In one study (Jenkins & Heinen, 1989), however, 686 second-, fourth-, and fifth-grade children were asked about service-delivery preferences. Half of the children were currently receiving services for mild impairments (primarily learning disabilities) in either pull-out or in-class settings, and half were regular education classmates of the first group who had observed the special service models of their peers but had not participated in them. Both groups were asked about where they would rather have help if they were having problems with reading (pullout room or in class), and who they would rather have help them (their regular teacher or the building reading specialist).

In this study, children who had experience with pull-out services (either for themselves or their classmates) indicated a preference for that model over in-class programs, whereas children with in-class experience did not show a significant preference for one model or the other. Grade level also played a significant role in influencing choices. Older children indicated a preference for pullout services significantly more often as a way of avoiding embarrassment. However, avoidance of embarrassment was listed as a reason both for preferring the pullout model and the in-class model. Other reasons given for preferring the in-class model were the convenience of not having to walk to another room and preferring to stay with classmates. Another reason for preferring the pullout model was the perception that specialists can give more and better help in a pullout room (Jenkins & Heinen, 1989).

Although these results cannot be generalized to situations involving language intervention and language specialists, they do provide insights that can be brought to the decision-making process. Elementary school children with mild disabilities are primarily concerned with getting help relevant to their needs to succeed in the regular classroom, but they wish to avoid embarrassment while doing so. They are not averse to going to pullout rooms if it can be done without embarrassment and if the help provided is relevant to their needs to succeed in their regular classrooms.

Parents' Preferences.   There are probably as many parental preferences for types of service delivery as there are parents. Because of the heterogeneity of children's language impairments, associated disabilities, family histories, and community options, it is difficult to generalize about parental preferences (see Personal Reflection 5.10). In addition, if professionals cannot agree on which service-delivery models are best, and if research has not offered clear-cut answers as to which models work best, how can parents be expected to agree on a preference for one model over another?

Parents are experts on their own children. They are usually the most sensitive observers of the intervention setting's influence on their children's self-perceptions, and sometimes they assume strong advocacy roles to obtain services that they feel their children need. When their role as experts on their children is respected, they are valuable members of the team.

Hanline and Halvorsen (1989) studied parental preference by investigating parents' perceptions about their children's transitions from segregated to integrated educational placements. Parents of fourteen children from

---

PERSONAL REFLECTION 5.10 _____

"Sometimes I feel overwhelmed. How can I evaluate this program? How do I know this is best? Then I remember that it's a team approach. I'm not in it alone. It's just my job to get the specialists I trust to talk to each other about it. I remind myself that they know the programs and I know Wilson. . . . Thinking of myself as Wilson's 'case manager' makes it easier to ask for the things that he needs."

Barb Buswell, talking about her relationships to professionals and school systems, quoted by Robin Simons (1987, p. 54) in her book *After the Tears.*

thirteen families in the San Francisco Bay Area were interviewed regarding their perceptions of the experience. The children ranged in age from 4 to 22 years and exhibited a variety of impairments (e.g., Down syndrome, cerebral palsy, communicative disability with motor delay, and multiple disabilities) with eleven children classified as having severe disabilities.

Parents' reviews of the process varied with the roles they had to play to accomplish the transitions. Parents who fought for their child's integration against opposition were the least satisfied, and they were resentful that they had had to play such a major role in the process. "As one parent asked, 'Why wasn't it done by the people whose job it is to do it?' " (Hanline & Halvorsen, 1989, p. 489).

When asked about their perceptions of the advantages and disadvantages of the integration model of service delivery for their children, five parents stated that there was no disadvantage to integration, and none of the parents reported regret about placing their child in an integrated setting. Parents' concerns were related to worries about their children's reduced ability to establish friendships within the community of persons with disabilities (who might serve as role models), about whether they would establish friendships with their nondisabled peers, and about their lack of experiences to prepare them for the social demands of regular schools. When asked about advantages, most parents spoke about skill enhancement, particularly in the area of social skill development, about their children's enhanced self-esteem and confidence, and about the presence of normally developing role models and increased stimulation in integrated settings that would prepare them for living in mainstream society (Hanline & Halvorsen, 1989).

Parents also reported that their own expectations for their children had been raised, along with their "admiration" for their children, and that they now had hopes that their children would lead more interesting and independent lives as adults. Parents of half of the children reported that their children had established friendships with nondisabled peers that extended outside of school hours, and several parents also noted the benefits in increased understanding of disability by nondisabled students. An added benefit to families mentioned by two parents was reduced concern about long-term care expressed by nondisabled siblings (Hanline & Halvorsen, 1989).

SUMMARY

When designing programs for individual children, the specialist should consider public policy at federal, state, intermediate, and local levels. Public policies are intended to guide service provision to children with special needs in positive ways, but it is up to professionals to see that they work. When service provision is ineffective, professionals must work together with parents and other professionals to ensure positive changes.

No one answer can apply to difficult questions about establishing a service-delivery context for an individual child. Answers can only come out of the collaborative process involving parents, teachers, health-care professionals, and other individuals. Multiple good answers may be possible for individual children. Comprehensive planning includes consideration of the multiple contexts in the child's life. The caution in putting together patchwork schedules, however, is that children like Barbie (see Personal Reflection 5.5) may get lost in the shuffle.

Finally, one more caution. In this chapter, I have considered only the obvious variables related to context. As S. F. Warren (1988) noted, "Context is more than who is present, when, with what objects, and in what environmental setting" (p. 295). In addition, context includes the linguistic context established not only in a current piece of specific discourse but also in the discourse history shared by the partners. Context also includes the social, emotional, and event interactions that become a part of the system that evolves when two or more people interact. Those are the variables that daily occupy the attention of language interventionists and are the variables that occupy much of the discussion in Part II.

REVIEW TOPICS

- Federal policymaking laws, including Section 504, PL 94–142 (Part B: preschool [optional] to school-age [required], FAPE, LRE, IEP, parent notification and assessment requirements); PL 99–457 (Part B: Preschool Grant Program; Part H: Infant and Toddler Program, developmental risks, IFSP); PL 100–407 (Technology Related Assistance for Individuals with Disabilities Act, defined assistive devices and services); PL 101–476 (renamed law as IDEA, added autism and TBI categories, added transition service requirement); PL 102–119 (added assistive devices to Part H; 3- to 5-year-olds may have either IFSP or IEP; changed "case management" to "service coordination"); PL 105–17 (changed Part H to Part C and added emphasis on general education)

- Part B of IDEA (school-age): parent notification, comprehensive evaluation, determination of disability and eligibility, IEP meetings, development of the IEP, IEP content, review and revision of the IEP, transition services, periodic reevaluation, due process.
- Part C of IDEA (infants, toddlers, preschool-age): evaluation and eligibility, individualized family service plan (IFSP)
- Other federal policy influences (REI, full inclusion, assistive technology interpretation)
- State, intermediate, and local policy influences
- How to influence policy development
- Service delivery issues, including:

  setting variables (pullout rooms, center programs, special classrooms in home schools, regular education classrooms, home and family contexts, social contexts, vocational contexts)

  people variables, including professional roles for language specialists (direct service provider, consultant, teacher, co-teacher, mixed models), peers (cooperative learning), and parents and siblings (as language intervention aides, primary intervention agents, and incidental intervention agents)

  scheduling variables, including session frequency, session length, program duration

REVIEW QUESTIONS

1. What components must be included in an IEP?
2. What are the differences between an IEP and IFSP?

3. Outline the steps you would use if you wanted to provide services in a way not currently permitted by public policy in the school district where you work. What options might be available for resolving this conflict?
4. What do we know about parental and student preferences and concerns about service delivery models?
5. What is the recommended maximum caseload size for speech–language caseloads? What conditions would justify caseloads lower than this number?

ACTIVITIES FOR EXTENDED THINKING

1. Develop the points for both sides of the debate on full inclusion. On one side, take the position that children with severe disabilities are best served in facilities that are tailor-made to meet their needs; on the other, take the position that children with severe disabilities should be educated in regular education classrooms and never be pulled out for any special services. Then state your own position, and why.

2. Visit a school speech–language pathologist and learning disabilities specialist. Ask to see IEP forms used in their schools. Interview them about what they like and do not like about the federal legislation. Ask them what requirements are added at the state and local level to the federal requirements. Ask to see policy and guideline documents that guide their practices.

3. Interview specialists in early childhood special education and speech–language pathology about Part C requirements for serving infants and toddlers. What do they like about the process? What strategies have they developed to facilitate the development of IFSPs and to make the process work as intended?

Making Assessment and Intervention
Work for Children

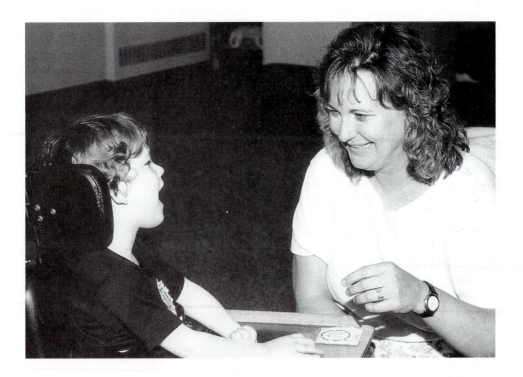

A SEQUENCE OF QUESTIONS

ASSESSMENT AND INTERVENTION AS
INTEGRATED PROCESSES

ASSESSMENT PURPOSES AND PRACTICES

INTERVENTION PURPOSES AND PRACTICES

How should children with language disorders be identified, described, and treated? Asking good questions is particularly important for guiding assessment and intervention. Chapter 1 considered the importance of questions not only about what is wrong (and right) about a child's communicative **processes** but also about the child's communicative **needs** and participation **opportunities.** Chapter 5 considered policy and service delivery issues. This chapter considers the more specific questions and strategies of language assessment and intervention across the age span from infancy through adolescence. In Part II, assessment and intervention approaches are made even more specific for children in the early, middle, and later stages of language acquisition.

A SEQUENCE OF QUESTIONS

Different questions are appropriate at different stages of the assessment and intervention process. The flowchart in Figure 6.1 offers a summary of the main decision points and assessment and intervention activities for children of all ages. The details of this flowchart are the subject of the chapters in Part II. The general principles that guide the decision-making processes of assessment and intervention are the focus of this chapter.

The intervention and assessment process starts with screening or referral activities that identify children with a problem that potentially involves language and communication. The process has several possible exit points, depending on the outcome of events and decisions, at which participants may decide that special intervention for language and communication development is no longer needed. Even when exit decisions are made, however, follow-up checks may indicate that further assessment and intervention are warranted when a child's skills do not match current contextual demands.

1. Does the child have a problem that might be related to a language disorder? The first question leads a child into the language assessment and intervention system. It generally arises either during screening or referral. One reason for preferring an entry system based on referral rather than screening is that others who know the child well may be best able to answer the question whether a child has a problem. Screening procedures tend to look for a problem where none may exist.

If a child scores below age norms on a screening test but no one in the child's environment thinks the child

has a problem, and if the child is functioning well when observed closely within those contexts, little can be gained by labeling the child as having a language disorder. Whatever wobbly language skills or processing behaviors are evident in formal assessment contexts, the child and participants in real-life situations must be compensating well enough to enable the child to function normally without special assistance. Premature introduction of assistance might remove the child from a natural context where he or she is apparently functioning well, and it might foster lowered self-expectations and lowered expectations by the adults in the child's environment. The ultimate result could be the "Pygmalion effect," in which lowered expectations are associated with lowered opportunities until the self-fulfilling prophecy comes true (Rosenthal & Jacobson, 1968).

On the other hand, low scores on screening tests might be interpreted as indicators that children should be monitored, and in some cases, preventive services (possibly in the nature of consultation or ongoing monitoring) should be offered. Decisions may depend on a variety of factors, including possible causative influences, stages of development, contextual expectations, and multicultural influences.

The group for whom services should be provided before a problem may be clearly apparent is the group of infants and toddlers known to be at risk for developing problems. This is the group for whom many of the requirements of Part C of IDEA were written (see Chapter 5). Preschool children are also often screened for language disorders and potential learning problems when they are ready to enter kindergarten.

2. Is the problem better explained as one of language difference rather than language disorder? It must be determined whether this is a case of language disorder, of language difference, or both.

Valid assessment procedures cannot be selected until professionals identify whether tests standardized on mainstream cultures and linguistic systems are appropriate. If a child has limited English proficiency because his or her family's cultural or linguistic backgrounds differ from those of formal testing procedures and tools, alternative methods and tools must be used to answer the remaining questions of assessment and intervention.

3. Does the child have a language disorder (possibly related to some other condition)? If this is an initial assessment, one of the first questions is whether a

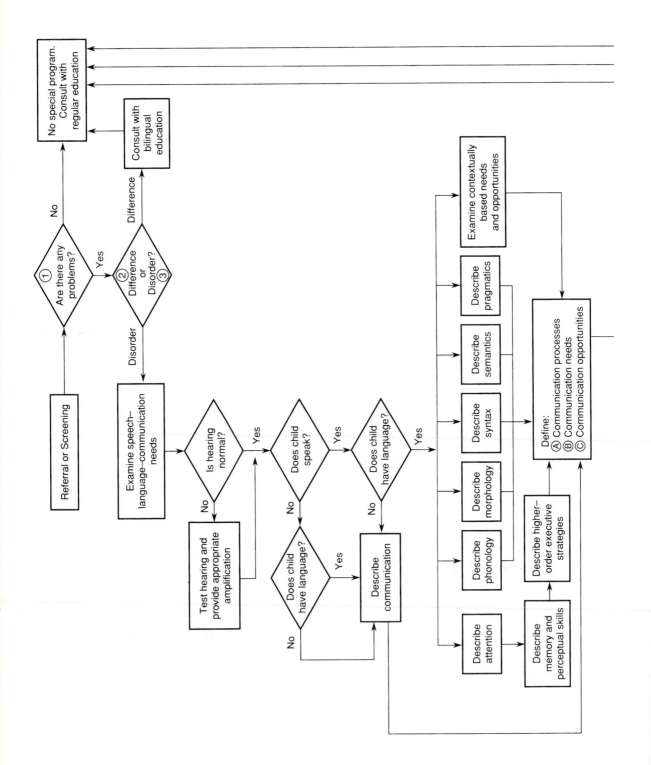

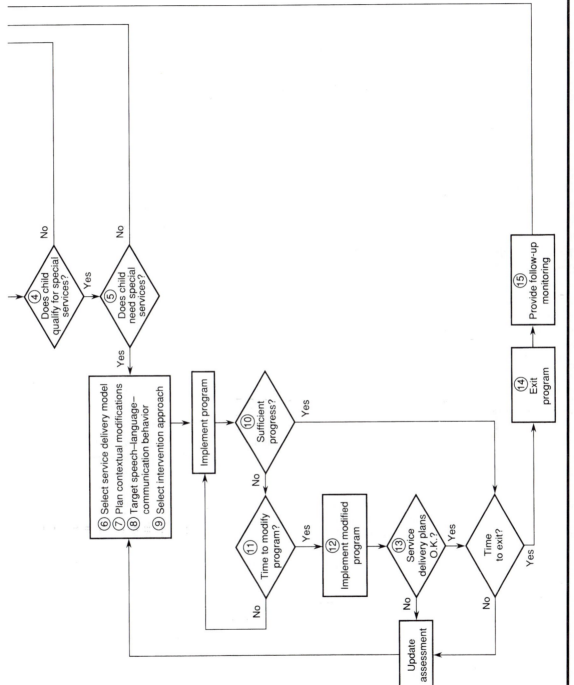

FIGURE 6.1 A decision-making flowchart for the primary steps of the language assessment and intervention process.

disorder of language development exists and whether some other causative condition might be active as well or instead. Although many disagree about the advisability of labeling impairment, labels are often needed for services to be reimbursed. For example, Wang & Reynolds in 1985 reported on a successful intervention program involving declassification of students. However, the program was terminated because it resulted in a net loss of revenue for the school district.

Diagnosis (and labeling) of impairment is one of the primary purposes of assessment, but as discussed later in this chapter, defining language disorder operationally is difficult. Two criteria frequently used to define language disorder are **discrepancy criteria** and **exclusion criteria.** Both are discussed in greater detail later in this chapter.

4. Does the child qualify for special services? To qualify for special services, a child usually must meet eligibility criteria established by some public or private agency (e.g., a state department of education or a third-party payer). Eligibility criteria may involve not only judgments about characteristics of the impairment (possibly including discrepancy and exclusionary criteria) but also procedures for diagnosticians and decision-making teams, even including the specific makeup of those teams.

5. Does the child need special services? The question of whether a child *needs* special services may not always be asked. Because a student qualifies for special services does not necessarily mean that he or she needs them. Conversely, a student may need special services but not qualify for them according to strict policy standards. Some have suggested that the question about need should be asked without spending so much time, effort, and money on whether those children qualify. This could happen if regular, special, and bilingual education were not viewed and funded as separate entities but as cooperative ways to meet the needs of all students having difficulty achieving, no matter what the cause, and as a result, bias against youngsters from minority cultural or linguistic groups might be reduced (Reynolds & Wang, 1983; Rueda, 1989; J. E. Ysseldyke et al., 1983).

6. What services does the child need? This question was a major topic in Chapter 5. Decisions about settings, people, and scheduling variables are used to select service-delivery models as part of transdiscipli-

nary planning. Later in this chapter, the emphasis is on creating appropriate matches between the problems and strengths identified in assessment and the purposes, types, content, and contexts of intervention.

7. Should specific contexts be changed or introduced? Answers to questions about appropriate service are integrally tied to answers about whether specific contexts should be modified during intervention. When a child cannot function in a particular environment, the two choices are to change the environment or to change the child. Most intervention programs involve a little of both.

When the ultimate goal is to assist children to participate successfully in society, education, and work as adults, it is important to identify contexts that may help them to develop those characteristics. The idea is to foster a closer match between the communicative demands of situations and the communicative abilities of children. Sometimes this match can be achieved through a special modified context that helps students gain access to learning not available in the regular classroom (e.g., G. M. Anderson & Nelson, 1988; L. P. Hoffman, 1990; N. W. Nelson, 1981a). Increasingly however, intervention planners are seeking ways to modify natural contexts with same-age peers to allow children with impairments greater opportunity to participate with peers who may or may not have impairments (e.g., N. W. Nelson, 1989b; W. Stainback et al., 1985).

8. Which speech, language, and communication behaviors and strategies should be changed? The other side of the intervention coin involves changing the child. When children's knowledge, skill, and strategies are insufficient to meet communicative demands, intervention efforts should target areas most in need of change that will make the most difference to the child. Goals are established, each with a set of operationally defined objectives targeting specific changes. The choices made in writing objectives are guided by one's theories of language acquisition, which are discussed in Chapter 3. Other guidance comes from interviewing parents, teachers, and children about the child's needs. A third source comes from individualized assessment, in which the youngster's abilities are compared with those of normally developing peers.

9. What intervention approach should be used? In addition to targets of intervention, procedures of intervention need to be selected. As discussed in Chapter 3, selection and implementation of intervention methods are theory driven. An eclectic approach (N. W. Nelson, 1981a)—in which professionals select one or more methods to accomplish a particular purpose—may be best for meeting individualized needs.

10. Is progress occurring? Integral to intervention is the ongoing measurement of change. The plan for measuring progress is established as part of the written objectives. Each objective includes a criterion statement indicating how participants will know when it has been accomplished. Participants also must regularly obtain a broader view of the child. Federal policy determines the timing of this process to be at least twice a year for Individualized Family Service Plans (IFSPs) (as required by Part C) and at least once a year for Individualized Education Plans (IEPs) (as required by Part B, IDEA, PL 105–17, 1997).

11. Has enough change occurred that it is time to modify the plan? To some extent, good plans become obsolete sooner than poor ones. If a plan works, the changes it specifies are made without taking forever, and thus, new targets are justified sooner. Of course, it is possible to write a plan targeting trivial changes that are easy to accomplish but make little difference to the child. The likelihood of this occurring is reduced if the progress-measuring plan includes measurement of outcomes in relevant contexts.

12. If not enough change is occurring, what modifications are needed? If no change is occurring, or very little, modifications are also needed in the plan. Perhaps the targets were too ambitious. Maybe they do not meet contextually based needs. The mismatch between the communicative expectations of the child's environment and the communicative abilities of the child simply may be too great. The procedures being implemented may not be appropriate for the kinds of changes sought. Regardless, if positive change is not occurring, the plan must be changed.

13. Does the current service-delivery model remain best for meeting the child's needs? At some point, an IEP team may decide that a basic change in the service-delivery model is needed. The occasion for this question may be a system-wide look at how the needs of all children with special problems are being met as a part of program accountability evaluation, or it may be asked on an individual basis. Parents of children served under IDEA have a right to ask for a formal review of service

delivery plans any time that they think that their children's needs are not being met. Part B specifies that at least once every three years children must undergo comprehensive reevaluation and their need for special education services must be reconfirmed. This is usually interpreted to mean that children must again meet local eligibility standards based on current formal assessment results.

One of the most difficult problems facing professionals occurs when they think that a child continues to need special services but formal test results indicate that the student no longer qualifies. In such cases, primary options are (1) to conduct further testing specifically to tap the remaining areas of impairment, (2) to conduct different kinds of assessment to determine whether the student can actually apply newly acquired skills in the classroom, or (3) to decide that the professional is being overprotective and that the student is actually ready to be more independent, particularly if sufficient support is available in the regular classroom. At one time or another, all three options may be needed.

14. Is it time for the child to exit formal intervention services? At some point, a particular child may be ready to exit formal speech and language intervention services. Federal policy set by IDEA specifies that this cannot be a unilateral decision by a single professional but must be part of the IEP or IFSP process.

15. Does follow-up monitoring indicate a need for direct attention to needs again? A point of the discussion of causes, categories, and characteristics in Chapter 4 was that disabilities evolve over time, both as a result of changing abilities of children and changing expectations of contexts. Results presented by Scarborough and Dobrich (1990) showed in particular that children who receive language intervention as preschoolers may appear to catch up with their peers when they first enter school but run into problems later when language and literacy demands of school contexts increase. This situation was also illustrated by Damico's (1988) case study in Chapter 1.

A little recognized requirement of IDEA is that follow-up monitoring is required after children leave special education. As professionals become more skilled in using the strategies of collaborative consultation and natural contexts for measuring outcomes of intervention, the student's transition from special intervention contexts to home, school, and work may be smoother. In systems in which the concept of a continuum of services is a reality, the view of service provision as all-or-none can become more flexible, with a mechanism in place to provide more or less intensive services as needed.

ASSESSMENT AND INTERVENTION AS INTEGRATED PROCESSES

Using Team Contributions Effectively

When children are seen as members of whole systems, they cannot be treated in isolation. When whole systems are the focus, assessment and intervention cannot be viewed as isolated processes.

Contributions of members from several professional disciplines may be needed, depending on the particular child, but most certainly, contributions are needed from parents and the children. When children are of school age, or even preschool age, members of the educational community are essential members of planning and intervention teams, and when children near the end of schooling, vocational planners may be appropriate team members.

How should teams be organized, and how should they function? Calling a group of people together does not ensure that it will function as a team. Understanding the various ways that teams can function can contribute to the development of a more effective team.

Three Models of Team Process

L. McCormick (1990c) defined a team as "a group of persons who have a shared goal and required actions to perform in order to reach that goal" (p. 262). Beyond that basic similarity, at least three different team approaches are available.

Multidisciplinary.   A multidisciplinary team is a team composed of representatives of different disciplines. The term implies nothing more about mode of organization or functioning. V. Hart (1977) identified several problems of a multidisciplinary approach in which a group of individuals works independently. Primary are the possibilities for conflicting recommendations, neglect of important information, and presentation of separate implications not reconstructed into a whole picture. The multidisciplinary mode also is more likely to result either in the kind of "competitive goal setting" or "independent goal setting" (D. W. Johnson & Johnson, 1975) discussed in Chapter 1.

Interdisciplinary.   An interdisciplinary team is distinguished from a multidisciplinary team by the formal communication channels between disciplines and a case manager or service coordinator acting as leader (McCormick & Goldman, 1979). Interdisciplinary models also often involve consultative relationships among professional "experts" and individuals who know the child well. Because consultation in such models tends to flow in one direction (e.g., from the consultant to the teacher), the team may have no mechanism for the teacher to play an equal role in decision making and for providing input for establishing the validity and reliability of assessment and intervention outcomes (L. McCormick, 1990c).

Transdisciplinary.   A transdisciplinary team encourages active sharing of information and skills across disciplines in multiple directions. The term **transdisciplinary** was introduced by Hutchinson (1974) to describe the collaborative relationship in a project for atypical infants and their families. The model was described further by Lyon and Lyon (1980) as having three key features: (1) **joint functioning**—team members perform service-delivery functions together whenever possible; (2) **continuous staff development**—members train and receive training from each other in reciprocal interactions; and (3) **role release**—team members not only share information with each other, but assist each other to perform functions usually reserved to their own disciplines. L. McCormick (1990c) summarized the relationship as follows:

> Team members are accountable for seeing that the best practices of their respective disciplines are implemented, monitoring program implementation, training others if necessary, and revising programs when evaluation data indicate that procedures are not working as well as intended. (p. 269)

The concept of role release was developed further by Woodruff and McGonigel (1988) to include the following dimensions: (1) **role extension**—members learn from each other; (2) **role enrichment**—members teach each other; (3) **role expansion**—members assume aspects of each others' professional roles, and (4) **role**

support—members provide the necessary backup support for each other as they assume the roles of other disciplines.

A truly transdisciplinary team cannot function unless members participate in cooperative goal setting. A program implemented as a single integrated service is less fragmented and potentially more effective than a team comprising a set of separate services with separate goals.

The transdisciplinary team process is not without its critics. Some have questioned whether teams can make better decisions than individuals and whether they are cost-effective (Yoshida, 1983; J. R. Ysseldyke & Algozzine, 1982). Efforts to conduct research on team process are complicated by the fact that different labels may not represent clear distinctions among functional relationships (Golin & Ducanis, 1985). Unidisciplinary approaches sometimes may be desirable, particularly at some points of development and when the child seems to have a relatively isolated impairment. Cooperative goal setting with family members remains desirable, however, and is always critical if programs are to be relevant to children's individualized needs.

ASSESSMENT PURPOSES AND PRACTICES

Diagnosing the Disorder

Defining the Disorder.   Diagnosis requires an operational definition of language disorder. In Chapter 4, I argued for a broad view of language disorders, including conditions beyond those known as "specific language impairment." Bashir's (1989) definition is repeated here:

> Language disorders *is a term that represents a heterogeneous group of either developmental or acquired disabilities principally characterized by deficits in comprehension, production, and/or use of language. Language disorders are chronic and may persist across the lifetime of the individual. The symptoms, manifestations, effects, and severity of the problems change over time. The changes occur as a consequence of context, content, and learning tasks. (p. 181)*

Although this definition has many strengths (discussed in Chapter 4), it is not specific enough for diagnosing a child as having a language disorder without further information. It begs the question "What are deficits in comprehension, production, and/or use of language?"

Another definition, proposed by the American Speech-Language-Hearing Association (ASHA) Committee on Language, Speech, and Hearing Services in Schools (1982), has similar problems being operationalized without further detail:

> *A language disorder is the impairment or deviant development of comprehension and/or use of a spoken, written, and/or other symbol system. The disorder may involve (1) the form of language (phonologic, morphologic, and syntactic systems, (2) the content of language (semantic system), and/or (3) the function of language in communication (pragmatic system) in any combination. (p. 949)*

This definition uses the form, content, and use ("function") categories suggested by L. Bloom and Lahey (1978), which are cross-referenced with the five systems, phonology, morphology, syntax, semantics, and pragmatics. It also mentions "comprehension and/or use" of these systems, and specifically refers to "spoken, written, and/or other symbol systems." The element of heterogeneity that Bashir (1989) emphasized is only hinted at in the phrase, "in any combination."

A third definition, suggested by Lahey (1988), clarifies the expectation that the disorder occurs while learning one's native language and that it involves discrepancy from developmental expectations based on chronological age:

> *Thus we can use the term* language disorder *to refer to any disruption in the learning or use of one's native language as evidenced by language behaviors that are different from (but not superior to) those expected given a child's chronological age. (p. 21)*

Many questions remain after all of these definitions. The primary one is the meaning of phrases such as "any disruption in the learning or use" (Lahey, 1988, p. 21), "impairment or deviant development of comprehension and/or use" (American Speech-Language-Hearing Association Committee, 1982, p. 949), and "deficits in comprehension, production, and/or use of language" (Bashir, 1989, p. 181). Exact meanings may be ignored when language disorders are defined in the abstract, but they must be addressed when answering the question "Does this specific child have a language disorder?"

When establishing operational criteria for determining language disorder, questions of deviance, disruption, or deficit are often defined by comparing observed abilities of one child against expected abilities for some comparison group. Most commonly, a child's language performance on formal tests is compared with children at the same (1) chronological age (CA) or (2) mental age (MA). Although IDEA requires nonbiased assessment, in practice this requirement is often ignored (Taylor & Payne, 1983). Children from minority groups should be compared with a group from a similar linguistic and cultural background.

Using Discrepancy Criteria.   Tallal (1988) expressed the rationale for using MA referencing as well as CA referencing as discrepancy criteria for diagnosing *specific* language impairment:

> It is essential that in addition to demonstrating that language abilities of a child are significantly below what would be expected based on the child's chronological age, it is important to establish that they are also significantly discrepant from what would be predicted based on the child's mental abilities. (p. 211)

A problem arises in practice because children's language abilities usually are not compared directly with those of local peers of either the same CA or MA. Rather, indirect comparisons are made psychometrically with a remote normative group of "peers" (a different group of remote peers is used for each test). That is, diagnosticians often administer standardized tests and apply a set of discrepancy criteria to determine disorder.

Chronological Age Referencing.   CA referencing occurs whenever a child's scores on language tests are measured against normative data for children of the same age group. Discrepancy can be expressed in terms of any of the standard scores that are provided with most formal tests (e.g., standard deviations or z-scores, percentile rankings, and age equivalent scores) and with normative data for some informal measures, such as mean length of utterance (MLU) (Miller, 1981).

Cognitive Referencing.   Cognitive referencing occurs whenever a child's scores on language tests are measured against the child's scores on intelligence tests. One or more language tests are typically used to determine language age (LA), and one or more intelligence tests (usually one) to determine MA. Then, the scores on those different measures are compared to see if they are discrepant enough to meet a standard established by a qualifying agency. For students with learning disabil-

ities, intelligence test scores are also compared with achievement test scores or other grade-level measures.

Several problems arise from this approach. First, psychometric problems are associated with attempting to directly compare scores from tests with different normative samples. Even standard scores are not directly comparable (Seashore, 1955). This problem is compounded by the fact that the children included in normative samples may be from cultural and linguistic communities different from the child being tested. Few tests have been standardized on children from diverse sociolinguistic groups, and simply averaging the scores of a small proportion of minority group children into the norms of a test designed to measure majority culture and linguistic knowledge does not remove this element of bias.

One reason for the lack of culturally fair tests may be the cost (in terms of both time and money) of test standardization. Another is that it would be difficult to establish national norms appropriate for all of the diverse geographic, ethnic, and socioeconomic demographic combinations in the United States, let alone other parts of the world.

An alternative is to establish local community norms. This is one of several possible solutions mentioned by Vaughn-Cooke to reduce bias in testing (1983). In practice, local norms are rarely established. Of course, there is good reason for this. A lot of time and a thorough knowledge of psychometric procedures are required to gather adequate samples of one child's language behavior to obtain an accurate picture of the child's functioning level. Practitioners cannot perform a community-based normative study every time they need a set of scores for comparative purposes.

A second problem is that, even if appropriate norms are available, scores earned on cognitive functioning tests cannot be assumed to be independent of scores earned on language functioning tests. The problem of confounding LA and MA scores is threefold. First, some cognitive assessment tools use tasks very similar to those used in language assessment. Thus, two ostensibly different scores compared for discrepancy may reflect the same impairment (this is particularly a problem with full-scale IQ scores). Second, cognitive assessment tools, although designed specifically to measure nonverbal cognitive skills, may tap only a limited aspect of nonverbal cognition. For example, J. R. Johnston (1982a) found that the test items for children under age

8 from the Leiter International Performance Scale (Leiter, 1959) tested primarily the ability to recognize physical characteristics of visual stimuli. Similarly, Kamhi, Minor, and Mauer (1990) showed that 15 items (30%) of the 50 items on the Test of Nonverbal Intelligence (TONI; L. Brown, Sherbenou, & Johnsen, 1985) required perceptual rather than conceptual processing. Furthermore, almost all of the perceptual items occurred early in the test, making it possible for most children up to the age of 11 to obtain normal range IQs without passing any of the conceptual items.

A third problem is that even when cognitive assessment tools use nonverbal stimuli and responses, children with language disorders may still be disadvantaged. The lack of verbal mediation strategies may make it difficult for them to encode key features of nonverbal stimuli. Yet, their scores are compared with normative scores that reflect normal use of verbal strategies to identify, retain, and manipulate nonverbal symbols. To appreciate this, consider the matrix problem that appears in Figure 6.2. As you solve this problem, notice how this and similar items from the TONI might lend

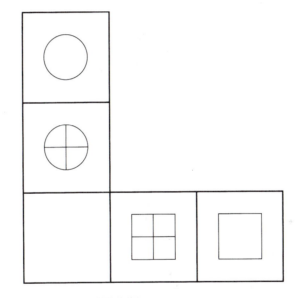

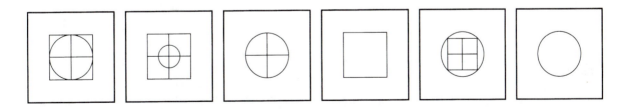

FIGURE 6.2   Matrix problem from the Test of Nonverbal Intelligence (TONI).

Note: From *Test of Nonverbal Intelligence* (p. A24) by L. Brown, R. J. Sherbenou, and S. K. Johnsen, 1997, Austin, TX: Pro-Ed. Copyright 1997 by Pro-Ed. Reprinted by permission.

themselves to linguistic encoding of forms and relationships to facilitate correct choices.

Other problems with discrepancy criteria, cognitive referencing in particular, were discussed in Chapter 3, including that (1) cognitive tests may reflect language deficits (Francis et al., 1996); (2) some combinations of language tests and cognitive tests may show a discrepancy for individual children when others do not, at some points in development but not others (Cole et al., 1990, 1992; Cole et al., 1994); (3) formal tests often yield biased results for children from diverse cultural and linguistic communities (Lahey, 1992; Seymour, 1992; Terrell & Terrell, 1983); (4) formal tests fail to assess needs for language intervention in everyday contexts (Westby et al., 1996); and (5) children can benefit equally from language intervention services whether or not they show discrepancies (Cole & Harris, 1992; Fey, Long, & Cleave, 1994). My own recommendation both in Chapter 3 and here is that professionals seek to limit their dependence on discrepancy criteria for diagnosing language disorder or learning disability. The evidence simply does not support the validity of such a criterion for clinical purposes (research purposes may be another matter), and discrepancy criteria may interfere with some children receiving service who need it and could benefit from it (Francis et al., 1996; also Personal Reflection 6.1).

Intralinguistic Referencing. Intralinguistic referencing looks for discrepancies among language abilities within the individual (Fey, 1986). It "involves the eval-

---

PERSONAL REFLECTION 6.1 _____

"There are numerous problems with the hypothesis that children who are deficient in language or academic skills relative to age and IQ scores are etiologically and phenotypically different from children who are different in language or academic skills relative to age but not IQ. Unfortunately, the notion that these subgroups are different is firmly embedded in public policy and clinical practice." (p. 133)

David J. Francis, University of Houston, TX; *Jack M. Fletcher,* University of Texas Medical School, Houston, TX; *Bennett A. Shaywitz* and *Sally E. Shaywitz,* Yale University School of Medicine, New Haven, CT, and *Byron P. Rourke,* University of Windsor, Windsor, Ontario (1996)

---

uation and comparison of a child's performance in expressive and receptive form, content, and use" (Olswang & Bain, 1991, p. 256).

In this approach, measures of different aspects of language are compared (see Figure 6.3). Thus, children's scores on a test that measures one aspect of language might be compared against scores from another test that measures another aspect of language. The rationale behind this approach is that it can reveal scattered patterns of developmental accomplishments, which have been reported for children with specific language disability (e.g., the "patterns of frequency of usage" differences, Leonard, 1980). Patterns in which more advanced behaviors co-occur with earlier developing behaviors provide an important piece of the diagnostic puzzle.

In fact, identification of this type of scattered intralinguistic pattern represents an example of an inclusionary criterion for determining who should be diagnosed as having a language disorder. Kamhi (1990) suggested that perhaps more time should be spent looking for inclusionary criteria and less for exclusionary criteria and that criteria for defining language disorder should shift with the child's age.

Using Exclusionary Criteria. Exclusionary criteria are established to determine whether the child's language-based symptoms are related to a specific language impairment or to some other disorder that includes language difficulties as part of a more complex picture. In some ways, this is a question about cause. To identify a child as having a language disorder, it is necessary to rule out that the child has some other kind of disorder. Or is it?

Maybe what is needed is an awareness that, in the heterogeneous category of children with language disorders, some have language disorders relatively isolated from other impairments, and others have language disorders thoroughly intertwined with other kinds of impairments. Both might need special education services related to their language disorders. But only one group might meet the definition of language disorder if it is based on discrepancy and exclusionary criteria for determining *specific* language impairment.

Here, the question of purpose comes into play. If the purpose of diagnosing language disorder is to select subjects for a research project to study specific language impairment, then Tallal's (1988) comments are perti-

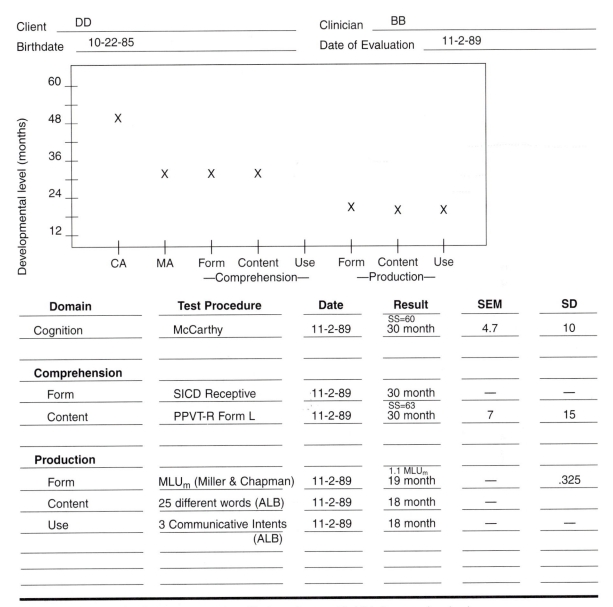

Client ___DD___   Clinician ___BB___

Birthdate ___10-22-85___   Date of Evaluation ___11-2-89___

Domain	Test Procedure	Date	Result	SEM	SD
Cognition					
Cognition	McCarthy	11-2-89	SS=60 30 month	4.7	10
Comprehension					
Form	SICD Receptive	11-2-89	30 month	—	—
Content	PPVT-R Form L	11-2-89	SS=63 30 month	7	15
Production					
Form	MLU$_m$ (Miller & Chapman)	11-2-89	1.1 MLU$_m$ 19 month	—	.325
Content	25 different words (ALB)	11-2-89	18 month	—	
Use	3 Communicative Intents (ALB)	11-2-89	18 month	—	—

FIGURE 6.3   Example of an assessment profile for a 4-year-old child diagnosed as having a language disorder.

Note: This profile illustrates an age discrepancy but not a cognitive discrepancy (at least in the area of language comprehension). An intralinguistic discrepancy between measures of comprehension and production also appears. Measures used to construct this profile included the *McCarthy Scales of Children's Abilities* (McCarthy, 1972), the *Sequenced Inventory of Communication Development-Revised* (SICD-R; Hedrick, Prather, & Tobin, 1984) the *Peabody Picture Vocabulary Test-Revised* (PPVT-R; Dunn & Dunn, 1981), *Assessing Linguistic Behaviors* (ALB; Olswang, Stoel-Gammon, Coggins, & Carpenter, 1987), MLU data from Miller and Chapman (1979; cited in Miller, 1981).

From "When to recommend intervention" by L. B. Olswang and B. A. Bain, 1991, *Language, Speech, and Hearing Services in Schools, 22,* p. 238. Copyright 1994 by American Speech-Language-Hearing Association. Reprinted by permission.

nent. In a presentation at the National Conference on Learning Disabilities, Tallal argued:

> The number one priority for research [is] the development of standardized inclusionary and exclusionary criteria and the encouragement of their uniform usage for subsequent federally funded or privately funded research in this area. (p. 206)

Stark and Tallal (1981) suggested standard exclusion criteria (meaning such a child would *not* be diagnosed with specific language impairment):

1. *Hearing level:* failure to pass 250- to 6000-Hz screening or to perform picture-pointing task at 25-dB hearing level.
2. *Emotional and behavioral status:* history of severe behavior or adjustment problems.
3. *Intellectual status:* performance scale IQ less than 85.
4. *Neurological status:* evidence of neurological deficit or lesion.
5. *Speech motor skills:* evidence of peripheral neuro-muscular or speech articulation impairment.
6. *Reading level:* reading age-level score more than 6 months lower than composite LA score.

This list was designed to determine whether children could qualify as research subjects, not whether they could qualify for clinical services based on language needs. These are two very different purposes. In the Stark and Tallal (1981) study, only one third of the 132 children originally identified by clinicians as meeting the loosely defined referral criteria for the study met the stricter operationally defined criteria for diagnosing specific language impairment.

Commenting on this 2:1 mismatch between clinicians' judgments and criteria-based determination of specific language disorders, Aram, Morris, and Hall (1993) noted that something must be wrong either with clinicians' assessments, with assessment criteria, or both.

Records and Tomblin (1994) also found imperfect agreement about which children should be considered language impaired. Records and Tomblin collected a set of hypothetical and real assessment profiles for children ages 4 to 9:11. They presented the profiles to a group of clinicians from diverse backgrounds and asked them to decide whether each child should be classified as lan-

guage impaired. Although the overall agreement among the 27 clinicians who responded was significantly greater than chance, the group agreed unanimously on only 17% of the cases, typically those at the extreme high or low ends of the ability range. There was, however, evidence of some consistency in the clinicians' integrated use of multiple test scores, with one score influencing the interpretation of another. This is the human factor in the diagnostic process.

Using Multiple Sources of Input to Define Disorder. Again, diagnosing language disorder for clinical purposes is not the same as diagnosing specific language impairment for research purposes, and the two should not be confused. In this book, I have argued repeatedly for a broader, more inclusive definition of language disorder (beyond specific language impairment) to include individuals who are different from their same-age peers, who show uneven patterns of language development, and who may have any of the "exclusionary" conditions that often cause language disorders of the non-specific kind. Language disorders can (and often do) co-occur with hearing impairment, emotional disturbance, mental retardation, autism, neurological impairment, speech–motor control impairment (apraxia or dysarthria), and reading difficulties. In Chapter 4, I also noted the strong overlap between definitions of learning disability and specific language impairment.

To make a diagnosis of language disorder and to tie it to decisions on whether a child needs and is eligible for language intervention service, it is critical to consider multiple sources of data, including input on functional limitations from those who know the child well. No definition of language disorder is adequate from a clinical standpoint if it fails to ask more than whether psychometrically determined inclusionary and exclusionary criteria can be met. Although a psychometric approach might be instrumental in identifying certain kinds of impairment, it has little to say about whether a child has a functional limitation or disability. That becomes evident when the child attempts to perform essential communicative or language-based tasks and cannot. To operationalize this part of a definition of language disorder, ethnographic as well as psychometric tools must be employed (Kovarsky & Crago, 1991). This requires contextually based observations and interviews of participants.

Comprehensive language assessment involves sampling a child's behavior in multiple relevant contexts and basing a diagnosis of language disorder on judgments of two types: (1) *judgments of degree,* children show more frequent and severe inability to meet communicative demands than their peers, and (2) *judgments of kind,* children have qualitatively different patterns of language development from their peers. In addition to asking psychometrically based questions about impairment and contextually based questions about functional limitations, specialists should ask socially based questions about opportunity to participate (Beukelman & Mirenda, 1988) and about risk for social disvalue (Fey, 1986; Tomblin, 1983, 1989). All these questions contribute to a diagnosis of disorder.

Determining Eligibility for Service

The Importance of Eligibility Criteria.   A second purpose of assessment is to determine eligibility for special intervention services. As noted previously, this purpose might seem indistinguishable from determining whether the child has a language disorder, but the two actually are separate.

Consider the possibility that a child's language skills are delayed relative to CA but commensurate with abilities across other delayed developmental areas. The language disorder then is often considered to be part of more general cognitive limitations. This child may or may not be identified as having a language disorder, depending on how the local community defines language disorder, but the child may still be eligible for language intervention services even if mental retardation is identified as the "primary" disorder. Conversely, a child may be diagnosed as having a language disorder according to accepted professional criteria but still not qualify for services based on a set of agency-specific eligibility criteria.

Rueda (1989) emphasized the importance of separating questions of eligibility and need, particularly for students from language-minority groups with "mildly handicapping conditions" such as communication disorders, learning disabilities, or mild mental retardation. Rueda's concern was that such individuals might either be over- or underidentified when decisions were made on the basis of psychometric measures alone.

Even though underclassification has been a much less visible issue than misclassification, there is a danger of exclusion from needed services because low-achieving students cannot meet specific criteria even though they need additional academic assistance. (p. 124)

Assessment to determine eligibility usually requires reference to official policy guidelines, and as noted in Chapter 5, state education agencies are most often the source of such criteria (although criteria may be established at intermediate and local levels as well). In addition to a set of standards to identify the child's language impairment, criteria for determining intervention eligibility may include a variety of required procedures as well as assessment of specific areas of language knowledge and use. Required standards might include discrepancy and exclusion criteria. Required procedures might include spontaneous language sampling and classroom observations. Specified areas of language knowledge and use might include requirements for demonstrated impairment in receptive and/or expressive language, based on an information processing theoretical model; or in one or more of the areas of language content, form, and use (or phonology, morphology, syntax, semantics, and pragmatics), based on linguistic and social interaction models.

Using Psychometrically Sound Practice to Guide Decisions.   The more liberal practice of using CA (Lahey, 1988) as the standard for determining discrepancy between expected and observed abilities is not without controversy. The basic objection is that it might result in classification of children with general developmental delays as having language disorders. Beyond that concern, CA-based eligibility criteria still require an answer to the question "How different must a child's language be from same-age peers before it is considered disordered?"

Answering this question requires both sound knowledge of psychometric principles and professional common sense. The normative relationships among standard test scores are illustrated in Figure 6.4. The exact middle of a normal distribution for a particular age group can be expressed as a standard score of 100, a percentile score of 50, or a z-score of 0 (based on standard deviations from the mean). How far should a child's own score deviate from that exact middle to be considered to be outside of "normal expectations"?

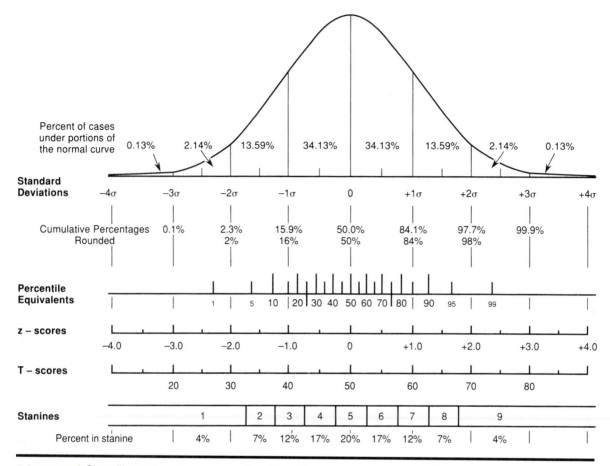

FIGURE 6.4   Chart illustrating normative relationships. The normal curve, percentiles, and selected standard scores.

Interpreting Standard Scores.   Raw scores, as numbers of correct or incorrect responses, by themselves mean nothing. Scores must be transformed before they can be used to compare children against a normative standard. This is usually done with tables provided in test manuals of (1) standard scores, (2) percentile scores, and (3) equivalent scores.

Standard scores and percentile scores function in similar ways. **Standard scores** may be expressed in several ways, e.g., as z-scores, T-scores, IQ-type scores, or stanines (see Figure 6.4). For example, when a child earns a raw score of 36 on a test, and the mean score for children of the same age is 48 with a standard deviation (*SD*) of 6, that child is scoring exactly 2 *SD* below the mean ($48 - 36 = 12$; $12 \div 6 = 2$). This can be expressed as a z-score of -2.

Percentile scores indicate the percentage of children in the normative sample in a certain age range who earned a raw score lower than that of the target child. For example, when a child earns a percentile score of 30, this indicates that the child scored higher than 30% of the children in the same age range who took that same test (this is why you can never score higher than the 99.9th percentile on tests; it is impossible to score higher than yourself). Percentile scores are not to be confused with percentage scores, which provide another way of expressing raw scores (i.e., as a proportion of items correct rather than as a straight frequency count).

Equivalent scores specify some level of functioning, usually grade level (often used in tests of reading or other academic skills) or age level (often used in tests of language to yield an LA or in IQ tests to yield an MA). Interpreting equivalent scores appropriately requires knowing how the scores are derived. Equivalent scores represent average scores earned by a particular group of children at an age or grade level. Thus, when you obtain a raw score for a child and look it up on a table to assign an age-equivalent score, you are actually identifying which group of children earned that score as an average. When you report this score for the target child, you are then comparing the child to a different age group, not to children of his or her own age.

Lahey (1988; also Hutchinson, 1996) pointed out the pitfalls of this approach. To illustrate its problems, Lahey described a 7-year-old child whose raw score on a language test was equivalent to the mean score for 5-year-olds. Because a two-year delay is often considered to be the standard for judging a child to have an impairment, such a result might lead to the conclusion that the child is indeed language disordered. Equivalent scores, however, are only central tendency measures; they represent mean scores for a particular limited age range. They do not represent the distribution of scores for that age group. Thus, depending on the test and the norm sample, distributions of scores across age levels may overlap considerably. In Lahey's example, when the distribution of scores for this test were considered for 7-year-olds (the same age as the child), his score was clearly within 1 SD of the mean for that group. When compared with his own age range, the child clearly scored within normal limits on this particular test. Any decision about the presence of a language disorder would have to involve additional evidence, including the reason for referral and evidence about the actual performance on language-related tasks in the classroom.

When specialists use formal tests to support eligibility decisions, their inferences are more likely appropriate when based on standard scores than equivalent scores. Lahey (1988) strongly recommended that assessment instruments should be evaluated on whether they include sets of standard scores, or at least standard deviations as well as mean scores. She also commented that "measures that report standard scores are more useful than measures that report only age equivalent scores; and when there is a choice between both types of reporting for an instrument, standard scores should be utilized" (p. 162).

Using Standard Scores to Make Eligibility Decisions. How should standard scores be used to make eligibility decisions? Different agencies use different criteria for standard deviations. Some agencies require children to score at least 1 SD below the mean on some measure(s) to qualify for services. More use a criterion of at least −1.5 SD. Others recommend a criterion of at least −2 SD, but that is probably too stringent.

Can you tell why it is too stringent by looking at the relationships illustrated in Figure 6.4? To answer this question, notice that when a test population is distributed normally, only 2.3% of the population scores more than 2 SDs below the mean. This suggests that only around 2% of a population of children would be expected to exhibit a language disorder.

What is the percentage of children actually expected to exhibit language delays significant enough to be considered disorders? You may notice that this is a circular question. It depends on the stringency of the inclusion criteria for the population of children studied, along with many other variables such as the children's ages, their cultural and socioeconomic matches to a standardization sample, and the philosophy of those who are defining what is important for the children to know.

Lahey (1988) summarized the results of eight studies, some of which used more than one set of psychometric criteria (some lenient, −1 SD, and some conservative, −2 SD) to identify the prevalence of language disorder. Estimates ranged from below 1% to over 12% of the population, with variation both within and between studies. As expected, the lowest prevalence percentages were found in studies using −2 SD as a criterion (Randall, Rynell, & Curwen, 1974), as well as those referring children between 5 and 14 years of age to special clinics (Rutter, Graham, & Yule, 1970). In one of the largest and most recent of the studies, Beitchman et al. (1986) conducted a two-tiered assessment of 1655 5-year-old kindergarten-age children in the Ottawa-Carleton region of Canada. The results showed that 6.4% of the group demonstrated evidence of speech disorders alone, 8.04% showed evidence of language disorders alone, and 4.56% showed evidence of mixed speech and language disorders. Even if the group of children with speech disorders alone is eliminated from this set, these results suggest that 12.6% of all kindergarten children show evidence of language disorder and that approximately a third of these demonstrate evidence of speech impairments as well.

These percentages are considerably higher than the 2.3% that represents the proportion of a normative sample scoring more than 2 *SD* below the mean. It suggests that the criterion of 2 *SD* is too stringent. Probably a criterion of 1.5 or 1 *SD* below the mean for the child's age group would be better, and probably more than one test or subtest should be used to support the child's need in this way. In their research, Records and Tomblin (1994) found that the majority of a diverse group of clinicians used –1.2 *SD* as the cutoff score for rating a child's diagnostic profile as "language impaired."

Varied criteria may also be used to define levels of severity. For example, Wiig (1989) recommended judging "total language scores" on the Clinical Evaluation of Language Fundamentals—Revised (CELF-R) (Semel, Wiig, & Secord, 1987) on the following criteria:

- Mild to moderate language disorder, between 1.0 and 1.5 *SD*s below the mean
- Moderate language disorder, between 1.5 and 2.0 *SD*s below the mean
- Severe language disorder, more than 2.0 *SD*s below the mean

The requirements for comprehensive evaluation established by IDEA make it clear that more than one test score and more than one person must participate in the decision to place a child in a special education program. Tests must also be valid for the purpose for which they are used. Consider that the same standard scores may mean different things at different ages. Developmental curves vary across age ranges (they usually decelerate, starting off steeply and then tapering off until old age when they begin to decline. Certain skills also vary in their contextually based importance for infants, toddlers, young children, and adolescents (Bishop & Edmundson, 1987; Rescorla, 1989; Scarborough & Dobrich, 1990). For example, children who are significantly behind age peers in language skills at age 3 years may appear to catch up at age 5, only to fall behind again when literacy learning demands become significant in the school-age years (Scarborough & Dobrich, 1990).

Discrepancies among scores may also have different implications depending on tests. For example, Aylward

(1987) described a problem with using a discrepancy between verbal IQ (VIQ) and performance IQ (PIQ) scores on the Wechsler Intelligence Scale for Children—Revised (WISC-R; Wechsler, 1974) as the sole criterion for diagnosing learning disability. Research has thus far yielded inconsistent data on the size and direction of VIQ–PIQ discrepancies on the WISC-R for children with learning disabilities. Aylward commented that, "Although learning-disabled students may show great subtest scatter (i.e., differences in performance among the various subtests) and VIQ–PIQ discrepancies, there are many children without learning disabilities who also show these abnormal patterns, and there are many learning-disabled students who do not show these patterns" (p. 48).

The Kaufman Assessment Battery for Children (K-ABC; Kaufman & Kaufman, 1983) has shown more consistency in demonstrating a directional difference between its "sequential" and "simultaneous" scales for children with learning disabilities. Kaufman & Kaufman (1983) noted that children with learning disabilities "performed consistently well on Gestalt Closure, one of the purest measures of Simultaneous Processing" and "tended to score most poorly on the Sequential Processing subtests" (p. 139). The point is that "a statistically significant discrepancy is not necessarily an abnormal one" (Aylward, 1987, p. 51). On the K-ABC, the average scatter between sequential and simultaneous scale composite scores is 12.3 points. Kaufman and Kaufman (1983) have suggested that a 22-point discrepancy must be reached before being considered unusual and denoting "marked scatter" (p. 194).

Using Dynamic Assessment to Support Eligibility Decisions.   Most eligibility criteria are stated in policy, but earlier in this chapter, I observed that not all children who need special services and can benefit from them qualify for them. What if a school district has a policy that children must show a discrepancy between cognitive abilities and language abilities to qualify for service? If a language impairment causes a student to need special intervention to benefit from education, the student has a right to receive that service as part of his or her FAPE according to IDEA (see Chapter 5). This raises a dilemma for the clinician. I believe that it is the clinician's responsibility to develop the case for eligibility.

Most of the methods discussed thus far in this chapter have been examples of **static assessment.** That is, they assess what a child knows about language at a given point in time. "During a static assessment, the child's performance is unassisted by the examiner, suggesting that the behaviors displayed by the child should be present in most natural contexts" (Olswang & Bain, 1991, p. 257). A more relevant question for determining whether a child should receive special language intervention services is whether the child shows potential to change, given such service. The tools for answering this question are those of **dynamic assessment.** "Dynamic assessment focuses on potential level of performance revealing a child's immediate ability to change or advance when provided with guided instruction from a more experienced person" (Olswang & Bain, 1996, p. 415). Using dynamic assessment techniques, which are based on Vygotsky's (1978) theory of the zone of proximal development (ZPD), clinicians strategically introduce scaffolding to frame relevant cues and mediate the learning process. Children who are able to perform better with the additional cuing are considered to have good potential for change (Palincsar et al., 1994) and to be good candidates for intervention.

All of this suggests that decisions about eligibility are very complex. The best way to guard against mistakes is for thoroughly educated professionals to collaborate with parents and others to make the best decisions possible to meet the needs of individual children. The age-related discussions of chapters in Part Two provide some additional information to facilitate the process.

Formal Testing

Selecting Valid Measures.   Validity is a relative concept. The concept of test **validity** refers to the "appropriateness, meaningfulness, and usefulness of the specific inferences made from test scores. . . . The inferences regarding specific uses of a test are validated, not the test itself" (American Psychological Association, 1985, p. 9). This is an important concept that is often overlooked. Test validity is not absolute, no matter how extensive the original test validation information. Unless a test is used for the specific purposes for which it was intended, the inferences drawn from it cannot be considered valid.

In judging the validity of a specific test for a specific purpose, three sources of evidence should be used:

1. Construct-related evidence indicates that the test is based on a sound theoretical construct embedded in a conceptual framework.

2. Content-related evidence indicates that the test items, tasks, or questions represent a defined domain of content. Part of judging the content validity of inferences drawn from particular tests involves determining whether the test measures what it purports to measure.

3. Criterion-related evidence shows that the test scores are related to some measure of outcome, such as predicting school performance, or performance on some other kind of criterion measure. When judging a test's criterion-related predictive success, it is helpful to determine how frequently the test results in false-positive or false-negative decisions. A *false-positive* decision selects a person as special in some way who is not special in that way; a *false-negative* result fails to select a person as special in some way who is special in that way.

In assessing the validity of a test for a particular purpose, the specialist must consider that purpose, the test construct and content, and the representativeness of the standardization sample relative to the needs and background of the child. Standardization data alone can suggest an illusion of validity, which is particularly dangerous when assessing children from multicultural backgrounds.

A test performance is only a valid representation of a child's ability if the child exerts optimal effort on the test. Experienced evaluators recognize the importance of establishing rapport before administering a formal test. They also know that standard administration procedures must be followed, because any significant variation may invalidate score interpretations. Usually, test instructions provide some information about how much encouragement can be given, but some children are simply bigger risk takers than others (see Personal Reflection 6.2). Any other alterations should occur only after the test is administered in the standard way and quantitative data have been gathered. Then, it may be possible to gather additional qualitative information by altering the demands of the task slightly. Just be careful to record what you do, and be sure to make your task alterations clear in your discussion of any qualitative differences that result.

The best approach may be to recognize the limitations and contributions of formal tests for what they are.

"Take a chance. Sometimes the brain knows more than you think it does."

Gloria Zeal Davis (1990, p. 4), Orton-Gillingham tutor, trying to urge a third-grader to take a risk after he had refused to attempt many test items.

They are highly structured observations of limited aspects of behavior in specialized contexts. Formal tests are useful to define a disorder's parameters relatively objectively. I use them minimally in my own practice, but I do use them, especially when diagnosing a child as having a language disorder and determining eligibility for service. They help me to validate my own less formal impressions of a child's functioning (I have found that spending a lot of time with children with special needs tends to result in warped internalized standards of "normal."). But I find the information that I obtain from informal assessment procedures much more useful in planning intervention efforts. I am also careful to use contextually based informal assessment information of varying types to assist me in judging the validity of the results from formal assessment.

Selecting Reliable Measures.   Given the heterogeneity of children with language disorders, it is surprising that we tend to treat a single score earned on a particular day as representing a child's "true" performance. Phenomenology involves recognizing the relativity of "truth" and the way the essential nature of a phenomenon varies depending on the tools used to observe it.

Tasks vary in how "tight" they are. Informal tasks are informal partly because the evaluator exerts less control over the context. This can lead to considerable variation from one observational occasion to another. One reason for giving a formal test is that the test maker has probably established its reliability. This is usually done in two ways: (1) **Test–retest reliability** is established by giving the test more than once to the same group of children. (2) **Split-half reliability** is established by comparing scores earned on items on one half of a test with the other. Both comparisons are usually expressed as correlation coefficients. (3) **Interscorer reliability** coefficients are computed by comparing scores assigned by more than one evaluator for the same behaviors.

Evaluators also need to be confident about what a score represents for a particular child. This is done by using information about the **standard error of measurement** (Hutchinson, 1996). Standard error provides a measure of reliability expressed as a range of score units within which a child's "true" score actually lies (the score that would emerge as the average of an infinite number of test administrations without any retest effects). Standard error varies for different confidence intervals, depending on how confident an evaluator wants to be that an actual score lies within a particular range. A confidence interval of 95% would include a wider range of scores than a confidence interval of 85%. Some test manuals report standard error values for different confidence intervals at different age levels.

Criterion-Referenced Testing.   Not all formal tests are norm referenced; some are criterion referenced (McCauley, 1996). As previously discussed, norm referencing involves judging performance relative to some larger standardization group. Norm referenced tests generally are required to determine eligibility for services. Criterion referencing involves judging performance relative to some predetermined level of performance, often for children of a particular age or grade level. Criterion-referenced tests are more frequently used to measure progress than to determine eligibility, but they also might be used to support eligibility decisions. For example, a child might be considered not to have a problem in reading if the child can read and can answer 85% of related questions correctly in a test using grade-level reading passages. Criterion-referenced testing is more closely related to answering the question about functional limitation than impairment. Criterion-referenced measures may be informal as well as formal. When a criterion is set, it stands as someone's estimate of what a child must do to succeed in a particular context.

By formal definition (American Educational Research Association, American Psychological Association, and National Council on Measurement in Education, 1985), a criterion-referenced test is:

> a test that allows its users to make score interpretations in relation to a functional performance standard, as distinguished from those interpretations that are made in relation to the performance of others. (p. 90)

Multicultural Perspectives for Guarding Against Bias

A test based on standard American English (SAE) provides a valid measure of true language ability only for children whose native language is SAE. Such tests are clearly not appropriate for children who are either non-English speaking (NES), also termed non-English proficient (NEP), or who have limited English proficiency (LEP). Bias also applies when a child is learning a variation of English based on rules of a system such as Black English Vernacular (BEV; sometimes called *ebonics*) or other nonstandard varieties of English, such as Appalachian English.

One area that has received considerable attention is the assessment of children learning BEV. More than 20 years have passed since serious challenges first addressed the validity of inferences drawn from administering standardized assessment instruments to children learning BEV (Baratz, 1969; Taylor et al., 1969; Wolfram, Williams, & Taylor, 1972). Yet, alternatives in the form of culturally fair, nonbiased assessment tools are still not available (Taylor, 1985; Taylor & Payne, 1983; Vaughn-Cooke, 1989; Washington, 1996; Wiener, Lewnau, & Erway, 1983).

Designing Culture-Fair Language Tests. As S. L. Terrell and Terrell noted (1983), "the development of dialect-sensitive or culture-fair language tests has not kept pace with the development of testing materials designed to assess the speech and language of standard English speakers" (p. 3). Reveron (in press) commented further that "there currently exists a dearth of valid language tests for speakers of non-mainstream English dialects, particularly BE" (p. 2), and Vaughn-Cooke (1989) noted that the situation still had not changed by the end of the 1980s. This is in spite of the fact that PL 94–142 (1977) mandated that selection and administration of all test materials and procedures must not be racially or culturally discriminatory. Partially because of the lack of tests to meet that mandate, Taylor and Payne (1983) commented that "If this stipulation were enforced today to its fullest intent, most school systems in the United States would be in violation of the law" (p. 8).

A variety of reasons explain the lack of appropriate measures, including challenges of test design. Vaughn-

Cooke (1983) listed and evaluated strategies for constructing culturally fair tests:

1. *Standardize existing tests on non-mainstream speakers.*
2. *Include a small percentage of minorities in the standardization sample when developing the test.*
3. *Modify or revise existing tests in ways that will make them appropriate for non-mainstream speakers.*
4. *Utilize a language sample when assessing the language of non-mainstream speakers.*
5. *Utilize criterion-referenced measures when assessing the language of non-mainstream speakers.*
6. *Refrain from using all standardized tests that have not been corrected for test bias when assessing the language of non-mainstream speakers.*
7. *Develop a new test which can provide a more appropriate assessment of the language of non-mainstream English speakers. (p. 29)*

My own attempt has involved working with Yvette Hyter (with consultation from Walt Wolfram) on an approach combining Vaughn-Cooke's (1983) recommendations 3, 4, and 7 in the development of Black English Sentence Scoring (BESS) (N. W. Nelson & Hyter, 1990a, 1990b). BESS is a tool for nonbiased assessment of the language of BE-speaking children between the ages of 3:0 and 6:11. It is used in conjunction with Lee's (1974) Developmental Sentence Scoring (DSS) to award points for grammatical features in eight categories (see Chapter 9 on Middle Stage Assessment).

J. G. Erickson (1981) urged a broader view of the language problems of bilingual bicultural children than one based on surface grammatical features. She noted that the answer may not lie in new tests modeled after old ones, which are often discrete point tests. These "reflected the thinking that language was a series of separate or discrete points which, when added up, made the whole. Language was not viewed as a synergistic and social phenomenon" (p. 4). Based on such thinking, some tests in English have simply been translated into other languages, a method that violates the statistical support for the test and results in questionable cultural and linguistic relevancy of test items.

In addition, Heath (1984) and Wolfram (1983) pointed out that not all children have the same frame of reference for taking formal tests. Heath noted that most formal tests are based on assumptions that normal language learners (1) know the routines of test behavior;

(2) are information givers, interpreters of pictures, and narrators; (3) know how to segment language into "words" and "meanings"; and (4) know how to identify the mainstream meaning of texts. Wolfram pointed out that testing is a social occasion with many specialized game-like rules, but that all players may not use the same rules. For example, he noted that in some cultures, children may have learned the relative values of silence and withdrawal in the presence of more powerful adults. Cheng (1989) gave the example of Japanese children, who may say "yes" when they mean "no" because it is rude in Japanese culture to say "no" in some contexts.

Developing Cultural Literacy.   Evaluating children from diverse cultures requires more than understanding the linguistic differences between the child's first language and standard English. An appreciation for the broader elements of cultural differences is required, including a self-awareness of how one's own cultural background influences communication as well as attributes one values as positive and evaluates as normal. Cultural literacy has been described as the "broad working knowledge of the traditions, terminology, folklore, and history of our [a] culture" (Bjorkland & Bjorkland, 1988, p. 144). It is a practical impossibility for professionals to be culturally literate in all of the different cultures they might encounter. Cultural diversity is rich even within "one" culture. For example, Cheng (1989) pointed out that hundreds of distinct languages and dialects are spoken in East Asia, Southeast Asia, and the Pacific Islands. G. A. Harris (1985) noted that Native American tribes in the U.S. Southwest are distinct and sovereign nations.

The best approach is to attempt to view the cultural milieu of a particular child or group from within the eyes of other group members. O. L. Taylor (1986) suggested that language disorder be defined for members of minority cultures when their communicative behaviors deviated sufficiently from the norms and expectations of that child's own language community. Other than gathering local norms on tests, the only way to find this out is (1) to ask people in the child's own community and (2) to observe the child's communicative behavior relative to that of other members of the child's own cultural group. Battle (1993) offered a set of "dos and don'ts to consider when treating persons from different cultures" (p. xxii) (see Box 6.1).

Alternative Referral and Assessment Criteria.   Seymour (1992) emphasized the need for alternative individualized assessment criteria for the diverse groups of "minority" students that now make up the majority of student enrollment in 25 major cities of the United States. He noted problems with two commonly recommended approaches: (1) developing different age norms for different language groups, and (2) developing norm-referenced tests that include a representation of minority groups within the standardization sample. The problem with the first approach is the diversity within language groups that may appear similar to outsiders. For example, a child learning a Cuban version of Spanish is not learning the same system as a child learning a Mexican version of Spanish. As Seymour noted, "Given that there are as many as 60–80 different language backgrounds in some school systems, the magnitude of this problem is indeed formidable" (p. 640). The problem with the second approach, which seems psychometrically acceptable on the surface, is that all children taking the test are not faced with a comparable task. Again:

> the important point here is that different language groups and different dialect groups have different grammars. Unless a test can capture the commonalities among language and cultural groups, so that the behaviors being tested are culturally and linguistically free of bias, test scores will reflect considerable group differences and large standard errors of measurement. (p. 640)

What is an acceptable solution then? The best approach seems to be one in which language samples (Seymour, 1986) are gathered "in naturalistic settings followed by probing of language in a criterion-referenced manner, with criteria for 'normalcy' based on language behavior indigenous to the child's cultural group and on language universals" (Seymour, 1992, p. 641).

Garcia and Ortiz (1988) also described a criterion-referenced approach. They recommended using referral criteria for students with limited English proficiency that are grounded in observations by teacher assistance teams (TATs) formed exclusively of regular educators, with speech–language pathologists or other special educators called in only as consultants. These teams would address a series of questions designed to prevent inappropriate referrals for special education services: (1) Is the student experiencing academic difficulty? (2) Are the curricula and instructional materials known to be ef-

Box 6.1 _____

Dos and Don'ts to Consider When Assessing and Treating Individuals from Cultures Other Than One's Own
(Excerpts from Battle, 1993, pp. xxii–xxiii)

1. In communicating with individuals from cultural groups other than one's own, *learn the name of that culture as assigned by its members—and use it.*

2. Avoid the use of generic terminology as substitutes or synonyms for more descriptive racial or ethnic terms such as *minority* to refer to African Americans, *bilingual* to refer to Hispanics, or *culturally diverse* or *multicultural* to avoid saying nonwhite.

3. Be aware of words, images, and situations that suggest that all or most members of a racial or ethnic group are the same without taking into account intragroup variations related to factors such as gender, age, socioeconomic status, and education.

4. Be aware that some terms have questionable or negative racial, ethnic, or socioeconomic connotations, such as *culturally deprived, at risk, minority,* and *culturally disadvantaged.*

5. Avoid using unnecessary qualifiers, clichés, and negative implications of color symbolic language that reinforce racial and ethnic stereotypes, such as articulate black student, Chinese fire drill, Indian giver, white lie, black sheep, yellow journalism, and black comedy.

6. Be aware of the nonverbal sources of miscommunication between persons from different cultural groups.

7. Be aware of verbal sources of miscommunication while communicating with persons from other cultures . . . In English, for example, *I* is the most commonly spoken word, and, unlike other pronouns, it is always capitalized. In Chinese, the most common word is *you,* and it is written with larger characters than the other pronouns. In English, the thought patterns and the communication style are linear—get straight to the point. In many Asian languages, the thought patterns are circular—talk around the topic. In Spanish and Portuguese, official occasions or business conversations are preceded by lengthy greetings, pleasantries, and other social talk unrelated to the point of business. Getting down to business in American style is considered rude and abrasive.

fective for students learning a second language? (3) Has the problem been validated through the collection of several kinds of information? (4) Is there evidence of systematic efforts to identify the source of the difficulty and to take corrective action within the regular education system? (5) Do student difficulties persist? (6) Have other programming alternatives been tried? (7) Do difficulties continue in spite of alternatives? If, at each of these steps, the answer is still affirmative, then students may be appropriately referred as having disorders that justify evaluation rather than simply having differences that should be addressed in other ways.

Damico, Oller, and Storey (1983) recommended using pragmatic elements in everyday communication (rather than surface grammatical criteria) to diagnose language disorder among bilingual children. They studied ten Spanish–English bilingual children who had been referred by bilingual classroom teachers for a special education evaluation by collecting language samples in both languages and scoring them in two ways: (1) using traditional morphological and syntactic structural criteria, and (2) using pragmatic criteria such as nonfluencies, revisions, and delays. As might be expected, the different criteria identified two different subgroups of children. The children were reevaluated seven months later, after they had all been mainstreamed in essentially monolingual English classroom settings. The results revealed that the pragmatic criteria were superior predictors of both academic achievement and teacher ratings. The authors concluded that traditional diagnostic criteria needed supplementation (not replacement) by pragmatic criteria.

Knowing the heterogeneity of language disorders, we might expect that multiple criteria are needed to identify all children with language disorders fairly. As summarized by J. G. Erickson and Omark (1981), culturally fair assessment should sample

> communication in a natural setting and [obtain] supportive information from integrative testing and interviews, including probes into specific functions and forms of language use. It is a model that encourages the use of criterion-referenced testing, and, when indicated, norm-referenced testing based on local data. (p. 7)

Informal Assessment Procedures

Informal assessment procedures are critical when making decisions about the needs and abilities of children from nonmainstream cultural and linguistic groups. Informal procedures also provide important insights and diagnostic information for all children with special needs. Ecological and ethnographic principles consistent with a system theory view of complex behavior in complex contexts was presented in Chapter 1. The specific techniques are considered further as they apply to each of the three developmental ranges in Part Two. The techniques include strategies for interviewing participants, using observational strategies, and gathering naturalistic samples and other artifacts.

Interviewing Participants. Interviews are used to gather information relevant to a child's needs and to reflect the perspectives and goal priorities of the various persons in the problem situation. The participant interview, borrowed from anthropologists, is an ethnographic technique for looking at a culture (in this case, the varied cultures of a child's home and school) through the eyes of the participants (Green & Wallat, 1981; S. Stainback & Stainback, 1988) (see Personal Reflections 6.3 and 6.4).

Although participant interviewing is related to the traditional practice of "gathering the case history," it is

---

PERSONAL REFLECTION 6.3 _____

"The goal in interviewing is to have the participants talk about things of interest to them and to cover matters of importance to the researcher [professional] in a way that allows the participants to use their own concepts and terms."

Susan Stainback and *William Stainback* (1988, p. 52), writing about uses of interviewing in qualitative research with application to clinical interactions.

PERSONAL REFLECTION 6.4 _____

"Don't put the other fellow in your shoes—wear his. 'Tis true, if 'I were you' I could use the logic that you espouse to solve my problem. But, since I am me, we must find a solution that fits well into the scheme of my mold. We must cloak the solutions of my problems in garments wrinkled by my needs and desires, otherwise, what you are saying to me is not, 'If I were you,' but 'If you were me'; and since I am not, your answers help me little."

F. Poyadue (1979), a parent of a child with a disability, quoted by Carol Westby (1990, p. 111) in an article entitled "Ethnographic Interviewing: Asking the Right Questions to the Right People in the Right Ways."

---

distinct in several ways. The interview is not just another method of gathering information. The interview begins the intervention. It is also often a key to moving an interaction into the cooperative goal-setting mode. The questions the interviewer asks influence the discourse elicited from interviewees, and it is desirable to elicit more than one kind of discourse. When I interview participants in a problem situation, I find it helpful to ask questions of two types. I ask for their lists and stories. First, I ask participants to tell about the problem. This kind of questioning usually elicits expository discourse, including labels for key aspects of the problem and a list of priorities as viewed by the participants themselves. A good probe for this part of the interview is, "If you could change just one thing for _____, what would it be?" Second, I ask participants to tell anecdotes about specific incidents to illustrate the problem. This usually elicits narrative discourse, including characterization of the interactions among the participants in a way that allows me to begin to form a more complete picture and to begin to apply my own labels and interpretations to stories about the problem. A good probe for this part of the interview is, "Think of a time when (you felt bored, you thought Shawn wasn't listening, etc.) and tell me about it."

When interviewing participants, the interviewer's attitude is especially important. If the participants' perspectives are to be understood, the interviewer must remain nonjudgmental about participants' comments. Although I may not think it productive to label a child who avoids a situation where he might fail as "lazy" (in fact, I might call that "smart"), it is important for me to know that this is how that child's problems appear to his teachers and parents. Accepting individuals' viewpoints as valid does not mean that the interviewer may not, at another time, encourage participants to shift those views. In fact, asking for the story of what was going on the last time the child appeared lazy may trigger parents and teachers to begin the reconstruction process themselves.

Where and when interviews occur may vary. In the early stages of assessment and intervention, separate interviews with each important participant (parents, teachers, and students) may yield clearer pictures of individuals' views of the problem. Group interviews, however, also have advantages, because participants can learn from each other and can begin the process of cooperative goal setting as a natural outcome of identifying current abilities, needs, and opportunities. For example, I once consulted regarding a child who had a patchwork schedule requiring him to spend time with several different special education and regular education teachers each day. Just asking each teacher to describe the child's responsibilities in that setting led to teachers' spontaneous problem solving to consolidate aspects of several different curricular expectations.

Even in ongoing programs, it is important to update the picture regularly because children and contexts change. Annual review IEP meetings can be used for this purpose, if they are small enough, but update interviews held before IEP meetings may be more productive. Then, the formal meeting can be used to summarize the priorities established in earlier interviews so that mutual goal setting and planning can proceed efficiently at the meeting.

Participant interviews can be used to satisfy several different assessment purposes. They can be as helpful in determining the presence of a problem. Particularly

when children have cultural differences that make the validity of standard assessment procedures questionable, I rely heavily on input from people in the child's own cultural and home environments for diagnosing language disorder. It is easier to feel confident that a child has a problem requiring attention when parents respond with immediate and definite confirmation when asked, "Have you noticed this child being different from your other children in learning to talk?" The speed and quality of the verbal and nonverbal responses you receive to this type of questioning should allow you to tell whether this has been bothering interviewees or whether you have suggested a new possibility that they have to mull over. It is also helpful when participants offer to back up their evaluative judgments with specific examples. If they do not volunteer their stories, request them. This kind of inquiry is particularly useful when questions of linguistic or cultural difference are involved, but it can be just as useful for children from mainstream-culture homes.

If a parent seems hesitant to identify this child as different in development, and if others who work with the child regularly seem to have no concerns until the possibility is raised to them, caution should be exercised in finding the child to have a language disorder, even if some formal test results support such a conclusion. Several options are available, including further testing, further naturalistic observation, or a scheduled recheck. Usually rechecks occur at 6 months to 1 year, depending on the child's age, with younger children checked more frequently.

Bear in mind also that an interview style that is appropriate with members of one's own culture may have different connotations for members of other cultural groups (Battle, 1993; Kamhi, Pollock, & Harris, 1996; Saville-Troike, 1993). For example, Westby (1990) suggested caution in the use of *why* questions in ethnographic interviews because they have a judgmental tone. They also "presume knowledge of cause–effect relationships, an ordered world, perfect knowledge and rationality" (p. 106). Rather than asking *why* questions, ethnographic interviewers ask participants to describe what they have experienced, how they feel, and what they know. For example, rather than asking parents what they mean when they describe their child as "hyper," parents should be asked to describe what their child does when acting that way. This is similar to the request for stories, described previously. When parents are bilingual, they may also be asked to use the words of their first language to describe their child, so that the interviewer can seek to understand what those terms mean to the parents. If the interviewer does not speak that language and no translator is immediately available, translation should be sought from the taped interview transcript, interpreting cultural as well as literal meanings.

Using Onlooker and Participant Observation.   Onlooker observation can be conducted in situations that participants have identified as important, such as during particular class times or on the playground. Of course, part of an ecological perspective is that, as soon as an outside observer enters a context, the context changes. Not only is the child probably different when being observed by an outsider, but the child's parents, siblings, teacher, or peers are probably different as well. This fact needs to be taken into account. The primary objective of onlooker observation is to obtain a contextually bound view of the linguistic demands of naturalistic contexts and how the child uses language when intervention is not provided intentionally.

Participant observation differs in that the language specialist using this approach makes direct contact with the child and communicative partners. This process has two purposes: (1) to find out how the participants interpret events during the events (by asking them) and (2) to determine how interactions might change if the variables are purposefully shifted (by using strategic questions and probes). Participant observations in classrooms should be arranged in collaboration with teachers to address their goals and concerns.

Gathering Naturalistic Samples.   Basing decisions about language disorders on naturalistic language samples is not new (see, e.g., W. Johnson, Darley, & Spriesterbach, 1952; McCarthy, 1930, 1954; Templin, 1957). Whole books and monographs (e.g., Hubbell, 1988; Lund & Duchan, 1993; J. F. Miller, 1981) have been written about gathering and analyzing naturalistic samples of language and communicative behavior. Language samples, including mean length of utterance measures, serve as common criterion-referenced assessment measures (McCauley, 1996). I will not attempt to review language sampling techniques extensively here. Specific suggestions for analyzing spontaneous language

samples relative to developmental expectations at early, middle, and later stages are given in Part Two.

Some elements are basic to all types of spontaneous sampling. James (1989) identified the process as consisting of two basic steps, both of which require special considerations: (1) collecting and recording the sample and (2) analyzing it.

The choice of audio or video recording of the sample is important (generally, the younger the child, and the more nonverbal the communication, the more critical is the use of video equipment), but the primary concern is whether the collected sample truly represents the child's language ability. Because of the importance of gathering samples of children's best performances, it is helpful to know what kinds of conditions tend to foster those. Hubbell (1988) identified three major influences on children's talking: (1) their language knowledge and skill, (2) their purposes and motivations, and (3) the contexts in which they are talking.

Although adequate samples can be obtained by clinicians acting as conversational partners in clinic rooms (Olswang & Carpenter, 1978), children produce longer utterances in samples gathered by their mothers at home than gathered by clinicians in clinical settings (Kramer, James, & Saxman, 1979). Recognizing the influence of different environmental contexts and conversational partners, researchers often recommend (e.g., Lund & Duchan, 1988; J. F. Miller, 1981) that clinicians use multiple contexts and conversational partners to obtain more representative, contextually based samples.

Emphasizing the importance of human factors in determining how much a child talks, Hubbell (1988) reviewed literature suggesting that three interrelated human relationship factors can work together to create a context that elicits maximum talking from children: (1) "Children are likely to talk more when they have equal or greater power in a relationship than the listener does," (2) "The more limits there are on children's behavior, the more their activities are constrained, the less freely they communicate," and (3) "Children talk more when the topic is of immediate interest to them" (p. 10).

The necessary length of samples has also been studied. Generally, samples of 50 to 100 utterances are adequate for most purposes (L. Bloom & Lahey, 1978). The amount of time required to gather the sample varies depending on the child. Younger or more reticent children may require longer than one-half hour to produce a sample of this length, but a gregarious child may produce a sample of more than 100 utterances in less than 30 minutes (James, 1989). To investigate several questions about length and number of language samples, K. N. Cole, Mills, and Dale (1989) used test–retest and split-half reliability techniques on language samples gathered from ten children between the ages of 52 and 80 months. Cole and colleagues interpreted their results as having four implications: (1) Collecting more than one language sample yields more representative information about a child's productive language. (2) Contrary to traditional wisdom, "children do not necessarily produce more complex or longer utterances during the second half of a language sample due to a 'warm-up' effect." (3) "Two shorter examples taken on different days may yield slightly more information about a child's lexical production." (4) "A 50 utterance sample may yield 73–83% of the lexical information found in a 100 utterance sample" (1989, p. 266).

Different sampling strategies also work better for children of different ages. Toys with multiple pieces associated with well-known cognitive play scripts (such as playhouses, barns, and fast-food restaurants) tend to work better with younger children. Complicated or broken toys may also elicit questions or negative comments. Less effective are stacks of pictures, which tend to elicit stilted language with little cohesion, and art or building activities (clay molding, drawing, or blocks), which may cause children to get so involved in the activity that they are less likely to talk. School-age children and older preschool children are less reliant on props and are more likely to use narrative discourse as well as conversation in their samples. Samples that include varied discourse types as well as varied sentence structures are more likely to be representative.

Gathering Elicited Samples. Spontaneous samples may not allow sufficient opportunity to observe certain language forms. Relatively more structured elicitation techniques can be used to draw them forth. The most frequently used elicitation strategy is a direct request for imitation. Because of the control possible when using such a strategy, it has been a frequent choice on formal standardized tests. It also has been recommended for use as a nonstandardized assessment technique (Menyuk, 1968; J. F. Miller, 1981), but problems have been identified in its use. Some evidence suggests that it

may underestimate spontaneous language performance (L. Bloom, Hood, & Lightbown, 1974; Connell & Myles-Zitzer, 1982; Prutting, Gallagher, & Mulac, 1975; Weber-Olsen, Putnam-Sims, & Gannon, 1983), whereas other evidence suggests that it may overestimate that performance (Kuczaj & Maratsos, 1975; C. Smith, 1970).

Recall earlier discussions about metalinguistic versus linguistic contexts and their different processing demands. Elicitation tasks, such as patterning or puppet modeling, almost always involve some metalinguistic elements. Children must grasp that they are playing a language "game." I remember one preschooler who went along with our requests for imitation just fine, until we came to: "Say, 'Do frogs jump in the grass?' " She answered "no" and nothing we could do persuaded her to repeat the question rather than answer it.

Other elicitation tasks for judging knowledge of linguistic rules are reviewed in Chapter 2. As illustrated there, elicitation tasks vary in their naturalness. Some fall so close to spontaneous language sampling on the naturalness continuum that they are hard to distinguish. For example, Dollaghan, Campbell, and Tomlin (1990) described video narration as a context for sampling "spontaneous expressive language." They gathered these samples by having clients produce on-line descriptions of the cartoon events while watching videotapes they had seen before. This procedure has the particular advantage of increased consistency across samples.

Assessing Comprehension Informally. Most language-sampling techniques are aimed at assessing language production rather than comprehension, although transcripts of language-sampling events can provide information about both processes. Because language comprehension is relatively more difficult to observe directly, it is often overlooked during informal assessment activities. Information about language comprehension, however, is critical to understanding a child's language abilities and needs. In contexts such as classroom participation, language comprehension may play an even greater role in meeting children's needs than does language expression.

Perhaps the biggest problem associated with measuring language comprehension informally arises from the difficulty in separating the child's comprehension of a particular situation, based on nonverbal cues, from the child's comprehension of language, based on linguistic cues. James (1989) suggested use of the terms **communication comprehension** and **linguistic comprehension,** respectively, to recognize the distinction. Typically, formal testing procedures are more likely to measure linguistic comprehension because they are designed to present isolated examples of particular language structures out of context. The usual strategy is for the evaluator to read a sentence to a child who is looking at a set of pictures so that the child can select the picture that best matches the sentence. This strategy fails to provide a way to observe comprehension of discourse connected to other linguistic and nonverbal information. Using this approach, it is also quite difficult to estimate how well the child comprehends complex language of the type found in school curricular experiences.

Informal comprehension assessment measures vary with the client's age. Miller and Paul (1995) described different informal comprehension assessment procedures for three developmental levels: (1) the emerging language stage (8–24 months); (2) the developing language stage (24–60 months); and (3) the language for learning stage (5–10 years). With older children and adolescents, assessing language comprehension informally using curriculum-based language assessment techniques is essential to understanding possible interaction of their language and academic difficulties. With younger children, comprehension usually can be assessed informally in play with the children as spontaneous language samples are gathered. With infants and toddlers, comprehension almost always must be assessed through observation of their interactions with their caregivers during familiar routines.

A frequent problem that I have observed when speech–language pathologists and special educators assess comprehension informally is that they tend to overestimate children's linguistic comprehension abilities because these professionals are such facilitative communicators. Having learned well the strategies for helping children with limited language abilities to communicate, they often unconsciously use those strategies during assessment. They may sometimes employ nonverbal cues like pauses and eye gaze to facilitate their listeners' comprehension without being aware of using those cues. It is fine to vary the contextual cues consciously to observe their varied effects, but a problem occurs when language comprehension skill is attributed to listeners when the children actually are exhibiting communicative comprehension.

With younger children, these problems can be overcome if clinicians design specific requests for either verbal or nonverbal behaviors that cannot be understood based on context alone and then refrain from using nonlinguistic or paralinguistic cues to augment the message. I almost sit on my hands sometimes to avoid gesturing when asking a child to retrieve a particular toy from a particular place in the room. My goal is to sample comprehension of a variety of content words, including nouns and verbs, as well as prepositions and other locative terms, and a variety of sentence types.

With older children, comprehension may be measured by asking questions about a story they have heard or a text they have read. Another strategy is to ask students to paraphrase a sentence or short paragraph. That is a particularly good way to find out whether they have acquired traditional meanings of complex sentences. For math story problems, language comprehension can be measured by asking students to sketch what they think a problem means. This is a good way to see how they transform language symbols to other modalities. Such strategies are tools of curriculum-based language assessment when conducted using materials drawn from the student's own classroom.

Curriculum-Based Language Assessment. When a criterion-referenced approach uses success in activities related to the academic school curriculum, it is curriculum-based. Idol and co-workers (1986) defined curriculum-based assessment (CBA) as "a criterion-referenced test that is teacher-constructed and designed to reflect curriculum content" (p. vii). Not all CBA is criterion referenced (Marston, 1989); nor does it involve the construction of specific tasks (N. W. Nelson, 1989b). More generally, CBA is defined as the use of the student's progress in the local school's curriculum to measure success in education. Tucker (1985) used this definition, adding, "Curriculum-based assessment includes *any* procedure that directly assesses student performance within the course content for the purpose of determining that student's instructional needs" (p. 200). Other sources (Shinn, 1989) support this flexibility inherent within different CBA models.

CBA may be modified to be used primarily for curriculum-based *language* assessment (CBLA). The focus then is not so much on whether the child is learning the course content but on whether the child is using language knowledge, skills, and strategies effectively when attempting to learn the course content. I have suggested that this approach be defined as the "use of curriculum contexts and content for measuring a student's language intervention needs and progress" (N. W. Nelson, 1989b, p. 171). Particular areas of language strengths and needs then can be identified without assigning a single numerical value to the performance, or even a pass–fail judgment.

Data from curriculum-based language samples can be quantified, however, to act as baseline and progress-marking samples of **reading, writing, speaking,** and **listening.** For example, in a sample of a student **reading aloud** from a classroom text, numbers and types of miscues (showing match or mismatch with graphophonemic, semantic, or syntactic features of the original text) can be counted to give an idea of which cuing systems the student is using or ignoring. In a sample of **story writing,** words and sentence types (simple or complex, with or without syntactic or morphological errors) can be counted, and even compared with stories written by classmates. Narrative maturity can be judged and other qualitative descriptors can describe the student's writing processes (e.g., Did the student do any planning or organizing before writing? Was there any evidence of reflective revision or editing?). In **oral samples** of cooperative learning group discourse, number of bids to enter a conversation can be counted, and the types of contributions can be described. If **oral direction following** is a problem, the child can be observed in a classroom activity. Data collection might involve keeping a three-column account of what the teacher says, what the target child does in response to each direction, and what an average child in the class does to the same directions.

Quantitative and qualitative data from curriculum-based language samples can be used to select intervention target areas and intervention methods. Such samples can also be used to observe quantitative and qualitative changes in performance over time.

Gathering Other Artifacts.   When the language comprehended or produced is written, artifacts may be gathered. The difficulty in using written language artifacts such as class assignments or writing portfolios such as journals is that the evaluator is often uncertain of the context in which the assignment was explained and the processes the student used in producing this product. This problem can be addressed by interviewing the teacher or child about the item as well as looking at it, and by combining these perspectives with participant observation of current processes.

Other methods for gathering artifacts include audiotaping and videotaping of naturalistic verbal and nonverbal interactions. The value of audio and videotapes is that they can help in analyzing current systems as well as providing a historical record for marking progress. Tapes can also be made without an outside observer present and thus may provide a clearer picture of the influence of natural context.

Establishing Prognosis

When using assessment to establish a prognosis for improvement, the specialist may need some different strategies. Accurate determination of prognosis in the decision-making process has considerable importance for children. It can influence decisions made in the present and the future.

For preschool children with specific language impairments, Bishop and Edmundson (1987) characterized problems related to establishing prognosis as follows:

> On the one hand, it might seem desirable to initiate therapy as early as possible to give the child the best opportunity of overcoming the impairment before starting school. On the other hand, the disorder might resolve naturally, and treatment could create more problems than it solves by producing low expectations in teachers, anxiety in parents, and self-consciousness in the child. The parents of a language-impaired child want to know what the future holds, in particular, whether the child will be able to cope with regular schooling. Should one offer reassurance or a guarded prognosis? This is an area where even experienced clinicians find it hard to make decisions. (p. 156)

As these comments acknowledge, despite the importance of prognosis, establishing it is an inexact process, relying on a combination of professional expertise, experience, and knowledge of factors that influence language development among children with language disorders. Expertise is a broad concept; experience comes only with time and opportunity, but information about factors influencing language development can come from a review of the results of scientific inquiry.

Prognostic Data from Longitudinal Studies for Children with Specific Language Impairments.   Longitudinal studies of change among children with language disorders provide one of the best sources of information about factors influencing prognosis. Longitudinal studies and clinical reports both suggest that language disorders persist as children grow older but change in their expression (Aram et al., 1984; Aram & Nation, 1980; Fundudis, Kolvin, & Garside, 1979; S. E. Maxwell & Wallach, 1984; Stark et al., 1984).

Symptoms of oral language deficit that are obvious when children are preschoolers become less obvious during the school-age years. Then, the most obvious symptoms may be difficulty in learning to read. Although basic language impairments persist, they are often hidden by the fact that children with early language disorders tend to make fewer errors in their expressive language as they grow older (perhaps partially as a result of development and partially as a result of intervention). When speaking, children can select among a variety of ways to express their ideas. When listening or reading, they have no choice. They must process whatever is presented. That is, children may choose to speak primarily in simple sentences, rarely using complex connectives, or even misusing them from a logical semantic perspective (e.g., a language-impaired child might say, "I fell off my bike because I hurt my arm"), but still sound OK to teachers and adults whose ears are tuned to hear articulatory or syntactic *errors*. In the school-age years, and in academic contexts particularly, language comprehension needs are critical (perhaps even more critical than language expression skills). The difficulties that some language-impaired children experience in such contexts may be masked by their apparently error-free oral language productions. Thus, instead of language weakness being identified as the root of the problem for such children, other reasons may be invoked (e.g., not paying attention, not trying, laziness). A language specialist, by asking the right questions, can contribute to the process of sorting out the potential contribution of the language disability to the child's problems. Failure to consider the prognosis for academic risk that may persist after surface features of language improve is failure to learn from the case study presented by Damico (1988), which was reviewed in Chapter 1.

Evidence that can be used to make prognostic judgments has been gathered by many researchers in a variety of longitudinal studies. Table 6.1 summarizes the major characteristics of those studies in terms of sample size, time at longitudinal follow-up, and whether an evaluation or interview method was used to measure outcome. The results of the studies on prognostic variables are also summarized. Most of these researchers selected their samples using criteria to exclude conditions such as hearing loss, mental retardation, and frank neuromotor impairments. Readers should keep in mind that Table 6.1 generally represents findings regarding only a very narrow section of the entire realm of children with language disorders for whom they may need to establish a prognosis.

Another caution regards variables that may not be reported in Table 6.1 as being significant based on existing research but yet may be significant to a child. For example, environmental conditions such as socioeconomic status and child abuse and neglect are not mentioned.

Schery (1985) investigated the usefulness of socioeconomic status variables in determining prognosis for children with language disorders. Noting that such variables are "usually very strong predictors of performance in language and educational research with nonimpaired children" (p. 81), Schery was surprised to find that neither socioeconomic status nor socioemotional variables predicted *initial* levels of language functioning in her study of 718 children with specific language disorders in the Los Angeles County schools. (This public school sample population is important because it is probably more representative of the broader population than that group of children whose parents make special efforts to bring them to university or community clinics.) As Schery summarized, "Indeed, the children showed pervasive problems that were unrelated to family background characteristics such as parents' education, occupation, and cultural/ethnic ties" (p. 81). On the other hand, the *improvement* made by children in the two- to three-year study period was affected by many variables related to social status, including the children's own socioemotional status and personality characteristics, their mothers' levels of education, and the presence of physical discipline in the home.

Establishing a Prognosis When Language Disorder Is Mixed with Other Conditions.   When language disorder is mixed with other impairments (e.g., hearing loss, mental retardation), or when disorders stem from acquired brain injuries, the prognostic picture becomes even more complicated. As a general rule, the level of

TABLE 6.1 Prognostic factors identified in research studies associated with better and poorer outcomes for children with speech and language disorders. (*Note:* These prognostic indicators are not organized by strength of prediction—initial language scores and nonverbal IQ measures tend to be the best prognostic indicators—some factors listed are rather weak.)

BETTER PROGNOSIS	POORER PROGNOSIS
No family history of language and/or reading disability[a,b]	Significant family history of language and/or reading disability[a,b]
Low-risk birth[b]	High-risk birth[b]
Reported to be communicative as infant[b]	Reported to be noncommunicative as infant[b]
Younger (<6:6 years) when first identified[c]	Older (>6:6 years) when first identified[c]
Younger when still having difficulty[b]	Older when still having difficulty[b]
Less severe when identified[b,c,d]	More severe when identified[b,c,d]
Higher nonverbal IQ[a,b,d,e]	Lower nonverbal IQ[a,b,d,e]
No associated deficits (e.g., hearing, mental retardation)[b,d,e]	More associated deficits[b,d,e]
Fewer language components involved[b,d,e,f]	More language components involved[b,d,e,f]
Problems limited to articulation[f]	Problems with language or mixed articulation/language[f]
Able to retell story with picture at 5 years[d]	Unable to retell story with pictures at 5 years[d]
High score on exp. Northwestern Syntax Screening Test (NSST) as preschooler[e]	Low score on expressive NSST as preschooler[e]
Child prefers to participate in groups[b]	Child prefers to be alone[b]
Parents say positive things about child[b]	Parents rely on physical discipline[b]

POTENTIAL PROBLEMS FOR CHILDREN AS THEY GROW OLDER

Persistent language and speech problems
    Proportions vary: 40%,[g] 50%,[f] 56%,[d] 80%[c]
    Continue to develop speech and language skills but at slower rate than peers[c,h]
    Broader problems tend to give way to narrower ones[b]
Difficulty learning to read/persistent reading difficulty
    Proportions vary: 40%,[g] 75%,[a] 90%[c]
    For some, severe reading problems may follow a period of illusory recovery at age 5[a]
Other limitations of academic achievement
    Proportions vary with inclusion criteria for study:
        In one follow-up study[e] of preschoolers with nonspecific language disorders when they were adolescents, 20% were in classes for students with mild retardation, and 69% of the remaining needed tutoring, grade retention, learning disability classroom placement
        In another study,[h] only 24% received grades below a B or C level, but 52% had some academic difficulties and needed some tutoring
Few or mild problems with social interaction
    One study reported only a small proportion of 8%[h] having significant social-emotional difficulties
    Parents may rate child as showing significantly less social competence, but comparable to normal adolescents in involvement in activities[e]

POTENTIAL FOR EXCELLENCE

(Few studies have investigated areas of excellence)
Some excel in communication-related activities (e.g., debate, organization leadership, drama activities)[h]
Some attend college, finish a BA or BS degree, and attend graduate school[f] (all of the 18 young adults in the Iowa study[f] either finished high school or were still attending)

---

[a]Scarborough & Dobrich (1990). 4 children, evaluated at 2:6 years; 5 years; end of grade 2.

[b]Schery (1985). 718 children, originally identified at 3:1–16:4 years. At 8 years, records reviewed. Correlates of improvement over 2- to 3-year period studied.

[c]Stark et al. (1984). 29 specifically language-impaired (SLI) children, identified at 4:6–8 years; evaluated at 8–12 years.

[d]Bishop & Edmundson (1987). 68 SLI children (19 more with low nonverbal IQs and "general delays"), evaluated at 4; 4:6; 5:6 years.

[e]Aram, Ekelman, & Nation (1984). 20 adolescents originally identified as preschoolers with language disabilities, evaluated +10 years later.

[f]Hall & Tomblin (1978). 18 adults with language impairments (LI) evaluated in early elementary years (compared with 18 adults with articulation impairments evaluated in early elementary years); 13- to 20-year follow-up interviews with parents.

[g]Aram & Nation (1980). 63 children, identified at <5 years; evaluated at 9 years (included children with multiple problems).

[h]R. R. King, Jones, & Lasky (1982). 50 adolescents (did not exclude motor, hearing, intellectual deficits); identified as preschoolers; +15-year follow-up interviews with mothers.

language functioning observed when children are first identified may be the best indicator of their ultimate outcome, perhaps in concert with levels of cognitive functioning in other areas, as well as consideration of causative factors (both past and ongoing).

When Language Disorder Accompanies Pervasive Developmental Disabilities, Including Autism. The importance of level of language functioning in determining ultimate outcome for persons with severe disabilities has been repeatedly confirmed, particularly with regard to autism. Schreibman (1988) noted that "It is widely accepted that the single most important prognostic indicator (for autistic and other handicapped children) is language ability" (p. 147). Yet, the expectations for advanced language development among children with autism are usually quite limited.

One longitudinal study of children with autism involved a seven-year follow-up of 85 autistic boys and 34 autistic girls (with a control group of 36 children). DeMyer and colleagues (1973) found that only a few of the children with autism learned to use spoken language more complex than that needed for making simple requests. Those who remained seriously detached from their social environment and who were loners tended to have the worst prognosis. Other negative indicators were cognitive functioning below the educable level of mental retardation and the failure to develop functional language by age 5. (This cutoff of 5 years is commonly cited as the point beyond which speech is unlikely to develop in children with autism; this does not mean, however, that augmentative and alternative communication techniques should not be used with nonspeaking autistic children before the age of 5.)

In a review of other studies concerning prognosis for children with autism, Ornitz and Ritvo (1976) reported that 7% to 28% of these children develop seizures before age 18 and that 75% are likely to be assessed as mentally retarded throughout life. They also found that severe social and interpersonal problems were likely to continue even among those persons with autism who made considerable improvement.

The prognosis for other children with severe cognitive and multiple handicaps is also limited. DeMyer, Hingtgen, and Jackson (1981) summarized the results of six longitudinal studies of children with severe and multiple disorders (including autism) and found overall outcome judgments reported with the following ranges of proportions: 5% to 19%, "good outcome" (defined as borderline normal): 16% to 27%, "fair outcome"; and 55% to 74%, "poor outcome."

Not all sources agree that the picture is so bleak for children with autism. For the most part, the picture emerging from the literature is highly consistent with a limited prognosis determined largely by the individual's cognitive function level and especially by the language function level in the preschool years. Although most children with autism grow up with continued severe disabilities, some exceptions do occur (Lovaas, 1987). The Lovaas approach is based on the behaviorist model described in Chapter 3 with intensive one-on-one sessions for 40 hours per week. In our own clinic, we have also seen success with early intervention for children with autism using a social-interactive approach and strong parental involvement.

When Language Disorder Accompanies Hearing Impairment. Discussions of prognosis for language development among children with severe to profound hearing loss are thoroughly intertwined with debates about language systems and educational methods. "Deafness-as-culture" advocates (Lane, 1992, p. 19) argue that there is no disability when deaf children grow up as members of Deaf culture. Indeed, children (both hearing and deaf) whose deaf parents communicate using American Sign Language (ASL) start signing in their infancy and move through typical stages of babbling in sign and using "baby signs" (Pettito & Marentette, 1991). They rarely need intervention to learn this language.

The fact is, however, that the parents of about 90% of deaf infants do hear (P. M. Brown & Gustafson, 1995), and many of them, as well as some deaf parents, do view deafness as a disability. The "deafness-as-disability" model (Lane, 1992 p. 19) includes the notion that deafness can result in functional limitations and reduced ability to communicate in the mainstream. According to this model, the best way to reduce the disability is to teach English language skills (ASL is not English). A key element is to provide early amplification or a cochlear implant to enhance the person's ability to hear. Home programs and educational programs in this model emphasize the optimal use of residual hearing, extensive opportunities to listen and talk in the context of deliberately enriched English language environments, and specialized speech reception and production training. Some programs emphasize auditory-verbal skills and others use Total Communication strategies with visual-manual components, such as Signing Exact English.

Regardless of educational approach, language skill plays a significant role as a prognostic indicator of general education outcome for children with hearing impairment. Goldgar and Osberger (1986), in a multivariate analysis of 150 students (90 boys and 60 girls) from a state school for the deaf, found that "language, particularly expressive language, is the major determinant of academic achievement in the sample studied" (p. 87). Those authors also noted that receptive language plays a role as well, and that their study provided further statistical evidence for the interrelation of expressive and receptive skills. Nevertheless, expressive measures correlated more highly with academic achievement than receptive measures. Two factors that did not correlate highly with academic achievement were speech intelligibility and degree of hearing loss, but visual perceptual skills did. Some children with profound hearing losses also have learning disabilities, but Goldgar and Osberger noted the difficulty of separating the influences of hearing loss and learning disability.

Geers and Moog (1989) confirmed that English language competence is the highest predictor of achievement in the acquisition of advanced literacy skills for students in oral/aural programs. Most studies have shown that students with profound hearing loss reach a plateau in reading at about the third-grade level (Schildroth & Karchmer, 1986) or fourth-grade level (Osberger, 1986). Geers and Moog, however, found students in their study to have a mean reading level of eighth grade. Other positive prognostic indicators for this group included "at least average nonverbal intellectual ability, early oral education management and auditory stimulation, and middle-class family environment with strong family support" (p. 84).

One of the most significant questions facing families and teachers of children with profound hearing impairments is their prognosis for acquiring functional spoken language. For some families, decisions are guided by strong philosophical stances either for an exclusively oral or a total communication approach or a deafness-as-culture model. Others seek professional guidance about methods that might be best for their child. To es-

tablish a prognosis for the acquisition of spoken language and to select the most appropriate communication modes for educating a particular hearing impaired child, Geers and Moog (1987) devised a Spoken Language Predictor (SLP) Index. They designed the SLP to overcome some of the limitations noted in the more commonly used Deafness Management Quotient (DMQ; Northern & Downs, 1984). To aid decision making, points are assigned in each of five areas: (1) hearing, further subdivided into ratings of speech reception capability and aided articulation index; (2) language, assigned a percentile ranking on a test standardized on hearing impaired children; (3) a nonverbal intelligence quotient; (4) family support, rated subjectively; and (5) the child's own speech communication attitude. Based on points assigned in these five areas, a recommendation is made either for speech emphasis, provisional speech instruction, or sign language emphasis.

When Language Disorder Follows Acquired Brain Injury. It is also difficult but important to determine prognosis for children with acquired brain injuries. As discussed in Chapter 4, the prognosis for children with well-defined lesions of cerebrovascular origin is usually quite good (although some children may have persistent reading difficulties). The prognosis for children with acquired seizure disorders, however, varies widely, and the picture for children with traumatic brain injuries is not clear at all.

Summarizing the literature regarding the prognosis for expressive language recovery following traumatic brain injury in childhood, T. F. Campbell and Dollaghan (1990) found it to be limited in several ways, including: (1) a lack of longitudinally gathered detailed data, (2) a relatively narrow range of verbal abilities sampled (usually in nonnaturalistic contexts), and (3) a lack of information about concomitant variables that may affect outcome such as age, cause, associated neurological disturbance, duration of coma, and preinjury cognitive and academic status. Campbell and Dollaghan, using multiple measures of language recovery, found that children and adolescents with severe brain trauma, as a group, improved on the majority of measures, but individual variability was considerable, and only a few reached the levels of their control subjects. The authors concluded that the prognosis for clinically significant improvement among children and adolescents with severe acquired brain injuries is quite good, but some deficits in expressive skills may remain apparent up to at least 12 months following injury.

Remembering Individual Differences. The contrasts reported for children with various problems show that the apparent prognosis for a large group of children may not accurately represent the actual prognosis for a particular child. These contrasts also suggest that prognosis can be influenced by more than variables within the child. Remember the refrain, *problems are not just within children, and neither are the solutions.* Notice that a critical question concerns how the mode or frequency of treatment influences the prognosis for a particular child or group of children.

This question is more easily answered for individual children than for groups of children. That is one reason why no large-scale research studies of treatment efficacy have appeared in the literature. As Bishop and Edmundson (1987) pointed out, it is virtually impossible to interpret research results from large-group studies that attempt to correlate amount of treatment with the degree of improvement. For example, consider how decisions are made about who gets how much treatment. In most cases, children with the most severe language problems receive more intensive language intervention treatment (except, perhaps, for children with severe multiple impairments, whose programs are discussed in Chapter 13). The children with the most severe problems also tend to have the worst prognosis. Therefore, imagine how thoroughly confounded the two variables must be in most large-scale longitudinal studies. Also because of the questionable ethics associated with withholding a desirable treatment, demonstration of treatment efficacy will continue to rely primarily on individual and small-group studies with single-subject designs.

Parting Advice. Establishing prognosis is more than a scientific endeavor, or even a clinical one. It brings a lot of emotional baggage, for both the professional and the family. Although establishing a prognosis is particularly challenging for new professionals, the significance of the process rarely escapes the attention of even the experienced practitioner. Even after many years of experience, I still view the establishment of prognosis as one of the most challenging parts of my professional practice, whether I am giving a legal deposition about a child who was head injured in a vehicular accident or talking privately with parents. Perhaps this is because I am aware of the potential that prognosis not only may predict the future but also may influence it.

Based on my own philosophy about the more subjective elements of establishing a prognosis, I offer advice in two areas. Both relate to the general theme of focusing on the overall picture and not only on the close-up. The first has to do with hope, and the second with quality of life.

Whenever a person makes an educated guess about prognosis for a particular individual (and that is all it really is), the foremost concern should be the needs of the real people involved in a real-life situation. Perhaps one of the worst things you can do is take away a person's hope. Therefore, a portion of this parting advice is to use the data presented here for what they are, but not to give them more credit than they deserve. This requires a careful balancing of what we usually think of as "objective realism" with positive expectation. None of us knows for sure the outcome for a particular child or even an adolescent. It does no harm to acknowledge this, especially when one must convey a discouraging prognosis to parents. In those cases, I try to give parents the most honest picture I can in a way that leaves a window of hope. All of us can hope for a better outcome than we expect.

The same philosophy applies when children have mild-to-moderate disabilities. It is illustrated in this sample of clinical discourse (based on evidence in Table 6.1) that might be used when talking to the parents of a preschooler with moderate language difficulties:

You asked about the future. Based on experience with other children like Jeremy, we find that at least half of them continue to have some problems with their language all the way through school. We also know that learning to read is especially difficult for many children who have had language disorders like Jeremy's, even when their speech starts to sound better. So we will have to watch out for that and try to do some things to prevent problems as much as we can.

But you should also know that, even with continuing language problems, most kids like Jeremy can graduate from high school and even go to college. A lot depends on the things that all of us, including Jeremy, do from now on. And the better Jeremy feels about himself, the more he'll be able to give all he has at each step along the way. The challenge we all will face is to keep expectations high without placing unrealistic pressure on Jeremy. The most important contribution that parents can *make to this whole procedure is to convey to their child a sense of their unconditional love. He also needs to know that you respect his efforts.*

Too often professionals get the idea that they are being unprofessional unless they are absolutely objective (usually interpreted as conservative) about the prognosis for improvement. They fail to acknowledge that prognosis involves subjective elements based on value judgments. It is a value judgment, for example, that leads "good outcome" to be defined as "normal functioning." Who is to say that the set of values used for judging outcome should not be redefined in terms of qualify of life? Then a person who can act appropriately and participate in society can be valued as having a "good outcome."

INTERVENTION PURPOSES AND PRACTICES

Selecting Goal Areas

Assessment and intervention are thoroughly integrated processes. Evaluating language and communicative skills in contexts ranging from formal tests to naturalistic samples provides a wealth of information that can be used to establish goals. Sometimes such a comprehensive approach can yield so much information that it becomes overwhelming. I then remind myself that I do not need to know everything there is to know about a child to be relevant to his needs. It is enough to have a clear idea of the child's present functioning in a variety of areas, to have a sense of the priorities of others who know the child well, and to have an idea of how much the child can participate in those contexts identified as important. At this stage of the process, knowing the priorities is more important than knowing the details.

Shifting Focus When Writing Goals and Objectives. Difference in scope is one of the major distinctions between goals and objectives. Goals nail down the essential elements of the big picture. Objectives specify aspects of change targeted within it. To keep the scope appropriately broad when establishing goals, I often encourage speech–language pathologists to think of goals as *goal areas* (N. W. Nelson, 1988b) for laying out the horizontal scope of a program, whereas sequences of objectives define aspects of a program's vertical dimensions, or the sequential steps to take in accomplishing

the goal. Goals address the question "What should we work on?" Objectives address the questions "What steps should we take?" and "How will we know the program is working?"

Goals are established first. Hopefully, they emerge as a result of the collaborative process encouraged throughout this book. Deciding on goal areas requires a group of people to meet to identify areas most in need of focus. The meeting may also validate areas that might have been identified by particular professionals as part of the more general assessment process.

A variety of strategies can be used for selecting goal areas. Decisions often involve selecting areas that are (1) most impaired, (2) most obvious, (3) earliest in a developmental sequence, (4) most amenable to treatment, (5) most functional, (6) most critically needed at the moment, or (7) identified as highest priority by the parent, teacher, or child.

Although the application of varied criteria may yield slightly different recommendations about potential goals areas, usually some fairly strong convergence results. Remember that it is fine to think about goals as relatively broad areas. Goals may be expressed as loosely as expecting "improvement" in a particular area (a looseness that would not pass muster for operationally defined objectives). For example, a group of participants might decide that a child needs to work on listening comprehension and direction following, vocabulary acquisition (relational terms in particular), and narrative organization. These then become the specific goal areas for the language intervention programs designed to complement comprehensive programming efforts to help this child become more successful in school.

Another reason that it is advisable to state goals simply is that they are easier to remember. I believe that clients should know what their own goal areas are. If possible, they will have participated in establishing them. I often ask clients, "Now what are we working on here?" "What are you trying to get better at?" Then, I help them to rearticulate their goals in a way that is meaningful to them. I find that this kind of metacognitive strategy helps them to feel a sense of control and responsibility for their own improvement. In the Language-Based Homework Lab in our clinic (Nelson, 1997; Nelson & Van Meter, 1996), students have their goals written in "kid language" in their Tool Books. They open the looseleaf notebooks to these pages and discuss which language goals they can work on before starting homework assignments.

Objectives must be stated more precisely than goals. They are sometimes called **behavioral objectives** or **performance objectives** because they operationally define performance to measure change. Although some objective writing systems require as many as six or seven components, a three-component model can suffice. Using this approach, each objective specifies (1) what the child will do, (2) under what conditions, and (3) how well.

The *do* **statement** is especially important. It must be written in terms of the child's behavior (not the clinician's); it is not a description of procedure (although it may imply procedure); and it must be written in terms of observable behavior. Although writing a *do* statement in behavioral terms might seem to predispose the intervention process to a behaviorist model, the statement can be consistent with any of the theoretical models. Even "hidden processes" can be targeted; if they are, some plan must be established to identify when they have occurred based on observable indicators. For example, a *do* statement may indicate that a child will "answer questions to demonstrate comprehension," or "keep his body and eyes oriented toward the teacher to demonstrate attention." In a sequence of objectives, the *do* statements may be written to specify behaviors of increasing variety, length, fluency, complexity, abstraction, or sophistication as the program proceeds. The type of shift specified will depend on the type of knowledge, skill, or strategy being targeted. Sometimes, rather than shifting the *do* statement over time to indicate progress, the conditions statements or criteria statements are shifted to document changing expectations.

The **conditions statement** establishes the context in which the desired new behavior will be demonstrated. I have repeatedly emphasized the importance of context. When specified in a sequence of objectives, context may be a major element in determining whether a child will be able to demonstrate a desired behavior. Both linguistic (e.g., "in words," "in complex sentences") and social interaction contexts (e.g., "in social conversational with friends," "when reading aloud in the classroom") may be specified. The conditions statements in a series of objectives will likely reflect the outcome of assessment activities that have identified linguistic and social interaction contexts in which the child appears more or less limited.

The **criterion statement** specifies *how well* a child will perform a particular skill, demonstrate knowledge, or use a strategy. How it is written will depend on the nature of the targeted change and how much evidence the language specialist feels is necessary to be confident that the objective has been met. The criterion statement should be written with enough precision to allow the professional to identify when it has been met. Frequently used choices are (1) percentages, (2) ratios, (3) frequencies, and (4) duration. Each has advantages for specifying different kinds of change.

Objective Organization Strategies.   Objectives can be implemented vertically, horizontally, or with a cyclical attack strategy. In a **vertical** strategy, objectives are introduced one at a time as the child reaches a criterion on the current objective. Either the *do* statement or the conditions statement can change as the child advances in skill. A usual procedure is to sequence objectives so that contextual demands become increasingly intense over time.

Part of the influence of social interaction theory, however, has been to suggest that it is counterproductive to remove a desired behavior from natural contexts in the early stages of intervention with the intention of targeting more natural contexts later. Such a strategy contributes to widely recognized problems of generalization or "carry over." Although some theorists might argue that a behavior should never be targeted outside its natural context, a less radical alternative is to specify a target behavior within its linguistic context, and then identify several social interaction contexts in which the desired behavior may be targeted at the same point of the program.

This results in a **horizontal** arrangement of objectives rather than a **vertical** one. This strategy, illustrated in Figures 6.5 and 6.6, may involve the expectation that the child will use the targeted communicative skill in an individual interaction with the language specialist, and in the same day, will use the skill when interacting socially with peers. This differs from the vertical approach of attempting to perfect a new skill under one set of conditions before moving to another. Instead, the assistance of other participants is enlisted to monitor change beyond the walls of the isolated speech room from the beginning.

A third objective organization strategy is to use a **cyclical** approach. This approach, which is recommended by Hodson and Paden (1990) for phonological

FIGURE 6.5   A set of short-term instructional objectives.

LANGUAGE USE: CONVERSATIONAL DISCOURSE

Date: _____

CHILD: _____ AGE: _____ SCHOOL: _____ GRADE/LEVEL: _____

SPEECH-LANGUAGE PATHOLOGIST: _____

OTHERS IMPLEMENTING OBJECTIVES: _____

GOAL: The child will demonstrate skill for taking conversational turns, and for initiating, maintaining, changing, and concluding topics and conversations.

PRESENT LEVELS OF PERFORMANCE:

PART A. CONVERSATIONAL STRUCTURE

SHORT-TERM OBJECTIVES: THE CHILD WILL	CONVERSATIONAL CONTEXT										COMMENTS TECHNIQUES/ EVALUATION
	Practice conv. with speech-language pathologist		Spontaneous conv. with speech-language pathologist		Conv. with adult other than speech-language pathologist		Conv. with peer		Conv. with group of 2 or more peers		
	Date In.	Date Accom.	Date In.	Date Accom.	Date In.	Date Accom.	Date In.	Date Accom.	Date In.	Date Accom.	
1. demonstrate ability to initiate, and to respond appropriately when others initiate *conversational openings,* by demonstrating each of the following skills (each behavior observed in 3 separate conversations):											
a. give attention when it is requested with verbal and nonverbal cues, by establishing eye contact, moving into proximity (if necessary and appropriate), and orienting body toward speaker;											
b. get attention from prospective listener by using appropriate verbal (such as *Hi! Got a minute? What are you doing?*) and nonverbal cues along with proximity and orienting strategies;											
c. maintain attention during a 2- to 3-turn exchange;											
d. maintain attention during conversation on several topics of 2 to 3 turns each;											
e. maintain attention during an extended conversation on a topic (at least 7 turns);											
f. maintain attention during a conversation in which the topic is changed at least 2 times.											

Note. From *Planning Individualized Speech and Language Intervention Programs* (p. 274), Revised and Expanded, by Nickola Wolf Nelson, copyright 1988 by Communication Skill Builders, Inc., The Psychological Corporation. Reprinted by permission.

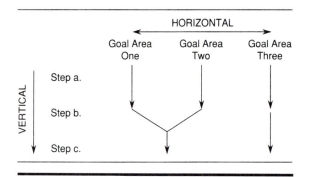

FIGURE 6.6   Combined horizontal and vertical organization of goals and objectives.

intervention, has also been used successfully for other language targets by Fey and colleagues (1993). In this approach, the clinician targets one objective (e.g., one phonological process or one grammatical structure) for a predetermined amount of time, perhaps one week. At the end of this period, the clinician moves on to the next clinical target, whether or not the first has been acquired, and then perhaps to one or two more, before beginning the cycle again. The cyclical approach probably works best when the targeted skills have something in common, although to my knowledge, no research has addressed this question.

Gathering Baseline Data

Establishing Baselines.   After identifying goal areas (and often before writing objectives), the language specialist should explore each in more detail than the initial evaluation may have permitted. In my experience, three goal areas are about right for most children. Of course, more or fewer areas may be targeted. Unless they are closely related, however, four areas become a little hard to manage.

A baseline is established by carefully describing a problem area as it exists before intervention or before a particular phase of intervention. The description usually is both quantitative and qualitative. The qualitative description is parallel to the statements included in performance objectives, except the baseline statements specify *what is* rather than *what is desired*. Baseline statements are written in terms of observable behaviors (again, possibly used as indices of deeper processes), and they describe both linguistic and nonlinguistic context variables. Several different descriptions of the appearance of a targeted communication skill in several different contexts therefore may be required. The specialist should quantify the targeted knowledge, skill, or strategy.

Naturalistic observation is the only way to develop a baseline for judging progress in using language knowledge and strategies in "real-life" situations. A more formal test–retest approach can be used to measure progress, particularly when targeting a skill, such as sound–symbol association. When formal procedures are used, however, the language specialist must keep in mind psychometric concerns about how frequently the same test can be readministered.

Professional judgment is required to decide how much time should be spent in gathering baseline information. Cost–benefit analyses must be made. Although scientific procedure dictates that baseline data should be gathered over several observation points until reliability (stability over time) can be established, it is usually neither feasible nor desirable to spend too much time gathering extensive assessment data before beginning intervention. Some baseline information, however, must be gathered (usually in more than one context), and the data should provide a valid representation of the targeted behavior.

The method of gathering baseline information sets the stage for similar observations at the end of the intervention period. Perhaps at the end of a school grading period or as specified in an IFSP or IEP, the targeted behavior will be observed again under similar conditions to judge progress. The new description should compare favorably with the old in that the newly established behavior represents an advance, appears under new more demanding conditions, or appears more (or less) frequently, depending on how desirable it is. For example, one student may need to *increase* the number of turns taken in group interaction. Another may need to *decrease* the frequency of interruptions.

Identifying the Developing Edge of Competence.
Part of the intent in gathering baseline information is to identify what I call the *developing edge of competence*. Finding it can assist the professional to know where to begin to focus, or how to arrange contextual conditions, when attempting to facilitate change. In almost any goal area, children can already demonstrate some behaviors (or linguistic rules) that are so firmly established that they are unlikely to disappear even under the most de-

manding conditions. At the other extreme, some behaviors or linguistic rules in the same domain are simply beyond the child's current capabilities. Somewhere in the middle is a developing edge of competence in which abilities wobble. In this area of complexity, the child can either demonstrate only part of the desired behavior or can demonstrate it only under some conditions. It is highly contextually dependent performance. Remember Sheldon White's (1980) description of children with wobbly competencies:

> A child is not a computer that either "knows" or "does not know." A child is a bumpy, blippy, excitable, fatiguable, distractible, active, friendly, mulish, semicooperative, bundle of biology. Some factors help a moving child pull together coherent address to a problem; others hinder that pulling together and tend to make a child "not know." (p. 43)

Earlier in this chapter, principles of dynamic assessment (Olswang & Bain, 1991, 1996; Palincsar et al., 1994) were introduced as a strategy to identify potential to change under guided instruction. Those strategies are related to Vygotsky's (1978) **zone of proximal development,** which is the range within which an individual child can vary given mediational support. This concept is similar to my suggestion that you use strategic probes and scaffolding techniques to find a child's developing edge of competence within goal areas.

In some cases, finding a place to start may involve looking across domains. I have criticized cognitive referencing when it is used as a gatekeeper for keeping children with language disorders from receiving special intervention services. Looking for intraindividual patterns of discrepancy between cognitive and linguistic abilities, however, can help identify areas that offer rich possibilities for growth. For example, Olswang and Bain (1991) suggested that "if a child at the one-word stage of development is exhibiting play behaviors reflecting his knowledge that objects can exist in relationship to each other in particular ways (e.g., locative relationships), one might argue that he is demonstrating cognitive skills that would support the comprehension and production of two-word semantic relations coding location" (p. 256). A clinician could use this knowledge to design dynamic assessment activities to encourage such phrases as "Ball chair," "Cookie floor," and see whether the child responds to modeling in situations with heightened linguistic and nonlinguistic cues.

Intervention efforts are most likely to bear fruit at the developing edge of competence. It is part of a contextually based intervention program to identify factors that tend to help a child pull together a new behavior or set of behaviors and make them work and then to use those factors as part of the intervention plan.

Developing an Intervention Plan

Designing and implementing an intervention plan requires a careful juggling of many factors. A major premise of this book is that no one type of intervention plan is right for all children. The chapters in Part Two discuss assessment and intervention content and contexts specific to early, middle, and later stages of language acquisition.

To achieve flexible programming to fit children's needs, it helps to remember that objectives and activities are not in a one-to-one relationship. Several activities may be used to work on one objective, and one activity can be used to work on several objectives. The degree of structure and adult control may also vary.

Decisions may be easier to make when they are visualized as moving in one direction or another on a continuum. Box 6.2 summarizes several different continua that involve decision making about service provision. Although my personal bias is toward using strategies form the left side of Box 6.2, a mixture of variables should be considered when making decisions for individual children and adolescents.

Box 6.2 _____

Decision-Making Continua That Influence the Choice of Intervention Methods, Targets, and Contexts When Designing Programs for Children

Contextually based needs ....*Developmentally sequenced tasks*	
Child-centered ....*Adult-centered*	
Nurturant-naturalistic ....*Highly structured*	
Constructive learning ....*Direct instruction*	
Holistic/ interactive ....*Discrete skills*	
In class services ....*Pullout sessions*	

Direct Control of Task Complexity. Pullout approaches have predominated traditionally partly because separation creates greater opportunity to control task complexity than that in relatively uncontrolled natural settings. Several variables can be manipulated to make a task more or less complex. They are illustrated in Figure 6.7. It is important to remember, however, that setting up communicative events with specially engineered contextual characteristics may remove events so much from their natural contexts that newly acquired behaviors may fail to generalize. Working within natural contexts, keeping experiences as intact as possible, and monitoring targeted changes within those more naturalistic experiences therefore are desired techniques.

Using Mediated Experiences and Scaffolding. The use of more naturalistic experiences is an alternative to designing special tasks for intervention. These experiences should be mediated for the child to intensify aspects targeted in the intervention plan. Intervention strategies of this type have been modeled, to some extent, on the parents' role in normal language acquisition.

Bruner (1978, 1983) described how parents build scaffolds by controlling linguistic and nonlinguistic

FIGURE 6.7   Task variables that can be controlled in direct treatment approaches.

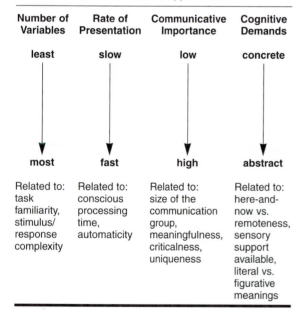

Number of Variables	Rate of Presentation	Communicative Importance	Cognitive Demands
least	slow	low	concrete
↓	↓	↓	↓
most	fast	high	abstract
Related to: task familiarity, stimulus/response complexity	Related to: conscious processing time, automaticity	Related to: size of the communication group, meaningfulness, criticalness, uniqueness	Related to: here-and-now vs. remoteness, sensory support available, literal vs. figurative meanings

contextual variables to make new information and behaviors accessible to their children. Snow (1983) noted that parents use similar interaction techniques when guiding their children through early book reading and other literacy experiences. Techniques include (1) semantic contingency strategies for staying on topics the child introduces, (2) scaffolding for structuring and constraining the demands of the activity, (3) accountability procedures for requiring that a child contributes at the child's level of capability, and (4) routines for presenting new content within predictable interaction patterns. Teachers also use mediation and scaffolding strategies when they help children individually with problems in completing assignments or when they read a passage from a textbook. They frame important content and focus attention by asking key questions before having children read the passage themselves (Applebee & Langer, 1983; Cazden, 1988).

The mediated approach differs from a stimulus–response–reinforcement approach typical of formal behavior modification sessions and classroom teaching. In mediated learning, the adult approaches the interaction with specific objectives in mind, but acts as a participant or co-learner in problem solving with the child, rather than as a traditional "teacher." The adult intentionally looks for opportunities within naturally occurring contexts to frame aspects of events and to focus the child's attention and efforts to elicit targeted behaviors that enable the child to master these behaviors.

Mediated learning strategies (Feuerstein, 1979) are based largely in the social interaction theory contributions of Vygotsky (1978). According to this view, children learn all psychological function through interaction with a more competent member of their culture who controls tasks to be consistent with the child's zone of proximal development. This adult, or a more competent peer, initially provides a great deal of support to ensure the child's success but gradually relinquishes control as the child assumes greater self-regulation capability for mediating his own behavior. Vygotsky defined this shift as transfer from interpsychological to intrapsychological functioning.

An advantage of the mediated approach is that it does not require analysis of tasks into small bits so that they can be presented in discrete units, later to be rebuilt into wholes. Instead, the adult may enter a naturally occurring holistic context with the child and make it manageable by framing certain aspects for the child's immediate attention and getting the child to begin to ask himself questions about what to do next.

When using this strategy, rather than preselecting all content for an intervention session, the adult follows the child's lead, making the approach more child initiated (Norris & Hoffman, 1990a, 1990b). For preschoolers, the adult may provide an interesting play setting with varied materials and areas and then let the child choose where to play. For school-age children, the adult may use the regular curriculum to provide the content and contexts for target skills work.

Using Different Methods for Different Problems.   In their content–form–use model, L. Bloom and Lahey (1978; Lahey, 1988) provided a way to organize language intervention efforts based on children's specific needs. They argued that it makes more sense to consider individual differences based on needs and abilities in these three interacting systems of content, form, and use than to treat children differently based on their presenting diagnostic conditions, such as learning disability or mental retardation. In their transactional model of child language, McLean and Snyder-McLean (1978) schematically illustrated (see Figure 6.8) the interactions of motivating factors, contextual experiences, and language content, form, and function.

A child with problems of language use needs a program that uses social interactions as a primary intervention context. A child with language content problems needs meaningful experiences to develop world and word knowledge. Other children—like Fey's (1986) active communicators and many children with the profile of specific language disorders, learning disabilities, and dyslexia (overlapping, not mutually exclusive categories)—have relatively more difficulty with language form than with its content and use. Some of these children seem to go merrily on their way, communicating fairly well with content words supplemented by gestures, but with syntax, morphology, and phonological maturity lagging behind. For these children, language intervention entirely in the context of natural communicative situations may not be the most efficient way to help them acquire needed skills. Proficiency in language form seems to require more practice than language content or use.

Somewhere along the line, however, *drill* became a dirty word, mostly for good reasons but not necessarily for reasons that apply in all situations. Drill is counter-productive when children have difficulty understanding language and communication, learning to express intentions, and learning to understand the meanings and intentions of others. When children have difficulty with motor control of word articulation, when they need to become more fluent and automatic in the inclusion of certain morphemes or syntactic structures, or when they have limited opportunity to practice those skills in natural contexts, then specialized, highly structured activities may be an important part of their intervention programs (see Personal Reflection 6.5). In my experience, children with intact cognitive abilities but specific expressive language impairments particularly may benefit from more focused and intensive practice sessions. Minidrills may also be embedded within more intact discourse events. Remember that an eclectic approach allows combinations of procedures, so that highly structured practice can be combined with more child-centered, naturalistic activities. New forms are first used for old functions (such as repetitive practice) and new functions (such as asking a question in class) are first served by old forms (Slobin, 1979). Expecting a child to combine both in the same activity may be unrealistic at first.

Keeping Purpose Clear

It is easier to adjust a program for a particular child along each of the continua outlined in Box 6.2 if the purpose of intervention for that child is kept in mind. Chapter 1 considered a broad purpose for language intervention; changes are targeted in the communicative systems of individuals and in the important contexts of their lives, relevant to their needs for social appropriateness, acceptance, and closeness; formal and informal

---

PERSONAL REFLECTION 6.5_____

"I am concerned about whether my 4-year-old daughter is getting the right kind of service. She can't talk (I've been told that she has developmental apraxia), but she can play quite well. Still, no one works directly with her speech. All they seem to do is work on teaching her to play."

Mother of a nonspeaking child expressing concerns about whether her daughter's needs are being met in her special education classroom.

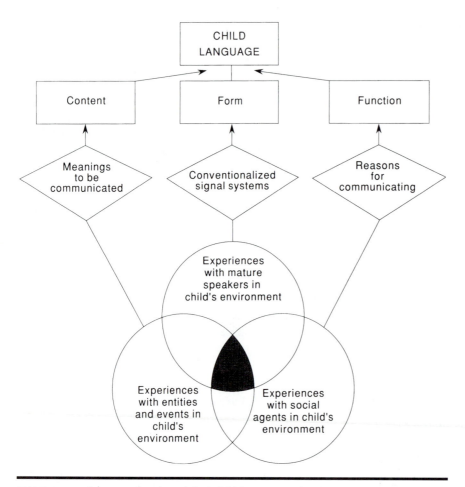

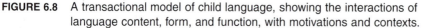

FIGURE 6.8   A transactional model of child language, showing the interactions of language content, form, and function, with motivations and contexts.

Note: From J. E. McLean and L. K. Snyder-McLean, *Transactional Approach to Early Language Training* (p. 213). Copyright © 1978 by Allyn and Bacon. Reprinted by permission.

learning; and gainful occupation (whether paid or unpaid).

Although the long-term outcome goal may be communicative competence, individual differences such as age, family constellation, causative conditions, needs, and abilities differentiate the programming decisions for individual children. Wilcox (1989) noted that some of the differences also center on whether the purpose of intervention is remediation, prevention, or compensation.

Traditionally, most goals of speech and language intervention and special education programs have been

remedial. The usual strategy in a remedial program is to identify one or more areas of impairment, often by measuring delay or disorder in development against normative expectations, and then to design activities to help the child either acquire a new desirable behavior, eradicate undesirable behavior, or mitigate the effects of some long-term impairment that cannot be corrected.

Sometimes, particularly in infant programs, the major focus of the intervention is prevention. A preventive focus is most likely to be appropriate when some unalterable biological condition, such as brain damage, Down syndrome, or sensory or motor impairment, places the infant at risk for developmental delay. Then, even though a disorder may not yet be apparent, services may be provided to influence other alterable aspects to reduce the likelihood that problems will develop or to lessen their severity (Wilcox, 1989). This focus might also be appropriate for preschoolers and kindergartners with specific language impairments who are at risk for reading disability, by intensifying their prereading "print literacy" (van Kleeck, 1990) experiences. (These might include additional experiences with story structure and phonological awareness activities and by deliberate exposure to print and writing, and perhaps by suggestions to watch Sesame Street with them, Mason, 1980).

Aspects of an impairment sometimes cannot be directly altered no matter how early services are provided and no matter how appropriate they are. For example, some persons with severe oral-motor deficits and some with profound hearing losses may never learn to speak intelligibly. These individuals, perhaps in addition to other remedial and preventive intervention efforts, need to be assisted to compensate for the areas of impairment. Compensatory efforts might include devices and strategies to meet needs in alternative ways. For example, an augmentative communication device for the child with cerebral palsy and an interpreter for the deaf child might enable them to participate in regular classrooms.

When the specialist considers all the ways that children's impairments, functional limitations, and disabilities might be reduced, planning is more likely to involve more than one of these purposes. It is also more likely to be relevant to the lives of children and those of their families and teachers.

Monitoring Progress and Measuring Outcomes

Many methods are available for marking progress during intervention. Progress is measured differently for different purposes. As part of the philosophical framework introduced in Chapter 1, I recommended taking both wide-angle and close-up views to build a comprehensive picture of effects in the child's life during intervention.

Keeping an Eye on the Forest (the Whole).   The big picture will stay in focus if the language specialist uses questions about functional limitation and disability (i.e., whether contextually based needs are being met), as well as about impairment (i.e., whether specific communicative processes are changing).

Relevant Change.   Professionals occasionally need to stand back and ask whether the changes occurring are relevant to the overall purposes of assisting clients to make changes relevant to their needs (needs to be socially appropriate and to have social closeness, to use language and communication skills for formal and informal learning, and to gainfully occupy their time). These questions are best addressed in collaboration with others in daily contact with the child who know the child well. The techniques used to answer these questions are usually interview and observation. It is difficult to use formal measurement techniques to get answers about relevance.

Functional Outcomes.   Functional outcomes are documented as improved functioning in natural contexts. The concept of functional assessment comes from specialists in rehabilitation and long-term care. "Simply described, functional assessment is a measure of a person's ability to function in his or her environment despite disease, disability, or social deprivation" (Frattali & Lynch, 1989, p. 70).

When functional outcomes are mentioned for persons with severe disabilities, people often think immediately of such activities of daily living (ADLs) as dressing, bathing, toileting, and feeding, but there is much more to being functional in life than having minimal physical care needs met. Although these needs are important, and communicative improvements may contribute significantly to improved ADL functioning, other functional outcomes also should be measured. For example:

- For business or social purposes, can the individuals attract the attention of someone other than persons who have been assigned to work with them, and can they maintain and terminate such transactions appropriately?
- Can individuals use language to get information and to give it (whether or not topics are complex or abstract)?
- Can individuals with severe disabilities use communicative and thinking skills well enough to keep themselves busy and entertained or for getting the resources they need to do so?

For students in school who can "almost but not quite" (ABNQ) succeed in the regular curriculum, a different set of functional outcomes may be sought. If changes in language and communicative behavior are significant and relevant, they should influence improved functioning in many contexts. For example, functional outcomes might be measured as increased participation in activities in the classroom and on the playground or in other extracurricular activities.

Existing academic measures also can represent functional outcomes for such students. Grades earned on report cards and individual assignments, projects, and tests can serve as criterion-referenced curriculum-based measures to demonstrate functional improvements.

Keeping an Eye on the Trees.　When children have significant needs, broad evidence of progress may not appear quickly. When a whole system does begin to change, it may be difficult to sort out the factors contributing to that change, but progress in specific areas can be monitored in several ways.

Keeping Log Notes.　After each direct or consultative contact regarding a particular child, it is helpful to keep dated notes on what happened. The log notes provide a running commentary about progress in several goal areas and associated qualitative comments. Generally, they should take no more than five minutes to write and should require no more than one fourth of a page. Log notes should also record quantitative data in the form of frequency information, percentages, or proportions to be entered on a progress chart later.

Charting Data.　The old adage that a picture is worth a thousand words is certainly true for monitoring progress. Almost any behavior that can be observed in natural (or formal) contexts can be quantified in some way, and quantities can be charted. Charts provide a clearer picture of growth than numbers presented in isolation (computer programs make the charting process easy).

Charting data is an important component of highly structured approaches with massed instructional trials of stimulus–response–reinforcement sequences. It also can be used for communicative behaviors occurring in more naturalistic contexts. These samples usually are not taken every session but once a week or once a month. More than one behavior can be quantified, either on-line or from audio or videotapes. Examples are the number of times a child looks in the direction of an adult who calls his name within a standard block of time, and the number of times the child initiates communication within the same time frame.

Figure 6.9 presents a different method for charting data from a communication sample gathered in a session with a child with autism (L. Watson, Lord, Schaffer, & Schopler, 1989). It illustrates how a single chart

may record naturalistic observations coded for context and the actual linguistic and nonlinguistic forms the child produced. It permits qualitative judgments about the functions and semantic categories encoded and categorizes aspects of the sample for subsequent quantitative analyses.

Keeping Running Language Samples.　Another way to keep a more qualitative running record is to keep a separate piece of paper at hand to record on-line bits of language produced daily in interactions with a child. This is not a formal language sample, and it cannot be used for formal analysis, such as for computing MLU, but it is useful for keeping track of unusual things the child says. I usually enter a new date at the beginning of each contact and write down particular utterances as the child says them. I select utterances that are especially long and complex, that demonstrate a peculiar use of a linguistic rule, or that provide unexpected evidence of miscomprehension. This can also be used to keep track of new vocabulary for children in the early stages of language development. Writing down only exceptionally good or unusual productions biases the sample, but over time, a pattern of increasing length, complexity, and appropriateness of utterances will emerge if the intervention is working. The examples of restricted language also can provide a window into the child's current language processing, keeping assessment up to date and helping to plan future sessions with the child.

Noting When Objectives Are Accomplished.　Well-written instructional objectives include criteria for knowing when they have been accomplished. When a sequence of objectives is arranged vertically, dates can be entered whenever a new objective is initiated or accomplished in a particular context. Figure 6.5 illustrates a combination of vertical and horizontal aspects of programming (N. W. Nelson, 1988b).

Using Exit Criteria

At some point, a decision may be made that enough treatment has been provided and that the child should be dismissed from specialized language intervention. It is not always easy to know when to quit. Fey (1986) noted that decisions about exiting are usually made because one of three situations has occurred:

　1. The child has reached all stated objectives and is no longer considered to be at risk for social disvalue (i.e., the child can no longer be viewed as language impaired).

2. *The child's progress toward stated goals has plateaued and efforts made to modify the intervention plan, including goals, procedures, activities, and goal attack strategies . . . have not led to notable gains in the child's performance.*
3. *The child exhibits continued progress toward basic goals, but there is no evidence that the intervention program is responsible for these gains. (p. 47)*

These situations are identified in response to three questions: (1) Is more change needed? (2) Is more change possible? (3) Is the attempt to bring about more change through special services justified by a cost–benefit analysis?

The question "Is more change needed?" may be answered by using some of the previously discussed strategies to justify a need for special services. IDEA requires that this question must be asked at least once every three years for school-age children as a part of their comprehensive three-year reevaluations.

The question "Is more change possible?" may be answered by using the goals and objectives and progress monitoring techniques of individualized programming. When I gather data failing to support progress in the child, showing a plateau effect rather than a positive slope, my first question is not whether the child might no longer need service. Rather, it is, "What am I doing wrong?" That is followed by the question "How can I do things better?" The child may need a different

Student: Ralph
Observer: Warren
Date: 1/17
Time began: 9:30
Time ended: 11:30

		FUNCTIONS							SEMANTIC CATEGORIES				
CONTEXT	WHAT STUDENT SAID OR DID	Request	Getting Attention	Reject	Comment	Give Information	Seek Information	Other	Object	Action	Person	Location	Other
① Makes mess while making breakfast	towel (signs)	✓							object wanted				
② Work-folding clothes	finish (signs)				✓					own action			
③ Free time-R. walks into kitchenette	touches teacher's arm		✓										
④ "	hands teacher a cup	✓											
⑤ T: "What ?"	drink (signs)	✓							object wanted				
⑥ T. hands R. orange juice	pushes jar away			✓									
⑦ R. opens refrigerator	drink (signs)	✓											
⑧ T: "Drink what?"	R. picks up cola bottle												
	+ signs drink	✓							object wanted				
⑨ R. stands up T.: "What do you want?"	bathroom (signs)	✓										own location	
⑩ R's shoe untied; to T.	shoe (signs)	✓							object acted on				
⑪ " "	shoe (signs) + holds								object acted on				
	up untied shoe	✓											
⑫ finishes playing with comb	finish (signs)				✓					own action			

FIGURE 6.9 Illustration of a charting method that combines qualitative and quantitative observations of a naturalistic communicative interaction between a teacher (observer) and a student with autism.

Note: From *Teaching Spontaneous Communication to Autistic and Developmentally Handicapped Children* (p. 29) by L. Watson, C. Lord, B. Schaffer, and E. Schopler, 1989, Austin, TX: Pro-Ed. Copyright 1989 by Pro-Ed. Reprinted by permission.

service-delivery model or service provider rather than release from treatment.

Other children who still need special education may no longer need speech and language intervention services. For example, a child with cognitive limitations might need a boost to get going in communicating, but when growth in speech, language, and communication level off and are commensurate with other developmental domains, this child may no longer need direct service. In Chapter 13, a Michigan Decision-Making Model (N. W. Nelson et al., 1981) is described. It advocates a strong language component in every child's regular or special education curriculum, but it suggests different levels and modes of service to be delivered by language intervention specialists depending on individualized need.

The costs implied in the question "Is the attempt justified by a cost–benefit analysis?" are not usually monetary. In fact, the regulations of IDEA clearly state that decisions must be based on the child's needs rather than what a district can afford. There are other costs to consider. For example, being pulled out for special services may cost a student time in the regular classroom; being seen by multiple specialists may cost a student needed consistency. Cost is always relevant to the expected benefits. If potential benefits are high enough, more cost is acceptable, but if the benefits have been shown to be minimal, a child's time may be better spent in other ways.

Exit decisions are not easy. They can be guided by asking the three preceding questions, but they should never be made without using the collaborative processes (required by federal policy in United States) discussed throughout this book.

Judging Program Accountability

In an earlier discussion on establishing prognosis, I acknowledged the difficulty of judging program effectiveness on a large scale. Program accountability may be judged in more than one way, however.

In a complex program serving varied children with multiple service-delivery models, it may not be feasible to measure the effectiveness of the program as a whole. All professionals, however, need well-organized strategies for keeping data on the number of their clients and sessions, as well as session type and length. They also need categorical data about assessment and intervention outcomes (e.g., in terms of numbers of individuals evaluated and diagnosed as needing service, numbers re-

ferred, numbers receiving follow-up monitoring). Most agencies have a specific method for collecting these data, a regularly scheduled period for reporting them, and a monitoring system.

Numerical accountability is important, and usually is required, but increasingly agencies also want evidence of quality assurance. A danger of simple number crunching is that it may obscure efforts to demonstrate that children are indeed making progress as individuals. Regardless of an interest in quality assurance when assessing program accountability, program monitors and administrators may fail "to see the trees for the forest" (just the opposite of the danger sometimes facing individual clinicians working alone). Administrators may seem to focus exclusively on the question "Can we afford it?" when professionals wish they would ask, "Does it work?" Professionals may find that administrators are more likely to find a way to afford a program if they can be given some hard evidence that it works, and even more so, that it works better than old, or different, or less (or more) expensive methods.

It is essential to prepare a plan to demonstrate that a project is effective in meeting its objectives efficiently (i.e., it meets efficacy requirements) when advocating for special funding. More than one method usually is described to measure the accomplishment of objectives. A test–retest plan or a set of criterion measures might be used to evaluate how many individuals in the special program reach criteria. It would be helpful to show that clients are either progressing farther or reaching desired goals faster than they did under an old approach. Qualitative measures, such as interviews, also can document program effectiveness, and functional outcome measures are critical for demonstrating program relevance. I know of one group who assembled a slide-tape show to demonstrate the continuing need for a classroom for severely language impaired children. Perhaps its most effective elements were audiotaped language samples of children in the program illustrating their significant needs (of course, with their own and their parents' permission). Board members heard those needs better than they could see them, and they maintained the program.

SUMMARY

This chapter has covered a lot of ground, beginning with the steps required to meet the needs of an individual with language disorders. Fifteen questions were listed to correspond with the flowchart of Figure 6.1. Questions of problem, language difference, language disorder, eligibility for service, and need for service were differentiated. Three models of team process—multidisciplinary, interdisciplinary, and trandisciplinary—were discussed, and the advantages of transdisciplinary teamwork to collaborative problem solving were described.

Criteria for diagnosing disorder and establishing eligibility for service were described. Operationalizing the definition of language disorder usually involves application of discrepancy criteria (CA referencing, MA referencing, and intralinguistic referencing) and exclusionary criteria (factors to rule out for diagnosing specific language impairment). For clinical purposes, I argued for a broader, more inclusive definition of language disorder (beyond specific language impairment) to include individuals who are different from their same-age peers, who show uneven patterns of language development, and who may have confounding conditions of mental retardation, hearing impairment, autism, or any of the other conditions described in Chapter 4. In making a diagnosis and determining the need and eligibility for service, I emphasized the need to consider multiple sources of data, including input regarding functional limitations from those who know the child well. For determining eligibility, the implications of using standard deviation cutoffs of −1, −1.5, and −2.0 were considered. Other standard scores, such as percentiles and age- and grade-equivalent scores, were described, and the limitations of age-equivalent scores were mentioned. Aspects of formal testing to be considered relate to test validity (construct-related, content-related, and criterion-related), reliability (test–retest and split-half), and standard error of measurement. Criterion-referenced tests were differentiated from norm-referenced tests.

Multicultural testing strategies were discussed, including strategies for designing culturally fair tests, for developing cultural literacy, and for using alternative referral and assessment criteria. The value of informal assessment procedures for identifying relevant goal areas and developing collaborative strategies was emphasized. Data and procedures for establishing a prognosis were discussed, including factors related to autism, hearing impairment, and acquired brain injury. Different implications were considered for describing communicative processes, needs, and opportunities.

Intervention planning was discussed, starting with the difference between broader goals and more specific oper-

ationalized objectives. Strategies for gathering baseline data and finding a child's developing edge of competence were described. Vertical (sequential) and horizontal (simultaneous) elements of program planning were described and variables to be controlled in the planning process. Exit criteria were considered for use when no more change seems needed, possible, or justified. On an individual basis, strategies were described for monitoring progress and measuring outcomes. On a programmatic basis, strategies were discussed for measuring accountability.

REVIEW TOPICS

- Fifteen questions for guiding language assessment and intervention: (1) A problem? (2) Language difference? (3) Language disorder? (4) Eligible for service? (5) Need for service? (6) What service(s)? (7) Which contexts should be modified or introduced? (8) Which speech, language, communicative behaviors should be changed? (9) What intervention approach? (10) Is progress occurring? (11) Does change justify new plan? (12) Does lack of change justify new plan? (13) Should service delivery model change? (14) Ready to exit services? (15) New need indicated by follow-up monitoring?

- Three models of team process: multidisciplinary, interdisciplinary, transdisciplinary

- Diagnosing disorder: discrepancy criteria—CA referencing, MA referencing, intralinguistic referencing (and their limitations); exclusionary criteria (and their limitations); comprehensive criteria that include questions about impairment, functional limitation, and disability; distinctions between broad clinical definitions of language disorder and research definitions of specific language impairment

- Eligibility criteria: problems of cultural bias (over- and underidentification), methods and criteria for interpreting standard scores (standard deviations, percentiles, age- and grade-equivalent scores), static versus dynamic assessment

- Formal testing: validity (construct-related, content-related, criterion-related); reliability (test–retest, split-half, SEM); criterion-referenced tests

- Multicultural testing strategies: designing culturally fair tests, developing cultural literacy, alternative referral and assessment criteria

- Informal assessment procedures: participant interviews (lists and labels, stories); onlooker observation;

participant observation; gathering naturalistic samples; eliciting samples; assessing comprehension informally (preschool-age; school-age); curriculum-based language assessment; artifacts
- Longitudinal studies and prognosis: Establishing prognosis—with autism; with hearing impairment; with acquired brain injury (focal CVA; seizure disorder; TBI); considering individual differences and sensitivity to family concerns in establishing prognosis
- Goals, objectives (*do* statement, conditions statement, criterion statement), establishing baselines, developing edge of competence
- Developing an intervention plan: controlling task complexity (review factors in Figure 6.7); mediation and scaffolding techniques; variations for problems of content, form, and use; targeting social, learning, and occupational purposes; compensating for functional limitations or reducing disability by working with communicative partners
- Monitoring progress and measuring outcomes (broader and more specific): relevant change, functional outcomes, keeping log notes, charting data (numerical, categorical), running language samples, documenting accomplishment of objectives
- Exit criteria: more change needed? more change possible? more attempt justified by more benefits than costs (e.g., best use of time)?
- Program accountability

REVIEW QUESTIONS

1. What is the difference between asking (a) whether there is a problem, (b) whether a language disorder might exist, (c) whether a child is eligible for service, and (d) whether a child needs service?
2. Which team process model is used:
   a. When members of different disciplines function jointly to perform a number of service-delivery activities, and instruct each other in how to carry out aspects of their roles?
   b. When members of different disciplines see a client separately, but send each other copies of their reports and recommendations?
   c. When members of different disciplines see a client separately, but come together in a team meeting to

generate recommendations that will be conveyed by the client's case manager to those working with the client on a daily basis?
3. What information from Table 6.1 would be associated with (a) better prognosis, (b) poorer prognosis, and (c) expectation of educational and social risks? What would you say to an adolescent with language-learning disabilities who wants to go to college?
4. If you were planning intervention for a preschooler who is having difficulty with communicative functions and another who is having trouble learning morphological rules, which would be more likely to need a program involving relatively structured and intensive practice? Which would be more likely to need a program involving coaching to interact socially with peers in play?
5. When a child has an impairment that cannot be fixed, what should be the targets of intervention? *Hint:* How could a plan target compensations for functional limitations or reducing disability by working with communicative partners?

ACTIVITIES FOR EXTENDED THINKING

1. Prepare to debate both sides of the issue of discrepancy criteria. Write points in favor of using discrepancy criteria and in opposition. Are there some situations in which such criteria might be appropriate? Are there others where they would not?

2. If you were devising eligibility criteria, what standard deviation cutoff would you establish and why? What proportion of children would you expect to be identified with your cutoff?

3. If you are a student and have a practicum client with language disorders, consult with your supervisor about using participant interview strategies with the child, parent, and teacher (if available) about their priorities for language intervention. When you have elicited lists and labels, ask for stories.

4. Evaluate your goals and short-term objectives to see if they are consistent with the recommendations of this chapter. How could you design an approach to be more relevant to contextualized needs raised in the interview process?

PART TWO

Balancing Ages and
Developmental Stages

This section provides specific information and strategies for working with infants, toddlers, children, and adolescents with language disorders and communication deficits. Of course, ultimately, we do not work with groups but with individuals. The view of clients as individuals participating in broader systems is central to successful practice. To a large extent, the successful practitioner can call on past experience and general knowledge about language disorders and related conditions, while never losing sight of the need to learn about the present client, an individual with unique abilities, needs, and opportunities.

Questions of organization of topics related to ages and stages of development assume more than technical importance in Part Two. These chapters convey information about the content and contexts of early, middle, and later stages of language acquisition. Each chapter provides information about developmental expectations, typical partner interactions, and usual communicative contexts. Also included are suggestions for using the information in assessment and intervention with youngsters at that particular stage of language acquisition.

This strategy raises a major question. Where should one discuss older children who stay at earlier stages of language development? For the first edition, I solved this question differently than I have for this edition. In that edition, I wove discussions of treatment for severe communicative abilities into each of the chapters on early, middle, and later stages. For this edition, I decided that the unique needs of individuals with severe communication impairments could be understood best in a chapter dedicated to the topic. Yet, I continue to see parallels in the intervention approaches. When one focuses on intervention as fostering normal development, and the discussions are not entirely separate. I also decided to separate discussions of assessment and intervention for the early, middle, and later stages, even though I view assessment and intervention as thoroughly integrated processes. The reason was, pure and simple, to make the chapters more manageable for readers.

Juggling many important concerns is the real life business of multidisciplinary and transdisciplinary teams, including students and parents, as well as professionals. The organization of Chapters 7 to 13 is designed to facilitate perspective juggling that will permit consideration of children's needs within the contexts of one or more developmental levels, while not forgetting the contexts of their chronological levels. This approach still leads to commentary on older children with earlier stage abilities in multiple sections. My hope is that this approach will seem not redundant but, rather, will facilitate decision making that will work for children of all kinds of ages and abilities.

Considerations of other special concerns are also woven throughout the chapters rather than being consigned to special chapters or sections of their own. Topics such as the need for multicultural sensitivity and uses of augmentative and alternative communication technology and strategies are discussed throughout Part Two. The purpose of this approach is to encourage the use of mutual goal-setting and problem-solving methods that are consistent with a collaborative model of consultation rather than an expert one. Although varied participants bring varied expertise to problem solving, aspects of problems cannot be ignored or passed on to someone else if the child is to be treated as a whole person participating in a whole system. The philosophy that *problems are not just within children, and neither are the solutions* continues to guide the discussions of this book.

7

Early Stages: Identification and Assessment for Infants and Toddlers

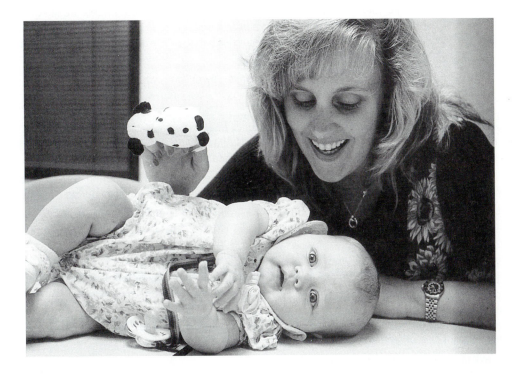

IDENTIFYING INFANTS AT RISK FOR
DEVELOPMENTAL PROBLEMS

CONTEXTS FOR EARLY-STAGE ASSESSMENT
AND INTERVENTION

A FAMILY SYSTEMS APPROACH TO EARLY-
STAGE ASSESSMENT

TOOLS AND STRATEGIES FOR EARLY-STAGE
ASSESSMENT

IDENTIFYING INFANTS AT RISK FOR DEVELOPMENTAL PROBLEMS

Risk Factors and Early Identification

Risk factors in infancy are often differentiated into three categories: (1) **established risk,** related to a diagnosed medical disorder of known cause, such as Down syndrome or deafness; (2) **environmental risk,** related to life experiences, such as abuse or neglect, that place an infant who otherwise may be biologically sound at risk for developmental delay; and (3) **biological risk,** related to a history of prenatal, perinatal, neonatal, and immediately postnatal events that might insult the developing central nervous system, compromising further development, but the effects of these events are yet to be established (Liebergott, Bashir, & Schultz, 1984; Ramey, Trohanis, & Hostler, 1982; Tjossem, 1976). These categories are not mutually exclusive, and the same child may demonstrate more than one kind of risk.

Factors related to **established** and **environmental** risk were discussed in Chapter 4. **Biological risk** may be associated with prenatal and perinatal factors such as environmental toxins and infections such as cytomegalovirus (D. A. Clark, 1989). Other factors associated with biological risk at birth include prematurity, asphyxia, and intracranial hemorrhage. The concerns about infants born with acquired immunodeficiency syndrome (AIDS) from their infected mothers continue to grow (Odom & Warren, 1988). Mothers who consume alcohol or use other drugs during their pregnancies also put their infants at biological risk. Sparks (1993) reviewed the literature on communicative development after-effects of Fetal Alcohol Syndrome (FAS) and Fetal Alcohol Effect (FAE) and cocaine exposure. These are summarized in Table 7.1. (See also Personal Reflection 7.1.)

Premature infants are those born at less than 37 weeks of gestation, with the percentage of prematurity in the United States remaining constant at around 7% to 8% of all newborns over recent years (D. A. Clark, 1989). Not all premature infants are at equal risk. The birth weight of 2500 g is frequently cited as a threshold of risk based on size. Babies below that weight may be at

TABLE 7.1   Research implications for understanding risks faced by children whose mothers used alcohol or cocaine while pregnant (summarized from Sparks, 1993)

RISKS FROM FETAL ALCOHOL EXPOSURE	RISKS FROM FETAL COCAINE EXPOSURE
• Low scores on standardized receptive language scales	• Irritable and stiff as newborns (transient effects that tend to disappear)
• Marked discrepancy between high verbal skills and inability to communicate effectively	• More difficulty with verbal and nonverbal reasoning than nonexposed children during childhood
• Poor judgment (difficulty predicting consequences of behavior) and common sense	• Self-regulation difficulty, more distractibility, increased activity level, more difficulty with sound discrimination (symptoms tend to last into childhood)
• Lower academic achievement and adaptive skills than expected based on intelligence and achievement test scores	• Most children exposed prenatally are unaffected; affected children do not appear to have mental retardation or learning disabilities
• Overlapping symptoms with Attention-Deficit Hyperactivity Disorder (difficulty sustaining attention, impulsivity) and Oppositional Defiant Disorder (frequent loss of temper; out of control)	• Early intervention is effective
• Neurobehavioral symptoms may be as severe for Fetal Alcohol Effect (without the physical appearance symptoms) as for Fetal Alcohol Syndrome (eyes widespread, long face, flat philtrum, thin upper lip, and small head)	
• Symptoms remain lifelong	

PERSONAL REFLECTION 7.1 _____

"The exciting thing about intervention is that we never know how far we can take a particular child. The following letter [excerpts here] written in response to published research about children and adults with fetal alcohol syndrome, points out the dangers of thinking that we know all there is to know."

Shirley N. Sparks (1993, p. 175), in her book, *Children of Prenatal Substance Abuse.*

"As the parent of a child diagnosed at birth as FAS, who is now in a preschool speech and language class in our school district, I have become increasingly alarmed at the fatalism being spread regarding the learning 'capacity' of my child from school district employees. . . . Our dentist made an FAS diagnosis of our son two minutes after meeting him. Anxious to share his wealth of information, he was quick to point out physical characteristics commonly associated with FAS, and proclaimed "he's hyperactive too, isn't he?" A look of condescension and disbelief pouted his face when I responded that the child was not hyperactive. Neither his speech therapist of one year, his occupational therapist of two years, nor we as parents, have ever noted anything but an average amount of activity in our son . . .

   "Don't give [relatives and educators] a message of fatalism. Instead, throw down the gauntlet of challenge to your audience to seek better methods of teaching these children . . . Don't allow the children of the 1990s to be limited to the accomplishments of those born two decades earlier."

Phyllis Tugman-Alexander, parent (Sparks, 1993, pp. 175–177)

---

greater risk than premature infants who weigh more. Other babies who are full term but small for gestational age, possibly as a result of FAS, are also at risk. A birth weight of less than 1500 g is considered to be **very low birth weight.** Technological advances have now led to increased survival rates for infants with **extremely low birth weights** of less than 1000 g (2 lb, 3 oz) and even for infants less than 750 g (1 lb, 10 oz) (Hack, Klein, & Taylor, 1995). Children with very low birth weights tend not to show signs of specific language impairment (Aram, Hack, Hawkins, Weissman, & Borawski-Clark, 1991). They do show increased rates of language disorders related to cognitive deficits and deficits in percep-

tual performance skills, however, and these increase with lower birth weights. The incidence of subnormal intelligence (IQ 70 to 84) is 8% to 13% for children weighing less than 1000 g, but 20% for children weighing less than 750 g at birth. The incidence of cerebral palsy and other sensory-motor deficits starts at 6% to 8% for children with birth weights of 1500 g to 2499 g; increases to 14% to 17% for children with birth weights of 1000 g to 1500 g; and to 20% for children with birth weights of less than 1000 g (Hack et al., 1995).

   Additional risk factors, such as sensory deficits or adverse environmental factors, multiply the risk of developmental difficulty. "Sick" premature infants—who experience complications such as asphyxia, respiratory distress syndrome, metabolic disorders, and intracranial hemorrhage—therefore are at greater risk for developmental problems than "healthy" premature infants (Field, 1979).

   Infants and toddlers with special needs or risks for developmental disorders usually enter the service-delivery system through medical referral, some after extended care by medical professionals. Ensher (1989) noted that very premature infants (born at 24 to 28 weeks of gestation) typically require hospital stays of at least 3 to 4 months and are often discharged with such technological dependencies as oxygen assistance. When an infant leaves the neonatal intensive care unit (NICU), or even while still in it, a speech–language pathologist may evaluate the neonate's current status and consult with the family about their concerns such as feeding and the best ways to encourage initial communication and to enjoy social interactions with their infant (Dunn, van Kleeck, & Rosetti, 1993).

Auditory Screening of Infants

Infants should undergo auditory screening before leaving the hospital, with follow-up whenever hearing status is in doubt. A few states require hearing screening of all newborns, and others require screening and follow-up for any infant who meets criteria of a high-risk register (see Box 7.1), but any child whose birth is associated with risks should undergo careful and early assessment of hearing status.

   Hearing sometimes is screened merely by using a special sound-generating device to present sounds of known frequencies and intensities under semicontrolled conditions. The infant's ability to hear these sounds is

Box 7.1 _____

Criteria Recommended by the American Speech-Language-Hearing Association (1991) for Identifying Infants at Risk for Hearing Impairment

1. Family history of childhood hearing impairment.
2. Congenital perinatal infections.
3. Anatomical malformations of the head and neck.
4. Birth weight less than 1500 g.
5. Hyperbilirubinemia at a level exceeding indications for exchange transfusion.
6. Ototoxic medications.
7. Bacterial meningitis.
8. Severe asphyxia, which may include infants with Apgar scores of 0 to 3 who fail to institute spontaneous respiration by 10 minutes and those with hypotonia persisting to 2 hours of age.
9. Prolonged mechanical ventilation.
10. Findings associated with a syndrome known to include sensorineural hearing loss.

inferred by a physician or nurse observing the eyeblink response (called the **auropalpebral response** [APR]). However, this method relies on fairly subjective observation, and it is not highly reliable. More objective methods are available but not universally; they are also more expensive. One relatively objective method uses a "Crib-o-gram," a specially designed crib with sensors connected to a polygraph recorder to measure changes in newborns' movement patterns from before introduction of a 92-dB complex tone to immediately afterward (for at least 20 trials) (Kinney, Ouellette, & Wolery, 1989). Another objective method, **auditory brain stem response** (ABR) audiometry, uses surface electrodes placed on an infant's head during a normal sleep state (no sedation required) to sense potentials evoked by controlled auditory stimuli (Amochaev, 1987). When there is any doubt about an infant's hearing sensitivity, early hearing assessment should be conducted and interpreted by an audiologist. Even among audiologists, agreement is not universal about how extensive screening and diagnostic measures must be to assess the hearing of infants at risk (Turner, 1990).

It is widely agreed, however, that informal means such as parental report, hand clapping, and noise mak-

ers are not sensitive enough. They are too easily contaminated by uncontrolled circumstances and may lead to false-negative decisions about hearing risks (Kinney et al., 1989). Furthermore, intact peripheral hearing is too critical to the infant's further development, particularly in the area of language, to risk delaying identification of a hearing loss, especially because early amplification can make an important difference in ultimate auditory and linguistic functioning.

Child-Find Efforts and Screening

Some infants may have developmental risks that are not identified while they are still in the hospital but show up later in infancy. Referrals from public health facilities and well-baby clinics to other service agencies provide an important avenue for identifying infants with risks such as these. The amendments to IDEA require interagency agreements so that health, educational, and other social service agencies communicate with each other.

Nursing professionals provide a particularly important link in this network because their knowledge crosses medical and family systems concerns, One study that spanned eight disciplines (Bailey, Simeonsson, Yoder, & Huntington, 1990) showed that nurses and social workers tended to receive more specific information about family assessment and intervention than professionals in any of the other disciplines studied. Part of a transdisciplinary service-delivery model calls for role release and the funneling of information through one professional acting as service coordinator. Often, particularly when physical care needs are involved, the case manager may be a nurse. When a service-coordinator approach is used, families are less likely to be overwhelmed by a set of fragmented and possibly conflicting interactions with many different professionals. Of course, many factors enter into decisions regarding what kind of person qualifies best as case manager for a particular child. As always, such decisions should be individualized.

States are required by IDEA to identify children who might need special services but who might not otherwise come to the attention of service agencies. **Child Find** is a "systematic process of identifying infants and children who are eligible for enrollment in intervention programs, tracking those individuals and making them known to appropriate service providers" (Wolery, 1989,

p. 120). Serious Child-Find efforts are complicated, involving many components, such as defining the target population, screening and prescreening, public awareness, and referrals, to keep track of children and to provide services.

The need for public awareness cannot be taken for granted. When I was employed in the schools, I once had to explain to my supervisor why a speech–language pathologist should be involved in the interdisciplinary team seeing infants. He could not imagine such a professional being of any use before a child began to talk! One of the things I learned from that experience was that "public" awareness efforts conducted on several levels would be needed to make appropriate early intervention services available to all children who needed them.

Screening in the Child-Find programs consists of activities used to answer the question "Should this child be given a thorough diagnostic assessment?" Many screening efforts involve preliminary assessments of large groups of children using published screening instruments designed to identify children who might have impairments or who are at risk for demonstrating disabilities.

Formal screening instruments should meet all of the psychometric standards discussed in Chapter 6, and they should yield as few false-positive (overreferrals) and false-negative (underreferrals) errors as possible. It is also helpful if screening procedures for young children are appropriate for serial use. Wolery (1989) noted that serial screening during the preschool years is useful because it "allows delays that occur later in the toddler and preschool years to be identified, allows better decision making because of the multiple data points, and assists in providing parents with information about child development and rearing" (p. 129).

Sparks (1989b) recommended serial assessment, as well, based on the rationale that infant behavior changes so strikingly, particularly during the first 18 months of life. She also noted that multiple observations permit better inferencing about environmental influences, and that serial observations can reveal whether the child is developing faster in one domain than in another (e.g., motor skill faster than language or vice versa). However, because no instrument has yet been shown to predict with much certainty which infants will exhibit developmental delays—even when their births have involved seemingly overwhelming complications—Sparks also recommended that professionals should not rely on neonatal screening results to predict later behavior for babies who have difficult beginnings. The picture is relatively hopeful for the majority of survivors of neonatal intensive care units, because the majority are found not to demonstrate severe or even moderate disabilities. (M. C. McCormick, 1989).

Several screening tools appropriate for use with infants and toddlers are identified in the Chapter Appendix A, Early-Stage Assessment Tools. They vary in their standardization characteristics and also in whether they are appropriate for screening comprehensive developmental domains or are intended for identification of communication problems primarily. Two of the instruments used most frequently for general assessment of neonatal status were developed by T. Berry Brazelton, M.D., and his colleagues. The Neonatal Behavioral Assessment Scale (NBAS) (Brazelton, 1984) is credited with heightening the awareness in the medical community of the newborn's behavioral capabilities and individual differences when it was introduced in its first edition in 1973. The instrument included the traditional evaluation of neurological reflexes and developmental milestones but extended beyond it (O'Donnell & Oehler, 1989). Widespread use of the NBAS over subsequent years demonstrated that small-for-gestational-age and premature infants were less well organized than their full-term peers. This led to the development of the Assessment of Preterm Infant Behavior (APIB) (Als, Lester, Tronick, & Brazelton, 1982) to assess low-birth-weight infants (Sparks, 1989b).

CONTEXTS FOR EARLY-STAGE ASSESSMENT AND INTERVENTION

The most valid and comprehensive assessments of children in the earliest stages of language acquisition are based on multiple methods of data gathering, including observations of communicative interactions in multiple contexts with more than one partner (Crais, 1995; Westby, StevensDominguez, and Oetter, 1996). For infants at risk, serial assessments may be conducted to monitor and document changes over time. Neisworth and Bagnato (1988) argued that outcomes are more comprehensive, reliable, and valid when based on a multidimensional assessment model that employs multiple measures, derives data from multiple sources, surveys multiple domains, and fulfills multiple purposes.

Hospital

When established risks, biological risks, and marked environmental risks are evident at birth, assessment and intervention are appropriate while the infant is still in the hospital. Sparks (1989b) listed essential assessment components: (1) the prenatal and perinatal birth history, (2) factors that seem to influence the infant's ability to maintain physiological organization (called *homeostasis*), (3) oral–motor status and feeding needs, and (4) the infant's hospital environment, including the amount and kinds of stimulation to which the infant is exposed (e.g., ambient noise), as well as nurturing opportunities for communication.

In response to a survey (Dunn et al., 1993), 45 speech–language pathologists commented on their multifaceted roles in neonatal intensive care units across the United States. Communication specialists working in these units provide assessments and intervention that are focused on feeding and communication interaction, as well as education to medical professionals, team members, and parents. When asked about team models, almost half (49%) reported working on a multidisciplinary team; "only 31% were functioning as an interdisciplinary team" (p. 60). None reported working on a transdisciplinary team even though the choice was available.

Home

In the broadest sense, home-based services are defined simply as services delivered in the home of a target infant or toddler rather than in a center. Bailey and Simeonsson (1988) noted that the rationale for providing assessment and intervention in the home is twofold. First, homes can provide natural contexts for facilitating the roles of parents as primary interventionists for their children. Second, homes may be preferred for assessment and intervention, based on practical considerations such as increased access to children in rural areas and the relative economy of providing services in homes compared to the expense of setting up a large center-based facility. Parents in remote sites can videotape a child during key events and an assessment team can use the videotape to assess areas of concern. "The major disadvantage of this approach is that the assessment cannot be easily dynamic, that is, the team members cannot interact with the child in order to see how quickly the child learns or how the child responds if activities are

presented in different ways by different persons" (Westby et al., 1996, p. 150).

Communication specialists may find that periodically seeing children, parents, and siblings interacting in their own home, with the materials available there, may yield a better understanding of home routines and ways to use them during intervention. Clinical recommendations then may be expressed relevant to everyday opportunities in the standard routine at home. The specialist should emphasize assisting parents not only to improve things for their children but to make things easier for themselves. A professional might assist a mother to position her child in an infant swing (in which the infant rarely fusses or cries) so that the mother can see the child's face (and vice versa) while she folds laundry, talking to her child about the clothing—whose they are, their size, and their softness.

Disadvantages of providing home-based assessment and intervention services also may be evident. These include the reluctance of some parents to be cast in the role of primary teacher for their young children (Crais, 1995), limited access to different professional specialists, limited opportunities of children for social and communication interactions with peers when isolated at home, and limited access to a wide range of toys and specialized equipment in many homes (Bailey & Simeonsson, 1988).

Infant Center or Clinic

Among the advantages of center-based programs, Bailey and Simeonsson (1988) mentioned the following: (1) the availability of early childhood education teachers with proficiencies for facilitating learning, communication, and development; (2) the availability of related service personnel such as speech–language pathologists, occupational therapists, and physical therapists, and (3) opportunities for infants to engage in social and communicative interactions with peers with and without disabilities.

In addition, Wieder and Findikoglu (1987) mentioned that their urban infant center allowed mothers with special needs to experience a responsive and nurturing environment. The center also offered individualized therapeutic programs for both infants and caregivers; therapy groups for mothers and children; workshops on nutrition, birth control, toys, and driver's education; a high school equivalency program; trips; and celebrations of birthdays and holidays.

Disadvantages associated with providing services to infants and toddlers in center-based programs concern the potential reduction of parental time spent with their infants and opportunities to establish attachments in one-to-one interactions. In addition, advances made in center-based programs may not generalize back to home environments, and travel to centers may be impractical for some families (Bailey & Simeonsson, 1988).

A FAMILY SYSTEMS APPROACH
TO EARLY-STAGE ASSESSMENT

The influence of context should be considered whenever assessment and intervention services are provided to children with language disorders. Context should be considered during planning for every child, but it is particularly important when planning for infants and toddlers. Crais (1991) emphasized the distinctions between "parent involvement" and truly **family-centered services.** Teams that are family-centered listen more than they ask questions and involve family members directly in all major planning activities.

The system theory perspective (developed in Chapter 1) is ideal for working with infants in the contexts of their families. A family systems perspective of the assessment process addresses many factors that influence the availability of family resources for dealing with the problem, not only in the present but over the long haul (Barber, Turnbull, Behr, & Kerns, 1988). These factors include characteristics of the exceptionality; characteristics of the family (e.g., family size and form, cultural and religious backgrounds of the members, socioeconomic factors, and geographic location); and personality characteristics of the individual family members. Family interactions are influenced not only by the parental subsystem of the mother–child dyad, which has been studied most extensively, but other family subsystems, such as the marital and extrafamily subsystems.

How individuals cope with infants with disabilities may also be influenced by where families are in the "family life cycle." Family life cycles are typically divided into six or more stages defined in terms of the ages of children, particularly the oldest child. Six common stages are (1) birth and early childhood, (2) elementary school years, (3) adolescence, (4) young adulthood,

(5) empty nest, and (6) elderly years (Barber et al., 1988). Stepfamilies and single-parent families can bring added complexities to family life cycles, sometimes resulting in repeats and recycling through the stages.

No matter when babies with special needs arrive in their families' life cycles, they can foster stresses that surpass those normally associated with having a baby (which does not suggest that families cannot enjoy a child with special needs and feel positively influenced by the experience) (Barber et al., 1988). When parents have special needs themselves, suggesting influences of environmental risk factors in conjunction with established and/or biological risk factors, it is particularly important for the specialist to consider parental mental health concerns and the parents' possible need for support in caring for and interacting with their infants.

For multirisk families, the picture may be even further complicated by the parents' lack of organizational skills, trust, or motivation to seek professional assistance. Wieder and Greenspan (1987) found that the staff of their clinical infant development program had to develop special techniques for engaging and working with such families (see Personal Reflection 7.2); the staff needed to be persistent, respectful, and sensitive when offering services to multirisk families who had never been able to take advantage of special services, but who clearly needed them.

Assessments in infancy should address the infant, primary caregivers, and interactions between them (Sparks, 1989b). According to Part C of IDEA, they should identify "the child's unique needs; the family's concerns, priorities, and resources (often called CPRs)

PERSONAL REFLECTION 7.2 _____

"In most cases, continued reaching out by an interested person willing to hear about and try to understand the difficulties a mother, father, or family was experiencing eventually met with a response, however slight, indirect, or cautious it might be. We learned that each family, like each baby, could respond if our overtures were persistent, respectful, and sensitive."

Serena Wieder, Ph.D., and *Stanley I. Greenspan, M.D.* (1987, p. 11), writing about the staffing, process, and structure of a clinical infant development program developed to provide preventive intervention for infants in multirisk families.

regarding the child's development; and the nature and extent of intervention services needed by the child and family" (Crais, 1995, p. 47). When assessing parental resources and the potential need for services to support parental efforts, Wieder and Greenspan (1987) recommended thinking in terms of primary and secondary maternal functions. As primary maternal functions, they included "the ability to provide physical care and protection, the basic ability to read an infant's signals of pleasure or displeasure, and the minimum emotional basis for a human attachment between mother and infant" (p. 11). As secondary maternal functions, they included "the ability to discern a child's changing developmental needs during the course of the first two years of life and the capacity to respond promptly, effectively, and empathically to the signals" (p. 11).

With the shift toward more family-centered approaches, less emphasis is placed on evaluating the family and more on evaluating *with* the family. Westby and her colleagues (1996) suggested using an open-ended ethnographic interview style, in which the interviewer asks the parents to describe a typical day with the child, following their lead to probe for more specific information:

> *You said that Ian doesn't talk, but he's good at letting you know what he wants. Tell me what he does to let you know what he wants. (p. 150)*

TOOLS AND STRATEGIES FOR EARLY-STAGE ASSESSMENT

Some measurement methods appropriate for children in the earliest stages of development are designed to diagnose disorder, but many instruments act primarily as gross screening devices. Some are so imprecise that they fail to differentiate among children diagnostically, particularly at the youngest ages. For example, a 3-month delay, which might be ignored for a 5-year-old, could be highly significant for a 5-month-old child.

Very young children are eligible for services when they are at risk and not only when it is possible to diagnose a frank disorder. Some assessment instruments designed for screening and diagnosis in the earliest stages of language acquisition are presented with brief abstracts in Chapter Appendix A, Early-Stage Assessment Tools. A select few are discussed more fully in the following sections.

Formal Assessment Tools

Some tools focus on general developmental concerns, and some are aimed more specifically at the assessment of communication and related developmental advances. Examples of cross-domain assessment tools include the Assessment, Evaluation, and Programming System (AEPS; Bricker, 1993a), the Ages and Stages Questionnaires (ASQ; Bricker, Squires, & Mounts, 1995); and the Transdisciplinary Play-Based Assessment (TPBA; Linder, 1993). Examples of language-specific instruments include Assessing Linguistic Behavior (ALB; Olswang et al., 1987); Communication and Symbolic Behavior Scales (CSBS; Wetherby & Prizant, 1993), the Infant-Toddler Language Scale (Rosetti, 1990), the Language Development Survey (Rescorla, 1989), and the MacArthur Communicative Development Inventories (Fenson et al., 1993). The TPBA and CSBS are described here to illustrate some of the principles of formal assessment appropriate to the prelanguage and early language stage of development.

Transdisciplinary Play-Based Assessment. The TPBA (Linder, 1993) is an example of an approach that represents combined elements of cognitivist and social interaction theoretical perspectives. It is designed for children functioning developmentally between the ages of 6 months and 6 years, using a play interaction context to provide opportunity for developmental observations in four domains: (1) social–emotional, (2) cognitive, (3) language and communication, and (4) sensorimotor. This truly transdisciplinary approach involves a team of parents and representatives of disciplines who release their varied professional roles to a single play facilitator who works directly with the target child while the others observe, in **arena fashion.** During the 1 hour to 1½ hour of videotaped play interaction, the team also observes the child interacting with her parents and a peer. No standardized scores are computed with the TPBA, but the outcome is a criterion-referenced analysis of developmental level, learning style, interaction patterns, and other relevant behaviors that can become an integral part of intervention planning. Linder reported that "Communication between the parents and other team members, prior to and during the assessment, is the key to ongoing dialogue that will continue throughout the child's involvement in an intervention program" (p. 1). The outcome of assessment using the TPBA is a description of current levels of performance and a set of recommendations such as those illustrated in Box 7.2.

Communication and Symbolic Behavior Scales.   The CSBS (Wetherby & Prizant, 1993) has some features in common with the TPBA, but it includes normative data. The CSBS also differs from the TPBA in that, although it includes items addressing cognitive and social–affective behaviors, it aims primarily to assess communicative behavior. The CSBS is designed to be used with children whose functional communication ages are between 9 months and 2 years.

The CSBS (Wetherby & Prizant, 1993) procedures include a caregiver questionnaire, direct sampling of verbal and nonverbal communicative behaviors, and observation of relatively unstructured play activities. In the manual, Wetherby and Prizant indicated that the caregiver questionnaire can be completed before the assessment, which takes about 1 hour and is videotaped for analysis and scoring (videotaping is optional for TPBA). The videotape scoring is also reported to take a little more than 1 hour for trained evaluators.

The sampling procedures of the CSBS resemble natural, ongoing child–adult interactions, using a continuum from structured to unstructured contexts. The procedures start with a warm-up, followed by a series of "communicative temptations" based on earlier work by Wetherby and Prutting (1984). For example, the examiner winds up a toy or blows up a balloon, then lets it wind down or deflate and waits for the child to request reactivation.

In addition to the communicative temptations, the CSBS provides a book-sharing preliteracy activity, and materials and strategies for symbolic play probes, language comprehension probes, and combinatorial play probes. At the conclusion of the CSBS session, caregivers are asked to help validate the results by rating

---

Box 7.2 _____

An Example of Results and Recommendations Based on the TPBA

An evaluation determined that Melody enjoyed and initiated dramatic play. She was capable of putting together a 3-step sequence of activities with objects in relation to a doll. She poured "milk" in a cup, fed the doll, and burped it. The evaluation also found that Melody had difficulty taking turns with adults and peers. Her language was intelligible about half the time and was limited to 2-word approximations ("a o," for "want more"). Melody was able to label familiar objects, but did not attempt to imitate new words.

Program recommendations for Melody should include:

1. Encouraging Melody's dramatic play and modeling 3-step sequences in new behaviors with the doll, in order to promote generalizations (washing the doll's hair, drying it, and combing it);
2. Expanding her existing 3-step schemes by adding one more step (after burping the doll, putting it to bed);
3. Helping Melody to generalize her vocabulary by presenting variations of common objects (different shaped and colored combs, brushes, socks, etc.) every day. Also, adding one common object not presently in her expressive vocabulary each week was recommended (deciding with the parents which common objects are most relevant in her life). (p. 18)

Note: From *Transdisciplinary Play-Based Assessment: A Functional Approach to Working with Young Children* (p. 18) by T. W. Linder, 1993, Baltimore, MD: Paul H. Brookes Publishing Co. Copyright 1993 by Paul H. Brookes Publishing Co. Reprinted by permission.

their child's behavior in several areas in terms of how typical it was during the session.

Box 7.3 is an outline of the sampling procedures and instructions used in the CSBS. Scoring of the CSBS is accomplished by assigning a rating of 1 to 5 for each of 20 separate scales, including 16 communication scales (subdivided into the four areas of communicative function, communicative means, reciprocity, and social-affective signaling) and four scales for rating symbolic behavior (subdivided into two areas).

Parent Report Measures

An assessment format that is unique to the early stages of development is the parental report. Tools include vocabulary checklists that parents use to indicate the receptive and expressive vocabularies of their infants and toddlers (e.g., Fenson et al., 1993; Rescorla, 1989; Rosetti, 1990). Using such tools, parents go down lists of words commonly used in early childhood and check off those their child can produce or comprehend spontaneously. Miller, Sedey, and Miolo (1995) noted two advantages of these approaches: "(a) They use a recognition format rather than relying on parents' ability to recall vocabulary items, and (b) they provide a means of documenting the child's entire lexicon via parents' knowledge of their child's language use across a wide range of contexts and speaking partners" (p. 1037). Miller and his colleagues found that the MacArthur Communication Development Inventory (CDI; Fenson et al., 1993), which provides normative data and scores, had concurrent validity (significant correlations between .70 and .82) with a set of laboratory measures of vocabulary for 44 children with Down syndrome and 46 typically developing children with mental ages from 12 to 27 months.

Parents may also be involved in using such cross-domain tools as the Ages and Stages Questionnaires (ASQ; Bricker, Squires, & Mounts, 1995), which include normative data and scores, and the Assessment, Evaluation, and Programming System (AEPS; Bricker, 1993a). Parent report tools save time and increase the ecological and sociocultural validity of procedures conducted with children's own toys and in natural contexts, as long as parents understand this role and want to take a formal part in the assessment process (Crais, 1995)

Informal Procedures: Blurring the Boundaries Between Assessment and Intervention

Whenever children are suspected of having language disorders, formal assessment procedures should be augmented by informal ones (Roberts & Crais, 1989). For many reasons, however, informal procedures, and procedures blending assessment and intervention goals beyond labeling, are especially appropriate in the early stages of communicative development. First, a diagnostic label may not be an appropriate or a fruitful goal of infant and toddler assessment because children change rapidly in the first months and years of life; a label assigned one month may not be appropriate the next. Second, policies that encourage preventive intervention approaches enable the specialist to postpone the differential diagnosis of specific disorders in very young children without jeopardizing the family's access to services. Third, more can be learned about the child's abilities and needs through working with the child to encourage further development and noting how the child learns than by presenting isolated tasks and assessing whether a particular kind of skill or knowledge is already present.

This process-oriented assessment is not new. In 1977, DuBose, Langley, and Stass identified the following assumptions underlying a process-oriented approach to assessing children with severe disabilities: (1) Children are "active agents" operating on their environments. (2) The learning process can be measured and modified within the contexts of the assessment. (3) Children's learning potential is best assessed by observing their performance in learning tasks, for which corrective feedback can be provided.

A major distinction between formal and informal assessment procedures is the degree to which an adult evaluator controls the sequence of events, selects the stimulus materials, and prescribes the responses. Norris and Hoffman (1990a) differentiated adult-initiated approaches from child-initiated strategies for interacting with children at prelanguage stages of development (see Table 7.2). Although the approach advocated by Norris and Hoffman was relatively informal, it was not without direction. Their Infant Scale of Nonverbal Interaction, which is provided as an appendix to their article (Norris & Hoffman, 1990a), outlines target behaviors in the three domains of vocalization, limb actions, and fa-

Box 7.3 _____

Outline of Sampling Procedures and Instructions

 I. Warm-Up (10–15 minutes)

I am going to begin by asking you some questions about how [child's name] communicates. You can hold [child's name] on your lap or let him [her] play on the floor.

 II. Communicative Temptations (10–20 minutes)

We want to get a sample of how [child's name] communicates with sounds, gestures, or words. First, I am going to present some situations that will encourage [child's name] to communicate. Please try not to direct [child's name] or tell him [her] what to do. Also try not to ask him [her] questions. Wait for [child's name] to initiate. If [child's name] communicates to you, try to respond naturally, by helping him [her] or noticing what he [she] is playing with. Remember, don't tell [child's name] what to do.

1. Wind-Up Toy
2. Balloon
3. Bubbles
4. Peek-a-boo
5. Walk Mouse, Creep Mouse
6. Blocks in Box
7. Jar
8. Toys in Bag

 III. Sharing Books (5 minutes)

Now we want to see what [child's name] does when looking at books. Try to avoid telling [child's name] what to look at or asking [child's name] to label the picture. Follow [child's name]'s lead by noticing or labeling the picture that he [she] directs your attention to.

 IV. Symbolic Play Probes (10 minutes)

Now we want to see how [child's name] plays with different sets of toys. Again try to avoid telling [child's name] what to do or asking [child's name] questions. Follow [child's name]'s lead by commenting about what [child's name] is doing.

1. First Toy Set (Feeding Set or Grooming Set)
2. Verbal Instructions and Modeling
3. Second Toy Set

 V. Language Comprehension Probes (5 minutes)

1. Comprehension Response Strategy

Now we want to see how [child's name] understands words by asking him [her] to point to body parts. What body parts does [child's name] know?

2. Body Parts
3. Agents
4. Possessor–Possession Combinations

 VI. Combinatorial Play Probes (5 minutes)

Now we want to see how [child's name] combines objects in play. Again try to avoid telling [child's name] what to do or asking [child's name] questions. Follow [child's name]'s lead by commenting about what [child's name] is doing.

1. Blocks
2. Stacking Rings
3. Nesting Cups

 VII. Caregiver Perception Rating Form

cial and body postures. Based on observations in these three areas, Norris and Hoffman rated children's levels of interactive behaviors as being at one of five levels designed to characterize shifts at 3-month developmental intervals:

Level I (1 to 3 Month Rating). These behaviors occur in response to general stimulation and are usually in reaction to the adults' actions or the general environment.

Level II (4 to 6 Month Rating). These behaviors occur in response to play between people, generally reflecting turn taking but not specific control over others.

Level III (7 to 9 Month Rating). These behaviors occur when the infant initiates control in the in-

teraction, by imitating actions and reacting as participants share interactions with objects.

Level IV (10 to 12 Month Rating). These behaviors include imitations of actual functional actions and conventional gestures or vocalizations; their meaning is usually clear in context.

Level V (13 to 18 Months Rating). These behaviors are directed at getting the adult to share objects or to control the game so the adult keeps playing. (pp. 34–35)

The results of the research conducted by Norris and Hoffman (1990a) using these techniques supported the use of child-initiated strategies for assessment and intervention with children in the early stages of development. The child-initiated approach yielded a greater

TABLE 7.2   Differences between adult-initiated versus child-initiated interactions

ADULT-INITIATED	CHILD-INITIATED
Specific semantic, phonological, syntactic, or pragmatic skills are targeted.	A level of communication is targeted: content, form, and use are indivisible.
Adult design an activity to elicit targeted behaviors with high frequency.	Activity is designed to allow for a variety of communicative behaviors to occur; adult interprets.
Specific forms are taught receptively (pointing to exemplars) and expressively (shaping productions).	Adult imparts meaning on child's behavior by interpreting it as a request, comment, protest, and so on.
The adult form is used as the standard for an acceptable response.	Adult adds complexity to spontaneously occurring behavior.
A one-to-one relationship is established between a word and its referent.	Communications are interpreted variably to create novel effects with limited communicative behaviors.
Imitation and shaping are used to elicit closer approximations to a target behavior.	Adult provides models; the highest communicative behavior the child produces is responded to each moment.
Nontargeted behaviors are considered irrelevant and interfere with elicitation of targeted responses.	Any behavior is interpretable as communication; adult imparts contextually appropriate meaning.
Adult feedback focuses on the correctness of the child's response.	Adult responds with contextually appropriate action and words to indicate what child had communicated.
Secondary reinforcers (claps, praise, tokens) reward the occurrence of target behavior.	Behaviors are reinforced through their effects—controlling the actions of the adult and toys.

Note: From "Comparison of Adult-Initiated vs. Child-Initiated Styles with Handicapped Prelanguage Children" by J. A. Norris and P. R. Hoffman, 1990. *Language, Speech, and Hearing Services in Schools, 21,* p. 29. Copyright 1990 by American Speech-Language-Hearing Association. Reprinted by permission.

frequency and higher developmental levels of communicative behaviors than the adult-initiated approach.

Some informal assessment tools for early stages of communicative development have been devised specifically to look at the interactions between caregivers and their children. One of these, the scale for Observation of Communicative Interactions (OCI; M. D. Klein & Briggs, 1987), was designed specifically to measure caregiver responsivity to the infant's communicative cues. It includes a continuum of ten categories of responsiveness, ranging from basic caregiving responses to more sophisticated efforts to facilitate language and conceptual development. It can also be used to guide intervention efforts. Another scale that can be used for combined assessment and intervention is the Parent-Infant Interaction Scale (G. N. Clark & Seifer, 1985). The areas this scale addresses include caregiver interaction behaviors, caregiver and child social referencing, caregiver and child reciprocity, and caregiver affect. It can be used to rate the caregiver's relative sensitivity to the infant's cues along a continuum in which physical restraint or forced head turning by parents is rated as least sensitive and most intrusive, and expansion or elaboration of a child's behavior, such as comments on the child's focus of attention, is rated as most sensitive.

Another consideration is whether the procedures used in assessment offer broad enough samples of early language, speech, and communication to provide evidence (in the prelinguistic or one-word stage) that a child might need intervention services. Broader views of communicative processes are needed, particularly to illuminate uneven profiles of intralinguistic abilities associated with specific difficulties in language acquisition.

Recognizing this need, A. M. Wetherby, Yonclas, and Bryan (1989) explored the possibilities for using a varied set of indicators in the early stage of language acquisition. They tested the procedures with children who demonstrated three different kinds of causative conditions, including four children with Down syndrome (ranging in age from 30 to 35 months), four children with specific language impairments (19 to 29 months), and three children with autism (30 to 52 months), all of whom functioned in the prelinguistic and one-word stage. Wetherby and co-workers used indicators in the following four categories: (1) communicative functions, (2) discourse structure, (3) communicative means, and (4) syllabic shape (note that these categories relate

closely to the observational categories of the CSBS by A. M. Wetherby & Prizant, 1993, outlined previously).

The results of the measures in these four areas varied for the different groups of children. Outcomes for children with Down syndrome fell in the normal range in all four areas; those for children with specific language impairment demonstrated deviance only in the area of syllabic shape; and results for children with autism fell outside the normal range in all areas except adequate rates of communicating (A. M. Wetherby et al., 1989).

Based on their results, A. M. Wetherby and her colleagues (1989) made some preliminary recommendations for using information about these four parameters in making clinical decisions about children's relative needs in language, speech, and communicative development. They also noted that the prognosis for a particular child might be worse if more parameters are affected and if certain parameters are affected (e.g., the absence of consonants might be less worrisome than the absence of joint attention acts). Another important factor in establishing prognosis may be the amount and rate of change observed in a child's profile with advancing age.

Miller and Paul (1995) emphasized the need to assess language comprehension separately from language expression (see Personal Reflection 7.3). They described the goals of comprehension assessment for children in the early stages of language acquisition:

> Children in the emerging language stage, which corresponds in typical development from about 8 to 24 months of age, understand very little of the language spoken to them. Our task is to document how much true linguistic comprehension is present. In addition, though, we want to examine the extent to which nonlinguistic and discourse-level strategies are used to aid comprehension of more advanced forms. (p. 23)

Techniques for assessing language comprehension by children in the early stages of language acquisition involve the parents in selecting vocabulary and familiar toys and objects that might be in the child's emerging lexicon. Miller and Paul (1995) described procedures for assessing children's nonlinguistic comprehension within familiar routines (e.g., peekaboo, "I'm-gonna-get-you") and joint reference activities, and for assessing language comprehension for object and person names, action words, words for absent persons and ob-

PERSONAL REFLECTION 7.3 _____

"It seems that the traditional wisdom that 'comprehension precedes production' is not operating—at least for some structures and during some developmental periods. To us, as clinicians, this is more than an interesting empirical finding. It means that we cannot make assumptions about language comprehension on the basis of a child's production or vice versa. It also means that in order to get a picture of a child's language competence, each modality of language will have to be assessed independently." (1995, p. 1)

Jon F. Miller, University of Wisconsin-Madison, and *Rhea Paul,* Portland State University, setting the stage for their discussion of informal approaches to assessing language comprehension in their book, *The Clinical Assessment of Language Comprehension.*

jects, and for early two-word relations. Strategies are considered further in Chapter 8 as they relate to the intervention process.

SUMMARY

This chapter addressed identification and assessment for infants and toddlers at risk for language development problems. Risk factors include **established risks** such as Down syndrome and hearing impairment and **environmental risks** such as child abuse and neglect. In this chapter, **biological risks** related to low birth weight and related factors were also discussed. The increased risks associated with increasingly low birth weight were noted, especially for cognitive delays and sensory-motor impairments, such as cerebral palsy. Risks associated with fetal alcohol syndrome, fetal alcohol effect, and fetal cocaine exposure were also noted.

Auditory and developmental screening procedures were described, and Child-Find requirements of IDEA were discussed. Hospital neonatal intensive care units, as well as homes and infant centers, were considered as assessment contexts. The unique family-centered and family systems needs of infants and toddlers were emphasized. Techniques of ethnographic interviews and other culturally sensitive procedures were described.

Three forms of assessment discussed were: formal, parent report, and informal. Transdisciplinary Play Based Assessment (TPBA; Linder, 1993) was described as an example of cross-domain arena assessment in which a group of professionals from multiple disciplines observe (with the parents) the same set of interaction activities. The Communication and Symbolic Behavior Scales (CSBS; Wetherby & Prizant, 1993) tool was described as an example of norm-referenced assessment focused on nonverbal and verbal communicative abilities. Parents provide input to the CSBS and are asked to validate its results. Parent report measures include language-specific vocabulary measures, such as the MacArthur Communication Development Inventories (Fenson et al., 1993), and cross-domain measures, such as the Ages and Stages Questionnaires (Bricker et al., 1995). Informal procedures, which are introduced here and discussed further in Chapter 8, are especially useful for gathering baseline measures in relevant goal areas. Child-initiated approaches were distinguished from adult-initiated approaches, and their advantages were described. The need to assess comprehension as well as expression and to consider nonlinguistic as well as linguistic comprehension strategies was emphasized.

REVIEW TOPICS

- Risk factors (established, environmental, biological) and early identification, especially the implications of various degrees of low birth weight
- Objective auditory screening techniques, such as ABR audiometry, and behavioral techniques, such as the APR and the crib-o-gram
- IDEA Child-Find requirements and requirements from Part C for involving parents in developing IFSPs (including CPRs—concerns, priorities, resources)
- Hospitals, homes, and centers as contexts for assessment
- Family-centered and family systems philosophies, ethnographic interview techniques
- Formal assessment tools (cross-domain and language specific; TPBA and CSBS as extended examples)
- Parent report tools (MacArthur CDIs; ASQ, AEPS)
- Informal procedures (child-initiated; adult-initiated)
- Comprehension assessment within familiar routines and joint reference activity, and for object and person names, action words, words for absent persons and objects, and early two-word relations

REVIEW QUESTIONS

1. Does a child with extremely low birth weight have more serious risks than one with very low birth weight? Would you be more likely to see specific language impairment or language problems in conjunction with cognitive and perceptual-motor limitations in a child born with low birth weight? What is the tiniest neonate who might survive in today's NICUs: (a) 1500 g, (b) 1000 g, (c) 750 g?

2. What are some techniques used in screening the hearing of infants? What other types of screening are performed? In what contexts?

3. What risks are associated with fetal alcohol syndrome and fetal alcohol effect? What risks are associated with fetal cocaine exposure?

4. Are neonatal intensive care unit teams more likely to be multidisciplinary, interdisciplinary, or transdisciplinary in the way they function?

5. From the TPBA and CSBS: What are communicative temptations? What is arena assessment? Which tool(s) emphasized a transdisciplinary team approach? Which tool(s) use play as an assessment context? Which tool(s) cross multiple domains? Which tool(s) emphasize verbal and nonverbal communication? Which tool(s) involve parents in observing and validating the process?

6. What characteristics distinguish adult-initiated and child-initiated interactions with prelanguage children?

ACTIVITIES FOR EXTENDED THINKING

1. Visit a speech–language pathologist who works in a neonatal intensive care unit and observe the role; accompany a professional on a home visit; interview a member of an early childhood intervention team; or view a sample IFSP. What are the unique challenges and benefits of working with infants and toddlers and their families?

2. Consider how you would start an ethnographic parental interview for a toddler who has been referred to you. What would you do to establish rapport before beginning the interview? What is the first question you would ask? What follow-up question could you use if a parent tells you something like, "Meals are the worst time for us"?

3. Compare and contrast the TPBA and CSBS. List the advantages and disadvantages of each. What are their different purposes? What features would you include if you were designing a test for infants and toddlers?

4. Spend some time with a normally developing infant or toddler. What can you say about the child's expressive language development? What evidence do you have that the child is comprehending language? What evidence do you have of nonlinguistic comprehension strategies? (Use Miller and Paul, 1995 to support your observations of comprehension.)

CHAPTER APPENDIX A
ANNOTATED BIBLIOGRAPHY
OF EARLY-STAGE
ASSESSMENT TOOLS

Ages and Stages Questionnaire (ASQ): A Parent Completed, Child-Monitoring System. Bricker, D., Squires, J., Mounts L., Potter, L., Nickel, R., & Farrell, J. (1997). Baltimore, MD: Paul H. Brookes Publishing Co. Identifies children ages 4 mos. to 4:0 years who might have, or be at risk for, developmental delays. Actively involves parents and family members in assessment, intervention, and evaluation.

Assessing Prelinguistic and Early Linguistic Behaviors in Developmentally Young Children. Olswang, L. B., Stoel-Gammon, C., Coggins, T. E., & Carpenter, R. L. (1987). Includes five scales of cognitive antecedents to word meaning, play, communication intention, language comprehension, and language production. A training videotape is also available. Based on 3-year longitudinal study of prelinguistic and early linguistic behaviors of 37 normally developing children.

Assessment in Infancy. Uzgiris, I. C., & Hunt, J. C. (1975). Chicago: University of Illinois Press. Six scales are used to assess sensorimotor behaviors expected in the range from birth to 2 years.

Assessment of Children's Language Comprehension (ACLC). Foster, R., Giddan, J., & Stark, J. (1983). Palo Alto, CA: Consulting Psychologists Press. Establishes recognition of single-word vocabulary,

Note: Background sources include Crais (1995); Sparks and Clark (1990); Hill and Singer (1990); Roberts and Crais (1989).

then uses this vocabulary to test comprehension of 2-, 3-, and 4-word phrase (e.g., "Happy little girl jumping), using picture-pointing task.

Assessment of Premature Infant Behavior (APIB). Als, H. (1984). Boston: The Children's Hospital. Behavioral evaluation scale (adapted and expanded from Brazelton's 1984 *Neonatal Behavioral Assessment Scale*) for rating behaviors in visual, auditory, tactile, organization, and reflexes categories. Used with medically stable neonates until they react to environment similar to full-term infants.

Autism Screening Instrument for Education Planning (ASIEP). Krug, D. A., Arick, J. R., & Almond, P. J. (1980). Portland, OR: ASIEP Education Company. Assessment and educational planning system for persons with autism, severe handicaps, and developmental disabilities who are between 18 months and adulthood but have low language abilities. Includes five components: autism behavior checklist; sample of vocal behavior; interaction assessment (including self-stimulation, crying, laughing, gesturing, manipulation of toys, conversation, and tantrums); educational assessment; and prognosis of learning rate.

Battelle Developmental Inventory (BDI). Newborg, J., Stock, J. R., Wnek, L., Guidubaldi, J., & Svinicki, J. (1984). Allen, TX: DLM. Comprehensive, standardized assessment (requiring 1 to 2 hours) for children from birth to 8 years in the domains of personal-social, adaptability, motor, communication, and cognition. Spanish version is available.

Battelle Developmental Inventory Screening Test. Newborg, J., Stock, J. R., & Wnek, L. (1984). Allen, TX: DLM. Screens personal-social, adaptive, motor, communication, and cognitive areas from birth to age 8 years.

Bayley Infant Neurodevelopmental Screener (BINS). Aylward, G. P. (1995). San Antonio, TX: Psychological Corporation. Screens infants aged 3 to 24 months who are at risk for neurological impairment or developmental delay. Assesses neurological functions, auditory and visual receptive functions, verbal and motor functions, and cognitive processes.

Bayley Scales of Infant Development (2nd ed.) (BSID-II). Bayley, N. (1993). San Antonio, TX: Psychological Corporation. Includes Mental, Motor, and Behavioral Scales useful with children aged 1 month to 42 months for describing developmental levels and making placement decisions. It yields standard scores for 14 age groups. Requires 45 minutes to administer.

Birth to Three Developmental Scales. Bangs, T., & Dodson, S. (1979). Allen, TX: DLM. Observation, direction following, motor and verbal imitation, object and picture naming, and pointing are used to build a development profile for the age range 0:0 to 3:0 years.

Communication and Symbolic Behavior Scales (CSBS). [Research ed.]. Wetherby, A. M., & Prizant, B. M. (1990). *Communication and Symbolic Behavior Scales* [Norm-referenced ed.] Wetherby, A. M., & Prizant, B. M. (1991). Chicago, IL: Applied Symbolix. (Reviewed extensively in Chapter 7.) The CSBS is designed to be used with children whose functional communication ages are 9 months to 2 years. Uses a caregiver questionnaire, direct sampling of verbal and nonverbal communicative behaviors, and observation of relatively unstructured play activities. Scoring of the CSBS is accomplished by assigning a rating of 1 to 5 for each of 20 separate scales. Includes 16 communication scales (subdivided into four areas) and 4 scales for rating symbolic behavior (subdivided into two areas).

Denver Developmental Screening Test (DDST). Frankenburg, W. K., Dodds, J. B., & Fandal, A. W. (1969). (Manual revised, 1970). Denver, CO: University of Colorado Medical Center. Designed to screen children from the general population to identify children from birth to age 6 years in four areas, including language, who need further evaluation. Standardized on 1036 Denver children. Items are marked as to when 25%, 50%, 75%, and 90% of the normative sample passed them.

Developmental Communication Curriculum (DCC). Hanna, R. P., Lippert, E. A., & Harris, A. B. (1982). San Antonio, TX: Psychological Corporation. This curriculum is designed for children of developmental ages birth to 5 years. It includes an assessment component, the Developmental Communication Inventory, for assessing four levels: prelinguistic, symbolic, symbolic relationships, complex symbolic relationships. Uses play contexts to observe form, content, and function. Encourages teacher and parent input.

Early Language Milestone Scale (2nd ed.) (ELM Scale-2). Coplan, J. (1993). Austin, TX: Pro-Ed. In one to ten minutes this test screens the Auditory Expressive, Auditory Receptive, and Visual skills of children birth to 36 months. It is also useful with older children whose development falls within this range. Can be scored as pass/fail or with a point system. Yields percentile and standard score equivalents.

ECOScales. MacDonald, J. D., & Gillette, Y. (1989). Chicago: Applied Symbolix. Five separate scales are used to assess the five competencies of social play, turn taking, preverbal communication, language, and conversation. Results may be displayed on the competencies profiles or the interaction profile to address developmental goals or adult-child interaction patterns. Takes 10 to 30 minutes.

Environmental Language Intervention Program (ELIP). MacDonald, J. D. (1978). San Antonio, TX: Psychological Corporation. This assessment/diagnostic/remediation program includes the Oliver (Parent-Assisted Communication Inventory) test of prelanguage and early language skills. The Environmental Prelanguage Battery (EPB) is an assessment tool for children who have no oral language skills, designed to assess readiness behaviors (e.g., play) for learning language. The Environmental Language Inventory (ELI) assesses early language development (two or more word phrases) in conversation, imitation, and free play.

Evaluating Acquired Skills in Communication (EASIC) (Revised). Riley, A. M. (1984). San Antonio, TX: Communication Skill Builders, The Psychological Corp. This assessment can be used with severely impaired clients with skills in the 3-months to 8-years range. It can be used to rate behaviors at the levels: prelanguage, receptive I (noun labels, action verbs, and basic concepts); expressive I (emerging modes of communication); receptive II (more complex language forms); and expressive II (using more complex communication). Criterion referenced.

Hawaii Early Leaning Profile (HELP). Furuno, S., O'Reilly, K., Inatsuka, T., Hosaka, C., Allman, T., & Zeisloft-Falbey. (1979). Palo Alto, CA: VORT Corporation. Charts are provided for 650 skills developed from birth to 3 years in the six areas of cognitive, language, gross motor, fine motor, social, and self-help. A sequenced checklist can be used to select objectives.

MacArthur Communicative Development Inventories (CDI). Fenson, L., Dale, P. S., Resnick, J. S., Thal, D., Bates, E., Hartung, J. P., Pethick, S., & Reilly, J. S. (1993). San Diego, CA: Singular Publishing Group. Uses a parental checklist format to assess first signs of understanding, comprehension of early phrases, and starting to talk. Vocabulary checklist (for both understanding and saying) includes sound effect and animal sounds, animal names, vehicles, toys, food and drink, clothing, body parts, furniture and rooms, small household items, outside things and places to go, people, games and routines, action words, words about time, descriptive words, pronouns, question words, prepositions and locations, and quantifiers. Early gestures, play, pretending, and imitating behaviors are also probed. A "Words and Sentences" CDI also probes sentences and grammar, including morphological endings, and varied expressions of two-word meanings. Can be used with older children at early stages.

Neonatal Behavioral Assessment Scale. Brazelton, T. B. (1984). Philadelphia, PA: J. B. Lippincott. Behavioral evaluation scale for use with neonates. Requires 30 to 60 minutes to assess visual, auditory, tactile, organization, motor maturity, and reflexes.

Observation of Communicative Interactions (OCI). Klein, M. D., & Briggs, M. H. (1987). Los Angeles: Mother–Infant Communication Project, California State University, Los Angeles. Designed specifically to measure caregiver responsivity to infant's communicative cues. Includes a continuum of 10 categories of responsiveness ranging from basic caregiving responses to more sophisticated efforts to facilitate language and conceptual development. It can also be used to guide intervention efforts.

Oral-Motor/Feeding Rating Scale. Jelm, J. M. (1990). San Antonio, TX: Communication Skill Builders, The Psychological Corporation. This observational scale can be used for combined assessment and intervention purposes with persons of all ages to summarize oral-motor and feeding functioning in eight areas: breast feeding, bottle feeding, spoon feeding, cup drinking, biting (soft cookie), biting (hard cookie), chewing, and straw drinking.

Parent–Infant Interaction Scale. Clark, G. N., & Seifer, R. (1985). Assessment of parents' interaction with their developmentally delayed infants. *Infant Mental Health Journal, 6*(4), 214–225. The areas addressed by this scale include caregiver interaction behaviors, caregiver and child social referencing, reciprocity, and caregiver affect.

Preverbal Assessment Intervention Profile (PAIP). Connard, P. (1984). Austin, TX: Pro-Ed. This is a standardized Piagetian assessment of sensorimotor (stages I to III) prelinguistic behavior. It can be used with severely, profoundly, and multiply handicapped individuals of all ages.

The Receptive–Expressive Emergent Language Scale (2nd ed.) (REEL-2). Bzoch, K., & League, R. (1991). Austin, TX: Pro-Ed. Designed to help public health nurses, pediatricians, and educators identify children up to 3 years of age who have specific language problems based on interview of "significant others" (usually a parent). Results are presented as expressive, receptive, and combined language ages.

Reynell Developmental Language Scales. Reynell, J. K. (1985). Los Angeles: Webster Psychological Services. Uses observation, picture identification, object identification, and object manipulation to measure general language receptive and expressive skills among 1:0- to 5:0-year-olds.

The Rossetti Infant–Toddler Language Scale. Rossetti, L. (1990). East Moline, IL: LinguiSystems. Designed for infants and toddlers, birth to 3 years, this is a criterion-referenced assessment scale covering multiple developmental areas: interaction and attachment, gestures, pragmatics, play, language comprehension, and language expression. Includes three to seven items for each domain at each 3-month interval.

Sequenced Inventory of Communication Development (2nd ed.) (SICD). Hedrick, D. L., Prather, E. M., & Tobin, A. R. (1984). Seattle: University of Washington Press. Designed for children functioning between 4 months and 4 years of age. Includes receptive and expressive scales. Cuban-Spanish edition (by L. R. Rosenberg) is available.

Transdisciplinary Play-Based Assessment (Rev. Ed.) (TPBA). Linder, T, W. (1993). Baltimore, MD: Paul H. Brookes. This set of criterion-referenced informal assessment scales (reviewed extensively in Chapter 7) is designed for children functioning developmentally between the ages of 6 months and 6 years. It uses a play interaction context to observe four domains: social–emotional, cognitive, language and communication, and sensorimotor. A 1-hour to 1½-hour session of videotaped play interaction with facilitator, parent, and peer is observed and scored by multiple professionals. No standardized scores are computed with the TPBA. The outcome is an analysis of developmental level, learning style, interaction patterns, and other relevant behaviors that can become an integral part of intervention planning.

8

Early Stages: Goals and Intervention Strategies

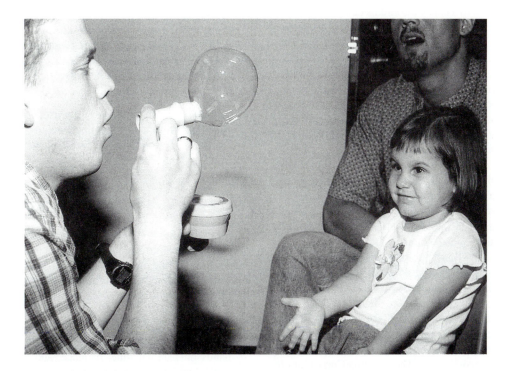

The goals and intervention strategies for the earliest stages of language acquisition are integrally tied to the relationships between children and the important adults in their lives. The sections that follow use the major events of early communicative development as a blueprint for intervention programs for infants and toddlers. This approach is based on the philosophy that language intervention works best when those who implement it view it as intensified efforts to foster normal development. In each section, a goal and outcome statement appears first to establish a focus for designing intervention activities. Planning requires that a team of specialists (defined under Part C of IDEA as a group that includes the parents and a service coordinator) consider the young child's current levels of performance (see Chapter 7). Next, the child's baseline functioning is described and quantified for each Goal Area. Intervention begins with the process of involving parents and other caregivers in these activities to identify the child's developing edge of competence. It intensifies with systematic attempts to arrange experiences, focus the child on cues that make sense, and respond to the child's current behaviors in ways that encourage the child to attempt higher level communicative interactions and acquire new language.

This approach assumes that all young children with communicative risks or identified disorders go through similar stages, regardless of etiological factors. Children with sensory deficits, such as hearing loss, and others with motor control problems may need specialized compensatory methods and technologies, but they too, need to be assisted to move as rapidly as possible through the normal developmental stages. Many organized curricula are available to encourage development of communication and other domains among infants and toddlers at risk because of known etiological factors.

Several curricula have been specially designed for infants with severe hearing losses and their parents, for example, the Ski–Hi curriculum (T. Clark & Watkins, 1985) and many others (e.g., Northcott, 1977; Sitnick, Rushmer, & Arpan, 1982; Statewide Project for the Deaf, 1982). Some curricula are designed to cross disability (and risk) categories (e.g., The Carolina Curriculum for Handicapped Infants and Infants at Risk, Johnson-Martin, Jens, & Attermeier, 1986). The INSITE Model (T. Clark, Morgan, & Wilson-Vlotman, 1984) is designed specifically to provide home intervention services to infants with sensory impairments and multiple handicaps.

The ECO Model, developed by MacDonald and his colleagues at the Nisonger Center in Ohio (described by MacDonald, 1989), focuses on establishing interactive communicative partnerships with infants and toddlers, no matter what their presenting conditions.

Curricula vary in organization and relative focus on certain aspects of development. Most now demonstrate an awareness that early development does not represent only acquisition of a set of isolated skills but reflects the nurturing and encouragement of communication as a cohesive, meaningful, and functional process.

GETTING THE BASICS TOGETHER

Goal: The infant will demonstrate strategies for gaining internal control, initiating positive social interactions, and engaging in vocal play facilitated by a sensitive caregiver.

- Organization and Early Sensing of Care and Safety
- Mutual Communication and Reciprocal "Dialogues"
- Early Vocal and Phonological Behavior
- Early Feeding Behaviors and Needs
- Early Comprehension of Routines and Sense Making
- Reciprocation and Imitation

Outcome: The infant will convey a sense of security and well-being, attachment, and openness to interactions and will thrive physically and emotionally.

Organization and Early Sensing of Care and Safety

Any physical problems that interfere with an infant's respiratory system, vocal tract, or feeding capabilities have implications for the development of speech and possibly language. They also have implications for many complicated expectations facing parents and the emotional bonding between the adult caregiver and the child with special needs. When parents must deal with technology to maintain their infant's health (e.g., tracheostomy tubes for breathing through a neck stoma or suctioning equipment for keeping the airway clear), the demands on parental time, patience, and stress levels multiply. Quality communication efforts may seem secondary to getting through the day with a baby whose life is at risk.

Objective 1: Facilitated by a caregiver's sensitive facilitation, the infant will become quiet and organized in circumstances that triggered loss of control during baseline observations.

Part of the early assessment of infants at risk relates to how well they can organize themselves. Thus, an important part of early intervention is to assist parents to provide a secure and stable environment that can support children's abilities to organize themselves. Some of the questions addressed by the Assessment of Preterm Infant Behavior (APIB) (Als et al., 1982) can be instructive toward planning these earliest stages of intervention. Sparks (1989b) summarized the questions of the APIB that have implications for developing intervention objectives for neonates:

- When, and with what help, does the infant function smoothly?
- How much and what kinds of stress and frustration are seen in the infant?
- How much handling can the infant tolerate before losing control?
- Is the infant's homeostatic balance easily disrupted?
- What strategies does the infant exhibit to avoid losing control?
- What support is necessary to help the infant maintain self-control? (p. 47)

The joint process of answering these questions constitutes some of the mutual goal setting and collaborative problem solving of early intervention. This kind of questioning may be used to guide initial IFSP discussions of child and family needs and strengths (see Chapter 5). Gillette (1992) discussed dealing with medical concerns within a comprehensive support system and showed how to develop IFSPs using a Coordinated Approach to the Transition for the Hospital to the Community and Home (CATCH).

Joint problem-solving attempts are also consistent with recent hypotheses about the earliest internal and external goals that seem to drive infant behavior (Tronick, 1989). For example, Tronick described early internal goals as being aimed at maintaining physiological homeostasis, establishing feelings of security, experiencing positive emotions, and controlling negative emotions.

Objective 2: The infant will increase the frequency of giving positive signals of wanting caregivers to be close (e.g., smiling, vocalizing, cuddling), as caregiver responds to both positive

and negative signals (e.g., crying, fussing), and will explore objects facilitated by caregiver.

Early external infant goals include interacting with others, maintaining proximity to caregivers, engaging in positive reciprocal interactions, and exploring objects (Tronick, 1989). In Greenspan's (1988) view, as parents assist their infants to achieve physiological and emotional regulation, they contribute to their children's ability to focus energy on the animate and the inanimate world, paving the way for them to establish emotional attachments and to develop in other ways.

Establishing Mutual Communication and Reciprocal "Dialogues"

The earliest forms of communication have been called **behavioral state communication** (Dunst & Lowe, 1986). In this preintentional stage of 0 to 3 months of age, whether an act will be considered communicative depends more on the interpretive abilities of adult caregivers than on the expressive abilities of children. The signals emitted by some infants are more "readable" than others', and the abilities of parents to read their infants' needs may vary as well. These mutual interactional abilities may become early targets of intervention efforts.

Objective 3: The infant will signal internal states in ways that the caregiver can recognize and respond to in synchrony.

To create a better match between the communicativeness of prelinguistic children at risk and the receptiveness of their parents or other caregivers, Prizant and Wetherby (1990) suggested using the transactional model of dynamic transactional interrelationships among the three variables of child characteristics, caregiver characteristics, and environmental influences (Dunst, Lowe, & Bartholomew, 1990; Sameroff & Chandler, 1975). Part of the power of transactions is that, over time, caregiver–child interactions build a sense of mutual efficacy by which bidirectional, contingent social responsiveness of caregiver and child together develop patterns of future communicativeness. Thus, an important part of the intervention process is to assist caregivers to accurately interpret their child's early social and communicative behavior so that the caregiver's response can meet the child's needs or support social exchange, contributing to this sense of mutual efficacy (Prizant & Wetherby, 1990). Contingent responsiveness of caregivers may also serve to teach the child the signal value of specific behaviors, such as crying and noncry vocalizations (Owens, 1996).

Schaffer (1977) described mother–infant influence on each other's behaviors during early infancy, with mothers looking for clues as to the amount of stimulation their infants can tolerate based on signals of infant attentiveness. By 3 months, because most infants can maintain fairly constant internal states (Owens, 1996), infants also can be attentive for longer periods. As Owens described it, "At any given moment the caregiver must determine the appropriate amount of stimulation based upon the infant's level of attention" (p. 165). At some points, infants may appear to be overstimulated (and need to be given time without stimulation), and at other points, they appear to be understimulated (and need enhanced input).

During this stage, the specialist may aim intervention to assist mothers and other caregivers to become more accurate in identifying the infant's internal states and being responsive to them (Brazelton, 1982). Lynch-Fraser and Tiegerman's (1987) book *Baby Signals* is designed to help parents learn to recognize their infants' states and varied learning styles and to encourage those, even at very young ages and when communicative styles are very different.

As noted in Chapter 4, efforts to teach synchrony, rhythm, and sensitivity to infant signals may be particularly important when infants have physical impairments or autism that make them respond to stimulation in unexpected ways. During intervention, the specialist should assist caregivers not to be discouraged by initial lack of infant responsiveness. Box 8.1 offers suggestions for intervention with families.

> *Objective 4:* The infant will participate in mutual dialogues, starting with initiation, and ending by turning away.

The specialist also may assist parents to look for opportunities to become synchronous with their infants in communicative cycles (Brazelton, 1982; Tronick, Als, & Adamson, 1979). These reciprocal **dialogues** include the following phases:

1. Initiation,
2. Orientation, which establishes the partner's expectations regarding interaction,

Box 8.1 _____

Sharing Information about Early Interactions with Families (Excerpts from Recommendations by Gillette, 1992, p. 74).

Effective professionals use simple comments to point out the things that make a difference in the way the family and child interact.

> *"The two of you seem to go after each other's attention with your eyes while he takes the bottle."*
>
> *"The more you wait, the more she seems to do."*
>
> *"You certainly have found a million ways to use that ball."*

Often, a verbal observation of something a professional considers beneficial yet sees only occasionally will increase the frequency of that behavior. . . . On the other hand, directives have a negative effect. Families may interpret directives as an indication that they don't do what they should. Avoid comments like:

> *"Make eye contact with your child each time you feed him."*
>
> *"Wait before you tell her to do that again."*

When you feel you must direct a family's behavior with a child, demonstrate what you mean. You might introduce your demonstration by saying, "Let me see how he responds when I try this." If it works, make a remark to point out what you did that worked.

> *"You might consider counting to ten and waiting before you give him another bite. It seemed to work for me."*
>
> *"I notice when I imitate her, she imitates me."*
>
> *"He really seems to perk up when I smile."*

_____

3. Acceleration to a peak of excitement,
4. Deceleration, and
5. Turning away. (Brazelton, 1982, p. 51)

Research in normal development has shown mothers to assist their infants to maintain attention and to engage in these early mutual "dialogues" by using a set of techniques (Schaffer, 1977):

1. *Phasing*—monitoring infant signals to time stimulation input to be most effective.
2. *Adapting*—using highly ordered, predictable input sequences to assist infants to assimilate new information.

3. *Facilitating*—structuring environmental routines to ensure infant success.
4. *Elaborating*—allowing their infants to indicate an interest and then elaborating on it gesturally, vocally, and verbally.
5. *Initiating*—directing their infants' attention to objects, events, and persons, and monitoring that attention.
6. *Controlling*—telling and showing infants what to do (emphasizing key words with pauses and gestures) and then assisting them to comply.

In normal development, caregivers use modifications such as these to increase their infants' opportunities to participate in mutual dialogues, with those prelinguistic dialogues reaching a peak of frequency at around 3 to 4 months of age (Owens, 1996). Similar strategies might be targeted directly for working with caregivers in the intervention process (N. W. Nelson, 1988b).

MacDonald (1989) presented many suggestions for helping caregivers and other communicative partners become more responsive to young children. He related them to a set of five principles for developing social and communicative partnerships: (1) Based on the **partnership principle,** parents should question whether they are sharing their child's learning in a balanced, give-and-take relationship. (2) Based on the **matching principle,** parents should question whether they are interacting and communicating in ways their children also can match. (3) Based on the **sensitive responsiveness** principle, parents should question whether they are responding to subtle behaviors that represent their children's developmental steps. (4) Based on the **child-based nondirectiveness principle,** parents should question whether they are allowing their children sufficient control over their own learning. (5) Based on the **emotional attachment principle,** parents should question whether their social attitudes are effective in helping their children to be social. MacDonald then presented a series of steps from the ECO model that parents can use to become play partners, turn-taking partners, communicating partners, language partners, and conversation partners with their children.

Early Vocal and Phonological Behavior

Objective 5: The infant will show increased frequency and variety of vocal play and other non-cry vocalizations compared with baseline measurements.

When normally developing infants begin to engage in mutual social interactional dialogues, they simultaneously exercise their vocal tract mechanisms. They extend their reflexive oral–motor abilities for sucking and swallowing into more sophisticated abilities under increasing voluntary control. They also begin to shape their vocalizations into productions that sound increasingly like phonemes, including greater proportions of varied consonants. As they move through these stages in the normal pattern, an increase appears first in the use of isolated vocal acts and vocal acts combined with gestures, then verbal acts predominate (rather than gestural or nonvocal acts) (Carpenter, Mastergeorge, & Coggins, 1983; A. M. Wetherby, Cain, Yonclas, & Walker, 1988).

Infants Who Are Medically Fragile. For some infants with motor impairments or medical complications, the process is particularly complex. Hill and Singer (1990) wrote about the problems that result when upper airway obstruction mandates the need for tracheostomy tubes. Such tubes allow infants to breathe but interfere with their ability to vocalize. For some, the tracheostomy tubes may need to stay in place for up to 30 months, extending this period of mechanically impaired vocalization far into the linguistic development stage. Expressive language delays may appear for some of these children as they advance into their elementary years (Hill & Singer, 1990). Children with limited cognitive abilities are particularly at risk (G. S. Ross, 1982). Communicative specialists therefore should work closely with medical personnel to minimize duration of intubation procedures as much as possible without jeopardizing the health and safety of children. They also should watch for the need to provide language intervention for expressive language difficulties as children with early tracheostomies advance in age.

Tube feedings may also be necessary but problematic to early communicative development. Jaffe (1989) described the use of tubes for nonoral feeding when required to prevent aspiration, malnutrition, and fatigue in biologically at-risk infants. The two major categories of feeding tubes are (1) those inserted down the pharynx and esophagus into the stomach through the nose (called *nasogastric* [N-G] tubes) or through the mouth (called *orogastric* tubes) and (2) those inserted directly into the stomach by means of minor abdominal surgery known as *gastrostomy,* implanting a gastrostomy tube (G-tube) or esophagostomy tube. Although physicians and parents may find it easier to accept N-G or orogastric tubes than gastrostomy tubes (at least until long-term eating problems are identified), the insertion of these tubes is associated with some clearly negative influences on early communicative development. Among these are negative social and emotional implications, preclusion of the association of oral eating with positive sensory experience, and the difficulty of encouraging feeding, nonnutritive sucking, and oral-motor stimulation and functioning (Jaffe, 1989).

Vocalization problems are sometimes associated with nonoral feeding tubes as well. I worked with an infant whose medical complications necessitated early feeding through an N-G tube. After this tube was removed, the child remained aphonic. Apparently the tube passing behind the vocal mechanism traumatized it. This baby produced both laughing and crying behaviors without voice. The aphonia was particularly unfortunate in his case because he was also blind. Thus, two peripheral communicative avenues were severely impaired. We had to work hard to find other ways to provide both receptive and expressive communication access for this infant, while still encouraging his attempts to produce noncry vocalizations.

Normal Expectations. Proctor (1989) reviewed research on normal noncry vocal development in infancy. She noted that different researchers use different theoretical models and measurement strategies to characterize those developments. Methods range from articulatory and phonatory methods to phonetic and acoustic approaches. Proctor compiled the major markers from each of these approaches into the five stages of early vocal and phonological development listed in Box 8.2. However, she also noted that "There are no normative values for the amount, quality, or type of noncry vocalizations during the infant's first year" (p. 33). Therefore, speech–language pathologists must use clinical judgment to interpret the results of early-stage vocal assessments. Stimulation of vocalization may not be the highest priority for intervention if other medical needs are great. Instead, it may be more appropriate to target increases in the infant's vocal output in the context of more general communicative intervention strategies (Proctor, 1989).

Box 8.2 _____

Primary Distinguishing Features of Early-Stage Vocal Development

STAGE 1 (BIRTH TO 2 MONTHS)
- More crying and discomfort sounds than noncry sounds
- Predominantly noncry sounds are vegetative (reflexive), neutral, and mainly vocalic (vowel-like) in nature

STAGE 2 (2 TO 4 MONTHS)
- Marked decrease in crying after 12 weeks
- Vocalic sounds predominate, but consonant-like sounds are introduced
- Combining of consonantal (C) and vocalic (V) segments (coo or goo)
- Glottal C's heard [g, h, ç, ʔ, X, k]

STAGE 3 (4 TO 6 MONTHS)
- Increased number of C segments produced
- More variation of V productions
- Consistent production of CV syllables
- Variation of intonational contours

STAGE 4 (6:7 TO 10 MONTHS)
- Canonical, repetitive, or reduplicated babbling (i.e., CV or CVC-like structure)
- Consistent variations of intonational contours
- Early nonreduplicated CV syllables
- Utterances produced with full stop

STAGE 5 (10 TO 12 MONTHS)
- Variegated babbling (advanced form of reduplicated babbling)
- Variety of CV and CVC combinations with sentence-like intonation
- Approximations of meaningful single words
- Variety of Cs overlaid on sentence-like intonation

Note. From "Stages of Normal Noncry Vocal Development: A Protocol for Assessment" by A. Proctor. Reprinted from *Topics in Language Disorders,* Vol. 10, No. 1, p. 32. © 1989, Aspen Publishers, Inc. Reprinted with permission.

Early vocal development stages are universal. No matter what language a child is exposed to, babies begin by cooing, then produce reduplicated consonant–vowel

(CV) syllables followed by "variegated" babbling with sentence-like intonation before producing words and word-like forms around the time of their first birthday (Oller, 1978, 1980). As children approach their first word productions, their babbling begins to sound more and more like the phonological patterns common to their own native languages—that is, if they can hear their native language adequately and can hear their own babbling.

Infants with Hearing Impairments.   Several studies have demonstrated more limited consonantal repertoires in the prespeech vocalizations of children with severe hearing impairments (R. Kent, Osberger, Netsell, & Hustedde, 1987; Oller, Eilers, Bull, & Carney, 1985). For example, Stoel-Gammon and Otomo (1986) and Stoel-Gammon (1988) analyzed a series of babbling samples gathered longitudinally over the 4- to 39-month age range from a group of infants and toddlers with normal hearing and with hearing impairments. Their results confirmed other indications that the babbling of children with hearing impairments differs, both quantitatively and qualitatively, from babbling by normal-hearing children. Consonantal inventories of normal-hearing children grew with age; inventories of hearing impaired children started smaller and decreased over the study period.

Daniel Ling (1976) devised one of the most widely used approaches for targeting early vocal and phonological development among children with severe hearing impairments. He based his approach on a view of speech acquisition as an orderly and sequential process in which developmental advances occur on two developmental levels in parallel. On the **phonetic level,** children learn to produce and to discriminate sounds but without assigning meaning to them. On the **phonological level,** children develop awareness of the meaningful use of speech sounds in their own speech and that of others.

This parallel organization is a departure from earlier programs designed on the basis of a progression from nonverbal to verbal stimuli. In Ling's (1976) approach, the seven stages of the phonetic level are to: (1) vocalize freely and on demand; (2) produce suprasegmental patterns (intonation and stress variations by shifting duration, intensity, and pitch relationships); (3) produce all vowels and diphthongs with voice control; (4) differentiate consonants by manner; (5) differentiate of consonants by manner and place; (6) differentiate consonants by manner, place, and voicing; and (7) produce initial and final blends.

Judgments of adequacy at the phonetic level are based on automaticity and speed as well as accuracy. The goal is to avoid the development of exaggerated, unnatural speech-production habits (Ling, 1976). To encourage natural functional speech production and perception, adults are cautioned to avoid providing exaggerated visual models during phonetic level interactions.

As speech sounds become part of the child's seven-stage phonetic repertoire and the child begins to demonstrate communicative functions using other means, seven parallel stages are introduced on the phonological level. These stages are based on objectives to: (1) use vocalization as a means of communication; (2) use different voice patterns meaningfully; (3) use different vowels to approximate words; (4) say some words clearly and with good voice patterns; (5) say more words clearly and with good voice patterns; (6) say most words clearly and with good voice patterns; and (7) produce all speech intelligibly and with natural voice patterns.

Although Ling's (1976) procedures and targets were designed specifically for children with peripheral hearing impairments, they are based on normal developmental principles. Other children with early phonological processing problems in both perception and production may also need more deliberate attention to the development of their sound systems, as well as perception and control of paralinguistic vocal features.

Infants with Autism.   Baltaxe and Simmons (1985) considered how prosodic development differs for infants with autism. They observed that some children with autism demonstrate seemingly advanced musical abilities and exact echoing of prosody, both of which require precise auditory perception, but simultaneously appear unable to attach linguistic value to prosodic indicators. Baltaxe and Simmons hypothesized that some of the mixed picture for children with autism arises out of difficulty in hemispheric switching and integrating prosodic and linguistic functioning. They noted that, in normal development, early use of prelinguistic prosody is affective. Subsequent linguistic use evolves from this initial affective basis. This suggests that early prosodic processing occurs largely in the right hemisphere. Then, as linguistic abilities unfold, processing moves increasingly to the left hemisphere. Baltaxe and Simmons hypothesized that "Autistic children may not be equipped to make an adequate switch, either because of deficits that directly or indirectly affect the dominant hemisphere or because of a possible maturational lag at the cortical level or both" (p. 117).

When making everyday clinical decisions for children with autism, I have sometimes faced the dilemma that these children seem to comprehend better when somewhat exaggerated prosody is used, but I wonder if I might have encouraged a maladaptive pattern when I hear my slightly exaggerated prosody echoed back stereotypically. I usually then vow to try to keep my own prosody more natural and attempt to enhance comprehension and attention through other nonlinguistic contextual support.

Some children with autism rarely echo or speak spontaneously. For them, intervention efforts often focus on training in the use of nonverbal communication methods, such as signing, rather than vocal development and speech. However, Koegel and Traphagen (1982) questioned the avoidance of a more deliberate focus on phonological development with nonverbal autistic children. Their research showed that two nonspeaking autistic boys (ages 7:6 and 9:11) learned to say simple CV words (CVC combinations were more difficult) fairly readily when the initial target words were selected carefully from CV combinations of phonemes already in the boys' nonverbal self-stimulatory phonetic repertoires.

Early Feeding Behaviors and Needs

Objective 6: The infant (with facilitative body positioning) will eat and drink successfully for nutritive and/or nonnutritive purposes (depending on technological accommodations).

Children who cannot use the oral-motor tract adequately for eating are unlikely to use it for talking. Adequate oral-motor foundation skills are necessary, but not sufficient, for the development of normal early speech.

As in the ability to vocalize, long-term mechanical disruptions may interfere with the development of oral-motor skill. Jaffe (1989) observed that "Infants who breathe through endotracheal tubes and eat nonorally via intravenous or gavage tubes for an extended period may eventually demonstrate decreased sucking and oral-motor function" (p. 18). When infants' oral-motor experiences are limited mechanically, they may be assisted nevertheless to associate oral movements with feeling full and contented by the caregivers' inducing

nonnutritive sucking on a pacifier, nipple, thumb, or finger during tube feedings. The encouragement of nonnutritive sucking at other times also may help normalize oral-motor behavior and oral sensation toleration.

The nurturing atmosphere of feeding is important to both mothers and children. When infants or children have feeding problems, their mothers' "feelings of concern, anxiety, frustration, resentment, anger, and failure are inevitable" (Jaffe, 1989, p. 13). Motor problems, in particular, may interfere with nonverbal communication signals during feeding:

> *Movement patterns of head extension, flexion or constant turning to one side may limit the child's ability to gain eye contact with the feeder. This, in turn, will make it difficult for the child to regulate the speed of feeding or the amount of food given. An abnormal tongue thrusting movement may push the food out of the mouth, whether or not the child wishes to eat it. A bite reflex on the spoon or nipple may be interpreted as teasing or misbehavior. The child may be unable to vocalize, reach, point, or in other ways indicate readiness to eat or cease eating. (S. E. Morris, 1981, p. 222)*

Such confusing biological signals may turn feeding sessions into negative experiences. The added stress for the child may lead to increased abnormal muscle tone, making eating yet more difficult.

The role of speech–language pathologists and other professionals to reverse this downward spiral is multifaceted. In addition to assisting with techniques related directly to feeding, the professional "facilitates communication between parent and child and enhances the child's language development" in the context of feeding (Jaffe, 1989, p. 24). This may include helping caregivers to recognize their children's subtle or overt cues that an approach is working (or not), which might be an important part of helping children develop feelings of competence and communicative control. It may also consist of giving caregivers support so they can relax and simply enjoy their child, not be their child's primary therapist.

One supportive technique may be to assist caregivers to identify the most facilitative feeding position for their child, encouraging efforts to hold their infants in a gently flexed position while feeding to enhance nurturing sensations for both. As the child grows, alternate positions may be explored in consultation with an occupational or physical therapist, and specialized techniques, such as jaw control, may be needed (e.g., see The Carolina Curriculum for Handicapped Infants and Infants at Risk by Johnson-Martin, Jens, & Attermeier, 1986).

Throughout the process, professionals and parents should avoid the trap of focusing on feeding difficulties to the exclusion of facilitating social and communicative growth at mealtimes. S. E. Morris (1981) noted how mealtimes provide opportunities to encourage communicative reciprocity, causality, or mean–ends behaviors, object permanence, and the communicative development of gaze behaviors. Mealtimes can also serve as a context for introducing early augmentative communication techniques.

Feeding assessment and intervention often involve complex decisions guided by fluoroscopic observation of swallowing to judge the safety of oral feeding. Table 8.1

is Jaffe's (1989) summary of normal, primitive, delayed, or abnormal feeding behaviors. Jaffe also provided specialized suggestions for children with neurological impairment, Down syndrome, or cleft palates.

Some relatively formal assessment tools address feeding concerns. One is the Pre-Speech Assessment Scale (PSAS; S. E. Morris, 1982), which facilitates observation of respiration, phonation, sound play, and meaningful speech behaviors that appear from birth through 2 years of age. Another is the Feeding Assessment by S. E. Morris and Klein (1987), which includes a questionnaire (administered either in Spanish or in English) and yields an analysis of the physical and communicative environment and of normal and limiting oral-motor skills relative to various treatment options.

TABLE 8.1   Major movement patterns related to feeding

PRIMITIVE PATTERNS USUALLY SEEN DURING THE FIRST 6 MONTHS OF INFANT DEVELOPMENT)	HIGHER DEVELOPMENTAL PATTERNS (USUALLY SEEN BETWEEN 6 AND 24 MONTHS)	ABNORMAL AND COMPENSATORY PATTERNS
Suckling: The early infantile method of sucking that involves extension–retraction of the tongue, up-and-down jaw excursions, and loose approximations of the lips.	*Munching:* The earliest form of chewing that involves a flattening and spreading of the tongue combined with up-and-down jaw movement.	*Tongue thrust:* An abnormally forceful protrusion of the tongue from the mouth.
Sucking: Characterized by negative pressure in the oral cavity, rhythmic up-and-down jaw movements, tongue tip elevation, firm approximation of the lips, and minimal jaw excursions.	*Chewing:* Characterized by spreading and rolling movements of the tongue propelling food between the teeth, tongue lateralization, and rotary jaw movements.	*Tongue retraction:* A strong pulling back of the tongue to the pharyngeal space.
Rooting reaction: Head turning in response to tactile stimulation applied to the lips or around the mouth.	*Tongue lateralization:* Movement of the tongue to the sides of the mouth to propel food between the teeth for chewing.	*Jaw thrust:* An abnormally forceful and tense downward extension of the mandible.
Phasic bite reflex: A rhythmic bite and release pattern, seen as a series of small jaw openings and closings when the teeth or gums are stimulated.	*Rotary jaw movements:* The smooth interaction and integration of vertical, lateral, diagonal, and eventually circular movements of the jaw used in chewing.	*Lip retraction:* Drawing back of the lips so that they form a tight line over the mouth.
	Controlled, sustained bite: An easy, gradual closure of the teeth on the food, with an easy release of the food for chewing.	*Lip pursing:* A tight purse-string movement of the lips.
		Tonic bite reflex: An abnormally strong jaw closure when the teeth or gums are stimulated.
		Jaw clenching: An abnormally tight closure of the mouth.

Note. From "Feeding At-Risk Infants and Toddlers" by M. B. Jaffe. Reprinted from *Topics in Language Disorders,* Vol. 10, No. 1, p. 15. © 1989, Aspen Publishers, Inc. Reprinted with permission.

Early Comprehension of Routines and Sensemaking

Objective: The infant/toddler will interact in familiar routines of play and daily living, taking turns appropriately and anticipating next actions.

By the time normally developing children are 3 to 4 months old, they incorporate early communicative dialogues into familiar feeding routines and game routines, such as "peekaboo," "this little piggy," and "I'm gonna get you." These routines include all the aspects of conversational communicative events (although each exchange might not include all of the components). Because of their similarity to conversational interactions, Bateson (1975) called them **proto-conversations.** Wells (1986) noted that, "By six months, then, a baby and his or her chief caregivers have established the basis for communication: a relationship of mutual attention" (p. 34). Encouraging parents to engage in these play routines when their infants show appropriate levels of sensitivity can provide an important strategy for engaging hard-to-reach children and extending their attention in social contexts.

K. Nelson (1986) proposed that early routines like these contribute to the development of **event knowledge,** which she viewed as a central feature of early cognitive development. Nelson defined an event as a dynamic incorporation of objects and relations into a larger whole that occurs over time. This view of cognitive development as shifting representation of events in the world departs from predominant views of cognitive development as changes in general processes, such as seriation, classification, inference, or inductive reasoning. It also differs from Piagetian views of cognitive development as shifts in schemas in which young children are thought to be incapable of accurately representing changes in the state of objects (Piaget & Inhelder, 1971). Rather, K. Nelson (1986) stressed that

> *even very young children represent events as complex and dynamic, that is, as holistic structures involving internal change over time. Both of these characteristics—holistic structure and internal variation in structural relations over time—are important in considering the implications of the content and structure of children's event representations for theories of cognitive development. The representation of a holistic structure implies a strong proclivity for structural organization in the mind of the young child. (p. 3)*

It is because the "young child's cognitive processing is contextualized in terms of everyday experience" (K. Nelson, 1986, p. 4) that children can exhibit greater cognitive competence in everyday activities than in artificial cognitive tasks. Nelson also noted that, whereas older children and adults may learn about the world through books and other media, such indirect knowledge sources are unavailable to young children who do not yet have the language skills to take advantage of them. Rather, "what young children know comes primarily from the analysis of their own experience rather than from mediated sources" (p. 5).

This is not to suggest that experience comes to the child as "raw encounters with a neutral physical world. Rather, in some important sense, all knowledge of the world is social or cultural knowledge" (K. Nelson, 1986, p. 5). Social and cultural agents, such as parents and interventionists (for children with disabilities), set the context for children's learning and scaffold their understanding. That does not imply, however, that adult agents determine the child's experiences. Children's experiences are influenced by the developmental state of their cognitive systems and current knowledge.

The interplay between current knowledge and new experience is often the focus of early-stage intervention. Professionals strive to help parents achieve this transactional balance by using reciprocation, imitation, and scaffolding procedures to move children to higher, more interactive developmental levels. Platt and Coggins (1990) offered a developmental hierarchy checklist for several early social-action game routines: Bye-bye, So Big, Peek-a-boo, Patty Cake, and Give Kisses. They described three levels of behaviors, including neutral signs of interaction (e.g., laughing and smiling), signs of inattention (e.g., moving away, looking at unrelated object), and conventional participation behaviors (e.g., waving for Bye-bye, clapping hands for Patty Cake).

The Canadian Hanen Program provides a variety of services and publications (including some in Spanish and French) to support this process. *Learning Language and Loving It* (Weitzman, 1992) is aimed at early childhood educators, with liberal drawings and examples. For example, recommendations for participating in early social routines include (1) get the child's attention; (2) play the game a few times in an animated way; (3) pause at an appropriate point, such as after blowing "raspberries" on a baby's stomach, and wait expectantly, as if to say, "It's your turn!"; (4) treat any reaction, such as a wriggle, smile, kick, burp, sound, or stare as if the child has taken his turn; and (5) take his turn for him if he doesn't respond; then continue the game (p. 107). Two other books are aimed primarily at parents, including one version for parents with higher literacy skills, *It Takes Two to Talk* (Manolson, 1992), and a second for parents with lower literacy skills, *You Make the Difference* (Manolson, 1995). Both use the mnemonic device, the "3a WAY" for: **A**llow your child to lead, **A**dapt to share the moment, and **A**dd new experiences and words.

Reciprocation and Imitation

Objective 8: The infant/toddler will participate in meaningful routines with adult scaffolding (e.g., imitating vocalizations, facial expressions, or gestures such as "bye bye").

Reciprocation suggests a balanced interaction; both children and adults bring something to the process. Early turn-taking and feeding exchanges between adults and children help to establish this kind of reciprocation.

Reciprocal interactions also incorporate a powerful tool for learning more—**imitation.** If children can acquire what MacDonald (1989) called "the rule of natural social learning: 'Do as others do' " (p. 132), they have access to innumerable incidental learning opportunities.

Infants show signs of imitation soon after birth, much earlier than originally credited by Piagetian models. By around 5 months, rather deliberate imitations of movements and vocalizations are possible, with a peak in frequency of imitation of hand and nonspeech imitation by around 6 to 8 months (Owens, 1996).

Imitation is far more than reproduction of surface structure, Wells (1986) commented that, "Children are not learning to talk in order to be able to behave like their parents for the sake of conformity, but rather to be able to communicate with them in collaborative activities in which the roles played are *reciprocal* rather than imitative" (p. 42).

Although intervention to improve imitative ability is not without caveats, children who cannot imitate, or who do so poorly, seem to be at a disadvantage in all aspects of learning. Again, normal development can serve as an intervention model. In early stages of normal development, it is easier for children to imitate behaviors that integrate components already in their spontaneous repertoires. Thus, interventionists encourage adults to imitate

something the child already does. This technique is especially useful for children who show little interest in reciprocal turn-taking interactions (Bullowa, 1979; MacDonald, 1989; Siegel-Causey, Ernst, & Guess, 1987). Adult imitation of infant behaviors occurs naturally in normal interactions. P. H. Wolff (1963) observed that from about the sixth week of normal development, parents can engage in exchanges of between 10 and 15 vocalizations by imitating their baby's sounds. Adult imitation of children can also maintain infants' play and contribute to their normal emotional development (Brazelton, Koslowski, & Main, 1974; Greenspan, 1985).

Tiegerman (1989) reported a case study illustrating a procedure for encouraging children with autism to acquire imitation and turn-taking skills in the context of social interaction. A clinician sits across the table from the child with autism with a matching set of objects. As the child selects and manipulates the objects, the adult selects the matching objects and imitates the child's behavior. This approach establishes a contingency relationship in which adult imitations are a function of the child's object manipulation, the activities are child-initiated, and the child has opportunities to control another person's behavior. In Tiegerman's case study, the procedure increased both gaze behavior and object manipulation for a child with autism.

MacDonald (1989) took the imitation strategy one step further in his **matching** process, which is a central principle of the ECO model. MacDonald related matching to Bruner's (1983) **scaffolding,** in which adults fine tune their expectations to what the child can already do but also challenge the child slightly:

> *Matching is perhaps the most effective strategy you can use with your child, regardless of his level. By matching we mean acting and communicating with your child in a way that he can do. Consider again the image of a staircase with your skills at the top and your child's at the bottom. To show him the next step, you must get to his step or a little step above his. There you do something that he can do and that he shows some interest in. What then? Wait. Think of MATCH AND WAIT as one extremely effective, natural teaching package for helping your child do more, stay with you, and become more like the people around him. (p. 126)*

Many mothers of late-talking toddlers are reasonably good at matching. Rescorla and Fechnay (1996) studied mother-child synchrony and communicative reciprocity in late-talking toddlers between 24 and 31 months. Most mothers and late-talking toddlers were as synchronous as normal-talking mothers and toddlers with matched nonverbal and socioeconomic status. The late-talking toddlers simply produced more unintelligible and nonverbal utterances. A few mothers of late-talking toddlers were high in control and low in synchrony, however. Their children were lower in both compliance and synchrony.

INTENTIONALITY AND EARLY COMMUNICATIVE FUNCTIONS

Goal: The child will communicate intentions, both nonverbally and with words, so that others can understand them.

- Preverbal Comments and Requests
- Communicative Functions: Preverbal and First Words

Outcome: The child will communicate and interact meaningfully with family members and others in daily routines, showing interest, fun, and growth in the process.

Preverbal Comments and Requests

> *Objective 1:* The infant/toddler will use conventional gestures to make intentional comments (e.g., point, hold, show, look, and verbalize) and requests (e.g., reaching or pointing and fussing or vocalizing while looking at object and adult to convey requests) more frequently than during baseline observations.

Normally developing children are generally credited with true intentional communication when they enter the **illocutionary stage** at around 8 or 9 months of age (see Table 8.2). During the illocutionary stage, gestural and nonverbal communication signals become increasingly conventional and clear to varied communicative partners, but children do not yet use words to communicate their intentions. By around 12 to 14 months, children who are developing normally begin to encode their intentions with words and enter the **locutionary stage.**

Caregivers who interpret their children's actions as communicative even during the **perlocutionary stage** (preintentional) play a critical role in helping children move from the perlocutionary into the illocutionary (intentional) stage. Therefore, frequent targets of assessment and intervention for young children involve the

transactional relationship between caregivers' sensitivity and children's signal clarity. Direct intervention may be needed partially because some signals of intention are rendered less "readable" by children's impairments, such as cerebral palsy or autism (S. E. Morris, 1981). Over time, if caregivers do not recognize the communicative messages of these behaviors, the danger is that children will become increasingly passive and both partners will lose the sense of the child's potential for communicative control.

To prevent that problem, the specialist must carefully observe children's early forms of communication, perhaps using formal assessment procedures and adult-elicitation techniques (Linder, 1990; A. M. Wetherby & Prizant, 1990) as well as naturalistic contexts that are largely child initiated (Coggins, Olswang, & Guthrie, 1987; Lund & Duchan, 1993; Norris & Hoffman, 1990a, 1990b). Regardless of the assessment and intervention strategy, it is important to consider how contextual variables and the child's stage of development interact to influence children's expression of intentions.

Table 8.3 outlines a set of observational criteria for identifying communicative intent in children at preverbal levels of communication. Coggins and colleagues (1987) developed this particular summary to study the effect of context on children's communicative functions. They divided the intentions observed in early childhood into comments and requests. Comments are used by infants to direct adult attention. Requests are used by infants to direct adult behavior. Different contexts tend to elicit different intentions. **Structured tasks** work better to **elicit requests** from young children, and **unstructured observations** work better to **elicit comments.** Age is also a factor. Nine-month-olds encode few intentions of either type in the clinical setting. Halliday (1975) also reported that requests were rare in his son's early communicative attempts. Such results should lead clinicians to reconsider their usual tendencies to encourage "wants and needs" as first communicative intentions.

When Coggins and colleagues (1987) observed the same group of normally developing 9-month-olds until they were 24 months old, intentional requests began to show up, however, particularly in structured elicitation contexts. By 15 months, two thirds of the children produced requests in structured contexts with tangible rewards. In contrast, by 12 months, two thirds of the children used comments to establish joint reference and

TABLE 8.2   Stages of additive intentional and linguistic communicative development

APPROXIMATE AGE (MONTHS)	STAGE	CHARACTERISTICS
0–8	**Perlocutionary**	Communicative intention is inferred by the adult
	Proactive perlocutionary	Active environmental exploration Vocal and gestural signals not directed at others Anticipates no contingent social outcomes No evidence of linguistic comprehension
8–12	**Illocutionary**	Child communicates intentions
	Primitive illocutionary	Signals directed at others expecting specific outcomes Signals may be subtle and only interpreted by immediate caregivers Signals apparently goal directed, as indicated by persistence or frustration if goal not reached Early apparently linguistic comprehension, but only in highly context-bound routines
	Conventional illocutionary	Evidence of clear concept of communication Conventional use of gestures and vocalizations to achieve specific outcomes Prelinguistic signals interpreted by wider range of people Greater persistence if communicative goals not met More evidence of linguistic comprehension, particularly in context, but some multiword utterances and some object labels may be understood out of context
>12	**Locutionary**	Child communicates intentions using conventional linguistic forms
	Emerging locutionary	Linguistic forms (words or signs) beginning to be used consistently for communication Word use is decontextualized Forms are conventional and understood by many others Some forms may be idiosyncratic and understood only by those close to the child Nonverbal devices (gaze, vocalizations, and gestures) may remain major part of repertoire Increased comprehension of single and simple multiword utterances, both in and out of context
	Locutionary	Language is primary means of sending and receiving messages Language knowledge (both receptive and expressive) extends beyond early multiword utterances to include varied sentence types, grammatical morphemes, and some complex sentences Language is used to talk about things that are temporally and spatially removed from the current context Most language is understood, except for some abstract and nonliteral uses

Based on Bates, Camaioni, & Volterra, 1975; Prizant, 1984.

to direct their parents' attention to interesting sights and sounds. Not until 21 months, were elicitation tasks as effective in obtaining comments as were unstructured interactions.

Other studies have supported the importance of working directly on early requesting with children with developmental risks. Down syndrome children, who are slower at acquiring nonverbal requesting than other

TABLE 8.3   General and operational definitions for intentional preverbal comments and requests

I. *Comments.* Intentional behaviors that direct the listener's attention to an object or the movement of an object.
  A. Extends arm to adult to show an object already in hand; may vocalize or verbalize (i.e., produce a single-word or multiword utterance).
  B. Picks up an object and immediately shows it to an adult; may vocalize or verbalize.
  C. Points to, looks toward, or approaches an object; may vocalize or verbalize.
II. *Requests.* Intentional behaviors that direct the listener to act on some object in order to make it move or to retrieve an unobtainable object.
  A. Stretches hand toward an object; whines or fusses while leaning toward object; may vocalize or verbalize.
  B. Stretches hand toward an object with ritual gesture; may vocalize or verbalize.
  C. Looks at an object that has ceased moving or has the potential to move or be moved; reaches or leans toward object; may vocalize or verbalize.
  D. Looks toward an object that has ceased moving, has the potential to move or be moved, and makes a ritual gesture; may vocalize or verbalize.
  E. Looks at or touches an object; points to or reaches toward object and produces a single-word or multiword utterance.
  F. Looks toward an object that has ceased moving, has the potential to move or be moved; may point toward the object or adult; may give the object to an adult and produce a single-word or multiword utterance.

Note: From "Assessing Communicative Intents in Young Children: Low Structured or Observation Tasks?" by T. E. Coggins, L. B. Olswang, and J. Guthrie, 1987. *Journal of Speech and Hearing Disorders, 52,* p. 46. Copyright 1987 by American Speech-Language-Hearing Association. Reprinted by permission.

cognitive skills, also tend to be slower in acquiring expressive language (Mundy, Kasari, Sigman, & Ruskin, 1995). Toddlers (between 18 and 33 months of age) with specific expressive language delay (SLI-E) seem to produce later symbolic gestures like their age/comprehension matched peers, but are lacking in the production of earlier communicative gestures such as pointing and showing (Thal & Tobias, 1994). Thal and Tobias recommended gesture imitation tasks as a tool for both assessment and intervention.

Yoder, Warren, Kim, and Gazdag (1994) reported on direct intervention with four toddlers, ranging from 21 to 27 months of age, with developmental delays. They worked with the toddlers in 25-minute sessions, 4 days per week in a clinical setting. These authors differentiated preintentional from intentional requests (an important difference). Intentional requests include three elements: a look at the desired object, a look at the adult, and a discrete requesting or vocalizing behavior. If the child just looks at an object and vocalizes or reaches, or just looks at the adult and vocalizes, the signal is preintentional. An example of an intentional request is for a child to look back and forth at an adult and at a ball the adult is playing with and to reach toward the ball. Yoder and his colleagues used a **milieu teaching approach** to

provide contexts for direct prompting of prelinguistic commenting and requesting by arranging the environment, by following the child's attentional lead, and by engaging in social routines. Within routines, the adult would stop and ask, "What do you want?" or "Do you want this?" while holding the object needed for continuing the routine. If the child left out one of the three components, the adult would assist it (physically or by saying "Look at me") before responding by continuing the routine. Yoder and his colleagues wanted to see if mothers would become more interactive when their toddlers started using more intentional gestures, so they kept the mothers from observing the intervention sessions, but had them play with their toddlers in the same room after each session. As hoped, the mothers did use more **linguistic mapping** behaviors (e.g., naming "ball" when the child looked and pointed; or saying "bye-bye" as the child waved while leaving) as their children used more intentional gestures. In this study, a technique that started as **adult-initiated** in a therapy context transferred to increased **child-initiated** opportunities in more natural contexts.

Norris and Hoffman (1990a) studied the differential effects of more structured (adult-initiated) and less structured (child-initiated) sampling contexts for toddlers with severe multiple disabilities. The children, between the ages of 2:6 and 2:10 years, all functioned at prelinguistic levels. To measure results, Norris and Hoffman used their Infant Scale of Nonverbal Interactions (described in Chapter 7). They found that "children would exhibit a higher frequency of communicative vocalizations, limb movements, and body postures when their spontaneously occurring behaviors were treated as initiations than when attempts were made to elicit communicative behaviors" (p. 29). They also found that the child-initiated condition was associated with higher developmental levels than was the adult-initiated condition.

The results of these varied studies support the importance of context and the value of an eclectic model of language intervention. Children with varied problems at varied developmental stages benefit differently from similar treatment approaches.

Communicative Functions: Preverbal and First Words

Objective 2: The infant/toddler will express *non-verbally* (with gestures and vocalizations) most or all of the communicative functions: attention-seeking (to self and other), requesting (objects,

action, information), greeting, transferring, protesting/rejecting, responding, acknowledging, informing.

Objective 3: The infant/toddler will express (with a combination of gestures, vocalizations, and *words*) most or all of the communicative functions: naming, commenting, requesting objects (present, absent), requesting action, requesting information, responding, protesting/rejecting, attention-seeking, greeting.

The preceding discussion centered around two communicative functions, comments, and requests. Many other categories of communicative intentions have been proposed (e.g., Bates, Camaioni, & Volterra, 1975; Coggins & Carpenter, 1981; Dale, 1980; Dore, 1974; Greenfield & Smith, 1976; Halliday, 1975). Roth and Spekman (1984) compiled them into three sets of categories for children at (1) preverbal levels, (2) the single-word level, and (3) the multiword stage of language development. The first two developmental levels, which pertain to the early stage of language acquisition, are reprinted here (see Tables 8.4 and 8.5). The third level is shown in Chapter 10.

TABLE 8.4 Preverbal communicative intentions

INTENTION	DESCRIPTIVE EXAMPLE
1. Attention seeking	
a. to self	Child tugs on mother's jeans to secure attention.
b. to events, objects, or other people	Child points to airplane to draw mother's attention to it.
2. Requesting	
a. objects	Child points to toy animal that he wants.
b. action	Child hands book to adult to have read.
c. information	Child points to usual location of cookie jar (which is not there) and simultaneously secures eye contact with mother to determine its whereabouts.
3. Greetings	Child waves "hi" or "bye."
4. Transferring	Child gives mother the toy that he was playing with.
5. Protesting/Rejecting	Child cries when mother takes away toy.
	Child pushes away a dish of oatmeal.
6. Responding/Acknowledging	Child responds appropriately to simple directions/child smiles when parent initiates a favorite game.
7. Informing	Child points to wheel on his toy truck to show mother that it is broken.

Note: From "Assessing the Pragmatic Abilities of Children. Part I: Organizational Framework and Assessment Parameters" by F. Roth and N. Spekman, 1984. *Journal of Speech and Hearing Disorders, 49,* p. 4. Copyright 1984 by American Speech-Language-Hearing Association. Reprinted by permission.

TABLE 8.5 Communicative intentions expressed at the single-word level

INTENTION	DEFINITION	EXAMPLE
1. Naming	Common and proper nouns that label people, objects, events, and locations.	"Dog," "Party," "Table
2. Commenting	Words that describe physical attributes of objects, events, and people, including size, shape, and location; observable movements and actions of objects and people; and words that refer to attributes that are not immediately observable such as possession and usual location. These words are not contingent on prior utterances.	"Big," "Here," "Mine"
3. Requesting object		
a. present	Words that solicit an object that is present in the environment.	"Gimme," "Cookie" (accompanied by gesture and/or visual regard)
b. absent	Words that solicit an absent object.	"Ball" (child pulls mother to another room)
4. Requesting action	Words that solicit an action be initiated or continued.	"Up" (child wants to be picked up), "More"
5. Requesting information	Words that solicit information about an object, action, person, or location. Rising intonation is also included.	"Shoe?" (Meaning "Is this a shoe?") "Wadæt?" "What's that?")
6. Responding	Words that directly complement preceding utterances.	"Crayon" (in response to "What's that?"), "Yes" (in response to "Do you want to go outside?")
7. Protesting/Rejecting	Words that express objection to ongoing or impending action or event.	"No" (in response to being tickled), "Yuk" (child pushes away unwanted food)
8. Attention seeking	Words that solicit attention to the child or to aspects of the environment.	"Mommy!" "Watch!"
9. Greetings	Words that express salutations and other conversationalized rituals.	"Hi," "Bye," "Nite-nite"

Note: From "Assessing the Pragmatic Abilities of Children. Part I: Organizational Framework and Assessment Parameters" by F. Roth and N. Spekman, 1984, *Journal of Speech and Hearing Disorders, 49,* p. 4. Copyright 1984 by American Speech-Language-Hearing Association. Reprinted by permission.

Children who can express multiple communicative intentions are in a stronger position to continue their development than those who express a limited variety. Communicative intentions are valid targets of early intervention efforts in themselves, but they also offer contexts for encouraging the development of other forms and content. Requests for objects, actions, and information can provide both the motivation and the method for acquiring new vocabulary. Greetings and attention-seeking behaviors can keep children in social interaction contexts that are rich with language learning possibilities.

Three steps may be used to increase functionality of early communicative behaviors: (1) start by selecting forms that can be used frequently in contexts in which the child already participates; (2) encourage functionality by training gestural, vocal, and other forms (e.g., by using imitation and shaping techniques) during opportunities to display particular intentions (e.g., greeting, making choices, requesting); and (3) attend to the child's forms and respond to them functionally as if they were intended to be communicative (Kaiser, Alpert, & Warren, 1987).

EARLY WORDS

Goal: The child will express communicative meanings with one-word utterances and demonstrate linguistic comprehension at the word level.

- How Children Learn First Words
- Documenting Early Word Knowledge
- Producing Single-Word Utterances
- Addressing Problems with Early Word Acquisition

Outcome: The child will use words (or other symbols) to communicate and interact meaningfully with family members and others in daily routines, showing interest, fun, and growth.

The preceding discussion concentrated mainly on social interactions and communicative functions in the early stages of language acquisition, along with some early aspects of learning to vocalize and to control the oral-motor mechanism. The social aspects of communicative development are highly pragmatic. They focus on language use more than its content and forms. For children to move beyond prelinguistic communicative stages, they must begin to acquire linguistic content and forms. Around the age of one year, normally developing children begin to combine varied components of prelinguistic behaviors into the production of true spoken words.

Children need to hear words to learn them. But children need to do more than hear words to learn them. They need to hear words in meaningful contexts. I have a friend whose daughter was born with a profound severe hearing loss. My friend tells the story of how her daughter learned her first word. Having been told that hearing-impaired children needed to hear words hundreds of times before learning them, the family devised a plan to encourage learning of the word *ball*. They did this by hiding balls of various sizes and colors all around the house (including the refrigerator drawer). Then, they would feign surprise and make a production out of labeling the balls when any one of them was discovered. Although the child seemed to enjoy the fun, she did not learn the word. Instead, some weeks into the program, as the family pulled into the driveway in their car, my friend and her husband heard a small voice from the back seat say, "Home." Their daughter's first true word was heard, not in the contrived context of the teaching situation (even though it was spread throughout the day), but incidentally in the real-life meaningful event of "coming home."

How Children Learn Early Words

The preceding story illustrates several aspects to keep in mind when providing assistance to children learning early words. Again, information from normal development can be instructive.

K. Nelson (1985) proposed that learning to talk involves entering into a system of shared meanings. Children learn to use words that have the power to evoke in others a conceptual representation that, ideally, matches the one children intend to express. This ability does not emerge suddenly but develops through stages to which several interrelated components contribute: (1) the communicative context, (2) the current status of the child's cognitive system, and (3) cognitive, linguistic, and social developments that change the parameters of the overall system over time. Efforts to encourage the development of a child's semantic system when it does not proceed normally must recognize these three elements as well.

In the earliest stages of linguistic learning, context is particularly important. As K. Nelson (1985) explained it, early words are often inseparable from the contexts in which they appear; they are embedded in particular contexts and are only understood or used within those activities. For example, a child might crawl to the high chair when his mother says, "Do you want to eat?" It is not the words that the child understands so much as the activity, partially because, at this point in development, "the child's representational system is largely organized around events that are undifferentiated, unanalyzed schemas without separable elements of concepts" (p. 121). K. Nelson argued that children's first spoken words are also grounded in the actions of **familiar routines** and are thus "pure performatives." "Even when the parent and child are focused on an object, the protolanguage form seems to be *part* of the activity rather than *referring* to the object of the activity" (p. 121). At this transitional point, K. Nelson considered the child's use of words to be prelexical activity language and not yet representative of activities.

Bruner (1977) offered a similar explanation for the transition from prelinguistic to linguistic communication in the context of **joint action routines (JARs).** He emphasized the role of social interaction factors over cognitive ones, however. "Communication is converted into speech through a series of behavioral advances that are achieved in highly familiar, well learned contexts that have already undergone conventionalization at the hands of the infant and his mother (or other caretaker)" (p. 274).

Bruner (1975) also identified **joint reference** as a critical aspect of early word learning. It develops out of earlier stages when **joint attention** is established. In the earliest joint-attention exchanges, parents follow their infants' leads, using gaze cues such as the child's line of regard to identify objects of the child's attention. This way they may label, comment, or elaborate on those objects (see Box 8.3).

For infants at risk, intervention might encourage early communication along a similar sequence. Especially when motor problems preclude the production of clear gestural and vocal signals by children, parents need to learn to interpret their children's intentions through alternative indices. Parents also may be encouraged to stay with each stage for longer periods than expected in normal development. In addition, they may need to be more deliberate in labeling the objects of their children's attentions. Even in normal development, labeling and pointing can sustain infants' attention to objects and may help them map relationships between words and objects (Baldwin & Markman, 1989). Early word learning occurs best within meaningful contexts and familiar routines. Clinical consultants can help parents recognize these opportunities.

Documenting Early Word Knowledge

A baseline can be established for intervention by documenting word knowledge at the single-word stage of expressive language development. A. M. Wetherby and colleagues (1989) reported on language-sampling techniques appropriate for this stage that are similar to those used in the Communication and Symbolic Behavior Scales (CSBS; A. M. Wetherby & Prizant, 1990, described in Chapter 7).

Rescorla (1989) developed the Language Development Survey (LDS) as a screening tool to identify language delay in 2-year-old children. The survey, which can be completed by parents in about 10 minutes, is a vocabulary checklist that includes 242 words arranged in 17 semantic categories. Parents are asked to check off any words that their children say but are advised not to include any words that their children can understand but not say or say only in imitation. Rescorla found that the results of the LDS were highly correlated with the results of other commonly used language assessment tools and that it showed both good sensitivity and good speci-

Box 8.3

The Age-Stage Relationships in the Establishment of Joint Reference

- By 4 to 6 weeks, parents may bring objects in closer, shaking them, and saying "Oh look!"
- By 8 weeks, the infant can follow the parents' movements visually.
- By 3 months, the infant can distinguish utterances addressed to the infant and attend to them.
- By 4 months, the infant can follow the parents' line of regard, and soon, the infant's response quickens to the parents' directive, "Look!"
- By 6 months, the infant may respond to the parents' use of the object or event name and intonational pattern to establish joint reference.
- With the onset of intentional communication, the infant may assume a more direct role in establishing the topic by reaching for desired objects, but without looking at the caregiver to see if the message was received.
- By around 8 months, two reaches may be distinguished, a "reach-for-real" and "reach-for-signal," in which the infant shifts gaze from the object to the parent and back again.
- This is followed by gradual replacement of the full hand reaching grasp with a finger point, at which time, the communicative function of *comment* begins to be distinguishable from the communicative function of *request,* in that the child's point may be used to direct attention, and not just to request the object.
- At this point, parents begin to increase their labeling of objects identified by the child.
- When children begin to use true words themselves, the strategy shifts somewhat, and for a time, parents attempt to get their infants or toddlers to look, point, and verbalize within ongoing dialogues.
- As children's discourse skills advance, they assume more control of the dialogue, and parental questioning decreases.

(Based on Bruner, 1975, 1977; Owens, 1996)

ficity (low false-negative and false-positive rates). The screening criteria that proved appropriate for defining language delay were fewer than 50 words or no word combinations at 2 years of age. As described in Chapter 7, the MacArthur Communication Development Inventory (CDI; Fenson et al., 1993) is a similar parental checklist, asking for report of both receptive and expressive vocabulary, including gestures. It provides normative data and scores.

Early word comprehension can also be documented by sorting out linguistic comprehension from situational comprehension (Chapman, 1978). Unless the influence of

comprehension strategies is taken into account, clinicians may overestimate or underestimate a child's level of word comprehension (Edmonston & Thane, 1992). Children are particularly likely to use comprehension strategies in response to relational words. The outline in Box 8.4 summarizes recommendations by Edmonston and Thane for

---

Box 8.4

Nonlinguistic Strategies to Consider When Targeting Comprehension of Relational Words by Toddlers, with Assessment/Intervention Techniques
(Summarized from Edmonston & Thane, 1992; More in Chapter 10 for Preschoolers)

1. **Spatial terms** (*in, on, under, over, beside*)

   Probable location strategy (normal for toddlers). Put object where you expect to see it in real life (e.g., child will more likely put boat *under* the bridge than *on* it).

   To assess and instruct:

   - Use a story to make all choices equiprobable for acting out (e.g., doll goes *in* truck to load it, *under* the truck to check the tires, and *on* the truck to clean the window).

   - Use tasks so that each choice is consistent with real-world occurrences and relationships (e.g., "Put butterfly *over/under/beside* a picnic table").

   Preference for containers and surfaces strategy (normal for toddlers). If a container is available, put the object *in* it; if no container, put the object *on* a surface (this makes the child appear to understand *in* and *on*, but not *under*).

   To assess and instruct:

   - Make multiple containers available and require correct placements of *under, on,* and *in* using the same set of materials before crediting linguistic comprehension of *in* or *on* (I use a cigar box or paper bag, and small objects).

   Motor ease strategy (normal for toddlers). Do the easiest thing (e.g., pointing is easier than lifting a lid to put something *in* or wrapping it *in*).

   To assess and instruct:

   - Make all response choices equally easy to accomplish.

   Preferred location strategy (normal for toddlers). When hearing *here, there, this, that,* or *close, far,* always pick the object closest to self (child-centered strategy) OR speaker (speaker-centered strategy)

   OR designated reference point (e.g., "far from the doll" interpreted the same as "close to the doll").

   To assess and instruct:

   - Credit lexical comprehension only when child can demonstrate both ends of the contrast.

   Fronted (versus nonfronted) reference object strategy (normal for toddlers). When hearing *in front, behind, back, side, behind* or *beside,* look for the object to have a face or clear front (e.g., people, animals, cars) to aid comprehension (young children can show comprehension with fronted objects before they can with such nonfronted objects as *tree, table, trash can*).

   To assess and instruct:

   - Use nonfronted objects to test true comprehension of relational terms.

2. **Amount terms** (*more, less, long, short*)

   Preference for greater amount strategy (normal for toddlers to preschoolers).

   To assess and instruct:

   - Use antonym pairs and only credit comprehension when both ends are understood (e.g., only give credit for pointing to "*more* ladybugs" if the child also points to "*less* ladybugs").

3. **Dimensional adjectives** (*thin, short, low, thick, wide, tall, long*)

   Big, little synonym strategy (normal for toddlers to preschoolers). Treat words like *thin, short,* and *low* as *little;* and words like *tall, wide,* and *thick* as *big.*

   To assess and instruct:

   - Use test objects that differ in more than one dimension (e.g., ask for the *thick crayon, but make it shorter* than the *thin* one).

documenting early relational word comprehension. Similar contexts can be used for intervention.

Producing Single-Word Utterances

Objective 1: The child will use words representing a variety of content categories—nominals (general and specific), action words, modifiers (states, locatives, attributes), personal, social, and function words—to perform a variety of functions—naming; commenting; requesting objects, action, and information; responding; protesting/rejecting; attention-seeking; greeting.

An important issue for the specialist is selecting words to target early in the language process. Perhaps it is easier to select a lexicon for young children than for children at later stages of language development, but in either case, it is an ominous task when one considers the rapidity of word acquisition in normal development and the huge number of possible choices. Crais (1990) noted that children between 1.5 and 6 years of age add an estimated five word roots daily and that the comprehension vocabulary of the average 6-year-old is around 14,000 words.

How then should we select among all of the possibilities to find the best target words for children—in order, from easiest to more difficult to learn? The best answer to this troublesome question probably is *let the context and the child be your guide.* When identifying target words in early language intervention, MacDonald (1989) suggested to parents that they should select (1) words to code their child's knowledge, (2) words to code their child's communication, (3) words to code their child's interests, (4) words with high communicative utility, and (5) "language for communication, not for storage" (p. 198). To reinforce these ideas, MacDonald told parents that the words should come from the adults' matched words, the child's communications without words, the child's current knowledge, and the child's own interests.

The first words of normally developing children generally have two types of meaning: (1) **Referential** meanings with words that stand for things such as objects (*milk*), events (*up*), and conditions (*hot*). (2) **Functional** meanings with words that accomplish things such as drawing attention (*hi*) or rejecting undesirable actions (*no*). Intervention to assist children to acquire first

words may be most successful if these dual levels of content and function are kept active and relevant to the child's needs. Box 8.5 is a summary of a first lexicon for intervention suggested by Lahey and Bloom (1977). It is based on a normal developmental model of language content, form, and use.

When encouraging early word learning, it is also important to remember the "linguistic universal" (Ingram, 1974) that children generally comprehend words before they can produce them. Benedict (1979) confirmed this expectation when he analyzed the first words of eight normally developing children who comprehended 50 words before they produced 10. Box 8.6 is a list of word-types Huttenlocher (1974) identified as comprehended by the four 10- to 18-month-old children she studied. She also noted that the phonological complexity of words that children comprehended often exceeded the phonological complexity of words they produced. Recognition of this discrepancy may be useful in intervention.

When K. Nelson (1973) inventoried the first 50 words produced by children, she noted that the highest

Box 8.5

A First Lexicon: Suggested Content and Forms (in Parentheses) Based on Normal Development
(Adapted from Lahey & Bloom, 1977)

- Rejection (*no*)
- Nonexistence or disappearance (*no, all gone, away*)
- Cessation of action (*stop, no*)
- Prohibition of action (*no,* or content word with negative head shake)
- Recurrence of objects and actions on objects (*more, again, another*)
- Noting the existence of objects, people, or animals (*it, this, that, there*)
- Identifying objects, people, or animals (*Mama, Daddy, doggie, baby, sock*)
- Actions on objects (*give, do, make, get, throw, eat, wash, kiss*)
- Attributes or descriptions of objects (*big, hot, dirty, heavy*)
- Persons and pets associated with objects (as in possession) (relevant proper names)

Box 8.6 _____

Categories and Examples of Words Comprehended by Normally Developing Children between 10 and 18 Months
(Based on Huttenlocher, 1974)

- Name of a family member or pet (*Mommy, fish*)
- Label for a game or social ritual (*bye-bye, peek-a-boo*)
- Manipulable object/toy (*blanket, telephone, shoe*)
- Body parts (*hair, nose, belly button*)
- Food related (*cookie, bottle*)

proportion, 65%, was made up of names of either general or specific things. R. Schwartz and Leonard (1984) also found that the twelve toddlers they studied acquired object words and concepts more rapidly than action words and concepts. K. Nelson's (1973) findings for the expressive lexicons of the eighteen children she studied showed the following proportions of early words:

1. **General nominals,** including objects (*ball*) 31%; animals and people (*doggie, girl*) 10%; substances (*milk*) 7%; and letters and numbers (*e, two*) 2%
2. **Specific nominals,** including people (*Mommy*) 12%; animals (*Fluffy*) 1%; and objects (*car*) 1%
3. **Action words,** including demand–descriptive (*up, bye-bye*) 11%; and notice (*look, hi*) 2%
4. **Modifiers,** including states (*hot, dirty, all gone*) 6%; locatives (*there, outside*) 2%; attributes (*big, pretty*) 1%; and possessives (*mine*) 1%
5. **Personal–social,** including assertions (*no, yes, want*) 4%; and social-expressions (*please, ouch*) 4%
6. **Function words,** including questions (*what, where*) 2%; and miscellaneous (*is, to, for*) 2%.

When planning intervention (N. W. Nelson, 1988b), the specialist might use this information to set up events to encourage toddlers to interact in what Roger Brown (1958) called "The Original Word Game." This is the normal developmental interaction in which an adult "tutor" supplies the label for an entity, and the child "player" then forms hypotheses about the named entity. The player tests these hypotheses by applying the label to other entities that appear to be members of the same

conceptual set. The tutor then evaluates the accuracy of the fit and provides evaluative feedback.

Potential Problems with Early Word Acquisition

Even when developing normally, children may differ in the things they talk about and the classes of words they acquire most easily. K. Nelson (1973) described **referential children** as those who use substantive words primarily to talk *about things* and **expressive children** as those who use words and formulaic phrases primarily to *direct social interactions*. Horgan (1979) called such children **noun lovers** and **noun leavers** respectively.

> *Objective 2:* The child will show an appropriate balance of content words to refer to things and routinized words and phrases to interact socially.

When specialists identify individualized learning patterns, they may use them to select intervention content and contexts but view them as normal variations. On the other hand, when proportions are extremely out of balance—such as when a child seems to have no substantive words, except perhaps a few glued into stereotypic phrases—concern is appropriate. The specialist then should design some intervention strategies to help children learn the symbolic value of words (Prizant, 1983). A little later in development (during what I call the **middle stage**), children with specific language impairments may begin to use multiple-word phrases but continue the telegraphic pattern of producing mostly content words without morphological inflections or function words. A different kind of concern then is justified; intervention is needed to help children with these specific impairments learn to use grammatical markers in their language.

> *Objective 3:* The child will show appropriate flexibility in word learning by using new vocabulary strategies to replace baseline overextensions (e.g., calling a cow "moo" rather than "woof woof") or underextensions (e.g., using "cookie" to refer to all varieties; not just one).

Another area that is expected to vary normally, but may represent pathology in the extreme, is the difference in the size of receptive and expressive vocabularies. Both

overextensions (i.e., applying a word to a category larger than the conventional one, such as calling horses *doggie*) and **underextensions** (i.e., applying a word to a category smaller than the conventional one, such as calling only Oreos *cookie*) may occur in normal development either in comprehension or expression. These misapplications may be viewed as signs of developmental adjustments in semantic systems and not necessarily matters of concern, as long as they do not persist for extended periods of time or after new learning opportunities are presented.

Most young children can differentiate varied words in their receptive vocabularies (e.g., *motorcycle, bike, truck*) that they cannot yet use expressively (e.g., the same children who can point to pictures representing each kind of vehicle may call them all *car*). K. Nelson, Benedict, Gruendel, and Rescorla (1977) offered an explanation for this disparity, suggesting that early word-learning strategies differ during three different stages of early word development. (1) From 10 to 13 months, children seem to match adult words to preexisting concepts in comprehension. (2) From 11 to 15 months, they acquire a small number of words in production that are constrained in use only to a particular context or to the action-function component of the concept to which they are bonded. (3) From 16 to 20 months, they acquire new productive words for old concepts, form new concepts to match novel words, and begin to use words to categorize new instances. According to this view, comprehension and production involve different processes at different stages, and "errors," such as calling all vehicles *car,* may actually indicate more about a child's positive ability to draw inferences and to form categories than about limitations of expressive vocabulary.

Children with AAC Needs.   For children who are nonspeaking and whose communication boards can hold only so many symbols, the ability to overextend a limited set of expressive symbols may be critical to their ability to communicate. At the same time, their parents should be urged not to fall into the trap of limiting the vocabulary that such children hear. Parents may need to relate several different words for the child by pointing to the same symbol on the communication board. For example, parents may talk about *jets* and *helicopters* when the child notices them flying overhead, while pointing to the symbol for *airplane* on the child's board.

Children with Hearing Impairments.   Parents of children with hearing impairments face a slightly different dilemma. These parents must strike a careful balance between keeping vocabulary to a level that will permit recognition and comprehension without overly limiting lexical input and preventing the child from learning a rich vocabulary. As Ling (1976) noted, parents must present natural speaking models to their children without exaggerating critical features if they want their children to have more natural speech. On the other hand, because of their reduced sensory input, children with severe hearing losses may have difficulty abstracting enough phonological information to segment words along their boundaries and to recognize the same words in different contexts.

A variety of strategies has been suggested for helping children to compensate for this deficit. In addition to total communication (Ling, 1984b)—the simultaneous use of multiple modalities including sign language symbols to communicate meaning—tactile stimulation devices (Lynch, Eilers, Oller, & Cobo-Lewis, 1989) may be used to assist children to feel some characteristics of sound they cannot hear. Cued speech (Cornett, 1967, 1972) is another tool (proponents stress that it is not a method or a philosophy) that involves a set of four hand positions and eight hand shapes that can be used near the mouth to accompany spoken words and to supplement speech reading information already available to the "listener" (Ling & Clarke, 1975, 1976). However, the technique is not without controversy (Moores, 1969). In particular, Wilbur (1976) suggested that cued speech may be more appropriate for later stage speech instruction than for initial language learning.

Children with Autism.   Other children with central language processing problems, such as those with autism or with apparent word-retrieval deficits, may need specific attention to prevent their semantic systems from getting stuck in inflexible or weak processing patterns. Particularly, children with autism are likely to develop semantic underextension, insisting on using certain words to refer only to specific exemplars of a concept rather than to all exemplars.

Underextensions and overextensions that occur in autism also seem to arise out of cognitive and linguistic difficulties that these children have in isolating the set of features characterizing referents for one word and separating that semantic concept from others. "To produce a word in a variety of contexts, the child must first separate the word from the context to which it was first attached. Once this major feat is accomplished, the child can use the word as a symbol for, rather than a feature of, its referent" (Pease, Gleason, & Pan, 1989, p. 114).

I once worked with a 6-year-old boy with autism who had learned to use the word *in* to refer either to containment ("in") or support ("on") relationships with a particular kind of container and used *on* to refer either to containment or support relationships with a different kind of container. The critical feature that he had apparently abstracted for using *in* and *on* was nonconventional. He focused on the type of container rather than on the discriminating feature of containment or support as the key to the meanings of those two words. He needed many examples of *in* and *on* with the same container (a clear plastic box), as described in Box 8.4, over many sessions before he could abstract the critical semantic features of containment and support and could separate them from association with the physical characteristics of particular containers (N. W. Nelson, 1988b).

ENCODING SEMANTIC RELATIONS AND COMBINING TWO WORDS TO DO MORE

Goal: The student will use two-word utterances to communicate sentence-like meanings for a variety of functions.

- Specialized Assessment Techniques for Early Multiword Utterances
- Producing Two-Word Utterances

Outcome: The child will participate in varied communicative interactions, producing and responding to a variety of multiword utterances.

First words are acquired in normal development as children become increasingly interested in what things are called and in the functional uses of words to communicate. At around 18 months, when single-word lexicons include a small core of words, normally developing children begin to combine words to communicate more elaborate meanings. However, children continue to mix two-word constructions with many single-word utter-

ances throughout the latter half of the second year (Owens, 1996). During R. A. Brown's (1973) first stage of language development, as MLU grows from 1.0 to 2.0, most of children's utterances are two words long, although a few may be as long as three or even four words.

Before the appearance of the first true two-word combinations, several transition behaviors may appear. These include combinations of nonmeaningful "empty" CV and CVCV combinations with meaningful words (e.g., *ma baby, beda baby*); reduplication of single-word utterances (e.g., *doggie doggie*); and production of successive one-word utterances made up of two words, both produced with falling intonation (e.g., *mommy, laugh*) (Owens, 1996). Children may also appear to use generative rules to construct two-word utterances by imitating formulaic or gestalt units before they actually do so. Common examples are *all gone, go bye, so big, go potty* (Owens, 1996, p. 260).

Documenting Early Multiword Utterances

Language comprehension continues to develop while children move toward producing two-word combinations. One procedure for documenting comprehension of two-term semantic relations (Miller, Chapman, Bronson, & Reichler, 1980) involves using sets of objects to represent **action, location, possession,** and **attribution.** First, the examiner teaches the child (to 80% criterion) to show, demonstrate, look toward an object, or perform an action following the examiner's request. Then the examiner presents the child with four examples of each of the relational categories. For example, the action category might be tested with the four exemplars *throw block, open door, baby drink,* and *boy ride.* Results are expressed as the proportion of times comprehension (or production) is demonstrated out of four trials for each semantic category.

When children reach the stage of being able to scan pictures that represent various word combinations and to point (or to eye-point) to those being named, specialists may use more formal procedures to assess early-stage comprehension of semantic–grammatical relationships. The Assessment of Children's Language Comprehension (Foster, Giddan, & Stark, 1973) presents sets of pictures representing single words that children select to demonstrate a basic one-word vocabulary level. Then the examiner asks the child to point to appropriate pictures (from contrasting foils) in other sets that represent two-word (e.g., *broken cup*), three-word (e.g., *cat under table*), and four-word (e.g., *happy little girl jumping*) combinations.

Special analytical techniques have also been recommended to assess whether children really are demonstrating creative, rule-based strategies in their production of two-word utterances (rather than just repeating language they have heard as unanalyzed chunks). Leonard, Steckol, and Panther (1983) suggested that two approaches could be used for this purpose. Using the **interpretive approach,** the specialist collects many spontaneous utterances over several sessions and then judges utterances as rule-based if they meet these criteria: (1) a high degree of positional consistency of elements and (2) some degree of creativity in word combinations. For example, the utterance, *hug mommy,* would qualify as being based on the semantic–grammatic rule **action + object** if *hug* and *mommy* both appeared also individually or combined with some other word and if other word combinations also representing **action + object** relations appeared. Using the second method, the **relevant component approach,** the specialist constructs specific probes, attempting to elicit a wide variety and range of possible semantic segmentations, in which the child combines the same words in various ways (e.g., *Doggie bone, Doggie bite, Big Doggie, Doggie bye bye*).

Stockman and Vaughn-Cooke (1986) presented data supporting the use of early spontaneous language sampling with young children in working-class families who speak nonstandard dialects of English. They recommended gathering at least 50 to 100 utterances in natural interactions using a variety of stimulus materials, then assigning the utterances to semantic categories to compare with developmental data. Stockman and Vaughn-Cooke recommended that by 30 months of age, working-class nonstandard speakers should "(a) use mainly two-word combinations, and (b) encode the following types of semantic categories: *existence, action, locative action, state, locative state, negation, possession, attribution, notice, intention, and recurrence*" (p. 23).

Stockman (1996) updated this research and offered a set of Minimal Competency Core criteria for African American children based an analysis of features that distinguished language samples of seven children between ages 33 and 36 months who were developing normally from the language produced by a child with language development difficulties. The language samples were gathered while the children played with a race car set or looked at books they had chosen. The full set of Minimal Competency Criteria are discussed in Chapter 9 regarding analysis of the language samples of middle-stage children. The data on semantic roles are summarized here because they make appropriate targets for early-stage children who are learning to encode early developing meanings. The categories "used by every child included a common core consisting of five major verb categories (*existence, state, locative state, action,* and *locative action*) and four minor or coordinated categories (*specification, possession, time,* and *negation*)" (pp. 360–361).

Producing Two-Word Utterances

Objective 1: The child will combine two words to represent a variety of semantic–grammatic relations, including most of the following: agent + action, action + object, agent + object, entity + attribute, possessor + possession, recurrence, nonexistence, disappearance, demonstrative + entity, entity + locative, action + locative.

A matrix training approach has been suggested for helping children with disabilities acquire early two-word combinations (e.g., Bunce, Ruder, & Ruder, 1985; Stremel-Campbell & Campbell, 1985; B. Wetherby & Striefel, 1978). A matrix provides a system for pairing a variety of content words representing a targeted semantic role with another set of content words representing a related semantic role. The instructor combines a limited set of words in one semantic category with another set in a related semantic category to help children maximize their abilities to recombine lexical items in unique and generative ways. Figure 8.1 shows a set of stimuli for an agent–action matrix suggested by H. Goldstein (1985). Other matrices have been designed to teach productive action–object sequences (Stremel-Campbell & Campbell, 1985) and the comprehension of preposition–object phrases (Bunce et al., 1985).

Early semantic relations appear to be universal from culture to culture. L. Bloom's (1970) observations of se-

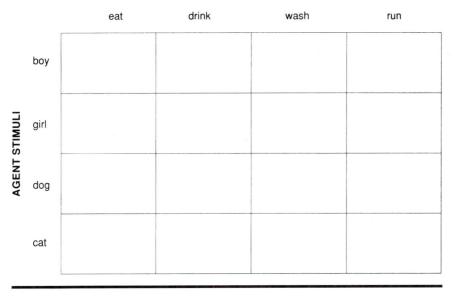

FIGURE 8.1   An example of stimuli for an agent–action language matrix.

Note: From "Enhancing Language Generalization Using Matrix and Stimulus Equivalence Training" by H. Goldstein in *Teaching Functional Language* (p. 228) edited by S. F. Warren and A. K. Rogers-Warren, 1985. Austin, TX: Pro-Ed. Copyright 1985 by Pro-Ed. Reprinted by permission.

mantic relations observed among the productions of three American children were similar to those that Roger Brown (1973) reported among children learning Finnish, Swedish, Samoan, French, Russian, Korean, Japanese, and Hebrew. Stockman and Vaughn-Cooke (1986) also described similar semantic category acquisitions for African American children in working-class families.

Brown (1973) suggested that this commonality in early semantic rules appears among toddlers worldwide because all toddlers appear to be preoccupied with objects, people, and actions at about the time they begin to combine words. Brown noted that these are the concepts that children have been developing during the immediately preceding Piagetian stages of sensorimotor development. When children talk about objects, they point out things (demonstrative) and name them (nominative), talk about where objects are (location), where they are not (nonexistence), what they are like (attributive), that they have disappeared (disappearance), who owns them (possession), who is acting on them (agent–object), and

having more of them (recurrence). In talking about actions, children comment on the actions that people perform (agent–action), actions performed on objects (action–object), and actions oriented toward certain locations (action–location). Table 8.6 includes listings of the two-word semantic rules identified by R. A. Brown (1973) and L. Bloom (1970, 1973) as most common. Intervention involves setting up contexts as opportunities to talk about such things.

Olswang and Carpenter (1982a, 1982b) studied how young children acquire the concept of *agent*. They observed three children in their homes once per month from age 11 months to 22 months and described a five-level developmental sequence. The first three levels are antecedents of the mature cognitive notion of agent: (1) in single-recipient acts, toddlers might act on an object *or* a person (e.g., when a wind-up toy runs down) but will not directly signal the adult (a potential agent) to help with object; (2) in nondirective multiple-recipient acts, toddlers might act on both objects and people in

TABLE 8.6   Commonly observed early two-word semantic–grammatic rules with examples

R. A. BROWN (1973)	L. BLOOM (1970, 1973)	EXAMPLES
Agent + action	Agent + action	Mommy come; Doggy sit
Action + object	Action + object	Drive car; Eat cereal
Agent + object	Agent + object	Daddy sock; Baby book
Entity + attribute	Attributive	Crayon dirty; Big doggy
Possessor + possession	Genitive	My bead; Mommy dress
Recurrence	Recurrence	More cookie
Nonexistence	Nonexistence	Allgone milk
Disappearance	Disappearance	Bye-bye car
	Rejection (of proposal)	No eat
	Denial (of statement)	No wet
Demonstrative + entity	Demonstrative + predicate nominative	There potty
Entity + locative	Noun + locative	Mommy stair
Agent + locative	Verb + locative	Go pool; Sit chair
	Noticing + locative	Me here

turn but do not direct the adult's attention to the need to fix the toy; (3) in directive multiple-recipient acts, toddlers begin to direct the adult's attention to the toy but do not yet use the adult in unique ways, only in familiar helping roles. Olswang and Carpenter describe the last two levels as representing a mature cognitive notion of agent; (4) in new adult recipient acts, toddlers request help efficiently and effectively from adults for agent roles that they have not previously seen the adults perform; and (5) in unobserved-adult recipient acts, they seem to realize that an adult agent must have been needed to activate a new toy that runs down even if the adult was not there when the original activation occurred. When the mature cognitive notion of agent did emerge, the children began to code the agent in agent–action–recipient events using single-word utterances. Before the age of 22 months, two of the normally developing children also began to use two-word utterances to code two of the elements in agent–action–recipient events.

The clinical implications of this research (Olswang & Carpenter, 1982a, 1982b) are that efforts to teach children to use words to encode semantic relationships can benefit from experiences designed to teach the concepts along with the words. Dynamic assessment techniques (Bain & Olswang, 1995) may also identify when children are especially open to learning two-word utterances and may help to jumpstart the process.

Clinical procedures for teaching two-word semantic relations have been described for young children with specific expressive language impairment (SLI-E; Bain & Olswang, 1995), autism (Scherer & Olswang, 1989), borderline to moderate retardation (S. F. Warren & Bambara, 1989), and hearing impairments (Schirmer, 1989). In all cases, the scaffolding behaviors of adults, including imitations, acknowledgements, modeling, and expansions, have seemed to play an important role in helping the children move forward in their word-combination production attempts.

Children with Specific Expressive Language Impairment (SLI-E). Bain and Olswang (1995) used dynamic assessment techniques to measure the readiness of 15 children (ages ranging from 30 to 36 months) to produce two-word utterances within their zones of proximal development (ZPD) (see Chapter 6). They set up a cuing (or scaffolding) hierarchy and examined the toddlers' responses to different levels of cues, from less supportive to more supportive: (1) general statement (GS) ("Oh, look at this"); (2) elicitation question (EQ) ("What's happening?"); (3) cloze or sentence completion (CLO) ("Look, the dog is sitting and ___," while making the toy dog walk); (4) indirect model (IM) ("See, the dog is walking; what is he doing?"); (5) direct model—evoking spontaneous imitation (DM-S) (spontaneous imitation to a direct model without an elicitation cue (Adult: "Dog walk"; Toddler: "Dog walk"); (6) direct model—plus elicitation statement (DM-E) (Adult: "Tell me 'Dog walk' "; Toddler: "Dog walk"). At baseline, many toddlers needed the more supportive cues to produce two-word utterances correctly. After a 9-week period, those who responded to the less-supportive early cuing strategies demonstrated greater language change. Bain and Olswang also found that children who could produce two-word utterances produced a greater variety in free-play language sampling than in the more highly constrained dynamic assessment activities.

Children with Autism.   In a study of children with autism, Scherer and Olswang (1989) allowed children to select objects for the intervention sessions from several boxes to provide the content for the constructions. The authors credited modeling and expansion procedures as being particularly instrumental, first in increasing spontaneous imitations of two-word utterances and, later, in increasing spontaneous productions of two-term utterances (with corresponding decreases in imitations).

Children with Mental Retardation.   S. F. Warren and Bambara (1989) embedded their training sessions with mentally retarded children in a **milieu approach.** They selected toys for each session according to a central play theme and used teaching techniques combined from the mand-model and incidental teaching procedures (described previously in this chapter). Warren and Bambara also noted differences in the relative skills with which the different teachers of their three subjects engaged the children in conversations with opportunities to learn the new structures. One teacher (whose student showed the greatest improvement and generalization, even though she was the most developmentally delayed and had the fewest sessions) was particularly good at using scaffolding utterances to assist children to climb to the next step. She presented models for the child to imitate but within a natural turn-taking exchange. The teacher might say, "I'm pushing the car," and push the car toward the girl, who would then push the car back and say "push car" with appropriate intonation and apparent pragmatic intent (see also Box 3.9 in Chapter 3).

Children with Hearing Impairment.   Schirmer (1989) also emphasized the importance of adult communicative partners who could provide appropriate interaction strategies and support with young hearing-impaired children. She noted that "Hearing-impaired children need the opportunity to interact linguistically in an environment structured to maximize appropriate-level language input and the freedom to take risks in experimenting with new language meanings, forms, and uses" (p. 87). Schirmer's recommendations extended across R. A. Brown's (1973) five linguistic stages and did not relate only to the period of two-word utterances. In assisting children to move from one level to the next, she noted the importance of matching children's current linguistic levels and stretching them slightly through modeling and expansion.

PARENTAL ROLES IN HELPING CHILDREN GO BEYOND THE HERE-AND-NOW

Goal: The child will talk about events of the past and things that are not present in the immediate context.

> *Objective 1:* The child will talk about remote events, people, and things in facilitative conversations with caregivers.

Outcome: The child will participate in conversations that include content relating to "there-and-then" events, people, and things.

At around 20 to 24 months of age, normally developing children begin to talk about objects and events from the past or in the future (Lucariello, 1990). This freeing of talk from the here-and-now is called **temporally displaced** talk. Its appearance is associated with the development of increasingly mature event knowledge, but its emergence is facilitated through scaffolding by parents.

Event knowledge (as discussed earlier in this chapter) includes concepts about frequently experienced sequences of actions, goals organizing the actions, and the actors, roles, and props associated with them. When Lucariello (1990) observed children aged 2:0 to 2:5 in varied contexts with their mothers, temporally displaced talk occurred far more frequently in highly scripted contexts about aspects of the child's routines than in nonscripted contexts. Scripted contexts included routines for getting dressed in the morning, having lunch, and bathing and getting ready for bed. Nonscripted contexts included free play and interactions with novel toys.

The second key to children's transitions from talk only about the here-and-now to talk about there-and-then is the scaffolding that parents provide to make temporally remote (but familiar) topics accessible to their children (Lucariello, 1990). One kind of scaffolding is illustrated in the following exchange:

M: You did get a boo-boo.
   Look at that foot.
   How'd you do that?
C: Door.
M: On the door?
C: Yeah. (Lucariello, 1990, p. 20)

It is important to note that most parental scaffolding attempts in normal development aim to help children *make sense* using language (either receptively or expressively) not to *elicit or teach* particular vocabulary items or grammatical structures. Although many middle-class parents conduct fairly direct vocabulary teaching toward the end of their child's second year, those efforts tend to be concentrated into a fairly short period of helping children learn the principle that everything has a name (Wells, 1986). As Gordon Wells noted, "Thereafter, only a minority of parents continue to teach vocabulary, and even then, this tends to be limited to common nouns and adjectives; verbs, adverbs, and other parts of speech are hardly ever explicitly taught at all" (p. 41). Furthermore, little evidence indicates that any parents engage directly in instruction of grammar. Yet children with normal developmental abilities continue to learn. Apparently, shared experiences, parental ability to mediate more difficult meanings, and positive social interaction elements all work together with increases in event knowledge to enable the cognitive and linguistic shift beyond the here-and-now.

For toddler-age children with disabilities, an important target of the intervention process may be assessment and enhancement of the facilitative characteristics of parental communicative interactions in naturally occurring contexts. Such efforts may need to occur in concert with efforts to change any maladaptive patterns that might have developed and to prevent development of any new maladaptive patterns.

Cross (1984) reviewed the literature on parent–child interaction in which interaction patterns of parents and their children with language impairments were compared with those of parents and their normally developing children. She noted many methodological problems with the studies but also summarized results that were fairly consistent across the studies in several areas. In the area of **discourse contingencies,** parents of children with language impairments (1) are less likely to use semantically or referentially contingent utterances; (2) are less likely to provide positive, accepting acknowledgments of their children's utterances; and (3) are more likely to produce exact repetitions of their own utterances. In the area of **sentence types** and associated functions, parents of children with language impairments (1) are more likely to use imperatives to control their children's verbal and nonverbal behaviors (a finding that correlates negatively with children's gains in syntactic development); (2) are more likely to use *wh-* questions, but less likely to use *yes–no* questions (parental recasts of children's utterances into *yes–no* questions have a high positive correlation with children's elaboration of the auxiliary verb system in normal development); and (3) are less likely to use declarative syntactic forms for the functions of commenting and stating. In the area of **input parameters,** parents of children with language impairments (1) are less likely to be verbally assertive and/or responsive with their children (although results in this area are mixed); (2) are more likely to use less complex speech (perhaps the reduction in complexity acts as an appropriate adjustment to children's communicative problems, but parents may need assistance to keep their input complexity low enough to facilitate their children's comprehension while high enough to encourage new language learning); (3) are more likely to speak rapidly to their children (although less evidence is available in this area, it may be appropriate to encourage parents to slow down); and (4) are more likely to be disfluent and unintelligible.

The irony of helping parents to appreciate the importance of their roles as primary language intervention agents with their young children at risk is that it may be counterproductive for them to feel this responsibility too keenly, because it may lead them to become tense and anxious about their language-teaching roles and to convey that anxiety to their children. This was one of the concerns expressed by S. J. White and White (1984) about interaction patterns of parents of children with hearing impairments. They cautioned that intervention efforts should aim not so much to encourage parents to bombard their children with talk, as to *interact with their children* in language. Van Kleeck (1994b) also cautioned against the cultural bias that can be involved with training parents as conversational partners with their children.

Although it is difficult to untangle patterns of cause and effect, a number of more recent studies continue to raise concern about parent–child interactions when children have language impairments. Donahue and Pearl (1995) studied mother–child interactions in a snack selection task and found that mothers of 4:5-year-old children who were born preterm were more likely to approach the task as a vocabulary lesson. These mothers produced less complex sentences and were more likely to name the snacks and test their children's knowledge than comparison mothers. Girolametto and Tannock (1994) found that the stress of parenting children with disabilities affects both mothers (more) and fathers (less) and influences their communicative interactions with their children. Fathers of young children who were developmentally less mature used greater turn taking and topic control; mothers used greater topic control for children who were less involved.

Conti-Ramsden, Hutcheson, and Grove (1995) compared mothers and fathers interacting with their children with specific language impairments (SLI) and then with their own younger normally developing children. Thus, these parents acted as their own controls. Fathers requested clarifications of their SLI children's utterances almost twice as often as mothers. Both mothers and fathers used fewer complex contingency recasts with their children with SLIs. SLI children were involved in simple, short sequence recast exchanges, such as:

FATHER: What are you making?
CHILD: Ship
FATHER: A big ship (p. 1299)

Younger typically developing siblings were involved in longer "looped" exchanges:

CHILD: Peeping
MOTHER: He is peeping
CHILD: He is peeping

MOTHER: Yeah, look! He is peeping
CHILD: Alex look
MOTHER: Alex, look he is peeping Yeah, look he is peeping

In intervention, Cross (1984) recommended that practitioners employ procedures to

(a) enhance the semantic contingency of parents' language on child's language; (b) reduce parents' directiveness; (c) increase their fluency, intelligibility, and tendency to question; and (d) generally encourage the parents of children with language impairments to talk with them more frequently than they do. (p. 12)

One intervention study (Tiegerman & Siperstein, 1984) aimed to modify parental styles of interaction by four mothers with their language-impaired children. The children ranged in age from 3 to 5 years, and had MLUs ranging from 1.0 to 2.0. None of the children had concomitant hearing, visual, or neurological problems. The procedure consisted of a series of pretraining videotapes and 6 weeks of group and individualized weekly training sessions in which parents were taught to become more child centered in their interactions and to focus on different aspects of semantic relatedness. They were also given "homework" assignments each week (e.g., transcribe a 5-minute sample of a father–child play session and identify features they had discussed). The results showed an increase in semantically related utterances and an expansion of communicative roles and behaviors used by the mothers, with more opportunities being given to their children to talk and to receive positive acknowledgments for that talk.

Children with Hearing Impairment

Specialized concerns arise when assisting parents of children with hearing impairments to enhance their simultaneous signed and spoken communication with their children (Moeller, 1989). Hearing parents of young children with profound hearing losses may be attempting to learn a new communication mode while they strive to provide facilitative linguistic input and to cope with all of the other stresses of having a child with a disability. Intervention, therefore, should help parents combine the trilogy of signing skills, parenting skills, and language stimulation skills. For example, they can learn signs that are helpful in managing their children's behavior.

EARLY LEARNING ABOUT LITERACY

Goal: The child will demonstrate concepts of emergent literacy while interacting with a variety of print sources.

- Interacting with Books
- Interacting with Other Print
- Emerging Awareness of Words and Sounds

Outcome: The child will show interest in learning to read and write, awareness of print and how words sound, and will be "ready" to learn to read when entering school.

Relatively direct but naturalistic teaching continues into the toddler and preschool years in homes where literacy is valued and books are available in the context of joint book reading activities (Heath, 1982; McGee & Richgels, 1990; Ninio, 1983; van Kleeck, 1990). These reading activities are useful not only for teaching new vocabulary but also for providing the context for conveying, either implicitly or explicitly, a variety of special rules for interacting with print.

Interacting with Books

Objective 1: The child will interact with books by holding a book upright, turning pages systematically, pointing differently to pictures and "words," listening and commenting while a story is read.

Snow and Ninio (1986) gathered transcripts of parents interacting with their young children using books. They found evidence that parents use direct and indirect instruction to help children learn that (1) books are for reading, not manipulating; (2) books control the topic in book reading; (3) pictures are not things but represent things; (4) pictures are for naming (especially at the single and two-word utterance stage); (5) pictures can represent events even though they are static; (6) book events occur outside of real time; and (7) books represent an autonomous fictional world.

Early book experiences offer a rich context for intervention in parent–child interactions (even children functioning at the 1- or 2-year-old level). By interviewing parents about this type of activity, professionals may be able to encourage more of it. Simply suggesting more book reading is not enough, however. Particularly when children have language delays and related disabilities, parents may have become discouraged about their initial attempts to "read" books with their children. Parents may need to be shown techniques to pace the page turning, to establish joint attention and referencing (e.g., pointing and commenting on the pictures), and to take turns in a naming game before asking many questions or trying to read the words printed on the pages. Remember that cultural differences may influence the strategies parents use. Anderson-Yockel and Haynes (1994) found that African American mothers used significantly fewer questioning behaviors than white mothers when interacting with their toddlers with books. African American children produced more spontaneous verbalizations. White children produced more question-related communications.

Remember also, that parents of children with disabilities may lead lives packed full of special meetings and appointments that make it difficult to spend time reading books with their children. Perhaps the best way to ensure that parents do find the time is to collaborate with parents to find literacy activities that will fit in with other activities (e.g., waiting in the physician's office) or as part of daily living (e.g., writing grocery lists, reading signs, taping notes to the refrigerator).

Interacting with Other Print

Objective 2: The child will interact with forms of nonbook print by scribbling lists, pretending to read forms and labels, recognizing highly familiar print symbols (e.g., Coca Cola, McDonalds).

Most of this discussion of parental roles in early language and literacy learning has focused on generalized expectations about middle-class mainstream families (regardless of ethnicity). Focus on book reading may be primarily a middle- and upper-class phenomenon, but books are not the only way that children are introduced to print early in life (McGee & Richgels, 1990; D. Taylor, 1983; D. Taylor & Dorsey-Gaines, 1987). Van Kleeck (1990) reviewed ethnographic studies with families in diverse geographic, cultural, ethnic, and socioeconomic situations. These studies "have found literacy artifacts and print-related events to be pervasive in all kinds of homes in literate societies" (p. 27). However, most print-related events in low-income families occur through activities of daily living, and not through books (D. Taylor & Dorsey-Gaines, 1987). Perhaps, intervention embedded in those naturally occurring practical activities is the best way to encourage early print experiences for young children with special needs in these homes.

When intervention teams work with families from cultures different from their own, the need for ethnographic sensitivity to different interaction styles and values also must be a part of the system. Prescriptive approaches that emphasize the "right" way to do things, only from the perspective of the professional, are doomed to failure. If parents and professionals work together to establish mutual goals and to develop interaction patterns that facilitate the child's development and are consistent with the family system, children may be able to consolidate gains in language and literacy and to continue to make new ones. Parents may also find that they like to learn new ways of interacting with their children if they can do so in a supportive and nonjudgmental context.

Emerging Awareness of Words and Sounds

Objective 3: The child will interact to show phonological awareness by responding to rhymes, songs, and spontaneous word play (e.g., making up lists like *car, mar, star*).

Infants and toddlers with communicative risks may seem too young for phonological awareness goals, but adults in their environment can provide low-key models for playing with words and sounds and can scaffold awareness in dynamic assessment tasks. Van Kleeck (1990) reviewed studies showing a developmental hierarchy for segmenting sentences into words, words into syllables, and words into phonemes. Abilities emerge as early as 3 years, or even earlier, for some children. Identifying words with the same **onset** (e.g., *play, plug*) or **rime** (e.g., *big, pig*) also emerges before most children can segment words into phonemes (Bird, Bishop, & Freeman, 1995). Having fun with the sounds of language in nursery rhymes before asking children to engage in metalinguistic assessment tasks may set the stage for literacy. Van Kleeck reminded us of the spontaneous crib soliloquies Ruth Weir (1962) provided from recordings of her son, Anthony:

Bink
Let Bobo bink
Bink ben bink
Blue kink (p. 105)

BUILDING MORE COMPLEX IDEAS THROUGH PLAY

Goal: The child will demonstrate complex understandings, symbolic thinking and pretending, and social skills through play.

- Assessing Play Skills
- Documenting Early Play Skills
- Decentering, Object Symbolism, and Social Relations in Play

Outcome: The child will fit well in play groups with peers, playing at their level, and sometimes leading the play.

Parental input and parent–child interactions contribute to the quality of children's early language and learning experiences, but they are not the only factors. The children themselves supply other factors. These relate to children's abilities to use their own current cognitive and linguistic abilities to help pull themselves up to the next step in the developmental process. (Recall the linguistic theory of "bootstrapping" from Chapter 3.) Continued advances in children's abilities to represent events and meanings symbolically are demonstrated in increasingly sophisticated play. Current understanding of the relationships of language and play do not permit a strong conclusion that play is a prerequisite of language (or vice versa), but the two abilities do seem to develop hand in hand.

Several theoretical explanations have been offered for relationships between language and play. Both Piaget (1962) and Vygotsky (1967) linked the emergence of symbolic play to the development of representational skills. The ability to represent one thing with another (e.g., pretending that beads are food) provides evidence that a child can function symbolically. Bates and colleagues (1979) found a correlation among symbolic play, vocal imitation, and language production in normally developing children. Casby and Ruder (1983) found a strong correlation between symbolic play and early language development in children with mental retardation. McCune-Nicolich (1981) found preliminary support for hypothesized correspondence between language and play in four areas: "(1) presymbolic behaviors in both domains [language and play], (2) initial pretending and first referential words, (3) the emergence of combinatorial behaviors in both domains, and (4) hierarchically organized language and symbolic play" (p. 795).

Kelly and Dale (1989) also found play skills to vary significantly among normally developing 1- and 2-year-old children, depending on whether their language was at the level of no words, single words, nonproductive syntax (defined as gestalt two-word phrases produced as formulaic routines or stereotyped units), or productive syntax (multiword utterances produced with evidence of rule-based creativity). In addition, however, they found evidence that the attainment of particular skills might be relatively more advanced or delayed either in language or in play.

Play-based assessments can be used to obtain information about children's internalized scripts and event knowledge. They also offer a context for naturalistic intervention (Norris & Hoffman, 1990b). In an ecological perspective, children's play may be viewed as an external context that the child creates by bringing together certain objects and roles, thus making play an outward expression of the way that the child perceives the world (Bronfenbrenner, 1979).

Documenting Early Play Skills

Many relatively formal assessment instruments, scales, and strategies have been constructed to take advantage of play as an indicator of early development in a variety of areas, including language (e.g. Linder, 1990; McConkey, 1984; McCune-Nicolich & Fenson, 1984; Norris & Hoffman, 1990b; Westby, 1980, 1988). Informal techniques can also be used to document varying patterns of sensorimotor, cognitive, linguistic, and social development through play.

These patterns may suggest specific goal areas (Linder, 1990). Particularly young children with specific language delays may demonstrate play skills that are relatively less impaired than their language skills (B. Y. Terrell, Schwartz, Prelock, & Messick, 1984). This finding suggests that play contexts might be used in intervention to target "verbal expressions of the meanings and relations already evidenced in play" (B. Y. Terrell et al., 1984, p. 428). When children make doll figures

cook food or drive a tractor, they demonstrate knowledge of the coordination of the concepts of agent, action, and object. The next step might be to help them to encode those relationships linguistically.

Westby (1980, 1988), in her Symbolic Play Scale, showed how cognitive and linguistic elements may correspond in the context of play. The first five stages in her scale are represented as Table 8.7. A set of expectations for categories of play and strategies for engaging others in play that are appropriate at the toddler level appear in Box 8.7.

Decentering, Object Symbolism, and Social Relations in Play

Objective 1: The child will play at a level commensurate with peers showing well-organized scripts and varied thematic content, using a variety of objects to symbolize other things, taking multiple roles, and using language functions, forms, and meanings consistent with the level of play.

Developmentally, pretend play may appear in primitive form as early as 18 months and possibly earlier. It is found in most normally developing children by the age of 3 years, and it increases steadily into middle childhood before disappearing (Chance, 1979).

During early-stage language development, assessment and intervention involving play might focus on three concerns (N. W. Nelson, 1988b). The first is the degree to which children can engage in pretend actions that are increasingly decentered from sensorimotor schemes (McCune-Nicolich, 1981). This includes evolution of play ability from a level of (1) presymbolic schemes (children can demonstrate function of real objects in real situations) through a level of (2) autosymbolic schemes (children can pretend by using objects in a nonliteral way but only for highly familiar schemes relating to the child's own body, e.g., "drinking" from a cup-like object), before reaching a level of (3) decentered symbolic games, marked by children's abilities to distance pretend actions from their own sensorimotor actions (e.g., using dolls for pretend).

A second assessment and intervention issue concerns the degree of similarity of pretend objects to the real objects they are supposed to represent. This focus is based on the work of Elder and Pederson (1978), who observed a developmental hierarchy in the following order: (1) similar substitute objects (e.g., a bristle block for a hairbrush), (2) dissimilar substitute objects (e.g., a plastic apple for a hammer), and (3) no object present. Elder and Pederson found that children under the age of 3 years were most dependent on the presence of similar substitute objects, but by the age of 3½, children could pretend equally well under all three conditions.

A third area of concern is the interaction of the development of social routines with the ability to pretend. Howes's (1985) research focused on this area and suggested that social play should be separated from social pretend play, which is more likely to appear after the child is around 23 months old. Howes suggested that substages for the development of **social play** might include (1) noninteractive parallel play, (2) simple social play with a turn-taking structure of at least three turns, and (3) complementary–reciprocal social play with reversal of play actions with another. Howes described three advancing types of **social pretend play:** (1) solitary pretend play, with a pretend action in the context of a social situation but not responded to by the partner; (2) simple social pretend play, in which both partners perform pretend actions that may be related temporally or using the same objects but not engaging in complementary roles; and (3) cooperative social pretend play, in which both partners engage in ongoing play with

---

Box 8.7

Categories of Play and Strategies for Engaging Others in Play
(Based on Categories Described by Howes, 1985)

SOCIAL PLAY. Tends to develop first and predominate up through the second year, with the child moving through stages of increasing maturity.

- *Noninteractive parallel play*
- *Simple social play* with a turn-taking structure of at least three turns
- *Complementary/reciprocal social play* with reversal of a play action of another

SOCIAL PRETEND PLAY. Tends to develop later; children above 32 months of age are observed to engage in all forms of social and social pretend play.

- *Solitary pretend play*—a fantasy action appears in the midst of social interaction but is not responded to by the partner
- *Simple social pretend play*—both partners perform fantasy actions that may be related temporally or using the same objects
- *Cooperative social pretend play*—-both partners engage in ongoing play with complementary pretend roles, such as mother and baby, or mother and father

STRATEGIES FOR ENGAGING OTHERS IN PLAY.

- *Imitation*—child A performs a fantasy action and does not direct it to the partner, child B; child B only imitates the action and does not verbally or nonverbally direct the action to A
- *Join*—child A performs a fantasy action and does not direct this action to child B, but B responds with a fantasy action and either directs the action to the partner, or names the pretend action to the partner as in recruitment
- *Nonverbal recruitment*—a child performs a fantasy action and directs the fantasy action to the partner by eye gaze, nonverbal gesture, or offering objects
- *Verbal recruitment*—a child performs a fantasy action and names the pretend action to the partner.

TABLE 8.7 Symbolic Play Scale—the first five stages (pp. 319–320)

DECONTEXTUALIZATION What Props Are Used in Pretend Play?	THEMATIC CONTENT What Schemas/Scripts Does the Child Represent?	ORGANIZATION How Coherent and Logical Are the Child's Schemas/Scripts?	SELF/OTHER RELATIONS What Roles Does Child Take and Give to Toys and Other People?	LANGUAGE Function	LANGUAGE Forms and Meaning
Stage I: 17 to 19 months Tool use (uses stick to reach toy) Finds toy invisibly hidden (when placed in box and box emptied under scarf) Uses common objects and toys appropriately in real and pretend activities; requires life-like props to pretend	Familiar, everyday activities (eating, sleeping) in which child has been active participant	Short, isolated schemas (single pretend action)	Self as agent (autosymbolic or self-representational play, i.e., child pretends to go to sleep, to eat from spoon, or to drink from cup)	Directing Requesting Commanding Interactional Self-maintaining Protesting Protecting self and self-interests Commenting Labeling (object or activity) Indicating personal feeling	Beginning of true verbal communication. Words have following functional and semantic relations: Recurrence Existence Nonexistence Rejection Denial Agent Object Action or state Location Object or person associated with object or person
Stage II: 19 to 22 months		Short, isolated schema combinations (child combines two actions or toys in pretend, e.g., rocking doll and putting it to bed, pouring from pitcher into cup, or feeding doll from plate with spoon)	Child acts on doll (doll is passive recipient of action): brushes doll's hair, feeds doll, covers doll with blanket Child performs pretend actions on more than one object or person, e.g., feeds self, a doll, mother, and another child	Refers to objects and persons not present	Beginning of word combinations with following semantic relations: Agent–action Action–object Agent–object Attributive Dative Action–locative Object–locative Possessive
Stage III: 2 years		Elaborated single schemas (represents daily experiences with details, e.g., puts lid on pan, puts pan on stove, turns on stove; or collects items associated with cooking/eating such as dishes, pans, silverware, glasses, highchair)			Uses phrases and short sentences Appearance of morphological markers Present progressive (ing) on verbs Plurals Possessives

TABLE 8.7 Continued

DECONTEXTUALIZATION What Props Are Used in Pretend Play?	THEMATIC CONTENT What Schemas/Scripts Does the Child Represent?	ORGANIZATION How Coherent and Logical Are the Child's Schemas/Scripts?	SELF/OTHER RELATIONS What Roles Does Child Take and Give to Toys and Other People?	LANGUAGE	
				Function	Forms and Meaning
Stage IV: 2½ years					
	Less frequently personally experienced events, particularly those that are memorable because they are pleasurable or traumatic Store shopping Doctor-nurse-sick child				Responds appropriately to the following *wh*-questions in context: What Whose Where What. . . . do Asks *wh*-questions (generally puts *wh*- at beginning of sentence) Responses to why questions inappropriately except for well-known routines Asks why, but often inappropriately except for well-known routines Asks why, but often inappropriately and does not attend to answer
Stage V: 3 years					
	Reenactment of experienced events, but modifies original outcome	Evolving schema sequences, e.g., child mixes cake, bakes it, serves it, washes dishes; or doctor checks patient, calls ambulance, takes patient to hospital (sequence is not planned)		Reporting Predicting Narrating or storytelling	Uses past tense, such as, "I ate the cake," "I walked Uses future aspect forms (particularly "gonna") such as, "I'm gonna wash dishes."

Note: From Westby, C., "Children's Play: Reflections of Social Competence," in *Seminars in Speech and Language,* Vol. 9, No. 1, New York, 1988, Thieme Medical Publishers, Inc. Reprinted by permission.

complementary pretend roles (e.g., mother and baby; daddy and mommy).

MAKING SPEECH MORE CLEAR

Goal: The child will speak clearly enough to be understood by unfamiliar partners.

Outcome: The child will have successful communicative interactions with multiple partners.

Children will not benefit much from having more ideas to communicate, or attempting to engage their peers in social pretend play, if they lack the means to articulate messages clearly enough to be understood by unfamiliar listeners. Stoel-Gammon (1987) pointed out that the normative information available for making judgments of children's phonological development at 2 years of age typically is based on extremely limited samples. For example, only about half of 21 subjects at this age in the normative study by Prather, Hedrick, and Kern (1975) could respond to direct metalinguistic prompts, such as "Say *fish,*" used to gather the data in that study. It also may be more useful to analyze children's speech patterns independently from adult models than to focus on "mastery" of adult speech pronunciation patterns, as done traditionally.

To add prior information and to correct earlier methodological problems, Stoel-Gammon (1987) analyzed the word and syllable shapes in conversational speech samples produced by 33 two-year-olds. She also inventoried the initial and final consonantal phones produced and the percentage of consonants correct in those samples. The results of these analyses are summarized in Box 8.8. Essentially, they show that normally developing two-year-olds can produce a range of sounds and structures and show evidence of synchrony in the developing sound system; children with larger initial inventories in earlier samples also tended to have larger inventories in later samples. Stoel-Gammon also found synchrony (in the form of a positive correlation) between the total inventory size for individual children and the percentage of consonants correct. She interpreted this as evidence "that phonetic abilities (as measured by the number of different consonants produced) and phonological abilities (as measured by appropriate use of consonantal phones in matching the segments of the

adult model) go hand in hand" (p. 326). The profile represented in Box 8.8 is also consistent with earlier research that has shown a preponderance of stops, nasals, and glides in early meaningful speech, as well as simple monosyllabic and disyllabic words, such as CV, CVC, and CVCV shapes, before 2 years of age. By contrast with typically developing toddlers, 24-month-old toddlers with specific expressive language impairment, vocalize significantly less frequently, have proportionately smaller consonantal and vowel inventories, and use a more restricted and less mature array of syllable shapes (Rescorla & Ratner, 1996). Box 8.9 summarizes phonological simplification processes that are normal in early development, but may persist among children with delayed language development.

These findings have implications for the kinds of words selected for early productive lexicon training with children who have severe phonological production deficits. The first priority in lexical selection for these children should be selecting words to map onto concepts that are already relevant and important. The child may also benefit if words are selected to approximate the phonological patterns prevalent in early normal development and/or in the children's existing phonetic repertoires (Koegel & Traphagen, 1982).

Box 8.8 _____

Phonological Abilities Demonstrated by the "Typical" Child by Age 2 Years
(Based on Stoel-Gammon, 1987)

- Produces words of the form CV, CVC, CVCV and CVCVC.
- Produces a few consonant clusters in initial position and maybe one or two in final position.
- Produces 9 to 10 different consonantal phones in initial position, including exemplars from the classes of stops (b/t/d/k/g), nasals (m/n), fricatives (f/s), and glides (w/h).
- Produces 5 to 6 different consonantal phones in the final position, mostly stops, but also a representative from the nasal, fricative, and liquid sound classes.
- Matches the consonant phonemes of adult words with at least 70% correctness.

Box 8.9 _____

Phonological Simplification Processes

Simplification processes are observed in the speech productions of normally developing children, but often persist among children with speech–language disorders beyond the ages when they usually disappear normally (based on Ingram, 1976; Shriberg & Kwiatkowski, 1980).

SYLLABLE STRUCTURE PROCESSES

1. Final consonant deletion—[bU] for *book*
2. Cluster reduction
   Initial—[baenki] for *blanket*
   Final—[poU:] for *porch;* [ba] for *bottle*
3. Unstressed syllable deletion—[naena] for *banana*

SUBSTITUTION AND ASSIMILATION PROCESSES

1. Velar fronting
   Initial—[bin] for *bring*
   Final—[teɪt] for *take*
2. Stopping
   Initial—[da] for *rock;* [ti] for *see*
   Final—[pit] for *piece*
3. Palatal fronting
   Initial—[toU] for *show;* [tu] for *shoe*
   Final—[put] for *push;* [wit] for *reach*
4. Liquid simplification
   Initial—[waebɪt] for *rabbit;* [wɪp] for *lip*
   Final—[ka] for *car;* [ba] for *ball*
5. Assimilation
   Progressive: consonant—[kɪki] for *kitty*
                vowel—[wawa] for *water*
   Retrograde: consonant—[bap] for *stop;*
                [keɪk] for *take*
               vowel—[bibi] for *baby*

Some attempts have been made to tie early phonological ability to imitation skill and other cognitive developments. R. Schwartz and Leonard (1982) studied the imitations of twelve normally developing children who were single-word users. They found that the children were better able to imitate words with characteristics already evident in their spontaneous phonological production systems than words with characteristics out-

side of those systems. The majority of this group had also not yet attained the means-end skills of Piaget's (1962) sensorimotor stage VI. This was in contrast to vocal imitation results obtained by Leonard, Schwartz, Folger, and Wilcox (1978) for slightly older children, all of whom had at least a 50-word vocabulary and most of whom had begun using two-word utterances. Most of the children in the older group demonstrated stage VI means–end ability. They also showed a tendency to imitate words whether or not the imitated consonants or syllabic shapes were part of their existing phonological systems.

More research is needed to guide decisions about selecting intervention targets and strategies for children who have specific speech and language impairments. As you may recall from Chapters 4 and 6, scatter among cognitive and linguistic indicators often is an identifying factor in diagnosing specific language and learning disabilities. Clearly, however, assessment and intervention of phonological skills should be incorporated into comprehensive programming for many young children with language and speech delays.

SUMMARY _____

This chapter considered intervention goals and strategies for infants and toddles. During this time, children and their caregivers exploit children's natural desires to communicate and to learn about their world and how it works. In the transactions of early-stage development, the seeds of language begin to grow in contexts that have shape, meaning, and purpose. Although the discussion did not dwell on the differences associated with various causative conditions, the chapter stressed that not all children learn in exactly the same ways (even in normal development) and that the same children may need different approaches at different stages of development.

Normally developing children smoothly and rapidly accomplish the transitions from the earliest stages of almost complete dependence on their caregivers' understanding, through emerging stages of expressing their own intentions, to using language symbols to create and communicate their own unique messages, starting with single words and moving to two-word utterances. It is easy to lose sight of how complex the navigation is until a child has difficulties. When children and their caregivers need assistance to move through the tiny steps and major stages of language acquisition, the process is no less marvelous if they pass the landmarks at slower rates and need extra scaffolding to do so. Evidence of positive outcomes does more than prove to agencies who provide funds for services that their money is well spent. It also provides occasions to survey a child's progress and appreciate the value of the journey to mature oral and written language development.

REVIEW TOPICS

- Infant–caregiver interactions, goals, and intervention strategies for: organizing and sensing care and safety; setting up mutual synchrony (behavioral state communication) and reciprocal "dialogues" (starting with initiation and ending with turning away); producing early vocal and phonological behaviors (including for medically fragile children and children with hearing impairments or autism); meeting early feeding needs (nutritive and nonnutritive); establishing play routines as a context for "protoconversations"; encouraging reciprocation and imitation
- Early intentional communication: gestural communication of comments (first) and requests (later); the role of structure in eliciting early functions; advantages of adult-initiated and child-initiated interventions; nonverbal and verbal expression of other communicative functions (attention-seeking, greeting, protesting, responding, informing)
- Early symbols: normal acquisition contexts (joint attention, joint reference, joint action routines); assessment strategies (comprehension and production); single-word utterances (expressing varied content/function relationships); early word categories—nominals (general and specific), action words, modifiers (state, locative, attribute, possessive), personal-social, function; different learning styles and potential problems (exclusively referential or expressive; over- or underextension; inflexibility in symbolic reference)
- Encoding semantic relations into two-word utterances: assessment techniques that acknowledge nonverbal comprehension strategies; producing a variety of two-word utterances to talk about—agent + action, action + object, agent + object, entity + attribute, possessor + possession, recurrence, nonexistence, disappearance, demonstrative + entity, entity + locative,

action + locative; intervention strategies (milieu teaching, dynamic assessment scaffolding cues); variations for children with specific expressive language impairment, autism, mental retardation, hearing impairment.
- Involving parents in helping their children develop temporally displaced talk; differences in the discourse of mothers and fathers with children with language delays
- Early emergent literacy; interactions with books and other print, sociocultural issues, early phonological awareness expectations
- Play as a context for assessment and intervention across cognitive and linguistic domains: decentering, symbolism, social relations, scripts, themes, pretending
- Phonological development concerns: differences in vocal and phonological behavior, relations to early word learning

REVIEW QUESTIONS

1. What goals and objectives would be appropriate for children with developmental risks identified in the hospital at birth or early in their infancy?
2. What published materials might help you develop IFSPs and plan for making the transition from hospital to home? For teaching parents to "match" their children's developmental stage? For teaching parents the "3a-way" to interact with their infants and toddlers?
3. When would an infant who is normally developing begin to show intentional but nonverbal communication? That is, when does the illocutionary stage begin? Would a child likely make intentional comments or requests first? What would they look like and what three criteria would you use to make sure they are intentional? Are structured elicitation contexts better for eliciting comments or requests? Which are more likely to show up in spontaneous play? How would one implement a milieu teaching approach to assist toddlers to make intentional gestural communicative attempts? What is linguistic mapping?
4. When are first words likely to appear? That is, when does the locutionary stage begin? What kinds of words do children produce in the early stages? What

words predominate for "referential" children? For "expressive" children? What word learning problems might be typical of children with autism? With specific expressive language impairments? With hearing loss? With mental retardation? What intervention strategies would be good for children with all of these special needs? What strategies might be unique to different groups?

5. What semantic relations might toddlers encode in their early two-word combinations? What are some early nonverbal comprehension strategies that toddlers might use for single relational terms and early multiword combinations? What assessment techniques could you use to be sure to measure linguistic comprehension rather than nonverbal comprehension? What intervention techniques could you use for encouraging the production of two-word utterances?

6. How do the discourse strategies of mothers and fathers differ when talking with children with language delays? How do parents of normally developing children help them learn to talk about the "there-and-then" as well as the "here-and-now" (e.g., consider the roles of routines and scaffolding)?

7. What preliteracy activities are appropriate for infants and toddlers (with and without books)? Does phonological awareness have a place in goals for toddlers? If so, how?

8. Using Westby's Symbolic Play Scale (Table 8.7), describe how you would use children's play as an assessment context by describing developments in thematic content (which schemas and scripts?), organization (how logical and elaborate are schemas and scripts?), self/other relations (who plays what roles?), and language (what forms and meanings are used to convey what functions?).

9. How might vocal and phonological behavior differ for children with communicative problems? How might a child's phonological inventory influence your selection of early vocabulary to emphasize in intervention?

ACTIVITIES FOR EXTENDED THINKING

1. Videotape an interaction between a parent and infant or toddler. Transcribe the nonverbal, vocal, and verbal aspects of the interaction. Code elements of the interaction using some of the developmental expectations discussed in this chapter or in articles referenced in it. Ask the parents if you can hold the infant (practice feeling comfortable doing so under parental guidance). Try different phasing and matching techniques to enter into a reciprocal dialogue if the infant seems receptive.

2. Watch a group of toddlers at play or participate with a toddler in pretend play with a doll or using some of the other props listed in Westby's Symbolic Play Scale. Is the child's play consistent with levels represented in the Scale? If your clinic opportunities allow, use the play scale with a child with special needs. How does this child differ from the first?

3. Engage in several shared book experiences with toddlers. How do they differ? With different books? At different times? If your clinic opportunities allow, do the same with a child with special needs. How do the experiences differ?

9

Middle Stages:
Identification and Assessment
Preschool Through Second Grade

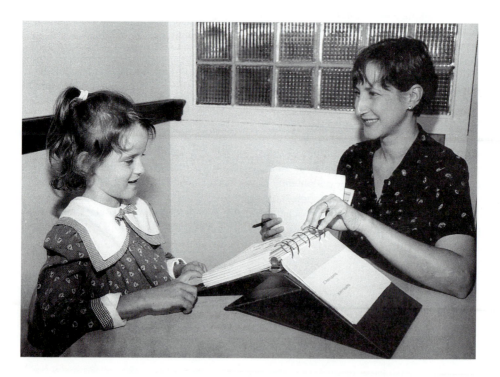

IDENTIFYING LANGUAGE DISORDERS IN
THE MIDDLE STAGES

CONTEXTS FOR MIDDLE-STAGE
ASSESSMENT AND INTERVENTION

TOOLS AND STRATEGIES FOR MIDDLE-
STAGE ASSESSMENT

The middle stage of language acquisition occurs quite early in normal development. It starts during the transition from toddlerhood to preschool age (at approximately 3 years of age)—when children begin to increase the number of multiple-word utterances in their expressive language—and it extends through ages 7 or 8 years (with no clear dividing line) into the threshold of preadolescence. Looking at the developmental process in this way, when children are in the middle stages, one observes that the primary feat is the acquisition of the grammatical code. Although, as considered in Chapters 11 and 12, much more recognition is now given to the developmental enrichments of the later stages of language development (those that normally occur during preadolescence and adolescence), the preschool and early elementary years still take the prize for dramatic language acquisition accomplishments, particularly in the area of grammatical development (language *form*) but also in expansion of concepts that children can talk about (language *content*) and in their resources for modifying their communications to be appropriate in particular contexts (language *use*) (see Personal Reflection 9.1).

PERSONAL REFLECTION 9.1 _____

"I am told that some remarkably high percentage of a child's learning—in language and other things—happens before the age of five. (I never can remember the percentage here, only that it is big). I have never understood how one could possibly give particular weights to particular learnings. How does one weigh the child's early acquisition of 'shoe,' 'hat,' 'key,' and 'mommy' against the child's later development of complex relational notions and the forms that express them: 'if-then,' 'although,' 'because,' 'unless'? How does one weigh the child's earlier interaction through talk, with her later development of ways of interacting through writing? How does one weigh the earlier simple, direct requests ('want juice') with her later development of more subtle and various ways of requesting—ways that take different partners and situations into account ('I just love orange juice' or 'I'll trade you my juice for your crackers')? I just don't know how anyone decides what each chunk of learning is worth (or even what a chunk is), and without knowing this, how does one total up the chunks and decide what proportion happened before age five and what proportion happened after that age? For me, this way of thinking about children's development doesn't make sense."

From Judith Wells Lindfors, 1987 (p. 217).

IDENTIFYING LANGUAGE DISORDERS IN THE MIDDLE STAGES

Child-Find Efforts and Preschool Screening

Children who need speech and language intervention services during the preschool years from ages 3 to 5 may be identified in several ways. The Child-Find efforts discussed in Chapter 7 are pertinent. Medical referral is also common during this period, particularly resulting from well-child clinics and follow-up monitoring of children who have had difficult births. Pediatricians and family practitioners in many communities increasingly appreciate the importance of early communication development and its relationship to later school success. As they become better informed, fewer adopt the well-known posture, "Don't worry, she'll outgrow it."

At the same time, more parents are aware of early developmental expectations, and they are not afraid of asserting concerns about their children's developmental needs. Thus, parental referral continues to be a common source of identification of children with speech and language delays throughout the preschool years. Preschool teachers also may refer children during this stage. If children have not been identified by the time they enter school, early elementary school teachers may refer them. In school districts with conservative eligibility criteria, concerned parents may seek out private speech–language intervention services when their children do not qualify for school services. Other public sector programs, such as Head Start, provide intervention as well.

Regardless of who makes the referral and where services are provided, the national priority of Child Find and IDEA (Parts B and C) is that any child who needs special services should receive them. Thus, it is important that all potential referral sources be informed about language and communication development danger signs. A listing of some of the danger signs that may signal the need for referral of 3- to 5-year-olds for speech–language evaluation appears in Box 9.1.

Some factors predict a child's need for special services better than others at certain developmental stages. In the early stage years from birth to 3 years, parental traits, such as maternal education, are better predictors of disabilities in adolescence than children's own behavior. In the middle stage years, from ages 4 to 7 years, child-centered skills are better predictors of later status than maternal education (Kochanek, Kabacoff, & Lipsitt, 1990).

Box 9.1 _____

Potential Danger Signals Related to Failure to Meet Developmental Milestones Expected of 3- to 5-Year-Olds. (Note: Few children at risk for language disorders would be expected to show *all* of these symptoms.)

- *Limitations of language expression.*   Is close to 3 years of age and produces few creative utterances that are three words or more in length.
- *Problems learning words.*   Has limited receptive or expressive vocabulary and has difficulty acquiring new words to express new ideas.
- *Problems comprehending language.*   Appears to rely too much on familiar contexts to understand language (shows difficulty comprehending language without gestural support or when produced by unfamiliar partners).
- *Limitations of social interaction.*   Shows little interest in social interaction, except perhaps to gain adult assistance to fulfill specific desires.
- *Limitations of play.*   Shows little interest in playing with peers or in combining toys and objects in imaginative symbolic play.
- *Problems learning speech.*   Has difficulty pronouncing words so that they are intelligible to unfamiliar adults (perfect articulation is not expected).
- *Difficulty with strategies for learning language and using language to learn.* Demonstrates unusual learning strategies for age level, such as either too much reliance on imitation (e.g., signs of echolalia), or inability to imitate the actions and verbalizations of others (e.g., signs of developmental apraxia or cognitive limitations). Shows little interest in using language to learn more about language and the world (e.g., does not ask "What's that?" questions early, or "Why?" questions, which become prevalent for most children around age 4 or 5).
- *Short attention span for language-related activities.*   Shows little interest in sitting with an adult and looking at a book while naming and talking about the pictures or in communicating with peers.

This suggests that screening tools that focus on children's developing speech–language, communicative, and cognitive abilities may be used appropriately during the middle-stage years. Many are available; some are broad, comprehensive screening tools, and some are aimed more exclusively at speech and language development (N. W. Nelson, 1981b; Sturner, Layton, Evans, Heller, Funk, & Machon, 1994). The most commonly used screening and assessment tools appropriate for this developmental level are listed in Chapter Appendix A Middle-Stage Assessment Tools.

Professionals are urged to be careful when selecting and interpreting screening tools. For example, Bailey and Brochin (1989) pointed out that the inclusion of items on a screening measure does not mean that they are necessarily important in a particular context or that they have been encouraged within a particular child's

cultural experiences. Different test makers also use different standards for assigning age levels to items. A common procedure is to place assessment items at a level at which they are passed by 50% of the children. Not all tests use this criterion, however. For example, the Battelle Developmental Inventory (Newborg, Stock, Wnek, Guidubaldi, & Svinicki, 1984) used as criterion the age at which 75% of the normative sample passed an item. It is important to be aware of these varying standards when interpreting screening test results and deciding which children should be given more comprehensive assessments.

A more serious problem is that some instruments allow the generation of developmental age scores even though they were never normed themselves (Bailey & Brochin, 1989). The problem with this approach is that the equivalence of measures gathered in different years and on different populations is uncertain, particularly because norms established on more recent populations tend to show developmental milestones being reached at younger ages than those reported on older measures (Bailey & Brochin, 1989).

A third concern is the degree to which a screening test is based on a normative group that can be considered representative of the population as a whole. Bailey and Brochin (1989) recommended that, "Ideally, the sample should be stratified, with proportionate representation of various racial groups, geographic regions, sex, income levels, and urban/rural distribution" (p. 28).

A fourth concern is whether the screening test's manual offers information about the test's **sensitivity** and **specificity** (Sturner et al., 1994). **Sensitivity** is the screening test's accuracy in identifying individuals who actually have disorders. It is quantified as a high percentage of correct fails. **Specificity** is defined in terms of the screening test's accuracy in identifying children who do not have disorders. A test with a high percentage of correct fails will show a reciprocally low percentage of **false positives** (incorrect fails), thus minimizing **overreferrals** of children who fail the screening test but do not have disorders. A test with a high percentage of correct passes will show a reciprocally low percentage of **false negatives** (incorrect passes), thus minimizing **underreferrals** of children who pass the screening test but later are found to have disorders (see Figure 9.1).

The Developmental Indicators of the Assessment of Learning (DIAL) is an example of a comprehensive

screening instrument that was standardized on 2447 children from geographical proportionate regions of the United States, with approximately equal numbers of boys and girls, and with a minority population of 44.5% of the group (Mardell-Czudnowski & Goldenberg, 1984, 1990). It can be used with children ages 2 to 6 years and provides statistical data based on three norming groups; 1990 census, white, and minority. The DIAL-R provides standardization data for the three screening cutoff points: ±1, ±1.5, and ±2 standard deviations. The DIAL has also been shown to correlate highly with the Boehm Test of Basic Concepts (Boehm, 1971) as a quick screening instrument to detect potential difficulties with basic language concepts in a young kindergarten population (Sarachan-Deily, Hopkins, & DeVivo, 1983). The language items include (1) articulation, (2) giving personal data, (3) remembering, (4) naming nouns, (5) naming verbs, (6) classifying foods, (7) problem solving, and (8) sentence length. An example of a screening test specific to speech and language development is the Sentence Repetition Screening Test (SRST; Sturner, Kunze, Funk, & Green, 1993). It is a brief (3 minute) elicited imitation task that is scored for articulation errors as well as syntax. Of the 51 measures reviewed by Sturner and colleagues (1994), it was the only one that met all of the evaluation criteria for screening tests, including quick administration, sensitivity, specificity, predictive validity, and reliability measured as agreement of interrater, test-retest, and split-half comparisons. Before selecting any screening test, the specialist should carefully examine the methods used for standardizing it and the validity of the constructs on which it is based (see Chapter 6).

FIGURE 9.1 Illustration of screening test results expressed as accuracy of fail criteria (sensitivity) and pass criteria (specificity) (based on Sturner et al., 1994, with modifications).

SCREENING TEST	DIAGNOSTIC CRITERION MEASURE	
	Fail	Pass
Fail	sensitivity	false-positive (overreferral)
Pass	false-negative (underreferral)	specificity

Prekindergarten Screening

Although screening may be conducted at any point throughout childhood, the practice of screening children before they enter kindergarten is particularly widespread. Two commonly used tools for this purpose are the Manual of Developmental Diagnosis for the Gesell Development Schedules (Knobloch et al., 1980) and the DIAL-R (Mardell-Czudnowski & Goldenberg, 1990). The screenings are used by school districts to identify children who are not ready to enter kindergarten. The outcome may be a recommendation to wait another year before starting a child in school, a referral for special education assessment, or placement in a developmental kindergarten program. Speech–language pathologists often participate in this screening activity.

The use of prekindergarten screening is not without controversy. Some see it as leading to an early form of ability tracking that may carry many of the detrimental effects associated with tracking throughout the grades, including (1) weaker learning environments, (2) lowered expectations, (3) cumulative losses compared to same-age peers, and (4) resegregation of children in minority groups (when busing and other methods have been used to achieve racial balance), particularly for children of lower socioeconomic status (Braddock & McPartland, 1990). On the other hand, when children have wobbly language and communicative skills and have had little exposure to preliteracy experiences, a strongly language-based developmental kindergarten experience may provide the boost they need to begin school successfully. More research is clearly needed in this area to understand what is best for children.

Early Elementary School Referral Criteria

When children are in the early elementary school years, teachers serve critical roles as referral sources. Some language-based, debilitating school problems are not, however, obvious to teachers. It is easier to notice errors such as misarticulations, pronoun substitutions, and morphological immaturities, than to notice the absence of important positive developments, such as later developing syntactic structures or adequate language comprehension.

Part of the problem is that most screening and referral criteria are based on expressive language and speech criteria alone. Exclusively spoken language criteria present problems for identifying children with language disorders in their school-age years for several related reasons. When individuals spontaneously express their own ideas, they can select lexicon and syntax from items and structures they know well. No one may notice that their linguistic formulations are not complex or abstract because they make few or no errors. On the other hand, the same luxury does not accompany language comprehension. It is well documented that children spend much more time in school settings listening than talking (e.g., Cazden, 1988; N. W. Nelson, 1985; Sturm, 1990; Wells,

1986). When children listen to others speak, or read what others have written, they have no choice except to try to understand that language. When they do have opportunities to speak in classrooms within the teachers' hearing, it is often as members of large groups, and their utterances are generally expected to be short answers to their teachers' questions. When a child fails to volunteer in class, he or she may not be noticed. When a child is called on and has difficulty answering, teachers might assume many explanations aside from linguistic impairment for not answering the teacher's questions (e.g., being inattentive, not listening, not trying, or being a slow learner). Language impairment is not usually one of the first explanations that occurs to teachers unless they are given specific guidance to identify the danger signs.

Damico and Oller (1980) studied varied referral criteria to discover which work best for children in the elementary grades. They provided inservice to two groups of teachers (54 teachers in grades kindergarten through fifth). Group S (surface-oriented) teachers were taught to use "traditional," superficial morphological and syntactic criteria, such as noun–verb agreement, possessive inflections, tense marking, auxiliary verbs, irregular verbs, irregular plurals, pronoun case or gender, reflexive pronouns, and syntactic transpositions as the basis for making referrals. Group P (pragmatically oriented) teachers were taught to use the criteria shown in Box 9.2. Following the inservice, a panel of judges reevaluated the referrals from both sets of teachers, using the state's criteria for determining speech–language impairment. The results showed that the teachers in Group P identified significantly more children and were more frequently correct in their identification than those in Group S. Both groups identified significantly fewer children as grade level increased.

Although whole-grade screening is much less common following the implementation of IDEA (because of the law's requirement that no child be placed in a special education program on the basis of screening results alone), speech–language pathologists may occasionally find widespread, whole-grade screening activities to be appropriate particularly in the early elementary years. A story-retelling procedure (see Box 9.3) was devised by Culatta, Page, and Ellis (1983) to perform this function. When Culatta and her colleagues compared this measure of integrated communicative performance

Box 9.2 _____

Pragmatically Oriented Referral Criteria for Elementary Education Teachers Suggested by Damico and Oller (1980).

- _Linguistic nonfluency._   Disruption of speech production by a disproportionately high number of repetitions, unusual pauses, and excessive use of hesitation forms.
- _Revisions._   Breakup of speech production by numerous false starts or self-interruptions; multiple revisions are made as if the child keeps coming to a dead end in a maze.
- _Delays before responding._   Pauses of inordinate length following communication attempts initiated by others.
- _Nonspecific vocabulary._   The use of expressions such as _this, that, then, he,_ or _over there_ without making the referents clear to the listener; also, the overuse of all-purpose words such as _thing, stuff, these,_ and _those._
- _Inappropriate responses._   The child's utterances appear to indicate that the child is operating on an independent discourse agenda—not attending to the prompts or probes of the adult or others.
- _Poor topic maintenance._   Rapid and inappropriate changes in the topic without providing transitional clues to the listener.
- _Need for repetition._   Requests for multiple repetitions of an utterance without any indication of improvement in comprehension.

Note: From "Pragmatic vs. Morphological/Syntactic Criteria for Language Referrals" by J. S. Damico and J. W. Oller, Jr., 1980, _Language, Speech and Hearing Services in Schools, 11,_ p. 88. Copyright 1980 by American-Speech-Language-Hearing Association. Adapted by permission.

---

with performance on two standardized screening tools that tested knowledge of discrete language rules, they found that the story-retelling measure was more stringent than the standardized discrete item tasks for kindergarten, for a transitional level between kindergarten and first grade, and for first-grade children. Although some of the children who scored adequately on the standardized measures—the Screening Test of Auditory Comprehension of Language (STACL; Carrow, 1973a) and the Evaluation of Language Scale (ELS; Vane, 1975)—were unable to relate events conveyed in a story, all children who performed poorly on the story-retelling task also had difficulty on the standardized measures. Because more children were identified at the kindergarten level than at the transitional first-grade or first-grade levels using this procedure, Culatta and her colleagues suggested that perhaps graded stories and sets of comprehension questions should be devised in the future. To my knowledge, no standardization of this kind of task has yet been accomplished for American children.

Bishop and Edmundson (1987) described a story-retelling task, called the Bus Story Test (Renfrew, 1969), used in England. It has standardization data with means and quartiles for children from 3 to 8 years. Using this procedure, the examiner tells a story about a naughty bus that runs away from its driver and ends up in a pond. The original telling is accompanied by four pages of cartoon pictures (three per page). After telling the story, the adult asks the child to retell it, starting with the prompt, "Now you tell me the story. Once upon a time there was a . . ." During the retelling, only general prompts are used, such as "Then what?", unless more direct questions are needed. Scoring is based on awarding two points for including main items (e.g., ran away, met train, alone, train in tunnel, into city/town, saw policeman, didn't stop, into country, tired of road, ran downhill, couldn't stop) and one point for subsidiary items (e.g., naughty/bad, made faces, policeman blew whistle, cow mooed, splash, stuck). Other diagnostic procedures for assessing the narrative productions of children in the middle stages are discussed later in this chapter.

Box 9.3 _____

Story Retelling as a Screening Tool
in the Early Elementary Grades

ADMINISTRATION

- Introduce the story-retelling task by saying, "I'm going to tell you a story. You listen and when I'm finished you tell me the same story."
- Read the story to the child.
- Say, "Now you tell me the story."
- If the child does not begin, say, "Can you tell me the name of the little boy in the story?" Provide additional open-ended prompts if necessary, such as: "That's OK, what's the rest of the story?" "What did Tommy want?" "Really—what else happened?"
- Present the ten comprehension questions.

MAKE ONE OF THREE DISPOSITION DECISIONS

1. *To enroll the child for language intervention.*   Legally, under IDEA, a comprehensive multidisciplinary evaluation should be conducted at this point—children cannot be determined to have a handicapping condition on the basis of a single procedure administered by a single professional. The story-retelling activity is judged to support a diagnosis of language impairment if the child is unable to relate the story or if the child's version deviates significantly from the original version in either sequencing or content.

2. *To re-evaluate the child's language.*   Children who seem to be "on-the-borderline" may be observed carefully in the regular education context or rescreened before receiving a comprehensive multidisciplinary evaluation if that seems more appropriate. This decision is made if the child tells a story that is sketchy but relevant and properly sequenced.

3. *To terminate contact.*   Children whose integrated language skills are clearly adequate may be considered to have passed the screening. This decision is made if the child tells a detailed version of the story that is properly sequenced.

STIMULUS STORY WITH NUMBER OF EVENTS

$\qquad\quad$ 1 $\qquad\qquad$ 2 $\qquad\qquad\qquad\qquad$ 3

Tommy was five years old, but his birthday was coming soon. He wanted a puppy for

$\qquad$ 4 $\qquad\qquad\qquad\qquad\qquad\qquad\qquad\qquad\qquad$ 5

his birthday, but his mother said he was too little to take care of it. Tommy didn't think

$\qquad\qquad$ 6 $\qquad\qquad\qquad\qquad\qquad\qquad\qquad\qquad$ 7 $\quad$ 8

he was too little. When his birthday came Tommy had a party. Five of his friends came

$\qquad\qquad\quad$ 9 $\qquad\qquad$ 10 $\qquad\qquad$ 11 $\qquad\qquad$ 12

to his house. They played games, ate animal crackers and cokes, and Tommy opened

$\qquad\quad$ 13 $\qquad\qquad$ 14 $\qquad\qquad$ 15 $\qquad\qquad$ 16 $\qquad\qquad$ 17

his presents. He got a GI Joe, a fire truck, some comic books, and a baseball bat. He

$\qquad\qquad$ 18 $\qquad\qquad\qquad\qquad\qquad\qquad\qquad$ 19

liked the presents, but he was disappointed because he didn't get a puppy. All of Tom-

$\qquad\qquad\qquad$ 20

my's friends were getting ready to go home when his daddy brought out another pre-

$\qquad\quad$ 21 $\qquad\qquad\qquad\qquad$ 22 $\qquad\qquad\qquad$ 23

sent for him to open. Inside was a little black puppy. Tommy was really happy because

$\qquad\quad$ 24

he got the present he wanted.

COMPREHENSION QUESTIONS

1. Who was the boy in the story?
2. How old was he?
3. Who said he was too little for something?
4. What was he too little for?
5. How many friends came to Tommy's house?
6. Why did the friends come over?
7. Name two presents Tommy got.
8. What did they eat at the party?
9. Who gave Tommy the puppy?
10. What color was the puppy?

Note: This is a nonstandardized procedure whose interpretation rests largely on clinical judgment. When the procedure is used within a particular school district, local norms might be established by quantifying some of the observations and performing statistical analyses to compute cutoff scores for children who fall more than 1 or 1.5 standard deviations below the mean for children when judged within the context of the normative group in their own linguistic and sociocultural community (see Saber & Hutchinson, 1990).

Note: From "Story Retelling as a Communative Performance Screening Tool" by B. Culatta, J. L. Page, and J. Ellis, 1983, *Language, Speech and Hearing Services in Schools, 14,* pp. 68, 73. Copyright 1983 by American Speech-Language-Hearing Association. Reprinted by permission from p. 73; adapted by permission from p. 68.

CONTEXTS FOR MIDDLE-STAGE ASSESSMENT AND INTERVENTION

The Continuing Importance of Family and Culture

Parents continue to play a primary role in the development of communicative ability throughout the preschool and early elementary years. It is largely through interactive experiences in the home that children come to understand their world and to have the language for mapping onto and extending their concepts.

By the time children leave toddlerhood, if their language and speech skills are noticeably limited, most parents begin to "do something." Depending on their own resources and community education efforts, parents may or may not be aware of the availability of professional help, but evidence shows that they modify their interactions with their children, consciously or subconsciously (e.g., Cross, 1984; Lasky & Klopp, 1982). To summarize research on parental interaction styles with children with language disorders (discussed at several points throughout this book), most evidence suggests that parents use more directive (even corrective) styles and less semantic contingency when their children have difficulty. Some parents appear to adopt strategies of asking test-like questions and making informal learning opportunities more like school. Others go the the opposite extreme, rarely asking questions (Cross, 1984). In either case, opportunities for experiencing the naturally rewarding consequences of meaningful interactions may suffer.

Family System Contexts. The evidence does not lead to the conclusion, however, that parents are to blame for their children's language delays. Both Cross (1984) and Leonard (1987) urged caution in concluding such a causative role. A better explanation seems to be one of interactive causative patterns (as described in the system theory discussion of Chapter 1). That is, children's communicative delays probably influence parental interaction strategies and vice versa. Acceptance of this explanation not only removes the need for blame, it also suggests possibilities for designing assessment and intervention to escape from downward spirals. Assessment within family systems (see Chapter 7) involves collaborating with parents to help them identify strategies for fostering development while communicating parental affection and disciplinary expectations in culturally consistent ways.

Cultural Contexts. Sensitivity to cultural differences continues to be an important feature of contextually based assessment activities in the preschool years. When a young child's communication is inconsistent with mainstream norms, professionals should never fail to consider whether the difference may be consistent with expectations in the child's nonmainstream culture rather than impaired performance. For example, Shirley Brice Heath (1983) described differences in adult expectations and interactions with young children in the African American working class community she called "Trackton." In this community, where Heath spent a considerable amount of time as a participant observer, babies and young children were constantly part of the adult communication scene. Children were not particularly encouraged to join in the conversations with adults, however, except when boys were coached in public "stage" presentations. Unlike the parents in mainstream middle-class cultures, the adults in this community did not assign meaning to babies' prelinguistic babbling noises. Nor did they address much of their talk directly to infants. As Heath put it, "Everyone talks *about* the baby, but rarely *to* the baby" (p. 75).

Differences in adult–child communication actions and interpretations were also found by Philips (1983) in the Warm Springs Indian Community in Oregon, where greater attention is given to the comprehension of language evidenced by young children than its expression. "Children are given many directions and then watched closely to see if they do what they are told. If they do what they are told, it is taken as evidence of comprehension" (p. 64).

Because professionals cannot possibly know all culturally based communication rules in our pluralistic society, they must often act as their own ethnographers, carefully observing children who seem to be developing normally in the same contexts as the children at risk. They may also find that interviewing participants in the culture can yield a critical perspective in helping to sort out whether a linguistic–cultural difference or a language disorder accounts for the behaviors they observe.

Increased Interactions with Peers

Children have varying opportunities to interact with other children during the preschool years from age 3 to 5 years. For many, their first opportunities are interactions with siblings. Efforts to make sense of the influences of sibling order and other factors on language development have met with limited success.

Wells (1986) followed 32 children through the final year of their elementary education in his longitudinal study of language development in Bristol, England. He found great variability among the developmental rates of siblings in the same families but no particular pattern for whether parents described their older or younger children as more advanced. Wells reported that interpretation of results was further complicated by varied age gaps between siblings and their differential prefer-

ences for interacting with younger or older siblings. The only generalization that seemed justified was that "there was a slight tendency for only children or those without a sibling close in age to develop more rapidly, due most probably to the more frequent opportunities these children had for interaction with their parents on a one-to-one basis" (p. 132).

In what context besides interactions with siblings at home do preschool children communicate with other children? One of the most important peer-interaction contexts is social play. As reviewed in Chapter 8, Howes (1985) found that social play tended to precede social pretend play in normal development, but that both were established by 3 years of age. Westby (1988) outlined the interwoven developmental pathways of play and language (preschool development of play behaviors is discussed in Chapter 10).

The Shift From Home to School

Although families continue to serve a primary role in children's development throughout childhood, when children reach the age of 3 years or so, their worlds begin to expand. Many enter a preschool setting, either Head Start, a private preschool, or a combined daycare–preschool setting. Some may enter a special classroom for children with communicative disorders. In classrooms, children are on their own as communicators as never before. For the first time, they may be expected to communicate with an adult in authority without a parent, grandparent, or familiar child-care worker to mediate the exchange. They also may be brought into large groups of peers for the first time.

Children's readiness to assume this relative independence as communicators follows on the heels of early-stage developments that rely on more dependent relationships with primary caregivers. When describing a toddler named Mark, for example, Wells (1986) noted that, "when he is talking with someone who knows him well and who is able to interpret his intention from the combination of his utterance and its context, he is successfully able to mean more than he can say" (p. 23). Wells likened the developmental accomplishments for Mark and his peers over the next few years of middle-stage development as an almost sheer climb up the face of a cliff. After the cliff, the rest of the mountain remains (i.e., the later stages of language development), but many routes are possible, and the going is somewhat easier.

Wells (1986) noted the continuity in the shift from home to school, as well as the discontinuity. He commented:

> As far as learning is concerned, therefore, entry into school should not be thought of as a beginning, but as a transition to a more broadly based community and to a wider range of opportunities for meaning-making and mastery. Every child has competencies, and these provide a positive base from which to start. The teacher's responsibility is to discover what they are and to help each child to extend and develop them. (p. 69)

The language of school does not always facilitate further language learning, however. Wells (1986) found that teachers were twice as likely as parents to develop meanings that they themselves had introduced rather than following the child's lead. He commented, "Small wonder that some children have little to say or even appear to be lacking in conversational skills altogether" (p. 87).

The Elementary School Classroom as a Context for Language Learning and Use

Classrooms play such an important role for school-age children that they warrant special consideration as assessment and intervention contexts. The formal interactions of classrooms have unique features. They differ considerably from the informal interactions of dyadic communication in homes and adult–child conversations. In classroom discussions, the power differential between teachers and students is usually obvious (Cazden, 1988; Lindfors, 1987). McDermott (1977) noted that "teaching is invariably a form of coercion" (p. 204). That is, teachers almost always fill the role of authority in the classroom, controlling topics and the allotment of turns, asking test-like questions to which they already know the answers, and establishing a variety of special communication rules (such as flipping the light switch to signal that children should stop talking).

Contrast this style with interaction in homes, where children establish topics and guide conversations with their own interests. J. N. Britton (1979) contrasted the **participant** mode of discourse in conversation, where both partners play an equal role with the **spectator** mode, in which one partner takes the lead and dominates the turns. Britton commented, "As participants, we use language to shape experience in order to handle it; as spectators, we use language to digest experience" (1979, p. 192). The spectator role (e.g., listening to stories, reading them) is assumed more often in classrooms.

As Cazden (1988) pointed out, teachers guide discourse in the classroom, both when they are in expressive control themselves and when their students are taking extended turns. For example, in sharing time, when teachers perceive that their students have begun to stray too far from announced topics, they say things like:

> OK I'm going to stop you // I want you to talk about things that are really very important // that's important to you but can you tell us things that are sort of different // can you do that? // (p. 13)

Problems arise for students when cultural differences in discourse styles learned at home do not match the expectations of their teachers. For example, Cazden (1988) pointed out that children from African American homes are more likely to use a narrative style involving an episodic structure, with one event tied sequentially to the next but no overall theme. Such narratives might be evaluated as the norm by adults in the child's culture, but may be evaluated as inferior by white mainstream teachers.

The debate about the degree of distinction between language in home and school is echoed in the debate about the distinction between oral and written language (Blank, 1982; M. M. Cooper, 1982; Tannen, 1982). The debate is about whether school and home language and oral and written language represent truly separate systems or merely different points on a continuum. Distinctions in lexical choices (more varied and abstract), sentence structure (more complex), and discourse organization strategies (more preplanned and cohesive) are associated both with written language and with formal spoken language, such as that used in classrooms. The differences in all of these linguistic dimensions can be traced to the influences of one key factor—the degree of **contextualization.**

As children shift roles from home to school and from oral to written modalities, increasing decontextualization occurs. Less meaning is available in the situation, and more must be gleaned from words. It is a shift from **situated meaning** to **lexicalized meaning** (Cook-Gumperz, 1977) (see Box 9.4 for a list of other terms

Box 9.4

HOME LANGUAGE AND ORAL LANGUAGE		SCHOOL LANGUAGE AND WRITTEN LANGUAGE
Heavy reliance on non-linguistic context		Heavy reliance on linguistically encoded meaning
Situated meaning	(Cook-Gumperz, 1977)	Lexicalized meaning
Restricted code	(B. B. Bernstein, 1972)	Elaborated code
Particularistic meanings implicit in text		Universalistic meaning explicit in text
Exophoric meaning	(Gregory & Carroll, 1978)	Endophoric meaning

Note: From "The Nature of Literacy" by N. W. Nelson in *Later Language Development: Ages Nine Through Nineteen* (p. 17) edited by M. A. Nippold, 1988, Austin, TX; Pro-Ed. Copyright 1988 by Pro-Ed. Adapted by permission.

for these shifts). When contextualization shifts occur, children whose linguistic comprehension skills are weaker than their nonlinguistic skills are at increasing risk for functional limitation and language disability.

For such children, several consequences are possible. One is that no one will recognize the problem as involving a language disorder. Going unrecognized and untreated for what they are, the language-related problems of these children may mount with the advancing language demands of classrooms. Such children may be at risk for problems of other types as well, particularly involving self-image. Another possibility is that the problem may be recognized as involving language disorder, with the result that the child is removed from the mainstream to a special education context to address the problem.

When children need help to make sense of instructional language, the best solutions may involve collaborative consultation with teachers to modify language expectations slightly (e.g., by adding redundancy or slowing speaking rate), while helping children acquire skills for processing increasingly complex language. Many teachers are willing to monitor a child's comprehension more closely and to engage in individualized communicative repair when they recognize that a child has failed, not because of lack of trying or inattention, but because the child did not understand the language. Language permeates all aspects of teaching and learning. "Language" is not something that happens from

9:00 to 10:00 on Monday, Wednesday, and Friday mornings. It happens all the time. It happens when teachers and children study math or science. It also happens when children learn the new rules of a game on the playground (see Personal Reflection 9.2).

The language of classrooms is used (1) for instruction in how to read and write language (fostering the acquisition of literacy); (2) to talk about language (much of school language is metalinguistic, from talking about words and sounds in kindergarten to talking about metaphor and simile in the later grades); (3) to use language to learn how to do other things (much of school language is used to convey procedure); and (4) to use language to learn about other things (in other cases, school language is used to convey content).

Table 9.1 shows the speech acts that teachers used in a study of formal classroom discourse (Sturm, 1990). Most frequent were questions to "solicit information" (SI). Correspondingly, the speech acts children used

PERSONAL REFLECTION 9.2

"Where children and teachers are doing real work, there is no way to separate out 'language' and what is sometimes called 'content.'"

Judith Wells Lindfors (1987), writing about the language of classrooms.

TABLE 9.1   Classroom speech acts

COMMUNICATION ACT VARIABLES	GRADE-LEVEL STUDENT MEANS			GRADE-LEVEL TEACHER MEANS		
	1ST	3RD	5TH	1ST	3RD	5TH
1. To convey content (CC)	0.6%	1.4%	2.0%	12.3%	14.3%	15.9%
2. To mark content (MC)	0.1	0.2	0.4	11.9	12.3	16.3
3. To call on specific child, "solicit other"(SO)	0.0	0.2	0.0	9.8	6.0	5.3
4. To convey procedure (CP)	0.0	0.0	0.2	14.7	13.5	13.8
5. To convey attitude (CA)	0.1	0.2	0.3	2.7	3.4	3.5
6. To acknowledge evaluate (AE)	0.2	0.1	0.2	5.2	4.0	3.3
7. To acknowledge modify (AM)	0.0	0.0	0.1	6.4	6.5	4.5
8. To ask questions or "solicit information or action" (SI)(SA)	0.7	1.8	2.4	22.1	17.0	17.6
9. To answer questions/read aloud "supply solicited info" (SSI)	10.1	13.0	10.0	0.8	1.0	1.7
10. Performatives (P)	0.1	0.2	0.2	0.8	0.8	0.5
11. Free responses (FR)	1.4	4.1	1.8	0.0	0.0	0.0
Totals	13.3%	21.2%	17.6%	86.7%	78.8%	82.4%

Note: Mean proportions of total speech acts produced at a grade level over the 3-day period in instruction–discussion discourse involving the class as a whole (total = 15 classes, 5 at each grade level, based on data from Sturm, 1990).

most often were to "supply solicited information" (SSI). Children showed extremely small proportions of any other kind of speech act in this type of interaction. Other speech acts that teachers frequently used were to convey content (CC) and to convey procedure (CP), each of which account for approximately 15% of speech acts across grade levels. These language functions require different linguistic abilities of children attempting to make sense of them.

Language used to convey procedure typically places greater demands on auditory memory and the ability to process language in sequence. Children often must reauditorize (D. J. Johnson & Myklebust, 1967) procedural language as they seek to carry out the teacher's instructions. The following is an excerpt from a sample recorded by Sturm (1990) in a first-grade classroom. It is coded for the variables represented in Table 9.1 and for analysis with the Systematic Analysis of Language Transcripts (SALT) program (Miller & Chapman, 1991) (including bound morphemes marked with a slash, e.g., "trade/ed"). The teacher is conveying a procedure about the transitions in a cooperative learning task involving

process writing. Notice the high demand on the ability to decode complex logico-grammatical (if–then) structures involving negative and temporal concepts and to remember the teacher's instructions (perhaps by reconstructing them) long enough to carry them out:

T: OK, if you have not trade/ed job/s, it is now time for the listener to become the reader and the reader become the listener [MC][CP].

T: If you have both had time to finish what you/'re do/ing, you/'ve read your story all the way, it is time to go back to your seat and make any correction/s that you need to make [CP].

S: XXX [SI?] [A question asked by a student was unintelligible on the tape].

T: Then she can read it as far as she is [SSI].

T: (People who are not done . . .) OK, then you can go back to your seat and work [MC][CP].

T: None of you need to be up here [CP][CA].

Teachers also use language to convey curricular content. Curriculum referents are often abstract and metalinguistic. An example is the following sequence, recorded in a first-grade classroom, where a teacher and students are editing the punctuation on a letter. The teacher has just called on an individual student, coded as "solicit other" (SO):

T: Chantel, what else should we do to our letter [SO][SI]?
= room silent waiting for an answer 00:10 seconds
S: Put a comma after "love" [SSI].
T: All right a comma after "love" [MC][AE+].
T: We call that our close/ing don/'t we [CC][SI]?
T: We/'d always put a comma whether it/'s "yours truly," or "love," or "sincerely" [CC][CP].

To successfully process language conveying the curriculum content (in this case, rules of punctuation and capitalization), children often must understand multiple-meaning words (e.g., *letter* in this context does not refer to a letter of the alphabet, and *closing* is used as a noun, rather than as a verb as in "closing a door"). If children can immediately recognize that the referent for closing in this case is the word *love*, but that the teacher is offering other exemplars from the same category in the listing, "yours truly," or "love," or "sincerely," they will have simplified the task of remembering the rule for when to use a comma. When children have trouble with the concrete vocabulary of everyday interactions, such abstract discussions make no sense.

TOOLS AND STRATEGIES FOR MIDDLE-STAGE ASSESSMENT

Gathering Background Information for Contextually Based Assessment

When the purpose of assessment is to determine eligibility for special education services, the basic question is whether the child has lower language abilities than same-age peers. This question is answered most readily by administering relatively formal tests standardized on an appropriate reference group.

Norm-referenced assessment activities are inadequate by themselves, however, for meeting other assessment purposes. Another is to determine whether a child *needs* special education services. The only way to answer this question is to interview those who know the child well and to observe the child's ability to meet everyday linguistic demands of key life contexts. Life

significant contexts are identified by collaborating with others who are concerned and knowledgeable about the child. A sequence for gathering this essential background information appears in Box 9.5.

Language Sampling and Other Informal Assessment Techniques

The *pièce de résistance* of most speech–language evaluations of children in the middle stages of language development is the spontaneous language sample. Although professionals use formal assessment tools to quantify aspects of a child's language and speech abilities, the spontaneous language sample affords the richest opportunity to observe a child's integrated communicative abilities.

Language-sampling techniques can be used to gather quantitative data to support a diagnosis of language disorder (Lee, 1974; J. F. Miller, 1981; Roberts & Crais, 1989), or they can serve as a source of qualitative data for the intervention-planning process (Fey, 1986; Lahey, 1988; Lund & Duchan, 1993; J. F. Miller, 1981; Roberts & Crais, 1989). Both purposes are important, and both can be approached in a variety of ways.

Language sample analysis is not new. It has been used as a diagnostic and research technique at least since McCarthy (1930) reported that 50 utterances of spontaneous speech "would give a fairly representative sample of the child's linguistic development in a relatively short period of time, without tiring the child with a prolonged observation" (p. 32). Many versions of language-sampling and analysis strategies have appeared since the early 1970s, including several computer software programs. These are listed and described in Box 9.6. Unfortunately, no one has developed a way to avoid human transcription of the recordings. For most experienced clinicians, that remains the most time-consuming part of the process. Following is a description of transcription and other aspects of the language-sampling process: (1) gathering the sample, (2) transcribing it, (3) analyzing language form variables, (4) analyzing language content variables, and (5) analyzing language use variables.

Gathering the Sample. When gathering a language sample, a question arises about control of contextual variables. Should one gather samples entirely through conversation or ask children to retell a story or give in-

Box 9.5 _____

Procedures for Gathering Background Information Essential to the Assessment of Children in the Middle Stages of Language Acquisition

1. Determine the **reason for referral** by interviewing the person who made the referral (or suggested that it be made). The fact that someone was concerned enough about the child's communicative development to make a referral is significant. If the child was identified through screening instead of referral, interview those who might have made a referral (but did not) to determine whether they have ever felt any concern about the child's communicative development.

2. Gather **history information** about the nature of the problem using the parents as informants, but also interview other informants who are significant in the child's life. Include questions about (a) the family and any communicative problems or disorders family members might exhibit (or may have exhibited as children); (b) the child's medical history and any significant injuries or illnesses; (c) the child's developmental history, especially related to major developmental milestones; (d) the child's educational history (if there is one), including any previous referral and/or enrollment in special services; and (e) the child's social history, including information about the child's interactions with peers and the effects on those interactions of the child's communicative behaviors.

3. Collaborate with other important adults to **identify contexts** where it is important that the child meet communicative expectations. Include questions about (a) places (e.g., home, school, day-care center); (b) people (e.g., parents, siblings, day-care playmates or friends); (c) communicative events (e.g., show-and-tell, understanding parental requests, free-play time at preschool).

4. Use multiple strategies to **identify aspects of communicative competence in each of these important contexts.** Include both (a) observational strategies and (b) interview strategies. When using observational strategies, attempt to use strategies of both onlooker observation (the mouse-in-the-corner strategy) and participation observation (dynamic assessment to explore the child's ability to be more effective when contextual conditions are modified). When using interview strategies, ask informants to list and prioritize areas of greatest strength and concern, and ask other questions that ask informants to give examples of what they mean by the way they choose to label behaviors.

5. Based on this initial compilation of background information, **form additional hypotheses about the child's relative areas of strength and difficulty** that can be tested in the remainder of the assessment process using both informal and formal assessment techniques.

_____

structions for playing a game? Should pictures or toys be used? Should professionals gather the samples or record children in interactions with other adults or peers?

These questions have no one best answer. The best answer to all of them is, it depends. It depends on the purposes of the assessment and on whether the clinician plans to apply an established set of quantitative analytic criteria. When quantitative comparisons are desired, one

must use methods recommended by the author of the analysis procedure. What looks like a standard procedure, however, may actually be experienced in unequivalent ways by different children. Depending on past experiences, what may be easy and familiar for child A may be hard for child B; in a different cultural milieu, the reverse may be true. Clinicians must be careful not to draw conclusions about a general lack of

Box 9.6 _____

Language Sampling and Analysis Strategies

Crystal, D., Fletcher, P., & Garman, M. (1976). *The grammatical analysis of language disability.* London: Edward Arnold. Describes their Language Assessment, Remediation, and Screening Procedure (LARSP): Both morphological and syntactic developments are tallied on a LARSP chart, arranged in order from earlier to later developing forms, which can be used to plan intervention.

Leadholm, B. J., & Miller, J. F. (1992). *Language sample analysis: The Wisconsin guide.* Madison, WI: Wisconsin Department of Public Instruction. Describes language sampling techniques and provides normative data for children from 3 years to 13 years from the Wisconsin Research Data Base (also included with the most recent versions of SALT).

Lee, L. L. (1974). *Developmental sentence analysis.* Evanston, IL: Northwestern University Press. Describes Developmental Sentence Types analysis for children not producing at least 50% complete sentences (defined as including a subject and verb) and Developmental Sentence Scoring (DSS) for those who are. DSS is based on grammatical analysis of eight categories for a 50-utterance sample, which yields a score that can be compared with normative data for 3- to 7-year olds.

Long, S. H., & Fey, M. E. (1991). *Computerized profiling* [computer program; Version 7.1]. Ithaca, NY: Computerized Profiling. Provides computer assistance for several other analysis systems, including LARSP.

Lund, N. J., & Duchan, J. F. (1993). *Assessing children's language in naturalistic contexts* (3rd ed.). Englewood Cliffs, NJ: Prentice-Hall. Serves as a reference text, summarizing multiple language sampling and analysis strategies.

MacWhinney, B. (1996). The CHILDES System. Described in *American Journal of Speech-Language Pathology, 5*(1), 5–14. To participate, researchers should send e-mail with computer address, postal address, affiliations, and phone number to *childes@cmu.edu*. Bulletin board participants should send information to *childes@andrew.cmu.edu*. CHILDES includes three integrated components: "(a) a system for discourse notation and coding called CHAT, (b) a set of computer programs called CLAN, and (c) a large database of language transcripts formatted in CHAT" (p. 5).

Miller, J. (1981). *Assessing language production in children: Experimental procedures.* Baltimore, MD: University Park Press. Serves as a reference text, summarizing multiple language sampling and analysis strategies.

Miller, J., & Chapman, R. (1991). *Systematic analysis of language transcripts (SALT)* [Computer program; A. Nockerts, Programmer]. Madison, WI: Language Analysis Laboratory, Waisman Center on Mental Retardation and Human Development. Available in both Macintosh and IBM versions, this computerized analysis system can accommodate more than one speaker. Samples are entered using slashes to indicate bound morphemes and using customized codes. Offers standard analyses (e.g., MLU, type-token ratios, word counts) and customized analysis.

Palin, M. W., Mordecai, D. R., & Palmer, C. B. (1985). *Lingquest 1: Language sample analysis software* [Computer program]. San Antonio, TX: Psychological Corporation. Available in both Apple and IBM versions, this software package yields type-token analysis, form analysis of eight grammatical categories, an error profile, structure analysis of 7 basic sentence types, 10 question types, and 12 complex sentence types. At least 50 utterance samples are typed in with glosses.

Stickler, K. R. (1987). *Guide to analysis of language transcripts.* Eau Claire, WI: Thinking Publications. A transcript guides readers through varied procedures for analysis of semantic, syntactic, and pragmatic features. Procedures are most useful with young children with language disorders, but many are also applicable with older students.

Tyack, D. L., & Gottsleben, R. H. (1977). *Language sampling, analysis, and training: A handbook for teachers and clinicians.* Palo Alto, CA: Consulting Psychologists Press. A sample of approximately 100 sentences is transcribed on a form. The professional counts words and morphemes, computes a word-morpheme mean to assign the child to one of five linguistic levels, compares the child's language forms to a developmental chart of those expected for the child's level, and uses these results to make clinical decisions.

communicative competence when the child may be demonstrating reduced competence *in a particular context.* For example, telling a story about a picture may be highly familiar and comfortable to one child but unfamiliar to another. Remember Crago's (1990) report in Chapter 2 of her surprise when an Inuk teacher perceived a verbal child as having a learning problem because "children who don't have such high intelligence have trouble stopping themselves" (p. 80).

When doubts are raised about the communicative competence of a child whose culture and ethnicity differ from that of the interactant, the professional should sample in other, more familiar contexts. Failure to observe the child's communicative abilities within his or her own language community may lead to biased assessment results.

The materials and discourse tasks best suited for gathering language samples vary based on children's ages and language levels as well as assessment purposes. As a general rule, the younger the child, the more toys and other props are needed to facilitate the language sampling interaction. Older children can interact when the context is established through linguistic rather than nonlinguistic means. Conversational interaction, in which children are allowed to set the topics, is desirable for all children. Yes–no questions and questions that can be answered elliptically should be avoided. When children are reticent, it is helpful to avoid questions altogether, engaging instead in joint focus or parallel play activity, gradually commenting on aspects of the environment to which the child is attending. This usually takes the pressure off talking and leads to more natural interactions. As Lund and Duchan (1993) commented, when clinicians insert their own opinions or comments occasionally, a more natural and less "testing" atmosphere may be created. Manipulable materials like play dough and puzzles are not particularly effective for gathering rich language samples. Many children with language impairments become so preoccupied with the motor activity, that they say little. Stockman (1996) used race car and book interactions to gather language samples from preschool African American children. She specifically avoided "interaction with objects or images that the child had to create" (p. 359) (e.g., block play or picture drawing).

Narrative discourse should also be probed for most middle-stage children. The appropriateness of probing the narrative genre, even for 3-year-olds, is supported by K. Nelson's (1989) report of "narratives from the crib." Even very young children, when conditions are right, can use connected discourse without heavy support from an adult. The probing of narrative discourse is useful because attempts at storytelling are generally associated with the production of longer and more complex utterances, the use of cohesive devices, and the opportunity to observe whether the child has a sense of story grammar (see sampling and intervention suggestions in Chapter 10).

Recording the Sample. Videotaping is essential to capture the nonlinguistic context for very young or physically impaired children. Audiotaping may suffice for most middle-stage language assessment purposes. When children produce mostly utterances of three words or more, enough context is usually encoded in language to enable judgment of their linguistic and communicative abilities from the language sample itself. In these instances, the clinician should transcribe the audiotape as soon as possible, so that contextual notes may be added.

Whenever professionals document clinical activities, it is important to keep in mind the absent audience for the written report of each activity, the purpose of the report, and alternative purposes to which the report might be put. In this case, the audience is most likely other professionals, and its primary purposes may be (1) to capture the essential qualities of the child's linguistic and communicative abilities, (2) to make quantitative judgments about normalcy and/or progress, and (3) to select target goal areas for the intervention process.

Transcribing the Sample. Aside from the time transcription takes, most problems in transcription arise around decisions for segmenting utterances. A second issue is what to do with the linguistic nonfluencies (false starts and revisions), fillers (*well, uh, ah, um, you know*), and repetitions that are inevitable features of oral conversations.

Utterance Segmentation. Decisions for utterance segmentation are particularly important because they influence measurements such as MLU that depend on utterance units. Recommended strategies depend on the child's linguistic and developmental level. J. F. Miller (1981) recommended that "Utterance segmentation should be based on terminal intonation contour, rising or falling" (p. 14). This **prosodic strategy** is especially appropriate when transcribing samples of children in the early stages of language acquisition. It is also the strategy Miller and his colleagues in Wisconsin used for constructing their Research Data Base (RDB), which comes as part of later editions of the SALT computer program (*Systematic Analysis of Language Transcripts;* Miller & Chapman, 1991) and in *Language Sample Analysis: The Wisconsin Guide* (Leadholm & Miller, 1992). The RDB is a set of normative data (including means and standard deviations for a variety of language sample descriptors, including MLU and mazes) for 266 typically developing children ages 3 through 13 years.

For children at middle stages of language development who are learning to elaborate and combine sentences, however, others believe that syntax-based segmentation rules are needed. The problem is how to give credit for compound sentence constructions without inflating the child's MLU from multiple run-on clauses, such as those conjoined with "and then" starters. Lee (1974) suggested a way to satisfy these concerns by allowing only two independent clauses per compound sentence. Lund and Duchan (1993) restated and elaborated this approach (summarized in Box 9.7).

An alternative strategy is to divide utterances into "T-units" or "C-units." These approaches are appropriate for children beyond Brown's Post Stage V (MLU = 4.50+). According to J. F. Miller's (1981) normative projections (see Table 9.2), the predicted mean for the age 60 months (5 years) ±1 month is 5.63 (±1 *SD* for MLU at this age is represented by the range 4.44 to 6.82). Traditionally, the MLU has been assumed to become less meaningful as a measure of children's development beyond the age of 5 years. At that point, advancing maturity begins to be marked by children's ability to say more in fewer words (Hunt, 1965), and a different criterion for dividing utterances for analysis then becomes appropriate.

Kellogg Hunt (1965) therefore proposed the **T-unit** as "one main clause with all the subordinate clauses attached to it" (p. 20). As Hunt pointed out, the advantage is that this method preserves all of the youngster's subordination and all of the coordination between words and phrases and subordinate clauses, but does not overcredit the less mature strategy of coordinating main clauses.

C-unit (for "communication unit") was the term Loban (1963, 1976) used for utterance division based on

Box 9.7 _____

Guidelines for Segmenting Utterances

Judgment of utterance boundaries must be made at the time of transcription, using contextual and intonation cues. Once the words are written down, the information is lost. Indicate pauses with a slash (/).

1. The end of an utterance is indicated by a definite pause preceded by a drop in pitch or rise in pitch.
2. The end of a sentence is the end of the utterance. Two or more sentences may be said in one breath without a pause, but each one will be treated as a separate utterance for syntax analysis.
3. A group of words, such as a noun phrase, that can't be further divided without losing the essential meaning is an utterance, even though it may not be a sentence.
4. A sentence with two independent clauses joined by a coordinating conjunction is counted as one utterance. If the sentence contains more than two independent compound clauses, it is segmented so that the third clause, beginning with the conjunction, is a separate utterance.
5. Sentences with subordinate or relative clauses are always counted as single utterances.

Note: From *Assessing Children's Language in Naturalistic Contexts* (3rd ed.) (p. 223) by N. J. Lund and J. F. Duchan, 1993, Englewood Cliffs, NJ: Prentice-Hall. Copyright 1993 by Prentice-Hall. Reprinted by permission.

a combination of syntactic and semantic criteria. The syntactic criterion was the same as for T-units (i.e., one main clause and any subordinated or embedded phrases and clauses). The semantic criterion was "a group of words which cannot be further subdivided without the loss of their essential meaning" (1963, p. 6). Most professionals use the term C-unit for utterance division in oral samples to allow for the fragments and elliptical responses to questions that are common in oral conversations. Loban reported on the oral language development of a group of elementary school students (starting with 338), which he followed from kindergarten through grade 12. Data from the 1963 report of the elementary school years are summarized in Table 9.3.

Box 9.8 illustrates how the same sample might be divided using the two different strategies proposed by

TABLE 9.2   Predicted MLUs and MLU ranges within 1 *SD* of predicted mean for each age group

AGE ±1 MONTH	PREDICTED MLU[a]	PREDICTED SD[b]	PREDICTED MLU ±1 *SD* (MIDDLE 68%)
18	1.31	0.325	0.99–1.64
21	1.62	0.386	1.23–2.01
24	1.92	0.448	1.47–2.37
30	2.54	0.571	1.97–3.11
33	2.85	0.633	2.22–3.48
36	3.16	0.694	2.47–3.85
39	3.47	0.756	2.71–4.23
42	3.78	0.817	2.96–4.60
45	4.09	0.879	3.21–4.97
48	4.40	0.940	3.46–5.34
51	4.71	1.002	3.71–5.71
54	5.02	1.064	3.96–6.08
57	5.32	1.125	4.20–6.45
60	5.63	1.187	4.44–6.82

[a]MLU is predicted from the equation MLU = −0.548 + 0.103 (age).
[b]SD is predicted from the equation SD_{MLU} = −0.0446 + 0.0205 (age).

Note: From Jon F. Miller, *Assessing Language Production in Children: Experimental Procedures* (p. 27). Copyright © 1981 by Allyn and Bacon. Reprinted by permission.

Hunt (1965) and Lund and Duchan (1993). It is the attempt of a child with a language-learning disability to retell the story of "Dumbo."

Setting off Mazes.   The sample in Box 9.8 also illustrates how to handle linguistic nonfluencies when transcribing language samples by placing in parentheses such devices as initial conjunctions, pause fillers (*um, ah, er, OK*), part-word or whole-word repetitions not intended for emphasis, and revisions. Revisions sometimes look like linguistic dead-ends and were labeled **mazes** by Loban (1963). Hunt (1965) called them **garbles.** Mazes are not counted as communication units. That is, they should not be included when counting morphemes to determine utterance length or when assigning credit for grammatical features (e.g., when performing Laura Lee's, 1974, developmental sentence analysis). When mazes are set off in parenthesis, however, "the remaining material *always* constitutes a straightforward, acceptable communication unit" (Loban, 1963, p. 9). Linguistic nonfluencies do provide important information about internalized processing efforts and should

be maintained in language sample transcripts (see Table 9.4).

Analyzing Language Form Variables.   The clinician's analysis of the language sample depends on the questions raised during the observations and interviews when gathering background information. Questions about **language form** may be divided into three types: (1) questions about inflectional morphology, (2) questions about syntactic construction and comprehension, (3) and questions about contextually based variation of language form.

First, questions about **language morphology** are usually guided by reference to information about the acquisition of the 14 morphemes studied by Roger Brown (1973) and by Jill and Peter De Villiers (1973). These are summarized in Box 9.9.

Mabel Rice and her colleagues (Rice & Wexler, 1996a, 1996b, 1996c; Rice et al., 1995) have also suggested that verb tense and number endings can serve a special diagnostic function for identifying specific language impairment (SLI). Their research has shown that

TABLE 9.3 MLU data (means and *SD*s) reported by Loban (1963) for elementary school children, using C-unit criteria to segment utterances (Note: This was a longitudinal study, starting with a group of 338 children in kindergarten that became smaller across the grades. These data are extracted from Loban, 1963).

	LOWEST GROUP		HIGHEST GROUP		TOTAL GROUP	
GRADE	*Mean*	*SD*	*Mean*	*SD*	*Mean*	*SD*
K	4.18 (N = 22)	1.29	5.76 (N = 30)	1.53	4.81 (N = 338)	1.33
1st	4.89 (N = 22)	1.36	6.89 (N = 30)	1.39	6.05 (N = 260)	1.37
2nd	5.49 (N = 22)	1.18	7.04 (N = 30)	1.18	6.57 (N = 261)	1.18
3rd	6.08 (N = 22)	1.82	7.73 (N = 30)	1.33	6.65 (N = 259)	1.81
4th	6.42 (N = 24)	1.20	8.77 (N = 25)	1.08	7.70 (N = 246)	1.26
5th	6.90 (N = 24)	0.93	8.85 (N = 25)	0.95	7.89 (N = 243)	1.10
6th	7.19 (N = 24)	0.88	9.48 (N = 25)	1.12	8.37 (N = 236)	1.25

TABLE 9.4 Data for mazes reported by Loban (1963, p. 33) based on the same samples as Table 9.3, for high and low subgroups and the total group.

	PERCENTAGE OF WORDS IN MAZES IN RELATION TO TOTAL WORDS			PERCENTAGE OF WORDS IN MAZES IN RELATION TO COMMUNICATION UNITS		
	High	*Low*	*Total*	*High*	*Low*	*Total*
K	9.17	11.92	12.30	22.55	32.07	25.38
1st	7.57	15.51	9.97	21.80	39.29	25.16
2nd	6.65	10.49	8.88	14.69	26.30	19.90
3rd	4.98	10.62	6.15	13.69	25.54	18.67
4th	5.43	9.74	7.11	23.82	31.63	28.33
5th	5.17	9.27	7.41	23.27	32.51	29.74
6th	5.17	9.49	7.53	25.75	32.09	32.06

children with SLI tend to extend the period of normal development in which children treat finite verbs (including *be* and *do*), which are typically marked for tense and number, as if they were not finite. To understand this distinction, consider that infinitive (nonfinite) forms of verbs (e.g., *to be, to do, to walk*) are not marked for tense or number. The Extended Optional Infinitive (EOI) interpretation of the unmarked verbs of children with SLI suggests that they are treating finite verbs as infinitives beyond the point at which most children figure out the morphological markers for tense and number. Yet, when children with SLI do use the markers, they usually use them correctly. That is, diagnostically, we might expect to see children with SLI and EOI grammar producing unmarked (infinitival) forms like "Patsy talk about her dog" and "She like her dog?" (for *"Does* she like her dog?"), but not erroneously marked forms like "She are happy" or "I talks about my dog." A critical reminder is that symptoms based on inflectional morphology are diagnostic only for children learning standard American English. Other dialects and language influences would invalidate assessment questions related to an EOI stage or development of Brown's 14 morphemes.

When analyzing morphological development, the clinician generally starts by computing MLU for a sample of at least 50 utterances. This MLU is used to assign the child to a developmental level (usually corresponding to one of R. A. Brown's, 1973, stages; also see Tables 9.2 and 9.3). Then the clinician looks for evidence that morphological developments expected for the child's age and MLU are occurring. J. F. Miller (1981) referred to the analysis of simple sentences as Assigning Structural Stage (ASS). His procedure compares the evidence from a child's language sample to a series of charts summarizing developmental expectations. In a similar procedure, Tyack and Gottsleben (1977) defined mastery of a particular structure as correct adult usage in 90% or more in obligatory contexts. Tyack and Gottsleben's system consists of constructing an outline of baseline forms (morphological developments) and

Box 9.8 _____

Two Methods of Utterance Segmentation

Excerpt from a language sample produced by a 9-year-old with a language-learning disability who is retelling the story of "Dumbo" (slashes indicate pauses).

so a circus was there and they had these other hands/he had these other people in it/so he first got in a train/and so he didn't get in the train cause he could fly/so he/Mr. Tyler wasn't/he was happy/he didn't care if the train was broke down/and so this little guy, Timothy, a little mouse, he gets on and they found a boat/so they sailed on the boat/and so hippopotamus/no/the elephant had to go up in a tiny bed/so the bed broke down and they try to XXX hippopotamus up there . . .

Method I.   Segmentation keeping the first two main clauses in coordinated compound sentences together (Lee, 1974; Lund & Duchan, 1993):

1. (so) a circus was there and they had these other hands/
2. he had these other people in it/
3. (so) he first got in a train/
4. (and so) he didn't get in the train cause he could fly/
5. (so he/Mr. Tyler wasn't/) he was happy/
6. he didn't care if the train was broke down/
7. (and so) this little guy, Timothy, a little mouse, he gets on and they found a boat/
8. (so) they sailed on the boat/
9. (and so hippopotamus/no/) the elephant had to go up in a tiny bed/
10. (so) the bed broke down and they try to XXX hippopotamus up there . . .

Method II.   Segmentation into T-units of one main clause with all subordinate clauses attached to it (Hunt, 1965); also called C-units (Loban, 1963, 1976)

1. (so) a circus was there
2. (and) they had these other hands/
3. he had these other people in it/
4. (so) he first got in the train/
5. (and so) he didn't get in the train cause he could fly/
6. (so he/Mr. Tyler wasn't) he was happy/
7. he didn't care if the train was broken down/
8. (and so) this little guy, Timothy, a little mouse, he gets on
9. (and) they found a boat/
10. (so) they sailed on the boat/
11. (and so hippopotamus/no/) the elephant had to go up in a tiny bed/
12. (so) the bed broke down
13. (and) they try to XXX hippopotamus up there . . .

_____

constructions (syntactic developments) that have been mastered (1) at and below the assigned level or (2) above the assigned level. The clinician then can propose intervention goals based on evidence about forms and constructions that are at or below the assigned level and either (1) do not appear or (2) appear inconsistently (i.e., in less than 90% of obligatory contexts).

Another similar approach, called language assessment, remediation, and screening procedure (LARSP), was described by Crystal, Fletcher, and Garman (1976).

Box 9.9 _____

Development of 14 Morphemes

BROWN'S ORDER		DE VILLIERS & DE VILLIERS'S ORDER	
-ing (no auxiliary verb)	(STAGE II)	*-ing* (no auxiliary verb)	(STAGE II)
in		regular plural, *-s*	
on		*in*	
regular plural, *-s*		*on*	(STAGE III)
irregular past (imitated)		possessive, *-'s*	
possessive, *-'s*		regular past, *-ed*	(STAGE V)
uncontractible copula, *be*	(STAGE III)	irregular past (imitated)	
articles, *a, the*		regular third-person singular, *-s*	
regular past, *-ed*		articles, *a, the*	
regular third-person singular, *-s*	(STAGE V)		
irregular third-person singular, *does, has*		contractible copula, *be*	
uncontractible auxiliary, *be*		contractible auxiliary, *be*	(STAGE V+)
contractible copula, *be*		uncontractible copula, *be*	
contractible auxiliary, *be*		uncontractible auxiliary, *be*	
		irregular third-person singular, *does, has*	

Note: Although the sequences of morphological development reported by R. A. Brown (1973) and De Villiers and De Villiers (1973) are quite similar, some differences are evident, especially in the order of contractible and uncontractible verb forms. (Brown also found some variation in order and stage of acquisition for his three famous subjects, Adam, Eve, and Sarah.) All 14 regular morphemes are acquired by Stage V+ (MLU 4.5+) by children acquiring standard English normally, but most children continue to sort out irregular forms into their school-age years. Children learning dialectal variants of English such as Black English Vernacular or Spanish-influenced English follow a different developmental pattern.

▬▬▬▬▬▬▬▬▬▬▬▬▬▬▬▬▬▬▬▬▬▬▬▬▬▬

Using the LARSP, the specialist summarizes evidence of both morphological and syntactic developments on a tally sheet, based on a 30-minute language sample. Crystal and his colleagues emphasized that positive evidence about the forms and constructions a child uses in spontaneous language is always more directly useful and reliable in defining a pattern than negative evidence. "The presence of a score is a positive indication of ability, whereas the absence of a score may mean only that the sample is biased" (p. 113). Once a child's sample is outlined on the summary chart, Crystal and colleagues defined the purpose of intervention as assisting the child to move "down the LARSP chart [from earlier to later developments] in as controlled a way as possible" (p. 117).

Perhaps the most complex aspect of morphological development in English is the acquisition of rules related to **auxiliary verb construction.** Auxiliary verbs are particularly important syntactic elements. They contribute, for example, to conveying **questions** (e.g., "He found it → Did he find it?"); **negation** (e.g., "He found it → He didn't find it"); **tense** (e.g., "He finds it → He will find it → He has found it"); and **mood** (e.g., "He can find it → He could find it"). Lee (1974) used Chomsky's (1957) auxiliary verb construction schema (see Figure 9.2) to design verb scoring for the Developmental Sentence Scoring (DSS) system (assigning credit ranging from 1 to 8) in the area of main verbs. Lee's procedure can give clinicians an internalized system for helping children to acquire more flexible strategies for conveying meanings using auxiliary verbs (see Chapter Appendix B).

Other important aspects of morphological development include **personal pronouns** and **articles.** Recall from Chapter 4 that persistence in pronoun case problems is one feature that distinguishes the performance of children with specific language impairments

FIGURE 9.2   Chomsky's (1957) auxiliary verb construction rule. C + (Modal) + (have + en) +
(be + ing) + MV as interpreted by Lee (1974).

SCORE	DEVELOPMENTAL VERB FORMS	CHOMSKY'S SCHEMA: C + MODAL + (HAVE + EN) + (BE + ING) + MV	TRANSFORMATIONS AND COLLOQUIAL FORMS
1 0	I *play.* It *is* good. It's good. He *play.* She *play.* It *play.*	V	
0	I *playing.* He *playing.*	ing V	
0 1	I *is playing.* You *is playing.* He *is playing.*	is + ing V	
2 2 2	He *plays.* He *played.* I *am playing.* He *was playing.* We *are* good. They *were* good.	C (be + ing) V prés. past am, are -s -ed was, were	

4
 	
4
4
4
	I *can play.* He *will play.*
	Transformations:
	I *don't* play. They *don't play.*
	Do you play? *Do* they play?
	They *do play.*
		C (M) V
		prés. can, will, may
			Transformations:
			Obligatory *do*
			  + negative
			  + question
			Emphasis

6
6
 	
6
6
6
	He *could play.* He *would play.*
	He *might play.* He *should play.*
	Transformations:
	He *doesn't play.* He *didn't play.*
	Does he play? *Did* he play?
	He *does play.* He *did play.*
		C (M) V
		past could, would
		        might, should
			Transformations:
			Obligatory *does, did:*
			  + negative
			  + question
			Emphasis

7 7 7 7 7	I *must play.* I *shall play.* (rare) I *have eaten.* I *had eaten.* Colloquial form: I'*ve got* to play. The music *was being played.* The music *could have been played.*	C (M) V prés. must, shall C (have + en) V prés. past Passives of all tenses are scored the same.	Colloquial form: *have got* Transformation: Passive
8 8 8 8	I *have been playing.* I *may have eaten.* I *might be playing.* I *might have been playing.* Etc.	C (M) (have + en) (be + ing) V prés. past	

C, an abstract symbol for markers indicating person (first, second, or third), tense, and number; MV, main verb.

Note: From *Developmental Sentence Analysis* (p. 13) by L. L. Lee, 1974, Evanston, IL: Northwestern University Press. Copyright 1974 by Northwestern University Press. Reprinted by permission.

(Leonard, 1980). When children have trouble including appropriate articles in their expressive language, they may have difficulty learning to recognize similar elements in written language and those opportunities may need to be probed as well.

Second, questions about **syntactic construction** and **comprehension** play an important role in language form analysis. When the analytical focus shifts from the level of inflectional morphology and function words to the level of sentence construction, the clinician should ask questions about children's abilities to construct well-formed simple sentences that include all essential elements in an acceptable sequence. A particular concern may be whether syntactic **subjects** (semantic "agents") are included when obligated by the linguistic context. This is because, as noted in Chapter 4, the omission of subjects may be a danger sign that a young child's language development is not proceeding normally. Development of **question** and **negative** forms have also been studied extensively, and data from that research may be used to analyze the target child's constructions as well (e.g., Crystal et al., 1976; Lee, 1974; J. F. Miller, 1981; Tyack and Gottsleben, 1977).

Beyond the simple sentence level, it is important to ask about children's abilities to construct and comprehend **complex sentences.** Rhea Paul (1981) suggested some strategies for analyzing complex sentence development to accompany J. F. Miller's (1981) ASS procedure. To perform this analysis, it may be helpful to make a listing transcript in which all of the sentences of a particular type are pulled out from the overall sample and listed. A set of criteria for analyzing complex constructions is summarized in Box 9.10. Some information about complex sentence development also may be obtained from the J. F. Miller and Chapman (1991) SALT program for computer analysis of language samples by asking the software program to list the number of different conjunctions and the number of times each conjunction appears in the sample.

Third, questions about **contextually based variation** related to language content and use guide assessment of the child's ability to adjust language form to represent language content and use. Children must know how to use rules for expressing language content–form interactions to make sense to their communicative partners and to express their ideas effectively (Lahey, 1988). A variety of assessment questions can be asked about

these abilities. For example, one might ask whether a child in the latter part of the middle stages has the syntactic flexibility to emphasize the importance of the object of a sentence by using a complex passive construction to move the object to the initial position (e.g., "The girl was chased across the parking lot"). Additionally, can the child understand passive-construction sentences encountered in teacher talk or in books? Can the child paraphrase individual or multiple sentences that encode multiple semantic relations in complex or embedded sentences? Can the child understand and use rules of complex pronominal reference that contribute to discourse cohesion?

What about language form–use interactions? For example, what happens when an adult or child conversational partner fails to understand something that the child has tried to communicate? What are the target child's syntactic resources for rephrasing the utterance and repairing the communication? Can anything be learned from the child's linguistic nonfluencies, such as revision and maze behaviors, about potential problems in language formulation? Do contextual variables (linguistic, situational, or emotional) co-occur with difficulty in formulating language? What are the child's syntactic resources for making polite, indirect requests (and understanding them)? Does the child use different syntactic styles appropriately when communicating with different partners in different settings? Does the child have syntactic resources for expressing and understanding deictic relationships of person, place, and time? (*Deixis* is reference to relationships that vary with the speaker's perspective, e.g., *your* book becomes *my* book when the person speaking changes; *here* becomes *there* when the speaker's relative position to an object changes; "We are going to the zoo *tomorrow*" becomes "We went to the zoo *yesterday*" when the relative temporal relationship to the event changes.)

An additional set of questions that should be asked about contextually based language form is whether variations represent dialect or language difference. Most analysis systems are based on the development of standard English rules, but not all children are learning standard English. For example, if the child hears a mixture of Spanish and English at home, or is learning English from parents who themselves learned English as a second language, it is likely that morphological development will not follow the expected developmental pattern

Box 9.10 _____

The Development of Compound and Complex Sentences

Developmental stage information is based on suggestions by R. Paul (1981) for the point at which 50% to 90% of children exhibit a structure and by Lee (1974) for assigning Developmental Sentence Scores (DSS). As a rule of thumb, whenever a sentence contains two verbs that are not related as auxiliary and main verb, a compound or complex sentence form is evident.

Catenative (semiauxiliary) forms *gonna* (in Black English Vernacular, children may use /fɪn tə/ "fixin' to"), *wanna, hafta.*   These forms appear early, and rather than representing infinitival embeddings, probably function more as auxiliaries in simple sentences.
(Stage II; scores 2 as secondary verb in DSS.)

   "I'm gonna make some."

Early forms *let's, let me.*   These forms also act similar to unanalyzed catenatives. Note that they involve obligatory deletion of the infinitival *to.*
(Early Stage IV; scores 2 as secondary verb in DSS.)

   "Let me do it."

Simple infinitives with equivalent subjects in both clauses.
(Early Stage IV; scores 3 as secondary verb in DSS.)

   "I have to see."

   "He wants to come."

Compound sentences conjoined by *and.*   These are sentences in which two independent clauses are joined.
(Early Stage IV; the conjunction *and* scores 3 in DSS.)

   "He looked out the door and he saw a big dog."

Full propositional complements.   Full propositional complements occur when a complete sentence is used as the object of another sentence, usually following verbs such as *know, wonder, guess, think, pretend, hope, show,* and *forget,* which name an action that brings something into existence. The clause may or may not start with *that,* but does not begin with a *wh-* word.
(Early Stage IV; if used, *that* scores 8 as a conjunction in DSS.)

   "I know (that) he did it."

   "I think (that) that's right."

   "He said (that) he might come."

Simple *wh-* clauses with finite verbs.   Other early subordinate clauses are introduced by the subordinating conjunctions *what, where, why,* or *how* (these were called *indirect* or *embedded questions* by R. A. Brown, 1973).
(Early Stage IV; some *wh-* words score 6 as relative pronouns, and others score 8 as conjunctions in DSS.)

   "That's why it happened."

   "That's what I thought."

   "She knows how it works."

(continued)

BOX 9.10 continued

Double embeddings. These forms are credited when one clause is embedded within another (one of which might include a catenative).
(Late Stage IV—Early V; all primary and secondary verbs score in DSS.)

> *"I'm gonna think about how to do it."*

> *"You hafta let me come."*

Infinitive clauses with differing subjects. In these sentences, the subject of the embedded sentence differs from that of the main sentence.
(Late Stage V; score 5 as secondary verbs in DSS.)

> *"I want you to be my friend."*

> *"How do you get this to work?"*

Subordinating conjunction *if* is used.
(Late Stage V; *if* scores 5 in DSS.)

> *"I can come if you invite me."*

Relative clauses. These modify noun constituents of main sentences. They are introduced by one of the relative pronouns *which, who, that,* or *what.*
(Late Stage V; relative pronouns score 6 in DSS.)

> *"It's the one that I want."*

> *"That's the dog who bit me."*

Unmarked infinitive clauses. These are embedded infinitive clauses that do not contain *to* in the surface sentence and usually follow verbs like *let, make, watch,* or *help.*
(Stage V+; score 5 as secondary verbs in DSS.)

> *"He made her fall down."*

> *"She'll let me go."*

***Wh-* infinitive clauses.** These clauses are introduced by a *wh-* word and include the infinitival *to.*
(Stage V+; score 5 as secondary verbs in DSS.)

> *"Do you know how to do it?"*

> *"Show me what to do."*

Coordinating conjunction *because* is used.
(Stage V+; *because* scores 6 in DSS.)

> *"The boy fell because his bike hit a rock."*

Gerund clauses. Gerunds are verbs with *-ing* endings that are used as part of a noun phrase.
(Stage V+; gerunds score 8 as secondary verbs in DSS)

> *"I like making noise."*

> *"He hurt me by pushing me down."*

Subordinating conjunctions *when* and *so* are used.
(Stage V++; *so* scores 5, and *when* scores 8 in DSS.)

> *"Tell me when it's time."*

> *"He whispered so she wouldn't hear him."*

for middle-socioeconomic-class native standard English speakers. Children whose primary home language is Black English Vernacular (BEV) also will learn different language rules as part of the normal developmental process. When professionals assess the language of these children, they must consider which features represent developmental delays or abnormalities and which represent legitimate rules of other linguistic systems. This requires knowledge of more than one linguistic system and the ability to apply contrastive linguistic analysis techniques to identify features representing language difference.

A system for differentiating language difference from disorder, called **Black English Sentence Scoring (BESS)** is illustrated in Figure 9.3. I have developed this technique over several years, most recently in collaboration with Yvette Hyter (N. W. Nelson & Hyter, 1990a, 1990b), and with consultation from Walt Wolfram of the Center for Applied Linguistics. BESS is not an independent assessment system. It is an analysis procedure that starts with the techniques of Lee's (1974) Developmental Sentence Scoring (DSS), with scoring criteria in Chapter Appendix B. Children who use features of BEV also use features predicted by rules of standard English. Therefore, when a child's language sample is analyzed using BESS, the child is given credit for all structures that score in eight grammatical categories analyzed with DSS (indefinite pronouns and noun modifiers, personal pronouns, main verbs, secondary verbs, negatives, conjunctions, auxiliary inversion in questions, and Wh- questions). In addition, the child receives credit for structures that are acceptable

according to the rules of adult BEV as represented in the scoring standards of BESS in Chapter Appendix C. By adding up the points awarded according to DSS and BESS standards (including sentence points given differentially according to DSS and BESS standards) and dividing by 50, a mean BESS is computed that can be compared to a set of preliminary normative data gathered based on samples from 64 normally developing children of African American descent (most were from Kansas and Michigan, but a few were from Florida, Texas, Chicago, and Washington, DC) between the ages of 3:0 and 7:0. All were learning BEV as a primary linguistic system (see Table 9.5). For Hyter's (1984) master's thesis research, we both scored the first 25 sentences from 17 transcripts and agreed on 90 percent of the 560 ratings (Nelson & Hyter, 1990a). This suggests that trained evaluators can achieve a high level of interrater reliability. Hyter's research also supported the predictive validity of BESS as a tool for diagnosing language disorder, and Reveron (1984) described its revised version as a tool that avoids the dialectal bias of most language assessment procedures.

Washington and Craig (1994) and Craig and Washington (1995) listed 17 African American English forms (AAE and *Ebonics* are synonyms for BEV) that speech–language pathologists should recognize as signifying dialect difference. Research has shown that increased frequency of these AAE forms is associated with increased use of complex sentences and prepositional semantic relations for a group of low-income, urban African American preschoolers (21 boys and 24 girls).

TABLE 9.5   Means and standard deviations for Developmental Sentence Analysis (DSS) and Black English Sentence Scoring (BESS) scores at 6-month intervals from normative studies

AGE RANGE	N	MEAN DSS	SD	MEAN BESS	SD
3:0–3:6	8	5.63	0.91	7.44	1.15
3:6–4:0	8	5.73	1.04	7.71	0.98
4:0–4:6	8	7.47	1.58	9.33	1.26
4:6–5:0	8	7.51	1.68	8.85	1.48
5:0–5:6	8	8.86	1.93	10.79	1.92
5:6–6:0	8	8.31	2.04	10.02	2.16
6:0–6:6	8	9.12	2.43	11.08	1.61
6:6–7:0	8	9.47	1.72	11.17	2.17

Note: From *Black English Sentence Scoring: Development and Use as a Tool for Nonbiased Assessment* by N. W. Nelson and Y. D. Hyter, 1990, unpublished manuscript, Western Michigan University, Kalamazoo. Copyright 1990 by N. W. Nelson. Reprinted by permission.

FIGURE 9.3   Example scoring form and partial sample for Black English Sentence Scoring (BESS) using Developmental Sentence Scoring (DSS; Lee, 1974) as a base.

Name   Eric

Age   4;0

Date   May 31, 1993 DSS 3.73 BESS 6.55

	Indef. Pron.	Pers. Pron.	Prim. Verb	Sec. Verb	Neg.	Conj.	Inter. Rev.	WH Ques.	Sent. Point DSS	Sent. Point BESS	Total DSS	Total BESS
1. That the food that grandma ate.	1	6	1 / –, 2						0	1[c]	9[a]	11 [b]
2. I goin' to nursery school.		1	1 / –						0	1	1	3
3. I putting my sister on a motorcycle.		1,1	1 / –						0	1	2	4
4. I listening.		1	1 / –						0	1	1	3
5. I watched him yesterday,		1,2	2						1		6	
6. I like these.		1,3	1						1		6	
7. I push all these buttons, ok?	3	1,3	4 / –			–			0	1	7	12
8. They try catch me.		3,1	2 / –	5 / –					0	1	4	12
9. I had a spoon.		1	2						1		4	
10. Who this on the phone?	1		1 / –				1 / –	2 / –	0	1	1	6
11. Where the gun?			1 / –				1 / –	2 / –	0	1	0	5

Total DSS for this partial sample: 41 divided by 11 = 3.73

Total BESS for this partial sample: 72 divided by 11 = 6.55

[a]Sentence total for DSS.

[b]Sentence total for BESS.

[c]Point earned for BESS but not DSS. (Numbers above DSS attempt markers (–) represent credit awarded for BESS but not DSS.)

Note: From *Black English Sentence Scoring: Development and Use as a Tool for Nonbiased Assessment* by N. W. Nelson and Y. C. Hyter, 1990, unpublished manuscript, Western Michigan University, Kalamazoo. Copyright 1990 by N. W. Nelson. Reprinted by permission.

That is, they are positive signs of language development. The 17 forms are: (1) zero copula or auxiliary—*The bridge out; How you do this?* (2) subject-verb agreement—*What do this mean?* (3) abbreviations of "fixing to"—*She fitna backward flip*; "supposed to"—*When does it sposeta go?* and "about to"—*This one bouta go in the school*; (4) "ain't"—*Why she ain't comin?* (5) undifferentiated nominative, objective, and demonstrative pronoun case—*Him did and him*; (6) multiple negation—*I don't got no brothers*; (7) zero possessive—*He just hit the man car*; *Kids just goin' to walk to they school*; (8) zero past tense—*And this car crash*; *And then them fall*; (9) zero "-ing"—*And the lady is sleep*; (10) invariant "be"—*And this one be flying up in the sky*; *If he be drunk I'm taking him to jail*; (11) zero infinitive "to"—*Now my turn shoot you*; (12) zero plural—*Ghost are boys*; (13) double modal—*I'm is the last one ridin' on*; (14) regularized reflexive—*He stands by hisself*; (15) indefinite article pronunciation—*Branda had to play for a hour, didn't he?* (16) appositive pronoun—*The teacher she's goin' up here*; (17) remote past been—although no examples appeared in the data reported by Craig and Washington, examples Hyter and I gathered in the research for BESS (see Chapter Appendix C) included *She been whuptin' the baby* and *I been wanted this*. BESS awards credit for all of the AAE structures recommended as positive developmental signs by Washington and Craig (1994) and Craig and Washington (1995).

Stockman (1996) recommended a different approach to analyzing the language samples of preschool-age African American children. She described a criterion-referenced assessment procedure, which involved looking for a **Minimal Competency Core** (MCC), as a sign of whether a child was developing language normally, depending on the presence or absence of the set of minimal core features from a 2-hour play interaction with race cars and books. She described the MCC as the "set of linguistic features that the least competent normal child should demonstrate" (p. 359) at a given age. This allows a clinician to conclude that "a child is at risk if even one minimal competence feature is absent, in the face of ample opportunity to observe it" (p. 359). MCC analysis involves gathering a language sample and looking across the five linguistic rule systems—phonology, morphology, syntax, semantics, pragmatics—for evidence of productive use of a set of key features (see Box 9.11). Stockman defined productive use as a mini-

mum of four different exemplars with at least two variants to show flexibility. For example, to be credited with productive use of the phoneme /s/, the child needs to produce at least four total words with the /s/ phoneme, with at least two of them being different. To be credited with productive use of a pragmatic function, the child needs to use it at least four times in two different situations or events. Box 9.11 summarizes the MCC based on the data Stockman reported for seven African American children who were normally developing, distinguishing their language from that produced by a child with language learning difficulties.

Nonbiased evidence about the development of language form can be added to other pieces of information about the child and his or her language to make quantitative as well as qualitative decisions about the child's need for special services and potential areas to be targeted by short-term objectives.

Analyzing Language Content Variables. Analysis of middle-stage language content should include description of (1) the child's lexicon at the word level; (2) semantic roles the child uses and understands at the sentence level; (3) topics and topic organization strategies available to the child at the discourse level; and (4) the child's ability to linguistically encode and decode information representing world knowledge at broader cognitive processing levels.

First, the clinician should attempt to characterize the **lexicon** in the spontaneous language sample. Lexical quantification for children beyond the stage of early vocabulary acquisition is difficult. Most language samples tap only a small portion of the total lexicon a child might be able to use. When a child does not use certain words in a spontaneous sampling context, it is difficult to know whether the child's lexicon is limited or whether the sampling context was limited. This problem may be particularly acute when children and clinicians come from different cultural backgrounds and world experiences.

A quantitative technique sometimes recommended for measuring vocabulary diversity is the **type/token ratio** (TTR). Type/token ratios are computed by dividing the total number of different words (types) in a speaker's sample by the total number of all words produced (tokens) by the speaker in the sample. The SALT program (J. F. Miller & Chapman, 1991) computes the TTR automatically, making it a fairly easy measure to obtain. The question is, what does the measure mean? A

Box 9.11 _____

Minimal Competency Core
(summarized from Stockman, 1996) **that should be expected in the language of normally developing African American children in the age range 33 to 36 months** (productive use defined as a minimum of four different exemplars with at least two variants).

PHONOLOGICAL FEATURES CORE: 15 CONSONANTS:

/m/n/p/b/t/d/k/g/f/s/h/w/y/l/r/
(/r/ not essential)

PRAGMATIC FUNCTIONS CORE: 8 FUNCTIONS:

- comments
- social interaction regulations: asking questions and requesting objects and actions
- responses to prior speech acts: spontaneous imitations, nonobligated responses (affirming or negating the prior utterance), and obligated responses (answering questions)
- repair functions: initiating repairs (saying "Huh?" or self-initiating repetition or revision of own utterances) and responding to requests for repairs (changing the phonetic and/or grammatic form)

SEMANTIC RELATIONS CORE: 10 CATEGORIES:

- five major verb categories: existence, state, locative state, action, locative action
- four minor or coordinated categories: specification, possession, time, and negation
- at least one superordinate category: usually causality

MORPHOSYNTACTIC CORE: MLU GREATER THAN 2.70

- *-ing* inflection
- four syntactic construction types: simple nonelaborated (*He eat food*), simple elaborated with an inflectional or lexical modifier (*He eating the food*), simple combined (*He eating food and she sitting*), complex (*Let me see the car*)

---

problem with the TTR is that it tends to be negatively related to increasing sample lengths, because, as sentence length increases, grammatical function words tend to make up a greater proportion of the total sample. Therefore, older children, who generally produce longer samples and use more complex grammatical constructions (with a higher proportion of function words), may in fact have relatively lower TTRs. If the sample length is not controlled, TTR comparisons may be meaningless, or even deceptive. However, as Loban (1963) commented, the TTR measure "can disclose important distinctions *when the size of the language sample is kept uniform*" (p. 22). It is also helpful to be aware of the gen-

eral rule of thumb suggested by J. F. Miller (1981) based on the data Mildred Templin (1957) gathered for 480 3:0- to 8:0-year-old children. Across this age range, across both genders, and regardless of socioeconomic status, Templin found TTRs of approximately 1:2, or 0.50. Miller suggested that "if a normal hearing child's TTR is significantly below 0.50 we can be reasonably certain the sparseness of vocabulary use is *not* an artifact of SES but is probably indicative of a language-specific deficiency" (1981, p. 41).

Because of problems with the TTR, alternatives have been proposed. Bennett (1989) developed Referential Semantic Analysis (RSA) as an alternative method to measure expressive vocabulary diversity. Rather than using a ratio that varies little with increasing age and vocabulary development, Bennett and Alter (1985) gathered normative data on the means for the total words and number of different words produced in 50 utterance samples by youngsters between the ages of 2 and 15 years. These data provide evidence of developmental advances. Bennett's original samples included 20 middle-class normally developing children (from rural and urban Virginia) at each age level. The children were grouped into 6-month intervals from ages 2 to 5 years, into 1-year intervals from 5 to 12 years, and into 2-year intervals for the age range of 13 to 15 years. In a follow-up study, Olson and Bennett (1987a, 1987b) studied test–retest reliability and possible geographic differences for a group of 24 children (6- and 7-years-olds) by comparing 12 children from Virginia with 12 children from North Dakota. Their findings showed no significant geographic differences and significant test–retest reliability coefficients of .68 for number of different words and .88 for number of total words. A computer software program (Bennett, 1989) facilitates the computation of RSA data and generates separate counts for the number of different words and total words coded as nouns, verbs, adjectives, adverbs, pronouns, conjunctions, prepositions, articles, and "other." The program can also generate the derived ages, as well as the overall number of different and total words for the complete sample, along with derived ages (age–equivalency scores).

Watkins, Kelly, Harbers, and Hollis (1995) also recommended using **number of different words** (NDW) rather than TTR to measure lexical diversity. They compared language samples, gathered by an adult interacting with a standard set of toys, from 25 children with specific language impairment (SLI), 25 age-equivalent children (AE), and 25 language-equivalent children (LE). The SLI and AE groups both had a mean age of 4:11. The LE group had a mean age of 3:2. All three groups earned the same TTR for 50-utterance samples (mean = .45; SD = .05) and almost the same for 100-utterance samples (mean = .35; SD = .05 for SLI and AE; mean = .34; SD = .04 for LE). Thus, TTR did not distinguish the SLI children even when sample size, in terms of numbers of utterances, was controlled. When sample size was controlled as number of tokens (total words), the NDW measure did differentiate the SLI chil-

dren from their AE peers, but found them not different from their LE peers, as expected. The mean NDWs for 100-tokens was 53 for both SLI (SD = 6) and LE (SD = 8) groups; whereas it was 60 (SD = 8) for AE peers. For a 200-token sample, the mean NDWs (and SDs) were: SLI 82 (9), LE 84 (11), and AE 93 (8).

Many other questions might be asked about the child's lexicon based on evidence from spontaneous language samples. For example, does the child have a variety of words to indicate fine shades of meaning or seem to have to make do with a limited set of nonspecific **"all-purpose" words** such as *stuff* and *thing?* Does the child create any new words using derivational morphemes that seem generative rather than merely imitative (e.g., "destoppable tank")? By the middle grades in elementary school, does the child understand many multiple-meaning words and figurative meanings? Does the child use appropriate memory and recall strategies to acquire the lexicon appropriate to key contexts of the child's life, such as preschool and early elementary school classrooms?

Second, questioning about language content might address **semantic roles** the child uses and understands at the sentence level. For example, does the child use words that fill a variety of semantic roles (e.g., actor, action, state, location, time), or does the child encode only a limited variety of semantic relations? A summary of four studies of the development of semantic relationships (Stockman & Vaughn-Cooke, 1986) showed that 11 major and 12 minor semantic categories were all represented in the language samples of children in Post Stage II (MLU > 4.0) by the age of 53 to 54 months. Even more important, these findings were consistent across the three subject populations, working-class black children, working-class white children, and middle-class white children. The 11 major categories were *existence, action, locative action, state, locative state, negation, possession, attribution, notice, intention, and recurrence.* The 12 minor categories were *Wh-questions, place, action + place, dative, instrument, quantity, time, mood, coordination, causality, epistemic,* and *antithesis.* Stockman's (1996) Minimal Competence Core for semantic roles produced by normally developing African American children at age 30 to 33 months appears in Box 9.11.

A third level of analysis might address **topics** and **topic organization** strategies available to the child at the discourse level. Brinton and Fujiki (1989) described this area as encompassing both what speakers talk *about* and how speakers *manage* what they talk about. In asking what children talk about, the clinician might ask whether particular categories or topics appear frequently and might ask questions about the nature of the topics. For example, does the child talk mostly about concrete things or about abstract topics as well? By the time children enter the middle stages of language acquisition, they should be able to talk about remote topics as well as the here-and-now (review discussion in Chapter 8). For children in elementary school the specialist may use language sampling to probe their understanding and ability to talk about curricular content.

Questions should also address overlapping language content and use issues regarding topic organization and manipulation. Brinton and Fujiki (1989) included questions about how topics are introduced, continued, changed, and recycled. They noted that topic manipulation strategies change with increasing age and linguistic maturity. Roots of topic management are found in the interactions of caregivers and infants with the establishment of joint reference (discussed in Chapter 8). Growth in topic management involves a reduction in the child's dependence on adults to construct and change topic sequences and a reduction in the number of different topics introduced in a particular time period. Five-year-olds are more likely to recycle previous topics in conversations than 9-year-olds are, but research has also shown considerable variability in several areas across different age groups (Brinton & Fujiki, 1984). The development of independent strategies to manipulate topics is observed well into middle childhood (Brinton & Fujiki, 1989). Many questions might be asked in this area. For example, can the child organize topics logically and follow topic shading strategies to connect one with another? Are there any unusual delays in responding or perseverative topics that might suggest emotional impairment or other processing difficulties? Does the child focus on tangential aspects of topics and seem unable to grasp the big picture?

A final level of analysis regarding language content might address the child's ability to linguistically encode and decode information representing **world knowledge.** At the information processing level, what can be hypothesized about the child's developing perceptual and cognitive abilities based on topics the child talks about? Are the child's word memory and recall strategies adequate? Children with specific language impairments have more difficulty repeating three- and four-syllable nonsense words than their peers, and such problems are correlated with difficulty comprehending longer sentences, suggesting a problem with phonological working memory (Montgomery, 1995). (Problems like this are also discussed in Chapters 3 and 4).

How do higher levels of language comprehension relate to broader understanding of the world? Milosky (1990) reviewed two language comprehension models. According to the traditional decoding model of language comprehension, listeners start by using semantic and syntactic decoding strategies to generate a small number of possible meanings for individual sentences. Then they disambiguate more than one possible meaning by using available contextual information and world knowledge. The alternative model suggests that almost every word has many possible meanings, and that to understand listeners must *start* the language comprehension process by drawing on existing world knowledge. Then they activate only relevant senses of words and information and attempt to make incoming information relevant to what they already know. Milosky described this top-down processing model (see Chapter 3) as more efficient:

> *The relevant information, or world knowledge, that is accessed and activated is, in part, determined by what knowledge is relevant given the speaker, the physical environment, the social occasion, the goals of the interaction, the affective variables, and the prior discussion. These all enable a listener to determine rapidly and selectively what a speaker is saying. (1990, p. 3)*

The implications of this alternative view are significant for guiding language assessment and intervention. Assessment and intervention goals shift from learning a set of words or structures to learning how "to call up relevant knowledge and to use language in order to interact and add to that knowledge in some coherent fashion" (Milosky, 1990, p. 4).

Analyzing Language Use Variables.   Analysis of middle-stage language use might include description of (1) the child's ability to use language to communicate a variety of intentions and to perform a variety of pragmatic functions (also called **speech acts**); (2) the child's ability to organize discourse of several types; and (3) the child's ability to use and understand contextually based variations in linguistic, paralinguistic, and nonlinguistic communicative features.

Questions about the adequacy of children's language use relate ultimately to definitions of communicative competence. The classic definition of communicative competence was provided by sociolinguist Dell Hymes (1972), who defined it as a language user's

> *. . . knowledge of sentences, not only as grammatical but also as appropriate. He or she acquires competence as to when to speak, when not, and as what to talk about with whom, when, where, in what manner. (p. 277)*

When assessing communicative competence, the first level of analysis might address the child's intentional use of varied **pragmatic functions.** This aspect relates to the first of three clusters Dollaghan and Miller (1986) suggested to guide observations of communicative competence. They identified it as the set of "communicative intents, communicative functions, or speech acts: the reasons for which speakers communicate" (p. 116).

This analysis is based on the question "What purposes do the child's utterances seem to serve?" It may be difficult to decide how to categorize the speech acts of a particular child. As noted in Chapter 8, taxonomies of communicative intentions have been proposed by various authors (e.g., Bates et al., 1975; Dale, 1980; Dore, 1974; Halliday, 1975). Some argue that no one taxonomy should be applied to all children because one set of categories may characterize development better at one point than another (Halliday, 1975; Lund & Duchan, 1993). Dollaghan and Miller (1986) also noted that taxonomies of normal development may "fail to capture numerous aspects of the performance of the disordered subjects" (p. 109). Variations of communicative intention were illustrated by the work of Prizant and his colleagues (Prizant, 1987; Prizant & Duchan, 1981; Prizant & Rydell, 1984) for the echolalic utterances of children with autism.

Taxonomies for organizing pragmatic functions into categories for children functioning at the preverbal and single-word levels were presented in Chapter 8 (see Tables 8.4 and 8.5), based on summaries by Roth and Spekman (1984). Here, Roth and Spekman's third level,

which summarizes categories appropriate to middle-stage multiword levels of production, is reprinted (see Table 9.6). The inclusion of this particular taxonomical set should not suggest, however, that these are the only categories to consider.

To be useful in intervention, speech-act analysis should surpass merely coding and counting pragmatic intentions. Fey (1986) proposed a decision-making matrix based on the relative use of **assertive** and **responsive conversational acts** by young children. In Fey's system, **assertive acts** include *requestives* of four types (for information, action, clarification, and attention); *assertives* of three types (comments, statements, and disagreements); and performatives (e.g., claims, jokes, teasing, protests, and warnings). **Responsive acts** include *responses to requests* of four types (for information, action, clarification, and attention), and *responses to assertives and performatives.* Fey used two other categories to classify individual utterances as **imitations** or as **other** (when they do not fit well into any of the other three categories). Beyond the utterance level, conversational acts are also coded at the discourse level, depending on whether they serve to **initiate, maintain,** or **extend** topics, or to **extend topics tangentially** (not adequately). Box 9.12 provides an example of this analysis procedure. Children who show a high rate of both assertive and responsive conversational acts are **active conversationalists.** Children who show a high rate of assertive acts but a low rate of responsive ones are **verbal noncommunicators.** Children who show a low rate of assertive acts but a high rate of responsive ones are **passive conversationalists.** Children who are low in use of either assertive or responsive acts are **inactive communicators** (see Figure 9.4). Children with these varied patterns of conversational speech acts are considered to have different intervention needs (see Chapter 10 for potential goals). Stockman's (1996) Minimal Competence Core for pragmatic functions produced by normally developing African American children at age 30 to 33 months appears in Box 9.11.

Another system for coding spontaneous social interactions among preschoolers was devised by Rice, Sell, and Hadley (1990). Called the **Social Interactive Coding System** (SICS), this is an observational tool that can be used "on-line" (i.e., while the events are occurring) to code social interaction behaviors in free play

TABLE 9.6   Communicative intentions expressed at the multiword stage of development

INTENTION	DEFINITION	EXAMPLE
1. Requesting information	Utterances that solicit information, permission, confirmation, or repetition.	"Where's Mary?" "Can I come?"
2. Requesting action	Utterances that solicit action or cessation of action.	"Give me the doll." "Stop it." "Don't do that."
3. Responding to requests	Utterances that supply solicited information or acknowledge preceding messages.	"Okay." "Mary is over there." "No, you can't come." "It's blue."
4. Stating or commenting	Utterances that state facts or rules, express beliefs, attitudes, or emotions, or describe environmental aspects.	"This a bird." "You have to throw the dice, first." "I don't like dogs." "I'm happy today." "My school is two blocks away." "He can't do that."
5. Regulating conversational behavior	Utterances that monitor and regulate interpersonal contact.	"Hey, Marvin!" "Hi," "Bye," "Please." "Here you are." "Know what I did?"
6. Other performatives	Utterances that tease, warn, claim, exclaim, or convey humor.	"You can't catch me." "Watch out." "It's my turn." "The dog said 'moo.' "

Note: From "Assessing the Pragmatic Abilities of Children; Part 1. Organizational Framework and Assessment Parameters" by F. P. Roth and N. J. Spekman, 1984, *Journal of Speech and Hearing Disorders, 49,* p. 5. Copyright 1984 by American Speech-Language-Hearing Association. Reprinted by permission.

(5-minute blocks are observed). These include the start time, play activity, addressee, verbal interactive status, script code (type of play area), play level (solitary, adjacent, or social interactive), and language used. Thus, this approach may be used with bilingual children. Verbal interactive behaviors coded include *initiation* (coded as repetition if repeated after the first initiation fails), *response* (coded as one-word verbal R-V-1, multiword verbal R-V, or nonverbal R-NV), and *ignore.*

After gathering information about speech act behavior the specialist might address a second level of analysis, the child's ability to organize and participate in the production of **discourse types.** This cluster was identified by Dollaghan and Miller (1986) as the pragmatic "rules for sequencing communicative acts, or for constructing and managing discourse" (p. 116). The major types of discourse to be probed include free conversation, narrative, and expository.

The usual discourse context for gathering language samples is free conversation with an adult. This is the genre of participant discourse (J. N. Britton, 1979), discussed previously. As examples of the kinds of rules used in structuring conversational discourse, Dollaghan and Miller (1986) listed (1) initiating and terminating conversational sequences, (2) exchanging speaker turns, (3) introducing and maintaining topics, and (4) identifying and repairing conversational breakdowns. A variety of potential problems have been identified in this area among children with specific language impairments. For example, Brinton and Fujiki (1982) found that children with specific language impairments who were between ages 5:6 and 6:0 years frequently ignored

Box 9.12

Two second grade children conversing in the context of an art activity in which they are tearing and gluing paper to construct pictures. This is a portion of a transcript formatted with the conventions of SALT (Miller & Chapman, 1991) and coded with Fey's (1986) Communication Acts Profiling (CAP) codes. Alex was identified as having a language problem that necessitated an Individual Program Plan (this sample was gathered in Newfoundland by Kim Rideout-Waller and Sheila Greene when they were graduate students at Western Michigan University). In the conversational sample, Rideout-Waller and Greene found Alex to be an active communicator. He used 24 assertive conversational acts, responded to all questions he was asked, and initiated 13 new topics.

Assertive Acts

RQIN = request information
RQAC = request action
RQCL = request clarification
RQAT = request attention
ASCO = assertive comment
ASST = assertive statement
ASDA = assertive disagreement
PERF = performative

Responsive Acts

RSIN = respond to request for information
RSAC = respond to request for action
RSCL = respond to request for clarification
RSAT = respond to request for attention
RSAS = respond to assertive
RSPF = respond to performative

IMIT = imitate
OTHER = uncodable in other categories

TOPIC CONTROL

IT = initiate topic
MT = maintain topic
ET = extend topic
ETT = extend topic tangentially

LANGUAGE SAMPLE IN SALT FORMAT WITH FEY'S CAPCODES

$[a] Alex, Peer, Kim (the clinician)
A: I'm gonna make a house [ASCO][IT].
P: I need some glue [ASST][ET].
P: You got the glue [RQIN][MT]?
A: I need to get a popsicle stick [ASST][ET].
=[b] for managing the glue
P: You gotta rip it [ASST][IT].
A: Here comes the glue [RSAC][MT].
= Alex responds to RQAC implied indirectly in peer's prior turn as the glue comes sailing
P: Oh no [ASST][MT]!
A: That's a nice roof [ASST][IT].

P: There, is that a nice roof [RQAT][MT]?
= Kim entered room bringing popsicle sticks
P: Look at the piece I got [RQAT][IT].
A: What's it for? [RQIN][MT]?
= A has glue on his stick and it starts dripping
A: I don't know where to put it [ASST][IT].
K: Do you want a paper towel [RQIN][MT]?
A: I got to [RSIN][MT].
A: My hands are go/ing to stick to it [ASST][MT].
A: Yah, I do need a paper towel [ASST][MT].
P: Oh, it's run/ing down the side [ASCO][MT].

[a]In SALT conventions, speakers are identified on a line that begins $.

[b]In SALT conventions, transcriber comments are made on a line that begins =.

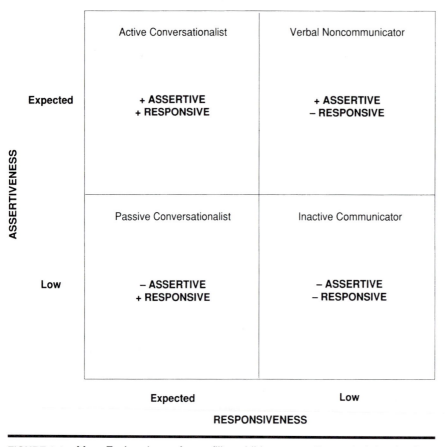

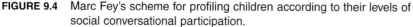

FIGURE 9.4   Marc Fey's scheme for profiling children according to their levels of social conversational participation.

Note: From Marc E. Fey, *Language Intervention with Young Children.* Copyright © 1986 by Allyn and Bacon. Reprinted with permission.

or responded inappropriately to conversational requests. However, some of their problems seemed to relate more to difficulty managing language content than language use. Some of the children showed skill in using strategies that facilitated the flow of conversations but showed no understanding of the content.

Brinton and Fujiki (1989) suggested questions to ask about conversational samples of children with potential language disorders: Does the child initiate topics or mostly respond to questions asked by the conversational partner? Does the child stay on topic or make frequent switches without preparing the listener? Does the child have presupposition skills to judge how much informa-

tion the listener needs? Does the child have strategies to repair communication when it breaks down?

Although conversational discourse provides an important context for judging communicative competence, it is not the only discourse genre to probe. As illustrated by K. Nelson's (1989) bedtime transcripts of 2-year-old Emily, not unusually, rather young children produce monologues that approximate the structure of narratives. By probing narrative discourse contexts, professionals can determine whether a child has internalized rules related to the genre of spectator discourse (J. N. Britton, 1979) involving longer turns, more organized structures, and domination by a single speaker.

Young children's earliest narratives appear as "heaps" of isolated information. As they increase in maturity, children become better at maintaining a central focus while relating a logical, temporally and causally ordered sequence of events that relate to the center (Applebee, 1978; Botvin & Sutton-Smith, 1977; Hedberg & Westby, 1993; Westby, 1984). The scoring criteria for analyzing narrative development with this approach (often identified as the Applebee approach) appear in Figure 9.5. McCabe and Rollins (1994) described a procedure for gathering personal narratives and performing "high point" analyses of preschoolers' narratives and for recognizing differences in narrative structure for children of different cultures.

When observing **narrative development,** the clinician can also ask questions about the child's apparent internalization of a narrative schema, sometimes referred to as "story grammar." Several variations of story grammar schemata have been proposed (e.g., N. S. Johnson & Mandler, 1980; Rumelhart, 1975; Stein & Glenn, 1979; Thorndyke, 1977). As shown in Table 9.7, most describe a discourse schema that includes one or more episodes with information about setting (e.g., person, place, and time), a problem, some action aimed at alleviating the problem (more complex story grammar

schemas include a plan by the protagonist before taking action), an outcome, and an ending, which completes the story by relating logically to issues raised in the beginning. A description of feelings, personality traits, and motives of main characters are also observed in more mature narratives (Westby, 1984, 1991). Scoring criteria for analyzing narratives based on their inclusion of story grammar structural properties (Hedberg & Westby, 1993) are shown in Figure 9.6.

Telling and comprehending narratives requires more than a knowledge of story grammar. Judith Johnston (1982b) suggested that professionals analyze narrative ability by looking for evidence that children (1) use **story grammar** (including both a setting and a coherent episode structure); (2) use **mature organization;** (3) use knowledge of common **event scripts** and sequences in constructing a plot; (4) operationalize linguistic **textual cohesion devices** (e.g., pronoun reference and complex sentences); and (5) demonstrate sensitivity to the **needs of the listener.** The ultimate test is whether the story was communicated clearly.

The third discourse type that the specialist might probe through spontaneous sampling is **expository.** Because of its importance in later stages of language acquisition, expository discourse is discussed more fully

TABLE 9.7   Comparison of four major story grammars to a simplified story grammar

THOMAS ET AL. (1984)	MANDLER & JOHNSON (1977)	STEIN & GLENN (1979)	THORNDYKE (1977)	RUMELHART (1975)
Setting	Setting	Setting	Setting	Setting
Problem	Beginning	Initiating event	Theme	Event
			Event	Episode, or
			+	Change of
			Goal	state, or Action,
				or Event + Event
Response	Reaction	Internal response	Plot	Reaction
	Attempt		Subgoal	Internal response
		Attempt	+	+
			Attempt	Overt response
			+	
Outcome	Outcome	Consequence	Outcome	
	Ending	Reaction	Resolution	

Note: From "Story Grammar Skills in School-Age Children" by J. L. Page and S. R. Stewart. Reprinted from *Topics in Language Disorders,* Vol. 5, No. 2, p. 18. © 1985, Aspen Publishers, Inc. Reprinted with permission.

FIGURE 9.5 Criteria for rating narrative maturity based on descriptions by Applebee (1978), Botvin
and Sutton-Smith (1977), Nelson and Friedman (1988), and Westby (1982, 1984).

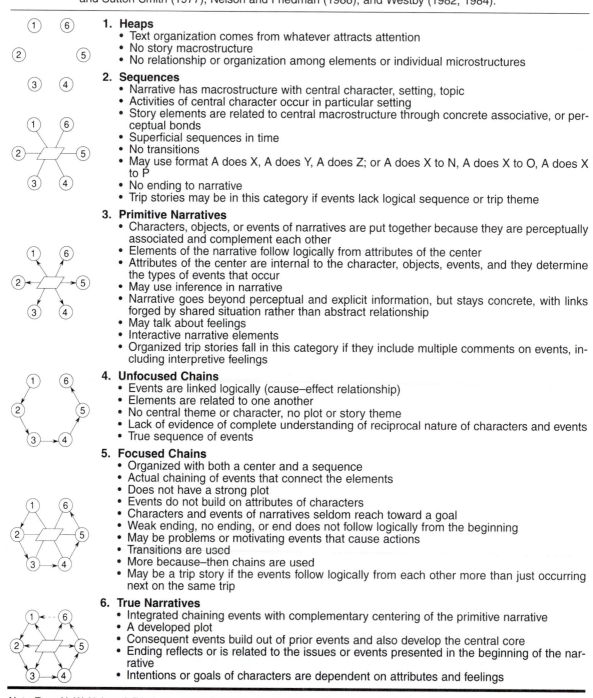

1. **Heaps**
   - Text organization comes from whatever attracts attention
   - No story macrostructure
   - No relationship or organization among elements or individual microstructures

2. **Sequences**
   - Narrative has macrostructure with central character, setting, topic
   - Activities of central character occur in particular setting
   - Story elements are related to central macrostructure through concrete associative, or perceptual bonds
   - Superficial sequences in time
   - No transitions
   - May use format A does X, A does Y, A does Z; or A does X to N, A does X to O, A does X to P
   - No ending to narrative
   - Trip stories may be in this category if events lack logical sequence or trip theme

3. **Primitive Narratives**
   - Characters, objects, or events of narratives are put together because they are perceptually associated and complement each other
   - Elements of the narrative follow logically from attributes of the center
   - Attributes of the center are internal to the character, objects, events, and they determine the types of events that occur
   - May use inference in narrative
   - Narrative goes beyond perceptual and explicit information, but stays concrete, with links forged by shared situation rather than abstract relationship
   - May talk about feelings
   - Interactive narrative elements
   - Organized trip stories fall in this category if they include multiple comments on events, including interpretive feelings

4. **Unfocused Chains**
   - Events are linked logically (cause–effect relationship)
   - Elements are related to one another
   - No central theme or character, no plot or story theme
   - Lack of evidence of complete understanding of reciprocal nature of characters and events
   - True sequence of events

5. **Focused Chains**
   - Organized with both a center and a sequence
   - Actual chaining of events that connect the elements
   - Does not have a strong plot
   - Events do not build on attributes of characters
   - Characters and events of narratives seldom reach toward a goal
   - Weak ending, no ending, or end does not follow logically from the beginning
   - May be problems or motivating events that cause actions
   - Transitions are used
   - More because–then chains are used
   - May be a trip story if the events follow logically from each other more than just occurring next on the same trip

6. **True Narratives**
   - Integrated chaining events with complementary centering of the primitive narrative
   - A developed plot
   - Consequent events build out of prior events and also develop the central core
   - Ending reflects or is related to the issues or events presented in the beginning of the narrative
   - Intentions or goals of characters are dependent on attributes and feelings

Note: From N. W. Nelson & Friedman, 1988. © 1988 by N. W. Nelson. Shared by permission of the author.

..

FIGURE 9.6   Scoring criteria for analyzing narratives based on their inclusion of story grammar structural properties.

STORY GRAMMAR STRUCTURAL PROPERTIES

Properties

Levels	Animated Character	Related Statements	Temporal Relations	Causal Relations/ Consequence	Resolution/ Ending	Goal	Attempt	Plan	Obstacles
1. Isolated Description	–/+	–	–	–	–	–	–	–	–
2. Descriptive Sequence	–/+	+	–	–	–	–	–	–	–
3. Action Sequence	+	+	+	–	–	–	–	–	–
4. Reactive Sequence	+	+	+	+	–/+	–	–	–	–
5. Abbreviated Episode	+	+	+	+	–/+	+	+	–	–
6. Complete Episode	+	+	+	+	–/+	+	+	+	–
7. Complex Episode	+	+	+	+	–/+	+	+	+	+

Note: Multiple episode stories may consist of episodes at the reactive sequence level or higher. The properties of each episode must be coded independently.

Note: From *Analyzing Storytelling Skills: Theory to Practice* (p. 134) by N. L. Hedberg and C. E. Westby, © 1993. Communication Skill Builders, Inc., a division of The Psychological Corporation. Reprinted by permission. All rights reserved.

and illustrated in Chapters 11 and 12. Expository discourse may be defined as discourse that conveys factual or technical information. This discourse is demanded when a child is asked to explain the rules of a game or how to make something, to describe the characteristics of an object, or to engage in "show-and-tell." Some expository discourse, such as that used to explain the making of a peanut butter sandwich, is ordered by temporal sequence. Other expository discourse, such as a discussion of pets, may be organized as a series of hierarchically or horizontally related categories, with definitions and examples of each. Most academic discourse produced by teachers and in textbooks is expository.

Questions to ask about expository discourse include: Does the child have enough cognitive control of the topic to organize an explanation logically? Does the child use linguistic cohesion devices, such as complex sentences and logical connectors? Does the child demonstrate excessive linguistic nonfluencies (e.g., mazes, tangles, and revisions) that suggest internalized processing and text formulation difficulties? Does the child show evidence of comprehending expository discourse produced by others orally or in textbooks?

The third level analysis of pragmatic aspects of language development asks about the child's ability to use and understand **contextually based variations** in linguistic, paralinguistic, and nonlinguistic form and content. This cluster of behaviors was identified by Dollaghan and Miller (1986) as "the ways in which speakers and listeners integrate linguistic and nonlinguistic information and includes rules for presupposing and foregrounding information" (p. 116). Dollaghan and Miller also included rules for selecting and maintaining speech register and for using cohesion devices and deixis (considered previously under issues of language form). Children with language impairments, especially those with specific language impairments, may not always show delays relative to their normally developing peers in these areas. When Fey and Leonard (1984) investigated discourse adaptation skills of 4:6- to 6-year-old children, based on whether they were talking to adults, age-peers, or toddlers, they found that children with specific language impairments performed at least as well as normally developing younger-age language-matched peers and below the levels of same-age peers in only a few areas (related to form variables such as MLU and the ability to ask internal state questions).

Many questions might be used to focus language sample analysis on pragmatic adaptation, including: Does the child seem to have ways of altering the delivery style to achieve a certain effect (e.g., teasing, polite forms)? Does the child seem to understand such variations? Does the child have any strategies for helping out if the listener fails to understand something the child said? Can this child participate appropriately in classroom discussions?

Formal Assessment

Although informal assessment of spontaneous language samples provides some of the most useful information about the nature of children's language abilities and disabilities, particularly in the middle stage, it is not sufficient for all assessment purposes. Formal assessment with standardized tests may be required to identify children as having a language disorder and being eligible for service. It may also help to check clinical impressions of relative strengths and weaknesses against the performance of normative groups.

Unfortunately, many formal standardized tests promise more than they can deliver. McCauley and Swisher (1984) applied 10 psychometric criteria for norm-referenced tests to a review of 30 language and articulation tests designed to be used with preschool children: (1) description of the normative sample, (2) adequate sample size, (3) item analysis used to promote test reliability and validity, (4) report of measures of central tendency and variability for relevant subgroups, (5) evidence of concurrent validity, (6) evidence of predictive validity, (7) estimate of test–retest reliability, (8) inter-

examiner reliability, (9) detailed description of administration and scoring procedures, and (10) specification of qualifications required of test administrators or scorers. They found that half of the tests met no more than two of the criteria (most often, numbers 9 and 10). Most frequently *unmet* criteria were those requiring empirical evidence of test validity and reliability. Table 9.8 summarizes the results for the 30 instruments that McCauley and Swisher reviewed. The full identification of these instruments appears in Chapter Appendix A with the summary of test instruments designed for the middle stages of language acquisition.

McCauley and Swisher (1984) noted the possibility that psychometric test-evaluation may discourage the use of standardized tests. Rather than avoiding formal test use entirely, however, they recommended that potential test users should become more sophisticated in recognizing psychometric flaws and should consider these limitations when interpreting test results and making clinical decisions. They also pointed out that "clinical decisions are never properly based on test results alone" (p. 41). Furthermore, they noted that, by being selective, consumers of standardized tests may influence premarketing development of these instruments.

A more recent update (Plante & Vance, 1994) shows continuing problems with lack of information in test manuals about whether instruments meet psychometric criteria. Plante and Vance replicated application of the 10 McCauley and Swisher (1984) criteria with 21 tests for preschoolers. They found that:

> *Thirty-eight percent of the tests met half or more of the criteria. Most tests met only four criteria, with the most frequently met criterion being adequate description of test administration and scoring. The criteria met least frequently concerned predictive validity, followed by adequate description of the normative population.* (p. 16)

Plante and Vance did note some improvements over the McCauley and Swisher review. Specifically, Plante and Vance found twice as many tests meeting criteria for reporting sample size, means and standard deviations, and concurrent validity as McCauley and Swisher did.

Plante and Vance (1994) studied four of the tests further in a validation study of test sensitivity and speci-

TABLE 9.8   Tests meeting psychometric criteria established by McCauley and Swisher (1984)

CRITERION	NUMBER OF TESTS	TESTS
1. Description of normative sample	3	ITPA, PPVT-R, TOLD
2. Sample size	6	BTBC, ITPA, PPVT-R, STACL, SOLST, TOLD
3. Item analysis	9	BTBC, EOWPVT, ITPA, PPVT, PPVT-R, QT, SICD, T-D, TOLD
4. Means and standard deviations	7	ICLAT, PAT, PPVT, T-D, TACL, TOLD, TTC
5. Concurrent validity	5	CELI, PLAI, PLST, TOLD, VLDS
6. Predictive validity	0	—
7. Test–retest reliability	1	TOLD
8. Interexaminer reliability	0	—
9. Description of test procedures	25	ACLC, BLST, BTBC, CELI, DASE, EOWPVT, ICLAT, ITPA, LAS, NSST, PAT, PLAI, PPVT, PPVT-R, REEL-scale, STACL, SICD, SOLST, T-D, TACL, TOLD, TTC, UTLD, VANE-L, VLDS,
10. Description of tester qualifications	14	BLST, ICLAT, ITPA, PLAI, PPVT, PPVT-R, QT, SICD, STACL, SOLST, TACL, TOLD, UTLD, VANE-L

ACLC, Assessment of Children's Language Comprehension; BLST, Bankson Language Screening Test; BTBC, Boehm Test of Basic Concepts; CELI, Carrow Elicited Language Inventory; DASE, The Denver Articulation Screening Examination; EOWPVT, Expressive One Word Picture Vocabulary Test; ICLAT, Illinois Children's Language Assessment Test; ITPA, Illinois Test of Psycholinguistic Abilities; LAS, Laradon Articulation Scale; NSST, Northwestern Syntax Screening Test; PAT, Photo Articulation Test; PLAI, Preschool Language Assessment Instrument; PLST, Preschool Language Screening Test; PPVT, Peabody Picture Vocabulary Test; PPVT-R, Peabody Picture Vocabulary Test—Revised; QT, The Quick Test; REEL-scale, The Receptive Expressive Emergent Language Scale; SICD, Sequenced Inventory of Communication Development; SOLST, Stephens Oral Language Screening Test; STACL, The Screening Test of Auditory Comprehension of Language; T-D, Templin-Darley Tests of Articulation; TACL, The Test of Auditory Comprehension of Language; TOLD, Test of Language Development; TTC, The Token Test for Children; UTLD, Utah Test of Language Development; VANE, Vane Evaluation of Language Scale; VLDS, Verbal Language Development Scale.

Note: From "Psychometric Review of Language and Articulation Tests for Preschool Children" by R. J. McCauley and L. Swisher, 1984, *Journal of Speech and Hearing Disorders, 49,* p. 40. Copyright 1984 by American Speech-Language-Hearing Association. Reprinted by permission.

ficity (review Figure 9.1). The four tests were the Clark-Madison Test of Oral Language (CMTOL; Clark & Madison, 1986), the Structured Photographic Expressive Language Test-II (SPELT-II; Werner & Kresheck, 1983), the Test for Auditory Comprehension of Language-Revised (TACL-R; Carrow-Woolfolk, 1985), and the Test of Early Language Development, 2nd edition (TELD-2; Hresko, Reid, & Hammill, 1991). Of these,

only the SPELT-II showed acceptable sensitivity and specificity. That is, it accurately identified 90 percent of a group of 20 children (half low income and half middle to high income; 12 white, 3 black, 4 Hispanic, 1 Native American) who were previously clinically diagnosed as having specific language impairment (showing good sensitivity) and 90 percent of a comparison group (similar in socioeconomic and racial makeup) as having normal language. None of the other three measures approached these levels of accuracy. Furthermore, "No combination of tests produced as accurate a discrimination as use of the SPELT-II alone" (p. 20).

Standardized tests are most useful when professionals select them to test diagnostic hypotheses. The first hypothesis tested may be rather broad. It may simply be that the child will score below normal limits on a broad comprehensive test of language abilities. For this purpose, tests that include a variety of sub-tests, such as the Clinical Evaluation of Language Fundamentals—Third Edition (CELF-3) (Semel, Wiig, & Secord, 1995) or the Test of Language Development-2 Primary (TOLD-2 P) (Newcomer & Hammill, 1988), may be used with children in middle stages of language acquisition. The best way to learn about the strengths and foibles of a particular instrument is to administer it to many children. No test is without its limitations, and it is important to remember that any standardized test may be either useless or harmful for children whose backgrounds differ from those of the normative group. For example, Washington and Craig (1992) recommended that the PPVT-R not be used with low-income, urban, African American preschool and kindergarten boys and girls. Their research with 105 of these children showed that most scored more than one standard deviation below the mean and that a scoring adjustment to the test was not adequate to make up for the bias.

Nevertheless, standardized batteries like the CELF-3 and the TOLD-2 P provide a profile of relative strengths and weaknesses for many children. Directions for giving a standardized test must be followed explicitly. Some adjustments, however, may be made when interpreting results of subtests that may be biased for particular children. As Taylor (1986) commented, "If

PERSONAL REFLECTION 9.3 _____

"Every professional must accept the challenge to resolve to acquire new attitudes toward cultural diversity and to learn more about cross-cultural communication."

Dolores E. Battle, State University College at Buffalo, in the Introduction to _Communication Disorders in Multicultural Populations_ (Battle, 1993, p. xxiv).

group comparisons are to be made, they must be made in the context of standards or norms derived from comparable individuals from the same cultural or linguistic group as the client" (p. 15). Washington (1996) described formal and informal procedures for assessing the language abilities of African American children (including BESS), but lamented the continuing lack of appropriate standardized measures. She also noted the absence of an adequate understanding of normal language development for African American children. Battle (1993) emphasized the importance of a clinician's attitude toward cultural diversity and willingness to take the time and effort to learn about particular cultures and linguistic systems (see Chapter 6; also Personal Reflection 9.3).

In addition to results of broad comprehensive tests, participant interviews and spontaneous communication samples can be used to refine hypotheses about probable areas of greater strength and difficulty for a particular child. Then, deeper tests of more narrow areas may be selected to evaluate those hypotheses. For example, if I am testing a kindergarten child whose primary difficulty seems to be in the area of language form, with relatively higher skills in the area of language content and use, I might use the Structured Photographic Expressive Language Test—II (SPELT-II) (Werner & Kresheck, 1983) to confirm and to round out the data from spontaneous sampling about expressive syntax. I might also administer the Boehm Test of Basic Concepts—Revised (BTBC-R) (Boehm, 1986) or the Bracken Basic Concept Scale (BBCS) (Bracken, 1984) to test my impression that this child can handle key relational concepts and vocabulary important for understanding school discourse in kindergarten and first grade. If I am evaluating a slightly older child, I might use The Word Test—R (Huisingh, Barrett, Zachman, Blagden, & Orman, 1990) and informal strategies of curriculum-based language assessment (discussed in Chapters 11 and 12) to identify problems related to difficulty in understanding written and oral instructions and stories.

A difficult but important decision to be made during the comprehensive initial assessment of a middle-stage child is just how much standardized testing to do. This is always something of a value judgment involving cost–benefit analysis. By constantly asking oneself whether the benefit of additional information outweighs the cost of time borrowed from intervention activities, professionals can avoid the trap of continued assessment that delays getting to the meat of intervention.

SUMMARY

This chapter considered a variety of methods for identifying language and other communicative disorders among middle-stage children. Both formal and informal methods were reviewed. Whereas large-scale screening programs using standardized instruments may be appropriate before kindergarten, the pitfalls of such programs should not be ignored, particularly for children from diverse cultural backgrounds. When children are in their early and middle elementary school years, a strong information dissemination program should be designed to solicit appropriate referrals based on observation of communication abilities in naturalistic and classroom settings. Teachers and parents should be interviewed to identify areas of concern, which can then guide decisions about contexts and communication needs to consider in the assessment process.

Informal language sampling techniques are a primary assessment tool of middle-stage development. In this chapter, methods were discussed for gathering, transcribing, and analyzing language samples. Strategies for segmenting utterances include those that are based on intonation and pause criteria (Leadholm & Miller, 1992; J. F. Miller, 1981) and others that are structurally based. Some approaches keep a maximum of two main clauses together (Lee, 1974; Lund & Duchan, 1993). My own opinion (see also Scott & Stokes, 1995) is that the best information about developmental advances in MLU comes from samples divided into T-units (Hunt, 1965, 1970) or C-units (Loban, 1963, 1976). Both approaches divide utterances into independent clauses and embedded or subordinated clauses and phrases. When making comparisons to a data base, however, it is important to use the same strategy as that used in constructing the data base.

When analyzing aspects of language form in middle-stage language samples, suggestions are to make comparisons with developmental expectations based on MLU, Brown's 14 morphemes, verb phrase structure, and syntactic construction and comprehension. Dialect differences are associated with different morphological rule expectations that must be considered when analyzing language samples for children in diverse dialect communities. For children learning Black English Vernacular (also called African American English or Ebonics) nonbiased assessment of spontaneous language samples should be done with reference to the 17 morphological rule differences listed by Craig and Washington (1995). Black English Sentence Scoring (Nelson & Hyter, 1990a; Chapter Appendix C) provides developmental credit for acquiring these rules and permits comparisons with data for 64 normally developing children.

When analyzing aspects of language content, consideration should be given to lexical diversity. Problems were acknowledged with the type-token ratio (TTR) measure. A better way of assessing lexical diversity is to count the number of different words in samples with 100 words total. (Watkins et al., 1995). Other language content variables include semantic roles, topics and topic organization, and children's ability to represent world knowledge with language.

When analyzing aspects of language use, consideration should be given to whether children can use a balance of assertive and responsive conversational acts. For this purpose, Fey's (1986) Conversational Act Profiling (CAP) system was described and illustrated. The Social Interactive Coding System (SICS) proposed by Rice and colleagues (1990) was also described as an on-line system for use in preschool settings. In the middle stages, particular consideration should be given to children's emerging ability to use the narrative discourse genre for storytelling and retelling. Two analytical systems that yield compatible but different pictures of the developmental process are Applebee coding (1978) and story grammar coding (e.g., Hedberg & Westby, 1993; Stein & Glenn, 1979). The expository discourse genre poses particular challenges for middle-stage children that should also be recognized.

Formal assessment procedures should take into consideration the qualities of formal tests. The results of two studies (McCauley & Swisher, 1984; Plante & Vance, 1994) were reviewed that used the same 10 criteria for judging standardized tests. Formal tests are most helpful in diagnosing disorder when they show qualities of both sensitivity (i.e., they are good at detecting a disorder where it exists) and specificity (i.e., they are good at finding normally developing children to be normal).

REVIEW TOPICS _____

- Identification systems for middle-stage children with communication risks: Child Find, medical referral, preschool screening, prekindergarten screening
- Principles of screening sensitivity (low proportion of false-negative results) and specificity (low proportion of false-positive results)
- Referral criteria for early elementary school children, including "pragmatically oriented" criteria
- Story-retelling tasks for screening (the "Tommy" story; the "Bus" story)
- Contexts for assessing communicative needs and abilities of middle-stage children: family systems, cultures, interactions with peers, beginning school, elementary school classrooms
- Informal assessment processes, including interviews about life significant contexts; language sampling (gathering, recording, transcription techniques) and utterance segmentation alternatives (prosody-based, two main clause maximum, T-units, C-units); language form variables (Brown's 14 morphemes, verb phrase structure, syntactic construction and comprehension; concerns related to dialect difference); language content variables (lexical diversity, TTR, number of different words, semantic roles, topics, topic organization, representing world knowledge); language use variables (assertive and responsive pragmatic functions, conversational act profiling, social interactive coding system, narrative discourse genre—Applebee coding, and story grammar coding, expository discourse genre)
- Formal assessment procedures, including 10 criteria for judging standardized tests, application of sensitivity and specificity criteria to diagnostic tests

REVIEW QUESTIONS _____

1. What strategies should be available for identifying children in the middle stages of language development with needs for special services?

2. Outline variables to consider when gathering, transcribing, and analyzing the language form, content, and use of spontaneous language samples.
3. What are some of the pitfalls of using TTR as a measure of lexical diversity and what is a better way?
4. How should you adjust procedures for analyzing the language samples of children from diverse linguistic and dialect groups?
5. What are 10 criteria that should be used to judge the acceptability of a standardized test?

ACTIVITIES FOR EXTENDED THINKING _____

1. Gather a language sample from a child who is experiencing developmental language problems. Analyze it and describe its characteristics in the areas of language form, content, and use as described in this chapter. What evidence do you have to support a diagnosis of language disorder? Is there evidence of relative strength in any of the systems that you looked at? What are the clearest signs of impairment that should be targeted in an intervention program? If you have access to parents or a preschool teacher, interview them about their areas of greatest concern. What recommendations can you make based on this process about specific targets and intervention contexts?

2. Gather a language sample from two children whose primary language system is Black English Vernacular—one developing normally, and one for whom concerns have been raised. Look for evidence of the 17 morphological markers described by Washington and Craig (1994). Analyze the two samples using BESS as shown in Chapter Appendix C. What differences can you describe for the two samples? Does this analysis support concern about language development reported for the child having developmental difficulties? What language development strengths can you describe for each child?

3. Ask a kindergarten-age child to retell the "Tommy Story" (Culatta et al., 1983) and answer the questions about it. Then ask the child to make up a story about a fantasy or action picture. What can you learn about the child's development of narrative story structure from the two approaches? What levels do you find when you

classify the child's narratives according to Applebee (1978) or story grammar (Hedberg & Westby, 1993; Stein & Glenn, 1979) criteria?

4. Pick two formal tests for this age range that were not included in the reviews by McCauley and Swisher (1984) and Plante and Vance (1994). What evidence can you find in their manuals that they do or do not meet the 10 criteria used in those two reviews?

CHAPTER APPENDIX A
MIDDLE-STAGE ASSESSMENT TOOLS _____

Note: Sources include Deal and Rodriguez (1987), McCauley and Swisher (1984), who reviewed tests summarized in Table 9.8, and Plante and Vance (1994).

Analysis of the Language of Learning (ALL). Blodgett, E. G. & Cooper, E. G. (1987). East Moline, IL: LinguiSystems. Provides standardized scores for 5- to 9-year-olds based on their ability to display metalinguistic knowledge of what a word is, a syllable, and a sentence, and understanding of directions. It is appropriate for nonreaders.

Assessment of Phonological Processes—Revised (APP-R). Hodson, B. (1986). Austin, TX: Pro-Ed. Can be administered in 15 to 20 minutes and scored in 30 minutes. Results in categorization of phonological processes that is useful for intervention planning.

Assessing Semantic Skills through Everyday Themes (ASSET). Barrett, M., Zachman, L., & Huisingh, R. (1988). East Moline, IL: LinguiSystems. Uses a thematic approach to assess receptive and expressive vocabulary for 3- to 9-year-olds in 10 tasks: understanding labels, identifying categories, identifying attributes, identifying functions, understanding definitions, expressing labels, expressing categories, expressing attributes, expressing functions, expressing definitions. Yields standard scores, percentile ranks, and age equivalencies.

Bankson-Bernthal Test of Phonology (BBTOP). Bankson, N. W. & Bernthal, J. E. (1990). Chicago, IL: Applied Symbolix. Assesses articulation and phonological processes among children ages 3 to 9 years.

Bankson Language Text (2nd ed.) (BLT-2). Bankson, N. W. (1990). Austin, TX: Pro Ed. In the revised

version, test results may be reported for children from ages 3 through 7 years as standard scores or percentile ranks. Organized into three general categories: semantic knowledge (body parts, nouns, verbs, categories, functions, propositions, opposites); morphological/syntactic rules (pronouns, verb tense, auxiliaries, modals, copulas, plurals, comparatives/superlatives, negation, questions); and pragmatics (ritualizing, informing, controlling, imagining). Standardized on 1200 children in 19 states.

Bilingual Syntax Measure I and II. Medida de Sintaxis Bilingue (BSM). Burt, M. K., Dulay, H. C., & Chavez, E. H. (1978). San Antonio, TX: The Psychological Corporation. Assesses mastery of basic oral syntactic structures in both English and Spanish. Provides a criterion-referenced measure of proficiency.

Boder Test of Reading-Spelling Patterns. Boder, E. & Jarrico, S. (1982). San Antonio, TX: The Psychological Corporation. This criterion-referenced test uses word reading and spelling tasks to identify students in elementary and secondary grades as having one of four types of reading disability: nonspecific, dysphonetic, eidetic, and mixed dysphonetic-eidetic.

Boehm Test of Basic Concepts—Revised (BTBC-R), and *Boehm Test of Basic Concepts-Preschool Version.* Boehm, A. (1986). San Antonio, TX: The Psychological Corporation. The preschool version is for children ages 3 to 5 years. It is individually administered to test comprehension of basic relational concepts. The BTBC-R is for children ages kindergarten to grade 2. It is group administered and tests concepts generally considered important for following teacher instructions. Yields percentile rankings.

Bracken Basic Concept Scale (BBCS). Bracken, B. A. (1984). San Antonio, TX: The Psychological Corporation. Designed to be used with preschool- and primary-age children and children with receptive language difficulties. Items require either short verbal responses or pointing. Eleven subtests of colors, letter identification, numbers/counting, comparisons, shapes, direction/position, social/emotional, size, texture/material, quantity, and time/sequence. Yields percentile ranks, z-scores, and standard scores with a mean of 10 and standard deviation of 3 based on national norms.

Carolina Picture Vocabulary Test (CPVT). Layton, T. L., & Holmes, D. W. (1985). Austin, TX: Pro-Ed. Norm-referenced test of receptive sign vocabulary for deaf and hearing impaired children between 4 and 11:6 years.

Carrow Auditory—Visual Abilities Test (CAVAT). Carrow-Woolfolk, E. (1991). Austin, TX: Pro-Ed. Norm-referenced test with 14 subtests to measure auditory and visual perceptual, motor, and memory skills for children ages 4 to 10 years. Entire test takes 1½ hours. Yields percentile ranks and T-scores.

Carrow Elicited Language Inventory (CELI). Carrow-Woolfolk, E. (1974). Austin, TX: Pro-Ed. Designed for children ages 3:0 to 7:11. This norm-referenced test uses elicitation tasks to assess productive use of imitated grammatical structures. Yields percentile ranks and standard scores.

Clinical Evaluation of Language Fundamentals—3rd ed. (CELF-3). Semel, E., Wiig, E., & Secord, W. (1995). Also *CELF-Screening Test* (1996) and *CELF-Preschool* (1992) by Wiig, E. H., Secord, W., & Semel, E. (1992). *CELF-Preschool* includes 6 diagnostic subtests for preschoolers. *CELF-3 Screening Test* yields criterion scores for ages 6 through 21 years in 10 minutes. *CELF-3* provides normative data for ages 6 through 21 years. Expressive subtests include Word Structure, Formulated Sentences, Sentence Assembly, Recalling Sentences, Word Associations, and Rapid, Automatic Naming. Receptive subtests include Sentence Structure, Concepts and Direction, Semantic Relationships, Word Classes, and Listening to Paragraphs. San Antonio, TX: The Psychological Corporation.

Communication Abilities Diagnostic Test (CADeT). Johnston, E. B. & Johnston, A. V. (1989). Chicago, IL: Applied Symbolix. Uses informal assessment tasks involving stories, a board game, and conversational contexts with children ages 3 to 9 to assess language development in the areas of syntax, semantics, and pragmatics. Yields norm-referenced language comprehension and expression scores.

Comprehensive Receptive and Expressive Vocabulary Test (CREVT). Wallace, G. & Hammill, D. D. (1994). Austin, TX: Pro-Ed. Assesses receptive and expressive oral vocabulary strengths and weaknesses. Identifies students 4:0 through 17:11 significantly below their peers in oral abilities. Scores from this test are correlated with scores from the TOLD:P–2, PPVT–R, EOWPVT–R, and the CELF.

Conner's Teacher Rating Scales (CTRS) and *Conner's Parent Rating Scales (CPRS).* Conners, C. K. (1989). Austin, TX: Pro-Ed. These scales provide both short and long versions to help identify hyperactive children. They can be used with children ages 3 to 17.

Detroit Tests of Learning Aptitude—Primary (DTLA P:2). Hammill, D. D. & Bryant, B. R. (1991). Austin, TX: Pro-Ed. Designed for ages 3 through 9. Includes 6 subtests measuring language, attention, and cognitive abilities. Yields standard scores, percentile ranks, and age equivalents.

Developmental Assessment of Spanish Grammar (DASG). Toronto, A. S. (1976). *Journal of Speech and Hearing Disorders, 41,* 150–171. Adaptation of Lee's (1974) Developmental Sentence Scoring technique for Spanish-speaking children.

Developmental Indicators for the Assessment of Learning—Revised (DIAL-R). Mardell-Czudnowski, C. & Goldenberg, D. S. (1990). Circle Pines, MN: AGS. A preschool and prekindergarten screening instrument that screens children ages 2 to 6 in three developmental skill areas (motor, concepts, and language) in 20 to 30 minutes. Includes statistical data from the three norming groups, 1990 census, caucasian, and minority. Results can be compared with cut-off scores at ±1, ±1.5, or ±2 SD.

Early Screening Profiles (ESP). Harrison, P., Kaufman, A., Kaufman, N., Bruininks, R., Rynders, J., Ilmer, S., Sparrow, S., & Cicchetti, D. (1990). Circle Pines, MN: AGS. Comprehensive screening instrument for children aged 2:0 to 6:11 years. Yields screening indexes or standard scores in cognitive/language, motor, or self-help social areas to identify at-risk or gifted children.

Expressive One Word Picture Vocabulary Test—Revised (EOWPVT—R). Gardner, M. (1990). Austin, TX: Pro-Ed. Assesses expressive vocabulary in children ages 2:0 to 11:11. (Can be administered with ROWPVT.)

The Expressive Vocabulary Test (EVT). Williams, K. T. (1997). Circle Pines, MN: AGS. Co-normed with the PPVT–III, this test measures expressive vocabulary and word retrieval for standard American English for clients 2:5 to 85+ years.

Goldman-Fristoe Test of Articulation (GFTA). Goldman, R., & Fristoe, M. (1972, 1986). Circle Pines, MN: AGS. Measures articulation of sounds-in-words, sounds-in-sentences, and stimulability. Yields percentile ranks for the sounds-in-words and stimulability subtests for children ages 2 to 16+.

Goldman-Fristoe-Woodcock Auditory Skills Test Battery (GFW-Battery). Goldman, R., Fristoe, M., & Woodcock, C. W. (1976). Circle Pines, MN: AGS. For persons 3 years to adult, this is a battery of four 15-minute tests: auditory selective attention, diagnostic auditory discrimination, auditory memory, and sound–symbol association. Yields age-based standard scores, percentile ranks, stanines, and age equivalents.

Goldman-Fristoe-Woodcock Test of Auditory Discrimination (GFW). Goldman, R., Fristoe, M., & Woodcock, C. W. (1970). Circle Pines, MN: AGS. To be used with persons 3 years old and up, this is a test of closed-set word identification in quiet and in noise. Yields standard scores and percentile ranks.

Grammatical Analysis of Elicited Language (GAEL). Moog, J. S. & Geers, A. E. (1980). St. Louis, MO: Central Institute for the Deaf. This test is used to elicit and evaluate important elements of spoken and signed English in children. It assesses 16 grammatical structures. The measure was normed on normal-hearing children ages 3:5 to 5:8 and on hearing-impaired children ages 8:2 to 11:11.

Illinois Test of Psycholinguistic Abilities (ITPA) (rev. ed.). Kirk, S., McCarthy, J. J., & Kirk, W. (1968). Urbana, IL: University of Illinois Press. This classic norm-referenced test includes 10 subtests (and two supplementary subtests) to evaluate auditory reception, visual reception, auditory association, visual association, verbal expression, manual expression, grammatic closure, visual closure, auditory sequential memory, visual sequential memory, auditory closure, and sound blending for children ages 2 to 10 years.

Kaufman Assessment Battery for Children (K-ABC). Kaufman, A. S. & Kaufman, N. L. (1983). Circle Pines, MN: AGS. Includes 16 subtests that examine sequential and serial processing, spatial tasks, reading and arithmetic, as well as vocabulary skills. Useful for evaluating a child's ability to apply mental processing skills to various learning situations. Ages 2:5 to 12:5.

Kaufman Survey of Early Academic and Language Skills (K-SEALS). Kaufman, A. S. & Kaufman, N. L. (1993). Circle Pines, MN: AGS. Nationally normed measure that assesses children's expressive and receptive language skills, preacademic skills, and articulation.

Khan-Lewis Phonological Analysis (KLPA). Khan, L. & Lewis, N. (1986). Circle Pines, MN: AGS. To be used with the Goldman-Fristoe Test of Articulation (G-FTA) to analyze articulatory responses for the presence of 15 phonological processes. Percentile ranks, speech simplification ratings, and age equivalents can be computed for composite scores for children ages 2 through 5:11 years.

Kindergarten Language Screening Test (KLST). Gauthier, S. V. & Madison, C. L. (1983). Austin, TX: Pro-Ed. Assesses expressive and receptive language comprehension by testing children's knowledge of name, age, body parts, and number concepts. Assesses children's ability to follow commands, repeat sentences, and produce spontaneous speech.

Language Processing Test—Revised (LPT-R). Richard, G. J. & Haner, M. A. (1995). Austin, TX: Pro-Ed. Useful with children 5:0 through 11:0 to identify processing problems and word retrieval errors. Assesses children's ability to organize information and make sense of auditory information.

Let's Talk Inventory for Children (LTI-C). Bray, C. M. & Wiig, E. H. (1987). San Antonio, TX: The Psychological Corporation. Helps identify preschool- and early elementary-age children who have inadequate or delayed social-verbal communication skills. Children are asked to formulate speech acts to go with pictured situational contexts. Items require formulation or association. Means and standard deviations are reported by age groups.

McCarthy Scales of Children's Abilities. McCarthy, D. (1972). San Antonio. TX: The Psychological Corporation. Used with children ages 2:6 through 8:6, subscales may be used for differential diagnosis in six areas: verbal scale, quantitative scale, perceptual performance scale, general cognitive index, memory, and motor development.

McCarthy Screening Test (MST). McCarthy, D. (1978). San Antonio, TX: The Psychological Corporation. Includes six scales that are predictive of a child's ability to cope with schoolwork in the early grades. Identifies children who may be at risk for learning disabilities.

Miller Assessment for Preschoolers (MAP). Miller, L. J. (1982). San Antonio, TX: The Psychological Corporation. This comprehensive preschool screening instrument can be individually administered to children between 2:9 and 5:8 years in approximately 20 to 30 minutes per child. It yields percentiles for six age groups based on a standardization of 1200 preschoolers across the United States.

Miller-Yoder Language Comprehension Test (MY). Miller, J. F. & Yoder, D. (1984). (Manual by G. Gill, M. Rosin, N. O. Owings, & K. A. Carlson). Austin, TX: Pro Ed. Includes three sets of pictures that can be used to assess comprehension of short simple sentences with a variety of grammatical structures. Can be administered to normally developing, developmentally delayed, or mentally retarded children. Results allow comparison to performance of same-age peers between 4 and 8 years.

Northwestern Syntax Screening Test (NSST). Lee, L. (1971). Evanston, IL: Northwestern University Press. Uses a picture pointing task to measure receptive language and a delayed imitation task to measure expressive language for children from 3:0 to 8 years.

Oral and Written Language Scales (OWLS). Carrow-Woolfolk, E. (1995, 1996). Circle Pines, MN: AGS. Offers a quick measure of receptive and expressive language through comprehensive examination of semantic, syntactic, pragmatic, and supralinguistic aspects of language for clients 3:0 to 21:0.

Peabody Picture Vocabulary Test (3rd ed.) (PPVT-III). Dunn, L. M., Dunn, L. M., & Williams, K. T. (1997). Circle Pines, MN: AGS. A quick measure of receptive hearing vocabulary for Standard American English for clients 2:5 to 85+ years.

Photo Articulation Test (3rd ed.). (PAT-3). Lippke, B. A., Dickey, S. E., Selmar, J. W., & Soder, A. L. (1997). Austin, TX: Pro-Ed. This completely revised measure uses 72 color photographs to assess initial, medial, and final position articulation errors in children 3:6 through 8:11.

Preschool Language Assessment Instrument (PLAI). Blank, M., Rose, S., & Berlin, L. (1978). San Antonio, TX: The Psychological Corporation. This is not a standardized test but can be used to assess a variety of language skills: labeling objects and actions, role play, responding to conversational interactions, describing object functions, solving problems, defining, and performing other language skills related to academic success. Can be used with Spanish-speaking children.

Preschool Language Scale—3 (PLS-3). Zimmerman, I. L., Steiner, V. G., & Pond, R. E. (1992). San Antonio, TX: The Psychological Corporation. Revised and standardized for use with children from birth to age 6:11. Takes 20 to 30 minutes and yields total language, auditory comprehension, and expressive communication standard scores, percentile ranks, and language-age equivalents. A Spanish-language version, with norms based on Spanish-speaking children throughout the United States, is also available.

Preschool Language Screening Test (PLST). Hannah, E. & Gardner, J. (1974). Northridge, CA: Joyce Publications.

Prueba del Desarrollo Inicial del Lenguaje (PDIL). Hresko, W. P., Reid, D. K., & Hammill, D. D. (1982). Austin, TX: Pro-Ed. This is a standardized test of the Spanish spoken language for children ages 3 to 7 years. It includes 38 items used to assess receptive and expressive language through a variety of semantic and syntactic tasks.

Raven's Progressive Matrices. Raven, J. C. (1990). San Antonio, TX: The Psychological Corporation. This test is designed for children aged 5:0 to 11:0 years, elderly persons, and mentally and physically impaired persons. Three nonverbal tests assess mental ability by presenting problem-solving tasks with abstract figures and designs.

Receptive One Word Picture Vocabulary Test (ROW-PVT). Gardner, M. (1985). Austin, TX: Pro-Ed. Assesses receptive vocabulary in children ages 2:0 through 11:11 years. (Can be administered with EOWPVT.)

Rhode Island Test of Language Structure (RITLS). Engen, E. & Engen, T. (1983). Austin, TX: Pro-Ed. This test of English language development emphasizes understanding of language structure. It was primarily designed for use with children with hearing impairments (ages 3 to 20 years) but can also be used with other children (ages 3 to 6 years), including those who have mental retardation or learning disabilities or who are bilingual.

Screening Kit of Language Development (*SKOLD*). Bliss, L. S. & Allen, D. V. (1983). East Aurora, NY: Slosson Educational Publications. Screening test that can be administered to 2- to 5-year-old children in 15 minutes by paraprofessionals. Assesses preschool language development in six areas: vocabulary, comprehension, story completion, individual and paired sentence repetition without pictures, and comprehension of commands. It is norm-referenced for both Black English- and Standard English-speaking children.

Screening Test for Auditory Processing Disorders (SCAN). Keith, R. W. (1986). San Antonio, TX: The Psychological Corporation. This test of auditory processing is designed for children ages 3 to 11 years. It consists of three subtests, which may be presented using a regular portable stereo cassette player: filtered words (two lists of 20 monosyllabic low-pass filtered words); auditory figure-ground (two lists of 20 monosyllabic words presented to the same ear as multitalker speech babble); and competing words (two lists of 25 monosyllabic words presented simultaneously to right and left ears).

Screening Test for Developmental Apraxia of Speech (STDAS). Blakely, R. W. (1980). Austin, TX: Pro-Ed. Designed to assist in the differential diagnosis of speech apraxia in children ages 4 through 12.

Uses eight subtests: expressive language discrepancy, vowels and diphthongs, oral-motor movement, verbal sequencing, motorically complex words, articulation, transposition, and prosody.

Slingerland Screening Tests for Identifying Children With Specific Language Disability. Slingerland, B. H. (1970). Cambridge, MA: Educators Publishing Service. Group-administered screening test for identifying specific language disability in reading, writing, and spelling in children in grades 1 through 6. (Spanish version by L. R. Strong, 1989.)

Smit-Hand Articulation and Phonology Evaluation (SHAPE). Smit, A. B. & Hand, L. (1997). Los Angeles: Western Psychological Services. Nationally norm-based measurement of speech sound acquisition for children ages 3:0 to 9:0. Uses photocards of common objects to assess the production of initial and final consonants and initial two and three consonant blends; grouped by semantic categories.

Stephens Oral Language Screening Test (SOLST). Stephens, M. I. (1977). Peninsula, OH: Interim Publishers.

Structured Photographic Expressive Language Test—Preschool (SPELT-P). Werner, E. O. & Kresheck, J. D. (1983). Sandwich, IL: Janelle Publications. Uses snapshots to elicit early developing morphological and syntactic forms including: prepositions; plurals; possessive nouns and pronouns; present progressive; regular/irregular past tense; contractible and uncontractible copula; negation. It can be administered in 10 to 15 minutes to children from ages 3:0 to 5:11. Guidelines are provided for analyzing productions from speakers of Black English.

Spanish Structured Photographic Expressive Language Test—Preschool (Spanish SPELT-P). Werner, E. O. & Kresheck, J. D. (1989). Sandwich, IL: Janelle Publications. This version uses snapshots to elicit early developing Spanish morphological and syntactic forms. It can be administered in 10 to 15 minutes to children from ages 3:0 to 5:11. The manual addresses issues in assessing children with limited English proficiency and provides developmental guidelines for Spanish morphology and syntax.

Structured Photographic Expressive Language Test—II (SPELT-II). Werner, E. O. & Kresheck, J. D. (1983). Sandwich, IL: Janelle Publications. This version of the test is for children ages 4:0 to 9:5. It elicits prepositions, plurals, possessive nouns and pronouns, reflexive pronouns, present progressive, regular/irregular past tense, future, contractible/uncontractible copula, contractible/uncontractible auxiliary, and secondary verbs. It also elicits syntactic structures: affirmatives, negatives, conjoined sentences, imperatives, *Wh*-questions, and interrogative reversals. Guidelines are provided for analyzing productions from speakers of Black English.

Spanish Structured Photographic Expressive Language Test—II (Spanish SPELT-II). Werner, E. O. & Kresheck, J. D. (1989). Sandwich, IL: Janelle Publications. This Spanish version of SPELT-II elicits articles; prepositions; plural and possessive nouns; possessive and reflexive pronouns; future, present, present progressive, and preterit (past) tenses of regular and irregular verbs; singular and plural present and past forms of copulas; secondary verbs; *Wh-* and *Y/ N* interrogatives; and negatives. It can be administered in 10 to 15 minutes to children from ages 4:0 to 9:5. The manual addresses issues in assessing children with limited English proficiency and provides developmental guidelines for Spanish morphology and syntax.

System of Multicultural Pluralistic Assessment (SOMPA). Mercer, J. R. & Lewis, J. F. (1978). San Antonio, TX: The Psychological Corporation. This assessment tool is used to measure a child's learning potential by considering sociocultural and health factors. It contains two major sections, a Parent Interview conducted in the home and a Student Interview conducted at school.

Templin-Darley Tests of Articulation (T-D) (2nd ed.). Templin, M. & Darley, F. (1969). Iowa City, IA: University of Iowa.

Test of Auditory Comprehension of Language—Revised (TACL-R). Carrow-Woolfolk, E. (1985). Austin, TX: Pro-Ed. The revised test provides age and grade norms for ages 3:0 through 9:11. Assesses auditory comprehension of word classes and relations, grammatical morphemes, elabo-

rated sentence constructions. Yields standard scores, percentile ranks, age equivalents. (A computerized scoring system is also available.)

Test of Auditory-Perceptual Skills (TAPS). Gardner, M. F. (1985) Burlingame, CA: Psychological and Educational Publications. This test can be administered in 10 to 15 minutes to children between 4 and 12 years. It assesses auditory discrimination, sequential memory, word memory, sentence memory, interpretation of directions, and processing (based on learning and thinking) and provides a measure of hyperactivity. Scores may be converted to stanines, percentiles, auditory age equivalents, and auditory standard scores for each subtest.

Test of Awareness of Language Segments (TALS). Sawyer, D. J. (1987). Austin, TX: Pro-Ed. A screening test that can be administered to children from 4:6 through 7 years. Includes 46 items distributed across three subtests: sentences-to-words, words-to-syllables, and words-to-sounds. Cut-off scores permit inferences about readiness to meet instructional demands of beginning reading programs, and which types of introductory reading approach might be easier for an individual child to master.

Test of Children's Language (TOCL). Barenbaum, E. & Newcomer, P. (1996). Austin, TX: Pro-Ed. Assesses aspects of spoken language, reading, and writing in approximately 30 to 40 minutes. Standardized for children 5:0 to 8:11. Identifies specific strengths and weaknesses in language components and in recognizing students who are at risk for failure in reading and writing.

Test of Early Language Development (TELD). Hresko, W. P., Reid, D. K., & Hammill, D. D. (1981). Austin, TX: Pro-Ed. Measures spoken language abilities of children ages 3:0 through 7:11 in the areas of semantics and syntax in about 15 minutes using 38 items. Yields standard scores, percentile ranks, and age-equivalent scores.

Test of Early Language Development (2nd ed.) (TELD-2). Hresko, W. P., Reid, D. K., & Hammill, D. D. (1991). Austin, TX: Pro-Ed. Measures the aspects of form and content of expressive and receptive language in children ages 2:0 to 7:11. Includes expanded diagnostic profile extended age range, and two alternative forms.

Test of Early Reading Ability—2 (TERA-2). Reid, D. K., Hresko, W. P., & Hammill, D. D. (1989). Austin, TX: Pro-Ed. Measures reading abilities of children between the ages 3:0 and 9:11. Items measure knowledge of contextual meaning, alphabet, and conventions. Standard scores with *M* = 100 and *SD* = 15 result.

Test of Early Written Language (TEWL). Hresko, W. P. (1988). Austin, TX: Pro-Ed. Measures emerging written language abilities of children ages 3:0 through 7:11. Standard scores and percentiles may be particularly helpful for identifying mildly handicapped students.

Test for Examining Expressive Morphology (TEEM). Shipley, K. G., Stone, T. A., & Sue, M. B. (1983). Tucson, AZ: Communication Skill Builders. Evaluates use of expressive morphemes by 3- to 8-year-olds (in 7 minutes). Assesses present progressives, plurals, possessives, past tenses, third-person singulars, derived adjectives. Norms based on more than 500 children.

Test of Language Competence—Expanded Edition (TLC-Expanded). Wiig, E. H. & Secord, W. (1988). San Antonio, TX: The Psychological Corporation. Identifies language and communication deficits in children ages 5 through 19 years. Includes two levels. Level 1 is designed for ages 5 through 9 years. It includes subtests: ambiguous sentences, listening comprehension (making inferences), oral expression (recreating speech acts), figurative language. Yields subtest and composite standard scores and age-equivalent scores.

Test of Language Development—Primary (3rd. ed.) (TOLD-P:3). Newcomer, P. L. & Hammill, D. D. (1997). Austin, TX: Pro-Ed. New normative data representative of the U.S. population and stratified by age for ages 4:0 to 8:11. Updated pictures, stimuli with diversity of gender and race. This test requires approximately 40 minutes. It yields standard and percentile scores. Nine subtests measure: picture vocabulary (understanding words); relational vocabulary (mediating words); oral vocabulary (defining words); grammatic understanding (understanding sentence structures); sentence imitation (repeating sentences); grammatic completion (using acceptable morphological forms); word discrimination (noticing sound differences); phone-

mic analysis (segmenting words into smaller units); and word articulation (saying words correctly).

Test of Nonverbal Intelligence—3 (TONI-3). Brown, L., Sherbenou, R. J., & Johnsen, S. K. (1997). Austin, TX: Pro-Ed. The administration of this test requires no reading, writing, speaking, or listening by the test subject. It measures intelligence, aptitude, and reasoning and may be used with individuals from age 5:0 through 85:11, including individuals with severe speech impairments, brain injury, and deafness or hearing loss. Requires 15 to 20 minutes.

Test of Phonological Awareness (TOPA). Torgesen, J. K. & Bryant, B. R. (1994). Austin, TX: Pro-Ed. In 15 to 20 minutes this test measures kindergartner's awareness of individual sounds in words. TOPA scores are related to reading growth in first grade.

Test of Pragmatic Language (TOPL). Phelps-Teraski, D. & Phelps-Gunn, T. (1992). Austin, TX: Pro-Ed. A comprehensive assessment of a student's ability to use pragmatic language in six core areas: physical setting, audience, topic, purpose, visual–gestural cues, and abstraction. Useful with clients from kindergarten through junior high school, as well as adult remedial, ESL, and aphasic populations.

Test of Pragmatic Skills—Revised. Shulman, B. B. (1986). *Computerized Test of Pragmatic Skills.* Shulman, B. B. & Fitch, J. L. (1987). San Antonio, TX: Communication Skill Builders/The Psychological Corporation. Assesses communicative intentions in 10 categories, including naming/labeling, reasoning, denying. Provides mean and percentile data.

Test of Problem Solving—Revised (TOPS). Bowers, L., Huisingh, R., Barrett, M., Orman, J., & LoGiudice, C. (1984). East Moline, IL: LinguiSystems. This standardized test for 6- to 12-year-olds assesses expressive reasoning in the areas explaining inferences ("How does the family know the electricity just went off?"); determining causes of events ("How did the boy's bike get a flat tire?"); answering "why" questions ("Why shouldn't he ride his bike with a flat tire?"); determining solutions ("The losing team has lost three games in a row. What could they do to improve the way they play?"); and avoiding problems ("The boy dripped all over his shirt. What could he have done to keep from getting his shirt dirty?").

Test of Word Finding (TWF). German, D. J. (1986; manual revised, 1989). Austin, TX: Pro-Ed. This is a standardized test of word finding skills for 6:6- to 12:11-year-olds with naming tasks organized into five sections: picture naming (nouns); sentence completion; description naming; picture naming (verbs); and picture naming (categories). A sixth section is used to assess comprehension or concept deficits. Analysis includes both accuracy and response time, yielding standard scores, percentile ranks, and grade standards.

Test of Word Finding in Discourse (TWFD). German, D. J. (1991). Austin, TX: Pro-Ed. In 15 to 20 minutes this test measures word-finding difficulties in students 6:6 to 12:11. Also assesses a child's language use in discourse. Yields a Productivity Index and a Word Finding Behaviors Index. Percentile ranks and standard scores can be obtained for both indices.

Test of Word Knowledge (TOWK). Wiig, E. H. & Secord, W. (1992). San Antonio, TX: The Psychological Corporation. This measure thoroughly evaluates a child's semantic development and lexical knowledge. Identifies children lacking the semantic skills forming the foundation of mature language and thinking.

Test of Written Language (3rd ed.) (TOWL-3). Hammill, D. D. & Larsen, S. C. (1996). Austin, TX: Pro-Ed. Uses spontaneous essay analysis and traditional test formats to measure written language skills in children age 7:6 to 17:11.

Token Test for Children (TTC). DiSimoni, F. (1978). Austin, TX: Pro-Ed. Used for children ages 3 to 12 years. Yields age and grade scores.

Test de Vocabulario en Imágenes Peabody (TVIP). Dunn, L. M., Lugo, D. E., Padilla, E. R., & Dunn, L. M. (1986). Circle Pines, MN: AGS. A test of receptive Spanish vocabulary (modified from the vocabulary of the PPVT-R to be culturally appropriate) for 2:6- to 18-year-olds. Separate and combined norms are available for children with either Mexican or Puerto Rican backgrounds.

Utah Test of Language Development—3 (UTLD-3). Mecham, M. J. (1989). Austin, TX: Pro-Ed. This revision can be administered to children from ages 3:0 to 10:11 years. It yields subtest standard scores with $M = 10$ and $SD = 3$ in the areas of language comprehension and language expression. It also yields a language quotient score with $M = 100$ and $SD = 15$.

Visual-Aural Digit Span Test. Koppitz, E. M. (1977). San Antonio, TX: The Psychological Corporation.

Wechsler Intelligence Scale for Children (3rd ed.) (WISC-III). Wechsler, D. (1991). San Antonio, TX: Psychological Corporation. This newly revised measure is designed to be unbiased for race and gender. The coding format has also been changed to benefit left-handed children, and stimulus items have been added to several subtests to provide better measurement of the youngest and oldest groups.

Wechsler Preschool and Primary Scale of Intelligence—Revised (WPPSI-R). Wechsler, D. (1989). San Antonio, TX: The Psychological Corporation. This assessment contains the original 11 subtests and a new Object Assembly measure that involves puzzles. The age range scale has been expanded to include children as young as 3:0 and as old as 7:3 years.

Wide Range Achievement Test—Revised (WRAT-R). Jastak, S. & Wilkinson, G. S. (1984). San Antonio, TX: The Psychological Corporation. Level 1 assesses reading (at the single-word level), spelling, and arithmetic abilities for children ages 5 through 11 years. Level 2 is for persons ages 12 through 75. Yields standard scores, percentiles, and grade equivalents.

Wiig Criterion-Referenced Inventory of Language (Wiig CRIL). Wiig, E. H. (1990). San Antonio, TX: The Psychological Corporation. This criterion-referenced assessment can be used as follow-up to norm-referenced testing to obtain baseline information and plan intervention in the areas of semantics, morphology, syntax, and pragmatics. For children ages 4 through 15 years.

Woodcock-Johnson Psycho-Educational Battery—Revised (WJPEB-R). Woodcock, R. W. & Johnson, W. B. (1989). Allen, TX: DLM. Includes two batteries: *Tests of Cognitive Ability and Tests of Achievement.* Based on extensive standardization information for persons in the age range 2 to 90+ years. It is a lengthy test, but it is divided into standard and supplemental batteries. The standard battery of the cognitive test can be used to yield a full-scale cognitive score in 40 minutes. The standard cognitive subtests are memory for names, memory for sentences, visual matching, incomplete words, visual closure, picture vocabulary, and analysis-synthesis. The supplemental cognitive subtests are visual–auditory learning, memory for words, cross out, sound blending, picture recognition, oral vocabulary, concept formation, delayed recall for names, delayed recall for visual–auditory learning, sound patterns, spatial relations, listening comprehension, and verbal analogies. The standard achievement subtests are letter–word identification, passage comprehension, calculation, applied problems, dictation, writing samples, science, social studies, humani-

ties. The supplemental achievement subtests are word attack, reading vocabulary, quantitative concepts, proofing, writing fluency, punctuation, spelling, usage, and handwriting.

Word Finding Referral Checklist (WFRC). German, D. J. (1992). Austin, TX: Pro-Ed. This checklist is used in cooperation with a classroom teacher to identify elementary, middle, or secondary school students who demonstrate word-finding difficulties. Specifically examines general understanding of language, word-finding skills, in single-word retrieval contexts, and word-finding skills in discourse.

The Word Test—R. Huisingh, R., Barrett, M., Zachman, L., Blagden, C., & Orman, J. (1990). East Moline, IL: LinguiSystems. This test is designed for 7- to 11-year-old children. It uses six subtests to assess associations, antonyms, synonyms, definitions, semantic absurdities, and multiple definitions. Standard scores, percentile ranks, and age equivalencies are provided for individual subtests and the total test.

	INDEFINITE PRONOUNS OR NOUN MODIFIERS	PERSONAL PRONOUNS	MAIN VERBS	SECONDARY VERBS
1	it, this, that	1st and 2nd person: I, me, my, mine, you, your(s)	A. Uninflected verb: I <u>see</u> you. B. copula, is, or 's: <u>It's</u> red. C. is + verb + ing: He <u>is coming</u>.	
2		3rd person: he, him, his, she, her, hers	A. -s and -ed: <u>plays</u>, <u>played</u> B. Irregular past: <u>ate</u>, <u>saw</u> C. Copula: <u>am</u>, <u>are</u>, <u>was</u>, <u>were</u> D. Auxiliary <u>am</u>, <u>are</u>, <u>was</u>, <u>were</u>	Five early-developing infinitives I wanna <u>see</u> (want to <u>see</u>) I'm gonna <u>see</u> (going to <u>see</u>) I gotta <u>see</u> (got to <u>see</u>) Lemme [to] see (let me [to] <u>see</u>) Let's [to] play (let [us to] play)
3	A. no, some, more, all, lot(s), one(s), two (etc.), other(s), another B. something, somebody, someone	A. Plurals: we, us, our(s), they, them, their B. these, those		Non-complementing infinitive: I stopped <u>to play</u>. I'm afraid <u>to look</u>. It's hard <u>to do</u> that.
4	nothing, nobody, none, no one		A. can, will, may + verb: <u>may go</u> B. Obligatory do + verb: <u>don't go</u> C. Emphatic do + verb: I <u>do see</u>.	Participle, present or past: I see a boy <u>running</u>. I found the toy <u>broken</u>.

5		Reflexives: myself, yourself, himself, herself, itself, themselves		A. Early infinitival complements with differing subjects in kernels: I want you <u>to come</u>.
				   Let him [to] <u>see</u>.
				B. Later infinitival complements:
				   I had <u>to go</u>. I told him <u>to go</u>.
				   I tried <u>to go</u>. He ought <u>to go</u>.
				C. Obligatory deletions:
				   Make it [to] <u>go</u>.
				   I'd better [to] <u>go</u>.
				D. Infinitive with wh- word:
				   I know what <u>to get</u>.
				   I know how <u>to do</u> it.

6		A. Wh- pronouns: who, which, whose, whom, what, that, how many, how much
		   I know <u>who</u> came.
		   That's <u>what</u> I said.
		B. Wh-word + infinitive:
		   I know <u>what</u> to do.
		   I know <u>who(m)</u> to take.
			A. could, would, should, might + verb: <u>might come</u>, <u>could be</u>
			B. Obligatory does, did + verb
			C. Emphatic does, did + verb	

7	A. any, anything, anybody, anyone
	B. every, everything, everybody, everyone
	C. both, few, many, each, several, most, least, much, next, first, last, second (etc.)
		(his) own, one, oneself, whichever, whoever, whatever
		   Take <u>whatever</u> you like.
			A. Passive with <u>get</u>, any tense
			   Passive with <u>be</u>, any tense
			B. must, shall + verb: must come
			C. have + verb + en: I've eaten
			D. have got: <u>I've got</u> it.
				Passive infinitival complement:
				With <u>get</u>: I have <u>to get dressed</u>.
				        I don't want <u>to get hurt</u>.
				With <u>be</u>: I want <u>to be pulled</u>.
				        It's going <u>to be locked</u>.

8			A. have been + verb + ing had been + verb + ing B. modal + have + verb + en <u>may have eaten</u> C. modal + be + verb + ing <u>could be playing</u> D. Other auxiliary combinations: <u>should have been sleeping</u>	Gerund <u>Swinging</u> is fun. I like <u>fishing</u>. He started <u>laughing</u>.

Note: From *Developmental Sentence Analysis* (p. 67) by L. L. Lee, 1974, Evanston, IL: Northwestern University Press. Copyright 1974 by Northwestern University Press. Reprinted by permission.

	NEGATIVES	CONJUNCTIONS	INTERROGATIVE REVERSALS	WH- QUESTIONS
1	it, this, that + copula, or auxiliary is 's, + not: It's <u>not</u> mine. This is <u>not</u> a dog. That is <u>not</u> moving.		Reversal of copula: Isn't <u>it</u> red? <u>Were</u> <u>they</u> there?	
2				A. who, what, what + noun: <u>Who</u> am I? <u>What</u> is he eating? <u>What</u> <u>book</u> are you reading? B. where, how many, how much, what . . . do, what . . . for <u>Where</u> did it go? <u>How</u> <u>much</u> do you want? <u>What</u> is he <u>doing</u>? <u>What</u> is a hammer <u>for</u>?
3		and		
4	can't, don't		Reversal of auxiliary be: Is <u>he</u> coming? Isn't <u>he</u> coming? Was <u>he</u> going? Wasn't <u>he</u> going?	
5	isn't, won't	A. but B. so, and so, so that C. or, if		when, how, how + adjective <u>When</u> shall I come? <u>How</u> do you do it? <u>How</u> <u>big</u> is it?
6		because	A. Obligatory do, does, did: <u>Do</u> <u>they</u> run? <u>Does</u> <u>it</u> bite? <u>Didn't</u> <u>it</u> hurt? B. Reversal of modal: <u>Can</u> <u>you</u> play? <u>Won't</u> <u>it</u> hurt? <u>Shall</u> <u>I</u> sit down? C. Tag question: It's fun, <u>isn't</u> <u>it</u>? It isn't fun, <u>is</u> <u>it</u>?	
7	All other negatives: A. Uncontracted negatives: I can <u>not</u> go. He has <u>not</u> gone. B. Pronoun-auxiliary or pronoun-copula contraction: I'm <u>not</u> coming. He's <u>not</u> here. C. Auxiliary-negative or copula-negative contraction: He wasn<u>'t</u> going. He hasn<u>'t</u> been seen. It couldn<u>'t</u> be mine. They aren<u>'t</u> big			why, what if, how come how about + gerund <u>Why</u> are you crying? <u>What</u> <u>if</u> I won't do it? <u>How</u> <u>come</u> he is crying? <u>How</u> <u>about</u> coming with me?
8		A. where, when, how while, whether (or not), till, until, unless, since, before, after, for, as + adjective + as, as if, like, that, than I know <u>where</u> you are. Don't come <u>till</u> I call. B. Obligatory deletions: I run faster <u>than</u> you [run]. I'm <u>as</u> big <u>as</u> a man [is big]. It looks <u>like</u> a dog [looks]. C. Elliptical deletions (score 0) That's <u>why</u> [I took it]. I know <u>how</u> [I can do it]. D. Wh- words + infinitive: I know <u>how</u> to do it. I know <u>where</u> to go.	A. Reversal of auxiliary have: <u>Has</u> <u>he</u> seen you? B. Reversal with two or three auxiliaries: <u>Has</u> <u>he</u> <u>been</u> eating? <u>Couldn't</u> <u>he</u> <u>have</u> waited? <u>Could</u> he <u>have</u> <u>been</u> crying? <u>Wouldn't</u> <u>he</u> <u>have</u> <u>been</u> going?	whose, which, which + noun <u>Whose</u> car is that? <u>Which</u> <u>book</u> do you want?

	INDEFINITE PRONOUNS OR NOUN MODIFIERS	PERSONAL PRONOUNS	PRIMARY VERBS	SECONDARY VERBS
1	–these/this: these many.	–mine's/my, you/your: That you book? –y'all (plural you) –me/I (in compound subj.): Me and my brother went in it.	–Ø copula is, am, are: That boy my friend. Or hypercorrect: I'm is six. –Ø aux be + Ving: The girl singin'. –locational go or existential it's: Here goes the dog. It's two dimes stuck on the table. –got as uninflected have: You gotta take it home.	
2		–he, she (in apposition): My brother, he bigger than you. –they/he: They my uncle. –he, he's/his: He's name is Terry. –she, she's/her	–third person singular and regular past tense markers deleted. It go fast. –have/has: It have money on it. –Regularization of -s and -ed: Trudy and my sister hides. –Aux was/were: We was gon' rob some money. –Irreg. past tense–Uninflected: He find the money; Past form as participle: We have went; Participle as past form: He done it first.	–I'm, I'mon, I'ma pronunciation of I'm gonna + V: I'm play. I'ma be tired. –go pronunciation of gonna: His nose go bleed. –fixin' to (used like gonna): I'm fixin' to take him to jail. (sometimes pronounced as /f^tə/)
3	–no (when 2nd or 3rd neg. marker): He don't like me no more.	–we, they (in apposition): The boys, they get in trouble. –they/their: They name is Tanya and Brian. –them/they or their: I know what them is. One of 'em name is Caesar. –them/those: them kids.		
4	–nothing, nobody, none, no one (when 2nd or 3rd neg. marker): Ain't nobody got none.		–Ø modal will or 'll: I be five when my birthday come. –don't + verb (3rd pers. sing.): My mama, she don't like it. –do uninflected: Do he still have it? (Score inc. in My sister do.) –Ø do in Qs: You still have it? –ain't (as copula or aux): Ain't no dirt in it. Nobody ain't got no more. –can't, don't, won't as preposed neg. aux.: Can't nobody do it. –could/can: He could climb that tree.	–participle with deleted -en: She has a state name Tennessee. (phonological cluster reduction rule) –I found the toy broke. (morphological difference)
5		–personal datives, me, him, her: I'm gonna buy me some candy. He make him a lot of 'em. –reflexives: hisself, theirselves, themself, theyselves		–deleted to in infinitival complements: My grandma tell me stay away from him. I like go shopping. My mommy used do it.
6		–what (in apposition): My voice gonna come out of here what I said on that book? –what/that or who: He's the one what I told you about. –Deleted relative pronoun: I saw a little girl was on the street.	–did + nt + verb (when 2nd or 3rd neg. marker: Nobody didn't do it. –could, would, should + nt + verb (preposed neg. aux): Couldn't nobody do it. –0 contracted could or would (phonol. deletions): You('d) burn your head off. –might/will: Who might be the baby?	
7	–many a: Many a people likes to give him a nickel.		–passive verb + en with getting (aux deleted): Leroy getting dressed. –passive verb ± be ± en: One is name Brick. They named Chief and JoJo. –done + verb + en (completive aspect): I done tried. –± (neg.) aux + supposed: He don't supposed to do it. What toy you supposed to play with? –± have ± verb + en: We seen him already. He have made him mad.	–passive with phonological deletions: I'm be dressed up real cute. I'ma be tired. She gonna be surprise, ain't she? I want it cut on.
8			–invariant be: My daddy know I skip school 'cause I be home with him. He be mad when somebody leave him home. –double modals: We might could come. –other expanded aux. forms: He be done jumped out the tub. He been going. (have has undergone phonological deletion) You shouldn't did that. –remote past aspect: She been whuptin' the baby. I been wanted this.	–gerund with go to, got to, start to: When I cry, she goes to whipping me. He started to crying. He got to thinking.

	NEGATIVES	CONJUNCTIONS	INTERROGATIVE REVERSAL	WH- QUESTIONS
1	–it, this, that + Ø copula/aux + not/ain't: That <u>not</u> mine. It <u>ain't</u> on?		–rising intonation with deleted or unreversed copula: You my friend? Where the gas at? What that is? –is/are: Derrick, is you?	
2				–who, what, what + noun (with deleted aux or copula) –where, how many, how much, what . . . do, what . . . for (with deleted aux or copula): Where the man? –Wh- Qs formed without interrogative reversal; What that is?
3		–and plus –Ø and (when intonation makes sentence combination clear): *He pointed his finger at him* (with rising intonation); *he pointed his finger at him* (with falling intonation).		
4	–don't (with 3rd pers. sing. as 2nd or 3rd neg. marker): He <u>don't</u> want none. No, nobody <u>don't</u> live with me. –can't, don't (as preposed aux): Can't nobody make me. –Ø copula/aux + not + V: My mama <u>not</u> gonna pick me up today. He <u>not</u> a baby. –ain't (as negative copula or aux. <u>be</u>): He <u>ain't</u> my friend.		–Ø auxiliary be: My voice gonna come out of here? You gonna tell my mama? –was/were: Was you throwin' rocks?	
5	–won't (as preposed aux): <u>Won't</u> nobody help him.	–for/so: The dog make too much noise for they won't catch many fish. –conditional <u>and</u>: You do that <u>and</u> I'm gonna smack you. –<u>if</u> with phrase deletions: He lookin' if he see the money. –aux. inversion in indirect Qs (instead of <u>if</u>): She ask me do he want some more.		–when, how (with deleted aux, copula or do): How you do this?
6		–or either, or neither (as disjunctives): He will go <u>or either</u> he will stay. He told her that he wouldn't be bad <u>or neither</u> get in trouble. –preposed why phrase (with because): Why he's in here, cause baby scared the dog.	–Ø do: You know that one with the tractor? Where you work? You got blue eyes? –do (with 3rd pers. sing.) Do he still have it? –Ø or unreversed modal: Now, what else I be doin? Why you can't talk on that? –Tag question with ain't: It gonna be fun, ain't it?	
7	–ain't (for have + not) ± uninflected V: I <u>ain't</u> taste any. –ain't (for did + not) ± uninflected V: Yesterday, he <u>ain't</u> go to school. I ain't found Marge in the school. –couldn't, wouldn't, shouldn't (as preposed aux). –wasn't/weren't: The brakes wasn't workin' right. –weren't/wasn't: There weren't no money. –uncontracted, uninflected neg. aux.: Lester <u>do not</u> like it.			–why, what if, how come (with deleted or unreversed aux, copula or do, or with got): Why she turn that way? Hey, why you got a dress on mama?
8		–less'n (for unless) –to/till: I didn't get to sleep to I had to come in the morning. –± as + adjective + as: He sock Leroy in the arm hard as he could.	–deleted have: He seen it? How you been? What you been doing? –have with 3rd pers. sing.: Have he seen you?	–whose, which, which + noun (with deleted aux, copula or do) –who/whose: Who this bed? Who baby is that?

10

Middle Stages: Goals and Intervention Strategies

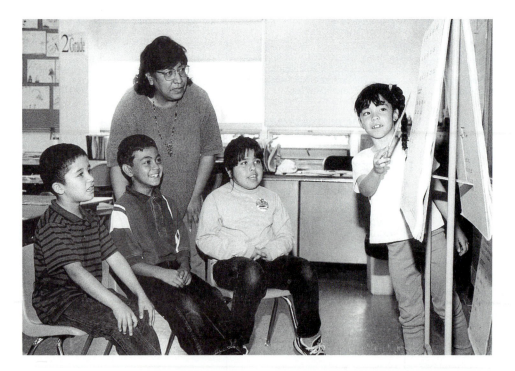

ROLES OF ADULT PARTNERS AND CONTEXTS IN LANGUAGE INTERVENTION

USING LANGUAGE TO ACCOMPLISH EXPANDED CONVERSATIONAL PURPOSES

PRODUCING AND COMPREHENDING SENTENCES

CONTINUED PHONOLOGICAL DEVELOPMENT

ACQUIRING AND RETRIEVING WORDS AND CONCEPTS

DEVELOPING SKILLS IN SYMBOLIC PLAY

PARTICIPATING IN STORYTELLING: EMERGING LITERACY

BEGINNING SCHOOL

The goals and intervention strategies for the middle stages of language acquisition are designed to build on the linguistic and nonlinguistic abilities the child has already acquired and to extend the child's development in areas not proceeding normally. The sections of this chapter highlight areas that pose problems for many children with middle-stage language acquisition needs. They also suggest ways that language specialists and others might assist children through a more normal development course. Although the discussion is organized by description of communicative targets rather than causative concerns, the latter often play a role in clinical decision making (e.g., when a child cannot hear). Special issues related to cause are, therefore, raised at a number of points throughout the chapter.

ROLES OF ADULT PARTNERS AND CONTEXTS IN LANGUAGE INTERVENTION

Although children in the middle stages of development are less tied to the home and primary caregivers than are infants and toddlers in the early stages, they nevertheless continue to learn much about language and communication through their interactions with adults. Therefore, part of the intervention process should continue to focus on adults' roles in encouraging more normal development.

Taking a conscious look at how best to facilitate language acquisition when it is not proceeding normally can help parents who are unsure how to assist their children's lagging communicative development. Such a deliberate process can address some of the concerns raised in Chapter 8 about language-learning environment modifications that parents seem to make subconsciously when they become concerned about their child's development. For example, some parents start to act more like vocabulary teachers than conversational partners (Donahue & Pearl, 1995). Some become more controlling and directive for children who are developmentally less mature (particularly fathers), and some exert greater topic control when their children are less involved (particularly mothers) (Girolametto & Tannock, 1994). Both mothers (Conti-Ramsden, 1990) and fathers (Conti-Ramsden, Hutcheson, & Grove, 1995) use fewer complex recasts contingent on what their children say, and fathers, particularly, ask for more frequent repeats for

clarification from their children with specific language impairments.

Modifying Parent Discourse as Part of Intervention

In discussing language intervention with young children, Fey (1986) noted that "needs to use language arise much more frequently at home and at school than in any clinical setting" (p. 291) and that some of the best opportunities for language learning seem to occur when children are the most motivated to communicate. Conditions under which these needs arise are often difficult to simulate in the clinic, and learning new skills in context can increase the likelihood that they will generalize. Therefore, Fey proposed that intervention with young children is most effective when it involves family members (see Personal Reflection 10.1).

Not all parents are equally prepared to assume intervention roles with their young children, however. Many need considerable preparation before they can act as language intervention aides or primary intervention agents for their children, and they may not always recognize opportunities to serve as incidental intervention agents (roles discussed in Chapter 5). Although the research reviewed in Chapter 5 suggests mixed results of formal efforts to involve parents in intervention, their role in helping their children learn to communicate and to know more about the world is critical. This should involve helping parents focus on their children's abilities as well as disabilities and helping them encourage the delight of informal discovery rather than formal teaching. Parents may also need assistance in focusing on areas presenting difficulties to their children. They may need some guidance in helping to build linguistic and nonlinguistic scaffolds, to intensify experience, to help frame and focus their children's attention (see Personal Reflection 10.2).

Parents as Primary Intervention Agents. Fey and colleagues (1993) compared implementation of a focused stimulation approach (see Box 10.1) by parents and speech–language pathologists. The children in the study were 30 preschool-age children with language impairments between the ages of 3:8 and 5:10, all with needs to develop more mature grammatical structures. Treatments ran for 4½ months. Children in a delayed-treatment group made no gains over their period of no treatment. Children in both the parent-treatment and clinician-treatment groups showed large treatment effects as measured by Lee's (1974) Developmental Sentence Scoring techniques (including significant improvements in the main verb and sentence point categories as well as the overall score). Some variability was noted in how well the parent intervention approach worked compared to the more consistently effective clinician intervention.

The parent intervention program Fey and his colleagues (1993) designed was not haphazard. It required a significant amount of both clinician time and parent commitment. Although approximately twice as many clinician hours were involved in the clinician treatment

---

PERSONAL REFLECTION 10.2 _____

When asked where the childlike expectation in her creativity came from, Jeannette Haien, concert pianist and novelist, responded:

"I credit my parents. One begins, or doesn't, with that. One of my first memories is of my father calling excitedly to say. 'Look.' He was looking up at the sky. I couldn't see what I was to look at. Then he said, 'Listen,' and I heard this peculiar sort of sound, very distant. He kept saying, 'Look higher, look higher,' and I did. Then I saw my first skein of geese and heard their call. He took my hand and said to me, 'Those are the whales of the sky.' I have never forgotten it. And I never look up at a sky without the expectation of some extraordinary thing coming—airplane, owls at night. I'm a great looker up to the sky."

Jeannette Haien, when interviewed by *Bill Moyers,* journalist, during his PBS series (quoted in Tucher, 1990, p. 53)

---

program as the parent treatment program, parents met in groups at the clinic for 2 hours per week for the first 3 months of the 4½ month intervention. In addition:

> *The investigators carefully observed and analyzed samples of the subjects' connected speech to determine a small set of specific goals. Parents observed clinician demonstrations, participated in role play exercises, and took part in group discussions of the procedures in 12 weekly group sessions and three home visits. They also received individually tailored feedback regarding their use of the techniques and follow-up to ensure that they were continuing to employ the procedures properly. (p. 154)*

Fey and his colleagues concluded that similar high levels of parent training and commitment, supported by direct clinician involvement, would probably be required to yield consistent treatment results from treatment programs administered by parents.

Parents Supporting Preschool Language Activities. When we developed a preschool language intervention program for children in Berrien County Intermediate School District, one of the devices we used to increase immediate contact with the children's parents was to send notebooks back and forth each day in the children's pouches. Each child had a colored symbol that identified his or her notebook, carrying pouch, storage "cubby," placemat, and other items at school. Each also had a carpet square of the same color to define where the child was supposed to sit during "circle time." (These strategies helped the children learn the concept of abstract symbols representing a person's belongings, built meaningfulness into abstract colors and shapes, and made it possible to talk about such concepts as "Who is *not* here today?" based on empty carpet squares.)

Not all parents were immediately anxious to write in the notebooks each night, however, and the usual problems with getting books returned each day were apparent in the early days of the program. The collaborating professionals soon discovered and modified a strategy that made all the difference. Each night, they asked parents to sit down with their children to sketch an event that had happened that day (professionals modeled extremely primitive stick figure drawings to reduce parental anxiety about drawing). They also instructed parents to write down what their child said about the

Box 10.1 _____

Focused Stimulation Procedures Used by Fey, Cleave, Long, and Hughes and the Parents They Taught to Act as Direct Language Intervention Agents with Their Preschool-Age Children

THE FOCUSED STIMULATION PROCEDURES EMPLOYED IN BOTH PROGRAMS

1. Activities were designed so that the child would have many opportunities to hear and to attempt productions of the specific grammatical targets. The actual frequency of opportunities for child attempts and interventionist models varied greatly depending on the target. For example, opportunities for the use of copular and auxiliary *is* occur naturally with far greater frequency than is the case for the relative pronoun *who.* Therefore, despite efforts to create more frequent opportunities for use of targets than might occur normally, pragmatic factors precluded maintenance of a standard number of models and opportunities for the use of targets by the subjects.
2. The target form or operation was modeled frequently under semantically and pragmatically appropriate conditions.
3. The child's attempts at the target were recast either through simple expansions or by changing the sentence modality (e.g., the child's use of a declarative sentence might be changed to a yes-no question to highlight the auxiliary form) or by buildups and breakdowns designed to put the child's target in a highly salient and informative context.
4. In general, the linguistic contest was manipulated so that the target was modeled for the child in contexts in which it was highly salient (e.g., sentence-initial position, elliptical contexts, informative contexts).
5. False assertions were used to encourage the children to produce sentences that obligate the use of the target (e.g., *That's not your cup* to evoke *Yes, it is*).
6. Contingent queries, especially requests for elaboration, were used frequently to force the child to code linguistically semantic details that were omitted from the child's original message (e.g., Child: *eating cookie.* Clinician: *Who is eating a cookie?* Child: *boy.*). The clinician then expanded the child's sentence using both the original message and the response to the query. This yielded a vertically structured production of the target (e.g., Clinician: *Oh, the boy is eating the cookie.*).
7. The child might be asked forced-alternative questions that provide a model of the correct use of the target (e.g., *You do like it or you don't like it?* to evoke *I don't like it.*).
8. These techniques were employed in stories that were created for the children on a weekly basis and given to parents to take home. The parents (or other caregivers) were required to read the story of the week at least once a day.

Note: From Fey, M. E., Cleave, P. L., Long, S. H., & Hughes, D. L. (1993). Two approaches to the facilitation of grammar in children with language impairment: An experimental evaluation (p. 157). *Journal of Speech and Hearing Research, 36,* 141–157. Used by permission.

event in the child's exact words. The parents learned to take mini-language samples of their child's words, to transcribe them exactly, to become sensitive to limitations of form, but also to tune into their children's interests and understandings. The professionals instructed parents *not* to correct their children's grammatical formulation errors but encouraged parents to show interest in their child's ideas and to model other ways to talk about the same topic and to extend it. Topics ranged from exciting visits to Grandmother's house to mundane teeth brushing.

Soon the children themselves (many with severe language limitations) were reminding their parents about their language books, because each child who brought the notebook spent some individual time talking about the picture with the speech–language clinician or the teacher during small-group time. During this time, the adult redrew the original sketch on larger paper and invited the child to fill in details and to recall and to talk about the event (a similar strategy could be used in pull-out sessions). When the group came back together in a circle, children with story pictures talked about them with their peers. The instructor also encouraged peers to ask questions of each other (something they rarely did spontaneously). This all made it highly desirable to take notebooks home and bring them back.

The notebook strategy also gave the professionals an opportunity to inform parents of the "concepts of the week" (we usually used three contrasting pairs) and to suggest some enrichment activities at home to reinforce those concepts during family routines (e.g., "accidentally" putting on both a *long* and *short* sock during dressing and waiting for the child to comment on it).

Parents Setting Contexts for More Complex Language. Exactly *how* parents communicate with their children with language impairments may not be as important as *that* they communicate with them. However, a key seems to be that language input be appropriately complex. Geers and Shick (1988) studied the language abilities of 5- to 8-year-old children who had either hearing parents or hearing impaired parents. The author hypothesized that the better language skills demonstrated by children of hearing impaired parents were related to the signing ability of their parents, which allowed the parents to provide consistent language stimulation, of appropriate advancing complexity, throughout the elementary school years. P. J. Yoder (1989) found that children with specific language impairments made greater improvement in mastering auxiliary verb use when their mothers used higher rates of information-seeking questions. As in all cases, scaffolding works best when implemented just at a child's developing edge of competence, but with challenges and assistance to move to the next higher step. Topic continuing Wh-questions, in which adults ask about what a child is saying or doing,

can have a facilitative effect on conversation for children with developmental disabilities at all levels (Yoder, Davies, Bishop, & Munson, 1994).

Modifying Teacher Discourse as Part of Intervention

As children enter school programs, adults other than their parents become significant interactants. As a result of IDEA Child-Find activities (see Chapter 7), children are identified with developmental problems at earlier ages, and more of these children may find their ways into specialized intervention programs. In such programs, teacher–child discourse has potential for influencing language development.

The principles of **incidental teaching, mand-model, or milieu instruction** were introduced in Chapter 3 and discussed further in Chapter 8. B. Hart and Risley defined this approach as the "interactions between an adult and a child that arise naturally in an unstructured situation, such as free play, and that are used systematically by the adult to transmit new information or give the child practice in developing a communication skill" (1975, p. 411). Some evidence supports the effectiveness of these strategies, which tend to be "brief, positive, and oriented toward communication rather than language teaching per se" (S. F. Warren & Kaiser, 1986, p. 291). For example, during free play in a preschool classroom, a child may point to a ball on a shelf, perhaps even saying the word *ball.* The teacher will follow this initiation by using a mand-model, saying, "Tell me, 'want ball.' " After the child does so, the ball is handed to the child (a natural reinforcer), and the classroom routine continues. Another possible use of the procedure would be for a teacher to approach a child engaged in an activity and to ask, with interest, "What are you doing?" (a mand). If the child responds verbally, the teacher says something like, "That's neat," or "Right." If the child fails to respond, the teacher produces a model for the child, such as, "Say, I'm coloring." If the child does so, social reinforcement is provided; if not, the interaction continues.

The effectiveness of incidental teaching was investigated by S. F. Warren, McQuarter, and Rogers-Warren (1984) in a university preschool for language-delayed children. Their results showed increased rates of total verbalizations, including both responses to questions and nonobligatory speech initiations. They also found evidence of increased MLU and generalization to other free-play situations.

The descriptions of milieu teaching or incidental intervention rely heavily on the terminology and technology of behaviorism (Kirchner, 1991). Relying more on a sociolinguistic theoretical perspective, Norris and Hoffman (1990b) described a set of naturalistic strategies for providing interaction-based language interventions for middle-stage children. They emphasized that even when language intervention is provided within naturalistic environments (in which language is treated more as a medium of communication than a system of rules to be learned), it must be organized. The naturalistic intervention steps suggested by Norris and Hoffman included the following: (1) organize the environment so that appropriate information is available and the child has opportunity to interact; (2) initiate and refine communication, encouraging the child to initiate, responding to the child's behaviors as if they are communicative, elaborating and expanding the child's topics, and using scaffolding to help the child reach the next level of complexity; and (3) provide consequences that are natural to the communicative event, emphasizing the criterion of communicative effectiveness, using clarification or repair strategies as necessary.

Kaiser and Hester (1994) studied an "enhanced milieu teaching" (EMT) approach, which was modified to incorporate features of more naturalistic approaches. They described it as a hybrid approach that included three key features. First, **environmental arrangement** was used to select materials of interest and to arrange them to promote requests in a context with an adult who mediated the environment and engaged in activities with the child. Second, **responsive interaction strategies** were used to follow the child's lead, balance turns, maintain the child's topic, map actions with linguistically and topically appropriate models, match the child's complexity level, expand and repeat the child's utterances, and respond communicatively to the child's verbal and nonverbal communication. Third, **milieu teaching techniques** included child-cued modeling, mand-modeling, time delay, and incidental teaching. Kaiser and Hester used a multiple baseline research design to study the approach and found that six children with significant language delays (CA 37 to 80 months, but language skills at the 18- to 36-month level) all acquired targeted language skills and maintained them after treatment.

In describing a **dialogue approach** to intervention, Marion Blank (1973) emphasized that the quality of adult–child interactive discourse depends on the degree to which it might encourage development of the "abstract attitude." Blank argued that, despite the fuzziness of the concept and breadth of phenomena subsumed under the rubric **abstract attitude,** advantages accrue from targeting its development rather than targeting the development of specific skills. Furthermore, Blank argued that the abstract attitude could best be developed in the context of extended, connected one-on-one dialogues between a child and an intentioned adult (not in discrete single-unit exchanges or group lessons). She emphasized the need for children to participate in contextually grounded sequences of discourse interactions, noting that, "The opportunity for the sustained pursuit of an idea is acquired" (p. 22). The notion that ideas can "attain their full potential only when embedded in context" (p. 22) is easier to understand when one considers that a sentence such as "The car is red" takes on entirely different meanings if it follows a question such as "How did he recognize the car?" or "How is the car different from the other car?" Consider how this kind of discourse interaction differs from common clinical discourse exchanges when clinicians ask a series of unrelated parallel questions such as "What color is the _____?" Such a series does not require children to make any cognitive connections beyond the surface ones. An example of Blank's scaffolding discourse appears in Box 10.2.

Haley, Camarata, and Nelson (1994) compared social responses of 15 preschool children with specific language impairment to intervention approaches that were imitation-based or conversation-based. The researchers found that both approaches were associated with a high frequency of such positive signs as smiling, laughing, and engagement in activities and a low frequency of negative expressions of boredom or dislike. However, the conversation-based treatment yielded significantly higher positive social ratings, as well as more verbal initiations by the children. Conversely, the imitation-based treatment yielded more negative social ratings and a significantly higher rate of quiet, passive participation. The conversation-based approach also had advantages in that fewer presentations were needed before targeted structures appeared spontaneously and spontaneous productions were more frequent. By contrast, elicited productions were more frequent in the imitation-based approach (Camarata, Nelson, & Camarata, 1994).

Box 10.2

The Pattern of Tutorial Discourse (Illustrating Scaffolding) Used in Storytelling in Which a Bit of Content Is Read and Is Then Used as a Takeoff Point for Posing a Series of Relevant Cognitive Questions

DIALOGUE

TEACHER: Where is this nest?

CHILD: On a tree.

TEACHER: And where is the nest in the tree?

CHILD: (No response.)

TEACHER: Near the ground?

CHILD: High up in the tree?

TEACHER: That's right! And if he just walks out high up in the tree what will happen to him?

CHILD: He'll fall out.

TEACHER: That's right. I guess he thinks he can fly. But why can't he fly? His mother can fly!

CHILD: He and the bird can fly.

TEACHER: You think he can fly? Let's see (turns the page).

CHILD: He fell.

TEACHER: Why did he fall? Why didn't he just fly?

CHILD: Cause, cause he took one foot off the nest!

TEACHER: Yeah. But his mother took one foot off of the nest and what did she do?

CHILD: She didn't fall out.

TEACHER: Why not?

CHILD: (Shrugs shoulders.)

TEACHER: Who's bigger and stronger? The mommy bird or the baby bird?

CHILD: The mommy.

TEACHER: And who can fly?

CHILD: The mommy.

TEACHER: That's right. But the bird cannot fly yet because he is not strong. His wings are not strong enough to help him fly. What could happen?

INTERPRETATION

This sounds correct but the child has still not shown that she has grasped the concept of height.

The posing of an incorrect alternative led in this case to the correct elaboration of the response.

The pictorial information told her that the bird would fall; her verbal associations to birds are that they fly. This is an illustration of how the child holds two opposing views without any awareness of their conflict.

A good use of memory, but still an incomplete answer to the question "why didn't he fly?" This question is to help the child realize that her initial response is obviously not correct.

While this question poses an alternative that may cause difficulty, the child's strong verbal associations make this a reasonable option to chance.

The teacher concludes the sequence since it would probably be too difficult for the child to do it, especially at the end of a lesson. Nevertheless, a question is left for the child to answer in order to make her use some of the information she has been given.

Cole and Dale (1986) found equivalent positive results for direct instruction and interactive instruction in preschool language intervention programs. After 8 months, children in both settings improved on syntactic and semantic measures, and there were no differences between the two groups as post-test.

For children at the school-age level, "teacher talk" may be a legitimate focus of intervention (N. W. Nelson, 1984, 1985, 1989b). At least, the specialist should ask questions about how the demands of classroom discourse intersect with the child's language abilities and disabilities. One can collaborate with teachers to consider discourse styles, speaking rate, and other variables, such as using more frequent comprehension checks and giving explicit directions, that facilitate particular children's language processing. Choices about the best classrooms and teachers for children might also be made on these bases.

Enhancing the Auditory Language-Learning Context

Amplifying the volume of adult speech is another way to modify the environment to encourage communicative development among middle-stage children (See Personal Reflection 10.3). A few investigators have used sound field amplification in classrooms to enhance the signal-noise ratio of teachers' language to background noise, even for children who have normal peripheral hearing (Flexer, 1989; Flexer, Millin, & Brown, 1990; Ray, Sarff, & Glassford, 1984; Sarff, Ray, & Bagwell, 1981).

> *Frequency-modulated sound-field FM amplification systems are similar to small, high fidelity, wireless public address systems that are self-contained in a classroom. Specifically, the teacher wears a small, unobstrusive wireless microphone; thus, teacher mobility is not restricted. His or her speech is frequency modulated onto a carrier wave that is sent from the transmitter to the receiver where it is demodulated and delivered to the students through one to five wall-or-ceiling-mounted loudspeakers. . . . The purpose of the equipment is to amplify the teacher's voice throughout the classroom, thereby providing a clear and consistent signal to all pupils in the room no matter where they or the teacher are located. (Crandell et al., 1995, pp. 4–5)*

The provision of amplification to children with language disorders but normal hearing is still experimental. In addition to sound field amplification, the use of amplification devices such as FM systems, auditory trainers, personal amplification devices, and other assistive listening devices has been reported with normal hearing children. For example, studies of classroom amplification provide preliminary evidence that amplification can help students with mild, fluctuating hearing loss (Carlson & Nelson, 1994) and with special education needs (Flexer, 1989; Sarff et al., 1981; Ray, Sarff, & Glassford, 1984). Children with developmental disabilities attending a primary-level special education class also made significantly fewer errors on a word identification task with amplification than without (Flexer et al., 1990). When they reviewed such studies, the American Speech-Language-Hearing Association (ASHA) Committee on Amplification (1991) cautioned that the work is preliminary and that more information is needed in the areas of efficacy, consumer safety, and professional liability before the procedures are considered a standard element in language treatment.

The provision of amplification for children with hearing impairments is, of course, another matter. The multiple considerations involved in providing amplification for children with hearing impairments exceed the boundaries of this text (see, e.g., Flexer, 1994). They involve the professional contributions of audiologists and other hearing health-care specialists. However, speech–language pathologists and other special and regular education professionals cannot afford to ignore those needs, or others that extend beyond amplification. "While the appropriate and effective use of FM units is essential for the classroom management of hearing impaired children, equipment use alone may not be sufficient for successful mainstreaming" (Flexer, Wray, & Ireland, 1989, p. 17). Other programming components for children with hearing impairments include specific training for using auditory skills in functional contexts, helping teachers and students maximize the auditory information available in educational activities, and providing intervention specifically related to understanding the language of the curriculum.

Friel-Patti (1994) described a series of six educational principles that could be used to guide decisions about children suspected of having central auditory processing disorders: (1) confirm the status of peripheral hearing, (2) observe the child in a variety of learning environments and record error patterns, (3) analyze task demands in terms of their linguistic and short-term memory expectations, (4) consider the child's attention and distractibility, (5) consider the child's comprehension abilities, and (6) develop strategies for effective learning and teaching.

USING LANGUAGE TO ACCOMPLISH EXPANDED CONVERSATIONAL PURPOSES

GOAL: The child will use appropriate conversational strategies with adults and peers.

- Maintaining an Assertiveness-Responsiveness Balance
- Making Requests
- Being Polite
- Taking Turns, Managing Topics, and Making Repairs
- Instructional Strategies for Conversation

OUTCOME: The child will interact appropriately in conversations and will be sought as a desired conversational partner.

Maintaining an Assertiveness–Responsiveness Balance

Objective 1: The child will adjust the frequency of assertive or responsive communicative acts to achieve an improved balance over baseline conversations.

In their preschool and early elementary years, children continue to expand the pragmatic functions they are able to accomplish with language. Children with language disorders, however, may be more limited in their communicative interaction patterns than their normal language-learning peers. In Chapter 9, patterns of communicative assertiveness or responsiveness were described (Fey, 1986; Figure 9.4). Different communicative function patterns justify different intervention goals. The intervention goals Fey suggested for children exhibiting communicative patterns as **active conversationalists, passive conversationalists, inactive communicators,** and **verbal noncommunicators** are summarized in Box 10.3.

Making Requests

Objective 2: The child will use appropriate linguistic forms to request actions, objects, and information, by: (1) getting attention, (2) communicating the request clearly, (3) being persistent, (4) being persuasive, and (5) making repairs using age-appropriate strategies.

It would be a mistake to think of intervention to expand communicative functions as affecting or targeting only single dimensions of communicative behavior. For example, one cannot simply target a function such as "making requests" without recognizing all of the kinds of knowledge and skills that must be integrated before a child can effectively do so. For example, Ervin-Trip and Gordon (1986) noted that a speaker must solve the five different problems of Objective 2 to make requests effectively. Developmental expectations in this area are summarized in Box 10.4.

Being Polite

Objective 3: The child will use polite conventions (*please, thank you, you're welcome,* and indirect forms) to make requests and join a conversation.

Box 10.3 _____

Suggested Intervention Goals Based on Conversational Speech-Act Analysis

GOALS FOR ACTIVE CONVERSATIONALISTS

1. Train [the child in] new content–form interactions to perform available conversational acts.
2. Facilitate the use of old forms to fulfill alternative conversational acts.

GOALS FOR PASSIVE CONVERSATIONALISTS

1. Increase the frequency of use of available assertive conversational acts in a variety of social contexts.
2. Increase the child's repertoire of assertive conversational acts, using existing forms when possible.
3. Train new linguistic forms that are useful in performing available assertive acts.

GOALS FOR INACTIVE COMMUNICATORS

1. Increase the child's rate of positive social bids (verbal and nonverbal) in a variety of social contexts.
2. When the child becomes more responsive and begins to initiate communication more frequently, goals for passive conversationalists probably will be appropriate.

GOALS FOR VERBAL NONCOMMUNICATORS

1. Increase the relatedness of the child's responses to the assertive acts (e.g., requestives, assertives, performatives) of the partner.
2. Facilitate the child's production of sequences of utterances that are topically related to one another.

Note: From Marc E. Fey, *Language Intervention With Young Children* (pp. 80–98). Copyright © 1986. Reprinted with permission of Allyn and Bacon.

_____

Most children in mainstream Western cultures begin to be held accountable for politeness by their parents during the preschool years. Being polite is more than a matter of being able to say *please* and *thank you* (as evident in the review by Ervin-Tripp and Gordon, 1986, summarized in Box 10.4). Nippold, Leonard, and Anastopoulos (1982) characterized development in production and understanding of polite forms as sensitivity to the function of these forms in an increasing number of sentence types related to increasing ability to assume perspectives of listeners. Intervention strategies might focus on the development of this perspective-taking ability by modeling and reinforcing it. Other strategies include directly modeling polite conversational behaviors and linguistic markers and requesting their imitation in appropriate contexts.

Taking Turns, Managing Topics, and Making Repairs

> *Objective 4:* The child will take and yield conversational turns, maintain topics over several turns, shade topics appropriately, and make successful conversational repairs when asked for clarification.

John Dore (1986) described growth in the development of conversational competence as context dependent. He also tied it to growth of **cohesion** (making sensible connections) and **coherence** (relating to a topic). During the one-word stage children begin to develop cohesion by choosing one word as a single option among several to fit the circumstances. This kind of cohesion is primarily lexically determined. Discourse cohesion across turns develops more slowly. At preschool level, Dore pointed out that children begin to work out new relationships with peers, school authorities, and others. While doing so, "the child explores the options for getting and constructing his turns at talk and for exploiting the conversational subsystems in negotiating his social power and solidarity" (p. 36). When children enter grade school, significant shifts in conversational influences are observed again:

> *The child's initiation into studenthood involves him with a much wider social milieu, a more structured authority system, an expansion of his relationship to others from peer to educational collaborator and a sense of being one among many, perhaps even of being an interchangeable member of a vast institution. Student membership brings with it many new responsibilities for "behaving like a good pupil." (Dore, 1986, p. 55)*

These efforts involve not only cooperation strategies but also competition strategies, such as in classroom attempts to get and to avoid turns to speak and read.

Much of the research on the conversational strategies of children with language-learning disabilities has been

Box 10.4 _____

Developmental Advances from Ages 2 to 8 Years in Skills Needed for Making Requests (Based on Ervin-Trip & Gordon, 1986)

GETTING ATTENTION

Ages 2 to 4: Children tend to make requests without first attempting to gain attention. By age 3, they improve in this regard, but tend to call "Hey" rather than the more specific, "Hey, Joe."

Ages 4 to 8: Children increase the specificity and effectiveness of attention forms.

CLARITY

Ages 2 to 4: Children learn a full array of basic forms for making instrumental moves, and clarity ceases to be their major problem. During this time, they learn to be specific about the agent, action, and goal in their requests.

Ages 4 to 8: Whereas young children are not good at attending to the cognitive needs of their listeners, this awareness increases in the early elementary years. During these years, interviewing shows that children are more explicit in their requests when they think the listener does not expect a request.

SOCIAL DISTINCTIONS

Ages 2 to 4: By age 2, children already show some distinctions in their speech for different listeners (e.g., on the basis of age, familiarity, and role). By age 2:6, they begin using auxiliaries that give them the possibility of adding polite questions to mark social contrasts, often combining requests with the word "Please." They also begin to use forms like "Can you," and "D'you wanna" when compliance cannot be assumed.

Ages 4 to 8: Children seem to become more sensitive to the effects of interruption on the listener. When they expect listeners to be compliant, children tend not to use imperatives. Polite forms are used more frequently when children interrupt their listeners. By age 8, children tend to be better at perspective taking.

PERSUASION

Ages 2 to 4: Spontaneous explanations or justifications for requests are rarely provided by 2- and 3-year-olds.

Ages 4 to 8: By age 4 or 5, children often supply reasons or check willingness when making requests of their peers. Older speakers eventually use the justification statements or reasons alone as indirect requests.

REPAIRS

Ages 2 to 4: Younger children are likely to attempt to make repairs by increasing their requests over and over with increasing urgency. By age 2:6, children who have developed politeness strategies will use them on second attempts if first attempts are unsuccessful.

Ages 4 to 8: When older children fail to have their requests met, they are more likely to use tactics of conveying obligation, justification, or bribery in addition to increased aggravation or urgency (as younger children tend to do).

done with children in the later grades. However, in her research review, T. Bryan (1986) noted that some children studied were as young as first graders. Although the children with learning disabilities were not inferior to their peers with normal language in all areas of conversational interaction, they were found to have difficulties in some. They had difficulties delivering bad news to peers tactfully, their messages were less informative, and they had difficulty asking clarification questions when given ambiguous messages. On the playground, they were less likely to give positive, encouraging remarks to their peers, such as "Good catch," and more likely to make negative, discouraging comments, for example, "Look, he can't even get up there" (p. 239).

Responses to requests for clarification by children ages 4:10 to 9:10 were studied by Brinton, Fujiki, Winkler, and Loeb (1986). They used a series of stacked responses from children with specific language impairments and children with normal language skills at three age levels. Brinton and her colleagues found that all children demonstrated the willingness and ability to respond to these neutral clarification requests. However, the quality of the responses differed. The language-impaired children produced more inappropriate responses than the normally developing children across age groups and clarification types. The children with language impairments showed particular difficulty repairing multiple times in stacked sequences. Perhaps this was because they had less linguistic flexibility, were less aware of their listener's needs, or interpreted the repeated requests for clarification as disapproval of the form or content of their messages.

Instructional Strategies for Conversation

Most clinicians agree that pragmatic functions can be targeted effectively only within the contexts of naturalistic communicative interactions. To some extent, such opportunities may be contrived, or enhanced with techniques of focusing and modeling, but the essential intervention strategy is to help children move through developmental sequences by giving them opportunities to practice their advancing skills in meaningful contexts.

In discussing intervention for problems related to conversational management, Brinton and Fujiki (1989) commented that clinical procedures must be devised to fit the child, the clinician, and the target. For example,

children with more severe impairments are likely to need more highly structured conversational contexts, whereas children with less severe impairments may benefit more from naturalistic exchanges. In either case, however, the final goal should be a set of integrated communicative abilities, "not to teach turn taking or topic mechanics per se but rather to facilitate the conversational management skills that enhance effective communication" (p. 142). Intervention objectives should be written to be consistent with this goal. Box 10.5 includes two kinds of objectives, one written in a way that Brinton and Fujiki considered to be more effective than the other.

Conversational contexts not only provide rich opportunities to observe and foster integrated language, speech, and communicative abilities, they also may be used to gain insights into possible factors contributing to communicative problems. Effective assessment during intervention involves identification of contributing factors to be addressed along with primary symptoms. For example, Brinton and Fujiki (1989) listed 10 related problems that might undermine smooth turn exchange and successful topic manipulation: (1) peripheral hearing loss, (2) selective attending difficulty, (3) language comprehension difficulty, (4) language production deficits, (5) problems with immediate memory span, (6) stuttering behaviors, (7) difficulty with relevance constraints, (8) being oblivious to the needs of other speakers, (9) being too easily intimidated, and (10) psychological disturbance.

Intervention strategies aimed directly at conversational interaction are implemented by first engaging children in conversations with enough environmental support to ensure success, starting with nonverbal ex-

---

Box 10.5 _____

Less and More Effective Ways of Designing Intervention Objectives for Topic Maintenance

Less effective objective: Teach the child to talk about any given topic for 30 seconds.

More effective objective: Facilitate the child's participation in topical sequences to share information when interacting in a dyad.

(From Brinton & Fujiki, 1989, p. 142).

---

changes or games if necessary. The support should be based on the child's needs. The strategy might include the use of such suprasegmentals as pause and stress to encourage children to notice cues for initiating turns, providing repair, or asking for clarification. Other strategies might involve direct or indirect modeling. Gradually, the clinician should reduce the environmental support to allow more equal responsibility for managing conversations (Brinton & Fujiki, 1989).

Remember that the best way to assist a child to improve functioning within a particular communicative event is to work within events that are as intact as possible (Duchan, 1995a). If you want a child's conversational language to improve, you have to engage the child in conversation (see Personal Reflection 10.4). The turn-taking structure of games may seem to provide the support that reluctant children need to get started, but it is not the same as conversation. Conversing with the child, perhaps with the support of the child's own drawings, or with parental drawings and comments about events from home is a more direct way to help the child improve conversational language ability than games. Children learn new words and forms as they need them for conveying desired meanings to interested conversational partners. For example, Nordenbrock (1995) found that children with severe-to-profound hearing impair-

ments benefited from conversing with their kindergarten teacher (certified as a teacher of hearing-impaired children) about their spontaneous drawings and labeling key features. Both the children's drawings and language, including beginning narrative structure, improved in complexity over the 2-month intervention period Nordenbrock studied.

Duchan (1995a) described three situational supports for helping children use several varieties of conversational discourse. The supports include **spatial arrangements, time allocation,** and **suggestive props.**

For example, a housekeeping corner can promote pretend conversations; Fisher Price play stations can promote play involving service encounters; sharing time can elicit event descriptions; story time or book time can elicit narratives; and an activity involving teaching peers how to do something is likely to promote event descriptions or expositions. Suggestive props provide children with support in initiations and enactments of discourse-based activities. For example, dress-up clothes can suggest particular roles to be played out, and objects such as toy foods or dishes can give the activity some needed structure. (p. 81)

Intervention may be delivered using a variety of service models. Conversational interaction strategies may be targeted in dyadic clinician-child conversations or in the contexts of small groups or special or regular education classrooms. The outcome of intervention should be legitimate conversation that is communicative and not distorted by intervention. For example, it would be a disservice to teach children to make multiple clarification requests when teachers find that behavior inappropriate without also teaching the children to recognize cues regarding appropriate timing of questions to the teacher. Teachers may also need to be assisted to appreciate the need for children to ask clarification questions through mutual goal setting and collaborative consultation.

PRODUCING AND COMPREHENDING SENTENCES

GOAL: The child will produce and understand sentences.

- Sentence Production
- Sentence Comprehension
- Content, Contexts, and Strategies for Syntactic Intervention

---

PERSONAL REFLECTION 10.4 _____

The following sample was reported by *Bonnie Brinton* and *Martin Fujiki* (1989) in their book *Conversational Management With Language-Impaired Children.*

CHILD: What do you do at work anyway?
CLINICIAN: Well, I help kids who have trouble talking.
CHILD: What happens to them?
CLINICIAN: Sometimes they don't understand people, and sometimes people don't understand them.
CHILD: So how do you help them?
CLINICIAN: Oh, we do a lot of things. We help them to say things clearly. We help them to learn new words, and we help them to make sentences.
CHILD: But how do they learn to talk to people?
CLINICIAN: We work on that too.
CHILD: Oh. (looks thoughtful) You gotta talk to people, you know.
CLINICIAN: I know. (pp. 214–215)

OUTCOME: The child will use language to convey and comprehend complex meanings at home, school, and in play.

Part of the process of gaining communicative competence involves making advances in producing and understanding complex content–form constructions. Although superficially, these developments may appear to be simply a matter of learning aspects of language form, meaningful uses of content–form constructions require sensitivity to semantic and pragmatic constraints as well. Choices about which language content and form structures to target should come from analyses of spontaneous language samples, using techniques such as those discussed in Chapter 9. Lee's (1974) Developmental Sentence Scoring procedure offers a useful tool for monitoring progress because it is sensitive to growth across a number of grammatical categories.

This section considers production aspects of syntactic and morphological rule use separately from comprehension. In actual communicative events, the two modalities are closely related but not necessarily mirror images of each other. This is because of the different processing demands associated with each.

Sentence Production

When children reach the beginning of the middle stages of language development, if they are learning language normally, they can combine such basic sentence constituents as agents, actions, and objects. In the middle stage, they acquire additional rules for elaborating the detail of those basic constituents, for making them agree with each other in number and tense, and for formulating variants of basic sentences, such as negatives and questions.

> *Objective 1.* The child will produce main sentence constituents (subject noun phrases and verb phrases) that show completeness, clarity, subject–verb agreement (*The boy is walking; The girls are walking*), and appropriate nominative pronoun case (*he, she, they* rather than *him, her, them*).

Subjecthood.   Learning some of the formal grammatical properties of subjecthood and subject–verb agreement appears to give many children with language disorders particular difficulty (Connell, 1986b). This is perhaps be-

cause the properties are not directly tied to meaning (Johnston & Kamhi, 1984). Properties to be learned relating to subjecthood include subject–verb agreement, the copula and auxiliary *be,* the third-person singular present-tense marker, the nominative case of pronouns, and the auxiliary inversion of questions.

An intervention strategy to teach multiple subject properties using a single procedure was devised by Connell (1986b). He tested the strategy with four children ranging from 3:4 to 4:2 who were diagnosed as having language disorders. The children were taught individually in ½-hour sessions three to four times per week. When the intervention procedure began, the children with language disorders were producing structures such as "Him walking," "Him walk," "Him big," or "Him a man." Connell described these as early topic-comment forms. Such forms do not, in the child's system, require subject–verb agreement or subjective (nominative) case on pronouns because they simply name a topic and comment on it. Connell designed the intervention procedure to move the children toward subject–predicate structures by "dislocating the topic." He modeled sentences with an accusative (objective case) pronoun placed before the nominative pronoun and the rest of the sentence. For example, children heard models like, "Him, he is walking." Such models use the accusative pronoun *him* to serve the topic function, followed by the nominative pronoun *he* to serve the subject function. The auxiliary *is* agrees with the singular subject. The children were taught to give this response when shown two contrasting pictures and asked, "Which one is walking?" Alternatively, the model "He is walking" was used with the question "What is the man doing?" presented with other pictures. By alternating the types of models and questions (with their corresponding stimulus pictures), Connell found that children could acquire the various aspects of subjecthood using a single set of varied models and questions.

> *Objective 2.* The child will use a variety of modal auxiliaries in present (*can, will, shall, may, must*) and past (*could, would, should, might, must*) tense forms in questions, negatives, and statements.

Modal Auxiliaries.   Elaborating the verb phrase depends heavily on the acquisition of rules for using the modal auxiliaries *can, will, shall, may,* and *must,* and corresponding past-tense forms *could, would, should,* *might,* and *must.* These forms have strong semantic, pragmatic, and syntactic implications (Bliss, 1987). Syntactically, the modal auxiliaries play important roles in forming negative and interrogative constructions, such as "May I have some?" and "I can't reach it." Semantically, they convey varied meanings: ability (*can*), intention (*will*), permission (*may, can*), obligation/necessity (*should*), probability/possibility (*may, might*), and certainty (*will*). Pragmatically, modals serve varied functions, such as making requests, especially polite, indirect requests, and performing other social interactive functions.

As discussed earlier in this chapter, problems with modal auxiliaries may be identified through language sample analysis. For example, Lee's (1974) DSS requires fairly elaborate analysis of modal auxiliaries and their contribution to forming negatives and interrogatives. The normal development of modal auxiliaries occurs over several years (Bliss, 1987), extending from the second year, when modals begin to emerge, until at least the age of 8. Bliss (1987) suggested intervention guidelines for working on modal auxiliaries that were based on the normal developmental sequence and included the following:

1. Focus on ability and intention early, as these are frequent and early acquired concepts [ability is expressed by the modals *can* or *can't,* intention is expressed by the modal *will*—"I'll show you how"].
2. Begin with *can* versus *can't.* Once these are mastered, wait several weeks to begin *will* and *won't.* The contrast eases learning. An interval is necessary to prevent confusion by the child.
3. Use self-reference early (first person pronouns or the child's name), as this form is the first to be associated with modals (Fletcher, 1979).
4. Link the modals with actions. Modals are initially used with an activity (Fletcher, 1979). An associated activity should facilitate learning. For example, "I *can* reach (it)." vs. "I *can't.*"
5. Initially, use short sentences with the modal occurring at the end of an utterance (Stimulus: "Can you reach the star?" Response: "Yes, I *can*" or "No, I *can't*"). This procedure increases the saliency of the form.
6. Make the words critical to a situation. Provide meaningful situations in which concepts are linked to the modals that have been targeted.
7. Generalization of modal usage to speakers other than the clinician is crucial for adequate carryover. Parents and teachers need to be involved in a successful intervention program.

Note: From " 'I Can't Talk Anymore; My Mouth Doesn't Want To.' The Development and Clinical Applications of Modal Auxiliaries" by L. S. Bliss, 1987, *Language, Speech, and Hearing Services in Schools, 18,* p. 77. Copyright 1987 by American Speech-Language-Hearing Association. Reprinted by permission.

> *Objective 3.* The child will use complex verb forms using present and past tense forms of modals, perfective forms (*have + en/ed*), progressive forms (*be + ing*), and main verbs to convey diverse meanings in questions, negatives, and statements.

Other Complex Verb Forms. Acquiring rules for modal auxiliaries is only one way that children learn to elaborate verb phrases. Even before children's earliest uses of *can't* and *don't,* auxiliary forms of *be* may begin to show up in children's present progressive (*is + Ving*) constructions. The auxiliary *is* appears as one of R. A. Brown's (1973) first 14 morphemes (see Box 9.9). Yet, perhaps because the grammatical rule, *is + Ving,* carries such a light semantic and pragmatic load, and perhaps because its acoustic qualities are often light as well, many children with form-based specific language impairments seem to need direct attention to acquire it.

Recall Chomsky's (1957) auxiliary construction rule (see Figure 8.1):

$$C + (modal) + (have + en) + (be + ing) + MV$$

In this rule, the C is an abstract symbol standing for the obligatory inclusion of markers indicating person (first, second, third), tense (present, past), and number (singular, plural) expressed on the first item in the verb string, which must agree with the subject of the sentence. The preceding discussion of *subjecthood* considered how intervention might help children acquire some of the subtleties of subject–verb agreement.

Except for the main verb (MV), all of the other items of Chomsky's (1957) verb construction rule, which appear in parentheses, are optional, depending on the linguistic context. As mentioned previously, modals may be used to shade meaning and to convey intention. The *be + ing* option of the rule is used to convey progressive action. When the auxiliary *be* is used in a present tense form (remember that syntactic tense can only be marked as present or past), such as "The boy is yelling," the semantic tense is present progressive, indicating ongoing action. When the auxiliary *be* is used in a past tense form, such as "The boy was yelling," the semantic tense is past progressive, indicating action that was ongoing during some past moment. When the *have + en* option is selected, the semantic tense of the verb changes to the "perfect" tense. When the auxiliary *have* is used in present tense, such as "She has arrived," it merely conveys that some action has been completed. This is called *present perfect* tense. When the auxiliary *have* is used in the past tense, such as "She had arrived by the time we got there," it conveys the past perfect semantic tense, meaning that the action was completed in the past.

Setting up situations that help children notice meaning contrasts like these may encourage them to use syntactic forms to convey similar shades of meaning in their own constructions (see Personal Reflection 10.5). For example, Fey (1986) noted that children are more likely to understand the use of perfective verb forms if children are placed in a context requiring their use, rather than if children simply form isolated sentence pairs primarily to please the clinician. Two of the sample discourse contexts he suggested for eliciting perfective verb forms appear in Box 10.6.

Children learning African American English (AAE), also called Ebonics and Black English Vernacular (BEV), have more options for forming semantic tenses than children learning standard English (SE) alone. According to the rules of the BEV linguistic system, including third-person singular present-tense markers and forms of the auxiliary and copular *be* is optional. When evaluating samples of spontaneous language or responses to test items, clinicians should not penalize the use of such "zero copula" and "zero auxiliary" forms by BEV speakers (Black English Sentence Scoring [BESS], N. W. Nelson & Hyter, 1990a, was designed for this purpose; see Chapter 9 Appendix C, Black English Sentence Scoring Criteria). Such forms should never be described as "incorrect" for BEV speakers. Children learning BEV also may use two later developing verb tenses that exist in BEV but not in SE: (1) the invariant *be* and (2) the remote time aspect with *been*.

The invariant *be* in BEV may be further subdivided into two uses: (1) as the uninflected main verb, or (2) as the distributive or nontense *be*. In BEV, unlike SE, in which forms of *be* must be inflected differently depending on the subject of the sentence (e.g., *is, are, am; was, were*), "the form *be* can be used as the main verb, regardless of the subject of the sentence" (Fasold &

Box 10.6 _____

Discourse Contexts Used to Evoke Past Perfect Verb Constructions

CLINICIAN: Suzy liked to bake chocolate chip cookies. One day, she decided to make some. She mixed the batter and spread the cookies on the sheet. Then she put them in the oven and turned on the timer. When the timer went off, Suzy got a big surprise. There was smoke everywhere and the cookies were black! What had happened?

CHILD (OR MODEL): She had set the timer wrong. She had left the cookies in too long. They had burned.

CLINICIAN: Basil, the dog, loved children. One day Karen decided that she would surprise the family with fried chicken for dinner. She laid the chicken on the table. Then, she remembered that she had no flour. She rushed to the store in her car. When she returned, she was surprised to find that her chicken was gone. Can you guess what had happened?

CHILD (OR MODEL): Basil had been hungry. He had jumped on the table and had eaten all of the chicken.

Note: From Marc E. Fey, *Language Intervention With Young Children* (p. 188). Copyright © 1986. Reprinted with permission of Allyn and Bacon.

Wolfram, 1970, p. 66). In one variation of this occurrence, phonological deletion causes *be* to appear to occur alone. Actually, the contracted auxiliary has been deleted phonologically (e.g., "He['ll] be here pretty soon" and "If you gave him a present he['d] be happy"). The other invariant *be* expresses a unique temporal meaning. The "distributive or nontense *be*" is used to indicate when an exact time cannot be clearly specified because the event is distributed intermittently in time (Fasold & Wolfram, 1970). Examples from a connected discourse sample spoken by a normally developing girl [age 6:3] illustrate this feature:

> *My mama don't like it neither. She be sayin' it stinks. My brothers be gettin' me in trouble. They be tellin' lies on me. [girl, 6:3]*

The remote time aspect with *been* is used in BEV to indicate that a "speaker conceives of the action as having taken place in the distant past" (Fasold & Wolfram, 1970, p. 62). For example, a boy [age 5:3] established his prior right to play with a toy airplane by saying "I been wanted this."

Intervention should not be designed to eliminate culturally acceptable forms from a child's communicative interactions, but intervention can appropriately target the addition of standard English options. Dialectal forms represent rich and meaningful expressions. As children learning different dialects or languages encounter SE forms through literacy activities and oral interactions in school, they may be more likely to acquire varied forms for varied contexts and purposes. Most children are more willing to try out different forms in speech and in writing if all of their communicative attempts are accepted and encouraged. When children whose first language experiences differ from SE demonstrate language impairments within their native systems, the collaborative planning process may be used to decide whether SE forms should be encouraged along with acceptance of forms of the child's first dialect or language. When making these decisions, the specialist should consider the language skills the child will need to participate in important life contexts.

> *Objective 4.* The child will produce: (1) compound sentences conjoined with *and, but, or*; (2) complex sentences with subordinate clauses conjoined with *because, while, when, although, since, if . . . then, before, after,* etc.; (3) complex sentences with embedded relative clauses and object complements introduced by *who, whose, that*; and (4) complex sentences with embedded infinitives, gerunds, and participles.

Complex Sentence Production.   In Chapter 9, a listing of expectations for complex sentence development was included in the discussion of language sample analysis (see Box 9.10). The acquisition of these forms may be an appropriate target when planning intervention for children who use complex forms rarely or incorrectly. Yet, such problems tend to be overlooked because it is easier to recognize misuse of a particular construction than to notice its absence. For example, when a kindergarten teacher hears a child produce sentences like "Me want to do it," or "Him coming to my house," the teacher is more likely to be alerted to the possibility that a language disorder might be present than when the child uses only simple forms for expressing ideas but makes few alerting "errors." Besides, short, simple utterances may be the expected norm in classroom group instruction (Sturm, 1990; Sturm & Nelson, 1997). On the other hand, the language of the curriculum itself is often filled with many complex sentence demands, and these show up from the earliest grades (N. W. Nelson, 1984). Children who have not learned to produce and comprehend such sentences in other contexts are then increasingly disadvantaged as grade level and linguistic demands increase.

Intervention plans targeting the acquisition of rules for forming complex sentences consider many variables. These were summarized by N. W. Nelson (1988b) as including developmental ordering and timing, relationships between comprehension and production, and recognition of the semantic and cognitive demands on speakers, listeners, readers, and writers. Infinitive embeddings are often the first complex forms to appear (Tyack & Gottsleben, 1986), and "at very young ages, as early as 2:6, children begin combining sentences to express complex or compound propositions" (Tager-Flusberg, 1985, p. 161). The first conjunction to emerge, *and*, appears even before children have mastered the grammatical morphemes (Laughton & Hasenstab, 1986; Tager-Flusberg, 1985). Other meanings of *and* are not acquired until much later. In one study, L. Bloom, Lahey, Hood, Lifter, and Fiess (1980) found that the meanings of the word *and* emerged in the following order (presented with the authors' examples):

1. Additive—"Maybe you can carry this and I can carry that."
2. Temporal—"Jocelyn's going home and take her sweater off."
3. Causal—"She put a bandage on her shoe and maked it feel better."

4. Adversative—"Cause I was tired and now I'm not tired."
5. Objective specification—"It looks like a fishing thing and you fish with it." (pp. 243–245)

Other conjunctions that can express varied conceptual relationships were summarized by N. W. Nelson (1988b) to include the following types:

1. Causal (*because, so, therefore*)
2. Coincidental (*while, during*)
3. Comparative (*as . . . as, . . . than*)
4. Consequential (*since, therefore, so*)
5. Conditional (*if, if . . . then*)
6. Disjunctive (*but, or, although, however*)
7. Temporal (*when, before, after, then*) (p. 171)

When teaching rules for combining and embedding sentences, it is important to ensure that children comprehend the conceptual relationships represented (Nelson, 1986b). Kamhi's (1982) research with normally developing 3:0- to 5:2-year-old children showed that children best acquire complex linguistic forms in contexts that encourage their own actions to represent compound and complex relationships in the presence of adult linguistic models.

> *Objective 5.* The child will detect and correct grammatical errors when editing dictated stories (produced by self, peers, or teacher) or when making puppets talk.

Metalinguistic Monitoring. Intervention approaches for young children of preschool and early elementary school age typically do not rely on metalinguistic awareness. However, whenever a child is asked to imitate a comment rather than respond to it, a certain amount of metalinguistic expectation is evident.

Metalinguistic awareness is also needed when children are asked to monitor their speech for grammaticality of their utterances. The research on syntactic awareness reviewed by Sutter and Johnson (1990) suggested that the identification of grammatical errors is most closely correlated to advancing chronological age; that it is not noticeably exhibited until around the age of 6 or 7 years; but that considerable variability is evident; and it can usually be attributed to contextual factors. Sutter and Johnson noted that focus on the early elementary school child suggests that "a relation may exist between tacit knowledge of grammatical rules and the ability to contemplate syntactic form" (p. 85). If this is

the case, one wonders about the advisability of asking children with language disorders to recognize grammatical errors in their own language or that of others. Strategies include raising their hands when they hear a grammatical problem or "correcting" grammatical sentences when acting with puppets or dictating stories.

The linguistic and cognitive processing demands of surrounding context influence children's ability to focus on surface-level features such as grammatical correctness. In their study of 6-, 7-, and 8-year-olds, Sutter and Johnson (1990) found that school-age children were less able to spot grammatical errors when the sentences with errors were embedded in a story than when the errors occurred in isolation. The authors hypothesized that this result might reflect children's efforts to focus their energy on getting the message of the story. They also found that children were more likely to spot errors involving auxiliaries and suffixes than adverbial constructions and that the normally developing 8-year-olds in their study were substantially better at identifying ungrammatical forms than their younger schoolmates.

At present, the wisdom of requiring explicit monitoring of grammatical errors in middle-stage children is still in question. The evidence suggests that this intervention time may be better spent on more implicit communicative avenues to build intrinsic linguistic proficiency. Explicit focus on grammar (i.e., talking about it) may be more appropriate in the middle grades, when children begin to monitor for grammaticality in their written work as well as in their oral language.

Sentence Comprehension

> *Objective 6.* The child will replace nonlinguistic comprehension strategies with age-appropriate language comprehension (shown by acting, pointing, or answering questions).

Although it might be assumed that once a child begins to produce a particular grammatical form, the child should also be able to comprehend it, that is not necessarily the case (Guess & Baer, 1973). Conversely, comprehension of language forms is usually assumed to precede production of language forms in normal development. Yet that also is not necessarily the case, as exemplified by children's use of forms such as *because* clauses before they can fully comprehend causal relationships (L. Bloom & Lahey, 1978; R. S. Chapman,

1978). Comprehension and production, although re-lated, do not seem to be fully reciprocal processes. The cognitive demands of recognition are not the same as those of recall, making comprehension a somewhat less demanding process in many respects, especially when other contextual variables support the child's ability to comprehend. Yet, the complexity of receptive processes needed to sort out the varied elements of content and form in compound and complex sentences results in production skills preceding comprehension skills for some structures at some intervals (Bates, 1976; Hood & Bloom, 1979). Comprehension is especially demand-ing when the nonlinguistic context does not support listening comprehension. In comparison, even without external contextual support, middle-stage speakers may choose to talk about things they know (in essence, bring-ing their own context to the task). Thus, production may be relatively easier than listening to someone else who controls both the topic and the linguistic complexity.

It is interesting to track development of a linguistic form in different modalities. For example, the sense of past time is understood at around 4 to 5 years of age, but production of these same forms is not fully mastered by 6 years of age (Sutter & Johnson, 1988), and the ability to monitor metalinguistically for errors in these verb forms is not very solid until around age 8 (Sutter & Johnson, 1990). Given this evidence, it may be inap-propriate to expect children with language impairments to exhibit evidence of similar forms of processing all in the same semester or year.

Some language intervention programs have been de-signed on the premise that comprehension facilitates production (Leonard et al., 1982; Winitz, 1973). How-ever, when Connell (1986a) tried to teach six 3-year-olds with language disorders both to produce and to comprehend semantic role distinctions, none of them learned word order through comprehension training alone. Furthermore, learning to produce word order ap-propriately in spontaneous speech did not help children learn to use word-order cues to decode semantically re-versible sentences on comprehension tasks.

Results of comprehension training on expression ca-pabilities may be rather confusing partly because lin-guistic comprehension is often confounded with world knowledge (R. Paul, 1990). Children also use different comprehension strategies at different developmental stages (R. S. Chapman, 1978; R. Paul, 1990; Wallach, 1984). Box 10.7 presents a summary of some of the

changes that can be expected over the years from 4 to 10.

Children with autism, specific language impair-ments, and hearing impairments use comprehension strategies similar to each other but different from younger, language-matched preschoolers (R. Paul, 1990). Children with all of these disabilities rely more heavily on canonical word-order strategies than on world knowledge or later developing syntactic strategies (Paul, 1990; van der Lely & Harris, 1990). All of the children with disabilities also used some knowledge of event probabilities and scripts to guide their responses.

R. Paul (1990) emphasized the need to evaluate both contextualized and decontextualized language compre-hension for all children referred for language problems, even if their parents report comprehension to be unaf-fected. She was less firm about a recommendation to help children acquire comprehension strategies when they have not learned them on their own. She suggested repetitive, highly ordered contexts, such as nursery rhymes and songs, to take advantage of word-order strategies common among many children with language impairments. She also recommended stretching chil-dren's comprehension capabilities by providing "oppor-tunities for the child to process sentences slightly above the current level of functioning" (p. 72). Most impor-tant, Paul noted, is to encourage children with language disorders to take risks in their attempts to comprehend. She believed this would prevent the later development of maladaptive patterns of nonresponsiveness.

When children have difficulty comprehending the language of others, their problems are often exacerbated because they do not realize that they did not understand. Thus, they fail to ask for clarification. Skarakis-Doyle and Mullin (1990) noted a symbiotic relationship be-tween primary linguistic comprehension and compre-hension monitoring. Although children with language disorders may have difficulty with both communicative and cognitive factors, Skarakis-Doyle and Mullin found a greater influence of communicative than cognitive factors in reducing comprehension monitoring by chil-dren with specific language impairments between the ages of 3:6 and 8:4 years. In a related study, language-impaired children distinguished ambiguous from un-ambiguous messages but did not always clearly signal that detection (Skarakis-Doyle, MacLellan, & Mullin, 1990). Alternatively, children with weak language skills may assume that everyone else understands, and that

Box 10.7 _____

Changes in Comprehension Strategies over the Ages 4 to 10 Years
(with Suggested Assessment Techniques)

1. Children move from almost exclusive reliance on **canonical order** (SUBJECT–VERB–OBJECT) strategies prior to age 4 (as infants and toddlers, their comprehension is largely context-determined), through **semantic constraints** and **probable event** strategies at age 4, to the ability to use **syntactic strategies,** at around age 5, for reversible passive sentences, in which the canonical order is violated (_The giraffe is kicked by the elephant_).

2. They also develop more mature strategies for comprehending **clause relationships** as they advance in age beyond 5, after which they learn to go beyond the **order-of-mention** and **pay-attention-to-the-main-clause strategies** that they have used earlier for processing clauses, and the **minimal-distance-principle** and **pronominalization strategies** that they have used earlier for determining reference.

   a. **Order-of-mention strategy** (normal from age 3 to 6 years). This strategy is to do things in the order you hear them (e.g., child responds the same to _After you brush the baby's hair, feed her_ and _Before you brush the baby's hair, feed her_ by brushing hair first).

   Assessment Technique

   Use varied presentation order for testing comprehension.

   b. **Main-clause-first strategy** (normal around age 5). This strategy is to respond to the main clause first (e.g., child responds the same to "Show me _he took a bath before brushing his teeth_" and "Show me _Before brushing his teeth, he took a bath_" by doing the bath part first).

   Assessment Technique

   Assess _before_ and _after_ as prepositions (e.g., _before school, after lunch_) rather than as subordinating conjunctions.

   Use two-event picture sequence choices, but with just one event named (e.g., Say "Show me _after the girl ate_" rather than "Show me _the girl ate her banana before she drank her milk._")

3. Children also advance in their abilities to use **cognitive constructive strategies** to comprehend complex meanings between the ages of 4 and 10. As early as age 4, children can demonstrate **integration strategies** by distinguishing semantically consistent pictures that belong in a sequence from those that are semantically inconsistent and do not belong. But not until between the ages of 7 and 10 do children develop **inferencing strategies** for reading beyond the words to fill in information that makes sense even though it was not explicitly stated. For example, after age 7, the word _broom_ can cue memory of the sentence, _Her friend swept the kitchen floor,_ even though _broom_ was never explicitly stated in the sentence.

4. Lexical categories associated with nonlinguistic comprehension strategies in the preschool years (summarized from Edmonston & Thane, 1992).

   a. **Preference for greater amount strategy** involves **amount terms,** e.g., _more, less, long, short_ (normal for toddlers to preschoolers).

(continued)

BOX 10.7   continued

Assessment Technique

Test antonym pairs and only credit comprehension when both ends are understood (e.g., only give credit for pointing to "*more* ladybugs" if the child also points to "*less* money").

b. **Judge by height strategy** involves **height and age** terms, e.g., *big, tall, short, small, young, old, -er, -est* (normal for 4- to 6-year-olds). When asked to pick the *tallest, largest,* or *oldest,* children using this strategy pick the *highest.*

Assessment Technique

Present assessment choices in which the greatest *height* does not coincide with *tallest, largest,* or *oldest.*

c. **Big, little synonym strategy** involves **dimensional adjectives** e.g., *thin, short, low, thick, wide, tall, long* (normal for toddlers to preschoolers). Children using this strategy treat words like *thin, short,* and *low* as *little;* and words like *tall, wide,* and *thick* as *big.*

Assessment Technique

Use test objects that differ in more than one dimension (e.g., ask for the *thick* crayon, but make it *shorter* than the *thin* one).

d. **Probable sequence strategy** involves **temporal terms,** e.g., *before, after* (normal for preschool children). This strategy is to do things in the order they usually occur in life (e.g., feed the baby, then put it to bed)

Assessment Technique

Use less predictable materials and events (e.g., "Before you feed the baby, give me the pencil")

Note. Summarized from Edmonston & Thane, 1992; with sections reprinted from *Planning Individualized Speech and Language Intervention Programs*—Revised and Expanded, by Nickola Wolf Nelson, copyright 1988 by Communication Skill Builders, Inc., San Antonio, TX. Reprinted with permission.

---

they are the only ones who do not. Or children with communicative deficits may feel too intimidated to ask for clarification. Or they may lack the linguistic prowess to do so. When any of these conditions is present, the clinician may facilitate language-related performance by directly teaching children to monitor their comprehension. Direct modeling and prompting may also be required to scaffold children to request clarification when they have not understood.

Dollaghan and Kaston (1986) taught four children with language impairments (ages 5:10 to 8:2 years) to recognize inadequate tape-recorded messages and to ask for appropriate modifications. The intervention was designed in stages so that children first learned to recognize, label, and demonstrate an active orientation to listening. Subobjectives include sitting still, looking at the speaker, and thinking about what the speaker is saying. Second, the children learned to detect and to react to messages that had "signal inadequacies," such as insufficient loudness or excessive rate that obscured the message. They were taught to say, for example, "I can't hear you," or "Slow down." Third, the children learned to evaluate and react to messages containing inadequate content, by saying, for example, "What do you mean?" or "Which one?" Finally, they learned to respond to messages that exceeded their comprehension owing to the presence of unfamiliar lexical items, excessive length, or excessive syntactic complexity. In this situation they learned to make requests such as "Say those one at a time" or "Can you show me?" Following the implementation of direct instruction, modeling, role playing, and guided discussions, these early elementary school children demonstrated increases in queries about inadequate messages and maintained high-level monitoring skills following a nontreatment interval of 3 to 6 weeks.

Content, Contexts, and Strategies for Syntactic Intervention

Goal and intervention method choices vary with theoretical positions. Approaches driven by linguistic rule induction or behaviorist theories tend to involve careful specification of target structures and intervention steps. Many were introduced in the 1970s when the psycholinguistic focus on grammatical rule acquisition was at its height, but instruction by speech–language pathologists and special educators was often behavioristic. Hence, many of the intervention approaches designed to teach language forms used the high structure that Fey (1986) labeled "**trainer-oriented**" programs. Using trainer-oriented approaches, clinicians select particular target structures; control stimuli and reinforcers (e.g., tokens to be turned in for small toys); and use strategies requiring children to make many responses of similar types (massed trials) in a short amount of time. The intended result is that children will induce rules under these focused conditions that they have not been able to induce from more random evidence in natural communicative interactions.

For example, Gray and Ryan (1973) designed a structured, highly controlled intervention program that gradually moved children from heavy dependence on imitative modeling and 100% reinforcement schedules, to more indirect modeling, and then no modeling. It included several subprograms for different grammatical structures with similar series of steps in which children learned first to imitate particular pieces of sentence forms. Subsequently, they learned to respond in the same way after the imitative prompts were removed. In the early stages of the program, the context and content for the practice sentences came from sets of pictures illustrating various situations (often cut from magazine advertisements) with interesting content. In the later stages of each subprogram, parents were taught to administer similar prompts and reinforcers to those used earlier by the clinician. Contexts for parent instruction at first were semistructured (looking at storybooks) and later unstructured.

Sensitivity to pragmatic functionality and context-dependence became more common in the 1980s. Programs such as Connell's (1986b) (described previously in this section) were designed to teach multidimensional aspects of language forms and to be sensitive to context and to conversational partners. However, even those approaches tended to remain highly structured and strongly dependent on operant methods, including such features as massed trials, gradually faded imitative models, and extrinsic reinforcers delivered on a preplanned schedule.

Structured, trainer-oriented approaches contrast with more "child oriented" (Fey, 1986) or "naturalistic" (Norris & Hoffman, 1990b) approaches. In less structured approaches, intervention is not focused on one target structure at a time. Although objectives may still be written that target the acquisition of particular structures, multiple structures may be targeted at once. The actual amount of practice on each target structure is determined more by the occasions that necessitate its use, based on the child's choices of context and topic, than on the basis of some predetermined sequence and number of productions. This approach is guided by social interaction theory more than by linguistic rule-induction theory. It is consistent with the view that children acquire a particular structure and generalize it to everyday use when they need it for real communicative purposes (rather than a contrived set of parallel sentences) (Duchan, 1995a).

Research comparing the results of imitative trainer-oriented approaches and conversational child-oriented approaches was discussed earlier in this chapter (in the section on teacher discourse). Some advantages were noted for conversational approaches in terms of a higher number of verbal initiations (Haley, Camarata, & Nelson, 1994), and more and quicker spontaneous use of targeted structures (Camarata, Nelson, & Camarata, 1994). Other research, however, found no advantage for either direct instruction or interactive instruction techniques. Both helped children acquire new semantic and syntactic skills (Cole & Dale, 1986).

One conclusion is that different children may benefit differentially from the two types of approaches. In my personal experience, children who are active conversationalists (using Fey's, 1986, terminology, see Figure 9.2) with relatively specific deficits of language form, benefit from an efficient, structured, trainer-oriented approach; however, children who are passive conversationalists, inactive conversationalists, or verbal noncommunicators need a more child-oriented naturalistic approach.

CONTINUED PHONOLOGICAL DEVELOPMENT

GOAL: The child will produce words with phonological clarity.

Objective 1: The child will reduce immature phonological processes and learn to articulate phonemes that are difficult to produce at the onset of intervention.

OUTCOME: The child will talk clearly enough to be understood by adults and peers, who will not have to ask for repetitions.

Phonology is one of the five rule systems (including morphology, syntax, semantics, and pragmatics) that children must acquire to become competent communicators. Consistent with system theory advocated throughout this book, it is impossible to consider other aspects of language development apart from acquisition of the phonological system (see Box 10.8). The influence of greater phonological complexity on reduced syntactic performance by children with language disorders has been demonstrated experimentally (Panagos & Prelock, 1982).

A problem in designing speech–language intervention is knowing how much time to devote to treating phonological impairment and how much to devote to other aspects of language treatment. Fey (1986) suggested that, as a rule of thumb, increasing intelligibility should be targeted as a basic goal within more comprehensive programs for children with language impairments. Signals for needing such intervention are when: (1) speech sound production deficits are a significant component of the child's communication problem, and (2) the child has at least a 50- to 100-word expressive vocabulary. Fey also noted that children in any of his four communicator categories (see Figure 9.4) might require direct attention to phonological development.

In a review of factors related to the classification, management, and severity of phonological disorders in children, Shriberg and Kwiatkowski (1982a, 1982b, 1982c) emphasized the need to consider individual differences when planning intervention for children with developmental phonological disorders. For example, some children might benefit most from a program with **mechanism emphasis.** Such an approach focuses on surface forms and speech motor control, using drill and drill-play modes early in treatment and structured play

and free-play modes later for transfer. Other children might need a more **cognitive-linguistic emphasis.** This approach focuses on underlying forms and phonological rules, using drill-play and structured play early for acquisition and the free-play mode later for transfer. A third group of children might benefit most from programs using a **psychosocial emphasis,** in which sociolinguistic forms serve as primary phonological targets; the play mode is used early for "acclimation," drill play and structured play modes are used later for acquisition, and play modes are used still later for transfer. This decision strategy is consistent with the eclectic approach advocated throughout this book.

Intervention for children with impairments of both grammar and phonology in the age range of 4- to 6-years was studied by Fey, Cleave, Ravida, Long, Dejmal, and Easton (1994). Noting the significant developmental relationship between grammar and phonology, Fey and his colleagues hypothesized that treatment focused on grammar might also result in improved phonology. Their research showed, however, that the children made significant improvements in grammatical output without changing their phonological production. The authors concluded that changes in phonology would require treatment that targeted phonology directly.

A relationship, although not a one-to-one correspondence, has also been demonstrated between expressive phonology and phonological awareness difficulties that predict difficulty in learning to read (Hodson, 1994) and spell (Clarke-Klein, 1994; Clarke-Klein & Hodson, 1995). These concerns are addressed later in this chapter in the section on beginning school.

ACQUIRING AND RETRIEVING WORDS AND CONCEPTS

GOAL: The child will: (1) use diverse vocabulary and acquire new words easily, (2) limit all-purpose words and empty phrases such as *this, that, thing, stuff, make* and *do,* and (3) retrieve words as needed in spontaneous communication.

- Building a Lexicon
- Intervention for Word-Finding Impairment

OUTCOME: The child will use language to convey and comprehend complex meanings at home, school, and in play without struggling.

Box 10.8 _____

Example of a Child with a Language Disorder Involving Phonological Difficulties

Lisa, a kindergartner with language-learning disabilities, was asked to retell the story of "Goldilocks and the Three Bears." The word *porridge* apparently was not in Lisa's expressive vocabulary (at least not in a way that she could retrieve it). Thus, when Lisa told the initial episode of the story, she told about how the mother bear had made *soup,* how the family of bears had decided to let it cool, and how Goldilocks had come into the house and had ended up tasting it. The interesting thing about Lisa's phonological rule system was the inconsistency with which she pronounced the word *soup.* At various times in the retelling, she pronounced it as *soup, thoup, thoot,* and *suit.* Although she did not demonstrate a typical pattern of consistent misarticulation in her speech (such as lisping), Lisa was certainly demonstrating wobbly concepts of the phonological shape of words. If we view this set of productions as being generated based on a rule system for differentiating sound classes, Lisa (at least in the context of the word *soup*) was behaving as if her rule system categorized /s/ and /th/, both initial voiceless continuant consonants, as members of the same phoneme class. She also seemed to have grouped two other English phonemes as one: the final voiceless stop consonants /t/ and /p/. It was no wonder that this kindergarten child was having such difficulty learning the sound–symbol associations that are an important part of most kindergarten curricula.

But was the problem even bigger? For her, it seemed to be. In another part of the story, after talking about the hot and cold characteristics of the bowls of soup that Goldilocks tasted, Lisa began to tell about the characteristics of the bears' chairs. When she began to talk about the Daddy Bear's chair, Lisa searched overtly for the correct word. "Haaard [drawing the word out in a questioning tone] . . . or cold?" she asked herself. And then, with confidence, answered, "I think cold." What happened here? Was Lisa treating the words *hot* and *hard* as if they were homonyms? It seemed that she was. Aside from demonstrating some healthy metacognitive strategies of self-questioning and some healthy metalinguistic strategies of word search using categorical opposites, Lisa seemed to be getting short circuited by her wobbly phonological concepts so that she confused word meanings as well. We wondered how much this difficulty might be associated with Lisa's other difficulties in learning pronoun case (she consistently substituted *him* for *he* and *her* for *she*), in pronouncing multisyllabic words with *metathesis* (she tended to mix up sound sequences, such as in the word *pasghetti*), and in learning the rules for inflecting verbs (she tended to leave out the auxiliary "*is*" in "*is + Ving*" constructions). Those problems with some of the other rule systems of language may have been intertwined with the phonological confusions that Lisa demonstrated in her word-production inconsistencies.

Building a Lexicon: Fast Mapping and Other Processes

Objective 1. The child will learn a set of new words that arise in the context of meaningful interactions in home, school, and play and will produce and comprehend them in novel contexts.

It is artificial to separate word learning from acquisition of the ability to produce and comprehend language constructions. Yet, it is sometimes helpful to focus relatively more on one domain or the other in intervention.

When children reach the middle stages of language acquisition, they already have a substantial vocabulary. From 18 months to 6 years of age, they can be expected

to add words at a rate unsurpassed at other stages of development. Crais (1990) summarized research showing that children add approximately five word roots per day during this time and comprehend around 14,000 words by the time they are 6 years old.

How do children accomplish such an amazing feat normally, and what differences might be expected for children with language disorders? As discussed in Chapter 8, infants and toddlers are heavily dependent on context and event-based strategies for learning word meanings. Developing more mature lexical acquisition strategies involves changing from solely event-based processing to multiple processing strategies. However, this does not mean that event-based strategies are abandoned. Even adults use event-based strategies to comprehend unfamiliar words and to recall less familiar words at times (Crais, 1990).

Establishing meaningful contexts that encourage children to add new words to their lexicons is one intervention strategy that can be used with children of all ages. This strategy draws on children's abilities to "map" information about words into memory. Carey (1978) described the mapping process as having two phases. In the first, called *fast mapping,* children map only a small portion of the available information into semantic memory by using episodic and contextual cues to form preliminary associations. The second phase is more gradual, involving subsequent encounters with a relatively new word, when additional information is mapped.

Fast mapping has been demonstrated for preschool-age children. Carey and Bartlett (1978) used the naturalistic context of snack time in a preschool to show that 3- and 4-year-olds could fast map a meaning of *chromium* when exposed only once in the context, "See those two trays? Bring me the chromium one, not the red one." A week later, more than half of those children demonstrated partial knowledge of the word *chromium* in comprehension and production tasks. As might be expected, however, the children's word concepts at that point were highly varied, supporting the idea of a second (perhaps indefinite) stage of mapping, in which word meanings continue to be clarified and amplified. This study also illustrates "the-rich-get-richer" phenomenon: In this example, children who already had solid control of the meaning of the word *red* and the syntactic construction conveying contrast were much more likely to have the tools needed to fast map.

Dollaghan (1985) designed a similar task. She asked 2- to 5-year-old children to hide three familiar objects and then to hide a *koob* (a novel plastic object). Later, a majority of the children comprehended the word sufficiently to select a *koob* from a set of five objects (two familiar and three unfamiliar) so they could feed it to a puppet. During a production task, when Dollaghan asked children to perform a phonetic reproduction of the word, more problems arose. Indeed, the production task in the *koob* procedure was the only one that discriminated performance of a group of 4- and 5-year-old children developing normally from a matched group with language impairments (Dollaghan, 1987a). Dollaghan was unsure whether the difficulty experienced by the language-impaired subjects (who were equally able to

choose a referent, to comprehend the word, and to store nonlinguistic information about it) was due to storage or retrieval difficulties. She suggested, however, that the breakdown probably involved retrieval, because four of the five children who could not name the object did recognize *koob* when given *soob* and *teed* as foils.

Rice, Buhr, and Nemeth (1990) identified several points in the fast-mapping process that might be vulnerable to language impairment: (1) attention to the stream of words, (2) identification of a novel item, (3) a quick assessment of the linguistic and nonlinguistic context for probable meaning, (4) entering the probable meaning into the appropriate slot in the available lexicon, and (5) storage for immediate or later use. Rice and colleagues found fast mapping by 5-year-olds with language impairments to be significantly poorer than fast mapping by MLU-matched and chronological age-matched peers. She and her colleagues noted that the most striking difference between the groups was the rate of fast mapping. Also, object words were discriminated best between groups. Perhaps this was because the normally developing children fast mapped them so readily, making the children with language impairments comparatively much poorer. Children with language impairments also performed more poorly on comprehension tasks. The researchers concluded that there was little support for attention deficits, limitations of lexical and grammatical knowledge, or the ability to store new lexical items in memory as primary explanations for the deficit.

In a later study, Rice and colleagues (Rice, Oetting, Marquis, Bode, & Pae, 1994) compared Quick Incidental Learning (QUIL) of new vocabulary by 5-years-olds with specific language impairments to learning by age-matched and MLU-matched peers. Their findings add to the support for intervention methods that give children with specific language impairments more time and support to infer word meanings from context as well as more frequent exposure. A clinical guideline based on this research is that children should hear new words in meaningful contexts at least 10 times. Some words, particularly verbs, may not stick well in long-term memory without additional intervention spread over multiple sessions. With sufficient support, however, children with specific language impairments can demonstrate QUIL for a variety of word types at the preschool level and in the early elementary years (Oetting, Rice, & Swank, 1995).

Perhaps the strongest implication of these collective studies is that children with language disorders need more time, more repetitions, and heightened focus on new words and concepts to acquire new meanings. They also may need more deliberate productive practice of novel words, modeled with slow speaking rate (Weismer & Hesketh, 1996), before making them their own. Such children are less apt to acquire new words in the context of completely naturalistic experiences.

The intervention techniques best suited for this kind of problem are scaffolding and mediation, including Blank's (1973) dialogue approach, in which adults interact with children in meaningful contexts, framing and focusing the children's attention on key relationships and highlighting contrastive details within existing knowledge structures and routines, giving them opportunities to use new words many times in appropriately varied ways.

For preschoolers, one should point out a meaningful contrast while naming it, but focus on the meaning, not the form of the word. In fact, a metalinguistic focus on word form may be counterproductive, particularly when introducing children with specific language impairments to the meaning of derivational bound morphemes. For example, Swisher, Restrepo, Plante, and Lowell (1995) found that children with specific language impairment generalized a novel name better when an indirect model (implicit-rule condition) was given than when an explicit rule explanation (explicit-rule condition) was given.

Indirect model (implicit-rule condition):

ADULT: *"Finally he reached the mud house and knocked on the door, knock, knock. The door opened. It was a pimu."*

ADULT: *"He is a pim [pointing to small figure]. What is he [pointing to large figure]?"*

CHILD: *"pimu"*

Explicit rule explanation (explicit-rule condition):

ADULT: *"The pimu was a big creature. When it is small, you say pim, but when it's big you have to say [u], pimu."*

ADULT: *"He is a pim [pointing to small figure]. What is he [pointing to large figure]?"*

CHILD: *"pimu"* (p. 170)

Intervention for Word-Finding Impairments

Objective 2. The child will retrieve words as they are needed to convey specific meanings, using strategies to assist in recalling words that cannot be retrieved instantly.

Relationships among processes of word comprehension, short- and long-term memory storage, retrieval, and production are difficult to sort out. Researchers have observed, however, that some children with language impairments and learning disabilities have difficulty "finding" the words they want to use in specific contexts. Such children have particular difficulty under stressful conditions, even when they appear to "know" those words under other conditions and at different times (Denckla & Rudel, 1976a; German, 1979; D. W. Johnson & Myklebust, 1967; Wiig & Semel, 1980). Stated most simply, word-finding difficulties (also called **dysnomia**) involve problems in generating appropriate words for particular contexts (Kail & Leonard, 1986). In some cases, children with these problems substitute unintended for intended words (German, 1982, 1983, 1993; see Personal Reflection 10.6), much like the paraphasic errors produced by adults with aphasia. German also described secondary characteristics: (1) talking around the intended word (circumlocutions), providing a description or function "you cut with it" instead of the word (*knife*); (2) using time fillers during long pauses (*um, er, ah*); (3) using empty words (*stuff*); (4) substituting indefinite pronouns (*something*); (5) producing attempts at self-correction ("fork, no, I mean knife"); (6) using gestures; and (7) producing extra verbalizations ("it's a, oh, I know it . . . ")

Following a series of experiments with school-age children between the ages of 7 and 14 years, Kail and Leonard (1986) provided an alternative explanation for retrieval problems. They concluded that retrieval problems experienced by children with language disorders were mainly a result of limited semantic elaboration. Kail and Leonard cautioned against intervention to teach processing strategies for word retrieval without confirming a child's knowledge about the meaning, use, and syntactic privileges of words to be retrieved.

PERSONAL REFLECTION 10.6

"Mary is seven and in the second grade. In her attempts to give specific responses to a set of picture cards, she made the following errors: 'question mark' for 'check mark,' 'head cover' for 'crown,' 'checkers' for 'jacks,' 'It's the thing you make a hole with' for 'drill,' and 'stool' for 'spool.'"

Description of a child with word-finding problems by *Diane German* (1983, p. 539).

German (1989; 1993) presented a slightly different explanation. She differentiated three groups of children with word-finding problems: (1) individuals with specific retrieval difficulty in the presence of good comprehension; (2) individuals with receptive language problems who have difficulty retrieving because their word meanings are unstable (this describes the group studied by Kail & Leonard, 1986); and (3) individuals with multiple challenges affecting both comprehension and retrieval. German's analysis suggested that some children have breakdowns of lexical representation in memory at the semantic level, and others at the phonological level. As German refined the Test of Word Finding (1989), she added tasks that can help sort out different levels of processing breakdown. She also developed procedures to analyze word-finding skills in other discourse contexts (German, 1991). German (1983) also noted that teachers can be the best sources for referring children with word-finding difficulties. A word-finding survey designed to be completed by teachers to aid in referral appears in Box 10.9.

Intervention for word-finding difficulties depends on whether a child's primary problem is lack of semantic elaboration, impaired phonological representation, or a specific retrieval processing deficit. In any of these cases, the process involves practice making rich associations and building stable semantic categories and word associations (in their auditory, oral, read, and written forms).

McGregor (1994) described a two-pronged treatment approach, which she used with two boys (ages 4:9 and 5:0) who showed similar communicative profiles. Both had mild to moderate expressive language delays involving morphology, syntax, and phonology identified when they were around 3 years old. Both had adequate receptive and expressive vocabularies but inconsistent and latent naming that suggested word-finding difficulties, and both exhibited disfluent speech. The first treatment focus was on phonological aspects of **word storage.** With clinician modeling and practice, the boys learned to identify first sounds and the number of syllables in target words. The syllabication task was facilitated by tapping out the number of syllables in a word and relating them to cards with numbers printed on them with a corresponding number of stickers. The second treatment focus was on practicing self-cueing to assist in the event of **retrieval breakdown.** This part of the treatment involved the instructions, "Think about the first sound in the word or how long the word is if you have

---

Box 10.9 _____

German's Word-Finding Survey for Use by Teachers

Teacher's Name _____

Child's Name _____

Does the child frequently (+ = yes, − = no)

1. Know the word he wants to retrieve, but can't think of it?
2. Show a delayed response time when he is trying to think of a word?
3. Talk around the word he wants to use?
4. Give word substitutions that have the same meaning as the word he wants to use?
5. Give the function of the word he wants to use?
6. Give a description of the word he wants to use?
7. Give a substitution that sounds like the word he wants to use?
8. Have difficulty finding the word he wants to use when he is trying to relate an experience to you?
9. Use such vague words as *they, stuff, you know,* in place of words he wants to retrieve?
10. Use filler words such as *um, er, ah,* when he is trying to retrieve a word?
11. Have difficulty retrieving a specific word, object name or fact?
12. Use gestures to pantomime the word he wants to retrieve?
13. State: "I know that word, but I can't think of it"?
14. Use incomplete phrases and self-corrections when describing an experience or event?
15. Have good understanding of oral language used in class?

Note: From "I Know It but I Can't Think of It: Word Retrieval Difficulties" by D. J. German, 1983, *Academic Therapy, 18,* p. 542. Copyright 1983 by PRO-ED. Reprinted by permission.

---

trouble remembering" (p. 1385). The treatment resulted in reduction of occasional phonological word-finding substitutions and also reduced the large number of semantic word-finding substitutions.

DEVELOPING SKILLS IN SYMBOLIC PLAY

GOAL: The child will demonstrate complex understandings, symbolic thinking and pretending, and social skills through play.

Objective 1: The child will use language to set the scene, actions, and roles for play.

Objective 2. The child will represent observed events and imaginative scripts in play.

Objective 3. The child will coordinate multiple objects and organize several children's roles in play.

Objective 4. The child will use language to perform a variety of functions in play.

Objective 5. The child will use a variety of language forms and relational terms while playing.

OUTCOME: The child will fit well in play groups with peers, playing at their level, and sometimes leading the play.

In the middle stages of language acquisition, play, especially role play, remains a valuable context for developing multiple aspects of language. By its nature, play offers particularly rich opportunities for encouraging children to develop the symbolic function of language. Other developments may come in the area of language content as it is embedded within the context of varied schemas and scripts, language forms as they are needed to express relatively complex meanings across integrated events, and social uses as they are required for setting up play with peers and acting out scripted roles.

Questions about the relationships of thought and language come to the fore in the context of child's play. Both Piaget (1962) and Vygotsky (1967) linked the emergence of symbolic play to the development of representational skills. Bates and her colleagues (1979) found early correlations among symbolic play, vocal imitation, and language production in normally developing children during infancy. But the relationships are far from clear.

Roth and Clark (1987) compared the symbolic play and social participation of six children with language impairments with eight children who were learning normally. They found that the children with language-impairments demonstrated "deficits" in symbolic play compared to their younger language-matched peers. For example, more than half of the language-impaired children failed to perform play behaviors such as putting a doll to bed or placing a toy figure in a tractor, items from the Symbolic Play Test (Lowe & Costello, 1976). Children with language impairments also demonstrated social participation difficulties. Roth and Clark noted that the social interaction difficulties may have resulted from pairing the normally developing children and the language-impaired children together as play partners. They also emphasized the heterogeneity of children with language impairments in their play interaction styles.

How might language interventionists encourage the rich imaginative and communicative skills needed for play with peers in the preschool and early elementary years? Opportunity seems to be one key. Children need to be in situations where they can feel included in their peers' games. The "Let's pretend" that comes only when a group of children decides to play "restaurant," "shoestore," "horses," or "jungle" (all fondly remembered from my own childhood) are hard to orchestrate (see Personal Reflection 10.7). But a possibility is enlisting the aid of an older child to figure out an appropriate role for the child in the wheelchair or one who can walk and run but not talk so well.

Part of the problem may be that children with language disorders do not know how to make appropriate social overtures to potential play partners. Some of this may be modeled for them. Older siblings or other interested peers can help instruct target children in how to join play groups. This differs from forcing the participation, and it takes quite a bit of groundwork by adults. Expectations for the play and communicative behaviors appropriate to middle stages of development are summarized by Westby (1988) in the last three stages of her Symbolic Play Scale, which appears in Table 10.1 (the earlier stages were summarized in Chapter 8).

Vivian Paley (1981, 1990, 1992) is a kindergarten teacher who used free play, storytelling, and play acting to learn what her students think and to help them

PERSONAL REFLECTION 10.7 _____

Play often provides wonderful opportunities for intersections of cognitive and linguistic development. My own family enjoys retelling the story of when, as a child, I was sent down the block during a cowboy game to bring back 100 head of cattle and returned lugging a heavy imaginary "bag" full of those 100 heads I had just lopped off with an imaginary sword. Besides being an embarrassing moment, this is an example of how play can be rich in idiomatic language use and how it is a normal part of childhood for younger children to learn from older, more advanced peers.

N. W. Nelson

TABLE 10.1   Symbolic Play Scale—the last three stages

DECONTEXTUALIZATION What Props Are Used in Pretend Play?	THEMATIC CONTENT What Schemas/Scripts Does the Child Represent?	ORGANIZATION How Coherent and Logical Are the Child's Schemas/Scripts?
Stage VI: 3 to 3½ years Carries out pretend activities with replica toys (Fisher-Price/Playmobile doll house, barn, garage, airport, village) Uses one object to represent another (stick can be a comb, chair can be a car) Uses blocks and sandbox for imaginative play. Blocks used as enclosures (fences, houses) for animals and dolls	Observed events, i.e., events in which child was not an active participant (policemen, firemen, schemas/scripts from familiar TV shows—Superman, Wonder Woman)	
Stage VII: 3½ to 4 years Uses language to invent props and set scene Builds 3-dimensional structures with blocks		Schemas/scripts are planned Child hypothesizes, "What would happen if . . ."
Stage VII: 5 years Can use language totally to set the scene, actions, and roles in the play	Highly imaginative activities that integrate parts of known schemas/scripts and develop new novel schemas/scripts for events child has never participated in or observed (e.g., astronaut builds ship, flies to strange planet, explores, eats unusual foods, talks with creatures on planet)	Plans several sequences of pretend events. Organizes what is needed—both objects and other children; coordinates several scripts occurring simultaneously

Note: From Westby, C., Children's Play: Reflections of Social Competence, in *Seminars in Speech and Language, 9*(1), p. 13, New York, 1988, Thieme Medical Publishers, Inc. Reprinted by permission.

SELF/OTHER RELATIONS What Roles Does Child Take and Give to Toys and Other People?	LANGUAGE	
	Function	Forms and Meaning
Uses doll or puppet as participant in play Child talks for doll Reciprocal role taking—child talks for doll and as parent to doll	Projecting: Gives desires, thoughts, feelings to doll or puppet Uses indirect requests, e.g., "mommy lets me have cookies for breakfast." Changes speech depending on listener Reasoning (integrates reporting, predicting, projecting information)	Descriptive vocabulary expands as child becomes more aware of perceptual attributes. Uses terms for following concepts (not always correctly): shapes sizes colors textures spatial relations Uses metalinguistic and metacognitive language, e.g., "He said . . . ," "I know . . ."
Uses dolls and puppets to act out schemas/scripts Child or doll has multi-roles (e.g., mother and wife; fireman, husband, and father)	Uses language to take roles of character in the play, stage manager for the props, or as author of the play story	Uses modals (*can, may, might, will, would, could*) Uses conjunctions (*and, but, so, if, because*) Note: Full competence for modals and conjunctions does not develop until 10–12 years of age Begins to respond appropriately to why and how questions which require reasoning Uses relational terms (*then, when, first, next, last, while, before, after*) Note: Full competence does not develop until 10–12 years of age

develop their thinking to higher levels. Her books are full of transcripts of the tape-recorded talk of play and storytelling, accompanied by reflection on children's meanings and her own role in facilitating the children's cognitive and social growth. Paley's conversations establish a model of scaffolding that balances respect for young children's opinions with expectation for growth in explaining the logic of those opinions or decisions. She also enlisted children in interpreting the language and play of their peers. Box 3.14 in Chapter 3 provided an example of how normally developing peers interpreted the play of a child with significant social and communicative disabilities and helped to normalize it.

In *You Can't Say You Can't Play,* Paley (1992) focused on increasing all children's opportunities to be included. She described the process that led up to enforcing the rule that all children (including those who were rejected previously) must be allowed to play:

> Clara has been one of the last to understand the procedural changes but now she is becoming a party to their workings. She comes upon Lisa and Cynthia as they cover the entrance to their dwelling with scarves and manages to narrate her way in without disrupting the play.
>
> "Pretend we're newborn baby princess mousies," Lisa says to Cynthia.
>
> "And pretend I'm a girl kitty that is lost and I see you," Clara offers hopefully.
>
> "Then you find your sister, Clara, in a different woods and you run away . . . "
>
> "No," Clara says firmly. "Me and sister see a trail of cheese and it's your cheese and we come to live in your mousie house."
>
> "But see, we're all running away," Lisa informs the new players. "Then we see the gold and then we find a haunted house." Lisa remains in charge. She can continue to feel she is in charge because the children welcome her leadership as long as she doesn't keep them outside the castle doors. (1992, pp. 121–122)

As this sequence shows, establishing and posting the rule, "You can't say you can't play," had a strong inclusionary effect. It also helped children throw off old role stereotypes in play and in acting out each other's stories. When roles were assigned based on who was next around the rug, rather than the storyteller's decisions about who was worthy and best for a part, surprising added benefits appeared for the children:

> They dare to take on implausible roles, shyly at the start, but after a while with great aplomb, as if accepting the challenge to eliminate their own stereotyped behaviors. Girls take on boys' roles and boys accept girls' roles. Not everyone to be sure, but enough children are willing to throw off their shackles to make these role reversals acceptable. Those who have never taken roles as bad guys, witches, and monsters are saying yes to such assignments, and the Ninja Turtles are agreeing to be newborn babies. (1992, p. 127)

PARTICIPATING IN STORYTELLING: EMERGING LITERACY

Discussion of language sample analysis for middle-stage children in Chapter 9 mentioned the need to consider varied modes of discourse, not only conversational interaction. As noted, even 2-year-olds may use some of the features of organized narrative discourse, such as longer turns, more organized structures, and domination by a single speaker, when they produce bedtime monologues (K. Nelson, 1989). A review of the literature on emerging literacy (Norris & Bruning, 1988) suggested that "the development of literate-style language begins as early as 2 years of age for children who have opportunities to engage in storybook reading and storytelling" (p. 416). Stories seem to have an organizing power that goes beyond their identity as a specialized discourse event (see Personal Reflection 10.8).

The importance of positive early literacy experiences on later language learning can hardly be overstated. Cullinan (1989) reviewed a series of studies, all of which supported the conclusion that children who have heard written language read aloud as preschoolers have dramatic advantages later in learning to read and understanding the world at large. For example, a child in Gordon Wells's (1986) longitudinal study who had never heard a story read aloud before entering school continued to lag behind the other students at the end of elementary school. Meanwhile a child who had heard more than 5,000 stories before starting school was at the top of the class in literacy-related activities. Although simple cause–effect relationships cannot be assumed, the need to experience good children's literature (see Cullinan, 1989, or Westby, 1985/1991, for selection suggestions) in positive social interactions with parents should never be ignored when programming for middle-stage children with language disorders.

"Why not divide the sand into separate sections and play alone?" I urge hoarsely. "There's too much arguing. I can't hear the stories."

"Angelo started it," Charlie says.

"They was fixin' to steal my sand," Angelo snaps angrily, "from my hill. Anyway, they's too nasty. I'm leaving!"

Wiping his hands on his pants, he makes a sand trail to the story table. Then, wearily, he puts down his head, closing his eyes. A moment later he springs up. "Can I tell a story teacher?"

"Good," I say, taking his notebook from the pile. "I'm in the mood for a story." The moment he begins a calm descends over this table, though the sand players are still noisy and quarrelsome at theirs. (Paley, 1992, pp. 25–26)

Vivian Gussin Paley (1992), in her role as kindergarten teacher at the University of Chicago Laboratory Schools, writing in her book, *You Can't Say You Can't Play.* Paley received the MacArthur Foundation Award for her pioneering work on the uses of storytelling in the classroom.

The need for literary experiences may be particularly acute for children with physical impairments. One example of the value of early literacy experiences for such children was reported by Butler (1980), who described the importance of books in the early development of Cushla, a girl with severe physical impairments. Cushla's parents used stories to calm her through long hospital stays and sleepless nights. Because she was unable to hold objects, crawl, sit up, or watch what happened around her, books became Cushla's chief means of learning, as well as her chief source of delight. Although Cushla's parents had been told to expect her to be mentally retarded, her intelligence was assessed as being well above average at age 3:8.

Providing opportunity to participate in varied literacy activities, such as hearing written language read aloud, looking at books, participating in storytelling, writing notes, and drawing pictures about stories, all may be part of reducing functional limitations and disabilities of children with language impairments and middle-stage needs. Not all children with disabilities have parents like Cushla's (Butler, 1980). Too often, delayed language skills and associated attention and cognitive deficits result in

children with language disorders receiving fewer opportunities to engage in positive narrative discourse activities with their parents and other adults.

Paley (1981) described one such child, Wally, who came to her kindergarten class after 2½ years in a daycare center:

> *Nothing in the school report suggests the scope of his imagination. It is a customary "bad boy" report: restless, hyperactive, noisy, uncooperative. Tonight the children will give their mothers a similar description: there's a boy Wally who growls like a lion; the teacher yells at him but not at me. (p. 5)*

Before Wally, Paley (1981) reported that story dictation had been a minor activity in her classroom, "even though books and dramatics had been high-priority activities" (p. 11). Most children chose other activities over telling stories. Thus, Paley said, "For years I accepted the 'fact' that no more than four or five children out of twenty-five enjoyed dictating stories, and most often they were girls" (p. 11). The event that brought story dictation and dramatization into Paley's classroom as a major daily activity, which also kept Wally from needing the time-out chair, is described in Personal Reflection 10.9.

To tell and to understand stories, children need at least two kinds of experience. First, they need to understand about the world and people. Second, they need to have an inner sense of how story structures reorganize and reconstruct reality.

Narratives do not spring forth fully formed. Rather, they undergo gradual development as children learn to create logical chains of events while keeping a central focus (see Figure 9.5; also Applebee, 1978; Botvin & Sutton-Smith, 1977; Westby, 1984). Many examples of children's literature parallel this developmental sequence. Professionals can seek to match literature selections fairly closely to children's own story grammar structure at first (see Figure 9.6). Cultural differences also should be honored (Cazden, 1988; Westby, 1994) (see Personal Reflection 10.10).

Gebers (1990) provided an annotated review of a range of children's books with suggestions about using them for varied speech and language intervention purposes. Norris and Hoffman (1993) showed how to use children's books in a whole language intervention approach. They recommended books with simple discourse events and predictable patterned language for facilitating

The first time I asked Wally if he wanted to write a story he looked surprised. "You didn't teach me how to write yet," he said.

"You just tell *me* the story, Wally, I'll write the words."
"What should I tell about?"
"You like dinosaurs. You could tell about dinosaurs." He dictated this story.

The dinosaur smashed down the city and the people got mad and put him in jail.

"Is that the end?" I asked. "Did he get out?"

He promised he would be good so they let him go home and his mother was waiting.

We acted out the story immediately for one reason—I felt sorry for Wally. He had been on the time-out chair twice that day, and his sadness stayed with me. I wanted to do something nice for him, and I was sure it would please him if we acted out his story.

It made Wally very happy, and a flurry of story writing began that continued and grew all year. The boys dictated as many stories as the girls, and we acted out each story the day it was written if we could.

Before, we had never acted out these stories. We had dramatized every other kind of printed word—fairy tales, story books, poems, songs—but it had always seemed enough just to write the children's words. Obviously it was not; the words did not sufficiently represent the action, which needed to be shared. For this alone, the children would give up play time, as it was a true extension of play. (Paley, 1981, pp. 11–12)

How Paley discovered that storytelling could replace the time-out chair.

_____

coordination of the multiple levels of language required for fluent reading. For example, in Cowley's (1990) *Jigaree*, the main character is first "jumping after me. Jumping here, jumping there. Jigarees jump everywhere"; then the Jigaree follows a similar pattern dancing, swimming, riding, skating, and climbing. When the focus is on more advanced discourse types, a book with an abbreviated episode structure, such as *Dragon with a Cold* (Cowley, 1988), may be a better choice.

Scott (1988a) emphasized the need to recognize different stories and storytelling contexts when analyzing

"The Garcia family also has found a special way of sharing books. Books are read in both English and Spanish. Raphael, age six, listens to the stories with his little sister, Maria, age two. When their mother, Carmen, begins reading the story of *Hester the Jester* by Ben Schecter, she starts in English. Raphael and Maria listen, and ask questions about the story. Carmen answers them, and then she gives a Spanish translation of the story. It is a family time, and the children enjoy listening to their mother as she reads and talks to them in the English and Spanish of their bilingual home."

Family literacy experiences described by *Dorothy Strickland* and *Denny Taylor* (1989, p. 31).

_____

stories told by children with language disorders. She noted that the same child may tell stories with different qualities, depending on the surrounding events and the degree of prompting the child receives before beginning the narration. The three types of narratives that have received the most attention in prior research include (1) personal narratives; (2) TV program, film, or book summaries; and (3) fictional tales. For stories retold from TV programs or books, Scott's review suggested that the medium in which children originally experience narratives might influence their later ability to retell them. Children's retellings of TV dramas and cartoons tend to lack explicit references to character's goals and discernible endings, perhaps because TV characters' motivations tend to be nonexplicit, and even normally developing 9-year-old children have difficulty answering inference questions about TV narratives (Collins, Wellman, Keniston, & Westby, 1978). Books that discuss characters' motivations and feelings explicitly may be better suited for modeling such considerations, particularly for children with language disorders. Their stories tend to include less information in the story grammar categories of internal response (Ripich & Griffith, 1985) and protagonist attempt (Roth & Spekman, 1986) than their peers who are learning language normally.

Schneider (1996) found different challenges and facilitative effects when pictures were used or not used to support story retelling. Children with language impairments in the age range 5:7 to 9:9 told the best stories (in terms of complete episodes and number of information units) when they retold stories they had listened to without pictures. When they told a story supported by pictures in a wordless picture book, their stories contained the most extraneous information and least story grammar information, but also the least evidence of formulation stress (shown as fewer linguistic mazes).

In my experience, when asked to tell or write personal narratives, many children use more story grammar elements when prompted to talk about a problem and how they solved it. When asked only to tell or write about something interesting that happened to them, the "narrative" they tell is far more likely to be a sequenced chain of events experienced on a vacation trip to an amusement park. Hearing examples of mature personal narratives modeled by adults may also help some children to incorporate more organized and thematically connected details in their stories. Telling stories with "sparkle" (Peterson & McCabe, 1983) may also be more likely to occur when children have some commitment (Perera, 1984) to the topic of the narration, as they do in a personal narrative involving themselves.

Assisting children to organize their narratives in mature ways may involve direct targeting of the inclusion of the key components of "story grammar" (N. W. Nelson, 1988b, Westby, 1984, 1985/1991). Research evidence suggests that children can learn to include more of the macrostructure elements as a result of training (Carnine & Kinder, 1985; Gordon & Braun, 1983). However, children need to be guided to do more than to make sure that they have something in each slot in the organizational schema. Westby (1984) emphasized the need for specific and sustained social interaction dialogue to support early narrative development, including discussions leading to knowledge of cause and effect and motives. Children with weak language skills, including poor readers, may be less likely to exhibit logical cohesion in their narratives (Norris & Bruning, 1988), and helping them to achieve better organization may depend as much on encouraging the development of complex ideas as the development of complex sentence structures. Indeed, mediated discussions about interesting stories may be the best way to target the acquisition of complex linguistic structures by children with wobbly language competencies.

Westby (1985/1991) described a scaffolding strategy in which a teacher led a discussion about a picture show-ing two children injured in an accident. The teacher guided the interaction by asking a series of focusing questions that led the children to describe a possible setting, initiating event, internal response, internal plan, attempts, consequence, and ending. These responses were outlined in separate columns on the chalkboard. Then the children constructed their story:

> *Angel and Michael got hurt in a car accident. An ambulance came real fast and took them to the hospital. Dr. David and Nurse Michelle washed their cuts. Then they put bandages on them. Officer Joe called Mrs. Chavez on the phone. He said, "Your children were hurt in a car accident. They are at the hospital. I'll pick you up in my police car." Mrs. Chavez was worried and scared. She asked Dr. David if she could take her children home. He said, "You may take them home. Give them soup and put them to bed." Angel and Michael got well and lived happily ever after. (reported by Costlow, 1983, in personal communication to Westby, 1985/1991, p. 200)*

Although learning to understand and to tell stories seems critical to the emergence of literate language during the preschool years, the importance of encouraging narrative discourse does not stop when children begin to learn to read. Narrative skills continue to develop into adulthood (N. W. Nelson, 1988c). Indeed, the best storytellers are rewarded handsomely for their novels and screenplays. Targeting narrative language skills for intervention in the later stages of language development may be as appropriate as in the middle stages. However, because of wide variations in narrative discourse among individual samples produced by the same children in different contexts, it may not be possible to separate issues of normal development (addressed through general education language arts) from special needs (addressed through special education and language intervention). Clearly, in this area, speech–language pathologists need to work closely with regular and special educators both in assessments and intervention.

BEGINNING SCHOOL

GOAL: The child will read and write at grade level using a combination of decoding–encoding (graphophonemic) strategies and comprehension–construction (semantic, syntactic, and script-level prediction) strategies to make sense of text, to produce stories and other written language, and to participate in classroom discussions.

- Learning to Read
- Learning to Write
- Using Language in Classrooms

OUTCOME: The child will participate in the literacy activities of school and use them for further learning.

Learning to Read

In the minds of children, parents, and teachers, learning to read is the crowning event of the middle stages of language acquisition. Learning to talk occurs so seemingly automatically that the oral language accomplishments of the preschool years appear far less dazzling than early elementary school accomplishments of learning to read. The difference is that learning to talk usually occurs without direct instruction, whereas learning to read is what children and parents in literate cultures talk about and look forward to as a primary motivation for going to school.

Becoming literate is not equally accessible to all children. Even in kindergarten, some children become so discouraged that they start each day with a stomachache. Children with a history of language acquisition difficulties are particularly at risk. Preventing such misery involves concentrated collaborative efforts of special and regular educators and speech–language pathologists. Working as a team, they seek ways to help children with language-learning difficulties crack the written language code.

To understand how to help these children, one must first understand the process of mature reading. Reading is more than pronouncing words on a page. Although acquisition of strategies for transforming text to speech certainly plays a role in obtaining meaning from print, reading involves much more than sounding out words. Mature readers focus their primary attention on decoding strategies only when they come to unusual or difficult words. Even then, good readers tend to sound out words syllable-by-syllable rather than sound-by-sound. Whether readers use phonemic, syllabic, or whole-word units to connect print with auditory and spoken word images, they use graphophonemic cues. These involve associations of graphemes to phonemes but not necessarily one-to-one correspondences between single graphemes and phonemes. Rather, they often require associating ir-

regular patterns such as *cough* and *through* with two- or three-phoneme sequences or directly with morphemic meanings, or they may involve associating irregularly spelled morphemes like *-tion* with other sound sequences and meanings.

Mature readers use two or three additional cuing systems, all based on knowledge of language and discourse, to form hypotheses about the messages they are attempting to get through print. K. S. Goodman (1969, 1973a, 1973b) proposed that mature readers use the three linguistic cuing systems (1) graphophonemic, (2) syntactic, and (3) semantic to form and test predictions as they read. In addition, it may be equally important to use (4) discourse knowledge and understanding of scripts to make sense of written language texts and to ensure that later and earlier parts of texts are integrated and connected (the pinball wizardry model of written language processing is introduced in Chapter 2 and discussed further in Chapter 9). In fact, mature readers rely heavily on their knowledge of language and the world to form hypotheses and to make predictions about the words on the page. They sample only enough perceptual data from the printed text to confirm that their predictions are accurate. If something does not make sense, they may backtrack to gather further perceptual data and relate it to what they know about how words sound and what words and sentence constructions mean, but only to the degree necessary to obtain meaning and to make sense.

The assumptions cannot necessarily be made about beginning readers. Chall (1983) proposed a developmental model of the stages of reading acquisition. She called the initial **prereading** period, **stage 0,** the stage from birth to 5 or 6 years of age, when children pretend to "read" familiar stories that they have heard read aloud many times. She noted that it was followed by **stage 1,** an initial reading or decoding stage, when children are **"glued to print."** During stage 1, occurring in 5- to 7-year-olds, Chall proposed that children devote a great deal of attention to the process of learning phoneme–grapheme correspondence rules. During **stage 2,** in 7- to 9-year-olds, children undergo the subsequent process of **ungluing from print.** They begin to rely more heavily on the redundancies of language and their knowledge of scripts and story structure to derive meaning more easily and fluently from text.

Focus on Whole Language.   Other theorists disagree with Chall's (1983) model. They argue that it only appears to be developmental because it is the way that adults traditionally have organized the curriculum for teaching children to read (K. S. Goodman, 1986; D. F. King & Goodman, 1990; Norris & Damico, 1990; Schory, 1990). Instead, this second group advocates keeping language whole in early literacy instruction. They argue that a better developmental explanation for early reading acquisition is that children are motivated to derive meaning from print (see Personal Reflection 10.11). They argue that fragmenting language to teach it is unnatural and counterproductive (Norris & Damico, 1990; Norris & Hoffman, 1993).

A whole language philosophy has guided language and reading instruction in New Zealand for more than 20 years, with considerable success (Mabbett, 1990). Mabbett articulated some of the principles of that approach:

- Reading, talking, and writing are inseparably interrelated;
- The foundations of literacy are laid in the early years;
- Reading for meaning is paramount;
- Books for children learning to read should use natural idiomatic language that is appropriate to the subject;
- There is no one way in which people learn to read. A combination of approaches is needed. (1990, p. 60)

Focus on Phonological Awareness.   When children with language-learning disabilities have difficulty learning to read, speech–language pathologists may identify weak language skills that contribute to the difficulty. Phonological processing limitations are often involved

(Blachman, 1994). Kamhi and Catts's (1989) review of the literature showed that children with reading difficulties frequently have deficits in encoding, retrieving, and using phonological memory codes. These problems tend to show up as deficits in performing metalinguistic tasks, such as rhyming and recognizing sound families. However, that does not necessarily mean that teaching children to rhyme isolated words is a particularly good intervention approach. A common recommendation of the 1970s and 1980s was that children with weak phonological skills should be taught to read by emphasizing visual patterns and whole-word recognition and by avoiding attention to phonics. In my experience, neither teaching phonics in isolation nor ignoring phonics entirely meets children's needs. Memorizing individual words places an immense load on memory and makes it difficult for children to decode words they have never seen. On the other hand, children with weak phonological processing skills may learn to make sound–symbol associations and to sequence them when reading and writing if deliberately assisted to make the associations.

Children who are developing normally often make such associations automatically in whole language contexts as they learn to read. The same may not be true of children with language-learning disabilities who find it difficult to induce such connections (Shapiro, 1992). They may need more "code emphasis" (I. Y. Liberman & Liberman, 1990) to become aware of the segments of language and the alphabetic principle by which artifacts of alphabet are associated with natural units of language. Although deliberate instruction may need special prominence, it should not be isolated completely from the top-down processes of obtaining meaning from text (see Personal Reflection 10.12).

PERSONAL REFLECTION 10.11 _____

"The term [*whole language*] originated in response to methods used in schools that fragment and tear language asunder. The subsystems of language are often the focus of useless, time-wasting, and confusing instruction. Speaking, listening, reading, and writing are often taught as if they were separable pieces of language, each composed of separable smaller units. We have had, in fact, a 'part-language' curriculum. The 'whole' in whole language emphasizes the integrity of language and the language process."

Dorothy King and *Kenneth Goodman* (1990, p. 222) writing about whole language as a philosophy about learners.

PERSONAL REFLECTION 10.12 _____

"Some readers of low skill appear to compensate for ineffective word-level processes by relying more on discourse-level information to identify words. Compared with skilled readers, such low-skill readers identify words much more quickly in context as long as the context is helpful. However, when context is misleading, such readers are slowed down more than skilled readers."

Steven Roth and *Charles Perfetti* (1980, p. 26).

Catts (1991) cautioned against using programs and activities to facilitate phonological awareness that might be above a child's cognitive and metalinguistic abilities. He described a hierarchy of phonological awareness activities. The first level involves **sound play** with nursery rhymes, finger plays, television jingles, poems, or stories. Carol Westby (personal communication, July 17, 1995), for example, introduced me to a set of song, story, and drawing materials with English and Spanish versions from J. Stone Creations (La Mesa, CA) called "The Animated Alphabet."™ The second level Catts recommended involves **segmentation and blending.** These activities explicitly require children to divide words into sound segments, syllables, and phonemes. The third level involves **sound manipulation tasks.** Activities at this level include: (1) deletion tasks ("Say *cowboy* without the *cow*"); (2) addition tasks ("Say 'at' with /f/ at the beginning"); and (3) substitution tasks ("Replace /f/ in fan with /m/"). Catts reviewed research suggesting that programs that facilitate phonological awareness can reduce early reading difficulties.

In my experience, children with language-learning difficulties benefit from a combination of bottom-up teaching strategies that focus on decoding in combination with top-down strategies that focus on the construction of meaning. My colleagues and I used an eclectic model of language intervention in classroom programs for children with severe language impairments. We instructed children in phonological analysis and synthesis skills, focusing on form, during part of the day, and helped them to construct and "read" their own personal news journals, focusing on meaning, during another part of the day (N. W. Nelson, 1981a). As children became stronger in both skills, we found they could integrate multiple components of the reading and writing process in the same context.

Learning to Write

Viewing literacy development as language development involves viewing reading, writing, and talking as integrated processes. This suggests that the best strategy for teaching writing is in conjunction with reading.

Learning to produce written language is a complex process involving the coordination of language formulation, phonological processing, graphomotor, and cognitive monitoring skills. Effective writers also use pragmatic knowledge to consider the needs of their imagined audience. One way that teachers encourage children to write is to serve as a real and interested audience for their messages (Calkins, 1983; Graves, 1983).

Written language, like spoken language, may serve varied sociolinguistic functions. In one classroom, students might use written language to label, remember, entertain, and learn academic content (McGee & Richgels, 1990). Children who have difficulty grasping the abstract nature of the writing process may need illumination of the communicative function by conversing with a real audience, such as the teacher or peers, through written notes. Parents can also be encouraged to exchange notes with their children. Teachers can allow children to write surreptitious social notes without appearing to sanction the process. Such spontaneous conversational writing is mapped onto early discourse functions, and the recipient almost always accepts and never criticizes it. Children who do not have access to the usual modes of writing because of motor deficits need augmentative systems that can support social notes as well as academic writing.

In the early stages of learning to write, children may lack sufficient knowledge to spell words they want to write. Box 10.10 lists strategies that children adopt as they learn to spell. Recognizing the normal variation that can occur in word-production strategies may prevent specialists in language and learning disabilities from becoming overly critical of the normal "errors" that children make when learning to produce words in writing.

As children develop more mature written language abilities, other discourse functions also may be encouraged. Children who have encountered written language in shared reading experiences may have more conceptual support for constructing stories of their own. In the early stages, a combination of printed words and drawings might be particularly effective for children who can more easily represent meanings in nonprint modes (Nordenbrock, 1995). In our Berrien County, Michigan, classrooms for children with severe language impairments, students either wrote or dictated personal narrative "news" each day in special booklets. They also illustrated their news and read it aloud for their classmates in the whole-group context later in the day. During the full-group interaction, the class decided together what news to record on the 4 × 6-inch cards that were later stapled to the bulletin board for each day of the month as a calendar. One child was selected to illustrate each bit of group news. At the end of the month, the daily cards were taken

Box 10.10 _____

A Description of Developmental Spelling (Word-Creation) Strategies

PHYSICAL RELATIONSHIP

Child tries to relate the number or the appearance of marks to some physical aspect of the object or person represented. The child might use three marks, for example, to write her name if she is three years old.

VISUAL DESIGN

Child accepts the arbitrary nature of words—that they do not resemble their referents physically. The child tries to recreate some designs. The first design attempted is often the child's name. Placeholders—other letters, circles, solid dots, or vertical lines—often are used in the place of those letters that the child cannot form.

SYLLABIC HYPOTHESIS

Child realizes there is a relationship between the oral and written version of words and also that spoken words can be segmented into "beats" or syllables. The child codes words syllabically, using one mark for each of a word's syllables.

LETTER STRINGS
(VISUAL RULES)

Children create words by stringing letters together so that they look like words. They use several rules. (1) Don't use too many letters. (2) Don't use too few letters. (3) Use a variety of letters, with not more than two of the same letter in succession. (4) Rearrange the same letters to make different words. Children ask, "What word is this?"

AUTHORITY BASED

This strategy often follows on the heels of the letter string strategy, apparently because children decide that it is more efficient to ask for spellings, since so many of their letter strings yield nonwords. Children ask for spellings of whole words, or they copy known words from environmental print or books.

EARLY PHONEMIC

Children begin to generate their own words by coding sounds they hear—an idea they might get as adults provide spellings and make letter–sound associations explicit when giving spellings during the time that children are using the Authority Based strategy. Independent spelling may be delayed in children who receive complex answers to their spelling questions during the early part of this stage. No known disadvantage is associated with delay of this kind.

TRANSITIONAL PHONEMIC

Children begin to realize that their sound-based spellings do not look quite like words they see in the environment and that specific spellings they generate are not always identical to ones they see elsewhere. Children often become dissatisfied with their own spellings and begin to ask again for whole word spellings, or they generate a spelling on their own and ask, "Is that right?" This strategy is not common among preschoolers, although children who read early often use it, presumably because they have more visual information about words than do typical preschoolers.

Note: The order of use for the strategies typically follows the order of this list, although different instructional supports can result in variations in children's word creation strategy development.

Note: From "The Place of Specific Skills in Preschool and Kindergarten" by J. A. Schickedanz, in *Emerging Literacy: Young Children Learn to Read and Write* (p. 103) edited by D. S. Strickland and L. M. Morrow, 1989, Newark, DE: International Reading Association. Copyright 1989 by International Reading Association. Reprinted with permission of Judith A. Schickedanz and the International Reading Association.

---

down and tied together with yarn to make a familiar book that any of these students with dyslexia could read. For children with physical disabilities, computer software programs (Beukelman, Tice, Garrett, & Lange, 1988) may help children learn to spell. Story frames (Stewart, 1985) may help children to see the structure of texts.

Using Language in Classrooms

Language plays many roles in classrooms. Language used to teach reading and writing is **metalinguistic.** When children have difficulty functioning in early elementary classrooms, they may need help acquiring metalinguistic talk about language. The focus of the intervention might be to help the children acquire the meanings of concepts such as *sound, letter, syllable, word,* and *sentence.*

A similar use of language in classrooms might be called **metapragmatic.** This is the language and non-verbal communication used by teachers to convey the rules for communicating in the classroom. For example, children need to learn to recognize when they must raise their hands to talk and when talking is permitted. See Chapter 12 (and Box 12.3) for further discussion of intervention focused on metapragmatic rules for school skills that children must infer.

A variety of other specialized uses of language occur in particular aspects of the curriculum. When teachers, parents, and students prioritize areas of the curriculum that present the most difficulty for a student, those areas should be the focus of investigation when performing curriculum-based language assessment activities (as described in Chapters 11 and 12).

Different curriculum content makes different language demands. For example, mathematics uses its own nonlinguistic symbol system. Some famous individuals, best exemplified by Albert Einstein, have shown great difficulty learning to talk and read but genius when manipulating mathematical symbols. Yet 4- and 5-year-old children with specific language impairment have difficulty with such tasks as oral rote counting of objects that seem to be related to a specific deficit in the rote sequential aspect of learning number words. In the elementary classroom, children who understand quantitative language concepts (*many, each,* and *all*) have a distinct advantage. So do children who are good at using verbal memory to remember teachers' instructions. These children can recall and paraphrase instructions to direct their own thinking. When children have difficulty using any of these language functions, they may find themselves in serious difficulty in classrooms.

What can be done about it? Different problems justify different intervention strategies. Verbal mediation can assist in many areas. For example, some children in first or second grade seem unable to remember whether to add or subtract when completing worksheets of mixed addition and subtraction problems. One possibility is that such students are not using verbal mediation strategies to label each problem before attempting to solve it. Metacognitive modeling of how to use "thinking language" to talk to oneself while completing problems might help these students. When verbal mediation

techniques are taught, language specialists and classroom teachers should collaborate to select labels that both can use to prompt the child. For example, if the speech–language pathologist uses the term *thinking language* in small group settings, the special or regular education teacher should use the same label. Teachers might later move the child toward "whisper thinking" as the new strategy becomes established.

When the problem relates most to limited conceptual vocabulary, the best assistance may be to target unfamiliar vocabulary within regular curricular materials. A three-part sequence might structure this curriculum-based language intervention. In the first step, the language specialist sits side-by-side with the student as the student attempts to complete a curricular assignment. The professional acts as onlooker-observer and analyzes the language demands of the activity and assesses the student's language skills and strategies without attempting to influence them. In the second stage, the professional begins to mediate the interaction between the demands of the task and the student's approach and asks questions to focus the student on key elements ("what are we supposed to do here?"); to paraphrase the instructional language ("what do you think that means?"); to identify the referent for a particular pronoun ("I wonder who the 'he' is in this problem?"); or to sketch the elements of a math story problem ("let's draw what we think that means").

The attitude is one of co-conspirator in unlocking the mysteries of the problem, not one of teacher who knows it all and is just testing the student. This is not to suggest that the adult should play dumb, but it does allow the adult to participate with the student in the problem-solving activity. The adult interjects scaffolding comments when appropriate, but primarily facilitates the child to make discoveries independently. When the child makes an "error," rather than correcting it, the interventionist frames inconsistencies between the child's response and the data of the problem ("When you call that word *saw* [the word is *was*], I expect it to start with the /s/ sound," or " 'The box *saw* full,' does that make sense?"). In the third step, the interventionist attempts the "question transplant" operation introduced in Chapter 1. In this step, the adult encourages the child to internalize the strategies and to become independent in problem solving. At this point, labels such as "thinking language" are helpful.

As children advance through the early grades, they are expected to use nonliteral language to think and to discuss abstract concepts. A review of almost any text-book or literature selection for the first few elementary school years yields examples where children must draw inferences, understand idioms and metaphors, and use analogical reasoning. One of the dangers of placing children with language-learning difficulties in special curricula is that they will have less exposure to such rich language uses. That is unfortunate for children who can almost but not quite handle the language demands of the regular curriculum. Although early elementary school children with language impairments have significantly more difficulty with analogical reasoning than their normal learning peers (Kamhi, Gentry, Mauer, & Gholson, 1990; Nippold, Erskine, & Freed, 1988), some evidence suggests that they can learn to use analogical language when assisted (Kamhi, Gentry, et al., 1990; N. W. Nelson & Gillespie, 1991).

The communication needs model advocated in this book suggests that professionals should use assessment to identify intervention targets based on needs for functioning successfully in key contexts. This differs from the more traditional approach of the communication processes model—basing target selection on weak areas identified on formal tests. When the communication needs model guides assessment, the professional is less likely to underestimate the communicative demands of contexts or children's potential to learn to meet those demands.

SUMMARY

This chapter considered the communicative contexts, abilities, and needs of children at middle stages of language development. During this period, children advance beyond one- and two-word utterances to formulating and comprehending complex sentences, weaving them into discourse events of many types, and accomplishing varied communicative purposes.

For middle-stage children, the spontaneous communicative sample is an essential assessment context, and methods were suggested for analyzing language form, content, and use in conversational contexts. Other types of discourse were also identified as important, including narrative and expository discourse in both informal and academic contexts.

Intervention targets and strategies related to problems of middle-stage development were discussed as they relate to interactions with adults, conversational management, developing knowledge of content–form

constructions, phonological production and processing capabilities (including relationships to early reading development), lexical development and recall strategies, play, storytelling, learning to read and write, and learning the language of school.

No one intervention approach was advocated as best for all abilities and all children. Some skills (e.g., phonological, morphological, and syntactic rule development) may be more amenable to direct, structured intervention approaches; whereas others (e.g., conceptual knowledge, pragmatic appropriateness, and contextually sensitive linguistic variations) may only be encouraged in meaningful, more naturalistic contexts. Finally, the underlying message throughout Chapter 10 (and the book) advocates identifying the child's current functioning levels in relationship to the communicative demands of important contexts of the child's life and then designing plans to help narrow the gap.

REVIEW TOPICS

- Roles of adult partners and contexts in language intervention, including roles for parents as intervention aides, primary intervention agents, or incidental agents; activities for involving parents in support of preschool activities; and strategies parents can use to scaffold more complex language production.
- Variation of teacher discourse approaches, including courses described as milieu instruction (also called mand-model or incidental teaching); a more naturalistic version called "enhanced milieu teaching" (with environmental arrangement, responsive interaction strategies, and milieu teaching techniques); and direct imitative approaches compared with interactive conversational approaches.
- Strategies for enhancing the auditory language-learning context, including sound-field amplification systems for normally hearing children, hearing aids for children with hearing impairments, and a series of steps for considering interactions between linguistic and auditory processing demands.
- Goals and methods for conversational language: maintaining an assertiveness–responsiveness balance, making requests, being polite, taking turns, managing topics, making repairs.
- Goals and methods for producing and comprehending complex content–form constructions: targeting sentence subjects, modal auxiliaries, multiple auxiliary

verb forms, dialectal verb forms, complex sentences, and metalinguistic monitoring; contrasts between trainer-oriented and child-oriented procedures.

- Goals and methods for continued phonological development: criteria for targeting phonology separately from language, expectations for grammatical treatment to influence phonological development, and expectations for children with expressive phonological problems to have phonological awareness problems.
- Goals and methods for acquiring and recalling words and concepts: fast mapping or quick incidental learning (QUIL), including expectations for children with specific learning impairments and variables that facilitate the process of word learning, as well as intervention strategies for word-finding problems (at storage and retrieval, phonological, and semantic levels).
- Goals and methods for facilitating language skills in the context of symbolic play.
- Goals and methods for facilitating storytelling and narrative elements in emerging literacy.
- Goals and methods for beginning school: learning to read (whole language philosophy, phonological awareness); learning to write (sociolinguistic factors, invented spelling); other uses of language in the classroom (discourse expectations, mathematical uses); metacognitive and metalinguistic concerns; expository discourse.

REVIEW QUESTIONS

1. What are some of the discourse differences that appear in interactions of parents and their children with language disorders compared with other parent–child dyads?
2. What are some of the features that characterize milieu teaching approaches? How does "enhanced milieu teaching" differ from earlier versions? What theoretical positions influence both versions of the approach? How do imitative and conversational approaches differ in their adult- or child-centeredness and their effects on social and grammatical aspects of language learning? Is there a clear advantage for either direct or interactive language intervention approaches? Which do you prefer? Why?
3. What are the relationships between phonological and grammatical development?
   a. Would you expect grammatical treatment to influence phonological development?
   b. Would you expect all children with expressive phonological problems to have phonological awareness problems? Are some of them at higher risk?
4. If you want to facilitate word learning by children with language disorders, what are three adjustments you would make in presenting the words from how they might appear in a completely natural environment? Should you point out rules to middle-stage children who are attempting to learn derivational morpheme meanings?
5. If you want to facilitate word storage and word retrieval by children having difficulty with word-finding problems, what strategies could you use?
6. What sampling contexts are most likely to elicit mature narratives with many story grammar features?
7. When children begin school, how might a whole language approach differ from a phonics-based approach? What strategies might facilitate a child's integrated approach to early reading development? What strategies might facilitate phonological awareness?
8. What are some of the problems that a child with a language disorder might experience when beginning school? How might the language disorder appear in mathematical learning contexts?

ACTIVITIES FOR EXTENDED THINKING

1. If you were asked to develop a preschool program for children with language development problems, what features would you include? How would you involve parents?

2. Engage in a shared book experience with two children who are in the beginning stages of learning to read—one who is learning normally and one having difficulty. What do you observe about the differences in their approaches? How can you scaffold the success of each child? Observe a reading specialist working with a child with special needs.

3. Read one or more of Paley's books (1981, 1990, 1992). What can you infer about how her classroom and schoolday were structured? What discourse strategies did she use to scaffold kindergarten-age children to higher levels of cognition and language? How did she use both play and storytelling to facilitate the process?

11

Later Stages: Identification and Assessment Third Grade Through High School

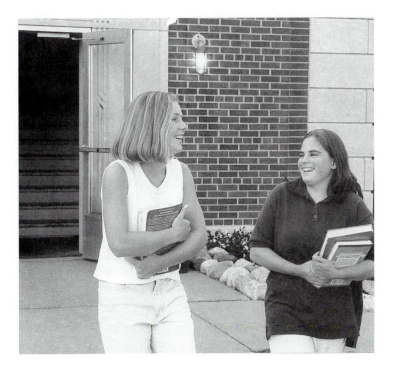

IDENTIFYING LANGUAGE DISORDERS IN THE LATER STAGES

CONTEXTS FOR LATER-STAGE ASSESSMENT AND INTERVENTION

TOOLS AND STRATEGIES FOR LATER-STAGE ASSESSMENT

The era called here the *later stages of language acquisition* covers the preadolescent period of later childhood (ages 8 to 12) through adolescence and the transition to adulthood (ages 12 to 21) (see Personal Reflection 11.1). This period of development was largely ignored in the early years of the psycholinguistic movement. In fact, Carol Chomsky's book, *The Acquisition of Syntax in Children From 5 to 10,* drew so much attention in 1969 partially because it was unusual to think that language acquisition of any consequence happened beyond age 5. The possibility that age-related changes in language might extend even into the geriatric years had barely been considered. As recently as 1986, Reed wrote that "there is no cohesive, integrated body of knowledge regarding normal language development during adolescence" (p. 229).

Now a considerable body of literature is available on the development of language in the later childhood years, and to a certain extent, across the age span. Nevertheless, the territory encompassing the later stages of childhood and adolescence is still less charted than that for the early and middle stages of language development. The shape of the developmental landscape also differs from that of earlier language acquisition. In the introduction to *Later Language Development: Ages Nine Through Nineteen,* Nippold (1988b) identified eight points of contrast that can be observed between earlier and later stages of language learning (see Table 11.1 for a summary).

PERSONAL REFLECTION 11.1 _____

"When the apostle Paul said, 'I put away childish things,' he reduced to five words a period of growth that psychologists and pediatricians eagerly study, parents anxiously anticipate and children inevitably undergo. This is the period called adolescence. Although Paul's description is admirably succinct, it hardly does justice to the process that begins with the early, subtle, biological stirrings of the 10- or 11-year-old and does not end until mature independence is achieved in the mid-20s. The course of adolescence can be orderly and serene, or it can be turbulent and unpredictable. So can the experience of working with adolescents."

Harry E. Hartzell (1984, p. 1), Clinical Professor in the Department of Pediatrics at Stanford Medical School, writing on "the challenge of adolescence."

Many of these factors make identification of clear indicators for normal language development more difficult in the later stages of childhood and adolescence than earlier. The gradual incline of the language learning curve, magnified individual variability, and increasing contributions of formal education and sociocultural variation all make it particularly difficult for specialists in language disorders to be clear about who should qualify for service in this age range. In addition, few formal assessment instruments have been designed to reflect the more subtle, abstract, and discourse-related nature of later-stage language acquisition (Nippold, 1988b; Stephens & Montgomery, 1985). The available tests tend to reflect exclusively a mainstream cultural and linguistic orientation. This factor, in the face of sociolinguistic variability that influences written as well as oral language acquisition, means that it is quite difficult to know who among the "almost but not quite" group should be identified as having a language disability and who should be considered "at risk" for school failure or dropping out for other reasons.

The purposes of this chapter are to outline developmental expectations for children and adolescents in the later stages of language development and to discuss assessment methods for the language problems associated with this developmental stage. Cultural and linguistic variations are considered important contextual variables, and their potential influence is highlighted through the chapter. Another undercurrent is the need to identify individuals' linguistic and nonlinguistic abilities in addition to their disabilities. Because the expression of language disorders may change over time (Bashir, 1989; S. E. Maxwell & Wallach, 1984), the same individual may need different services at different stages of development.

During adolescence, young people with and without disabilities redefine themselves. Particularly, youngsters who previously have been defined primarily as "special education students" may search out new peer groups or jobs as they move toward adulthood. In interviews, Hartzell (1984) noted that adolescents with learning disabilities "frequently said that their first feelings of self-confidence came from a work experience. School may have been frustrating, an experience in failure; but in a job, they perceive the possibility of a useful role for them in society" (p. 5).

Metacognitive and metalinguistic awareness increase in many adolescents and they can focus more consciously on their own abilities. Therefore, adoles-

TABLE 11.1   Contrasts between earlier and later stages of language development

CHARACTERISTIC	EARLIER DEVELOPMENT (AGES 0–9)	LATER DEVELOPMENT (AGES 9–19)
1. Speed of acquisition	Rapid change, with highly salient changes occurring year-to-year and even month-to-month in the earliest years.	Gradual change, with subtle changes noted only when sophisticated linguistic phenomena are analyzed in nonadjacent age groups.
2. Growth emphasis	Acquisition of spoken language skills.	Acquisition of written language skills.
3. Primary sources of input	Spoken communication.	Both spoken and written forms.
4. Degree of linguistic and cognitive freedom	Relative uniformity of developmental advances enable provision of reliable normative data.	Greater individualism and personal choice make it difficult to establish linguistic and cognitive norms.
5. Nature of settings and instructions	Most language learning occurs in nondirected informal settings.	Some language is learned in informal settings, but much language is acquired through formal instruction in grammar, spelling, etymology, literature, and composition.
6. The use of metalinguistics	Few requirements for metalinguistic focus on language as an object are made before school-age years.	Metalinguistic knowledge is required to learn to read and write, perform complex word analysis, and interpret figurative language.
7. The level of abstraction	Vocabulary and language interpretation are literal and concrete.	Newly learned words often represent abstract notions; nonliteral meanings are appreciated increasingly.
8. Social ability	Immaturity makes it difficult to take the perspective of another.	Increased perspective taking enables individual to adjust the content and style of language to an audience for conversation, story telling, and writing.

Note: Summary of "Introduction" by M. A. Nippold in *Later Language Development: Ages Nine Through Nineteen* (pp. 1–10) edited by M. A. Nippold, 1988, Austin, TX: Pro-Ed. Copyright 1988 by Pro-Ed.

cents can participate more actively in planning their own programs. They may exhibit a new readiness to reflect on their behavior and to adopt conscious strategies to reduce impairment or compensate for functional limitations. Approaches that involve modification of problem-solving strategies are often called **strategy-based intervention.** This differentiates them from **skill-based intervention** approaches, which are more typical of middle-stage programs that target basic abilities and naturalistic communication. Such changes may also influence roles played by interventionists such as speech–language pathologists and special educators, who may begin to function more as facilitators and less as direct instructors (Hoskins, 1990).

IDENTIFYING LANGUAGE DISORDERS IN THE LATER STAGES

School or health-care systems rarely implement screening programs to identify communicative disorders in the later stages of childhood. The majority of individuals who need services for language, speech, and other communicative disorders at this stage will have been enrolled in programs steadily since preschool. By the later elementary and secondary school years, it may not be in students' best interests for specialists to look for problems in the general population. Screening certain high-risk populations, however, may be appropriate to identify whether previously unrecognized language disorders might explain academic, social, or behavioral problems.

Information about the prevalence of communicative disorders among children and adolescents is difficult to interpret. According to IDEA, each person with a disability is counted only once. This "unduplicated count" means that many individuals with communicative disorders are not counted as having speech and language disorders but are counted in the categories associated with their other related disorders, such as learning disabilities or mental retardation. Prevalence figures also vary widely across regions, depending on philosophies about the need for services for older children and adolescents. The problem of identifying who qualifies for services therefore is circular; in some areas, children are not identified because no one provides services, and no one provides services because the need has not been identified.

Gillespie and Cooper (1973) estimated the prevalence of speech problems in junior and senior high schools in the United States to be around 5.5%. That figure is somewhat high compared to other estimates, which run closer to 1% to 2% (D. Fein, 1983); 3% to 5% is probably a fairly accurate prediction of the prevalence of language or speech disorders in the general population (Reed, 1986). In certain specialized settings, the prevalence may be considerably higher. For example, in 1969, Taylor (cited in Larson & McKinley, 1987) found that 84% of youth incarcerated in juvenile detention centers in Missouri had communicative disorders. A study reviewed by Ehren and Lenz (1989) found evidence of language disorders among 73% of a group of high-risk middle school students, including students in compensatory education and special education, with the figure jumping to 80% for students with learning disabilities.

Individuals may be at risk for learning and language disorders for a wide variety of reasons (see Personal Reflection 11.2). Frymier and Gansneder (1989) identified at least 46 different factors that can contribute to risk for educational dysfunction. Larson and McKinley (1987) described one portion of the at-risk population as including adolescents who

are not deviant enough for criminal justice services, not deprived enough for social service programs, and not disabled enough for special educational services. These students are described as having a high incidence of problems related to reasoning and communication skills,

PERSONAL REFLECTION 11.2 _____

"The term high risk in the educational literature is no longer confined to the consideration of preschoolers who may encounter language or learning difficulties on entering school. With the growing interest and concern for the adolescent who has a language learning handicap, we have come to examine more closely those children and youth in the middle and high school populations across the country."

Katherine G. Butler (1984a, p. iv), editor of the journal *Topics in Language Disorders,* in her introduction to an issue on "Adolescent Language Learning Disorders."

yet they may be receiving no help from established systems, including no speech-language services in the schools. (p. 8).

Screening

School-based screening programs at this age level are usually holdovers from earlier days when caseloads were reestablished following mass screenings each fall. With the implementation of IDEA and ongoing IEPS, that approach became inappropriate and, in many cases, impossible. IEPs must be implemented continuously, eliminating annual screening. Some practitioners continue to recommend testing all students at least once during their secondary education years, perhaps during their English classes in seventh, ninth, or tenth grades because of problems that may be overlooked (O'Connor & Eldridge, 1981; Tibbits, 1982). I agree with Larson and McKinley (1987), however, that more efficient alternatives to mass screening may identify individuals needing service at these levels.

Most alternatives involve encouraging referrals by informing potential referral sources—including teachers, parents, social workers, physicians, and students themselves—about the signs of a language disorder or other communicative impairment. Selective screening may also be used with high-risk groups. Larson and McKinley (1987) recommended screening (1) adolescents in special programs, such as programs for students with emotional impairment or mental retardation; (2) all seventh- and eighth-graders still receiving remedial reading services; (3) individuals about to drop out of high school; and (4) adolescents with academic difficulties not related primarily to attitudinal or motivational factors. Larson and McKinley also recommended selective screening as routine intake activities in juvenile detention centers and adolescent psychiatric institutions.

A few instruments are designed specifically to screen adolescents' language skills. The following individually administered instruments all measure language comprehension and production and recommend pass–fail decisions based on comparison with established norms: Adolescent Language Screening Test (ALST; Morgan & Guilford, 1984); Screening Tests of Adolescent Language (STAL: Prather, Beecher, Stafford, & Wallace, 1980), and Clinical Evaluation of Language Functions: Advanced Level Screening (CELF; Semel & Wiig, 1980).

Caution should be exercised when interpreting the results of formal screening measures. Some reflect earlier developing language skills and may not be sensitive to later language problems that impair "real-life" functioning. For example, the ALST (Morgan & Guilford, 1984) evaluates earlier developing skills and ignores later developing skills (Nippold, 1988b). The STAL (Prather et al., 1980) is too easy for students in middle-class suburban areas, so it does not identify problems among them; practitioners in lower socioeconomic districts, however, have found it useful (Stephens & Montgomery, 1985). Whenever students from racially or culturally diverse communities are assessed (from inner cities or isolated rural areas, such as Appalachia or Indian reservations), standardized screening instruments are probably inappropriate. They do not adequately allow for influences of nonstandard English dialects or other languages.

Referral

Informed referrals from individuals in close contact with older children and adolescents may be the most productive and efficient identification method. Referrals may come from parents, medical personnel, counselors, employers, or other adults. Teacher referrals are particularly important because of teachers' extensive opportunities to observe higher order language and thinking skills. This is where later language problems often appear. Older children and adolescents also refer themselves.

Accurate referrals generally result from strong information dissemination programs about the nature of

communicative disorders. In the later stages particularly, teachers need instruction to recognize communicative disorders when no overt speech impairments or obvious errors of grammatical formulation are evident. They also need to consider whether problems such as academic and social difficulties might signal the presence of previously untreated (or undertreated) communicative difficulties. The secondary-level referral form developed by Larson and McKinley (1987) includes observational signs of communicating disorders in the domains of thinking, listening, speaking, nonverbal communication, and survival language.

To make appropriate referrals, teachers need clear evidence that their students benefit from the time spent outside class for language assessment and intervention. Success stories provide the best stimulus for more requests for assistance. Magnotta (1991, p. 150) called it "invitation-by-success." On the other hand, if teachers refer students with suspected language-based problems only to be told that the students do not qualify for services, they are not likely to refer more students. When assessment involves only a limited set of standardized tests, it is difficult to be relevant to teacher and student needs. Constable (1987) described one teacher who commented on frustrating experiences with such an approach (see Personal Reflection 11.3)

As children reach adolescence, they also refer themselves, especially if they have adequate education about communicative disorders and are in the later stages of adolescence (Larson & McKinley, 1987). Self-referral is especially powerful because the student is motivated

---

PERSONAL REFLECTION 11.3 _____

I do not have the training that you people [speech–language pathologists] have. However, I've been in the business for a long time, and I think I know when I see a child with a language problem. So I make all the referrals. Now I don't know what happens in the 1:1 session, or what kinds of tests you give the kids, but my speech person keeps sending these children back to me saying they don't have a language problem. Finally I just said to her, 'then you get in the classroom and see what is wrong'."

Frustrated teacher, whose comments were reported by Catherine Constable (1987, pp. 347–348).

to change. Some individuals who refer themselves when provided a nonthreatening avenue to do so may have received speech–language intervention services in earlier grades. In the later grades, they may gain new appreciation of the value of strong communication skills and new insights into their own problems. They also may have increased access to professionals who understand the nature of later-stage communicative difficulties and how to work with them.

CONTEXTS FOR LATER-STAGE ASSESSMENT AND INTERVENTION

To understand the specialized needs of adolescents with developmental language disorders and related disabilities, consider that many of them have struggled for years to achieve the language and educational levels of their same-age peers but continue to fall further behind. Later-stage child development then may become increasingly complicated by self-image, identity, and motivational issues that are exaggerated in all adolescents, but perhaps excessively so in this group. It is sometimes difficult to differentiate problems associated with the special experience of growing up with a disability from those associated with simply growing up. As an aid, Box 11.1 outlines expectations for normal social-emotional development in early, middle, and later stages of adolescence.

Because adolescence may be confusing to teachers, clinicians, and parents, and to adolescents themselves, knowing that the period of maximum turmoil smooths out with time and maturity may be comforting to families. It is inappropriate to conclude, however, that just because some adolescents are rebellious, inconsistent, impulsive, or moody, most of them are. As Larson and McKinley (1987) pointed out, "the vast majority of adolescents are thriving, healthy beings who feel confident, happy, and self-satisfied" (p. 1) (see Personal Reflection 11.4).

This section addresses the multiple contexts in which later-stage children and adolescents participate. Of continued importance is the individual's family and primary culture, but the expanding world of adolescents beyond family also should be considered. Other important contexts for adolescents with language disorders include increased interactions with peers; participation in a variety of educational contexts that may represent cul-

tural and linguistic mismatches; participation in non-school contexts; and making transitions to employment or postsecondary schooling.

Changing Roles of Family and Continued Influence of Primary Culture

When children reach preadolescence and the onset of puberty, dramatic changes occur in their abilities and attitudes. Although families remain important, the role of family shifts. Moving into adolescence signals the beginning of the difficult work of distancing oneself from the primary influence of family. Many youngsters want desperately to be viewed as unique individuals and to be treated as adults by their parents, yet seek to be as much like their peers as possible in dress, action, music preference, and speech. The contrast is between striving for individuality and conformity.

When viewed from a distance, teenagers, in fact, may seem to share a culture of their own—one that cuts across ethnic and socioeconomic boundaries. When examined more closely, however, signs of cultural consistency with familial roots and the primary culture remain. Also evident is the continued importance of many communicative opportunities within family contexts (see Personal Reflection 11.5).

Perhaps no issue is more complicated than differentiating linguistic and cultural influence in language development, particularly as related to the potential for bias in the assessment of later-stage children and adolescents. Indicators of later language development are more likely to reflect a particular set of cultural and linguistic experiences and to be less predictable in time of

Box 11.1 _____

General Expectations for Change Occurring within the Early, Middle, and Later Stages of Adolescence

EARLY ADOLESCENCE

Period of rapid physical growth that precedes sexual maturity (ages 10–13 for girls and up to 2 years later for boys).

Gangly and awkward period; both boys and girls are uncomfortable with their new body images.

Problem solving is egocentric and concrete.

Self-consciousness leads to the formation of intense relationships with peers based on similarities (e.g., in dress), but home and family remain the most important emotional and social factors.

Approval of peers is important, with a strong yearning to be normal and average. Those in special education become strongly sensitive to its symbols (e.g., riding a different schoolbus, being called out of class, or working in a resource room).

Emotional lability may appear in the form of wide mood swings from depression to elation.

Moral outlook for most is at the conventional level (individual conforms to authority and obeys laws and social rules).

MIDDLE ADOLESCENCE

Period that begins after the physical changes of maturity are complete (ages 13–16 in girls and 14–17 in boys).

Boys show great interest in their bodies; girls diet and exercise to lose weight; both show dissatisfaction with their bodies and worry that they may not be normal.

Psychosomatic complaints may appear, and some need reassurance that stress and worry can cause physical symptoms like headaches and stomachaches.

Thinking is more abstract, theoretical, and idealistic. Interest in outside world and introspection both increase.

Beliefs persist in simple solutions for complex problems (from world hunger to fad diets and cures for acne).

Feelings of rebellion may be exhibited in dress styles, hair styles, adolescent slang, and fascination with rock music and rock stars. Extreme forms may involve drugs, alcohol, vandalism, and early pregnancy.

Social life is primarily with peers; dating becomes more common.

First jobs and participation in sports may make important contributions to self-confidence and maturity.

By end of the period (last 2 years of high school), begin to move beyond the self-consciousness and spirit of rebellion that characterize this stage.

LATER ADOLESCENCE

Period by which full adult growth and strength are reached (begins about age 16–17 and may extend into the mid-20s).

Comfort with body maturity increases.

Period of partial dependence on parents is often extended, compared to previous generations, owing to longer career preparations and postsecondary education.

Personal identity is developed with greater reliance on friends than family for social contact.

Sexual intimacy increases, as does ability to deal with interpersonal complexities.

Personal value systems are adopted, leading to the ability to make mature, independent judgments (in spite of earlier rebelliousness, most older adolescents adopt value systems similar to those of their parents).

Sources: Hartzell, 1984; Larson & McKinley, 1987

"In addition to knowing (something about) the rules for conversation, a typical child will be faced with a variety of conversational tasks in the course of growing up—engaging in dinner table conversation with parents, chatting on the phone to relatives, amusing oneself and one's siblings during long car rides, perhaps even being asked to entertain parental dinner guests while cocktails are being prepared. Performing effectively in these various tasks requires considerably more than knowing the language-specific rules for conversation. It requires integrating that rule-knowledge with the systems for syntax, morphology, lexical retrieval, and so forth. It requires analyzing the social and cognitive demands of the specific situation. It may depend very heavily on having practiced components of the skills required to perform the task, so that the processing load is reduced."

Catherine Snow (1991, pp. 122–123), writing about her task-analysis approach to understanding language proficiency.

---

development than indicators of early development, which tend to be more universal.

Socialization involves "the process of growing up in a particular society," a process that involves the transmission, primarily by parents and other adults, of Cultural knowledge required to operate Successfully and appropriately in the everyday world (D. C. Cooper & Anderson-Inman, 1988, p. 225). The specialist's need to recognize socialization factors and to be culturally sensitive during assessment and intervention has been emphasized by Crago and Cole (1991):

> The socialization of children to their culture is, indeed, an important and delicate process in which language and communication patterns have an integral and crucial role. The violation of minority cultures' cultural and socialization practices by a lack of awareness of the importance of this relationship prevents the formulation of appropriate assessment and intervention strategies for these populations. (p. 106).

Increased Interactions with Peers

Although families maintain an important role in the lives of older children and adolescents, peers occupy an increasingly important position. As D. C. Cooper and

Anderson-Inman (1988) pointed out, individuals may exhibit widely different levels of communicative competence in school and other environments:

> For example, children who are judged linguistically deficient in the school environment sometimes display sophisticated and competent communication skills in the home, neighborhood, or peer group situation. Vernacular forms of speech, or ways of talking that are appropriate for the speaker's group, may not reflect the standards of the preferred speech norms but can be judged competent because of their appropriateness for some of the situations in which they are used. It must be noted, however, that not all situationally competent communicative performances have the same influence in terms of social power, nor are they equally acceptable across a range of social contexts. (p. 232)

Language assessment and intervention for preadolescents and adolescents should involve consideration of communicative competence within multiple contexts including peer groups.

Influences of Cultural and Language Mismatches at School

School continues to be a critical context for children and adolescents in the later stages of language development, but it is often a place of mixed blessings. For many individuals with language disorders, school is simultaneously a place where they find satisfying social contacts, hopes for the future, and considerable frustration. As Trapani (1990) noted, even individuals with so-called "milder impairments" experience increasing stress:

> Youths with learning disabilities encounter increasing difficulties as they progress through the school system because their poor skills do not enable them to meet the demands of an increasingly demanding curriculum. The intensity of the current high school curriculum often overwhelms the adolescent with learning disabilities who cannot read textbooks and has poor writing skills. (p. x)

The high complexity and fast pace of middle school and secondary school communicative environments can be confusing whenever language skills are wobbly, but when cultural mismatches are thrown into the mix, the risks for dropping out, low self-esteem, and reduced employment potential are magnified. As children advance in school, problems of differential diagnosis related to cultural difference increase (see Personal Reflection 11.6). It is particularly difficult to sort out the interacting influences of cultural, linguistic, educational, and economic variables that contribute to widening differences in performance on formal and informal measures of cognitive and communicative development for individuals in lower socioeconomic groups, many of whom also belong to minority groups with limited English proficiency or who speak a nonstandard dialect of English.

Whereas societal indicators and formal assessments of communicative maturity tend to be tied to a specific, standard sociolinguistic system, not all individuals are equally likely to learn that particular system. In schools, the "rich get richer" metaphor (called the "Matthew effect" by Stanovich, 1988) refers to the observation that children who are good at the school "game" tend to get even better as they advance through the grades. All too often, in fact, the metaphor becomes literal. Because of differential success in formal education settings, individuals from different socioeconomic groups have varied opportunities for postsecondary education and, eventually, differential access to high-paying jobs. The problems related to this discrepancy extend far beyond problems associated with differential proficiency in the language use valued in school and business. They reach into the depths of societal problems involving poverty, racism, urban living conditions, drug culture, and other sociological complexities.

PERSONAL REFLECTION 11.6 _____

"After the first few years, mismatch between the child's communication skills and the teacher's demands tend not to be attributed by the teachers to the child's cultural and linguistic background. This is especially true for English-speaking minority children. The problems children in higher grades encounter are more often attributed to low intellectual capacity and/or to a communication disorder. What teachers at this level often fail to realize is that the communicative demands of their classrooms are different from those of earlier grades, and that many of these children have not been taught, either at home or in their previous classes, the particular skills required for success in the higher grades."

Aquiles Iglesias (1985, p. 37), writing about communicative mismatches between school and home.

Periodically, someone observes that people whose language systems differ from those of mainstream society are not actively involved in it. A federal judge in Ann Arbor, Michigan, for example, ruled that the district must consider the language differences of a group of African American children whose primary language was Black English when educating them (*Martin Luther King Junior Elementary School Children et al.,* v. *Ann Arbor School District Board,* 1978). Furthermore, Orr (1987) hypothesized that language mismatches might explain problems in learning the science and mathematics curriculum for some African American students from inner-city Washington, DC, who were enrolled in her private school. Both the Ann Arbor court ruling and Orr's book have been controversial. In 1997, a national debate was raging about a decision by the Oakland, California, public schools to recognize Ebonics (also called African American English and Black English Vernacular) as a legitimate language system.

It is seductive, but dangerous, to link language variation too closely to indices of success in settings such as school and the workplace. It is dangerous, because it may lead to a renewed acceptance of the old, discredited **deficit theory** of language variation, in which sociolinguistic variation was equated with social disadvantage and inferiority, ignoring the more preferred **difference theory,** in which no language system or dialect is seen as inherently superior or inferior to another (see Personal Reflection 11.7).

The emphasis here is on accurate and fair, nonbiased assessment so that all the children with language disorders, and only those children, will be identified as having language disorders. Although issues related to the effective education of minority individuals who do not have language disorders may be of interest to language specialists, they are beyond the scope of this book. Here, we consider the demands of the language of school and whether mismatches between the current abilities of students with language *disorders* and the expectations of written and oral language processing in classrooms might explain their academic and social interaction difficulties. Potential language differences that might complicate the picture for these students also should be considered.

Avoid the trap of equating racial or ethnic difference with language difference. As discussed in Chapter 2, minority group membership and linguistic difference are not isomorphic. The relative independence of the

"As far as I can see, technical answers of the type that Orr [1987], the Ann Arbor judge [*Martin Luther King Elementary School Children et al.,* v. *Ann Arbor School District Board,* 1978], and others offer no way out of the present situation in which the gap between the educational achievements of the African American poor and other poor minority groups and those of the white majority correlate so strongly with other gaps: IQ and SAT scores, dropout rates, unemployment rates, malnutrition rates, infant mortality rates, serious illness and longevity rates, violent-death rates, and so on. An understanding of the grammar of Black English will explain none of this. Perhaps the recent work that sees these differences to be the result of a caste-like structure of our society will lead to an explanation of its present disgraceful state. But still better explanations will not eliminate the Third World conditions that characterize much of urban existence in the United States."

Wayne O'Neil (1990, p. 87), linguist at Massachusetts Institute of Technology.

"Minority students who came from securely affluent home backgrounds did not show up in the low proficiency groups. The problem is poverty, not ethnic affiliation."

Walter Loban (1976, p. 23).

two elements was highlighted by Loban (1976) in his classic longitudinal study of language development in school-age children from kindergarten through grade 12 (see Personal Reflection 11.8). Loban's results demonstrated that socioeconomic status, and not racial or ethnic diversity, correlated highly with school success. Specifically, Loban found strong correlations between both high socioeconomic status and high language ability and low socioeconomic status and low language ability. He concluded that minority group membership alone was not predictive of school success or failure.

Participating in Nonschool Contexts

Not all services to adolescents are provided in school. In many communities, adolescents receive services from private practitioners and community service agencies. Hospitals and rehabilitation centers also may provide services following traumatic brain injury or other medical crises. Other youths may be admitted to residential treatment settings or juvenile detention centers for emotional or behavioral problems.

When services are provided in acute-care centers, several factors influence assessment and intervention.

If the reason for admission is crisis (e.g., vehicular accident, a suicide attempt, or delinquent behavior), the initial focus of the assessment may be on many factors other than communication. The speech–language pathologist and other learning specialists may need to focus the team on potential involvement of communicative, language, and learning impairments as well. Because of short admissions, more attention may be given to assessment than intervention. The transdisciplinary team then should review prior records, conduct tests including dynamic assessment of outcomes within modified communicative contexts, and generate transition plans for discharge.

When treatment is provided in long-term care centers, team members must consider individuals' needs to participate in contexts beyond the center. Many rehabilitation centers for individuals with traumatic brain injury have "community reentry" programs with systematic strategies to help patients return to functioning in the community as much as possible. Communication specialists should play an active role, analyzing communicative demands of those contexts, the patient's current abilities in them, the potential for (and desirability of) changing contextual demands, the potential for changing the individual's abilities, and the best strategies for doing so.

In some communities, alternative school programs also are available to students who cannot make it in the regular educational system. Taff (1990) described the population from which the DeLeSalle Education Center in Kansas City, Missouri, recruits:

> To enter the school, a student must be a confirmed educational failure. We recruit from juvenile court, mental health programs, school districts that have permanently expelled students, and the inner-city streets. Our students come from neighborhoods with the highest crime rates and the lowest family incomes. Some are from families who have been unemployed for generations and on wel-

fare for most of that time. Most have been abused. Many have a pattern of drug abuse. (p. 71)

In alternative school programs such as this, change is fostered through a combination of small class sizes; strong counseling programs with individualized goal setting; rules about attendance, drugs, and fighting; and specialized remedial programs using materials relevant to the students' interests (e.g., state driving manuals, pop music, and magazines). These programs also provide appropriate contexts to help students develop more effective communicative and language abilities and strategies.

Transitions to Higher Education, Employment, and Other Postschool Activities

Whether individuals participate in school programs or other settings, as they enter the middle stages of adolescence, the intervention team should begin deliberate planning for transitions to later adolescence and adulthood. Depending on the resources and goals of individuals and their families, transition services might focus on higher education, job training, and supported or competitive employment.

The implementation of IDEA requires the development and evaluation of transition services as part of educational programs for special education students age 16 and older. The history of special education in helping students make transitions beyond secondary education is not strong (Trapani, 1990). In a summary of the literature on individuals with learning disabilities, Trapani reported that "it cannot be assumed that adolescents with learning disabilities will become independent upon their graduation from high school" (p. 93). Deliberate plans to consider communicative needs in consultation with academic advisers, vocational educators, vocational counselors, and job coaches during transition have increased with IDEA. The potential for improved service delivery in this area is still ripe.

TOOLS AND STRATEGIES FOR LATER-STAGE ASSESSMENT

Gathering Background Information for Contextually Based Assessment

The specialist should gather a variety of background information when assessing problems of later-stage lan-

guage acquisition. As in early and middle stages, assessment questions related to impairment, disability, and handicap can be answered only if multiple sources of information are considered.

Information-gathering procedures for later-stage assessment parallel those of middle-stage assessment. Box 11.2 presents several modifications for procedures originally introduced in Chapter 9 (Box 9.5). Primary distinctions relate to the degree to which older children and adolescents act as informants about their own problems and participate actively in formulating plans for their future. Direct observation in classrooms may also be used less frequently in middle schools and secondary schools, partially because these students tend to have multiple teachers and to be more easily embarrassed. At these levels, interviews may be more helpful to professionals and less embarrassing to students. I have also enlisted the collaborative help of high school and junior high school teachers to audiotape record their classroom lectures. I let them know that I need samples of curricular language to gauge its complexity and to identify key vocabulary.

Formal Assessment in Later Stages

As in selecting screening instruments for later-stage language disorders, a variety of problems may arise when selecting standardized instruments for later-stage assessment. Problems relate to inadequate representation of later acquired language features (Nippold, 1988b), a lack of standardized instruments for measuring extended discourse production or comprehension (Constable, 1987; Launer & Lahey, 1981), and a lack of instruments that are demanding enough to be sensitive yet open-ended enough to be fair in terms of cultural and educational variation.

As pointed out by the practitioner in Personal Reflection 11.9, formal tests are mandated in schools to determine eligibility for services (Stephens & Montgomery, 1985). Third-party-pay requirements and other policies may dictate the need for formal tests in other settings as well.

In addition to meeting the need for norm-referenced tests to determine eligibility, formal testing may serve other purposes. It may identify multiple dimensions of a language disorder and related impairments, may suggest areas to address in intervention, and may identify potential strategies for doing so. Formal tests may also

Box 11.2 _____

Procedures for Gathering Background Information Essential to the Assessment of Children and Adolescents in the Later Stages of Language Acquisition

1. Determine the **reason for referral** by interviewing the person(s) who made the referral (or suggested that it be made). Also find out how the person being referred feels about the referral. If an older child or adolescent makes a self-referral, explore the reasons why and investigate whether others (including parents, teachers, and employers) think it was a good idea (or perhaps suggested it).

2. Gather **history information** about the nature of the problem by interviewing the adolescent as well as others who play important roles in the individual's life (e.g., parents, teachers, employers), being careful to obtain the appropriate permissions before contacting anyone beyond the person's immediate family. Information should be gathered regarding (a) family history, (b) medical history, (c) developmental history, (d) educational history, (e) social history, and (f) employment history.

3. Collaborate with others, including the client, to **identify contexts** that are particularly important in the client's life. These may be called "zones of significance." Include questions about (a) places (e.g. school, social settings, or work); (b) people (teachers, employers, romantic partners, or friends); and (c) communicative events (e.g., classroom interactions, note taking, homework, tests, social conversations, business conversations, asking assistance of strangers).

4. Use multiple strategies to **identify aspects of communicative competence in each of these important contexts.** Include both (a) observational strategies and (b) interview strategies.

5. Consider building a **profile of areas of proficiency, strength, and preference that do not involve language.** For example, *The Smart Profile* (L. Miller, 1990) might be used to guide interviews with the target individual and significant others to build a profile based on strengths (rather than deficits). Miller based this profiling procedure on Gardner's (1983) theory of multiple intelligences. Using ethnographic interviewing procedures, she recommended probing for evidence of strength in each of the following eight areas (Gardner proposed seven): linguistic, musical, logical, mathematical (Gardner combined these as logical-mathematical), spatial, bodily, intrapersonal, and interpersonal.

6. Based on this initial compilation of background information, **form additional hypotheses about the child's relative areas of strength and difficulty** that can be tested using both informal and formal assessment techniques.

_____

be used to provide ongoing assessment, particularly for documenting a continuing need for services. Norm-referenced tests, however, are generally not sensitive enough to measure changes resulting from intervention (McCauley & Swisher, 1984).

Formal tests need to be chosen based on their ability to address later-stage assessment concerns. These include assessment of (1) written and oral language, (2) language processing and language knowledge,

(3) higher order and basic language skills, and (4) the production and comprehension of connected discourse. Although similar assessment concerns are present in earlier stages of development to varying degrees, they become the hallmark of later-stage assessments.

To some extent, the preceding objectives may be met with formal tests selected from Chapter Appendix A. Formal assessment works best when conducted by multidisciplinary teams working collaboratively. Mutual

planning can spread the evaluation workload but more
importantly can result in mutual consideration of assessment results. Language specialists then can administer only a few formal tests but will have access to
results of tests administered by other educational consultants and psychologists and will have their insights
about language assessment results. Particularly helpful
may be the results of reading tests, processing tests (e.g.,
the Woodcock-Johnson Psycho-Educational Battery—
Revised, Woodcock & Johnson, 1989), or academic
achievement tests. If language specialists train collabo-
rators to record verbal responses exactly, they may have
a rich data source. Insights about language processing
might come from qualitative reviews of test responses
(not just quantitative scores). No formal test, however,
can meet all assessment needs. Informal methods also
must be used.

Informal Assessment in Later Stages

Identifying Zones of Significance. When one attempts to understand children with language disorders
within the framework of dynamic system theory, the
selection of relevant contexts is central to designing assessment and intervention activities. **Functional limitation,** by definition, is context dependent (see Chapter
1). It is defined relative to difficulty in meeting contextual demands. Therefore, reducing functional limitation
is based on the question "What does this individual need
to be able to do (communicatively) to succeed in important life contexts?"

When children reach the later stages of language development, they are expected to use language compe-
tently in a wide variety of modalities and contexts.
Therefore, to be comprehensive, language sampling for
most older children should include oral and written language samples (both reading and writing) and evidence
of the ability to use language to think and communicate.

Some prudence in selecting sampling contexts is wise,
however. If all relevant contexts and modalities were
sampled independently, comprehensive assessment
would demand prohibitive amounts of time. Streamlin-
ing the evaluation process as much as possible therefore
is important to allow assessment goals to be met without cutting into valuable intervention time. A minimal-
ist approach involves devoting only as much time as
necessary to meet goals of (1) establishing eligibility,
(2) outlining critical dimensions of the problem,
(3) identifying appropriate goal areas, and (4) designing
appropriate intervention strategies.

The time problem may also be addressed by viewing
"assessment" not as something to be completed before
beginning intervention but rather as an ongoing and integral part of intervention. For most purposes, it is useful
to see informal assessment and intervention as thoroughly integrated processes. When professionals adopt
this attitude, they learn how to gather only as much pure
assessment information as they need to make initial decisions. Then they shift to an intervention mode, implementing mediation and scaffolding strategies to assist
the person to process language, and then assessing the
client under the modified conditions. This "mediate and
measure" approach, sometimes known as **dynamic assessment** (Feuerstein, 1979) (see Chapter 6), is a key
strategy of contextually based assessment. It is a critical
part of keeping intervention plans updated and relevant.

Another way to narrow the sampling focus is to
consider background information gathered using interviews, review of records, and observation. By identifying "zones of significance," professionals may gather
in-depth information about areas particularly significant
for the individual (N. W. Nelson, 1994). Zones of significance are identified through participant interviews
with the target person and important others (particularly
parents, teachers, school administrators, and employers). Significance may stem from relevance to an individual's personal goals or to outstanding areas of ability
or disability. The specialist may use the ethnographic
technique of triangulation—confirmation of the same
observation by interviewing several sources—to validate the selection of assessment contexts as relevant.
To assist in the interview process, Table 11.2 presents
some of the areas that should be probed with parents,
teachers, and students. These sample questions are to be
used merely as guides for areas to probe. They should

TABLE 11.2   Starter questions to be asked of the key participants in the curriculum-based language assessment process

TEACHER INTERVIEWS	PARENT INTERVIEWS	STUDENT INTERVIEWS
Objective information about the student's academic performance, both from achievement tests and classroom levels of performance.	Early development (Did they suspect a problem early)?	The student's description of what is hardest about school.
Descriptions of the student's classroom strengths.	Medical history (especially middle ear problems)	The student's description of what is best about school.
A prioritized review of the problems the teacher identifies as most important.	Educational history	The student's prioritized list of changes to be made.
Anecdotal descriptions of recent classroom events with which the student has experienced difficulty.	When did problems first show up at school? Did decoding problems show up early? Or did the problems show up in third or fourth grade when it became more important to read longer texts for meaning?	Anecdotal evidence—accounts of recent classroom events that made the student feel really bad. The student's ideas about the future.
Descriptions of aspects of the curriculum that present the greatest difficulties to the student and the most concern to the teacher.	Anecdotal evidence of specific problems within the past year or so.	
The teacher's view of the student's potential within the current school year and in the future.	A prioritized review of the problems the parents view as most critical. The parents' goals for their child's future.	

not be asked verbatim, nor should they be turned into a form to be filled out in writing. If a young person has a primary concern about social interactions or employment settings, the interview participants and questions should shift accordingly.

Once the professional has identified zones of significance, he or she selects specific sampling contexts to probe different aspects of those areas. During sampling, the examiner should probe an individual's language skills and strategies in certain contexts and also clarify the communicative demands and opportunities associated with those contexts. This information is used to understand the problem and to design intervention.

If the specialist identifies impaired conversational skills and social interaction as particularly handicapping owing to social penalties from peers, he or she might gather a sample of social interaction discourse (i.e., the target student conversing with a peer, either a friend or someone recruited by the language specialist). If such an approach is objectionable to potential conversational partners or not feasible for other reasons, a variety of role-playing contexts may be used to set up discourse events between the examiner and the target individual (e.g., "I'm going to try to pick a fight with you, and I want you to show me what you would say in such a situation." or "How would you start a conversation with a girl you wanted to meet?"). If an adolescent is having trouble getting a job, the sampling process might involve filling out standard job applications (written language samples) or engaging in simulated job interviews. The important thing is to sample a variety of contextually based language uses relevant to the concerns of the client and others who care about him or her.

Organizing an Approach to Later-Stage Sampling and Analysis.   The nature of later-stage language developments differs sufficiently from early- and middle-stage developments that specialized language sample analysis techniques are required. As in earlier stages, the advantages of naturalistic samples relate to their relevance to real-life circumstances and their opportunities for observing holistic and interactive aspects of real communication. Later-stage naturalistic language sampling and analysis, however, may be especially complex because of all of the factors in the sampling process.

Professionals need an organizational system to observe multiple variables associated with mature communication in naturalistic contexts. The system should be open enough to avoid reductionism (i.e., fitting complex behavior into a limited set of predefined categories). It should allow inference about aspects of internalized language processing as well as direct observation of oral and written language products. It should relate to appro-

priate contextual aspects of an individual's educational, vocational, and social world. It should address linguistic knowledge of the five basic rule systems—phonology, morphology, syntax, semantics, and pragmatics—as well as metalinguistic and other "meta-" abilities. It should be based on samples that represent multiple modalities, including listening, speaking, reading, writing, and thinking. It should allow focus on a variety of sizes of linguistic units, from phonemes and graphemes to whole texts, and in particular, it should be appropriate for long and complex utterances. Finally, it should accomplish all of this within a variety of conversational, narrative, and expository discourse events that hold particular significance for the individual.

Table 11.3 represents an outline of most of these variables. It is an open outline, subject to revision and expansion or abbreviation, or to adaptation to allow

TABLE 11.3 Organizational framework of assessment variables and contexts for later-stage language sample analysis

		METASKILLS[a]		
CONTEXTS	RULE SYSTEMS	PROCESSING MODALITIES	LINGUISTIC UNITS	DISCOURSE EVENTS
School Curricula	Phonology	Listening	Sounds	Conversational
Official	Morphology	Speaking	Syllables	Informal classroom talk
Cultural	Syntax	Reading	Words	Playground or cafeteria talk
De facto	Semantics	Writing	Sentences	Peer tutoring
School culture	Pragmatics	Thinking	Simple	Peer social interaction
Hidden			Complex	Narrative
Underground			Discourse	Stories from reading texts or literature
Vocational				Stories teachers read aloud
Social				Stories students write
				Personal narratives (show and tell; oral reports)
				Expository
				Procedural directions and explanations
				Lectures
				Most textbooks
				Most worksheets and textbook assignments
				Informational papers
				Oral reports/speeches/(some show and tell)
				Note taking

[a]"Metaskills" include metalingistic skills for talking about and manipulating linguistic symbols, metacognitive skills for monitoring and controlling thinking, and metapragmatic skills for awareness of classroom discourse rules.

nonbiased consideration of proficiency in more than one system. For example, Adler (1991) presented an analysis system to compare aspects of language features in multiple discourse samples. He suggested rating competence separately for the individual's native language (L1), English as a second language (L2), and nonstandard dialect (D).

The organizational system presented in Table 11.3 represents observable language **products** better than it represents internalized language processing activities. **Processes,** which draw on several sources of knowledge, skill, and strategies are illustrated in the pinball wizardry model, which first appeared in Chapter 2 (see Figure 2.3), and is shown here as Figure 11.1. Professionals may use these two organizational frameworks together to organize the multiple factors to consider when gathering and analyzing later-stage language samples.

The Pinball Wizardry Model of Oral and Written Language Processing.

The primary accomplishments of later-stage language acquisition are associated not so much with learning new things as with putting together known pieces in new and more complex ways for new and more varied purposes in new and more demanding contexts. When attempting to analyze later-stage language processing, the specialist must do more than simply look at a limited sample of oral conversation. To understand how an adolescent's language disorder might be contributing to difficulties in the classroom or on the job, more is needed than a computation of mean length of utterance (MLU). To contribute to problem solving, language specialists need to consider the individual's internal processes as he or she attempts to process language. That is the value of the pinball wizardry model of complex oral and written language processing.

Figure 11.1 presents a model of competent, mature language processing in terms of four different but interrelated, synergistic contributions, which are explained in Chapter 2.

They include:

1. **Six kinds of knowledge structures** including three linguistic (graphophonemic, semantic, and syntactic) and three additional cognitive, pragmatic, and discourse rule systems (the boxes).
2. **Peripheral processing skills** for interacting with the environment to get information in and out (the bottom arrow).

3. **Central processing skills** for performing functions such as holding information in short-term memory, analyzing it, encoding it, associating it, storing it in long-term memory, and retrieving it when appropriate (the small black arrows).
4. **Conscious metacognitive strategies** for guiding attention and for directing and organizing all of the other processes and making them work efficiently (the top arrow).

Contextually Based Language Assessment.

Educational, vocational, and social contexts are all relevant to the later stages of language learning. Depending on areas identified as "zones of significance" for particular individuals, some contexts may be more critically in need of attention. For school-age children and adolescents with language disorders, however, school is almost always significant.

In school, where young people with language disorders spend the majority of their time, they encounter some of the most pressing language-based learning demands, and they are at great risk for failure and for damage to their self-esteem. **Curriculum-based language assessment** therefore is often the most critical form of contextually based assessment for older children and adolescents with language disorders. It is the method of focus in this section, with the expectation that readers will adapt its techniques to other contexts as appropriate when individual needs arise.

In my previous writing about curriculum-based language assessment and intervention (N. W. Nelson, 1989b, 1990, 1992b, 1994), I have been careful to differentiate it from general curriculum-based measurement (CBM). To understand the distinctions, first consider a description of general curriculum-based assessment (CBA):

> *Curriculum-based assessments are teacher-constructed tests designed to measure directly students' skill achievements at specified grades. The assessments are criterion-referenced, and their content reflects the curricula used in general education classrooms. (Idol, Nevin & Paolucci-Whitcomb, 1986, p. v)*

Tucker (1985) commented, in addition, that CBA "includes any procedure that directly assesses student performance within the course content for the purpose of determining that student's instructional needs" (p. 200). Deno (1989) noted that "CBM is a systematic set of procedures that produces a data base for making special ed-

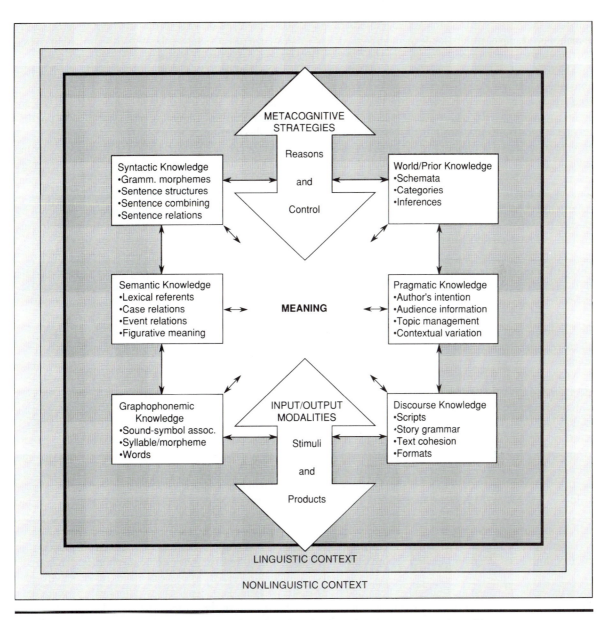

FIGURE 11.1   A model showing the interaction of oral and written language processing with external linguistic and nonlinguistic contextual factors to guide curriculum-based language assessment.

© 1992 N. W. Nelson. Shared by permission of the author.

ucation decisions" (p. 1). General forms of CBM address the question "Has the student learned the curriculum?"

In contrast, curriculum-based *language* assessment refers to the more specific "use of curriculum contexts and content for measuring a student's language intervention needs and progress" (N. W. Nelson, 1989b, p. 171). It addresses the question "How does the student use language in attempting to learn the curriculum?"

Although the primary distinction between the two approaches is one of specificity, some methodological distinctions also apply.

The two approaches complement each other. Questions about how well the curriculum has been learned (and which aspects are problematic) usually serve as a prelude to more specific questions about language processing. Conversely, specialists may use the in-depth probing strategies of curriculum-based language assessment to determine why a student is having difficulty learning the curriculum. It is wise, however, to keep some aspects of the two approaches separate. To understand why, consider an example: Student, parent, and teacher interviews about zones of significance for one high school student with language-learning disabilities make it fairly clear that he is competent in learning some aspects of the physical education (PE) and industrial arts curricula but that his performance is inadequate on paper and pencil or textbook tasks. He seems gifted as an athlete and when using his hands to make things. However, his language and reading deficits make it difficult for him to read the course textbooks, to answer questions on written assignments, and to take written tests.

Members of a diagnostic team attempting to implement general CBA for this adolescent might collaborate with the PE teacher to construct multiple-choice examination questions to assess the student's knowledge of sports rules studied and with the industrial arts teacher to construct a test with diagram labeling and true–false questions to assess knowledge of tools and methods for use in woodworking (see examples of these instruments in Idol et al., 1986). This team, recognizing probable negative effects of reading deficits, might design alternative forms of assessment to the paper and pencil tasks, perhaps administering the test orally, or allowing unlimited time and accepting spelling approximations. They might use the test results to draw conclusions about the extent to which the student has benefited from the regular classroom activities, whether placement should continue in those classrooms, and whether compensatory methods should be designed for note taking, textbook reading, and test taking.

A language specialist using curriculum-based language assessment would take a slightly different approach to these same problems that complements the first. This professional might work with the rest of the interdisciplinary diagnostic team to analyze the outcome of teacher designed tests but more likely would use samples of the real curriculum rather than specially designed tests to analyze the student's curriculum-based language processing abilities.

Curriculum-based **language** assessment involves several kinds of data collection. The primary tools and strategies, in addition to ethnographic interviews, are **artifact analysis, onlooker observation,** and **participant observation.**

Artifacts are products created by students in the process of regular curricular activities. For the high school student described, artifacts include classroom lecture notes and written assignments. These could be compared with class notes and homework produced by other classmates who are not having difficulty. In particular, language specialists might look for evidence of semantic organizational strategies, word knowledge, linguistic sophistication, completeness, and detail. Other artifacts that might be examined include actual responses to real classroom examinations and portfolios of representative work that classroom teachers collect for all of their students (e.g., Rief, 1990).

Onlooker observation involves sitting in the classroom with the student at a distance and observing signs of participation, including evidence of attention, listening, and communicative expression. Onlooker observation is not particularly appropriate at secondary levels because of student embarrassment, but tape recordings of classroom lectures might be used as indirect observation to gauge the level of linguistic complexity and other language demands of the classroom.

Participant observation is a somewhat more intrusive form of observation. The specialist sits beside the student while the student attempts a targeted curricular task (this can occur in an isolated therapy room, if appropriate). In participant observation, the adult acts not as traditional teacher, but as co-conspirator or co-learner, attempting to figure out the demands of the activity with the student. Participant observation involves more than observation of the current status of the situation. This dynamic assessment is a deliberate exploration of the effects of facilitative scaffolding on the student's ability to recognize relationships, comprehend the language of an activity, and formulate appropriate responses to it (Nelson, 1995; Palincsar et al., 1994; Silliman & Wilkinson, 1994a, 1994b). Participant observation is based on Vygotsky's (1962) observation that "with assistance, every child can do more than he can by himself—though only within the limits set by the state of his development"

(p. 103). Vygotsky labeled this range the zone of proximal development.

Bruner (1978) used Vygotsky's ideas to introduce the concept of scaffolding. Scaffolding techniques, as mentioned throughout the preceding chapters, are used by parents, teachers, and supervisors at all levels of the child's development, from infancy through adulthood. Scaffolding enables individuals to reach levels of processing efficiency and success that they might not be able to reach otherwise; even more importantly, particularly in the later stages of language development, it encourages independent use of strategies after they have been modeled (Applebee & Langer, 1983; Bruner, 1978; Cazden, 1988).

An example of a scaffolding technique that might be used with the high school student described previously is modeling of "thinking aloud" or self-questioning, verbal mediation strategies. When completing assignments involving questions in the shop manual, the student is encouraged to ask a series of questions, such as "What am I supposed to do here? How many different kinds of tools am I supposed to learn this week? What are the main types and subtypes of tools? What is the function of each?" In responding to such questions, the student is taught to draw a semantic map to show major headings, subheadings, definitions, characteristics, and examples of particular types of tools. Then the student could be taught how to study with peers, using notes and diagrams to ask questions of each other and themselves.

Unique contributions by language specialists in dynamic assessment contexts come from description of students' current language knowledge, skills, and strategies when attempting to process language of the curriculum. Concurrently, language specialists informally analyze the language demands of the curriculum. The first effort might be considered an inside-out approach, and the second might be considered an outside-in approach. These assessment concerns are summarized by the two questions (outside-in and inside-out, respectively):

1. What are the external contextual demands that influence how the student processes the information?
2. What are the internal language and communicative processing abilities that the student currently brings to the task?

These two questions—oriented relatively more toward assessment—are balanced by two more questions—oriented relatively more toward intervention The intervention-oriented questions also have an inside-out and outside-in balance:

3. What new language knowledge, skills, and strategies might the student acquire that would improve the situation in the future?
4. What modifications in context might facilitate the student's processing success?

The goal of curriculum-based language assessment and intervention activities is to facilitate the student's use of language and communicative skills and strategies for real purposes, in meaningful, functional contexts, and, as much as possible, to keep the student in the regular curriculum (Nelson, 1994). In planning to meet this goal, the question "What is the regular curriculum?" arises. I broadly define curriculum to include the official course of study for a school system and other less direct and less obvious aspects of school-required study. Six curricular types are summarized in Box 11.3.

Assessing Linguistic and Metalinguistic Knowledge. In the later stages of language acquisition, the importance of assessment questions about knowledge of rule systems for phonology, morphology, syntax, semantics, and pragmatics continues. (The categories of language content, form, and use remain preferred for some purposes, particularly for communicating with teachers and parents who might be overwhelmed by linguistic labels.) Two shifts in emphasis, however, differentiate later-stage language assessment from that of earlier stages. First is a greater emphasis on using linguistic knowledge to process language in multiple modalities (including written as well as oral), and second is a recognition of metalinguistic and other "meta-" abilities as primary targets of assessment.

First, consider the need to look for consistent patterns of competent or incompetent rule use across modalities (Scott & Stokes, 1995). Descriptions of rule-use patterns may help an interdisciplinary team understand how a student's language disorder interacts with other processing deficits. A language specialist might observe that an adolescent with a history of severe oral language delay tends to omit and transpose the same kinds of grammatical function words when reading aloud as when speaking. The team might then notice that the student ignores similar grammatical elements when listening and writing. The identification of consistency in cross-modality patterns is particularly helpful when

Box 11.3 _____

A Summary of Six Curricula Students Must Master
to Succeed in School

Official Curriculum	The outline produced by curriculum committees in many school districts. May or may not have major influence in a particular classroom. To find out, ask the teacher to show you a copy.
Cultural Curriculum	The unspoken expectations for students to know enough about the mainstream culture to use it as background context in understanding various aspects of the official curriculum.
De Facto Curriculum	The use of textbook selections rather than an official outline to determine the curriculum. Classrooms in the same district often vary in the degree to which "teacher manual teaching" occurs.
School Culture Curriculum	The set of spoken and unspoken rules about communication and behavior in classroom interactions. Includes expectations for metapragmatic awareness of rules about such things as when to talk, when not to talk, and how to request a turn.
Hidden Curriculum	The subtle expectations that teachers have for determining who the "good students" are in their classrooms. They vary with the value systems of individual teachers. Even students who are insensitive to the rules of the school culture curriculum usually know where they fall on a classroom continuum of "good" and "problem" students.
Underground Curriculum	The rules for social interaction among peers that determine who will be accepted and who will not. Includes expectations for using the latest slang and pragmatic rules of social interaction discourse as diverse as bragging and peer tutoring.

© 1992 N. W. Nelson. Shared by permission of the author.

attempting to identify basic rule system deficits that should be considered when planning intervention.

In the area of metaprocessing abilities, later-stage language learners meet particular challenges. Four types of deliberate multilevel processing should be considered: metalinguistic, metapragmatic, metatextual, and metacognitive.

Metalinguistic abilities are used to reflect consciously on language, to process it on more than one level at once, and to know the labels of formal education that are used to talk about language. Metalinguistic abilities must be probed through somewhat artificial tasks, because these tasks require language users to reflect on language and not just to use it for communication.

Another approach might be to observe evidence of metalinguistic ability (or the lack thereof) within regular curricular tasks. Opportunities to recognize anomalous language forms arise naturally during participant editing activities. If the student fails to recognize syntactic errors independently, the language specialist might read anomalous sentences aloud to see if the student can then identify and fix difficulties.

Other metalinguistic abilities are probed more readily as responses to texts written by others. Complex and ambiguous sentences, in particular, may arise in curricular texts. For example, after a student reads a sentence such as "The teacher told us to stop talking," a participant observer might probe to determine if the student can identify "Who did the telling?" and "Who was told?" Similarly, following the reading of an ambiguous sentence such as "The fat farmer's wife cooks all day long," the observer might ask, "Who was fat?" and "Could it have been anyone else?"

The ability to paraphrase (and to recognize syntactic synonymy in paraphrases) is a metalinguistic skill that is particularly important in the middle and later school-age years. It permits students to find answers to questions at the ends of chapters when the information in the text is worded differently, and it helps them to take notes without worrying about writing a teacher's words verbatim. Therefore, observers should look especially for opportunities to probe this skill. For example, the observer might ask the student to paraphrase complex sentences such as "His mother was waiting when he arrived." The ability to define words is another example of decontextualized language use that is appropriate for assessing the metalinguistic abilities of later stage students (Nippold, 1995). To conduct this analysis, a variety of formal language subtests and informal tasks might be used. Nippold listed five formal tests that include word definition: Test of Language Development-2: Primary (TOLD-2; Newcomer & Hammill, 1988); Word Test-R: Elementary (Huisingh et al., 1990); Word Test: Adolescent (Zachman, Huisingh, Barrett, Orman, & Blagden 1989); Test of Word Knowledge (TOWK; Wiig & Secord, 1992); and Comprehensive Receptive and Expressive Vocabulary Test (CREVT; Wallace & Hammill, 1994). Nippold also advocated for additional norms for word definition and for informal analysis procedures that look for differences across word categories and possible reasons for students' inaccurate responses.

Metapragmatic abilities may be probed by asking students to describe the rules of communicative interactions. The professional might ask a student how

the rules for entering a conversation politely differ from rules for taking turns in an argument. To probe metapragmatic awareness of the school culture curriculum, students might answer direct questions about classroom routines and rules (Creaghead & Tattershall, 1985; Tattershall, 1987; Wilkinson & Milosky, 1987). A set of questions suggested by Creaghead and Tattershall is reprinted in Box 11.4. These are appropriate to ask either at the middle or later stages of language development. A set of ten unspoken rules for participating in

---

Box 11.4 _____

Questionnaire Regarding Classroom Routine and Rules

1. What does your teacher do or say when he or she is angry with the class?
2. What really makes your teacher mad or angry?
3. What is the most important thing you should always do in class?
4. What is the most important thing you should never do in class?
5. How do you know when it is time to go inside after recess? [This question could be adapted at the secondary level to ask about the school's policy regarding tardiness.]
6. What is the first thing you should do when class begins?
7. What does your teacher do or say before he or she says something really important?
8. What is the last thing you should do before you go home at the end of the day?
9. When is it OK to talk aloud without raising your hand at school?
10. How do you know when your teacher is joking or teasing?
11. What does your teacher do when it is time for a lesson to begin?
12. When is it all right to ask a question in class?

Note: From "Observation and Assessment of Classroom Pragmatic Skills" by N. A. Creaghead and S. A. Tattershall in *Communication Skills and Classroom Success: Assessment and Therapy Methodologies for Language and Learning Disabled Students* (p. 110) edited by C. S. Simon, 1991, Eau Claire, WI: Thinking Publications. Copyright 1991 by Thinking Publications. Reprinted by permission.

TABLE 11.4 Average T-unit length for youngsters in 3rd through 12th grades

| | RESEARCH PROJECT | | | | | | | | | |
GRADE	a* S†	a W	b S	b W	c S	d S	e W	f W	g W	h W
3	7.62	7.60	8.73	7.67					7.45	
4	9.00	8.02				8.52	8.60	5.21		
5	8.82	8.76	8.90	9.34					8.81	10.70
										11.40
6	9.82	9.04			9.03	8.10		7.32	8.53	
7	9.72	8.98	9.80	9.99						
8	10.71	10.37					11.50	10.34	11.68	
9	10.96	10.05								
10	10.68	11.79			10.15			10.46		
11	11.17	10.67								
12	11.70	13.27					14.40	11.45		

*(a) Loban (1976): N = 35 at each grade. Data also available for high and low language ability groups. Ages unavailable. Spoken: adult–child informal interview. Written: school compositions.

(b) O'Donnell and colleagues (1967): N = 30 at each grade. Ages available. Spoken and written: retelling/rewriting of silent fable (narrative).

(c) Klecan-Acker and Hedrick (1985). N = 24 at each grade. Retelling of a favorite film (narrative).

(d) Scott (1984). N = 25 10-year-olds, 29 12-year-olds. Retelling of a favorite book, TV episode, film (narrative).

(e) Hunt (1965). N = 18 at each grade. School compositions.

(f) Hunt (1970). N = 50 at each grade. Sentence combining exercise.

(g) Morris and Crump (1982). N = 18 at each age (9.6, 11.25, 12.54, 14.08 years). Rewriting of silent film (narrative).

(h) Richardson and colleagues (1976). N = 257 11-year-old boys, 264 11-year-old girls, School compositions.

†S = spoken; W = written. The d, f, and g projects reported data for age only. The data were entered in the table using the following formula: Grade = Age—6 Years.

Note: From "Spoken and Written Syntax" by C. M. Scott in *Later Language Development: Ages Nine through Nineteen* (p. 56) edited by M. A. Nippold, 1988, Austin, TX: Pro-Ed. Copyright 1988 by Pro-Ed. Reprinted by permission.

formal classroom discourse (Sturm & Nelson, 1997) appears in Box 12.3.

Metatextual abilities may be probed by asking children to talk about the structure of stories or other discourse forms, such as expository texts. When conducting curriculum-based language assessment using samples of narrative texts, the professional might ask the student to talk about the "plot" of the story; to identify parts of the story such as the main characters, the setting, and the ending; or to tell about what makes a story a story. Asking for overt identification of story features differs from asking an individual to retell a story. When analyzing a student's ability to understand the language of expository text, the examiner might probe for the student's ability to recognize the organizational structure, for example, as involving temporal sequence or hierarchical categorical relationships.

Metacognitive abilities involve self-awareness and executive control of problem-solving strategies. One of the best ways to probe for metacognitive abilities is to ask students to "think aloud" as they attempt particular curricular tasks. Davey (1983) described how adults might model "think-aloud" reading comprehension techniques to make predictions, visualize meanings, develop analogies to things they already know, identify confusing points, and use repair strategies when comprehension fails. Students also may be taught to use "thinking language" during mathematics exercises. Similar metacognitive approaches involve asking students to reflect on reasons for reading certain texts and asking them questions such as "What do you have to do to get a good grade in this course?" (Burke, 1980; Westby, 1991; Wixson, Boskey, Yochum, & Alverman, 1984).

Assessing Language in Multiple Modalities. In the later stages of language development, literacy activities gain increased importance. Language development in the later stages involves all the modalities, listening, speaking, reading, writing, and thinking.

The importance of speech awareness related to phonological processing and word segmentation has been documented for some time as a key to normal acquisition of early reading ability (Blachman, 1994; Ehri, 1975; Holden & MacGinitie, 1972; I. Y. Liberman, Shankweiler, Liberman, Fowler, & Fischer, 1977; Massaro, 1973; Venezky, 1970). Impairment of phonological awareness has also been identified as a primary factor when children have difficulty learning to read (Kamhi & Catts, 1989; Stanovich, 1985). Recent theories, however, have emphasized the construction of meaning for social purposes as the primary link that connects different modalities of communicative processing and thinking (see Personal Reflection 11.10).

Tierney (1990) reviewed four major developments in theories of reading since 1970. First, Tierney noted that, "as part of a cognitive revolution in the 1970s," a constructivist or "schema-theoretic" view of reading comprehension became dominant. This theoretical shift was based on evidence that a reader's background knowledge is a better predictor of recall than factors such as verbal intelligence, word recognition, overall reading ability, and vocabulary knowledge. Second, in the 1980s, a view of "reading as writing" began to emerge. This shift occurred largely as a result of the work of Emig (1971), Flower and Hayes (1980), and Graves (1978, 1983), which led to emphasis on writing as process rather than product. As students began to compose, read, edit, and revise more of their own and each

PERSONAL REFLECTION 11.10 _____

"The days when reading comprehension skill was equated with reading speed or the ability to regurgitate the text have thankfully given way to a broader view of reading. Overly text-based accounts of comprehension have been displaced by multifaceted considerations of the subjectivity of meaning-making, shared understandings held by communities of readers, and reading as the flexible orchestration of problem-solving strategies in conjunction with the thoughtful consideration of ideas. Further, inference and evaluation are regarded as essential to achieving basic understanding as they are to the critical thinking that grows with interpretation and the ability to recount literal detail. In other words, a mechanical view of reading has given way to a view of reading as creative enterprise."

Robert J. Tierney (1990, p. 37), reading theorist at The Ohio State University about "Redefining Reading Comprehension."

other's texts, it became apparent that their attitudes and approaches toward reading and thinking about texts in general changed concurrently. Reading and writing came to be viewed as activities during which students could evaluate issues, explore possibilities, adopt various perspectives, experiment with ideas, and discover new insights. Third is a recognition of "reading as engagement. . . . views of reading that connect readers to their imaginations and that reach beneath the surface to a fuller consideration of the reader's emotional, affective, and visual involvement" (Tierney, 1990, p. 39). Fourth is the recent emphasis on "reading as situation-based," moving away from the view that "comprehension processes are neatly prepackaged to the view that they are ill-structured, complex, and vary from one context to another" (p. 41).

These four views of listening, speaking, reading, writing, and thinking as interactive processes can influence diagnostic teamwork. These views move teams away from territorial beliefs that only certain professionals should assess certain modalities (e.g., speech–language pathologists should assess oral communication only). They also remove the illusion that it is possible to adequately examine different modalities in isolation. In particular, the theoretical perspective that reading is situation based is consistent with the emphasis on context throughout this book. Largely because comprehension processes are constructive and "vary from one context to another" (Tierney, 1990, p. 41), participant observers can modify contexts by what they say and do. Techniques of dynamic assessment permit identification of contextual variables that help individuals with language disorders make sense when listening, talking, reading, writing, and thinking.

Points of divergence between oral and written processing modalities also should be recognized. As Rubin (1987) noted, "Writing and speech are not merely alternative and equivalent ways of encoding language. Oral and written communication differ profoundly in both functional and structural properties" (p. 2). Rubin cited studies of written language acquisition of speakers of Black English Vernacular (BEV), which showed them to include a lower frequency of BEV features in their writing than in their speech, and to produce writing errors that were, for the most part, indistinguishable from those made by standard English (SE) speakers learning to write (see Personal Reflection 11.11).

Pragmatic distinctions also create divergence between oral and written texts. When narrative texts are written rather than spoken, differences occur in the levels of interactions and involvement of communicative partners (J. N. Britton, 1970, 1979; Westby, 1984). Literate text is structured differently from oral text partially because literate language does not involve spatial and temporal commonality, immediate ability to interact, or ability to convey meaning through prosody and gesture. In written texts, nonverbal context, prosody, and gesture are replaced by greater lexicalization of concepts (Emig, 1977) and by punctuation and other writing conventions

that assist readers to parse texts and construct meanings. Intelligible spelling in written communication serves the role of intelligible speech articulation in oral communication. Writers unable to keep literate language distinctions in mind, or lacking the technical skill to execute them, may experience greater difficulty in producing written than oral language narratives.

Moran (1987) found divergence of oral and written language abilities in writing samples produced by three groups of 14- to 16-year-olds with learning disabilities, low achievement, or normal achievement. In particular, the students with learning disabilities produced more and better elaborated structures orally than in written form. Their oral language was also similar to peers with low or normal achievement in terms of syntactic, morphologic, and semantic measures. Their written language samples differed from their low-achieving peers primarily in lower spelling performance, and from samples of normal-achieving peers in lower frequency of optional words, such as adjectives. They also performed significantly lower than normal-achieving students on spelling and punctuation conventions.

Other research suggests that oral language skills of normally achieving and reading disabled children may relate differently to reading comprehension abilities at different age levels. Snyder and Downey (1991) compared word retrieval, phonological awareness, sentence completion, and narrative discourse skills of 93 reading disabled and 93 normally achieving students between the ages of 8 and 14 years. They found that variance in the younger children's reading comprehension scores was best explained by performance on sentence-completion and word-retrieval tasks. Variance in older children's reading comprehension scores was better explained by higher order inferencing skills. These results support the notion that bottom-up processing skills play a more critical role in the earlier stages of learning to read, whereas top-down processing skills play a more critical role in the later stages of written language acquisition.

The techniques for informal assessment of language in varied modalities include a combination of holistic and analytic strategies. This section presents three informal approaches for assessing reading, writing, and thinking: (1) miscue analysis for samples of oral reading, (2) procedures for analyzing written language sam-

PERSONAL REFLECTION 11.11 _____

"No one is a native speaker of writing, not SE speakers and not BEV speakers. All novice writers must learn to switch into the written code, and nonstandard dialect speakers are about as successful (or unsuccessful) as any others."

Donald L. Rubin (1987, p. 3), at The University of Georgia, from an article entitled "Divergence and Convergence Between Oral and Written Communication."

ples, and (3) strategies for observing the ability to think aloud.

Miscue analysis was proposed originally by K. S. Goodman (1973a, 1973b) as a system for analyzing "errors" individuals produce while reading aloud. Goodman proposed that **observed responses,** which differ from **expected responses,** are not accidents or errors. Rather, they represent the outcome of active internal processing strategies based on the "sum total of prior experience and learning" that a reader brings to the reading process (1973a, p. 160).

Miscue analysis is based on a theory of reading that suggests that mature readers use three types of cues to predict textual meaning: semantic, syntactic, and graphophonemic. Because mature readers have considerable knowledge about language, they continually form hypotheses as they read about what they expect texts to say. First, they use **semantic cues** to predict words that fit textual meaning; second, they use **syntactic cues** to predict words that fit syntactic contexts; and third, they use **graphophonemic cues** to check whether the words they have predicted fit visual perceptual information sampled from the print. In this way, they confirm or disconfirm hypotheses about what the print says. If the perceptual evidence does not fit what they have predicted or if in reading on, they find that they have produced a sentence that is syntactically or semantically anomalous, mature readers retrace their steps, sample additional perceptual information, check their multiple cues against their internal knowledge systems, and correct their miscues. Miscues that maintain semantic and syntactic acceptability are usually left alone. A fourth level of cues implied by this model, although not originally discussed by K. S. Goodman (1973a), consists of **discourse-level cues.** Readers must monitor not only whether elements of individual sentences maintain semantic, syntactic, and graphophonemic acceptability but also whether sentences they produce make sense within the context of the whole discourse they have been reading—and within the context of their knowledge of the world.

To conduct miscue analysis, the specialist selects appropriately challenging, unfamiliar, and unpracticed reading material (Y. M. Goodman, Watson, & Burke, 1987). When using miscue analysis in curriculum-based language assessment, material comes from the regular curriculum. The language specialist asks students to read aloud directly from an original source "as if they were reading alone," while following along on a photocopy of the text, marking miscues as indicated in Figure 11.2. Students are also told that they should try to understand what they read because they will be expected to retell it or answer questions about it.

Miscues are then analyzed to determine their acceptability in terms of each of the four cuing systems. Miscues that violate graphophonemic, syntactic, semantic, or textual acceptability suggest that readers have weak rule systems for recognizing cues in one or more of those language areas (corresponding with four of the six knowledge modules in Figure 11.1). Alternatively, readers may have rule-based knowledge but lack proficiency for using it in complex contexts. Self-correction of miscues provides evidence that the reader is actively using at least one cuing system to construct meaning. Some problems involve integration among systems. For example, a miscue that maintains semantic sense but violates syntactic acceptability suggests that a reader is relying on the semantic rule system at the expense of the syntactic one. Other readers may demonstrate contrasting patterns.

By definition, all miscues violate graphophonemic acceptability to some degree because they are speech productions that do not match print. Therefore, analysis procedures address the degree to which a reader's miscues are graphically or phonemically similar to the words in print. When many observed words diverge graphophonemically from expected ones, the reader probably needs help with basic decoding skills. When readers ignore minor graphophonemic miscues that do not violate semantic, syntactic, or textual meaning, they have adopted appropriate strategies to promote efficiency. These are signs of strength.

The process of analyzing miscues may be more or less formal, depending on the time available. Particularly when learning to use the procedure, professionals may wish to use formal analysis procedures and recording forms such as those published by Y. M. Goodman and colleagues (1987). These authors suggest that examiners base their miscue analyses on either word-level or sentence-level units, with relatively more abbreviated or extensive detail. For example, the following set of questions was adapted from those suggested by Y. M.

Omissions   (circled)   He made ⓐ kite...

Substitutions

1. Text item substitutions

   Her
   She didn't want him to be sad.

2. Involving reversals

   said
   "Why?" asked⟍Jane.

3. Involving bound morphemes

   ing
   ...and make kites⊙.
   ^

4. Involving nonwords

   Kansas   /kɔend/   /kakoni/
   A city is a special kind of community.

5. Misarticulations

   $pecific
   He had a specific thing in mind.

6. Intonation shifts

   récord
   He will record her voice.

7. Split syllables

   You should try cut|ting hair.

8. Pauses

   ⸢ 15 sec.
   Cities are/crowded.

Insertions   (indicate with a ∧)

   her
   Jane wanted to help ∧Grandfather.
              ∧

Repetitions and **corrections**

   ‖One day, Grandfather was sad.

Dialect and other language variations

   like ⓓ
   ...just about everybody likes babies.
                               Kansas

Assistance from the examiner

   There are four special things about a⌈city.⌉

FIGURE 11.2   Codes for marking miscues on oral reading transcripts.

Sources: K. S. Goodman, 1973; Y. M. Goodman et al., 1987. © 1992 N. W. Nelson. Shared by permission of the author.

Goodman and colleagues to guide analysis at the sentence level:

1. **Syntactic acceptability.** Does the miscue occur in a syntactically acceptable structure in the reader's dialect? [Answer yes (Y), no (N), or partial (P), depending on the degree of acceptability.]
2. **Semantic acceptability.** Does the miscue occur in a semantically acceptable structure in the reader's dialect? [Answer yes (Y), no (N), or partial (P), depending on the degree of acceptability; cannot be coded higher than syntactic acceptability.]
3. **Meaning change.** Does the miscue change the meaning of the text? [Answer yes (Y), no (N), or partial (P), depending on the degree of acceptability; Question is asked only if the miscues are both syntactically and semantically acceptable.]

4. **Correction.** Is the miscue corrected? [Answer yes (Y), no (N), or partial (P), depending on the degree of acceptability.]
5. **Graphic similarity.** How much does the miscue look like the text? [Answer high (H), some (S), or none (N), depending on the degree of similarity.]
6. **Sound similarity.** How much does the miscue sound like the expected response? [Answer high (H), some (S), or none (N), depending on the degree of similarity.]

Insights about a child's approach to the reading process can also be gleaned from analyzing how each miscue relates to the language that precedes and follows it (Weaver, 1994a). Children whose miscues fit syntactically and semantically with preceding text can be assumed to be using linguistic prediction strategies.

Children who go back to correct miscues that do not fit with text that follows them can be assumed to be using linguistic monitoring strategies.

Language specialists who use miscue analysis should also use evidence from other formal and informal assessment procedures to formulate and test assessment hypotheses. The outcome should be a fairly comprehensive picture of which rule systems are basically weak across modalities, which are relatively more weak in a particular modality, and which are fairly strong when used in highly controlled contexts but tend to be ignored when complex tasks demand integrated processing that draws on multiple cuing systems at one time.

Written language samples may be analyzed using a variety of strategies, including holistic qualitative scoring, analytic scoring, or quantitative scoring of countable indices (C. R. Cooper & Odell, 1977; Moran, 1987; Tindal & Parker, 1991). All three types of techniques have relative advantages and disadvantages.

Isaacson (1985) suggested a set of procedures that mixed all three. Where available, he provided normative guidelines for judging the five components (1) fluency, measured as total number of words written; (2) syntactic maturity, measured as numbers of fragments, simple, compound, and complex sentences, or as average T-unit length; (3) vocabulary, measured by counting unusual or infrequently used words that do not appear on lists of frequently used words, or by computing type-token ratios; (4) content, measured by rating global aspects of text organization, and (5) conventions, measured by counting errors in writing conventions using a checklist.

Writing is similar in many respects to speech production. It is, above all, a form of verbal expression. As noted, however, it also differs from speech in some important ways. An obvious difference is that writers must remember how to spell, which involves a complex set of cognitive linguistic processes (Frith, 1980) as diverse as sounding out words by syllable or recalling words' appearance holistically.

Mature writers also must use pragmatic knowledge about communicating with absent audiences. This involves complex decision making about how much information to encode in the text. Writers can do this well only if they have the world knowledge and metalin-

guistic flexibility to meet their particular purpose, the metapragmatic skills to be aware of that purpose, and the metacognitive strategies to review and revise until the purpose is met. All of this requires abstract, high-level, integrated thinking.

A more informal approach for analyzing written language samples might involve questions and strategies from oral reading miscue analysis. Language specialists might observe both the writing process and products to find evidence of internalized language knowledge, skills, and information processing strategies. To guide the comparisons of observed and expected responses, examiners might use the pinball wizardry model of written and oral language processing illustrated in Figure 11.1.

Language specialists may use adapted forms of miscue analysis to assess written language samples by analyzing written language evidence that the writer is actively using information from all six rule systems shown in Figure 11.1. Sample targets of observation for each of the six knowledge modules might include the following:

1. **Graphophonemic knowledge,** which shows up primarily as spelling accuracy
2. **Semantic knowledge,** which shows up as well-chosen lexical items and appropriate representation of case and event relations, use of semantic cohesion and transition devices, and use of figurative meanings
3. **Syntactic knowledge,** which shows up as syntactic acceptability, appropriate subject–verb agreement, parallel sentence structure, and appropriate use of syntactic cohesion and transition devices
4. **Discourse knowledge,** which shows up as broad text organization, formatting, and cohesion
5. **Pragmatic knowledge,** which shows up as adequate consideration of the audience's informational needs, clear management of topics, and demonstration of the ability to use different writing strategies for different communicative purposes
6. **World and prior knowledge,** which shows up as the provision of accurate and appropriately organized and elaborated information about the world

Professionals also might observe evidence of processing deficits in input–output modalities, such as fine motor coordination deficits that may influence hand-writing legibility, or phonological analysis and synthesis deficits that may influence the ability to spell unfamiliar words. Examiners may select formal assessment tools to check hypotheses about language processing formed during informal assessment. The Boder Test of Reading–Spelling Patterns (Boder & Jarrico, 1982) may be used to determine the language user's ability to use both analytic (sounding out) or eidetic (visual memory) strategies to recall and to spell words. Analytic strategies work well for words spelled phonemically, but eidetic strategies are necessary for reproducing irregularly spelled words.

The written language samples gathered and analyzed will depend on the comprehensive purposes of assessment, with selections representing zones of significance identified in the interview. Samples from the student's classroom portfolios produced as regular assignments may be particularly helpful because they can be compared with those of classmates that were presumably produced under similar conditions. In other cases, the language professional may make special writing assignments to observe the writing process more directly.

Examiners and teachers must be careful when using analytical strategies to evaluate student's written language and to select intervention targets to avoid producing a fragmented picture of the student as a writer and as a communicator. As Moran (1987) commented, "The process of surveying, analyzing, and selecting priorities is abused by limiting objectives to what is readily isolated, measured, and plotted on a profile" (p. 53).

Thinking language analysis is an informal approach for evaluating internal uses of language for thinking. Evidence of the ability to use language for thinking may be gathered simply by asking individuals to report what they are doing or thinking while performing a task. Their ability to do so without modeling may indicate the ease with which they use verbal mediation strategies. If examinees have no idea how to talk themselves through a problem-solving activity, the examiner may model the process during participant observation. It may be a direct target of language intervention (see discussion in Chapter 12).

Some examples of verbal mediation language that might appear when the student is attempting to process elements of the social studies curriculum might include the following:

"First, I have to read the directions. Then I read the first question. [Reads question aloud.] Now I have to find the part of the chapter that talks about this. Here it is. [And so forth.]"

The rationale for assessing thinking language is based on Vygotsky's (1934/1962) views of abbreviated "inner speech." Vygotsky contrasted his own views with those of Piaget that were prevalent at the time. Whereas Piaget (1926) viewed overt self-talk as immature "egocentric speech," which needed to be replaced by social interaction discourse as the child matured, Vygotsky saw self-talk as a way of supporting mature thought, which, as the child matured, merely went underground. Vygotsky made the distinction between Piaget's position and his own explicit in the following comments:

Our experimental results indicate that the function of egocentric speech is similar to that of inner speech: It does not merely accompany a child's activity; it serves mental orientation, conscious understanding; it helps in overcoming difficulties; it is speech for oneself, intimately and usefully connected with the child's thinking. Its fate is very different from that described by Piaget. Egocentric speech develops along a rising, not a declining, curve; it goes through an evolution, not an involution. In the end, it becomes inner speech (Vygotsky, 1934/1962, p. 133).

Assessing Different Sizes of Linguistic Units. Comprehensive language sample analysis involves focus on varied sizes of linguistic units. This does not mean that separate samples are gathered but that different analysis methods are used to focus on varied sizes of units within the same samples, particularly as they are gathered in the process of curriculum-based language assessment. Table 11.3, earlier in the chapter, lists the levels as sounds, syllables, words, simple sentences, complex sentences, and texts. In the later stages of development, analysis should involve looking for evidence that the individual has basic skills for using each of these units in naturalistic communication samples but also that the individual has metalinguistic awareness of them as entities.

Sound-level analysis continues to be important in the later stages of language development. The official curriculum of a school district helps to determine the degree to which language is parsed explicitly into linguistic units as small as sounds, particularly in the early grades. Whole language theorists avoid fragmenting language into individual units during the initial teaching of reading (K. S. Goodman, 1986), but others emphasize the need to segment words into sounds (I. Y. Liberman & Liberman, 1990; Sawyer et al., 1985). By the time children reach the later stages of language development, they should be able to analyze and synthesize complex phonological sequences across modalities. When children exhibit phonological problems involving sequencing, phoneme (or grapheme) omissions, additions, or transpositions in oral or written samples, the examiner should describe these problems across modalities.

Syllable-level analysis involves consideration of students' abilities to use syllable awareness in meeting curricular processing demands. The importance of syllabic complexity in the later grades is illustrated by readability formulas that use syllable counts to assign grade-level designations to written language samples (e.g., Fry, 1968). Some upper grade-level texts also show breakdowns of words into syllables in pronunciation guides. Indeed, when mature readers "sound out" words, they do not do it sound by sound but syllable by syllable. Without syllabication strategies, students with language-learning disabilities are more likely to panic when they see polysyllabic words in print. The analysis procedure for curriculum-based language samples should, therefore, involve identifying whether students can segment long words into syllables and whether they can recognize frequently recurring syllable patterns and the underlying meanings of syllables that encode derivational morphemes such as *pre-, dis-, -tion,* and *-ture.*

Word-level analysis is required in many later grade curricular tasks. Older students must recognize common meanings of words in complex contexts, recall words when they need them, consider alternative meanings of words when appropriate, compare and contrast word meanings, and think of alternative words for the same concept. They also must produce and understand words with abstract and figurative meanings.

Sentence-level analysis in the later stages of language development, as in the earlier stages, must determine whether students have control over a variety of simple sentence patterns, both in expression and comprehension, and with inflectional morphemes within those patterns. Especially critical in the later stages is

the ability to produce and understand a rich variety of complex sentence structures with multiple embeddings and with referential and logical connections across sentence boundaries. To succeed in school, older students must be particularly good at using their sentence level skills to recognize "syntactic synonymy" (van Kleeck, 1984). Many curricular tasks require students to recognize paraphrases of what they have read, to paraphrase material themselves, to infer the relationships between two different sentences with the same or almost the same meaning, to take true–false and multiple-choice tests that require sophisticated sentence analysis strategies, and to find alternative structures for saying the same thing when revising their own written compositions. Later-stage students are also expected to have the metalinguistic skill to reflect on and to formally discuss varied syntactic operations.

During the later-stage development, MLU remains a valid indicator of increasing syntactic ability in both oral and written expressive language samples (Scott & Stokes, 1995). In the later stages, however, the unit for dividing discourse into individual utterances should not be a sentence, because advancing maturity is not always evidenced by longer sentences. Some of the longest sentences by middle-stage language learners may be formed by the relatively immature "run-on" strategy of stringing multiple independent clauses together loosely with multiple *and then* connectors. More mature language learners generally expand utterance length by adding a variety of nonclausal structures, using embedding and phrase elaboration strategies, which allow them to say more in fewer words (Hunt, 1965, 1970, 1977).

Increasing syntactic maturity is best represented by dividing spoken or written discourse into analysis units that leave elaborated structures intact but divide immature add-on formulations into separate units. For this purpose, "communication units" (C-units) were devised by Loban (1963) and "T-units" were used by Hunt (1965, 1977) in their classic studies of language development by school-age children. As discussed in Chapter 9, Loban's (1963, 1976) C-unit strategy was more semantic than syntactic. He defined a C-unit as "a group of words which cannot be further subdivided with the loss of their essential meaning" (1963, p. 6). Loban provided the following example to illustrate how three C-units would be identified within a piece of oral discourse. He marked the end of each C-unit with a slant line (/) and each phonological unit with a pound sign (#):

I'm going to get a boy 'cause he hit me.#/ I'm going to beat him up an' kick him in his nose/ and I'm going to get the girl, too.#/ (p. 7)

Because semantic segmentation strategies are subjective, reliability may not be as easy to achieve with C-units as with Hunt's (1965) more syntactic "minimal terminable units" (T-units). Hunt defined a T-unit as "one main clause plus all the subordinate clauses attached to or embedded within it" (1965, p. 141). Hunt also described T-units are "the shortest grammatically complete sentences that a passage can be cut into without creating fragments" (1977, p. 93). Hunt's research showed T-units to be a better index of syntactic maturity than sentence length, clause length, or subordination indices (see example of T-unit segmentation in Box 9.8 in Chapter 9). Average T-unit lengths for youngsters in third through twelfth grade (as compiled by Scott, 1988c) appear in Table 11.4. Normative data for MLU for C-units and for mazes in language samples for children in the elementary grades (from Loban, 1963) were presented in Tables 9.3 and 9.4. Leadholm and Miller (1992) and Miller and Chapman (1991) are additional sources of normative data for language samples of school-age children.

Scott and Stokes (1995) provided an example of how to divide a written language sample into T-units and perform a clause density analysis. The calculation of clause density involves summing the number of clauses and dividing by the number of T-units. The following T-units are excerpts from the illustration provided by Scott and Stokes (numbers in parentheses are words, clauses):

1 (12,2)	Most people think of deserts as being dry hot areas of wasteland/ [embedded clause with gerund]
2 (4,1)	That is partly true/
3 (12,2)	but there are a lot of other things that happen in deserts [relative clause]
4 (10,1)	there are many life forms such as plants and animals
14 (8,1)	There are many food chains in the desert/
15 (26,3)	For example, the fly gets eaten by the frog, who gets eaten by the weasel,

who gets eaten by a big lizard—and on and on/
[relative clauses]

16 (15,2)	The top members of the food chains are the scavengers, who feed on dead animals/ [relative clause]
17 (9,1)	There is not always abundant rainfall in the desert/
18 (9,2)	but when it does rain, it rains very heavily/ [left-branching subordinate clause] (p. 317)

For the total sample, the computation was 46/27, yielding a clause density index of 1.70.

Both Hunt (1965) and Loban (1963) recommended separate analysis of linguistic nonfluencies that intrude in the language formulations of even mature speakers and writers. Loban (1963) called linguistic nonfluencies "mazes" and described the category as including initial revisions, conjunctions, pause fillers (*um, ah, er, OK*), and part-word or whole-word repetitions not intended for emphasis. Hunt (1965) called the same kinds of behavior *garbles*. Transcribers should maintain linguistic nonfluencies in transcripts of oral or written samples because they provide evidence of internalized processing conflicts. Words in mazes or garbles, however, should not be counted when computing syntactic complexity, because they would inflate the quantitative measurements.

Box 11.5 provides a sample of discourse from a normally developing 16-year-old tenth-grader reported by Squire (1964) from his study of adolescents' responses while reading short stories. The sample primarily illustrates the marking of T-units and linguistic nonfluencies and the ability of later-stage language users to talk about abstract concepts, draw inferences beyond what is stated explicitly in text, and focus consciously on how language is used to convey ideas. The number of mazes in this sample of discourse produced by a normal language user is also remarkable but not unusual. Loban (1963) found that during the first four years of schooling, individuals who were rated as skillful with language did reduce both their incidence of mazes and number of words per maze, but that the average number of words in mazes increased in a group of lower skilled but normally developing subjects. Similarly, Sturm (1990) found that

TABLE 11.5   Variations among discourse types

CONVERSATION	NARRATIVE	EXPOSITORY
Social	Story grammars	Description
Partners take equal turns	Setting	Definition
Negotiate topics as they go	Episode structure	Division and classification
Structured with rules for:	Problem or conflict	Comparison
Initiation	Goal and intention	
Topic introduction	Plan	Illustration
Maintaining topics	Action and event	Analogy
Contingent queries	Ending	Example
Clarification requests	Other structural elements	
Contingent statements	Foreshadowing	Sequence
Changing topics	Flashback	Process
Presupposition (adapting to	Repetition	Cause and effect
listeners' knowledge)	"Once upon a time"	Temporal order
Termination		
	Qualities	Argument and persuasion
Instructional	Have plots made up of:	Deductive reasoning
Partners unequal	Goals	Inductive reasoning
(teachers dominate)	Actions	Persuasion
Teachers control behavior and talk	Affective states	
Functions include:	Theme	Functional
Attract or show attention	Point	Introduction
Control amount of speech	Point of view	Transition
Check understanding		Conclusion
Summarize	Types	
Define	Fairy tale	
Edit or acknowledge but modify	Short story	
Correct	Mystery	
Specify topics	Western	
Predictable structure	Science fiction	
Initiate	Biography, diary, journal	
Respond	Drama, light or serious	
Evaluate	Parable	
Students take few and short turns	Fable	

Sources: Calfee & Curley, 1984; Cazden, 1988; Fitzgerald, 1989; Slater & Graves, 1989. *Note:* From "Performance is the prize: Language competence and performance among AAC users" by N. W. Nelson in *Augmentative and Alternative Communication* (p. 15), *8*, 3–18. Copyright 1992 by ISAAC. Reprinted by permission.

fifth graders produced significantly more mazes in formal classroom discourse than first graders and that increases were observed in the discourse both of students and teachers as grade increased. The incidence of mazes was the only discourse variable on which the teachers and students did not differ significantly from each other.

Discourse-level analysis in the later stages involves looking at students' abilities to use knowledge of a variety of kinds of discourse structures (conversational, narrative, and expository) and pragmatic rules to produce and understand complex texts in multiple modalities. Because this is such an important part of informal

Box 11.5 _____

Sample of Oral Discourse Produced by a 16-Year-Old Normally Developing Tenth-Grade Girl Who Was Describing Her Response to Reading *Reverdy* by Jessamyn West (Reported by Squire, 1964, p. 61; parentheses around mazes, including unfilled pauses (..), and slashes (/) dividing T-units have been added)

S: I don't like her mother.

Q: Why?

S: I don't like her one bit./ I think (her mother is an..jealous ah..) Reverdy's mother is jealous of her because (..perhaps she's..) her beauty is (..) so great and everything/ Maybe her mother didn't have boys over at her house or something/ but (ah..to me it just seems like her mother..) it said here that she didn't hate her actually/ but I think it was just plain old fashioned jealousy/ and I feel sorry for the girl for that and her mother thinking she's boy crazy/ and..I can kinda see how she'd feel about it when she was perfectly innocent and really wasn't because I have a girl friend myself that was just about in the same predicament/ (And ah..) I found out here that it was a little sister talking instead of a brother [laugh].

_____

assessment in the later stages of language development, it is discussed in greater detail in the following section.

Assessing Discourse Events. Discourse-level language processing abilities are critical determinants of school success (e.g., Roth & Spekman, 1989; Scott, 1989; Westby, 1989), but they are assessed minimally by formal language testing devices. Therefore, designing informal assessment tasks to analyze students' communication capabilities within a variety of discourse events is particularly important. The text used in discourse events may be categorized as one of three broad types: **conversational, narrative,** and **expository.** Some of the characteristics and examples of each are summarized in Table 11.5.

A major advance in language processing by older children and adolescents is their ability to manage larger units of discourse, enabling them to process both oral and written texts as coherent linguistic units (Hillocks, 1986; Pitcher & Prelinger, 1963; Scinto, 1986; Scott, 1988a, 1988c; Westby, 1982, 1984). Scinto (1986) defined text as a "functional unit of complex meaning, an extended predication that involves elaboration of ensembles of sentences by a process of composition and concatenation" (p. 108). Coherence is the distinguishing feature of organized texts. It involves three aspects: (1) **microstructures** are semantic representations of propositions, sentences, and sequences of sentences; (2) **macrostructures** are global textual structures; and (3) **coherence** results from the application of strategies for relating microstructures and macrostructures (T. Van Dijk & Kintsch, 1978). To produce written or oral extended texts, the individual must generate goal-directed intention to communicate meaning, organize meaning into appropriate information units, and integrate units into a coherent linear surface form. This discussion of connected discourse is organized under the three macrostructure headings **conversational, narrative,** and **expository.**

Conversational discourse is the primary context in which young children learn language, starting when they are infants engaging in protoconversations with caregivers. Because conversations are shared with partners who can help bear the communicative load, they are usually the earliest form of discourse in which children experience communicative success. In the later stages of language development, conversations continue to play an important role, but they become more demanding.

In schools, the underground curriculum involves learning to participate in social conversation with peers, and less frequently, with teachers. Social conversations tend to follow the usual conversational discourse rules, summarized in Table 11.5, involving balanced turn taking and negotiation of topics by the participants. Somewhat different conversational rules operate in the formal atmosphere of academic discussions (Sturm & Nelson, 1997; see Box 12.3) and some business transactions.

Classroom conversations, in particular, with their topics and turn allocations controlled tightly by teachers, have been the object of considerable research, The well-known initiate–respond–evaluate (IRE) pattern (Mehan, 1979) has been described as "the most common pattern of classroom discourse at all grade levels" (Cazden, 1988, p. 29). The teacher takes a fairly long conversational turn to initiate a topic (I), often in the form of a question, the student takes a much shorter turn to respond (R), and the teacher follows with an evaluation (E).

The rules for this stylized form of academic conversation differ from those of more natural social conversations in three primary ways: (1) the high frequency of test-like questions (to which the teacher already knows the answers), rather than sincere questions; (2) the lack of balance in talking time by the communicative partners; and (3) the direct evaluation of what one partner says by the other, establishing a clear imbalance of power. Some business conversations between employees and employers and between service persons and customers also are influenced by a power differential. As older students with language disorders make the transition to adulthood, it is important to sample their abilities to communicate appropriately in a variety of contexts that show their sensitivity to these concerns and to sophisticated applications of the other rules of conversational interaction rules (e.g., turn taking, interrupting, topic shading, and making polite exits from conversations). They also need to manage variations on these rules depending on the discourse's context (e.g., making a new friend, flirting, disagreeing with a teacher, apologizing to an employer).

Narrative discourse also occurs frequently in the oral and written language interactions of classrooms and some social settings. As noted in Chapter 10, most children know quite a bit about narrative discourse before they enter school (e.g., Applebee, 1978; McGee & Richgels, 1990; Strickland & Taylor, 1989). In oral production, narrative and conversational forms share some of the same functions (e.g., relating personal experiences, retelling sequences of events, allowing participation by conversational partners in the recall and organizational processes). Narratives also differ from conversational forms in their expanded units of discourse, styles of introductory and closing statements,

and inclusion of sequenced events leading to a conclusion (Roth & Spekman, 1986; Westby, 1984, 1985/1991).

Definitions and concepts of story grammar and narrative structure vary, but when mature language users tell what makes a story a story, certain elements—settings, beginnings, attempts, and outcomes—are always included. Other elements, such as complex reactions and endings, are reported less often (Fitzgerald, 1989). Cultural differences in story structure have also been found. Different strategies for opening and closing stories have been found among individuals of African American, Chinese American, Euro-American, and Hispanic American descent (Heath, 1982, 1983, 1986; McClure, Mason, & Williams, 1983; Westby, 1994). Japanese folktales tend not to have goal-oriented main characters such as those appearing in Western stories (Matsuyama, 1983). When the story grammar standards associated with Anglo-Saxon culture are used to evaluate the discourse of children whose familial history is filled with influences from other native cultures (whether or not English is the first language of these children), teachers and speech–language pathologists run the risk of misidentifying multigenerational cultural differences as problems (Westby, 1991).

Most information about the normal development of narratives comes from research on the oral production of stories (Applebee, 1978; Botvin & Sutton-Smith, 1977; Peterson & McCabe, 1983; Roth & Spekman, 1986). In studying the developmental progressions of oral narratives, Applebee (1978) and Botvin and Sutton-Smith (1977) proposed separate, but similar, schemes for rating narrative maturity. The criteria for making judgments of narrative maturity that appeared in Figure 9.5 are based primarily on Applebee's (1978) research. Scoring criteria for analyzing narratives based on their inclusion of story grammar structural properties appeared in Figure 9.6 (Hedberg & Westby, 1993; Stein & Glenn, 1979). This is the narrative scoring approach that we have used in our research on computer software feature effects on written story development by children of middle-school age (Bahr, Nelson, & Van Meter, 1996; Bahr, Nelson, Van Meter, & Yanna, 1996).

Lahey (1988) proposed a similar developmental sequence for rating children's narratives on four levels: additive chains, temporal chains, causal chains, and multiple causal chains. Lahey suggested that this rating system could be used to analyze content-form interactions in self-generated narratives and to establish goals for language intervention. She emphasized that in normal development, children are concerned with more than just making sense when they tell stories, quoting Kernan (1977) (see Personal Reflection 11.12). In addition to looking for evidence of logical–temporal structures in narratives, Lahey recommended that examiners should seek evidence that narrators can entertain, adapt to listeners' needs, and express their feelings about events they are narrating.

As discussed previously, specialists should seek evidence of cross-modality influences when conducting informal analyses of children's discourse capabilities. Research on normal development demonstrated that patterns of acquisition for oral production of narrative structures for young children are analogous to text structures in material read to them (Applebee, 1978; Botvin & Sutton-Smith, 1977). By age 5 or 6 years, children can begin to produce structurally complete fantasy narratives in oral storytelling, but they reach a peak in the ability to tell narratives that use episode structures embedded within stories by 11 to 12 years of age (Botvin & Sutton-Smith, 1977).

In our research on normal development of story writing (N. W. Nelson, 1988c; N. W. Nelson & Friedman, 1988), we rated written personal narratives produced by fourth-, seventh-, tenth-graders, and college freshmen, with a scoring system from 1 to 6, using categories based on Applebee's (1978) stages with criteria shown in Figure 9.5. We found that writers in regular classes still produced personal narratives with average story scores of 3.77 and 3.74 in fourth and seventh grade, respectively (63% of the seventh graders still produced primitive narratives that scored 3); the mean story score (5.11) for the tenth graders was significantly higher (46% of the tenth graders produced focused chains, and 39% produced *true narratives*; by the time they were college freshmen, the majority of the writers spontaneously produced true narrative texts (25% focused chains and 75% true narratives).

Although it would be desirable to have better normative data for narrative development in the later stages, the issue is problematic. C. J. Johnson (1995) noted, in particular, problems with the substantial range in storytelling ability associated with particular ages, situational differences, and narrative genres. McFadden and Gillam (1996) described holistic scoring as one method for establishing local norms and evaluating sets of narratives. Holistic scoring "takes into consideration the sum of quantifiable elements such as grammar, vocabulary, and episodic organization, as well as less quantifiable elements like charm, interest, and clarity" (p. 48). A group of raters demonstrates reliability for using a particular set of "rubrics" by practicing on an example set of "anchor stories." McFadden and Gillam recommended this approach as one that might be used by a group of speech–language pathologists and educators who could collaborate to develop the system and rate a group of stories for a single school or district.

Expository discourse competence is critical to success in school because expository text structure is used in most content textbooks and teacher lectures to give directions or to present information about theories, predictions, persons, facts, dates, specifications, generalizations, limitations, and conclusions. "Expository text assumes an increasingly greater amount of background knowledge with each grade level" (Norris, 1995, p. 347). Students who cannot understand the complex language of expository discourse are at great risk for school failure.

During a comprehensive curriculum-based language assessment, students may read a selection aloud, sound out complex words syllable by syllable, summarize the text, paraphrase selected passages, answer factual and inferential questions about it, and formulate questions that could be asked about the discourse on a test. The examiner's level of focus may shift fluidly from sound, to word, to sentence, to passage, to discourse level, and back again. Examiners might ask some students specific questions designed to elicit evidence about processing ability on one or more levels, or examiners might draw inferences about unit processing from holistic behavior.

Examiners also might observe multiple contexts. Students might be observed as they listen to lectures and take notes in class or as they listen to a tape-recorded lecture that simulates the classroom experience. Some

---

PERSONAL REFLECTION 11.12 _____

"Narratives, however, are concerned with more than making sense. They are also concerned with being appreciated, being amusing, being considered well done, and so on."

Keith T. Kernan (1977, p. 100), writing about "Semantic and Expressive Elaboration in Children's Narratives."

examples of expository contexts and discourse events to be used for varied purposes (depending on the student's own zones of significance) include the following:

1. Oral classroom discourse related to procedure and material presented in lectures (e.g., following directions, taking notes, making transitions between activities)
2. Expository discourse from textbooks, worksheets, and handouts (e.g., science textbook, social studies textbook, written homework assignments)
3. Mathematics discourse activities (e.g., self-talk while solving computational problems, sketching referents while solving story problems)

To probe for internalized models of text organizational structure and for comprehension of the complex semantic and syntactic relationships represented in expository text, the examiner might ask students to use visual–spatial strategies to outline or sketch organizational relationships they detect in examples of expository text. Most students are unlikely to be able to do this unless the process is modeled for them first (dynamic assessment). The examiner might select text excerpts from the student's curriculum that provide clear examples of two or three different organizational structures of expository text. A variety of expository text structures are diagrammed in Figure 11.3 (Calfee & Chambliss, 1988; Meyer, 1975; Pehrsson & Denner, 1988; Richgels, McGee, Lomax, & Sheard, 1987; Westby, 1991). Elements of hierarchical structure (with each organizational scheme having at least two or three levels) and sequencing may become evident to

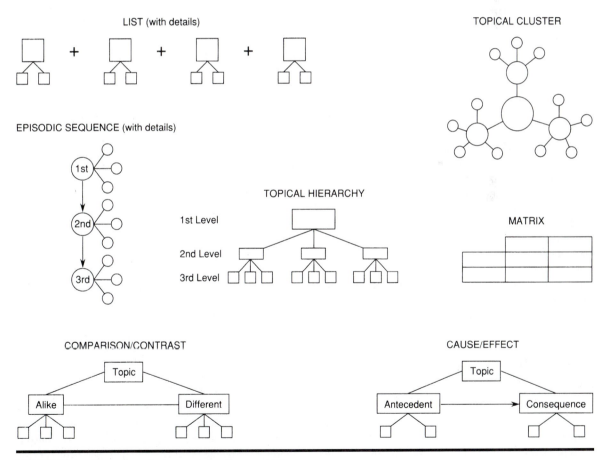

FIGURE 11.3   Expository text macrostructures used.

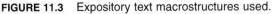

Sources: Calfee & Chambliss, 1988; Meyer, 1975; Pehrsson & Denner, 1988; Richgels et al., 1987; Westby, 1991.

students only when these elements are diagrammed spatially. "The reader who is able to uncover the author's top-level structure can organize ideas in ways that more or less match the pattern used by the author" (Pehrsson & Denner, 1988, p. 27).

The primary objective when assessing knowledge of expository text structure is to observe whether the student can grasp the concept of mapping elements of factual information from texts into spatial organizations. For example, it the examiner sets up the structure, can the student fit additional pieces of text information into the arrangement? If so, the examiner may infer that the student has some internalized recognition of common text organizational strategies and needs only to acquire more metatextual ability to use those strategies consciously for comprehending, studying, and remembering text-based information. If not, the student may need some basic instruction about how language is organized in different texts, using examples from the student's own curriculum.

The language of mathematics represents a special case of expository discourse. Across grade levels, some of the language in mathematics textbooks and much of the language in oral explanations by teachers is organized as direction-giving language. These directions sometimes are given primarily in words but often also include mathematical symbols that students have to learn to "read." The ability to use their short-term memory span and reauditorization of the teacher's directions (facilitated by visual memory) to maintain instructional steps in proper sequence is particularly critical when attempting to understand directional expository discourse. The ability to use verbal mediation strategies to "read" mathematical symbols to oneself may also be an important key to performing steps in the correct sequence when attempting to solve similar problems later without assistance. Verbal mediation comes into play particularly when a set of problems does not require application of the same operation but requires varied operations (e.g., multiplication, subtraction, division). In these cases, the student cannot work on "automatic pilot," without thinking about what a particular problem demands. Requesting the student to use thinking language may help the examiner observe whether the student misreads symbols (either linguistic or mathematical) or fails to use verbal mediation strategies in problem solving.

When Crouse (1996; Crouse & Nelson, 1996) studied the self-talk of fifth grade students with specific language impairments she found differences from same-grade peers for both math computation and story problem processes. The areas of difference suggest quantitative and qualitative variables that might be documented when conducting baseline measurements and measuring progress for language intervention involving math. Students with language impairments used fewer total words, fewer different words, and fewer personal pronouns. They also completed fewer problems per minute even though they talked less. When making choices about problem-solving approaches, the self-talk of students with language impairments was more often off-track and less often on-track. When students with normal language were off track, it was often linked to making a computation error or failing to complete a problem although a correct approach was selected. Students with language impairments made evaluative and confirming comments less often than their peers, suggesting they may need practice to reflect on their work. They also more frequently produced words while reading and talking that did not match the referents in the problems.

Other investigational strategies may be appropriate for assessing the ability to solve story problems. Asking the student to sketch the elements of the problem may allow the examiner to see whether the student comprehends the language of the problem sufficiently to picture its referents. Accurate understanding of the elements of story problems and their relationships is a key to setting up strategies to solve the problems. During this part of curriculum-based language assessment, the examiner asks the student to read the problem aloud (and observes for reading miscues and self-correction strategies) and then asks the student to show what he or she thinks the problem means by drawing a very rough sketch of the important pieces in it (the examiner may need to model this for the student to demonstrate that the quality of the drawings is not important). Often, story problems require the student to represent referents in two stages: first, before the mathematical operation is applied, and again afterward, to show how the situation has changed. If the student either misreads or misrepresents the meaning of language of the problem, the examiner should probe further whether the student did not understand the meaning of individual words (e.g., *each, neither, most*) or whether the student misunderstood the relationship represented by the word combination. See Box 11.6 for example.

Box 11.6 _____

Curriculum-Based Language Assessment for a Fifth-Grade Girl Having Difficulty Understanding the Language of Math Story Problems

She read aloud the language of the problem without error:

"There are seven bike racks. If each bike rack has eight bikes, how many bikes in all?"

She thought briefly, then said, "eight."

When asked to sketch the problem, she first drew representations of the seven bike racks correctly:

─── ── ── ── ── ── ──

But then, she drew only one cross mark (representing one bike) on each of the racks:

| │ │ │ │ │ │

How might language processing difficulty have interfered with her understanding of what the language of the problem meant? How could dynamic assessment be used to probe her understanding further?

_____

Language specialists who conduct curriculum-based language assessment should remember that their role is not to assess the child's understanding of mathematical principles and operations (that role belongs to the academic diagnostician) but to assess whether the student has the language capabilities and strategies to understand the language of the text and to direct his or her own thinking. It will be easier to design relevant intervention plans if the dimensions of the problem are better understood.

SUMMARY _____

This chapter presented the measurement of later-stage needs and abilities and covered a wide range of topics. To focus on later-stage needs, the discussion addressed various contexts for later-stage assessment and intervention. Family and cultural concerns are still important in the later stages, but interactions with peers are increasingly important as well, as is increased participation outside school and home. The culmination of the later stages of child development are marked by transi-

tion to higher education, employment, and other post-school activities.

A wide variety of tools and strategies particularly suited to later-stage assessment were discussed. Most initial diagnostic evaluations and 3-year comprehensive reevaluations involve a combination of formal and informal assessment procedures. If the assessment process is to be relevant to individualized needs, the first step must be to gather contextually based background information. This procedure leads to the selection of appropriate formal assessment devices and to the design of informal assessment activities tailored to the individual's needs.

Informal assessment in the later stages is based on the philosophy of dynamic assessment, which suggests that abilities are not found in static, identifiable quantities that can be labeled and numbered but are fluid, variable, interactive, and contextually sensitive. Abilities may be facilitated (scaffolded) to reach higher levels by certain contextual conditions but may be impeded by others. A major goal of the dynamic assessment process is to identify the conditions that result in these varied outcomes. The goals and activities of assessment and intervention are at times indistinguishable.

Because informal assessment of later-stage language developments can become quite complex, I suggested several organizational strategies. Examiners need to keep in mind at least three factors: (1) their plan to set up and administer participant assessment tasks, (2) a complex model of oral and written language processing that allows examiners to infer intactness and operation of internalized language processing abilities by guiding observations of external evidence, and (3) a system for organizing observations so that examiners can cover all of the bases without spending forever gathering evidence piece by piece.

Suggested procedures of contextually based language assessment included asking multifaceted questions about contextual demands and examinees' current functioning in those contexts and about the potential for modifying language learning contexts and individuals' basic abilities and strategies through intervention. Ethnographic interviewing, artifact analysis, and onlooker and participant observation techniques may be used to gather data. These data include information about linguistic and metalinguistic processing; the use of language in multiple modalities (through miscue analysis, written language sample analysis, and thinking language analysis); the ability to process different sizes of linguistic units (sounds, syllables, words, sentences, and texts); and specialized processing strategies for differing discourse types (conversational, narrative, and expository).

REVIEW TOPICS

- General developmental expectations for early, middle, and later adolescence.
- Screening and referral procedures for grades three through high school, in school and nonschool contexts (e.g., psychiatric hospital, juvenile detention center)
- Changing contexts: families, culture, peer groups, transitions to work and post-secondary education.
- Interview strategies; formal assessment; informal assessment (identification of zones of significance); the pinball wizardry model (six knowledge systems; peripheral input–output processes; central information processes; metacognitive reasons and control; the centrality of meaning construction); four questions of curriculum-based language assessment; artifact analysis; onlooker observation techniques; participant observation techniques; analysis of metalinguistic, metapragmatic, metatextual, and metacognitive abilities; miscue analysis of oral reading samples; analysis strategies for written language samples; analysis of thinking language using think-aloud protocols while performing academic tasks; assessing knowledge of different sizes of linguistic units (sounds, syllables, words, sentences, complex sentences, discourse); assessing varied discourse genres (conversational, narrative, expository)

REVIEW QUESTIONS

1. What stage of adolescence is most associated with distancing oneself from parental rules and values?
2. Explain why difference theories of language diversity replaced deficit theories.
3. Outline a procedure for curriculum-based language assessment, starting with interview techniques and the four questions you would use to guide the process. Which two questions have more of an inside-out focus? Which two have more of an outside-in focus?

Which two are more oriented toward assessment? Which two are more oriented toward intervention?
4. What are the cuing systems a mature reader brings to the reading processes? How can miscue analysis shed light on how a student's language disorder influences the reading process?
5. What are some of the strategies you could use for analyzing a written language sample at the sound, syllable, word, sentence, and discourse level?
6. Describe at least two approaches for analyzing narrative maturity.
7. Describe and sketch a variety of expository text structures (e.g., list with details, episodic sequence with details, topical hierarchy, topical cluster, matrix, comparison/contrast, cause/effect).

ACTIVITIES FOR EXTENDED THINKING

1. Interview a later-stage student about his or her primary concerns. Are concerns centered in academic or social domains? What is hardest and easiest about school and social relationships? If the student could change just one thing, what would it be? Practice using questions that ask for the student's priorities and labels; then follow up with requests for anecdotes about recent illustrations.

2. Gather and analyze a set of oral and written language samples using curriculum-based language assessment techniques: read-aloud samples of narrative and expository discourse from textbooks (marked for miscues and followed by comprehension questions), an oral conversation with a peer, an oral story retelling, and a written language sample. Summarize your findings using the pinball wizardry model to organize the description of the student's strengths and needs.

CHAPTER APPENDIX A
ANNOTATED BIBLIOGRAPHY OF LATER-STAGE ASSESSMENT TOOLS

Note: Sources include Deal & Rodriguez (1987), McCauley & Swisher (1984), and Plante & Vance (1994).

Adapted Sequenced Inventory of Communication Development for Adolescents and Adults with Severe Handicaps (A-SICD). McClennen, S. E. (1989).

Seattle: University of Washington Press. Retains theoretical basis for SICD-R but uses tasks, materials, and interactions appropriate for adolescents and adults, including those with severe hearing loss, legal blindness, epilepsy, spastic-quadriplegia, and nonambulation.

Adolescent Language Screening Test (ALST). Morgan, D. L. & Guilford, A. M. (1984). Austin, TX: Pro-Ed. Requires less than 15 minutes to screen speech and language for 11- to 17-year-old students. Includes seven subtests: pragmatics, receptive vocabulary, concepts, expressive vocabulary, sentence formulation, morphology, and phonology.

Assessing Asian Language Performance: Guidelines for Evaluating Limited-English-Proficient Students (2nd ed.). Cheng, L.-R. L. (1991). Oceanside, CA: Academic Communication Associates. Provides information about nonbiased assessment, cultural values, and communicative behaviors for individuals who are Vietnamese, Korean, Chinese, Japanese, Filipino, and members of other Asian populations.

Boder Test of Reading–Spelling Patterns. Boder, E. & Jarrico, S. (1982). San Antonio, TX: Psychological Corporation. This criterion-reference test uses word reading and spelling tasks to identify students in elementary and secondary grades as having one of four types of reading disability: nonspecific, dysphonetic, eidetic, and mixed dysphonetic-eidetic.

Classroom Communication Screening Procedure for Early Adolescents (CCSPEA) (rev. ed.). Simon, C. S. (1987). Tempe, AZ: Communi-Cog. Designed for screening large groups of upper elementary students before their entering junior high school. It is recommended for students who score below the 40th percentile on standardized reading assessments and other students whose underachievement might stem from oral language deficits. Assesses abilities to scan an assignment for answers, follow oral and multipart written directions, use metalinguistic and metacognitive skills, and match vocabulary items with definitions/synonyms.

Clinical Evaluation of Language Fundamentals—3rd ed. (CELF-3). Semel, E., Wiig, E., & Secord, W. (1997). San Antonio, TX: Psychological Corporation. Standardized for children ages 6 through 21 years. [Described in Chapter 9 Appendix A] (A screening test is available.)

Conner's Teacher Rating Scales (CTRS) and *Conner's Parent Rating Scales (CPRS).* Conners, C. K. (1989). Austin, TX: Pro-Ed. These scales provide both short and long versions to help identify hyperactive children. They can be used with children ages 3 to 17.

Detroit Tests of Learning Aptitude—3 (DTLA-3). Hammill, D. D. (1991). Austin, TX: Pro-Ed. Designed for 6- through 17-year-olds. Includes eleven subtests: word opposites, sentence imitation, design sequences, word sequences, story construction, design reproduction, object sequences, symbolic relations, picture fragments, story sequences, and reversed letters. Yields nine composite scores of specific abilities in linguistic, cognitive, attention, and motor domains.

Evaluating Communicative Competence: A Functional Pragmatic Procedure (rev. ed.). Simon, C. S. (1986). Tempe, AZ: Communi-Cog. Uses 21 informal evaluation tasks to assess the skills of 9- to 17-year-olds as communicators. Includes tasks to measure language processing, metalinguistic skills, and functional uses of language for varied communicative purposes. A videotape is also available.

Expressive One Word Picture Vocabulary Test: Upper Extension (EOWPVT-UE). Gardner, M. & Brownell, R. (1983). Austin, TX: Pro-Ed. Assesses expressive vocabulary in children ages 12 to 15 years. (Can be administered with ROWPVT-UE.)

Fullerton Language Tests for Adolescents (2nd ed.) (FLTA). Thorum, A. R. (1986). Austin, TX: Pro-Ed. Measures receptive and expressive language skills. Identifies students who are language impaired and diagnoses strengths and weaknesses.

Goldman-Fristoe-Woodcock Auditory Skills Test Battery (GFW-Battery). Goldman R., Fristoe, M., & Woodcock, C. W. (1976). Circle Pines, MN: AGS. For persons 3 years to adult, this is a battery of four 15-minute tests: auditory selective attention, diagnostic auditory discrimination, auditory memory, and sound–symbol associations. It yields age-based standard scores, percentile ranks, stanines, and age equivalents.

Goldman-Fristoe-Woodcock Test of Auditory Discrimination (GFW). Goldman, R., Fristoe, M., & Woodcock, C. W. (1970). Circle Pines, MN: AGS. To be used with persons 3 years old and up, this is a test of closed-set word identification in quiet and in noise. It yields standard scores and percentile ranks.

Gray Oral Reading Tests—Diagnostic (GORT-D). Bryant, B. R., & Wiederholt, J. L. (1991). Austin, TX: Pro-Ed. This test is designed for children in kindergarten through grade 6 who have trouble reading print. The first subtest requires the student to orally read passages and respond to comprehension questions. If the student performs poorly on this subtest, the remaining subtests are administered: decoding (consonant/cluster recognition, phonogram recognition, blending); word identification (word recognition and vocabulary); word attack, morphemic analysis; contextual analysis; and word ordering. Scores are reported as grade equivalents, standard scores (*M* = 100; *SD* = 15), and percentiles.

Gray Oral Reading Tests (3rd ed.) (GORT-3). Wiederholt, J. L. & Bryant, B. R. (1989). Austin, TX: Pro-Ed. This revisions yields a passage score and standard scores and percentile rankings for oral reading comprehension for students' ages 7:0 through 18:11. The manual provides a system for performing a miscue analysis. Analysis provides information in the following four areas: meaning similarity, function similarity, graphic/phonemic similarity, and self-correction.

Let's Talk Inventory for Adolescents (LTI-A). Bray, C. M. & Wiig, E. H. (1982). San Antonio, TX: Psychological Corporation. Helps identify inadequate or delayed social-verbal communication skills among 9-year-olds to young adults. Probes ability to formulate speech acts appropriate for pictured situational contexts for the functions: ritualizing, informing, controlling, feeling. Pictures represent interaction both with adolescent peers and with an authority figure. Means and standard deviations are reported for 2-year intervals.

Lindamood Auditory Conceptualization Test (LAC). Lindamood, C. & Lindamood, P. (1971). Austin, TX: Pro-Ed. Criterion-referenced test for ages preschool to adult. Measures auditory discrimination and perception of number and order of speech sounds in sequences. Takes 10 minutes. Spanish cue sheets are available.

Matrix Analogies Test—Short Form and *Expanded Form.* Naglieri, J. A. (1985). San Antonio, TX: Psychological Corporation. This test can be used with students ages 5 through 17 years. It uses a task in which a missing element must be selected from six options to fit into an analogical matrix. Yields percentile ranks, stanines, and age equivalents by half-year intervals.

Oral and Written Language Scales (OWLS): Listening Comprehension Scale (LCS); Oral Expression Scale (OES). Written Expression Scale Carrow-Woolfolk, E. (1996). For ages 3 to 21. Provides standard scores, percentile ranks, and age equivalents.

Picture Story Language Test (PSLT). Myklebust, H. R. (1965). San Antonio, TX: Psychological Corporation. Used with children ages 7 to 17, this test is used for differential diagnosis of learning disabilities, mental retardation, emotional disturbance, reading disability, and dyslexia. Individuals are asked to write the best story possible about a picture. Five scores are obtained: total words, total sentences, words per sentence, syntax, abstract-concrete meaning.

Prueba de Lectura & Lenguaje Escrito (PLLE). Hammill, D. D., Larsen, S. C., Wiederholt, J. L., & Fountain-Chambers, J. (1982). Austin, TX: Pro-Ed. This is a standardized battery of reading and writing in Spanish for children in grades 3 through 10. Its six subtests measure reading vocabulary, paragraph reading, thematic maturity, writing vocabulary, writing style, and spelling.

Pupil Rating Scale—Revised. Myklebust, H. R. (1981). San Antonio, TX: Psychological Corporation. Can be used to screen for learning disabilities with students ages 5 to 14. Teachers complete the scales, using a 5-point scale, in 5 to 10 minutes in five areas: auditory comprehension and memory, spoken language, orientation, motor coordination, and personal-social behavior.

Raven Progressive Matrices. Raven, J. C. (1986). San Antonio, TX: Psychological Corporation. Designed for age range 8 to 65 years. Assesses mental ability by requiring the examinee to solve problems in abstract figures and designs that assess nonverbal analogical reasoning ability. Percentiles are available for British children and adults.

Receptive One Word Picture Vocabulary Test: Upper Extension (ROWPVT-UE). Gardner, M. & Brownell, R. (1987). Austin, TX: Pro-Ed. Assesses expressive vocabulary in children ages 12 to 15 years. (Can be administered with EOWPVT-UE.)

Ross Information Processing Assessment (2nd ed.) (RIPA). Ross-Swain, D. (1996). Austin, TX: Pro-Ed. Quantifies cognitive-linguistic deficits, determines severity ratings in 10 communicative and cognitive areas, and assists in the development of goals and objectives for clients 15 through 90.

Speech and Language Evaluation Scale (SLES). Fressola, D. R. & Hoerchler, S. C. (1989). Columbia, MO: Hawthorne Educational Services. Includes a teacher rating scale and speech and language scale, which can be completed in approximately 20 minutes and used for screening, referral, and follow-up in areas of articulation, voice, fluency, form, content, and pragmatics.

Stanford Diagnostic Reading Test (3rd ed.) (SDRT). Karlsen, B. & Gardner, E. F. (1984). San Antonio, TX: Psychological Corporation. Provides diagnostic reading tasks at four levels (red, green, brown, blue) to measure specific strengths and needs in reading. Yields standard scores, percentile ranks, stanines, and grade equivalents.

Test of Adolescent and Adult Language (3rd ed.) (TOAL-3). Hammill, D. D., Brown, V. L., Larsen, S. C., & Wiederholt, J. L. (1994). Austin, TX: Pro-Ed. Examines listening, speaking, reading, writing, spoken language, written language, vocabulary, grammar, receptive and expressive language skills in clients ages 12:0 to 24:11.

Test of Adolescent/Adult Word Finding (TAWF). German, D. J. (1989). Allen, TX: DLM. This is a standardized test of word-finding skills for adolescents from 12 to 19:11 years, and adults from 20 to 80 years. It also includes a 10-minute brief test. Naming tasks are organized into five sections: picture naming (nouns), picture naming (verbs), sentence completion, naming, description naming, and naming categories of words. Analysis includes both accuracy and response time,

yielding standard scores, percentile ranks, and grade standards.

Test of Language Competence—Expanded Edition (TLC-Expanded). Wiig, E. H. & Secord, W. (1989). San Antonio, TX. Psychological Corporation. Identifies language and communication deficits in children ages 5 through 19 years. Includes two levels. Level 2 is designed for ages 9 through 18 years. It includes the following subtests: ambiguous sentences, listening comprehension (making inferences), oral expression (recreating speech acts), figurative language, remembering word pairs (supplemental subtest). Yields subtest and composite standard scores, and age-equivalent scores.

Test of Language Development—Intermediate (3rd ed.) (TOLD-I:3). Newcomer, P. L. & Hammill, D. D. (1997). Austin, TX: Pro-Ed. To be used with children ages 8 to 12:11, this test requires approximately 40 minutes to give. It yields standard and percentile scores. Has six subtests that measure different components of spoken language: sentence combining (constructing sentences); vocabulary (understanding word relationships); word ordering (constructing sentences); generals (knowing abstract relationships); grammatic comprehension (recognizing grammatical sentences); and malapropisms (correcting ridiculous sentences).

Test of Nonverbal Intelligence—3 (TONI-3). Brown, L., Sherbenou, R. J., & Johnsen, S. K. (1997). Austin, TX: Pro-Ed. The administration of this test requires no reading, writing, speaking, or listening by the test subject. It measures intelligence, aptitude, and reasoning, and may be used with individuals from ages 5 through 85:11, including individuals with severe speech impairments, brain injury, and deafness or hearing loss.

Test of Problem Solving—Adolescent (TOPS-A). Zachman L., Barrett, M., Huisingh, R., Orman, J., & Blagden, C. (1991). Austin, TX: Pro-Ed. A diagnostic tool for use with students 12 through 17:11. Assesses problem-solving and critical thinking skills in 30 to 40 minutes.

Test of Reading Comprehension (3rd ed.) (TORC-3). Brown, V. L., Hammill, D. D., & Wiederholt, L. J. (1995). Austin, TX: Pro-Ed. This is a multidimensional test of silent reading comprehension for students ages 7 through 17 years. The four major subtests measure general vocabulary, syntactic similarities, paragraph reading, and sentence sequencing. Five supplemental subtests measure abilities to read the vocabulary of math, science, and social studies, and the language of written directions.

Test of Written Language—(3rd ed.) (TOWL-3). Hammill, D. D. & Larsen, S. C. (1996). The revision provides two forms and new stimulus pictures for the spontaneous writing task that are analyzed for thematic maturity, contextual vocabulary, syntactic maturity, contextual spelling, and contextual style. Contrived writing tasks are also used to assess vocabulary, style and spelling, logical sentences, and sentence combining. Normative data are available for students ages 7:0 through 17:11 years.

Wide Range Achievement Test—(3rd ed.) (WRAT-3). Wilkinson, G. S. (1994). Austin, TX: Pro-Ed. Assesses reading (at the single-word level), spelling, and arithmetic abilities for ages 5 through 75 years. Yields standard scores, percentiles, and grade equivalents.

Woodcock-Johnson Psycho-Educational Battery-Revised (WJ-R). Woodcock, R. W. & Johnson, W. B. (1989). Allen, TX: DLM. Includes two batteries: *Tests of Cognitive Ability* and *Tests of Achievement.* This battery is based on extensive standardization information for persons in the age range 2 to 90+ years. It is a lengthy test, but it is divided into standard and supplemental batteries. The standard battery of the cognitive test can be used to yield a full-scale cognitive score in 40 minutes. The standard cognitive subtests are memory for names, memory for sentences, visual matching, incomplete words, visual closure, picture vocabulary, and analysis-synthesis. The supplemental cognitive subtests are visual–auditory learning, memory for words, cross out, sound blending, picture recognition, oral vocabulary, concept formation, delayed recall for names, delayed recall for visual–auditory learning, sound patterns, spatial relations, listening comprehension, and verbal analogies. The standard achievement subtests are letter-word identification, passage comprehension, calculation, applied problems, dictation, writing samples, science, social studies, and humanities. The supplemental achievement subtests are word attack, reading vocabulary, quantitative concepts, proofing, writing fluency, punctuation, spelling, usage, and handwriting.

Woodcock Language Proficiency Battery, English Form and *Spanish Form.* Woodcock, R. W. (1980). Allen, TX: DLM. This battery measures oral language, reading, and written language for persons ages 3 to 80+. It uses eight subtests in areas of oral language (picture vocabulary, antonyms and synonyms, analogies); reading (letter–word identification, word attack, passage comprehension) and written language (dictation, proofing, punctuation and capitalization, spelling, usage). The English form can be used with students for whom English is a second language if the Spanish form is also administered.

Woodcock Reading Mastery Tests—Revised (WRMT-R). Woodcock, R. W. (1987). Circle Pines, MN: AGS. This test may be used with persons ages 5 to 75+. Form G includes the following subtests: visual–auditory learning, letter identification, word identification, word attack, word comprehension (antonyms, synonyms, analogies), and passage comprehension. Form H includes word identification, word attack, word comprehension (antonyms, synonyms, analogies), and passage comprehension. Test scores are combined to form five clusters, with age and grade based on standard scores, percentile ranks, and equivalency scores.

The Word Test—Adolescent. Zachman, L., Huisingh, R., Barrett, M., Orman, J., & Blagden, C. (1989). East Moline, IL: LinguiSystems. This is a norm-referenced test for 12- to 17-year-olds that uses four tasks to assess semantic knowledge tapped by academic expectations and everyday life: brand names (explaining why a semantically descriptive name of a product is appropriate); synonyms; signs of the times (telling what a sign or message means and why it is important); and definitions. Yields standard scores, percentile ranks, and age equivalencies for both subtests and total test.

12

Later Stages: Goals
and Intervention Strategies

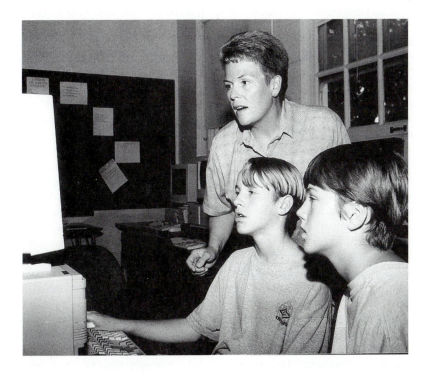

MODIFYING LANGUAGE-LEARNING
CONTEXTS

FOSTERING "METASKILLS" AND OTHER
EXECUTIVE STRATEGIES

DEVELOPING COMPETENCE IN DISCOURSE
GENRES AND EVENTS

ENCOURAGING LATER-STAGE
SYNTACTIC–SEMANTIC DEVELOPMENT

DEVELOPING ABSTRACT AND NONLITERAL
MEANINGS

FACILITATING TRANSITIONS

427

The goals and intervention strategies for the later stages of language acquisition encourage the integrated and complex use of language knowledge and skills. Most of these have been acquired to some degree in earlier stages. The later stages are a time for consolidating and fine-tuning foundation skills, for acquiring conscious strategies for using language for academic and vocational purposes, and for developing the automaticity and experience to communicate with confidence in a variety of modalities and circumstances.

Language processing and language strategies, as well as more basic aspects of language knowledge, are all appropriate targets of later stage intervention. The pinball wizardry model of complex oral and written language processing presented in Figure 11.1 represents these varied factors. Competent performance, according to this model, depends on synergistic contributions from four different but interrelated elements: (1) background knowledge to recognize and manipulate six kinds of linguistic and nonlinguistic units, rules, events, and relationships; (2) peripheral processing skills to interact with the environment and to get information in and out; (3) central processing skills to encode, store, remember, and retrieve information; and (4) conscious strategies to guide the processes efficiently. Mature communicative competency depends on partnership among these elements, and intervention strategies should be designed accordingly.

Discussions of intervention in this chapter are consistent with the view that language processing differs somewhat when using different units in different modalities. This discussion is also consistent with the view that boundaries are easily blurred during real-life communicative events, and it is not always clear what kinds of symbols (e.g., auditory word images, graphemes, or phonemes) a person is manipulating internally. Intervention that improves processing in one modality may facilitate processing in another (D. J. Johnson, 1985; N. W. Nelson, 1981a). For example, when a student acquires strategies for sounding out words syllable-by-syllable and for spelling from memory, the student may also hear sequences of syllables and remember new multisyllabic words during a lecture better. This, in turn, may help the student take notes during class and recall important words when responding on a test.

MODIFYING LANGUAGE-LEARNING CONTEXTS

When most children reach the later stages of language development, parents play a relatively minor role in fostering their development compared to teachers and peers. Even when children and adolescents in the later stages of child development have language disorders, most have acquired sufficient language for communicating basic meanings and performing most communicative functions, but their developmental pathways are considerably rockier than for individuals developing normally.

Summaries of longitudinal studies of individuals with developmental language impairments (P. S. Weiner, 1985) point to continued limitations in understanding and producing the complex language of regular classrooms; frequent problems with social–emotional development and behavioral adjustment; and many cases of special classroom placement with concurrent diagnoses of mental retardation and learning disabilities. Many adolescents with severe hearing losses experience academic struggles (Geers & Moog, 1989). Individuals with a history of impaired language development from any cause, in fact, have exaggerated risks for coping with the demands of adult work settings and independent living (Records, Tomblin, & Freese, 1992; Tomblin et al., 1990).

Professionals use a variety of strategies to help individuals with language weaknesses meet daily communicative demands. The traditional focus has been on "fixing" communicative processes. Newer approaches recognize the critical importance of designing language-learning contexts to help students improve their competence as communicators. Educational and intervention approaches designed to foster development by providing facilitative learning contexts are often called *mediated learning approaches.* Teachers and speech–language pathologists using these techniques act more as facilitators than instructors, leading students to make their own decisions and draw their own conclusions as they learn. The unique contribution of language specialists to this approach is their ability to be cognizant of the interactions of the activity's language demands with the student's language abilities and to design scaffolding questions and cues accordingly. Language demands of tasks, however, must be considered within even larger sociocultural contexts.

Respecting Sociocultural Backgrounds of Learners

Mediational techniques start when one or more key adults in a young person's life communicates respect for the individual as a learner and as a person who brings strengths to the learning process. This respect should extend to the participant's sociocultural background.

In the United States, more than one in five school-children come from families living in poverty, and despite commitment of federal and local resources, many of these children continue to experience disproportionate failure at school (Knapp, Turnbull, & Shields, 1990). Although some poor children have language disorders, many do not. Knapp and colleagues (1990) noted that traditional explanations for discouraging educational outcomes for poor children tend to locate the problem in the learner and his or her background. The child's language system may be implicated as the primary problem, which is inappropriate when the problem is language difference, not language disorder. Knapp and colleagues proposed an alternative view that locates parts of both the problem and the solution in the attitudes and practices of adults in school. Students whose families are poor are better able to meet the academic challenges of school when

- Teachers respect the students' cultural/linguistic backgrounds and communicate this appreciation to them in a personal way;
- The academic program encourages students to draw and build on the experiences they have, at the same time that it exposes them to unfamiliar experiences and ways of thinking;
- The assumptions, expectations, and ways of doing things in school—in short, its culture—are made explicit to these students by teachers who explain and model these dimensions of academic learning. (Knapp et al, 1990, p. 5)

Regardless of whether they come from poor, linguistically different, and/or culturally different families, students with language disorders will likely also benefit from these educational principles. A part of the intervention process for all students with language disorders involves helping them, in collaboration with classroom teachers, to consciously recognize aspects of classroom communication expectations that many more "typical" students acquire without explicit assistance.

Being sensitive to cultural differences also means that professionals should design learning contexts to take advantage of children's and adolescents' strengths from their home cultures. For example, Kawakami and Au (1986) noted that Hawaiian children, and particularly those from lower income families, were more likely to have participated in group interaction commu-

nication at home than in dyadic interactive experiences with adults. A talk-story format strongly facilitated reading and language development in these children.

Mediational Discourse in Curriculum-Based Language Intervention

One technique for assisting students to make more sense of varied classroom language is to teach them verbal mediation discourse for self-talk.

In our Language-Based Homework Lab (explained later in this chapter), we designed a Self-Talk Sheet, which we explain in a group minilesson (see Box 12.1). Then students keep it in front of them as they complete homework assignments or do practice problems as they learn to use self-talk to mediate their own work.

Box 12.1 _____

Student "Tool Book" Reminder for How to Use Self-Talk

SELF-TALK

About Self-Talk:

1. Self-talk is a learning *strategy* or *tool.*
2. People use self-talk when they think out loud.
3. Students can use self-talk to help guide their thinking about school problems by asking and answering questions one step at a time.

Some Ideas for Asking Myself Questions One Step at a Time:

Do I understand what this problem is about?
How can I solve this problem?
What information will help me to solve this problem?
What is the first step I need to do?
What is the next step?
Does the answer seem right?
Am I done?

Note: This self-talk sheet was designed by Adelia Van Meter as a handout for a minilesson on Self-Talk, which was conducted as part of the Language-Based Homework Lab (Nelson, 1997; Nelson & Van Meter, 1996). It was then incorporated in students' looseleaf notebooks, which we call "Tool Books." When a student started working on a school assignment, he or she would open the Tool Book to this page and use it to assist the process of talking himself or herself through each step of the process. © N. W. Nelson and A. VanMeter, 1996. Shared by permission of the authors.

Mediational discourse is a special form of scaffolding to facilitate "inner speech," as Vygotsky (1962) discussed it, to support mature thought. To some extent, the ability to use self-questioning strategies may depend on maturation. In a 3-year longitudinal study of students in first, second, and third grades, Bivens and Berk (1990) found that, in accordance with Vygotsky's theory, private speech moved from externalized to more internalized task-relevant forms as students worked on their math seatwork. These results suggest that children above third grade should be reasonably adept at using self-talk. Language intervention using verbal mediation is a top-down processing approach. Students are taught to process language better by using their world knowledge and sensemaking expectations to direct their other attentional and perceptual processes.

Psychologist Reuven Feuerstein (1979) defined mediated learning as an interactional process between a developing individual and "an experienced intentioned adult"; the adult mediates the world to the child by "framing, selecting, focusing, and feeding back environmental experiences" to produce in the child "appropriate learning sets and habits" (p. 179). The mediational strategies developed by Feuerstein, Rand, and Rynders (1988) for work with mentally retarded individuals, which they called instrumental enrichment (IE), have been adapted for persons with other problems.

For example, Haywood, Towery-Woolsey, Arbitman-Smith, and Aldridge (1988) reported a study using Feuerstein's IE methods with 53 deaf adolescents in residential schools. The results showed that the children who had received the experimental approach made significant gains (and greater gains than control subjects) on most measures (Haywood et al., 1988).

Haywood and his colleagues (1988) emphasized that the teacher's role during IE shifts from being a giver of information to being the mediator of experiences for children:

> *Mediational teachers elicit understanding from the children by asking guiding questions, supplying needed information, directing activity, challenging answers, requiring logical evidence for conclusions, and, most important, emphasizing the processes of thinking, learning, and problem solving rather than the products (answers). (p. 27)*

When applying these techniques, mediational teachers often respond, even to correct answers, with more

questions. They might ask the children how they knew which one to select, why that choice was better than another one, and what they had to do to solve the problem—also whether there might be another way to approach the problem. In addition, mediational teachers elicit "bridges" from the children. Teachers ask children to think of analogous contexts in which the same thinking operations and strategies might be used. Finally, mediational teachers seek to engage children in understanding that the universe has an order, structure, and predictability that they can grasp by applying generalized principles of thinking.

Because question-asking is central both to traditional classroom discourse and to mediated learning interactions, a closer look at the use and misuse of questions in mediation is appropriate. Marion Blank and her colleagues have contributed to understanding uses of questions to facilitate language and cognitive development, both in the preschool years and beyond (Blank, 1975; Blank, Rose, & Berlin, 1978; Blank & White, 1986). Blank and White (1986), however, also pointed out that questions might be misused in instructional discourse, leading to confusion and bad feelings. They commented that a "situation that is unfortunate for any child is almost unbearable for learning-disabled children, given the insecurities and failures that they face elsewhere" (p. 11).

Blank and White (1986) noted the failure of teachers to provide scaffolding questions appropriate to the individual's level of development. Teachers may have learned, as a general principle, that higher order, open-ended processing questions are best to elicit elaborate answers (e.g., *how* and *why* questions), but this strategy may go astray in a couple of ways. First, it may suggest to students that a wide range of responses is acceptable when a teacher has a very specific topic or response in mind. Only students who are tuned into the "hidden curriculum" of the teacher's own pet topics and peeves then can infer what the teacher really wants. For example, one teacher asked older students simply to talk about current events, suggesting that the topic was wide open, but then ignored a student's mention of Pablo Casals, the famous cellist, while accepting another student's topic of war in the Middle East. Blank and White commented that it would have been better for the teacher to state directly that she wanted to talk about the war in the Middle East in the first place. (Indirect communication of teachers' personal preferences make up a large part of the "hidden curriculum" described earlier in Box 11.3.)

A related problem may result when higher order questions require abstract reasoning at levels beyond the student's capabilities. Then, higher order questions are likely to result in unacceptable responses, putting teachers in a dilemma about whether to correct errors. Again, teachers may have learned well the lesson not to criticize directly anything students say. As a result, teachers may consequate inappropriate or incorrect responses from students with vague and ambiguous evaluative comments. For example, they may ask the same question of another child, or they may ask the same child again, perhaps repeating the child's erroneous response in an incredulous tone. This is what happened in the following example, reported by Blank and White (1986) from an exchange between a teacher using a poster of a jungle consumed by fire:

> **TEACHER:** *How could grass in a jungle get on fire?*
> **CHILD:** *Cause they* (referring to animals) *have to stay in the jungle.*
> **TEACHER:** (in an incredulous tone) *You mean the grass gets on fire because the animals stay in the jungle?*
> **CHILD:** *Yeah. (p. 4)*

A common teaching strategy is to identify areas a student does not understand and ask about them. In the preceding situation, this student was known to have difficulty with causal reasoning. The strategy of focusing on the area of deficit, in this case, only led to frustration for both the student and the teacher. After a few more attempts to get the student to identify causal relationships, the teacher abandoned the effort. A better strategy might have been to provide more concrete product-oriented questions, such as "What is happening in the picture?" or "What are the animals doing in this picture?" (Blank & White, 1986). Then the student could have experienced some success in answering and would have been assisted in focusing on the topic. The teacher then could have asked the entire group to brainstorm possible causes of fire in jungles. By using such strategies, skilled teachers can work with heterogeneous groups of students so that all can participate in constructing meaning at levels appropriate to their own ability.

Mediational strategies are appropriate across communicative modalities. For example, Hoskins (1990) described common guidelines for acting as "facilitator" for oral language conversation groups and written language mediation:

> *These same principles are relevant in facilitating print literacy: (a) intervention is based on the participant's communication; (b) language is learned in interaction; and (c) the facilitator acts as a metalinguistic guide. (p. 55)*

Facilitative strategies to guide written language production were studied formally by Bernice Wong and her colleagues (Wong, Wong, Darlington, & Jones, 1991). They reported two studies of **interactive teaching** (another term for **mediated learning** or **scaffolding**) aimed at helping adolescents with learning disabilities revise their written compositions. Written language problems of such students include "lower-order cognitive problems in spelling, punctuation, and grammar, and higher-order cognitive and metacognitive problems in planning, writing fluency, revising, and awareness of audience" (Wong et al., 1991, p. 117). Interactional teaching uses oral discourse with adolescent writers to help them identify ambiguities in their essays and to make their themes salient. An example of this strategy appears in Box 12.2.

Mediated Reading and Miscue Analysis

Mediated reading is a special case of mediational language intervention (Norris & Hoffman, 1993). The educator frames and focuses students' attention, first, on whether their reading of the text makes sense, and second, on whether it matches the printed data. This approach uses the basic principles of miscue analysis presented in Chapter 11, coupled with mediational instruction designed to teach self-questioning strategies.

The general technique involves repeating a piece of text the child has just read when the child has produced an observed response that does not match an expected response. The purpose is to focus the child on one or more key features of the mismatch.

Questions about bigger units of text, for example, might include the following:

- Does this make sense?
- Does this fit with what we have been reading?
- Does it fit with what we see on the page?
- When you say _____, I expect to see _____. Is that what you see?

Box 12.2 _____

An Example of Interactive Teaching Strategies to Help an Adolescent with Language-Learning Disabilities Develop an Awareness of Audience Informational Needs

This student was writing about the most scary event of his life, which concerned his daredevil antics on his mountain bike. He wrote, "I hit the ramp so hard my XKJ475 fell off." Upon reading this sentence, the experimenter-teacher stopped and hummed and sighed loudly. With a puzzled expression on her face, she turned to the student and said: "What on earth do you mean here? You're writing nicely and all of the sudden, you got this chunk of capital letters and numbers!" The student quickly inspected the offending sentence and with surprise exclaimed: "That's the license of my mountain bike!" "Oh, I see," said the experimenter, now totally demystified, "You mean to say your mountain bike hit the ramp so hard, it got its license plate knocked off. You see, it's all clear in your own head what you intend to say to the reader. You know what it's about, you understand what you have written. But I didn't! I don't know a thing about mountain bikes or their license numbers, so I wouldn't know what you were writing about! You see now, when you write, you've got to make yourself clear so people know what you mean, O.K.? So how can we fix this part so readers would understand what you want to say?" The student returned to the screen and added "my mountain bike license XKJ475 fell off.' "

(*Note:* Wong, Wong, Darlington, & Jones, 1991, p. 120)

_____

Depending on the individual students' needs, some mediational efforts may be designed to develop bottom-up abilities for decoding smaller units of text, perhaps by drawing students' attention to mismatches involving graphophonemic miscues at the word level. For example, when a student reads *was* for *saw,* the language interventionist might attempt to get the student to focus on the graphophonemic nature of the miscue by saying, "When you read this word as *was,* I expect to see a /w/ at the beginning of this word; Is that what you see?" If attempting to help the student focus on syntactic cues, the adult mediator might say, "Listen to what you read, 'The boy *was* a huge truck'; Does that make sense? Can we say that?" When students with speech–language impairments have significant and ongoing difficulty making sound–symbol associations, they may need highly systematic multimodality practice in articulating, tracing, writing, reading, and sequencing more isolated bits of print and related speech sounds and syllables before they can use graphophonemic cues reliably in contextual reading.

Decisions about which miscues to point out, which to let go, and how often to interrupt are not easy. If the student reads along fairly smoothly and appears to comprehend the text, it may be most appropriate to ignore the minor graphophonemic miscues. Letting the student read past a rough spot without correction may also leave the student more in charge of the process of creating meaning and more likely to self-correct. Cazden's (1988) review of the literature on correction showed that teachers tend to interrupt poorer readers more immediately and frequently than better readers. When language interventionists see themselves as guides and facilitators of the language acquisition process, rather than as individuals who must monitor for errors and let none get by, they can relax about jumping in too frequently and can begin to enjoy reading with the student for the central purpose of constructing meaning.

Strategies for Modifying the Language-Learning Contexts of Classrooms

Some methods for modifying learning contexts focus on one-on-one interactions between adult facilitators and students with special language-learning needs. Others focus on modifying broader aspects of classroom contexts or coordinating them with therapy room contexts.

Hughes (1989) provided suggestions for helping students with language-learning disabilities generalize newly acquired linguistic abilities from therapy room to classroom. She emphasized the need for speech–language pathologists and classroom teachers to collaborate to accomplish mutually set goals in slightly different ways. For example, when a student's problem has been identified through the collaborative process as failing to comprehend or follow the teacher's multistep directions, the following therapy room objectives and activities might be used:

> *Objectives: to increase comprehension of multistep directions that include terms used in classroom instructions; to increase readiness to listen; to teach compensatory strategies, such as writing down page numbers, problem numbers, due dates.*
>
> *Activities: in small groups, students take turns role playing teacher, giving common classroom directives that require multiple steps; verbal rehearsal of listening strategies for particular teachers, subject periods, or assignment. (p. 226)*

The corresponding strategy for modifying classroom contextual demands might include the following:

> *Teacher asks student chosen at random to orally repeat directions; writes specific details on the board; reinforces direction following specifically; cues student to write down details. (p. 226)*

Similarly, Maxon and Brackett (1987) pointed out how contextually based solutions might be designed for students with hearing impairments by analyzing specific problems (called zones of significance in Chapter 11) and their probable causes. Areas they identified as frequently problematic for students with hearing impairments included exchanges in the hallway, changes in teachers, spelling, language-based subjects such as social studies and science, class discussion, test taking, reading groups, classroom lectures on specific content material, independent desk work, group projects, peer-to-peer social interactions, homework, and announcements over the loudspeaker. Possible problems occurring in the hallway might include taking off amplification after every class and giving no response to greet-

ings. Possible causes might include embarrassment about wearing amplification and inability to hear in noisy, reverberant hallways. Possible solutions might include provision of less obvious amplification along with consultation with peers and teachers to teach them about the function and purposes of amplification and the importance of being in close proximity when conversing in hallways.

The critical steps of all of these curriculum-based language intervention strategies are to (1) identify zones of significance (contextually based needs); (2) analyze the communicative demands of the event or situation; (3) observe the individual's current attempts to meet those demands; (4) provide intervention to assist the individual to acquire new knowledge, skills, and strategies; (5) mediate the contextual demands to make them more accessible; and (6) keep in mind the desired outcome of independent functioning in the real world to avoid "the forest and the trees problem" (raised in Chapter 1).

Alternative Contexts for Practicing School Skills

In upper elementary, middle school, and high school, school days are packed with academic learning that uses complex language skills and develops language further. Integrated service delivery models are those that involve direct partnerships between classroom teachers and special service providers. Indirect, or consultative, models are also a possibility (Cirrin & Penner, 1995). Other classroom-based approaches are relevant to classroom concerns but are provided in contexts other than the classroom (Hoskins, 1997).

Integrated In-Class Programs.   Elksnin & Capilouto (1994) described seven versions of in-class integrated service delivery models. These models represent arrangements in which a speech–language pathologist (SLP) or other special educator (SPEC) and classroom teacher (CT) work in a single classroom at the same time: (1) **one teach, one observe,** gathering onlooker observation data that may be useful in future planning; (2) **one teach, one "drift,"** which involves assisting individual students who need help; (3) **station teaching,** with movement of students among stations to work with both the SLP and CT at different times; (4) **parallel teaching,** with the SLP and CT each teaching the same content to half the class; (5) **remedial teaching,** in which one adult works with the students who have not mastered a concept to remediate its meaning for them; (6) **supplemental teaching,** in which one adult provides extra support to students who have not mastered key material; (7) **team teaching,** in which adults share responsibility equally for lecturing and experiential learning.

Cirrin and Penner (1995) reviewed the research evidence on programs like these, which they called **classroom-based direct** service delivery models, as well as **classroom-indirect** service options. Indirect options include consultative models in which the clinician interacts primarily with teachers and others who work directly with the student (see Chapter 5). They noted that "direct language intervention procedures implemented in classroom settings have not been put to any adequate test to determine their effectiveness in facilitating development of specific language abilities in school-age children" (p. 345), although studies at the preschool level are encouraging. Consultative models also have been rarely investigated. Some studies have suggested positive effects for students with autism and with learning disabilities. Cirrin and Penner noted that service delivery options should occur along a continuum, and that "no comprehensive language intervention plan can be considered complete without a plan that will enable the student to use newly learned target skills in the classroom and other natural environments" (p. 358).

After-School Programs.   At Western Michigan University, we have experimented with two service delivery approaches in after-school activities, a **computer-supported story writing lab** and a **language-based homework lab.** Either of these service delivery models also could be provided as part of a regular school day. We provided both labs two days per week for an hour each after school. Both used a combination of individual and group activities. Individual time provided opportunities to work on specific language goals within the contexts of the students' own stories and homework with support from a mediational teacher (all graduate students in speech–language pathology or special education). Group minilessons were used to introduce and discuss topics related to the middle school students' (Grades 3 through 8) language learning needs and to introduce parts of the writing process. A group project was also an important component of both service delivery approaches. It provided the opportunity for students to spend extended time creating a product that displayed their own language for an authentic audience, giving purpose to processes of reflection and editing to make language clear and interesting. (Favorite editing questions for self and peers were "Is it clear?" "Is it interesting?" "What's good about it?" "How could the author make it better?") At the end of each semester a "publishing party" or "performance party" for parents and students provided opportunity for performance, celebration (cheese and crackers mandatory), and conferences with students and parents to set goals for what to work on next. Products of the writing lab were booklets of student stories. Group projects in the homework lab have included a newspaper full of students' stories, skits about school problems written and acted by students, and a TV newsprogram, with stories written and produced on videotape by students. Group projects set up a learning context that permits focus on both product and process. All students have objectives that target changes in their language products (such as mean length of utterance [MLU] for T-units or proportion of complex sentences, measured with pre- and postintervention samples of their oral and written language) and language processes (such as number of contributions to group discussions or willingness to attempt more challenging learning tasks, measured with quantitative and qualitative observational data).

The difference between the two service delivery models is that the **computer-supported story writing lab** was organized entirely as a writing workshop (using procedures described by Atwell, 1987; Calkins, 1983; Harris & Graham, 1996b; Swoger, 1989). It provided extended opportunities for students to work on the narrative genre, and within it, the sentences, word choices, and graphophonemic understandings to support their writing. The students wrote creative stories and interacted with mediational teachers, who looked with them at their own language on a computer screen, expressing appreciation for the students' ideas while scaffolding them to higher levels of language competence. Students learned to talk about three stages of the writing process: (1) planning and organizing, (2) writing your story, and (3) revising and editing, as they practiced it. In the schedule for this model, author groups provided opportunities for students to work on oral and social-interaction skills for approximately 15 minutes, students wrote at their own computers in a laboratory for at least one-half hour, and they conferred with their instructors about the writing process for approximately 5 minutes per session. Students also spent 10 to 15 minutes per session working independently through keyboarding software programs with minimal support from instructors. We developed the computer writing lab with support from the U.S. Department of Education, Office of Special Education and Rehabilitation Services (Grant No. H180G20005, "Linking Text-Processing Tools to Student Needs," Christine Bahr & N. W. Nelson, Principal Investigators) to conduct research on features of commercially available computer writing software and their ability to support the written language development of students with special language-learning needs. Some of the six research studies have been published (Bahr et al., 1996; Bahr, Nelson, Van Meter, & Yanna, 1996). Others are in the works, as is a book describing the intervention approach (Nelson, Bahr, & Van Meter, in press).

The **language-based homework lab** (Nelson, 1997; Nelson & Van Meter, 1996) maintained as many of the features of the writing lab as time permitted (regrettably, we had to give up the keyboarding practice and extended time writing at computers), while adding more individualized focus on the students' curriculum-based language intervention needs. Development of the language-based homework lab was supported with a personnel preparation grant from the U.S. Department of Education, Office of Special Education and Rehabilitation Services (Grant No. HO29B40183, "Project CONNECT: Preparation of Speech-Language Pathologists with Special Competencies for Making Connections," N. W. Nelson & M. J. Clark, Project Co-Directors). The instructors are graduate student trainees in Project CONNECT. We have experimented with several plans for getting maximum benefit from our three major learning activities, group minilessons, group project, and individualized intervention based in students' own curricula. One schedule that works fairly well is to spend 20 to 30 minutes on a minilesson in the Monday session, following with 30

minutes for individual intervention. Then on Wednesday, we start with individual time and spend the last half hour on the group project. We connect this work to the students' school curricula by visiting their schools and interviewing their teachers, as well as the students and their parents, about their curriculum-based language needs. We also communicate weekly with their teachers using the Teacher Talk sheets that appear in Figure 12.1.

Alternative Language Classrooms. The **alternate adolescent language class** (AALC) was developed by Gloria Anderson (Anderson & Nelson, 1988). It was an in-school program that Anderson implemented as a regularly scheduled course offering (in Michigan, Teachers of the Speech and Language Impaired are certified classroom teachers). The alternative language class became the source of the students' language arts credit for the one or two years they needed it. That is, students were scheduled for the alternative class in place of their English or language arts class. They attended five days per week and worked on student skills for all of the other classes in their curriculum, in addition to addressing the objectives of the general education curriculum for the middle-school grade levels in their district. Students who were enrolled had a variety of diagnostic labels, including hearing impairment and emotional impairment as well as language impairment and learning disability.

Special Topic Workshops. A **fourth-grade transition workshop** is another alternative service delivery model for later-stage students. It was developed by Sandra Tattershall (personal communication, July, 1996; in preparation) to meet a community need within her private practice. Tattershall designed the summer program for the students preparing to enter the fourth grade where they would for the first time change classes and teachers each hour and be expected to work more independently. Tattershall helped the students develop basic language and metapragmatic skills necessary to cope with the expectations for added independence and organization facing them. All of these alternative service delivery models have elements to address the students' needs to understand themselves as learners as well as their strengths and needs.

FIGURE 12.1   Teacher Talk sheet used to communicate with teachers of middle school students attending a language-based homework laboratory.

Note to teachers: The purpose of this form is to support our communication with you about your student's language-learning needs. We complete the Language Lab and student portions with the student at each Wednesday session. If possible, have your input ready for the student to return for our Monday sessions.

Student: _____   Speech–language specialist: _____   Phone: _____

Week of: _____   Teacher: _____   Phone: _____ (and best time to call)

SCHOOL:
Please provide an explanation of the classwork areas of emphasis for which your student may need support in the current and upcoming weeks. Include any suggestions for aiding your student's homework/learning efforts:

LANGUAGE LAB:
In Language Lab, we have been working on the following homework and study skills to meet both group learning and individual goals:

STUDENT INPUT:
1. Things at which I've been successful:

2. Things I want to work on more:

Note: From Nelson, N. W. (1997). Implementing a language-based homework lab: A plan for curriculum-based intervention. In N. W. Nelson & B. Hoskins (Eds.), *Strategies for supporting classroom success: Focus on communication.* San Diego, CA: Singular Publishing Group, Inc. © 1996 by N. W. Nelson. Used by permission of author.

FOSTERING "METASKILLS" AND OTHER EXECUTIVE STRATEGIES

GOAL: The student will use conscious strategies to guide interactions at school, to remember academic material, and to plan, organize, and implement approaches to academic tasks.

- Learning Strategy Models
- Metapragmatic Strategies and School Survival Skills
- Metacognitive Strategies for Improving Memory and Higher Order Thinking
- Metacognitive, Metalinguistic, and Metatextual Strategies for Focusing on Process as well as Product
- Summary of Metaskills and How to Teach Them

OUTCOME: The student will function independently in classroom contexts and will devise new strategies as new challenges arise.

The acquisition of mature strategies for directing one's own behavior is an important contributor to adult independence. The adoption of systematic "strategies" can enable learners to order input, make sense of it, remember it, and recall it. Such individuals have learned how to learn a particular kind of information. Language plays an important role in this process. Metaskills are an appropriate focus of later-stage intervention (van Kleeck, 1994a).

Learning Strategy Models

Prevalence.   The current emphasis on learning strategies in intervention programs for students with language-learning disabilities in secondary school programs (Ehren, 1994; Larson & McKinley, 1987; Schumaker, Deshler, Alley, Warner, & Denton, 1982) replaces older models. A review of earlier programming approaches in a large school district (Deshler, Lowrey, & Alley, 1979) showed: basic skills remediation (45%), tutorial approaches (24%), functional curriculum approaches (17%), and work–study approaches (5%). Learning strategies approaches accounted for only 4% of the programs.

Intervention programs that target the development of deliberate processing strategies are more common now than in 1979, when Deshler and his colleagues conducted their original study (Deshler et al., 1979). However, obtaining data about current programming is

difficult, even for high-incidence disorders such as learning disabilities. McKenzie (1991) surveyed all 50 states; Washington, DC; the Bureau of Indian Affairs; the Virgin Islands; and Puerto Rico to ask questions about the degree to which the service-delivery system in a particular state or territory was based on a model of "basic skill" instruction or "content area" instruction. McKenzie defined the **basic skill model** as *instruction to students with learning disabilities* "to improve their basic reading, writing, computational, and social skills for the purpose of improving their performance in mainstream content area classes" (p. 116). McKenzie described the **content area model** as instruction

> in core content areas such as English, math, social studies, science, etc., to those students who are assumed unable to benefit from inclusion in one or more mainstream content area classes. (p. 116)

McKenzie differentiated both the basic skill and content area models from a third, **learning strategies model.** He indicated that

> although instruction in "learning strategies" may occur within either model, a program focused exclusively on learning strategies should not be considered representative of either a "skill" or a "content" model. (p. 116)

McKenzie (1991) found wide variability by geographic region, as well as evidence that many state directors of special education were not sure about instructional methods used in their states. He did find that of 49 respondents, 41 reported that content area instruction occurred within their state or territory. Unfortunately, he did not ask about strategy instruction. McKenzie concluded that "although the question of 'which approach is better' may never be adequately answered, there is a pressing need to identify the efficacy of each." (p. 121)

Rationale.   Most aspects of purposeful "executive control" are acquired normally in the later stages of childhood (Forrest-Pressley & Waller, 1984; Nippold, 1988a; Pressley & Harris, 1990). They enable young people to become increasingly organized and self-directed as they move toward adulthood.

Executive control strategies often rely on the use of "metaskills." A variety of metaprocessing skills were described in Chapter 11, with suggestions for assessing individuals' conscious awareness of language (metalinguistic knowledge), pragmatics (metapragmatic knowledge), texts (metatextual knowledge) and their own cognitive processes (metacognitive knowledge). A primary reason for assessing these areas relates to the role they play in determining whether individuals can succeed in school and other formal communication contexts (Chabon & Prelock, 1989; Ehren & Lenz, 1989; Silliman, 1987; Wallach, 1989).

Although executive control involves systematic, strategic approaches to problem solving, not all strategy learning is highly conscious or deliberate; some is relatively automatic and unconsidered (Chabon & Prelock, 1989). The seemingly automatic acquisition of strategy learning by normally developing children may make the process appear to occur unassisted. However, the need to teach strategic approaches to information processing and problem solving deliberately is currently recognized in the literature of general education as well as special education. Pressley and Harris (1990) noted that "We realize now that many students do not learn strategies automatically" (p. 31). Pressley and Harris pointed to research findings that even some adults do not use self-questioning strategies automatically when they need to learn a set of facts.

Children and adolescents with certain conditions associated with language disorders, such as attention-deficit hyperactivity disorder or traumatic brain injury (Ylvisaker & Szekeres, 1986), have exaggerated risks for failure to use executive strategies. Others, such as youths with hearing impairments or deafness, may try to use strategies but lack sufficient language skills to support them (Andrews & Mason, 1991). Individuals with language-learning disabilities also have difficulty using self-mediational language to direct their own behavior and thinking because of weak underlying language competencies (Hagen, Barclay, & Schwethelm, 1982; Torgesen, 1982).

Silliman (1987) ascribed some of the individual differences in classroom performance by language-impaired students to their strategic planning limitations. She contrasted **declarative knowledge** for knowing about things, and **procedural knowledge** for knowing how to do things and noted that "communicative strategies might be considered part of the procedural component" (p. 359). When children have difficulty in school, intervention should involve sorting out the degree to which problems may be attributed to each of several factors: inefficient processing, inadequate management of available processing resources, or insufficient content knowledge (Silliman, 1987). Wallach (1989) also proposed that "individual strategy preferences of language learning disabled students must be understood over a variety of contexts and discourse types" (p. 213).

Students who take passive approaches to learning have been described as "inactive learners" (Silliman, 1987; Torgesen & Licht, 1983). These individuals may have relatively intact intellectual abilities but fail to take advantage of them, particularly in school. Wallach (1989) also noted that many learners with language-learning disabilities are passive but argued that they could become "constructive comprehenders" if they were taught how to draw on existing background knowledge and to use learning strategies.

Metapragmatic Strategies and School Survival Skills

Objective 1. The student will show awareness of the unspoken rules for classroom interactions by talking about them and by demonstrating skills in simulated and real-class interactions that did not appear in baseline samples.

Success in school largely depends on knowing how to follow unspoken rules for classroom interactions. Box 12.3 summarizes ten rules Janet Sturm and I inferred from analyzing the discourse interactions of formal lessons (Sturm & Nelson, 1997). When students understand the school culture curriculum and have efficient strategies for getting organized, they have greater attentional and information processing resources to devote to understanding the official academic curriculum. When they do not, they risk being inefficient, disorganized, inappropriate, and "lost" during a major portion of the school day. The problem is that much of what I call the "school culture curriculum" and "hidden curriculum" is never explained to students. R. J. Sternberg and his colleagues called this *the tacit knowledge of school* (R. J. Sternberg, Okagaki, & Jackson, 1990; see Personal Reflection 12.1).

Tattershall (1987) noted that "Just as most students learn their syntax and phonology without explicit teaching, many students extract the critical rules of classroom participation without direct instruction. However, there

Box 12.3 _____

Ten Unspoken Rules for Participating in Formal Classroom Discussions

Rule 1.   Teachers mostly talk and students mostly listen—except when teachers grant permission to talk.

Rule 2.   Teachers give cues about when to listen closely.

Rule 3.   Teachers convey content about things and procedures about how to do things.

Rule 4.   Teacher talk becomes more complex in the upper grades.

Rule 5.   Teachers ask questions and expect specific responses.

Rule 6.   Teachers give hints about what is correct and what is important to them.

Rule 7.   Student talk is brief and to the point.

Rule 8.   Students ask few questions and keep them short.

Rule 9.   Students talk to teachers, not to other students.

Rule 10. Students make few spontaneous comments—and only about the process or content of the lesson.

Note: From Sturm, J. M., & Nelson, N. W. (1997). Formal classroom lessons: New perspectives on a familiar discourse event, _Language Speech and Hearing Services in Schools._ © American Speech-Language-Hearing Association. Reprinted by permission.

_____

are some students who have to be taught these classroom interactional/instructional rules" (p. 182). Tattershall emphasized the importance of the critical first month of school, when students begin to learn the routines of new classrooms. She commented that parents may be valuable partners in monitoring whether their children are learning school rules. They may do this by observing whether their children seem vague when asked about classroom routines. If so, parents may urge their children to be more assertive in determining teachers' expectations about homework, asking clarification questions, and talking in class (see Box 11.4). By discussing classroom expectations with their youngsters, parents may stimulate students to recognize classroom rules they might otherwise overlook. Conveying the ex-

**PERSONAL REFLECTION 12.1** _____

"Teachers have a wide array of expectations for students, many of which are never explicitly verbalized. Students who cannot meet these implicit expectations may suffer through year after year of poor school performance without knowing quite what is wrong. Their teachers expect them to know how to allocate their time in doing homework, how to prepare course papers, how to study for tests, how to talk (and not to talk) to a teacher—if they never learn these things, they will suffer for it."

Robert J. Sternberg, Lynn Okagaki, and _Alice S. Jackson_ (1990, p. 35), writing about the need for what they called "practical intelligence" to succeed in school. Sternberg, who is IBM Professor of Psychology and Education at Yale, proposed the triarchic theory of human intelligence, with componential, contextual, and experiential operations (R. J. Sternberg, 1985, 1988).

_____

pectation that children are in charge may avoid the pitfalls of becoming too dependent on (and resentful of) the parents' rescuing efforts. Parental intervention, which may have been appropriate at earlier grade levels, is not as appropriate later. When children appear uncertain of classroom expectations, parents may alert others who may be in a better position to make them explicit. This in turn may contribute to consultation between speech–language pathologists and teachers as they seek to recognize how language-learning difficulties influence inappropriate behavior. By identifying misunderstanding as the source for inappropriate behavior, it may be possible to "change a student's premature 'bad' reputation" (Tattershall, 1987, p. 183) and to avert a destructive spiral of negative feedback from teachers and increasingly sullen attitudes from students.

Without intervention, students with learning disabilities are at risk for increased problems with school culture rules as they advance in grade level. Schumaker, Sheldon-Wildgen, and Sherman (1980) found classroom rule violations by students with learning disabilities to exceed those for students without learning disabilities by 9% in seventh grade, 17% in eighth grade, and 26% in ninth grade. When teachers left the classroom, the students with learning disabilities engaged in rule-violating episodes during 92% of the intervals; whereas students without learning disabilities did not participate in a single rule-violating episode.

One possible reason for the increase at the secondary level is that the processing demands of the school culture curriculum become particularly intense during those years. Students must deal with changing classrooms and multiple teachers. Ehren and Lenz (1989; also Ehren, 1994) discussed the executive demands of secondary school settings in conjunction with the executive characteristics of many adolescents with learning disabilities.

1. Students are expected to work independently with little feedback.
2. Students are expected to apply knowledge across the content areas.
3. Students are expected to solve problems on their own.
4. Students are expected to organize information and a variety of resources independently to solve problems. (1989, p. 197)

A comparison of this list of expected characteristics with the corresponding set of observed characteristics that Ehren and Lenz (1989) noted among students with learning disabilities highlights the mismatch that gives so many of these students difficulty:

1. LD [learning disabled] adolescents often do not invent appropriate strategies or approaches that lead to successful task completion.
2. They have difficulty learning how to solve problems.
3. They often do not generalize what they have learned.
4. They often fail to take advantage of prior knowledge when facing new problems. (p. 198)

Lists of expected school survival skills provided by Ehren and Lenz (1989) are supported by other research. Schaeffer, Zigmond, Kerr, and Farra (1990) surveyed principals, school administrators, special education teachers, mainstream teachers, and over 4000 high school students to identify skills important to school success. Of a list of 69 items, they identified six skills as most critical to school survival:

1. Going to class every day.
2. Arriving at school on time.
3. Bringing pencils, paper, and books to class.
4. Turning in work on time.

5. Talking to teachers without using "back talk."
6. Reading and following directions. (p. 198)

Skills like these were targeted in the alternative adolescent language classroom described previously in this chapter (G. M. Anderson & Nelson, 1988). Students learned about teachers' "unspoken contract" with their students, such as "I will live up to my part of the bargain and will continue to support and encourage you if you will also live up to yours and *attempt* to do the work" (p. 349). The students learned that the most unacceptable form of student behavior was failure to turn in required work. To avoid that problem and to help them organize themselves, these students learned strategies involving notebooks and assignment sheets to keep track of their responsibilities. They also participated in metapragmatic exercises observing the "student-like behaviors" exhibited by the successful students in their regular education classes and emulating them. They observed, labeled, and practiced paying attention, acting interested, asking questions, and taking notes. While they were in the alternative language classroom daily (for which they received grades and credit), the students constantly repeated to themselves and to each other their main goal of acquiring the skills they needed so that they would no longer need the alternative class. Of the initial seven students enrolled in the classroom, only one was unable to meet this goal after 1 year in the program (two moved out of the district and four were successfully mainstreamed in regular education programs). That student needed an additional year in the more structured classroom. Anderson and Nelson reported:

> Teachers began to indicate both verbally and on report cards that the students were "doing better, making an effort, interested, working harder," and "catching on." In many cases, the teachers felt that the students had been immature and had suddenly matured. Teachers also perceived that the students' attitudes toward school had actually changed. (1988, p. 351)

Metacognitive Strategies for Improving Memory and Higher Order Thinking

Objective 2. The student will use preplanning and organizational strategies for talking and writing about what he or she knows, needs to know, and how to remember new information: (1) with heavy scaffolding, (2) with moderate scaffolding, and (3) independently.

Not all students learn equally well in the same ways. At least since D. J. Johnson and Myklebust (1967) published their classic text on learning disabilities, speech–language pathologists and other special educators have been aware of the need for becoming attuned to the varied learning strengths of individual students. However, professionals have now surpassed the simplistic models of "visual learners" and "auditory learners" (see Chapter 3) and the faddish models of "left-hemisphere learners" and "right-hemisphere learners" and recognized that many factors together determine how an individual learns specific content in a particular context.

Students in the later stages of child development may benefit from direct instruction in understanding their own intelligence and that of their fellow students. A school curriculum on "practical intelligence," with this purpose, was developed through collaboration between Howard Gardner, at Harvard, and Robert Sternberg, at Yale University (R. J. Sternberg et al., 1990) (see Table 12.1). Gardner and Sternberg developed separate but relatively compatible theories of intelligence (Gardner, 1983; R. J. Sternberg, 1985, 1988). Gardner's theory addresses the multiple relatively autonomous forms of intelligence, and his seven modular intelligence forms include linguistic, logical-mathematical (L. Miller, 1990, separated logical and mathematical), musical, spatial, bodily-kinesthetic, interpersonal, and intrapersonal. (See L. Miller's 1990, "Smart Profile" system for helping students recognize the different ways they are smart.) Sternberg's (1985, 1988) triarchic theory of intelligence includes **componential operations** (mental processes), **contextual operations** (practical applications), and **experiential operations** (transfer to new situations).

Langer (1982) suggested that teachers assist students to focus on their prior knowledge by using a prereading plan (PREP) before attempting to learn from written texts. For example, teachers ask students to "Tell me everything you think of when you hear . . . " Then they ask, "What made you think of . . . ?," to prompt students to reflect on their thought processes and organization of knowledge. Finally, teachers ask, "Do you want to add to or change your first response?" to prompt students to reformulate and refine their responses.

Based on Langer's work, Westby (1991) summarized response characteristics that teachers or language specialists might use to judge children's prior knowledge as *little knowledge, some knowledge,* or *much knowledge.* For example, *little knowledge* is judged when students respond to teachers' questions with associative tangential comments, with tangential first-hand experiences, or with no apparent knowledge at all. *Some knowledge* is judged when students respond with specific examples from the appropriate classification, with attributes subordinate to the larger concept, or by citing defining characteristics of the concept. *Much knowledge* is judged when students place the concept within a superordinate (higher class) category, provide precise definitions of it, explain it by analogy, or appropriately link one concept with another on the same level. Teachers and students can also collaborate to create a prereading chart with the headings "What We Think We Know," "What We Want to Know," and "What We Found Out" (Marzano, Hagerty, Valencia, & DiStefano, 1987).

Many approaches that relate language and thinking in the later stages of language learning use B. S. Bloom's (1956) taxonomy of educational objectives. Bloom's taxonomy has influenced efforts to teach thinking strategies in both regular classrooms (e.g., Lundsteen, 1979; Tonjes & Zintz, 1987) and language intervention programs (Boyce & Larson, 1983; N. W. Nelson, 1988b; L. Schwartz & McKinley, 1984; Simon, 1985; Westby, 1991). Westby (1991) gave examples of questions that might be used in a social studies lesson to probe each of the six levels of Bloom's taxonomy:

Knowledge: Where did the Alaskan oil spill occur? What company owned the boat that caused the spill?

Comprehension: Describe how the Alaskan oil spill occurred.

Application: What are some other ways that the wildlife could have been rescued?

Analysis: What types of problems were created by the spill?

Synthesis: What kinds of problems would occur if there were a chemical spill in our town?

Evaluation: Discuss who should be responsible for the cleanup and why they should be responsible. (p. 19)

TABLE 12.1   A "practical intelligence" curriculum for success in school

I. MANAGING YOURSELF	II. MANAGING TASKS	III. COOPERATING WITH OTHERS
A. Overview of Managing Yourself 1. Introductory Lesson 2. Kinds of Intelligence: Definitions and Principles 3. Kinds of Intelligence: Multiple Intelligences 4. Kinds of Intelligence: Academic or Practical Intelligence 5. Understanding Test Scores 6. Exploring What You May Do 7. Accepting Responsibility 8. Collecting Your Thoughts and Setting Goals **B.** Learning Styles 9. What's Your Learning Style? 10. Taking in New Information 11. Showing What You Learned 12. Knowing How You Work Best 13. Recognizing the Whole and the Parts **C.** Improving Your Own Learning 14. Memory 15. Using What You Already Know 16. Making Pictures in Your Mind 17. Using Your Eyes—A Good Way to Learn 18. Recognizing the Point of View 19. Looking for the Best Way to Learn 20. Listening for Meaning 21. Learning by Doing	**A.** Overview of Solving Problems 22. Is There a Problem? 23. What Strategies Are You Using? 24. A Process to Help You Solve Problems 25. Planning a Way to Prevent Problems 26. Breaking Habits 27. Help with Our Problems **B.** Specific School Problems 28. Taking Notes 29. Getting Organized 30. Understanding Questions 31. Following Directions 32. Underlining—Finding the Main Idea 33. Noticing the Way Things Are Written 34. Choosing Between Mapping and Outlining 35. Taking Tests 36. Seeing Likenesses and Differences in Subjects 37. Getting It Done on Time	**A.** Communication 38. Class Discussions 39. What to Say 40. Tuning Your Conversation 41. Putting Yourself in Another's Place 42. Solving Problems in Communication **B.** Fitting into School 43. Making Choices—Adapting, Shaping, Selecting 44. Understanding Social Networks 45. Seeing the Network: Different Roles 46. Seeing the Network: Figuring Out the Rules 47. Seeing the Relationship Between Now and Later 48. What Does School Mean to You?

Note: From "Practical Intelligence for Success in School" by R. J. Sternberg, L. Okagaki, and A. S. Jackson, 1990, *Educational Leadership, 48*(1), p. 37. Reprinted with permission of the Association for Supervision and Curriculum Development. Copyright 1990 by ASCD. All rights reserved.

N. W. Nelson and Gillespie (1991) devised three sets of "Analogies for Thinking and Talking" that can be used as a framework to encourage similar kinds of cognitive–linguistic interactions in a social learning context. We designed one set of figurative analogies to tap visual–spatial analysis and synthesis abilities; a second to tap the ability to recognize and talk about analogical word meanings; the third set was represented entirely by pictures. We conducted field tests with adults with acquired brain injuries and with students who had language-learning disabilities, mild mental retardation, emotional problems, and varying degrees of hearing impairment. With mediational teaching and practice, almost everyone improved in the ability to complete the analogies correctly and to tell why other choices were not as good. One of the nicest outcomes was the development of confidence and skill in talking about and evaluating ideas in cooperative learning groups. The ability to engage in verbal analogical reasoning is one of the hallmarks of later language development (Nippold, 1986, 1988e) and one that deserves further attention.

Does research evidence show that intervention approaches designed to teach meta-awareness of language and learning strategies work? An overview of research on "talking about talking" (metalinguistics) and "thinking about thinking" by Chipman, Segal, and Glaser (1984) suggested that it is possible to change problem solving, memory, and abstract thinking by focusing consciously on the steps and strategies used to accomplish them. Research evidence gathered in the process of implementing the practical intelligence curriculum (Table 12.1) with 100 seventh-grade students (R. J. Sternberg et al., 1990) (contrasted with a control group) also supported the conclusion that it is possible to teach tacit knowledge and learning strategies.

Making aspects of the school culture curriculum and the hidden curriculum part of the official curriculum, as Sternberg and his colleagues did (R. J. Sternberg et al., 1990), may be the best pathway to building increased metacognitive proficiency. For other students, acquiring purposeful strategies of "executive control" through the use of mediational strategies may be preferred (described previously in one-to-one interactions with an "experienced, intentioned adult"; Feuerstein, 1979, p. 179). The adult mediators influence the acquisition of metacognitive strategies by modeling the language of mediated learning and then systematically assisting children to acquire self-mediating functions. Instructional techniques such as these have even been shown to influence the thinking of individuals with mental retardation (Feuerstein et al., 1988; Hagen et al., 1982) and with hearing impairments (Haywood et al., 1988).

It is impossible to talk about thinking without drawing on concepts of **memory.** In the pinball wizardry processing model illustrated in Figures 2.3 and 11.1, two types of memory, short-term and long-term memory, are represented as different entities. Long-term memory is noted as the mechanism for storing knowledge about events, things, abstract ideas, symbols, and rule systems within six rather different schemata (represented as boxes). Short-term memory is represented by the small black bidirectional arrows connecting all of the other components of the model. Rohwer and Dempster (1977) described the different kinds of storage functions this way:

> *Short-term memory represents information on a temporary basis and long-term memory represents information on a permanent basis. Moreover, since the contents of short-term memory are transitory, information can be continuously added and deleted in order to meet changing task demands. For example, in attempting to solve a problem it is often necessary to store and discard one partial result after another, while simultaneously coordinating these changes with the resources of long-term memory. Given these functions, it is clear why short-term memory is commonly referred to as the system's "working memory." By contrast, long-term memory plays a passive role in information processing; its primary importance arises from the fact that it represents the products of the individual's experience. These products range from the particular, such as individual letter codes, to the general, including strategies for processing and transforming new information. (p. 410)*

The trick in using metacognitive resources for intervention is to get learners to draw more actively and deliberately on experiential resources stored in long-term memory. Lahey and Bloom (1994) called this the limited capacity model (see Chapter 3). Because short-term memory is marked by a limited storage capacity, the learner must use storage and retrieval strategies while working on more complex and extensive sets of information. **Storage** is a person's mental representation of information in long-term memory. **Retrieval** is the process of returning to that information. The load on short-term memory capacity can be reduced by collapsing the number of units the person must remember. This can be done by applying conscious efforts to chunk or group together isolated bits of information into patterns that are easier to remember. Encoding information by using language or associating it with other information may facilitate long-term storage. Teachers and other professionals can encourage this process by arranging and organizing information to encourage the discovery of organizational processes, by instructing students directly in how to use such strategies, and by providing opportunities for practice (Rohwer & Dempster, 1977). B. Britton, Glynn, and Smith (1985) suggested that teachers could reduce the processing load associated with reading and remembering expository texts by (1) using titles, outlines, abstracts, and explicit descriptions to increase predictability; (2) priming students to pay attention to certain structure and content; (3) signaling transitions from phrase to phrase; and (4) controlling the number of concepts presented at one time.

Wiig (1984) compared the development of memory and memory strategies for academically achieving students and students with language-learning disabilities (see Table 12.2). She drew on descriptions of concept formation proposed by Bruner, Oliver, and Greenfield (1966), including (1) discrimination of the salient properties of objects, actions, and events; (2) categorization on the basis of those properties; (3) formation of superordinate concept for the category; and (4) generalization of this superordinate concept to other cases or contexts. Wiig noted that students with language-learning disabilities differ from other students because of inadequate memory capacity. Thus, they rely excessively on impulsive approaches, even though they often lead to blind alleys.

Instruction aimed specifically at teaching students to tie new information to old as a way to facilitate retrieval is called **mnemonic instruction.** Scruggs and Mastropieri (1990) described mnemonic techniques, including *key-word strategies* (using acoustically and semantically similar words, such as viper, to remember vituperation); *peg-word strategies* (using rhyming words to facilitate recall of numbered or ordered information); *acronym strategies* (using acronyms such as HOMES to remember the names of the Great Lakes, Huron, Ontario, Michigan, Erie, and Superior); *reconstructive elaborations* (using familiar and concrete associations to build elaborations of concepts); *phonemic mnemonics* (using sound patterns to build associations); and *spelling mnemonics* (using spelling patterns to build associations).

L. Schwartz and McKinley (1984) agreed that students with language-learning disabilities benefit from mnemonic strategies but cautioned against teaching them as isolated skills and making assumptions about background linguistic and nonlinguistic knowledge. Mnemonic strategies often make use of culturally based knowledge, which is not equally available to all participants (I remember when my husband tried to teach our daughter to associate *Bismarck* as the capital of North Dakota with jelly doughnuts, but first he had to teach her to call jelly doughnuts *Bismarcks*).

Metacognitive, Metalinguistic, and Metatextual Strategies for Focusing on Both Process and Product

In arguing that adolescents with language-learning disabilities should be taught strategies rather than specific course content, McKinley and Lord-Larson (1985) emphasized the importance of learning how to learn rather than what to learn. They commented that programs built on strategy acquisition would be more likely to help such students "generalize basic skills across situations, settings, and curricula" (p. 4). This philosophy is consistent with current general educational approaches that emphasize the value of process over products in the development of mature reading and writing.

Processes of mature reading and writing are guided metacognitively (as represented by the large upper arrow in the model in Figure 11.1). Purves (1981) noted that literacy involves more than simply reading words off a page—"one doesn't just read; one has a purpose for one's reading, and one reads for many purposes" (p. 77). Similarly, Odell (1981) noted that effective writers have something to communicate and that the process of writing involves discovering what they wish to say and how to say it. Nystrand (1982) emphasized purpose and control as important pragmatic factors associated with reading and writing as communicative acts.

Theorists have varied in the degree to which they believe that cognitive awareness controls literacy processes. LaBerge and Samuels (1987), for example, emphasized that automaticity is important because it allows mature readers to focus on deriving meaning rather than decoding words. Other researchers, however, emphasized that metacognitive monitoring of process may be essential for constructing meaning (e.g., Baker & Brown, 1984). Perhaps different processes are important at different developmental stages and for different purposes.

Tharp and Gallimore (1988) diagrammed four stages that involve differing degrees of automaticity. First, teachers and parents mediate beginning capacity within the zone of proximal development (Vygotsky, 1962).

TABLE 12.2   Overview of memory and memory strategy developmental patterns, with notation about delays among children and adolescents with learning disabilities

AGE LEVEL	POPULATION	SELECTIVE ATTENTION/REHEARSAL	ORGANIZATION/SERIAL RECALL	METAMEMORY
7–9 yr	Academic achievers	Can be taught to label and rehearse verbal labels/items at 6–7 yr.	Phonologically similar (goat–boat) are more often misrecognized than categorically related words (goat–sheep) at age 7.	Recognize that something should be done to facilitate memory but do not employ strategies spontaneously at age 7.
	Language-learning disabled	Show developmental delays in selective attention and in the acquisition of rehearsal strategies.	Can benefit from external organization by semantic category of pictured stimuli.	Show approximately a two-year delay in the use of past experiences and/or present context (complementary relations) and in the shift using generic (semantic) category for grouping.
10–13 yr	Academic achievers	Demonstrate efficient cumulative rehearsal at age 10, and verbal labeling, rehearsal, and chunking strategies at age 11.	Categorically related words (goat–sheep) are misrecognized more often than phonologically related words (goat–boat) at age 12. Central recall increases while incidental recall decreases significantly between ages 12 and 14.	Recognize and spontaneously employ rehearsal and categorization strategies.
	Language-learning disabled	Rehearsal strategies can be induced by reinforcement and verbal direction. Spontaneous rehearsal occurs with greater frequency for monosyllables than for multisyllabic words. Selective attention abilities better among reflective children and high modelers than among impulsive and low modeler counterparts.	External grouping and categorization of pictured stimuli can facilitate recall. Show random shifts in recalling foods but use grouping strategies for recalling animals.	The shift from using complementary relations to using generic category for grouping (thematic to taxonomic) was not completed at age 11.

Note: From "Language Disabilities in Adolescents: A Question of Cognitive Strategies" by E. H. Wiig. Reprinted from *Topics in Language Disorders,* Vol. 4, No. 2, p. 46, with permission of Aspen Publishers, Inc. © 1984.

Second, the child learns to assist his or her own processing with overt or covert verbal monitoring (also within the zone of proximal development). Third, automatization occurs through internalization of the strategy (extending learning beyond the zone of proximal development). Fourth, the child deautomatizes the task, analyzing the strategy and using it to learn new concepts. The final three stages may occur in recursive loops in which the child can use current understanding to become an active participant in further learning.

Recursive development patterns are typical of later learning and language processing. Researchers have used "thinking aloud protocols" (Emig, 1971; J. R. Hayes & Flower, 1980) to get normally developing secondary students to talk while composing written language. They have found that writing does not occur as a solid, evenly paced, uninterrupted activity from planning to proofreading. Rather, writing has a recursive rhythm that involves bursts of fluency, interspersed with pauses and revisions (Emig, 1971). This research has led to the development of "process-oriented" (rather than "product-oriented") instructional models.

> *Objective 3.* The student will use writing processes of preplanning, participating in author group discussions, drafting, reflecting on audience needs, revising, and editing with more independence and maturity than during baseline observations.

Writing Process Intervention Models.   According to process-oriented instructional models, writers generate the best products when they have "authentic" purposes for writing. Based on this philosophy, programs have been designed for both general educational special education students using the multiple processing stages: planning, drafting, revising, editing, sharing, and publication—not as isolated exercises but for real communicative purposes (Bos, 1988; J. R. Hayes & Flower, 1987; N. W. Nelson, 1988a, 1988b, 1988c; Nelson, Bahr, & Van Meter, in press).

Providing the opportunity to complete writing process steps with classmates who read and edit each others' work may encourage written language development among most students. Students with special education needs may require more direct modeling and explanation, using language they can understand and clear steps for planning. In addition, acceptance and encouragement from teachers may encourage students who have experienced failure to risk expressing themselves in writing and to overcome learned helplessness (Winograd & Niquette, 1988). Individuals who have experienced failure in reading also need to experience literacy as a process with its own rewards rather than as a product evaluated for acquisition (see Personal Reflection 12.2).

A staff member of a high school special services team (Carignan-Belleville, 1989) demonstrated the potential power of interactive literacy approaches with a seventh-grade student named Jason. Jason was described as having "writing paranoia" and a hearing impairment when Carignan-Belleville was brought in as a teacher consultant to work with him for 1 hour/week. Jason had previously announced to his teachers and the hearing specialist that he did not plan to write any more journals, essays, or book reports. The reason he gave was that he simply could not do it. Carignan-Belleville started the intervention by discussing with Jason a game of baseball his team had recently won. She asked him to give her three reasons why his team had deserved to win. After he had done so orally, she said, "Let's put that in writing," and provided him with the following format for organizing his short essay:

> *Question: Who won Saturday's baseball game?*
>
> *Five-sentence paragraph*
>
> *1. Topic sentence: (Answer to the question)*
> *2. Reason #1*
> *3. Reason #2*
> *4. Reason #3*
> *5. Conclusion: (Restate topic sentence in different words.) (1989, pp. 57–58)*

The organizational strategy and oral language rehearsal of this approach gave Jason sufficient support to

---

PERSONAL REFLECTION 12.2 _____

"Poor readers who suffer from learned helplessness need to spend more time interacting with books that interest them. These children, in particular, need to understand that success in reading is defined as the fulfillment of one's own purposes, not as one's placement relative to others."

Peter Winograd and *Garland Niquette* (1988, p. 52).

---

write an acceptable essay. Over time, Jason's writing continued to improve. Carignan-Belleville (1989) gave him story starters (e.g., "If I had more money . . . "), and these made him willing to attempt the journal writing he had once hated. He also was encouraged to dictate his stories first into a tape recorder and then transcribe them. As Jason began to experience more success, he also began to want to read books. A particularly interesting aspect of Jason's case study for language specialists is the way that improved competency in one modality encouraged increased effort in others.

Objective 4. The student will use reading process strategies to talk about purposes, text organization, finding the answers to questions, and comprehension monitoring with more independence and maturity than during baseline observations.

Improving Reading Comprehension with Metacognition. Metacognitive techniques can improve reading comprehension (A. L. Brown & Palincsar, 1982; Palincsar & Brown, 1987; Palincsar & Ransom, 1988). Metacognition is a good predictor of mature reading in normal development. Forrest-Pressley and Waller (1984) studied third and sixth graders who were poor, average, and good readers. They found that only older and better readers employed metacognitive strategies effectively.

Metacognitive intervention to improve written language comprehension may take a variety of forms, some previously discussed in this chapter. Students might be taught strategies for using advance organizers, self-questioning, and self-monitoring of their own comprehension.

Providing students with objectives before they read is an example of an advance organizer. When objectives are provided in advance, students are more likely to learn targeted material (Tierney & Cunningham, 1984). Other advance organizers include pretests, prequestions, and the PREP described previously (Langer, 1982). These may also alert students to the nature of particular tasks and help them acquire strategies to evaluate, categorize, and generalize information as they read.

A related metacognitive technique involves guiding students to become conscious of the purpose of a particular reading activity. For example, Tierney and Cunningham (1984) summarized four steps found to increase reading comprehension:

Step 1: Establish purposes(s) for comprehending.

Step 2: Have students read or listen for the established purposes(s).

Step 3: Have students perform some task which directly reflects and measures accomplishment of each established purpose for comprehending.

Step 4: Provide direct informative feedback concerning students' comprehension based on their performance of that (those) task(s). (p. 625)

The metacognitive strategy of self-questioning relies on mediational techniques described previously. When using self-questioning approaches, remember that asking good questions may not come automatically, particularly for students with language disorders. These students may need intensive modeling before they can use self-questions effectively on their own. For example, Wong and Jones (1982) taught a group of 120 learning disabled eighth and ninth graders and normally achieving sixth graders to use self-questioning strategies to monitor their understanding of important textual units. They did this in five steps:

(a) What are you studying this passage for? (So you can answer some questions you will be given later); (b) Find the main idea/ideas in the paragraph and underline it/them; (c) Think of a question about the main idea you have underlined. Remember what a good question should be like. (Look at the prompt); (d) Learn the answer to your question; (e) Always look back at the questions and answers to see how each successive question and answer provides you with more information. (p. 231)

The results (Wong & Jones, 1982) showed an increased awareness of important textual units. Students with learning disabilities also learned to monitor their own understanding of text units and to formulate good questions about them. As a result, their comprehension performance improved. The procedure did not increase the metacomprehension or comprehension performance of the normally achieving sixth graders to a similar degree. Wong and Jones interpreted this as evidence that the normally achieving students were already processing the texts actively compared to the inactive approaches taken by the adolescents with learning disabilities.

A related strategy-based approach to enhance written language comprehension of expository texts is called **multipass** (Schumaker et al., 1982). It is based on an adaptation of a widely known procedure originally published in 1946 to train soldiers rapidly for specialized jobs during World War II (Robinson, 1970). The acronym SQ3R represents the five strategic steps of this approach. As summarized by Just and Carpenter (1987), readers should (1) **survey,** by skimming the table of contents, major headings, illustrations, and summary paragraphs to become familiar with the text's general outline, main topics, and organization; (2) generate **questions** based on headings and topics to learn to be attentive and to think about what is already known about the topic; (3) **read** one section of the chapter at a time, while trying to answer the question posed for that section; (4) **recite** possible answers to the questions, citing examples from notes or memory; and (5) **review,** by

going over main points with the help of notes, citing subpoints, and trying to memorize both the main points and subpoints.

Another self-questioning approach taught students to identify task demands to guide comprehension (Raphael & Pearson, 1982). Students learned to examine textbook questions and to label them differentially depending on whether they required the students (1) to locate an answer in the text (**right there**); (2) to derive an answer from the student's own background knowledge (**on my own**); or (3) to derive an answer that involved inferring relationships among text segments (**think and search**). (See Box 12.4 for an adaptation of this approach.)

Box 12.4 _____

Minilesson on Comprehension Strategies for Relationships within and across Sentences. (This minilesson was designed by Shannon Kersten, modified from suggestions by Raphael and Pearson, 1982).

ANSWERING QUESTIONS FROM TEXTS

(1) Right There   **(2) Here and There**   **(3) Think Questions**

My teacher this year is Ms. Jenkins. She is a great teacher. She loves to play games with us during inside recess and sometimes during outside recess. When it is cold out though, Ms. Jenkins doesn't even like to come outside during recess, so we play with some of the fifth-grade teachers. She gets lots of colds during the winter and sometimes tells us she wished she lived in Florida!

Ms. Jenkins is teaching us about plants and animals this week in school. Our class is going on a field trip on November 19th to learn more about plants and animals. We are going to Yellowstone National Park! We will be camping in tents for two nights. There will be 20 students and 5 adults including Ms. Jenkins. It is supposed to snow the last day we are there. That probably won't make Ms. Jenkins very happy!

QUESTIONS: Tell whether the question is: (1) a "Right There" question, (2) a "Here and There" question, or (3) a "Think" question.

1. When are the students in Ms. Jenkins' class going on the field trip?
2. Which of the following is Ms. Jenkins most likely to do if it snows while the class is on the field trip: (Underline the clues in the story that helped you find the answer.)
   a. make snow angels with her students
   b. take an extra long hike in the snow
   c. let the other adults take the children on the hike while she stays inside
   d. have a snowball fight with her class
3. What would be some other field trips the class could take when learning about plants and animals?
4. Where are some places that you have gone for school field trips?
5. How many students went on this field trip?

Monitoring one's own comprehension is a strategy that can be acquired. Research has shown that task demands may influence comprehension monitoring to appear as early as age 2 or as late as age 12 in normal development (Dollaghan, 1987b). As Dollaghan cautioned, "trying to understand a message requires effort on the part of the listener, and even normal listeners do not try to construct meaning representations for all the messages they receive" (p. 47). The failure to construct an adequate representation of message meaning cannot be detected unless a receiver has made an attempt to understand the message. (The comprehension monitoring program designed by Dollaghan & Kaston, 1986, was described in Chapter 10.)

Summary of Metaskills and How to Teach Them

This review has provided examples of intervention programs designed to teach students to use learning strategies. Strategies include **metapragmatic** strategies to manage expectations of classroom communication events, **metacognitive** strategies to learn, think, and remember, and **process** strategies to guide writing and reading tasks.

Professionals across disciplines may implement such programs. Speech–language pathologists or other language specialists contribute awareness of the unique relationships between language abilities and learning strategies. Particularly when task expectations include highly language-related components such as discourse knowledge and verbal mediation techniques, individuals with intrinsic language disorders may need deliberate instruction to analyze tasks and remember steps in problem-solving strategies. Westby (1991) reported that many young adults who have acquired strategies and *can* use them, nevertheless do not use them in real life. When she asked university students why not, they gave reasons that suggested that they thought the strategies might take too much time or that they liked doing it their old way better.

To overcome such barriers, Seidenberg (1988) suggested that strategy instruction should be systematic. She suggested seven steps for teaching cognitive strategies: (1) Introduce the strategy and review the student's current performance. (2) Explain the relevance of the strategy by using real-life examples. (3) Describe the strategy and provide a "help sheet" that lists its steps.

(4) Model the strategy and rehearse it with students as a group. (5) Provide opportunity to practice using controlled materials, with prompts and corrective feedback as necessary. (6) With the student, evaluate the data gathered during practice with controlled materials. (7) Provide further practice using textbook materials drawn from the regular curriculum. In my experience, children can use their own textbook materials for learning strategies. Starting at step 4 in this sequence and using the regular curriculum as the source of practice materials can stimulate motivation and facilitate carryover of new strategies.

DEVELOPING COMPETENCE IN DISCOURSE GENRES AND EVENTS

GOAL: The student will comprehend and produce language effectively using conversational, narrative, and expository discourse genres.

- Interacting for Business or Pleasure: The Conversational Genre
- Understanding and Telling Stories: The Narrative Genre
- Getting and Giving Information: The Expository Genre

OUTCOME: The student will communicate successfully in social interactions and will succeed academically in school.

Three kinds of discourse genres—conversational, narrative, and expository—were discussed in Chapter 11 as contexts to probe during informal assessment. Decisions to target language knowledge and skills within one or more of these discourse contexts are made when participants identify zones of significance that involve them.

Individualization based on interview reports is important. After reviewing the literature on conversational deficits among children with specific language impairments (SLI), for example, Brinton and Fujiki (1995) reported that "Many (but not all) children with SLI have difficulty with many (but not all) aspects of conversational behavior. For some of these children, conversational difficulty is relatively subtle; for others it is a primary concern" (p. 184). Windsor (1995) noted that "Although the degree of overlap between language skills and social skills is debatable, there is no question that the presence of language impairments is correlated with social skills impairments" (p. 214). She cited evidence from research on learning disabilities, behavior and emotional disorders, and behaviors, such as challenging behaviors (see Chapter 13), which elicit negative responses.

If getting along with and being accepted by peers is identified as an area of particular concern, the specialist may target social conversational discourse with peers. If a student has difficulty comprehending written language stories, the specialist may probe the student's intrinsic and explicit knowledge of narrative structure. If concerns expressed by students, teachers, and parents center around academic difficulties in science and social studies or mathematics, targeting new skills to understand expository texts about them may be most appropriate.

Development of intervention plans might also involve choices of communicative events using one or more discourse type. Contextually based language intervention involves analyzing the demands and opportunities of currently available communicative events and deciding whether new communicative opportunities should be provided. Communicative events involving one or more of the three discourse types may be found throughout the regular curriculum and as students make transitions into employment settings.

Interacting for Business or Pleasure: The Conversational Genre

Conversation may be defined broadly as uses of language for social interaction. Conversation is the primary context for all natural language learning and a key context for language intervention. Hoskins (1990; see Personal Reflection 12.3) pointed out that reading and

PERSONAL REFLECTION 12.3 _____

"We not only are continuously learning language, but, in our interactions in language, we are constantly developing the narratives that comprise who we are, how we think of ourselves, and how we present ourselves to others."

Barbara Hoskins (1990, p. 60), Language/Learning Disabilities Consultant in Pasadena, California.

writing are also social interactive phenomena. She noted that written language interactions between authors and readers may be targeted for intervention as conversational events, just as oral interactions between speakers and listeners are. Students may be encouraged to act as conversational partners, imagining the absent audience for a piece they are writing or imagining the author of the work they are reading. Some of the techniques described in the previous section on metaskills may help to encourage such perspective taking.

Strategies for targeting social conversation in assessment and intervention were discussed in Chapter 10 (e.g., Brinton & Fujiki, 1989). This chapter adds consideration of the specialized needs of later-stage language learners for interacting in classrooms, with peers, and in family conversations.

Objective 1. The student will participate in classroom conversations (large and small group), showing appropriate: (1) turn taking (signaling, frequency, length); (2) language formulation (on topic, brief); (3) clarification requests (frequency, situation, structure) and (4) comprehension (appropriate responses, direction following).

Conversing in Classrooms. Participating in classroom conversations, as considered earlier in this chapter, requires a special set of linguistic and social skills but not a uniform set of skills. Part of the complexity of knowing how to participate in classroom conversations stems from the fact the rules for conversational access vary across classrooms and across discourse events (Bloome & Knott, 1985). Even within a single event, individual children may experience communicative demands and opportunities differently (Cazden, 1988; F. Erickson & Schultz, 1981; N. W. Nelson, 1986; Silliman & Lamanna, 1986).

Some aspects of classroom discourse superficially might seem less demanding than other forms of social interaction discourse. If only syntactic demands are considered for explaining the demands of answering teachers' questions, the lack of complexity might seem remarkable at first. In her analysis of formal classroom discourse, Sturm (1990) found that MLU counts for students did not vary significantly among first- (mean = 3.7), third- (mean = 4.6), and fifth-grade (mean = 4.8) classrooms. None of these expressive language means surpassed a level of complexity expected for preschoolers, but looks may be deceiving.

To be appropriate in classroom conversations, students need to keep their responses short and to the point (see Box 12.3). As Leonard and Fey (1991) pointed out, ellipsis is one of the bulwarks of conversation. It allows speakers to converse without repeating information already contained in prior utterances. Considerable syntactic sophistication, however, is required for a speaker to analyze specific grammatical elements that should be retained and replaced during ellipsis processes. For example, when an adult asks, "Who eats worms?," and a child responds, "I don't," the child must have analyzed the verb phrase as the focus of the question and have selected the appropriate auxiliary verb to replace it. Children with language impairments may need special practice in making their responses accurate, relevant, and brief. Language specialists should take particular note of these classroom conversation demands because of their more natural tendency to require students to give complete and elaborated responses to questions. A minilesson discussion about the different purposes and styles of responding may help, followed by practice.

Not only expressive but receptive demands of classroom conversations must be understood. With advancing grade level, children are faced with advancing syntactic complexity in their teachers' language (N. W. Nelson, 1984). Both Sturm (1990) and Cuda (1976) found significant increments in syntactic complexity of teacher talk beyond third grade, and neither found significant differences between first and third grades (Sturm's data resulted in mean T-unit MLUs of 7.5, 7.9 and 9.7 for first-, third-, and fifth-grade teachers, respectively). Teachers use considerable figurative language even in the early grades (Lazar, Warr-Leeper, Nicholson, & Johnson, 1989; N. W. Nelson, 1984), but the demands on cognitive processing of teacher talk increase with grade level. Students must learn to listen, take notes, organize their own thoughts, follow classroom rules for talking and not talking, think about what they are hearing and relate it to what they already know, and imagine absent contexts and textbook authors as they try to understand classroom language.

When children in classroom conversations have opportunities to do more than answer teachers' questions, the demands on their pragmatic and syntactic systems increase accordingly. Ervin-Tripp and Gordon (1986) studied children's skill in making requests. They found that before the age of 8 years, children had sufficient control of advanced syntactic structures and politeness markers to modulate features such as urgency, force, friendliness, and demand. Children above third grade demonstrated clear advantages in classroom strategies for making effective requests, such as requesting marker pens and other supplies from busy adults. The younger children used direct strategies, conveying assumptions that adults had the materials and would comply:

> *I need a blue marker.*
> *Where's the marker?*
> *Can I have the letter to my parents? (Ervin-Tripp & Gordon, 1986, p. 87)*

The older children used more indirect strategies, acknowledging that the addressee might not comply with the request and might view the request as intrusion:

> *Are there any more markers?*
> *Do you have a green marker I could use?*
> *She told me to get a letter for my parents. (Ervin-Tripp & Gordon, 1986, p. 87)*

Wilkinson, Milosky, and Genishi (1986) observed different strategies for making classroom requests, depending on the cultural backgrounds of individual children. They expressed concern that therapeutic activities aimed at teaching students mainstream strategies for looking at an intended listener, addressing the listener by name, and waiting for attention before speaking may conflict with some students' cultural customs. Nevertheless, Wilkinson and her colleagues found more similarities than differences among small-group academic conversations between monolingual English-speaking and bilingual Hispanic students. They suggested that effective speakers could be defined by their ability to elicit a response from their partners. Box 12.5 summarizes general behaviors that might be targeted in the intervention process, as long as cultural differences are respected.

Silliman and Lamanna (1986) studied the strategies that elementary school children use to get and keep the floor in classroom discussion, including turn overlaps and interruptions. They noted that teachers may control these turn disruptions to some extent but that children need systematic opportunities to practice turn taking in the classroom.

Box 12.5 _____

Request Characteristics of Effective Speakers

A successful request is likely to be:

1. *Direct:* Use of linguistic forms that directly signal the speaker's needs. For requests for action, the imperative or *I want/I need* statements; for requests for information, the *Wh-, yes–no* or tag question.

   Direct requests: *How do you do this one?, I need a pencil;*
   Indirect requests: *I don't get this, Anybody have a pencil?*

2. *Designated to a listener:* Unambiguously indicates the intended listener through verbal or nonverbal means:

   C: Sally, where do you put the dollar sign? *or*
   C: (*looking at P*) Did you get that one?

3. *Sincere:* According to Labov and Fanshel (1978), a request is sincere if (a) the action, purpose, and need for the request are clear; for example, in a request for information, the listener believes that the speaker really wants the information and does not already know the information; (b) there is both an ability and an obligation of the listener to respond to the request; and (c) the speaker has a right to make the request.

   Sincere: "John, I can't find the price for hamburger."
   Insincere: "Well, slow-poke, what one are you finally up to now?"

4. *Revised if unsuccessful:* A restatement of a request previously made by the same speaker to the same listener who had not responded appropriately:

   A: "Bob, I need a pencil:"
   B: "Uh?"
   A: "Bob, can I borrow a pencil?"

5. *On task:* Related to the academic content or procedures and materials of the assignment.

   On task: "Is this one add or subtract?"
   Off task: "Whaddya gonna do at recess?"

6. *Responded to appropriately:* The requested action or information was given or else a reason was given why the action and/or information could not be given.

Appropriate response:	C: "Alice, what's five?"
	A: "I got 22 for that one."
Inappropriate response:	C: "Alice, what's five?"
	A: "What did you get for it?"

Note: From "Second Language Learners' Use of Requests and Responses in Elementary Classrooms" by L. C. Wilkinson, L. M. Milosky, and C. Genishi. Reprinted from *Topics in Language Disorders,* Vol. 6, No. 2, p. 59, with permission of Aspen Publishers, Inc., © 1986.

Teachers can increase the opportunity for private dialogue with individual students by interacting with them using dialogue journals. Lindfors (1987) noted that dialogue journals give students a chance to express their personal wanderings, opinions, grievances, anger, and anticipation. C. W. Hayes and Bahruth (1985) described a fifth-grade classroom where teachers interacted in a dialogue with a reluctant writer. On the first day, when the children turned in their journals, Larry's first page was blank. The ensuing written conversation:

T: *How can we answer you if you don't write?*
L: *I don't like writing.*
T: *Does anything bother you about writing?*
L: *I don't like to write because I can't not spell right. That's bother me about writing.*
T: *Don't worry about it right now. The more you read and write the better your spelling will get. Just worry about getting your ideas written down. (p. 99)*

Speech–language pathologists might use similar dialogue journals to interact with their students; using journals written during regular classroom experiences may be more advantageous (Swoger, 1989). The speech–language pathologist who is granted access to writing produced during the regular or special classroom might have a rich source of data about the child's continuing language development. The naturalistic quality of conversing with a known partner in writing might also provide a powerful context for learning more elaborate language forms and vocabulary when previous language learning experiences have not been positive.

Objective 2. The student will participate in conversations with peers, showing appropriate: (1) assertive and responsive balance; (2) age-appropriate slang; (3) topic continuation strategies; (4) conversation entering and exiting strategies; and (5) conflict resolution strategies.

Conversing with Peers. Wiig and Semel (1976) viewed social perception as a component language skill. Donahue and Bryan (1984) commented:

Perhaps in no other developmental phase is the relationship between communicative skills and peer group membership as apparent as in adolescence. (p. 11)

Donahue and Bryan (1984) particularly mentioned the importance of slang in identifying group membership and also noted its importance to language and learning disabled youth who are often cast as "outsiders" (learning from peers was identified as the "underground curriculum" earlier in Chapter 11). Based on informal observation (owing to a lack of research data on the topic), Donahue and Bryan reported that the use of slang by students with learning disabilities related to the amount of interaction of these students with students who had no disabilities and appeared to lag by about 6 months to 1 year.

Donahue and Bryan (1984) commented that this problem might be partially remedied by structuring social and academic experiences of students with learning disabilities to increase their opportunities to learn adolescent social skills through satisfying peer interactions. Those authors commented that peers make the best coaches and that "No adult could keep up with the rapid changes in slang nor fully appreciated the fine nuances of its meaning" (p. 19).

In summarizing approaches to intervention for peer interaction problems, T. Bryan (1986) recognized three types: direct instruction, structured situations, and group-training programs. The structured situations that involved peer modeling seemed to be the most effective (although it is difficult to generalize across studies). The problem with the direct instruction approaches was that practicing a verbal behavior in one kind of discourse event (direct instruction) was insufficient to encourage its generalization to others. Bryan concluded that, "Not only particular verbal skills must be taught but also the parameters of the situations in which the child is expected to display these skills" (p. 251). Structured situations in which peers served as models of the targeted behaviors (e.g., asking open-ended questions in the talk show format), however, were found to be highly effective. The fact that students with learning disabilities could abstract conversational rules by listening to very few examples suggested that the students already had elements of the conversational skills in their repertoires and only needed to be taught the parameters of social situations in which they were appropriate.

Several programs aimed at helping adolescents with communicative disorders to acquire social communication skills have now been published (Hazel, Schumaker,

Sherman, & Sheldon-Wildgen, 1981; Hoskins, 1987; LaGreca & Mesibov, 1981; Minskoff, 1982; Wanat, 1983; Wiig, 1982). However, clear evidence regarding their effectiveness is not yet available. To evaluate these programs, Donahue and Bryan (1984) suggested asking the following questions:

- Will the acquisition of these skills allow students to meet peer as well as adult norms for appropriate communicative style? It is important to recognize that target behaviors are likely to be selected because they appeal to adult expectations. For example, should educators be teaching rules for polite requests or how to engage in friendly exchanges of insults?
- Will this training program enable students to discern how and when to use their newly acquired skills in naturalistic settings?
- Will use of these communicative skills enhance the adolescent's social acceptance with peers and adults? (p. 19)

One modeling program successful in encouraging adolescent students to exhibit greater competence in conversations is the model, analyze, practice (MAP) approach described by Hess and Fairchild (1988). A group of adolescents with learning disabilities participated in six weekly, 1-hour sessions. The adolescents viewed videotaped models of desirable and undesirable interactions, analyzed the models, and practiced the targeted skills of topic initiation, topic maintenance, and using open-ended questions and follow-up questions and comments to sustain the dialogue. In one segment, the students observed a videotaped sample in which each exchange consisted of one utterance per participant and one turn exchange:

> **SPEAKER 1:** *What are your hobbies?*
> **SPEAKER 2:** *I like to build models and play basketball.*
> **SPEAKER 1:** *Do you go to movies?*
> **SPEAKER 2:** *Yes.*
> **SPEAKER 1:** *How is your marching band doing?*
> **SPEAKER 2:** *Okay.*

After analyzing this sample, the students were shown a version where more effective conversational strategies were used:

> **SPEAKER 1:** *What are your hobbies?*
> **SPEAKER 2:** *I like to build models and play basketball.*

> **SPEAKER 1:** *Do you play basketball for your school team?*
> **SPEAKER 2:** *No. I play for fun with my friends. I'm not tall enough for the school team.*
> **SPEAKER 1:** *I didn't think so. I play basketball on one of the YMCA teams.*
> **SPEAKER 2:** *Oh yeah. How did you get on that team?*

The students then were assisted to analyze and compare the two samples, writing down their observations. They were encouraged to return to the first videotaped sample when necessary to check details. The third step in the procedure was to practice the better conversational techniques and to analyze their effectiveness. They videotaped themselves conversing about self-chosen topics so that they could practice the desirable features they had identified and critique their own performance when finished. If they identified problems, they retaped their conversations, again attempting to incorporate the group's suggestions, and again, analyzing the improvement. This approach is consistent with many of the principles of mediated learning and of strategy acquisition discussed previously.

Problems with peer acceptance have been consistently noted in the literature on learning disabilities (e.g., Bruininks, 1978; J. H. Bryan & Sherman, 1980; C. L. Fox, 1989; Vaughn, McIntosh, & Spencer-Rowe, 1991), and occasionally for individuals with other disabilities, such as hearing impairment (Gagné, Stelmacovich, & Yovetich, 1991) (see Personal Reflection 12.4). Peer acceptance is a central problem of the syndrome of autism (e.g., Schopler & Mesibov, 1986). Gallagher (1991)

PERSONAL REFLECTION 12.4

"Peer interaction is an essential component of the individual child's development. Experience with peers is not a superficial luxury to be enjoyed by some children and not others, but is a necessity in childhood socialization. And among the most sensitive indicators of difficulties in development are failure by the child to engage in the activities of the peer culture and failure to occupy a relatively comfortable place within it."

William Hartup (1983, p. 220), child development specialist, writing in a chapter entitled "Peer Interaction and the Behavioral Development of the Individual Child."

noted that negative social consequences were among the first problems identified in the early literature on speech–language pathology. Gallagher also noted that despite this fact, and despite the centrality of language as the primary means of interpersonal contact and socialization of children, "the profession has been slow to develop assessment and intervention programs that deal with language disorders in social interaction terms" (p. 11).

To identify specific skills to target for an individual student, the specialist must thoroughly understand expected social interaction patterns within that child's culture and potential influences of the child's disability and should investigate peer reactions to current interaction behaviors. For example, Gagné and co-workers (1991) staged scenes in which a group of "hearing impaired" actors interacted with normal-hearing college students. Gagné and co-workers asked another group of students to rate the acceptability of the clarification requests dramatized by "hearing impaired" students. The researchers found that reactions were more favorable when the "hearing impaired" actors used specific rather than nonspecific requests.

Similar studies might be conducted on a smaller scale for individual students within their own communities. For both assessment and intervention, aspects of the MAP sequence (Hess & Fairchild, 1988, described previously) could be implemented. However, instead of providing the group experience only for children with disabilities, professionals could include normally developing peer volunteers as partners.

Peers may be enlisted in conversational skills intervention programs in a variety of roles. Gallagher (1991) noted that "they can become directly involved in the intervention program by serving as peer partners or be involved more indirectly through their participation in cooperative group experiences" (p. 32). Some training of peer partners is probably necessary to teach them to use verbal and nonverbal communication strategies to facilitate partner participation.

A conversational skills intervention program might be used in the regular curriculum in early adolescent life skills classes that tend to be taught at the junior high school level. Even youngsters presumably developing normally may benefit from direct instruction in social interaction skills. D. W. Johnson and Johnson (1990) found, for example, that before children could succeed

in working toward mutual goals in cooperative learning groups, they needed to

> (1) get to know and trust one another, (2) communicate accurately and unambiguously, (3) accept and support one another, and (4) resolve conflicts constructively. (p. 30)

To teach such skills, teachers need to help students see the need to work cooperatively and to believe that they will be better off if they know how to do so. Teachers can assist the process by making the use of strategies for encouraging participation explicit. For example, D. W. Johnson and Johnson (1990) suggested using a chart, with the heading "encouraging participation" across the top and two vertical columns labeled "looks like" and "sounds like." The cue for the nonverbal *smiles* may be paired with the verbal suggestion, "What is your idea?"; *eye contact* may be paired with "Awesome!"; *thumbs up* with "Good idea!"; and *pat on back* with "That's interesting" (p. 30). Figure 12.2 shows how we adapted these suggestions in a minilesson.

The occasion for a minilesson on the encouraging and discouraging things we say to ourselves and others arose with Marcie, a student with Down syndrome who was participating in our computer-based writing lab. Over and over Marcie made disparaging remarks to herself. Every day, we heard at least one of the following, "I'm so dumb," "I'm so ugly," "This is a stupid story." She was not the only student who made such remarks. Others teased and insulted members of their author groups instead of themselves, but the self-esteem problems were rampant, and our efforts to reassure seemed only to reinforce these damaging forms of self-talk and conversation. Always looking for ways to help students revise their stories of themselves while getting as much linguistic, communicative, and cognitive mileage as possible from our minilessons, we hit upon a strategy that we have reused with numerous other groups of middle-school students. It always has a positive effect. The lesson has several parts, illustrated in Figure 12.2, and it works best if connected to outside experiments involving conversations at home and school as well as in our writing and homework labs.

As Donahue and Bryan (1984) pointed out, not all peer interactions are equally appealing to adults. Normal social interactions among peers may include ritualized insults and dispute behavior as well as other kinds

FIGURE 12.2   Four-step minilesson on encouraging and discouraging.

Step One. Write the word "courage" in the middle of a chalkboard. Have the students brainstorm what the word means and add key words in a semantic web.

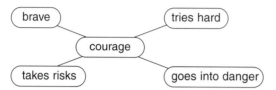

Step Two. Add the prefix "dis-" to the beginning of the word in a different colored chalk. Ask what happens to the meaning then. Students generally say things like, "It takes away your courage," and "You don't try." You can cross out related qualities out on the semantic web to dramatize the meaning.

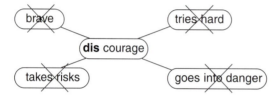

Step Three. Replace the "dis-" prefix with "en-," also in a different color. Ask the students what they think the word means now, and rebuild the semantic web.

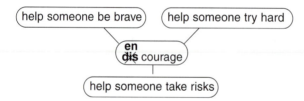

Step Four. Break into smaller groups of two to three students. Help the students list nonverbal and verbal ways they communicate messages to themselves and others in a chart with two columns:

Encouraging Things I Say and Do	**Dis**couraging Things I Say and Do

of exchanges. Although adults may not wish to encourage children's disputes because they seem to be mostly negative, learning to argue fairly and effectively can have positive outcomes and is part of achieving adult communicative competence.

Brenneis and Lein (1977) studied arguments among children in third- and fourth-grade classrooms who were all white, primarily middle class, and normally developing. The researchers categorized the content of 70 role plays of verbal arguments and found that a limited set of categories accounted for virtually all assertions or responses made by the children in disputes (see Box 12.6).

Although the examples in Box 12.6 are probably familiar to anyone who remembers childhood, such categories appear rarely if ever in assessment protocols, formal or informal. They serve here as reminders to consider the range of contexts in which children need to participate and the varied skills they need to become competent communicators. Another behavior Brenneis and Lein (1977) identified was the overt labeling of some speech acts, such as threats and insults (e.g., "Don't you threaten me"). This metapragmatic awareness might also be encouraged through direct modeling and role play. Children with disabilities could be taught to identify and to participate as more competitive partners in dispute discourse if they learn how to recognize it and label it, as well as how to use appropriate language and speech acts to participate.

Stevens and Bliss (1995) studied the conflict resolution abilities of third- to sixth-grade students with specific language impairments (SLI) compared with those of their normal language-learning peers. Students participated in two tasks, both of which might serve as language intervention contexts. The role enactment task was presented to dyads of children who were told:

> I will present some situations to you. I would like you to act out what you would do and say as if this was really happening to you. (p. 603)

For example, "Both of you sit, facing each other but not touching each other, and have an argument about who is the strongest" (p. 603). Students with SLI performed much like their peers on this task, except that they tended to have more difficulty using questions in the interactions, as well as using the higher level skills of persuasion, cooperation, and negotiation. The second task, hypothetical stories, was relatively harder for the students with SLI. Thus, it might be saved for later stages of intervention. The directions for this task were:

> I would like to know how boys [girls] like you think about things. I'm going to tell you some things that happen to a boy [girl]. Then I'd like you to think of all the things

---

Box 12.6 _____

Content Categories Observed in the Verbal Arguments of Third and Fourth Graders (Summarized from Brenneis & Lein, 1977, pp. 51–53)

1. Threats: "I'll kill you." "I'm going to tell the teacher on you."
1'. Bribes: "I'll give you a dollar if you can." "I'll give it right back to you."
2. Insults: "You dummy." "Your shirt is filthy."
2'. Praise: "You are smart." "You sure look pretty today."
3. Command: "Give it back." "Don't say that."
3'. Moral persuasion: "I had it first." "It's my brother's."
4. Negating or contradictory assertion: JULIE: "I'm the strongest."
                                          JOHN: "*I'm* the strongest."
4'. Simple assertion: "That's my shirt you're wearing." "I'm so strong I can lift you up."
5. Denial response: "No, you can't." "Unh-unh."
5'. Affirmative (often delivered ironically): "Yes." "Yes, I want it."
6. Supportive assertion: (It's mine) "Because I bought it." (I'm stronger) "Because I'm bigger than you."
6'. Demand for evidence: "Prove it." "How do you know?" "I bet you can't."
7. Nonword vocal signals: "Nyeeh-nyeeh." "Aaaargh."

he [she] can do about it. Tell me everything that comes into your head. Pretend that all the boys [girls] are [age of subject] years old. (p. 603)

When practicing such discourse events, the change process might involve targeting skills that are being addressed in the regular curriculum. Many schools today do include peacemaking and conflict resolution as part of the curriculum. In the summer program we operate in an inner-city school in Kalamazoo, for example, we posted and practiced strategies that students had been learning in the prior schoolyear to resolve the many real conflicts that arose. We used the "Win/Win Guidelines" [reducing the steps for some children who could not handle all of them] proposed by Drew (1987) to guide the process:

1. *Take time for cooling off, if needed. Find alternative ways to express your anger.*
2. *Using "I messages," each person states his/her feelings and the problem as he/she sees it. No blaming, no name calling, no interrupting.*
3. *Each person states the problem as the other person sees it.*
4. *Each person states how he/she is responsible for the problem.*
5. *Brainstorm solutions together and choose a solution that satisfies both—a Win/Win solution.*
6. *Affirm your partner. (p. 11)*

Another form of peer interaction discourse that is not often sanctioned by adults, but which may be a rich context for learning to communicate through writing, is surreptitious passing of social notes (Lindfors, 1987; N. W. Nelson, 1988c; see Figure 12.3). In Personal Reflection 12.5, Lindfors considers the rationale for discouraging the passing of social notes and recommends encouraging them (unless removing the forbidden aspect of the process lessens its desirability for children and adolescents, in which case it should just be ignored). Lindfors described the kind of rich communicative interactions in notes that she had been privileged to read, including a series of lengthy personal Eskimo-style ritual insults that the teacher had taught them. Do children with disabilities have the same kinds of opportunities for learning through written conversational exchanges where no red pencil is expected? If not, can we facilitate similar opportunities without spoiling their essence? It is worth a try.

PERSONAL REFLECTION 12.5 _____

"To me, one of the most intriguing types of personal writing that children seem to engage in so naturally is note passing. I find it interesting that we try so hard to stamp out this activity that is written personal communication at its very best! That it is so resistant to our stamping out efforts should tell us how meaningful this activity is to our children. Note passing is alive and well—thriving—in most of the classrooms I visit. And it should be! It involves everything we would ask of a communication experience; it is purposeful and relevant communication for the child; it is language used for a valid function (personal); it receives relevant and immediate feedback in the response of the receiver. Why, then, do we pounce with such zeal on the note being passed from hand to hand under the desks and across the aisles?"

From *Judith Wells Lindfors, Children's Language and Learning,* Second Edition. Copyright © 1987. Reprinted with permission of Allyn and Bacon.

We did a minilesson and follow-up activities using social notes in the Language-Based Homework Lab described previously in this chapter. Among a group of seven middle-school students, two had never exchanged social notes before that day. We discussed what a social note might say and, of course, demonstrated complex note folding patterns. One girl reported having considerable experience with social notes and using them to get back at people who made her angry. We suggested that she do an experiment. We asked her to find out what would happen if she wrote back something nice the next time someone wrote her an angry note. The next session she came in bubbling with the news that she had conducted the experiment. Another girl had written a negative note about feeling insulted. Our student experimenter wrote back that she had not meant to hurt her friend's feelings. The friend, in turn, wrote a friendly note and the friendship was patched. This active learning lesson was far more powerful than an adult lecture would have been about saying nice things in notes.

Objective 3. The student will participate in family conversations, showing appropriate: (a) assertive and responsive balance; (b) disclosure of

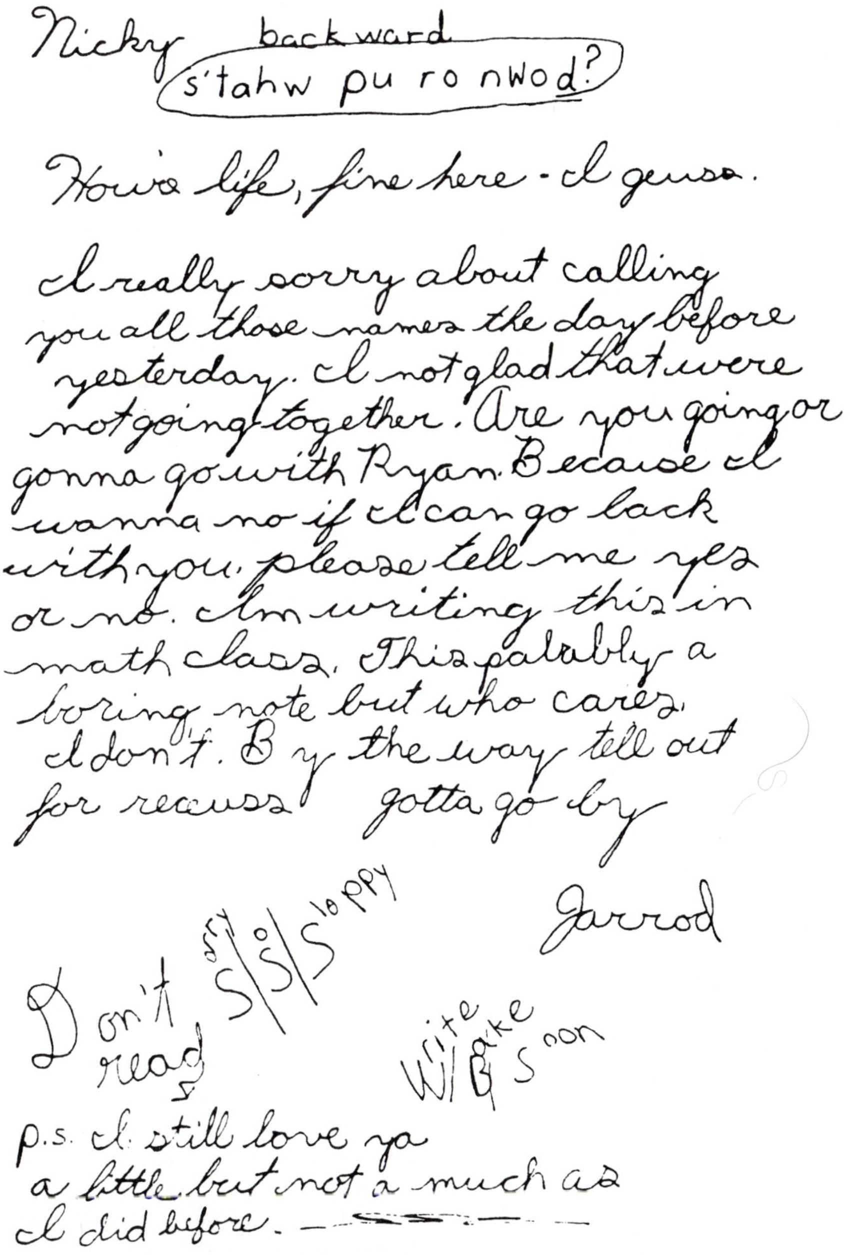

Nicky

backward

s'tahw pu ro nWod?

How's life, fine here - I guss.

I really sorry about calling you all those names the day before yesterday. I not glad that were not going together. Are you going or gonna go with Ryan. Because I wanna no if I can go back with you. please tell me yes or no. I'm writing this in math class. This palably a boring note but who cares. I don't. B y the way tell out for recuss! gotta go by

Jarrod

Don't read

S/S/S/S happy

Write me back soon

p.s. I still love ya a little but not a much as I did before. —————

FIGURE 12.3   Spontaneous personal writing by a fourth-grade boy, illustrating the dominance of fluency over correctness at this stage of writing development, and the high focus on metalinguistic play.

Note: From Nelson, N. W. (1988). Reading and writing (p. 104). In M. A. Nippold (Ed.), *Later language development: Ages nine through nineteen*. Austin, TX: Pro-Ed. Used by permission.

activities, interests, and feelings; and (c) topic contingent questions about other family members' interests.

Conversing in Families.   The quality of conversational contexts within and across families of children with disabilities is no more uniform than it is for any of us. Families' conversations are influenced by the age and gender relationships of participants, power and autonomy concerns, topics being discussed, the family's cultural history, and a large number of other variables.

Regardless of variability (and perhaps because of it), family conversations may provide a fruitful context for fostering later language learning. Intervention strategies for using family conversations might be two-pronged. Family conversations could help children acquire some of the middle-stage foundation skills they might have missed during therapeutic practice sessions (see discussion in Chapter 8 of conversational interaction strategies). They also could help parents acquire more deliberate scaffolding skills to ensure that their child participates actively in the conversation.

An example of suggestions for modifying family conversational contexts comes from research by Bodner-Johnson (1991). She studied 10 families, each of which included one deaf child between the ages of 10 and 12.75 years. All of the children had prelingual unaided hearing losses exceeding 70 dB in the range of 250 to 2000 Hz in the better ear and no other disability. The hearing parents and siblings of these youngsters used either a simultaneous method of signed and oral communication (four families) or oral–aural communication only (six families). Bodner-Johnson videotaped the families at home during their evening meals and found that deaf children were responsive participants in their families' dinner-table conversations. However, the deaf children participated significantly more often when the family member focused the topic with a two-question scaffold, such as "Did you like it? Did you like the street?" (p. 507). When the family asked *wh*- questions, children's responses tended to be more complex and elaborated, for example, "What was the favorite thing you did on the trip? Did you ride the roller coaster?" (p. 507). Although these deaf children tended to respond following sequences of two questions in family conversations, they were less responsive following a barrage

of questions. Intervention suggestions based on these findings appear in Box 12.7.

Understanding and Telling Stories: The Narrative Genre

Objective 4. The student will tell, retell, and answer questions about **stories** orally and in writing that show growth over baseline stories at four levels, including: (a) the **discourse level**—by planning adequately, including the major elements of story grammar structure (setting, problem, internal response, plan, action, outcome, ending); (b) the **sentence level**—by including a mixture of sentence types, mostly grammatically correct (subject–verb agreement, morphological inflections, function word inclusions, embedding and conjoining), but risking temporary grammatical "incorrectness" by attempting greater complexity, and using cohesive devices across sentences (lexical ties, pronoun reference, conjunctions); (c) the **word level**—by including interesting and appropriate word choices (some low frequency and multisyllabic words, some modifiers), avoiding all-purpose words (thing, stuff, make, do, put); and (d) the **sound level**—by spelling or articulating words clearly (syllabicating, sequencing, sound–symbol correspondence).

Previously in Part Two, narrative discourse was emphasized as an important language-learning context, relevant across the age span from infancy through adolescence. Milosky (1987) summarized the processing demands of narrative discourse:

> When narrating, the child must recall and organize content, take into account the listener by determining shared background, formulate new utterances, relate them to what has already been said, and introduce referents and distinguish unambiguously among them in subsequent utterances. The need to balance all these demands makes narration cognitively demanding and requires extensive mental resources. (p. 331)

As they enter the later stages of language development, normally developing children exhibit qualitative advances in their stories. In particular, "the sense of a

Box 12.7 _____

Suggestions for Encouraging Participation of Children Who Are Deaf in the Conversations of Their Families

- Conversation is a functional mechanism for facilitating the deaf child's access to an important aspect of family life. Families have their child's attention during dinnertime conversation. Children are at the ready for participation. Parents should make the most of that initiative by being responsive receptors, by paying attention to the flow of conversation, and by expressing interest and having fun.
- Mine the possibilities of questions but don't let go of a good idea. Questions seem to invite the greatest participation for the child—perhaps because their structure makes meaning clearer and, therefore, easier to respond to. Families should be encouraged to be their own researchers and observe how their children respond to comments/ideas they make versus questions they ask. Perhaps family members should rephrase or simplify the language of these comments to be sure the deaf child is understanding the content. The goal is to engage the child into more conversation on the same topic.
- "Mix it up" so that questions and ideas are integrated more evenly in conversation. The best strategy for encouraging participation in family conversation is to avoid a high rate of questioning relative to other conversation moves. Questions strung together seem to have a cumulative effect that diminishes the child's participation. (p. 508)

Note: From "Family Conversation Style: Its Effect on the Deaf Child's Participation" by B. Bodner-Johnson, _Exceptional Children, 57,_ 1991, p. 508. Copyright 1991 by The Council for Exceptional Children. Reprinted with permission.

plotted story becomes increasingly clear after the age of 8 years" (Sutton-Smith, 1986, p. 9), and mature narratives with multiple embedded episodes emerge in normal development at around 11 to 12 years of age (Botvin & Sutton-Smith, 1977). Older story tellers

> have all the verbal devices of turn-taking, argumentation, teasing, rebuttal, introduction, asides, giving background, summaries, morals, scandalous content, evaluations, dramatizations, and prosody to keep their audiences under control and in an appreciative state. When older children tell stories, they have control of both management and matter. (p. 9)

**Students with Language-Learning Disabilities.**   Children with language-learning disabilities and other language disorders, however, may not fare as well. Children with learning disabilities, in particular, have been shown

in many studies to have difficulty with various aspects of narrative comprehension and production. Garnett (1986) reviewed a series of studies showing that the original stories told by students with learning disabilities had more restricted vocabulary, less complex linguistic patterns, and more immature text construction. Data gathered by Roth and Spekman (1986) for children between the ages of 8 and 14 years confirmed that they were more like younger control subjects in that they tended to tell original stories that had fewer propositions and fewer complete episodes than did older and normally achieving students.

As Garnett's (1986) review showed, students with learning disabilities also tended to leave out key information about things such as settings (time, place, and characters) and endings when they retold stories. They often failed to use syntactic connectors to mark temporal and causal relations explicitly; they tended to produce sequencing errors; they were more likely to use a descriptive format tied to pictures; and they often had difficulty rephrasing when listeners failed to understand. When asked comprehension questions about stories, children with learning disabilities tended to have particular difficulty making use of cohesive ties that organize discourse and direct its flow. They were more likely to have difficulty identifying pronoun antecedents embedded in simple short paragraphs than their peers (Garnett, 1986).

Liles, Duffy, Merritt, and Purcell (1995) analyzed the results of several studies of narrative production by individuals with language impairments. The factor of global story organization contributed less to predicting membership in the language impaired group than a second factor, involving within- and across-sentence structure, measured as grammatical sentence structure, within subordinate clause productivity, and textual cohesion. On the other hand, McFadden and Gillam (1996) reported that textual-level measures were associated more reliably with judgments of the overall quality of narratives produced by students with language disorders than were measures of sentence-level complexity.

Students with Hearing Impairments. Children with hearing impairments perhaps have even greater difficulty with the narrative genre. Yoshinaga-Itano and Downey (1986) attributed a major portion of the difficulty to the limiting effects of severe hearing loss on incidental hearing and hence opportunities to gain a wide variety of language-based knowledge about the world. Components of stories that are not heard are missed, and then, a "child either fills in the gaps by making appropriate or inappropriate inferences, or simply stores incomplete information" (p. 47). As a result, hearing-impaired children often have underdeveloped concepts and verbal labels for those concepts. They also seem to have difficulty grasping the idea that scripts can be embedded within scripts and concepts within concepts. When they write stories, they tend to write primarily descriptive, immature sequence stories.

On the other hand, the basic concept of narrative structure seems to be relatively resistant to disruption across disorder types. Even in the studies reviewed by Garnett (1986) for children with learning disabilities, the findings on narrative structure tended to be subtle.

Garnett concluded that there seemed to be "no pervasive lack in these children's understanding of simple narratives" (p. 52). The narrative genre, because of its basis in universal human experience, may be a particularly appropriate context for language intervention with children with varied needs. As Heath (1986) pointed out, different cultures emphasize different subtypes and structures of narrative genre, but "the fundamental genres in every sociocultural group are narratives that capture verbally remembered or projected experiences" (p. 87).

Students with Traumatic Brain Injuries. Preliminary data suggest that the narrative genre may be a particularly useful intervention context for older children and adolescents with traumatic brain injury because of its relative resistance to the negative effects of brain damage. F. M. Jordan, Murdoch, and Buttsworth (1991) studied two groups of children in Australia who had been injured in accidents and were matched for age (8 to 16 years), sex (11 boys and 9 girls each), and socioeconomic status. One group of children had experienced closed head injuries in their accidents and the other had not. Jordan and colleagues examined both story grammar and intersentential cohesion by giving the children and adolescents a GI Joe figure and asking them to "tell me a story about this man—the sort of story you might write if you had to write a story for school; it can be a short story or as long as you like" (p. 575). Although the head-injured children had previously performed differently from their matched controls on standard measures of language, their story grammar and text cohesion skills did not differ significantly on the narrative measures.

Some intervention programs designed for children and adolescents with traumatic brain injuries have been aimed at remediating isolated perceptual and memory deficits. Focusing treatment instead on an area of integrated language and cognitive processing may be the most appropriate intervention for facilitating movement beyond the initial stages of confusion and fragmentation following brain injury (Ylvisaker, 1985).

Narrative Intervention Strategies. First, adult facilitators must thoroughly and explicitly understand narrative structure and cohesion (see Chapter 9) and the contexts in which narratives are normally found

(R. C. Anderson, 1985, Botvin & Sutton-Smith, 1977; Bransford & Johnson, 1972; Halliday & Hasan, 1976; Mandler & Johnson, 1977; Rumelhart, 1975; Stein & Glenn, 1979; van Dijk & Kintsch, 1978). In the pinball wizardry model that appears in Figure 11.1, the major subcomponents that contribute to the discourse knowledge module are (1) scripts, including nonlinguistic event knowledge whose predictability contributes to discourse knowledge as a form of shared experience; (2) story grammars (Stein & Glenn, 1979) and other ways of representing narrative text organizational maturity (Applebee, 1978); (3) text cohesive devices, including knowledge of both grammatical and semantic strategies (Halliday & Hasan, 1976) for building transitions and representing relationships among elements of texts (e.g., redundant, contrastive, or illustrative relationships); and (4) formats, including such variations as dramatic narratives in the form of plays and other subcategories, such as narrative jokes, science fiction stories, or murder mysteries. The question that remains is whether students also need explicit metatextual knowledge of scripts, story grammar, text cohesion, and formats to become competent adult language processors.

The essence of the argument that students need explicit knowledge is that individuals who can activate predictions to replay certain familiar scripts may be able to use those predictions to help them comprehend and produce texts structured similarly. Some of the advantages of encouraging individuals to use metacognitive awareness of text organization strategies were considered in the previous discussion of metaskills and executive control strategies. Familiarity with narrative structure through exposure to many stories with clear narrative elements may help prepare individuals to adopt such strategies (Page & Stewart, 1985). Quality literature for children and adolescents, rather than "controlled language" books and stories, may be particularly effective to help children "respond cognitively and aesthetically to the stories they hear and read" (Van Dongen & Westby, 1986, p. 80). Children may also be able to learn more about narrative structure by writing and acting in plays (Milosky, 1987), where plot and character motivations are central.

Once individuals are familiar with narrative structure through repeated exposure in different contexts, they can practice making predictions and drawing inferences

about characters, motivations, and events, based on a combination of world knowledge, discourse knowledge, and information gleaned from reading or hearing the initial parts of stories. Page and Stewart (1985) suggested a variety of techniques for helping students develop prediction abilities. One involves having students sequence parts of a scrambled story. Depending on reading level, students may use cut-apart paragraphs or pictures to complete this task. Milosky (1987) cautioned, however, that commercially available picture sequencing sets might be confusing to children because the sequences they depict are somewhat arbitrary and do not necessarily depict real cause–effect relationships driven by problem-solving efforts of characters with clear motivations (e.g., what does it matter whether a child washes his face or brushes his teeth first?). If children do need extra assistance to recognize narrative structure, other techniques involve "story frames" (Stewart, 1985) that provide fill-in tasks about story topics, main characters, motivating problems, first attempts, subsequent attempts, and problem resolutions. A story frame might include items such as "This story is about _____," and "The problem is solved when _____" (p. 351). Such structures and other "macrocloze" (fill-in-the-blank) techniques help children with language disorders focus on aspects of narratives they may not recognize on their own.

Many researchers have investigated instructional strategies that involve explicit instruction regarding story grammar structure. Stewart (1985), for example, recommended teaching children to use simplified outlines of story grammar elements (including setting, problem, response, and outcome) to help them organize their internalized schemas for reading and writing stories. B. L. Miller (1988) taught a group of severely to profoundly hearing-impaired adolescents the five parts of a "complete story." She taught the component labels **setting, problem, action, outcome,** and **ending.** She also taught that "*feelings* make a story interesting." Miller illustrated these components by displaying model personal narratives she had written with an overhead projector so groups of six or seven students could read and discuss them. The students used color-coded marking pens to identify parts of stories, using Miller's model stories (sometimes with key components deliberately omitted), stories they wrote themselves, and stories written by their peers. A matched control group spent the same amounts of time with Miller, learning about indefinite pronouns and noun modifiers and practicing written language only at the sentence level. The experimental group made greater improvement from pre- to post-test in the maturity of their written narratives than the control group. The experimental group also was able to use "metatextual" strategies at the conclusion of the study when asked to tell a friend how to write a story. In response to the same prompt, the control group tended to respond to the directions more directly, simply by writing about a friend.

Montague, Graves, and Leavell (1991) designed a similar program to teach junior high students with learning disabilities to write more mature narratives by providing them with a "story grammar cue card." When Montague and colleagues gave students the cue cards, along with sufficient planning time, the students wrote stories that did not differ along quantitative or qualitative measures when compared with stories of normally achieving students. When extra time and structure were not provided, the learning disabled students' stories were not as sophisticated.

Besides story grammar structure, other elements of narrative discourse may be drawn to the conscious attention of later-stage language learners. B. L. Miller (1988) taught her students to pay attention to feelings expressed in the stories they read and wrote. Westby (1985/1991) emphasized that discussions of narrative texts provide opportunities not only to build comprehension of factual elements but also to consider the feelings and motivations of characters. Lahey (1988) also reminded professionals of the need to help students appreciate uses of narratives to entertain.

An intervention program that uses narrative discourse as one context for targeting language change should encourage alive, shared, and communicative narratives. Children mostly need multiple opportunities to read, write, act out, and talk about stories. They need to work with interesting and entertaining stories, not sterile stories constructed to illustrate some grammatical feature, graphophonemic pattern, controlled set of vocabulary, or in response to a particular "story starter." As Hoskins (1990) commented (in Personal Reflection 12.3), narratives "comprise who we are, how we think of ourselves, and how we present ourselves to others" (1990, p. 60). This is not the same as completing exercises to please a teacher or a clinician.

Getting and Giving Information: The Expository Genre

Objective 5. The student will demonstrate strategies for comprehending, summarizing, studying, and producing **expository discourse** orally and in writing at: (a) the **discourse level**—by identifying discourse structure (how the student's textbooks are organized as well as how certain chapters and sections are structured) and diagraming key concepts or taking notes; (b) the **sentence level**—by paraphrasing, asking, and answering questions (single sentences, across sentences, and inferential); (c) the **word level**—by identifying and reproducing key words, unknown words, and words used a new way; and (d) the **sound level**—by using pronunciation keys, syllabication strategies, and sound–symbol correspondence to pronounce and spell.

A summary of research on expository text comprehension (Slater & Graves, 1989) showed that students (1) increasingly learn to use expository text structure to facilitate comprehension and recall from fourth grade through college; (2) remember more of what they read when they can identify and use text structures; (3) generally retain main ideas better than lower level ideas from expository texts; (4) can be taught to identify expository text structure and main ideas; (5) can benefit from training in the use of text structures and main ideas to improve reading comprehension; and (6) are particularly disadvantaged when they fail to use expository text structure to comprehend if the topic is unfamiliar.

When children and adolescents have difficulty handling the processing demands of expository texts, the problem may appear in several different classroom events. From at least third grade on, children are expected to spend considerable time reading, understanding, and recalling key facts from expository texts. They are also expected to discuss, describe, define, and use other expository discourse strategies to talk about ideas in whole class, small group, and individual learning, studying, and testing environments. As they listen to lectures, complete daily assignments, and prepare for tests, students might take notes from spoken lectures and from written work on the chalkboard. They might also review, outline, highlight, and answer factual and discussion questions from their textbooks. They may be expected to write expository texts of their own, doing research from multiple sources, and organizing information in an expository text format appropriate for the topic and purpose. Many of these activities require complex language and information processing strategies simultaneously on multiple levels, guided by an executive system to decide which questions to ask and strategies to use to understand the text, remember important parts, and recall them (using all the pinball wizardry illustrated in Figure 11.1).

Identifying Expository Text Structures to Assist Comprehension. Several authors recommend starting intervention for expository text problems by ensuring that individuals with problems can recognize different discourse structures, beginning with narrative structure (N. W. Nelson, 1988b; Scott, 1988a; Wallach, 1990; Westby 1985/1991, 1988). Then students may be taught to contrast narrative and expository structures. Those who have difficulty grasping the distinctions might be shown examples of their favorite narrative stories rewritten as expository texts (Piccolo, 1987, provided examples). When content is held relatively constant, some students may more easily recognize variations in form and talk about how different structures might be used for different purposes. Eventually, students might learn to recognize and diagram different expository discourse structures (e.g., those shown in Figure 11.3) and talk about why an author might have chosen to write in a particular style (Wallach & Miller, 1988).

Many researchers have demonstrated that reading comprehension improves when students learn to recognize text organizational structures (B. M. Taylor & Beach, 1984). Bos and Anders (1990) taught students with learning disabilities to build graphic representational "maps" of expository text structures and then to enter specific ideas from the text onto the text structure maps. P. L. Smith and Friend (1986) showed that training adolescents with learning disabilities to use a text structure–recognition strategy improved the students' ability both to recognize the structures and to recall instructional content, an effect that remained stable over at least 1 week.

Wallach (1990) pointed out that sensitivity to text structure is a skill that develops in interaction with other abilities and with demands of a particular text from the late elementary years through high school. Older students have advantages because of their greater familiarity with how textbooks are usually structured and because of their accumulated world knowledge and greater experience learning certain subject matter. Being able to "read better" involves more than just having better decoding and word-recognition skills.

The structure of math discourse has received less attention than the discourse of science and social studies textbooks. In fact, teachers, parents, and students do not always recognize that language impairments can be associated with deficits in mathematics processing, but math can be a major zone of significance for some students. Students with specific language impairments have difficulty not only with math story problems relative to their peers (Crouse, 1996; Parmar, Cawley, & Frazita, 1996), but also with computation processes (Conti-Ramsden, North, & Ward, 1995; Crouse, 1996; Fazio, 1996). In our interventions, we have often found it helpful to teach students with computational difficulties to engage in more deliberate, specific, and accurate self-talk for guiding themselves through computational processes. When story problems are at issue, examining the discourse demands may help. Parmar and her colleagues described three variables—directness, extraneous information, and number of steps—that place different demands on linguistic and information processing systems. They illustrated four types of word problems:

Direct Statement, No Extraneous Information, One-Step
A boy had 3 apples.
Another boy had 6 apples.
Together, how many apples do the boys have?

Indirect Statement
A boy had 3 apples left after he gave 2 apples to a friend.
How many apples did the boy start with?

Extraneous Information
A boy has 5 red apples.
A girl has 6 green apples.
Another girl has 7 red apples.
How many red apples do the children have?

Two-Step
A boy has 5 red apples.
A girl has 2 more red apples than the boy.
Together, how many apples do the children have? (p. 417)

One intervention strategy is to scaffold students to turn indirect statements into direct ones (Parmar et al., 1996). We have also found that it helps to have students represent the meanings behind the words with sketches. To scaffold this, we have provided worksheets for some impulsive students with a box for the sketch at the top of the page, and a self-talk strategy reminder, "First draw the picture" (printed above the box), "then do the math" (printed above the blank work space on the lower half of the sheet). This instruction is designed to overcome a common impulsive profile we have found among students with language impairments who have adopted partial strategies, sometimes as a result of well-meaning suggestions to pay attention to key words. Students with this profile tend to read a problem, extract numbers, and jump immediately to computation based on a key word they isolate from the problem (e.g., thinking that "left" in the indirect example above, must mean to subtract). Teaching students to sketch the variables of story problems from the regular curriculum provides a window on their inner comprehension and organization processes so that appropriate scaffolding can be provided.

If the textbooks in the students' curriculum are not written with explicit structure, and if the student has difficulty inferring the structure without assistance, the adult's job is not to rewrite the textbooks (although, sitting on curriculum committees and influencing textbook selection decisions is not a bad idea). Rather, the facilitator's job is to help frame existing cues so that the student can recognize them as independently as possible, to arrange opportunities to practice the strategies with scaffolding support, then to systematically withdraw that support until the student can use the strategies independently in the regular classroom.

Identifying Key Words and Other Text Cohesion Devices.

Westby (1991) pointed out that the framing and focusing process should help students recognize key words that may cue them to recognize different kinds of expository text. Key words in the form of conjunctions and logical connectors serve as one type of syntactic–semantic text cohesion device, which along with others such as pronoun reference, are particularly difficult for children with developmental language disorders (Liles, 1985; Norris & Bruning, 1988). Westby's summary of particular text functions, key words, and formats for

testing for six types of expository text appears in Table 12.3.

Curriculum-based language assessment and intervention process for students having difficulty with expository texts involves focusing students on key words to make sure students comprehend their meaning. The specialist can do this by giving students experience in noticing such words and highlighting them when they appear in texts. Another strategy is to teach students to use similar words and structures to write their own expository texts for similar purposes.

Writing Expository Texts.

Expository writing assignments may come fairly early in general education experience. Calkins (1983) provided an example of expository text written by a 5-year-old about how to make a robot in a kindergarten classroom. Several of the boy's steps, shown with his invented spellings, follow:

1. *get a hed*
2. *atuch one liot*
3. *atach the athr liot*
4. *get the boty*
13. *put a sekrt hand in the boty (p. 11)*

Children with language-learning disabilities should have similar opportunities to write expository texts, and they should be given similar latitude in meeting writing conventions (in my opinion). As students mature into the later stages of development, they benefit from explicit instruction in organizing their own writing like the macrostructures of texts they read. In turn, the explicit instruction and practice in writing expository texts may help them recognize similar structuring strategies used by other authors.

Englert and Raphael (1988) noted that successful writers seem to engage in both task-specific strategies and executive control functions simultaneously. Task-specific strategies include planning, monitoring, and revising, while carefully considering the needs and questions of the audience, using awareness of text structure to serve as a map to decide what information to include and what signals to use to indicate the relationships among various elements of the texts (e.g., cohesive devices, such as *in contrast to, but, like, different*). Executive functions used during expository writing include implementing, monitoring, and sustaining various

TABLE 12.3   Guide for monitoring expository texts

TEXT PATTERN	TEXT FUNCTION	KEY WORDS	TEST FORMATS
Description	The text tells what something is	is called, can be defined as, is, can be interpreted as, is explained as, refers to, is a procedure for, is someone who, means	Define . . . Describe . . . List the features of . . . What is . . . ? Who is . . . ?
Collection/ enumeration	The text gives a list of things that are related to the topic	an example is, for instance, another, next, finally, such as, to illustrate	Give example of . . . What is . . . and give some examples?
Sequence/ procedure	The text tells what happened or how to do something or make something	first, next, then, second, third, following this step, finally, subsequently, from here . . . to, eventually, before, after	Give the steps in doing . . . When did . . . occur?
Comparison/ contrast	The text shows how two things are the same or different	different, same, alike, similar, although, however, on the other hand, contrasted with, compared to, rather than, but, yet, still, instead of	Compare and contrast . . . and . . . How are . . . and . . . alike and different?
Cause/effect explanation	The text gives reasons for why something happened	because, since, reasons, then, therefore, for this reason, results, effects, consequently, so, in order to, thus, depends on, influences, is a function of, produces, leads to, affects, hence	Explain . . . Explain the cause(s) of . . . Explain the effect(s) of . . . Predict what will happen . . . Why did . . . happen? How did . . . happen? What are the causes (reasons for, effects, results, etc) of . . . ?
Problem/ solution	The text states a problem and offers solution to the problem	a problem is, a solution is	Describe the development of the problem and the solutions. What are the solutions to the problem . . . ?

Note: From *Steps to Developing and Achieving Language-Based Curriculum in the Classroom* (p. 12) by C. E. Westby, 1991, Rockville, MD, American Speech-Language-Hearing Association. Copyright 1991 by C. E. Westby. Reprinted by permission.

subprocesses. Mature writers self-instruct or ask themselves questions, consider and choose among various strategies and subprocesses, monitor performance, and make modifications or corrections as necessary. To teach students to develop skills at both levels, Englert and Raphael advocated a dialogic approach (referred to in this book as **mediational teaching,** or **scaffolding**). It included teacher modeling and "think sheets" to organize ideas. For example, students might use a series of four different think sheets for four different stages of the writing process:

STAGE ONE. *Plan think sheet* with categories and questions such as

Focus on audience—Who am I writing this for?

Purpose—Why am I writing this?

Background knowledge—What do I know about my topic?

Organization—How can I organize my brainstormed or collected ideas?

STAGE TWO. *Organize think sheet with categories and questions that change according to the type of text structure composed. For example, if a sequential–procedural text structure is being taught, the think sheet might ask*

What is being explained?

What are the materials you need?

What are the steps?

What do you do first, second, next, then, etc.?

STAGE THREE. *Self-edit think sheet with guides to focus students on both the content and structure of their work:*

First, star the parts I like best and put a question mark by something my readers might not understand.

Then, check whether I answered the text structure questions (rate this yes, no, or maybe); for example, Did I tell . . . what is being explained? . . . what materials are needed? . . . the steps? . . . what you do first, next, etc.?

STAGE FOUR. *Editor think sheet to be completed by a peer editor with the same categories on it as on the self-edit think sheet. Following its completion, the peer editor and author compare and discuss their observations, and revisions are made as needed.*

Note Taking, Summarizing, and Studying. Interactions among the language modalities—listening, speaking, reading, writing, and thinking—have been emphasized throughout this book. Nowhere is that relationship more apparent than in activities involving expository texts in classrooms. Learning to read and write expository texts involves opportunities to talk about expository texts, to ask and answer questions about them, and to take notes from written and oral presentations.

Williams (1988) pointed out that abstracting important points from larger units of text is a developmental skill that rests on the ability to categorize. Development data gathered by A. L. Brown and Day (1983) showed that text-summarizing rules are acquired over the years from fifth grade to college in the sequence (1) delete unimportant information, (2) delete redundant information, (3) substitute category names for lists, (4) select a topic sentence from the text, and (5) invent a topic sentence. Fifth graders could use only the delete strategy. College students were still not as competent as expert writers in using the strategy to invent a topic sentence.

Teaching students to take notes from material they read and hear involves helping them to make categorical decisions quickly. They also can be taught to build hierarchical and sequencing maps of important information for review, study, and recall on tests. Such intervention relates to information processing theories of language acquisition. Suritsky and Hughes (1991) pointed out that most studies of note taking ability have been conducted with college students without disabilities. Most also were designed to test one of two theories. The **level of processing theory** (F. I. Craik & Lockhart, 1972) is based on the idea that information retention is a function of the depth of cognitive processing applied to the input stimulus. The **information processing memory model** (Ladas, 1980) suggests that the preparation of information for long-term memory storage involves a series of processing steps: (1) giving attention in response to orienting stimuli; (2) using search and associate behaviors, such as differentiating relevant from irrelevant information and associating incoming lecture information with previous knowledge (this process may fail if the student possesses insufficient prerequisite knowledge); (3) coding the information, for example, by using shorthand notes, mnemonic devices, and varied levels of headings to represent superordinate and subordinate information; and (4) deliberately deciding which information to place in long-term storage in preparation for a test.

Intervention for note-taking problems may target changes in behavior of both lecturers and listeners. Through consultation, the language specialist may encourage lecturers to use strong orienting cues that a new topic is being introduced, to use strategically placed pauses to help students group together related pieces of information and to give them additional processing time at regular intervals, to write key words and to list outline headers and major subpoints on the chalkboard, and to review and summarize periodically. The professional might teach listeners to write down main points using abbreviations and other coding strategies, rather than to attempt verbatim encoding of the lecture, and, if possible, to paraphrase key points to ensure deeper cognitive processing of information. Because of their significantly slower "tool rates" (i.e., number of letters written per minute), most students with learning disabilities also need to learn shorthand abbreviations and symbols (Suritsky & Hughes, 1991).

Larson and McKinley (1987) noted that many adolescents with language disorders and learning disabilities, because of their slowness and other deficits, need compensatory support to compete in regular classroom settings. For example, lecturers might provide main points of lectures on preprinted "listening guides," to take some of the pressure off note taking. Students might use a "buddy system" to gain access to notes taken by a classmate who is a particularly proficient note taker, by using machine, carbon, or hand copying. My experience with the note-sharing approach at the university level suggests that students with disabilities still should be required to take some notes "on-line." Otherwise, they may assume a passive listening posture, knowing they will get the notes later. This observation is consistent with the research review by Suritsky and Hughes (1991) that showed that "students who record notes during lectures benefit more from the lectures than students who simply listen" (p. 14).

Tape recording has often been suggested for helping students with learning disabilities compensate for listening and note-taking deficits. Tape-recorded lectures are not automatically helpful, however, primarily because listening to taped lectures takes time, and time is often already a problem for students with learning disabilities. Some teachers also object to having their lectures recorded, although the right to listen to tape-recorded lectures may be interpreted as a reasonable accommodation under Section 504 (Larson & McKinley, 1987) (see Chapter 5 for a discussion of Section 504).

Note taking and review sheets may be constructed from analysis and review of tape-recorded lectures and written texts. Special arrangements may be made to allow students with learning disabilities to highlight key points in school textbooks as they read (not allowed for many regular education students in public schools). Again, however, students may need direct instruction to learn how to select pieces of text to highlight or underline as they read. Otherwise, they are likely to highlight everything! Larson and McKinley (1987) suggested that students might highlight main ideas in yellow, relevant details in blue, and new vocabulary words in green. They also recommended that teachers and clinicians

should collaborate to decide on one color-coding system so as not to confuse students and that early highlighting might be done by teachers in the students' books so that students will have their own teachers' models for identifying what is important.

Williams (1988) reviewed several studies in which students were given explicit instruction and practice to identify important points, using a variety of strategies, including rules for summarizing, and strategies for circling main topics and underlining details. All of the studies yielded some success in helping students to recognize main ideas and become more attentive to details (Figure 12.4 is a set of objectives from N. W. Nelson, 1988b, for guiding intervention in this area).

In the first chapter of this book and previously in this chapter, I identified questions as having a key function in orienting attention and higher order thinking skills. Knapczyk (1991) designed an intervention strategy to teach three ninth-grade students with learning disabilities better strategies for asking and answering questions in their regular education world geography class. The instructional program started with a series of sessions in the controlled environment of the resource room before moving into the regular classroom. From the beginning, however, the regular curriculum (in the form of videotape-recorded class sessions) provided the content for the intervention sessions. Knapczyk organized sessions for learning to ask questions as follows:

SESSION ONE. The student and resource teacher viewed the videotape together. The student was asked to identify places where he did not understand what the teacher said, was unclear about what was being asked, or was unfamiliar with the information being discussed. At that point, the tape was stopped and the student was directed to ask a question that met these criteria:

1. *Timed at a natural break where it is appropriate to ask questions, or*
2. *Timed following a teacher prompt that it is appropriate to ask questions*
3. *Formulated to solicit the desired information*
4. *Formulated to be relevant to the lesson content*

The resource teacher stopped the tape at several points and asked whether the student had any questions. Appropriately timed and formulated questions were reinforced. If problems arose, parts of the tape were replayed to demonstrate examples of appropriate performance.

FIGURE 12.4   A sequence of objectives for targeting note-taking ability.

OBJ WL2	WRITTEN LANGUAGE: LATER STAGES	Date: _____
	PART C. EXPOSITORY TEXTS	CHILD: _____

SHORT-TERM OBJECTIVES:	INTERVENTION SETTING						COMMENTS/ TECHNIQUES/ EVALUATION
	INDIVIDUAL THERAPY		MINICLASSROOM		CLASSROOM		
THE CHILD WILL: _____	Date In.	Date Accom.	Date In.	Date Accom.	Date In.	Date Accom.	
1. listen and take notes from expository lectures, showing the ability to detect organization and major points by using a variety of strategies adapted to lecture style, time available, familiarity with topic, and related variables, and the ability to use the notes for studying in order to answer test questions based on the lecture (notes should match major content of notes taken on the same lecture by a highly competent learner [such as the speech–language pathologist or a successful fellow classmate] and a passing percentage of questions based on the lecture must be answered correctly for 3 lectures in each target setting):							
a. by using listening skills, to abstract major point and organizational relationships in notes taken during the lecture;							
b. by developing and practicing a set of abbreviations and symbols for particular classes that the student can recognize and expand later;							
c. by recopying notes in a neater form, cleaning up their organization and detail in the process, asking clarification questions of fellow students or teacher as needed and appropriate, to make the notes complete;							
d. by referring to related written texts to fill in missing information, and to check spellings of key words;							
e. by referring to an audiotape of the lecture (if available) to check notes for completeness and accuracy;							
f. by using a highlighter pen or other color-coding strategy to box off information the teacher might emphasize on a test;							
g. by using the notes to ask a peer (or someone role-playing a peer) possible test questions, and to answer them, in a group study atmosphere;							
h. by taking an actual or contrived written test on material covered in the lecture.							

Note: From *Planning Individualized Speech and Language Intervention Programs* (Revised and Expanded) by Nickola Wolf Nelson. Copyright 1998 by Communication Skill Builders, Inc., P.O. Box 42050, Tucson, AZ 85733. Reprinted with permission.

SESSION TWO. The same tape was viewed again. The student was directed to stop the tape when appropriate and ask the clarification question, which the resource teacher answered.

SESSIONS THREE, FOUR, FIVE. Additional practice was provided using different taped lectures, with feedback about performance and additional demonstration as necessary.

LAST 2 DAYS OF TRAINING. These sessions consisted of regular classroom interactions. Before going into the classroom, students met with the resource teacher, who reviewed with them the major elements of asking questions. (In the research study, the teacher was not aware that the students had been working on question asking and answering.)

Knapczyk (1991) used a similar format for learning to answer questions but asked students to

(a) identify points in class activities where the teacher asked questions of the students, (b) repeat or paraphrase the question that was asked, (c) formulate an answer to the questions, (d) attend to examples of how other students recited answers, and (e) evaluate his and the other students' performance. (p. 78)

Knapczyk (1991) reported positive results in terms of numbers of questions asked and answered appropriately and in increased accuracy on assigned seatwork activities.

Combining Strategies for Complex Multimodality Processing.   An intervention approach might also combine many of the techniques discussed previously. One approach uses aspects of the procedure called "reciprocal teaching," in which students take turns acting as teachers to guide their own learning and that of their peers. In original descriptions, during reciprocal teaching (Palincsar & Brown, 1984) students led discussions about short sections of texts using the four strategies **predicting, questioning, clarifying,** and **summarizing.**

As developed further by Englert and Mariage (1991), text structure mapping and note-taking strategies are added. Englert and Mariage used the mnemonic acronym, POSSE, to represent the text processing steps **predict, organize, search, summarize,** and **evaluate.**

The researchers worked with fourth-, fifth-, and sixth-grade students with learning disabilities and their teachers. As part of the intervention, teachers modeled the strategies and then selected a student leader to guide aspects of the POSSE sequence. Student leaders were given cue cards to help them know what to ask:

PREDICT. Students learned to activate background knowledge by attending to cues in titles, headings, pictures, and initial paragraphs, prompting each other:
   "I predict that. . . ." "I'm remembering. . . ."

ORGANIZE. Students learned to brainstorm their ideas into a semantic map, prompting each other:
   "I think one category might be. . . ."

SEARCH–SUMMARIZE. Students read short segments of text and looked for text structure and predicted information, prompting each other:
   "I think the main idea is. . . ." "My question about the main idea is. . . ."

EVALUATE. Students learned to compare, clarify, and predict what the next section of the text would be about, prompting each other:
   "I think we did [did not] predict this main idea [compare]." "Are there any clarifications? [clarify]" "I predict the next part will be about . . . [predict]."

Teachers facilitated and scaffolded the discussions and decided which of and how the students' comments would be written in the group summary (see Figure 12.5), but gradually turned over as much control to students as possible.

Summary

This section presented a variety of strategies for using language to participate in different kinds of discourse—conversational, narrative, and expository. You have probably noticed that the discussions of this section have overlapped considerably with those of earlier sections in their joint focus on modifying the learning context, using mediational teaching approaches, and developing learning strategies and metaskills for processing different aspects of communicative events. That is no accident. These are common themes among many varieties of intervention systems used with later-stage language learners.

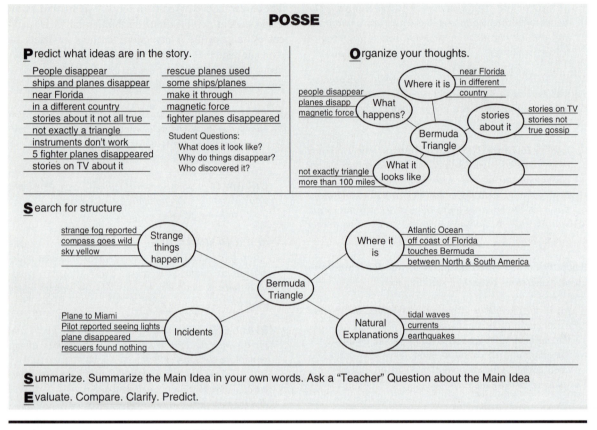

FIGURE 12.5   Partially completed POSSE strategy sheet.

Note: From "Making Student Partners in the Comprehension Process: Organizing the Reading 'POSSE'" by C. S. Englert and T. V. Mariage, 1991, *Learning Disability Quarterly, 14,* p. 129. Copyright 1991 by The Council for Learning Disabilities. Reprinted by permission.

ENCOURAGING LATER-STAGE SYNTACTIC–SEMANTIC DEVELOPMENT

GOAL: The child will produce and understand complex content–form constructions.

- Problems of Later-Stage Syntactic Development
- Judging Level of Syntactic Development
- Targeting Syntactic Comprehension and Production
- Targeting Sentence Combining and Paraphrasing
- Targeting Text Cohesion

OUTCOME: The child will use language to convey and comprehend complex meanings at home and school.

Most later-stage learners with language disorders need fairly direct instruction to acquire strategies to manage information and direct their own thinking and learning processes. Some individuals also struggle excessively with oral and written syntactic construction and comprehension. These students may need intervention that focuses specifically on complex syntactic structures and on syntactic–semantic strategies for comprehending and producing elements of text cohesion.

Problems of Later-Stage Syntactic Development

Klecan-Aker (1985) reviewed the research on the syntactic abilities of school-age children with language disorders. A summary of those findings includes evidence that (1) the syntactic abilities of adolescents with language-learning disabilities may plateau at levels expected for 5- or 6-year-olds; (2) children with language disorders are less proficient in paraphrasing than their normally developing peers, often repeating stimulus sentences rather than paraphrasing them; (3) children with language disorders are less proficient in using rules of linguistic cohesion; and (4) the linguistic cohesion problems they exhibit are characterized by a lower frequency of subordinating conjunctions (such as *which, after, where,* and *since*) and a higher frequency of ambiguous reference.

Judging Level of Syntactic Development

Several cautions should be observed when making developmental level decisions about later-stage needs. Scott (1988c) observed that although predictable schedules of morphological and syntactic development are established for the preschool years:

> it is much more difficult to construct comparable syntactic schedules for the 9 through 19 age range because the concern now is not with the presence or absence of high-frequency structures, but with the gradual acquisition of low-frequency structures and the ability to form unique combinations of structures. To uncover later syntactic developments, finer grained methods of analysis are needed. (pp. 50–51)

Later-stage syntactic developments are measured as changes in written and oral language samples. Individual differences exceed those of children in earlier stages, and the influences of both the immediate context and prior educational experiences must be considered in any quantification efforts. As Rubin (1984) noted, "research aimed at providing developmental descriptions of children's writing abilities must tread cautiously in formulating age-norm generalization that fail to provide for the effects of communicative context" (p. 227).

Appropriate, nontrivial indices of advancing maturity are difficult to identify (Scott & Stokes, 1995). Some syntactic characteristics of written language samples appear to represent developmental improvements but are not necessarily valid signs of greater language maturity. For example, Rubin (1984) noted that composition length often predicts judged quality, but under certain circumstances, mature writers seek to reduce verbosity rather than increase it (Rubin, 1982). Similarly, although syntactic complexity has often been used to measure composition quality (C. R. Cooper, 1976), complex syntax may not be appropriate in certain contexts (Crowhurst, 1980), and overly complex syntax may indicate that the writer has not judged the reader's needs.

Normal growth in child writers is often accompanied by errors involving both syntactic and semantic rules. As Weaver (1982) noted, when developing writers "start adding to or elaborating their ideas, they may produce fragments consisting of compound or explanatory phrases. And when they begin using a variety of subordinate clauses, they may punctuate some of these as if they were complete sentences" (p. 443). Based on a review of the literature on written language development, Brannon (1985) also concluded that "when writers push toward intellectual complexity in their work, their texts may not demonstrate the formal and technical competence of their previous, less complex texts" (p. 20). This is the form and function tradeoff, which operates across developmental stages.

Predicting the difficulty syntactic structures pose for individuals in receptive language also is not easy. Bransford and Nitsch (1985) reviewed studies exploring contextual or situational constraints on ease of comprehension and concluded that "the same sentence may differ in ease of comprehension depending on the contextual situations to which it refers" (p. 91). They also commented that "syntactic structure has semantic implications and that syntactic appropriateness is determined relative to the situation in which the sentence is uttered" (p. 91).

Syntactic knowledge is closely tied to strategies for representing meaning. Four subcomponents are represented in the syntactic module of the pinball wizardry model shown in Figure 11.1. Any of these might be targeted in language intervention. They include knowledge of (1) grammatical morphemes (including derivational bound morphemes and function words); (2) sentence structures (e.g., declaratives, questions, passives, imperatives, and negative sentences); (3) sentence combining (including phrasal and clausal embedding and other types of complex and compound sentences); and (4) relations among sentences (including syntactic elements that can be used to build text cohesion). See Scott's (1988b) summary of types of complex sentences in Figure 12.6.

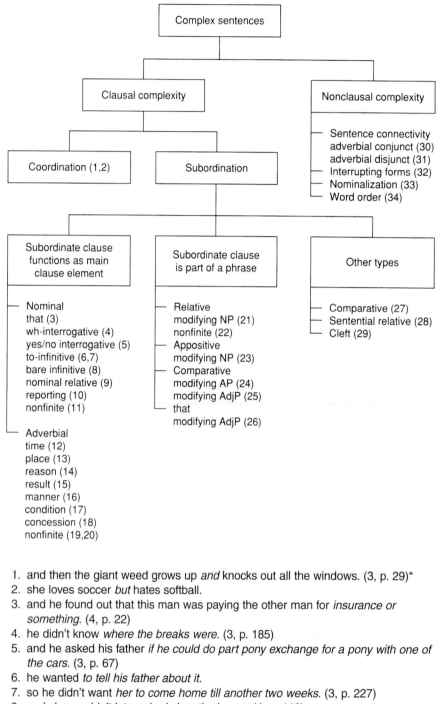

1. and then the giant weed grows up *and* knocks out all the windows. (3, p. 29)*
2. she loves soccer *but* hates softball.
3. and he found out that this man was paying the other man for *insurance or something.* (4, p. 22)
4. he didn't know *where the breaks were.* (3, p. 185)
5. and he asked his father *if he could do part pony exchange for a pony with one of the cars.* (3, p. 67)
6. he wanted *to tell his father about it.*
7. so he didn't want *her to come home till another two weeks.* (3, p. 227)
8. and she wouldn't let *anybody buy the house.* (4, p. 110)
9. and the hospital was *where the Zulus were waiting.* (3, p. 38)

10. then this boy goes *there's the brakes.* (3, p. 185)
11. the horse could hear *the boy shouting.* (4, p. 307)
12. *so when he got out* then they gave him the present of the pony. (3, p. 64)
13. they found nothing *wherever they went.*
14. and they couldn't get at him *because there was gates going round.* (3, p. 197)
15. he didn't pay any attention *so she left.*
16. she acts like *my mother did.*
17. *if you can't take me* I'll have to take the bus.
18. she tells good stories *even if sometimes they're too long.*
19. then in the end it was like they just sat there you know *getting everything out of the boat.* (4, p. 158)
20. *having tried the pizza before* they ordered spaghetti this time.
21. and there was this friend *that always brought cookies.*
22. it's this reporter *following the Hulk.* (3, p. 170)
23. and he took this vase thing *it was like an ornament* as proof and these papers from the safe. (4, p. 238)
24. she talks better *than she used to.*
25. you must have been sicker *than I was.*
26. she was sure *it was her lunchbox.*
27. they have more cookies in their house *than we ever did.*
28. the horse just disappeared *which made all the others very sad.*
29. it was in school *that they told him.*
30. I've never had nightmares/not as far as I know *anyway.* (4, p. 89)
31. *personally* I think I'm getting pretty good.
32. Harold *whose army had just marched across England after fighting an invading group of Norwegians back* was tired and sore.
33. the *development* of this beach makes me sick.
34. *there stood* a little tiger cub.

FIGURE 12.6   Structural relationships for categories of English sentence complexity. (Note: Numbers refer to examples of complex sentences under the figure)

*All sentences referenced with a page number have been taken from the Fawcett and Perkins corpus (1980) of spoken language of children 6 to 12 years.

Note: From "Producing Complex Sentences" by C. M. Scott. Reprinted from *Topics in Language Disorders,* Vol. 8, No. 2, pp. 47, 62, with permission of Aspen Publishers, Inc., © 1988.

Targeting Syntactic Comprehension and Production

Objective 1. The student will demonstrate: (a) competence for comprehending and producing a variety of sentence types with grammatically correct subject–verb agreement, morphological inflections, function word inclusions, and embedding and conjoining and (b) risk taking for attempting higher level sentences and making a few errors.

Some regular educators have recommended teaching grammar through written materials drawn from chil-dren's textbooks and writings (Vavra, 1987). For example, the educator might teach prepositions by deleting them from a textbook passage and then asking students to replace them in a cloze procedure. Alternatively, the instructor might ask students to place parentheses around structures such as prepositional phrases in their course texts or to highlight them. Students might practice adding complexity to their own writing by adding prepositional phrases where appropriate.

Individuals with written language syntax problems may have a history of oral language impairment. The comprehensive intervention program then should address problems of both oral and written syntactic knowledge. An advantage of using written language in intervention efforts is its relative permanence. Because written sentences are not transient, as oral sentences are, they may be reviewed and revised. When using regular curricular materials to foster syntactic knowledge, the instructor may give students practice in paraphrasing. Paraphrasing skill is often necessary to understand the questions at the ends of textbook chapters and to relate them to sections of the text where information for answering questions is found (N. W. Nelson, 1989b).

Moran (1988) recommended helping students be more productive in their writing by focusing on synthesis rather than analysis of sentences. She encouraged students to acquire new syntactic knowledge by starting with the smallest meaningful unit (the independent clause or proposition) and gradually adding length by expanding T-units (Hunt, 1970), "culminating in alternative arrangements of T-units to form paragraphs according to patterns dictated by expressive, descriptive, narrative, expository, or persuasive purpose" (Moran, 1988, p. 554). Moran's approach thus encouraged the activation of interactions among the various aspects of mature written language processing, with a focus on using syntactic knowledge to serve the construction of meaning.

Moran's (1988) approach started with small-group discussions, during which writers brainstormed topics, mentioning some person, object, place, or idea that they know. Teachers printed the student-generated topics on the left side of a chalkboard or overhead transparency and then guided the students to provide a comment about each. One student gave the comment, "lives next door," to go with the topic, "my friend Gloria." Another produced the comment, "is the best car," to go with the topic, "a Porsche."

In the next step, Moran (1988) helped students to expand the topics and to produce clauses, which she wrote on strips of paper without capital letters or end punctuation to mark their boundaries. This allowed students to reorder their sentence elements differently. When they learned to produce a variety of clauses, the students were taught to combine clauses into complex T-units using the set of subordinating terms *because, when,* and *after,* and the relative pronouns, *who, which,* and *that.* Finally, the students learned to generate additional T-units and to arrange them in paragraphs in more than one way, again to help them appreciate the flexibility of

being able to say basically the same thing in different ways. Ultimately, the students learned to produce paragraphs with expressive, descriptive, narrative, expository, and persuasive purposes.

Scott (1995) viewed discourse as a context that could be used either naturally or deliberately to assist students to develop higher level syntactic abilities. She categorized procedures like Moran's (1988) as sharing features with both direct and indirect approaches to teaching later developing syntactic forms. Scott noted that the written language modality offers special opportunities for developing the syntactic language skills of elementary and secondary school students. She recommended "writing programs that emphasize conscious awareness of text structure and metacognitive strategies," and noted that "children are motivated to write in order to convey particular meanings for particular reasons, not to produce impressive syntax" (p. 138).

Story retelling is another discourse context that can be used to encourage complex sentence use. Sutter and Johnson (1995) studied a process of normal development they called "borrowing verb forms from mature speakers" (p. 1074). They documented narratives as a context for three complex verb forms and found that normally developing 8-year-old third graders "borrowed" the forms in retelling at a higher rate than younger children. This suggests that retelling stories (with scaffolding) may provide a meaningful context for later-stage children. The verb forms loaded into the intervention stories Sutter and Johnson used were past progressive (e.g., "was feeling," "was shivering"), past perfect progressive (e.g., "had been wanting," "had been growing"), and past perfect (e.g., "had hoped," "had sent").

Gillam, McFadden, and Van Kleeck (1995) compared a whole language intervention approach with one that was based on direct intervention of language skills. They found that "spoken narratives produced by students in the whole language group tended to receive higher values on content measures and on holistic judgments of quality" (p. 173), whereas "the language-form properties of spoken and written narratives produced by students in the whole language group did not compare well with those of students in the language skills group" (p. 174). Their overall recommendation was to design a hybrid approach to intervention that would start and end with meaningful texts, but "focus on specific aspects of form when there is a pragmatically relevant reason for doing so" (p. 175).

Targeting Sentence Combining and Paraphrasing

Objective 2. The student will demonstrate competence for constructing meanings across sentence boundaries by: (a) constructing a complex sentence out of simple ones; (b) paraphrasing complex sentences into several simple ones; and (c) answering questions that can be found "right there" (in single sentences), "here and there" (across sentences), or "by thinking" (inferred from relating the text to background knowledge).

Sentence-combining strategies, such as those used by Moran (1988), are not new. Strong (1986) is credited with developing many of the modern approaches to sentence-combining exercises, but he pointed out that the fourteenth-century rhetorician Erasmus "showed how a single sentence could be expressed 150 ways by altering syntax or diction" (p. 3).

Strong (1986) noted that sentence-combining exercises come in a variety of formats, both oral and written. "Cued" formats have a limited set of right answers; "open" formats accept more divergent possibilities. Strong provided the following example of a cued exercise:

> *Sentence combining is an approach.*
> *The approach is for teaching.*
> *Some teachers find it useful. (THAT)*
> *Others regard as it dangerous. (BUT)*

This sentence, when combined, would yield "Sentence combining is a teaching approach that some teachers find useful but (that) others regard as dangerous" (p. 5). As an example of an open strategy, Strong provided this:

> *SC [sentence combining] is a means to an end.*
> *The end is clear syntax.*
> *The end is controlled syntax.*
> *SC is not an end in itself. (p. 5)*

This exercise is "open" because it allows several possible solutions, including, "SC is a means to an end, not an end in itself; that end is clear, controlled syntax," and "Rather than being an end in itself, SC is a means to an end: syntactic control and clarity."

The primary identifying characteristic of sentence-combining exercises is that they start with given language propositions, followed by play with the language to vary its form (see Personal Reflection 12.6). Sentence-combining exercises have been criticized as being artificial formula writing. Strong (1986) agreed:

> *SC works best when done two or three times a week for short periods, when students use exercises as springboards for journals or controlled writing, when teachers and students monitor problem sentences, and when transfer is made to real writing—either through decombined student drafts or marginal notations. (p. 22)*

Students who understand how sentences connect with each other within and across sentence boundaries have advantages for comprehending the complex sentence structures of their textbooks. They also produce stories that are judged more mature than those with weaker intra- and inter-sentence connections (Liles, Duffy, Merritt, & Purcell, 1995). Such skills assist students to paraphrase selectively, finding information for answering questions in their expository texts. Box 12.4 provided an example of a minilesson developed by graduate-student clinician Shannon Kersten for the Language-Based Homework Lab to help students develop awareness of how questions relate to information presented in a single sentence ("right there"), across sentences ("here and there"), and by drawing inferences with assistance from their background knowledge ("by thinking").

Targeting Text Cohesion

Objective 3. The student will demonstrate competence for comprehending and producing text cohesion devices within and across sentences, including: (a) lexical links, (b) pronoun reference, and (c) conjunctive links.

Writers must develop complex strategies to form a cohesive whole (Halliday & Hasan, 1976). As Halliday and Hasan defined it, **cohesion** is a semantic system of ties across sentence boundaries that bind a text together.

Cohesion strategies represent a true marriage between syntax and semantics. Halliday and Hasan (1976) described three cohesion processes: **Lexical cohesion** involves semantic linkage among vocabulary items. **Grammatical cohesion** involves the three syntactic–semantic operations of reference, substitution, and ellipsis. **Conjunction strategies** relate ideas with a cohesion process that is largely grammatical but also lexical (see Box 12.8).

The common feature among these strategies is that cohesion is established in words, so that linguistic items "point" to each other. Cohesive devices may be used to point backward to previously introduced lexical items (anaphora) or ahead to new information (cataphora). They can provide immediate cohesion between two linguistic items; be chained in a sequence of immediate ties; or be remote, separated by one or more sentences.

Text cohesion is built both within and between sentences (see Personal Reflection 12.7). Paragraphs may also be made more or less cohesive by arranging and rearranging clauses. Subordinating conjunctions (e.g., *because, when, after*) and relative pronouns (e.g., *who, which, that*) are examples of cohesive devices.

Irwin (1988) pointed out that most cohesion instruction occurs incidentally as teachers help students resolve

PERSONAL REFLECTION 12.7 _____

"The status of the sentence as the sole unit of analysis when studying complexity in child language has changed with the advent of discourse analysis."

Cheryl Scott (1988b, p. 45), Oklahoma State University, in an article entitled "Producing Complex Sentences."

their problems during normal reading and writing tasks. For example, teachers may help students to identify the correct referents for confusing pronouns as they read, or they may help students replace redundant nouns with appropriate pronouns when they write. Irwin noted that "there is general agreement that students need not learn the names for any of these devices; instead, instruction can be planned in which skills are explained to the students and modeled by the clinician, followed by guided practice" (p. 20). An example of the three steps of explaining, modeling, and practice is included in Box 12.9.

Tattershall (1994) illustrated scaffolding techniques (modeling to independence) for helping students tune into discourse cohesion as a means to increasing comprehension (using sentences from Hagans, 1985, p. 37):

> **JUST ME:** *The teacher or SLP reads from the text, "Earth is always moving. It moves in two ways." Let's see, "It," what is "It"?*
> **YOU AND ME:** *The teacher or SLP reads from the text, "Earth does not stand straight up as it moves around the sun. Instead, it leans to one side." "Instead"? "Instead of what?"*

Box 12.8 _____

Cohesive Devices

TYPE	EXAMPLE
Reference	*Jack* went to the park. *He* played ball.
Substitution	Jack *went*. Everyone *did*.
Ellipsis	The *roses* were red. There were twelve.
Conjunction	I left *after* he did.
	I left *because* he did.
Lexical reiteration	The *cat* was black. It was a good *cat*.
Lexical collocation	I had 50 *cents*. That made a *dollar*.

Note: From "Linguistic Cohesion and the Developing Writer" by J. W. Irwin. Reprinted from *Topics in Language Disorders*, Vol. 8, No. 3, p. 15, with permission of Aspen Publishers, Inc., © 1988.

Box 12.9 _____

Direct Teaching of Implicit Connective Inference

EXPLAINING THE SKILL

CLINICIAN: It is very important when you read to know how the sentences fit together. Sometimes there are things for you to infer that the author doesn't state directly. This is especially true when one sentence tells why the event in the next sentence happened. You will need to infer many of these in the story we are about to read.

MODELING THE SKILL

CLINICIAN: Let me show you how I do this. Read the first paragraph silently while I read it aloud (_read paragraph_). Now, let's see. The first sentence tells me that Janice loved the store. The second sentence tells me that it had a lot of pretty things. Now, I ask myself, how do these sentences fit together? Well, I know that most people love pretty things. So, she probably loved the store because . . .
STUDENT: It had pretty things!!

GUIDED PRACTICE

CLINICIAN: Good! Now, let's read the next two sentences. How do these fit together?
STUDENT: They sold the candy so they could get money.
CLINICIAN: Good! One thing was the reason for another. Now, let's read on until we find another place where we can find reasons like this.

Note: From "Linguistic Cohesion and the Developing Writer" by J. W. Irwin. Reprinted from _Topics in Language Disorders,_ Vol. 8, No. 3, p. 20, with permission of Aspen Publishers, Inc., © 1988.

_____

Student answers hopefully, "Instead of standing straight, the Earth leans to one side."
JUST YOU: _The teacher or SLP reads, "Every year around June 21, the North Pole leans toward the sun. When it does, the sun shines directly on the Northern hemisphere."_
TEACHER: _"Can you find a tie and tell what it ties back to?"_
STUDENT: _" 'When it does' means when the North Pole leans toward the sun." (p. 69)_

DEVELOPING ABSTRACT AND NONLITERAL MEANINGS

GOAL: The student will acquire and use new and abstract words in oral and written contexts.

- Acquiring a Literate Lexicon
- Targeting Lexical Learning
- Targeting Figurative Language
- Targeting Word Retrieval

OUTCOME: The student will have sufficient vocabulary to read and write at grade level.

As mentioned in Chapter 11, by traditional accounts, most language development was complete by the time children entered school. That notion has been countered throughout Chapters 11 and 12. Even in earlier accounts, semantic development was recognized through adulthood. In the later stages of development, acquisition of a mature literate lexicon and acquisition of figurative language are two major accomplishments (Nippold, 1988a, 1988b, 1988d, 1995).

Acquiring a Literate Lexicon

To describe the special characteristics of lexical acquisition in the later stages of language learning, Nippold (1988d) used the term **literate lexicon,** which acknowledges the symbiotic relationship between lexical growth and literate activities. Nippold explained that "whereas literacy requires knowledge and use of a wide variety of words, the process of lexical growth itself is facilitated by literate activities" (pp. 29–30).

This is part of the "rich-get-richer" phenomenon (Stanovich, 1988). Children who read have the means to acquire new words. Children who have large vocabularies like to read. Full capacity is never reached. The more words one knows, the easier it is to acquire additional ones. That is the good news. The bad news is that many individuals with language impairments are unable to hook into this positive spiral and instead, slip further and further behind.

Older children and adolescents with language disorders often fall short in acquiring a literate lexicon on two levels: (1) They have difficulty acquiring abstract words and concepts for basic comprehension and production, and (2) they may have difficulty using metalinguistic strategies to talk about meanings and definitions. Both levels are part of competent, mature language function-

ing and may be targeted appropriately in language intervention (N. W. Nelson, 1988b; Nippold, 1995).

Wiig's (1984) review of the literature in this area suggested that differences in semantic acquisition by children with specific language disabilities are primarily quantitative. Children with language-learning disabilities tend to know fewer words and have less elaborated meanings for them. Qualitative problems have also been found involving concept formation (reflected in restricted word definitions), categorization, semantic associations and contrasts, interpreting lexical ambiguities, and processing multiple meaning words. As in other areas, children with language disorders tend to perform more like younger children than their same-age peers. Table 12.4 includes Wiig's (1984) summary of the similarities between word definitions produced by adolescents with language-learning disabilities and younger children, based on their levels of cognitive development.

TABLE 12.4   Overview of cognitive stages and the acquisition of word meanings

STAGE/AGE	CHILD'S WORD MEANINGS	EXAMPLES OF AGE-EXPECTED DEFINITIONS	DEFINITIONS BY ADOLESCENTS WITH LANGUAGE-LEARNING DISABILITIES
Preoperational intuitive thinking (2–7 yr)	Meanings are tied to concrete actions. Child begins to compile a dictionary of word meanings.	Bird: "Something that flies in the sky." Bottle: "Where you pour something out." Mother: "She feeds me and gives me a bath."	Apple: "Something you eat." History: "Something you learn in school."
Concrete operational (7–11 yr)	Perceives more complex relationships and has broader meanings, has difficulties in conversing about events that are not visible. Word definitions are tied to sentence contexts.	Bird: "It's like an airplane only it's little and chirps." Bottle: "It's like a can only you can see through it." Mother: "She has babies and takes care of them."	Apple: "It's something you eat that grows on trees." History: "It's something you learn in school that tells about a long time ago."
Formal operational (11+ yr)	Word definitions are essentially at adult levels. Talks about complex processes from an abstract point of view.	Bird: "It's a warmblooded animal that uses its wings to fly." Bottle: "A hollow glass container that holds liquid." Mother: "A lady who is a parent."	

Note: From "Language Disabilities in Adolescents: A Question of Cognitive Strategies" by E. H. Wiig. Reprinted from *Topics in Language Disorders,* Vol. 4, No. 2, p. 45, with permission of Aspen Publishers, Inc., © 1984.

New words are generally acquired in normal development through direct teaching or contextual abstraction (Werner & Kaplan, 1950). The rate at which new words are acquired in normal development is incredible. G. A. Miller and Gildea (1987) estimated that the average high school graduate has learned the meanings of at least 80,000 different words. This rate of learning would be impossible if words were acquired only through direct teaching (18-year-olds would have had to acquire an average of 12 words per day, including during infancy, to reach this total). Therefore, the majority of words must be acquired by the majority of learners by abstracting their meanings from contextual uses rather than through direct instruction (G. A. Miller & Gildea, 1987).

Several factors complicate the lexical learning picture for all individuals, regardless of language disorder. Evidence from normal development suggests complex interactions between internalized organizational capabilities and externalized lexical learning opportunities. For example, the well-known **syntagmatic–paradigmatic shift** (Entwisle, Forsyth, & Muuss, 1964), which occurs between the ages of 5 and 9 years in the children's verbal responses to free-association tasks, suggests that children's semantic systems undergo semantic reorganization during these years. Younger children's responses to stimulus words, for example, *go,* are often **syntagmatic** words, for example, *home,* which might follow the stimulus word in a sentence; beyond age 7, older children's responses to stimulus words, for example, *go,* are often **paradigmatic,** categorically related words, including antonyms, for example, *come.*

During this period, methods for teaching words within the official curriculum shift. At around second grade, definitional learning begins to be emphasized as dictionary skills are introduced. By fourth grade, written language becomes a major source of new word learning (Nippold, 1988d). Official vocabulary lists often accompany reading assignments of formal textbook series (part of the *de facto* curriculum).

The second level of lexical learning then becomes obvious. Students talk about the meanings of words, look them up in dictionaries, write down varied definitions, and take tests on them. Learning new words and definitions places considerable demands on students' metalinguistic systems (Nippold, 1995). Crais (1990) studied children's and adults' comprehension of novel and familiar words in stories. She found that third and

fifth graders were the most likely to provide definitions when they were asked to tell what they remembered about common words. Four of 20 third graders and eight of 20 fifth graders did this, whereas none of the 20 first graders or adults did. Crais hypothesized that the difference was related to the educational emphasis on definition tasks in the middle grades.

Learning a common dictionary meaning does not mean that an individual has full adult understanding of a word with all of its multiple, abstract, and figurative connotations (see Chapter 2 for a discussion of these features). That takes time and exposure. Language learners must encounter new words in multiple contexts, must recognize new words each time they are encountered, and must be able to relate new shades of meaning to old, thus enhancing and modifying existing schemata as appropriate.

Targeting Lexical Learning

Objective 1: The student will demonstrate strategies for acquiring new vocabulary from curricular contexts by: (a) identifying new words or unfamiliar word uses in context, (b) using multiple strategies to figure out word meanings, and (c) defining words.

Wiig and Semel (1976, 1980) outlined several categories of words and lexical relationships to be probed and encouraged for older students with language-learning disabilities. N. W. Nelson (1988b) provided intervention objectives based on these categories including (1) varied parts of speech (verbs, adjectives, pronouns), with particular focus on subtle differences between exemplars (e.g., *strike, slug*); (2) abstract word relationships (e.g., antonyms, synonyms, homonyms); (3) semantic classification (e.g., functional word definitions, multifaceted word definitions); (4) verbal analogies; (5) words signaling logicogrammatical relationships of time (e.g., *when, while, after*) and space or order (e.g., "*John was in front of Bill.*"); (6) figurative language (e.g., idioms, metaphors, similes); and (7) semantic relationships (e.g., inconsistencies and absurdities).

Wiig and Semel (1980) provided a set of 12 principles to assist children and adolescents with language-learning disabilities to acquire new lexical concepts: (1) Use information from normal development to decide when to introduce words, concepts, and relational terms. (2) Introduce new words with their prototypical referents. (3) Introduce words with general meanings before those with specific meanings. (4) Introduce words that are less complex before those that are more complex semantically. (5) Introduce the positive member of antonymous pairs before the negative one. (6) Introduce new words in sentences with controlled syntax. (7) Use pictorial or concrete referents to illustrate the concept whenever possible. (8) Emphasize the critical components of meaning when illustrating a new concept with a picture or other means. (9) Use multiple (at least 10 typical but different), clear referential contexts to introduce and elaborate the new concept. (10) Extend the concept to at least 10 more specific and abstract semantic contexts. (11) Extend the range of application and control of newly established words, concepts, and relationships. (12) Extend the range of application and control of new concepts to curricular areas.

Crais (1990) summarized several methods for targeting lexical knowledge in language intervention programs. She noted that, although much lexical learning occurs in normal development through naturalistic contextual experiences, children with language-learning difficulties may not be able to benefit as readily from such experiences. They may need more explicit instruction, for which Crais reviewed the following options: (1) Conduct mediational discussions to build on existing vocabulary by finding out what a student currently knows about a word, helping the student to elaborate that knowledge and to correct any misconceptions. (2) Expand the characteristics students associate with a word, perhaps by filling in a grid that lists words on one axis and common attributes on another with plus (+) or minus (–) symbols for characteristics that are either present or absent on a semantic feature chart. (3) Introduce alternative meanings of words, particularly facilitating students' recognition that words can have different meanings in different contexts. (4) Teach students to use morphological strategies to recognize word roots and to modify them by adding derivational morphemes like *un-* and *-less*. (5) Introduce semantically related information.

In another source (N. W. Nelson, 1989b) I suggested that regular curricular contexts provide the most relevant source of new words to target. Targeting words in the regular curriculum provides a lexicon within a linguistic context shared with classmates, where alternative meanings and shades of meaning can be discussed and within a value system reinforced by the regular classroom teacher. A sequence of IEP objectives for a high school student might be written as follows (N. W. Nelson, 1988b):

- The student will recall target words and use them appropriately in structured intervention activities of the following types (at least 2 different tasks correct for 18 of 20 target words; 3 sets of target words):
  a. Fill-in tasks
  b. Synonym and antonym tasks
  c. Definition tasks
  d. Rephrasing tasks
  e. Alternate meaning tasks
- The student will use context to figure out meanings of words that are newly introduced in paragraph contexts and will define them or use them correctly in a related context (8 of 10 new words for 3 sets of new words). (pp. 248–249)

These are rather traditional-looking objectives. The content for meeting them, however, can be obtained from collaborative meetings with classroom teachers or online participant observations with the student and his textbooks. When new content words, descriptive words, derivational morphemes (e.g., *hypo-, hyper-*), connectives, or directional words (e.g., *discuss, compare*) are encountered within the context of curricular language, they can become the word sets mentioned in the objectives.

The reason for teaching new words in sets is that they tend to be learned better in association and contrast to each other. A notebook with divided sections might be used to organize aspects of the student's new word-learning and related information, such as semantic maps and study outlines. New words, concepts, and definitional characteristics may be added as they are encountered, and previously taught words may be reviewed periodically to make sure that they are still active. Other curricular activities may also provide rich opportunity for new vocabulary acquisition. When students engage in process writing activities with peers, the activities motivate them to need new words in a way that sterile exercises cannot (see Personal Reflection 12.8).

Semantic organizers (Pehrsson & Denner, 1988) or semantic mapping (Heimlich & Pittelman, 1986) techniques provide a graphic demonstration to help students conceptualize and remember categorical relationships among words and their definitive characteristics. Semantic organizers allow students to visualize superordinate and subordinate relationships, to identify defining

PERSONAL REFLECTION 12.8 _____

"One day, later in the year, he came to my desk and asked if there were two meanings of the word 'hospital.' He wrote: 'The friend's sister had a lot of people over to celebrate Mardi Gras. I met a lot of them and they were very hospitable.' Scott seemed to be noticing words. He needed words; he was a writer.

He also needed details. 'Scott notices everything,' his mother told me. His writing began to show this attention to detail. He wrote: 'It was the first time I ate crawfish. You suck the inside of the head and eat the tail. It was very spicy.' These details were certain to entertain his classmates."

Peggy A. Swoger (1989, pp. 62–63), Regular Education English Teacher, Mountain Brook Junior High School, Mountain Brook, Alabama, writing about Scott's gift, which appeared when he participated in a regular writing class.

---

traits and component parts, and to provide examples. They may be used as study sheets and to engage in question asking and answering exchanges with fellow classmates. Semantic maps may be used to organize semantic elements from a variety of discourse genre. Figure 12.7 is a semantic map that organizes information about a narrative, "Rattlesnakes," that had expository information embedded in the text.

Targeting Figurative Language

Objective 2: The student will demonstrate comprehension and production of nonliteral words and phrases in oral and written language, including: (a) idioms, (b) metaphors, (c) similes, and (d) proverbs.

Nippold (1985) commented that "learning the correct interpretation and appropriate use of figurative language is important to youths aged 10–18 in both the academic and personal–social realms" (p. 1). This acknowledges the need for older children and adolescents to learn teenage slang (see discussion of social interaction conversation with peers earlier in this chapter) as well as the figurative language of idioms, similes, and metaphors. Other authors (e.g., D. K. Bernstein, 1986; Lund & Duchan, 1993; N. W. Nelson, 1988b) have included humor among the categories of figurative language acquired in the later stages of language learning.

Figurative language requires the language user to recognize nonliteral meanings of words and phrases and to make metalinguistic judgments about multiple levels of meaning. Idioms, particularly, have a fixed or conventional meaning in the language (Ackerman, 1982). Hyperbole is a related figurative language strategy that is sometimes so stereotypic it becomes idiomatic. Because such meanings do not relate to referents in the usual ways, they generally require experience in a social context before their meaning can be discovered.

Metaphor and simile are closely related figurative language forms. They both compare two unlike entities on some shared quality. A metaphor typically has three parts that may be labeled *topic, vehicle,* and *ground.* For example, in the sentence, "After the new permanent, her hair was a rat's nest," *hair* is the topic, *rat's nest* is the vehicle, and *messiness* is the ground. Metaphors may be structured either as predicative metaphors (similarity) or as proportional metaphors. Predicative metaphors have one topic and one vehicle, with both stated, "Her eyes were deep blue pools." Proportional metaphors have two topics, but the second is only inferred, based on an analogical relationship in the ground (e.g., "The party was a balloon that never got off the ground"). Some aspects of metaphors may be perceptual, and some may be psychological.

Similes have much in common with metaphors, but differ in that the comparison between the literal and nonliteral meanings is explicit. Most studies have shown similes to be easier for younger children and children with language disorders than metaphors are, probably because of this explicitness (Nippold, 1985, 1988a).

Proverbs place varied demands on language-learning systems depending on the combined concreteness and familiarity of the items. Nippold and Haq (1996) studied these variables with a written forced-choice task, which they presented to normally achieving children in grades 5, 8, and 11. Four types of proverbs were presented: **concrete-familiar** ("A rolling stone gathers no moss"); **concrete-unfamiliar** ("A caged bird longs for the clouds"); **abstract-familiar** ("Two wrongs don't make a right"); and **abstract-unfamiliar** ("Of idleness comes no goodness") (p. 166). The study yielded the expected order of difficulty, with concrete being easier than abstract, supporting the "metasemantic" hypothesis that comprehension develops through active analysis, and familiar being easier than the unfamiliar, supporting the "language experience" hypothesis that

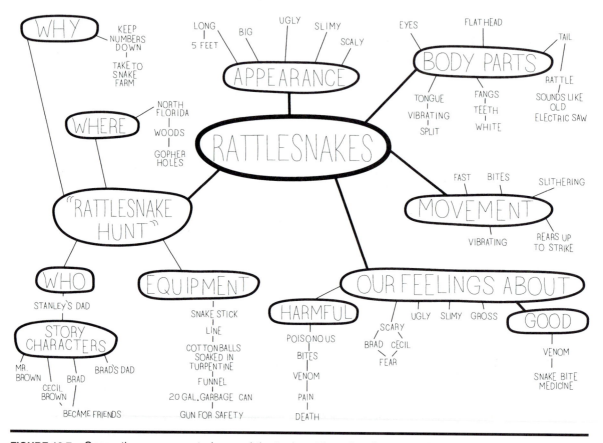

FIGURE 12.7   Semantic map generated around the topic *rattlesnakes,* in preparation for reading a story.

Note: From *Semantic Mapping: Classroom Applications* (p. 28) by J. E. Heimlich and S. D. Pittelman, 1986, Newark, DE, International Reading Assoc. Reprinted with permission of Joan E. Heimlich and the International Reading Association.

comprehension develops through meaningful exposure to proverbs. Both features might be built into intervention programs.

Familiarity (or frequency) also influences the interpretation of idioms. Children in grades 5, 8, and 11 responded more accurately about highly familiar idioms in tasks that required them to write what idioms mean (Nippold & Rudzinski, 1993) or to make a forced choice about meaning (Nippold & Taylor, 1995). An example of a more familiar idiom is "beat around the bush," and a less familiar one is to "take a powder." Students in both studies of Nippold and colleagues also were better able to respond accurately to idioms that were more transparent. Transparency is the degree of closeness between the

nonliteral and literal meaning. An example of a more transparent idiom is to "keep a straight face," and a more opaque one is to "talk through one's hat."

As this discussion suggests, many variables influence the relative ease or difficulty of understanding figurative language (Nippold, 1985; 1988a), including frequency, concreteness, transparency, syntactic complexity, semantic analyzability, and inclusion of linguistic and nonlinguistic context. If appropriate testing methods are used, preschoolers can understand some metaphoric meanings; first graders can give interpretations for some idioms; and figurative language skills continue to develop throughout the school-age years and into adulthood (Nippold & Martin, 1989).

Several studies have shown that children with language-learning disabilities in the later grades of elementary school and beyond do not fare as well as their normal-language-learning peers (Nippold & Fey, 1983; Seidenberg & Bernstein, 1986). They tend to process figurative language like younger children, needing additional contextual support and more explicit linguistic markers to understand the relationships conveyed. Nippold (1985) reviewed research that showed high correlations between figurative language proficiency, reading ability, and vocabulary development; experience seems to play a major role as well. Ezell and Goldstein (1991) found that a group of 9-year-old children with mild mental retardation performed worse than age-matched peers on an idiom-comprehension task, as expected. Surprisingly, however, they performed better than a group of younger children matched for receptive vocabulary age. The children with mental retardation did particularly well matching pictures to frequently occurring idioms such as "got cold feet" and "got carried away."

These results highlight an important intervention strategy for figurative language—*exposure.* Language specialists must ensure that older children and adolescents have the opportunity to hear examples of idiomatic and metaphoric language in meaningful and natural contexts. Older children also may need opportunities to practice telling jokes even before they fully understand them (Lund & Duchan, 1989). Studies of regular classroom environments show that even kindergarten teachers use figurative language (Lazar et al., 1989). However, teachers may not always provide the scaffolding necessary for all children to benefit. Children in special education classrooms are even less likely to hear figurative language in natural contexts, and their isolation from teenage slang has already been discussed. Newton (1985) compared the teacher talk of three groups of teachers, a group of teachers of the deaf who used oral communication strategies, a group who used total communication strategies, and a group of teachers of normal hearing students. She found no differences between the uses of idiomatic language in the teachers of oral-communicating deaf and normal-hearing children, but she found reduced idiomatic expression in both the oral and signed portions of communication in the total communication classrooms.

Many individuals with language disorders need to be shown how to abstract meaning from context through repeated exposure with mediation (Nippold, 1991). Learn-ing how to learn has been a major topic of this chapter. One might imagine a whole class of children becoming "idiom detectives" and creating a classroom master list of all of the idioms they hear or read, identifying the source, and noticing opportunities to reuse the idioms in their own exchanges. A language-rich environment is one of the enticements for including more children with language disorders in regular classrooms with students of mixed ability levels.

Computer software programs have been suggested as a context for providing both exposure and support targeting figurative language learning. Nippold, Schwarz, and Lewis (1992) reviewed four programs, Figurative Language (Abraham, 1984), Focusing on Language Arts: Figurative Language (Poirer, Jackson, & Boonyasopan, 1985), Figuring Out Figurative Language (Durgy, 1986), and Idioms in America (Esterreicher, 1986). Nippold and her colleagues provided a set of six standards for reviewing these and other programs: (1) reflects normal language development (all four did this minimally), (2) has clear theoretical rationale (none did this), (3) provides comprehensive instruction (none did this), (4) allows for customizing (Abraham did this, and Esterreicher minimally), (5) can bypass common learning problems (none did this), and (6) documents own teaching effectiveness (none did this). Although none of the four programs reviewed by Nippold and her colleagues met most or all of the criteria, computer software is no doubt an intervention context with a strong future.

Targeting Word Retrieval

Objective 3. The student will demonstrate multiple strategies and improved skill (over baseline measurements) for retrieving words in academic and social contexts and will advocate successfully for accommodations needed to compensate for the word-finding impairment.

Intervention procedures for targeting word retrieval were discussed in Chapter 10. As children enter the later stages of childhood and adolescence, the primary programmatic shifts are toward greater awareness, conscious control of strategies, and self-advocacy to obtain the accommodations for word-finding problems at school.

In her *Word Finding Intervention Program* (WFIP), German (1993) established five principles of intervention for word-finding difficulties. The first is to base the intervention on assessment of whether the individual's word-finding difficulty represents a problem of word storage (see also Casby, 1992a; Chapter 10), word retrieval, or weaknesses in both. The second is to individualize the intervention to match the unique word-finding profile of the learner, including (1) description of performance in both single-word and whole discourse contexts, and (2) whether the individual is slow or fast, accurate or inaccurate, in retrieving. The third principle is to design a program that is comprehensive in its focus and application. A comprehensive program includes remediation, self-advocacy instruction, and compensatory modification (more about those in the next paragraph). German's fourth principle is to integrate several programming perspectives in the intervention: direct instruction, application, co-teaching, cognitive modification, and collaboration. The fifth is to implement the program using several service delivery contexts, including the language room, the general or special education classroom, and the academic lesson. McGregor and Leonard (1995) agreed that "Intervention that does not take place in the classroom should at least involve a bridge to the classroom" (p. 91).

The three-pronged approach involving **remediation, self-advocacy instruction,** and **compensatory modification** relates to the three-level assessment and intervention strategy advocated throughout this book. **Remediation** is based on the communication processes model. It aims to reduce the word-finding impairment directly by improving the communicative processes of word storage and retrieval. German's remediation approach targets instruction in four strategies: (1) attribute cuing, (2) semantic alternates, (3) associate cuing, and (4) reflective pausing. Remedial procedures for developing these strategies include segmentation plus rehearsal, rhythm plus rehearsal, rehearsal, and rapid drill. Casby (1992a) described intervention aimed more at storage. **Self-advocacy instruction** is based on the communication needs model. It aims to reduce functional limitations by helping the individual develop an executive system based on self-awareness, self-assessment, and self-instruction. Students also learn to advocate for accommodations they need to perform successfully in the important contexts of their lives. **Compensatory modification** is based on a participation model to reduce disability (formerly called "handicap"). It involves changing learning and testing contexts to provide accommodations and to give students the opportunity to

show what they know (e.g., by using multiple choice tests instead of fill-in-the-blank).

Methods for measuring the outcome of intervention for word-finding deficits should consider changes in both structured tasks and naturalistic discourse. The two factors, speed (or latency) and accuracy, constitute the primary variables to monitor for change (Casby, 1992a). One approach is to measure the latency of single responses in milliseconds, but this approach is difficult without special equipment. Therefore, McGregor and Leonard (1995) suggested collecting sets of words into intervention sets and using a stopwatch to time how long it takes the student to name the whole set in a confrontation naming task, looking for change, and maintenance of change over time. They also cautioned, however, not to confuse testing with intervention, noting that "It is unlikely that naming drills in which words are neither elaborated nor practiced in connected discourse will improve word finding beyond confrontation-naming tasks" (p. 101). To document a reduction in naming errors, it may be best to track decreases within spontaneous discourse samples. Effects should also be considered in the broader domains of social interaction and academic performance.

FACILITATING TRANSITIONS

GOAL: The student will demonstrate self-advocacy and independence in discussing his or her educational, vocational, and social future.

- Transitions
- Independence

OUTCOME: The student will make successful adjustments at key transition points in later childhood and adolescence and will live independently as an adult.

Transitions

Objective 1. The students will participate in developing transition plans, helping to establish outcome goals, and will explain treatment objectives in terms that demonstrate understanding.

Language and communication are essential to every part of life. From the time students are 16 years old (and "when determined appropriate for the individual, beginning at age 14 or younger" §1401a.20, PL 101–476), their Individualized Education Plans (IEPs) must include a plan for transition services. Transition services, which were described in Chapter 5, are coordinated activities "based upon the individual student's needs, taking into account the student's preferences and interests, and shall include instruction, community experiences, the development of employment and other postschool adult living objectives, and, when appropriate, acquisition of daily living skills and functional vocational evaluation" (§1401a.19). They are designed to promote "movement from school to postschool activities, including postsecondary education, vocational training, integrated employment (including supported employment), continuing and adult education, adult services, independent living or community participation" (§1401a.19).

Often an initial need is to help students with communication disorders develop the skills and strategies for taking an active part in the planning process. They may need scaffolding to express their preferences and interests. If assessment and intervention from students' younger years have included interviews to establish their goals and priorities and procedures to develop their conscious awareness, they may be more likely to have ownership of those goals. Students may also need to learn how to advocate for themselves in a way that others respect and will get them the accommodations they need.

The first step of this process is for students to understand their own strengths and needs. Graduate-student clinician Elaine DeRoover used Lynda Miller's (1990, 1993) adaptations of Howard Gardner's (1983) theory of multiple intelligences to construct a Smart Profile with her 15-year-old client, Ken (see Figure 12.8). They constructed this profile together over several sessions, treating it as a modifiable representation of how Ken viewed himself as a learner. They also continued to gather data to support the view of Ken as an individual with many intellectual strengths, as well as language-learning needs. For example, in her daily report for the eighth session, DeRoover wrote:

MATHEMATICAL INTELLIGENCE. When Ken and clinician were "negotiating" a percentage for the objective to "decode all unfamiliar words, including all sounds present in the words," and the clinician said, "Let's just split the difference" between 55% [his idea] and 80% [hers], Ken continued to talk and respond appropriately to clinician comments, but then wrote 67.5% on his paper (exactly halfway between the two percentages).

LOGICAL INTELLIGENCE. Ken wrote a "key" at the end of his draft copy of semester therapy objectives, in

which he specified what his one-word comments and symbols by each objective meant.

DeRoover also worked with Ken directly on understanding his treatment objectives and the rationale for them. This involved active practice in expressing the essence of objectives, supported with scaffolding [steps and interpretations of Ken's responses in square brackets] to support greater understanding and independence. For example, in one session, Ken read the objective [framing]:

Ken will demonstrate improvement, as reported by his teachers and observed in therapy, of his reading-for-understanding strategies, including: (1) requesting help in decoding a particular word or phrase, (2) using "top-down" processing questions to ask if the passage makes sense, (3) attempting different syllable stress patterns on unknown words to find a match in his known vocabulary.

The discussion that followed illustrates how DeRoover used scaffolding techniques to frame, focus, guide, and feed back information to assist Ken to develop greater understanding, independence, and ownership of the change process. The discussion starts with Andew's attempt to paraphrase the objective:

/ = pause

K: *Basically, they write that I am using it or not / and like my reading strategies, if they improve or not or stay the same or whatever. Usually, it'll be just the same for all the teachers. [active processing—he understands the part about teacher feedback]*

D: *But this whole thing is about you improving what? [focusing]*

K: *My reading strategies, like reading bottom-up or top-down. [not clear whether Ken understands this distinction]*

D: *Reading so that you / what? [refocusing]*

K: *So you can say the word or whatever. [like many students with language learning disabilities who have had difficulty learning how to read, Ken thinks of reading primarily as "sounding out the words"]*

D: *(pointing to the line that starts "reading-for-understanding") Well, actually, what is this about? Is this reading so you can say the word or reading so you . . . [framing, giving feedback, and guiding]*

K: *(interrupting quickly) understand it [this is a heavily scaffolded response; it will be developed to a level of independence over the next few sessions].*

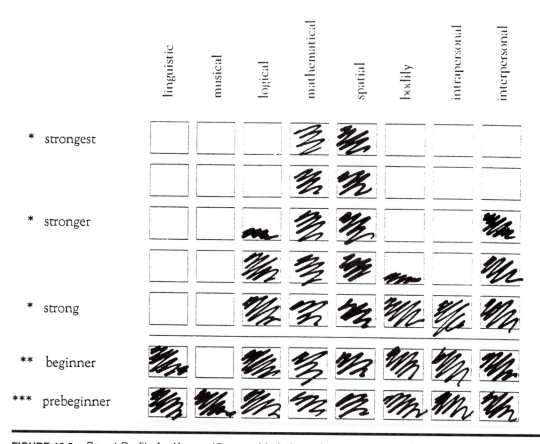

FIGURE 12.8   Smart Profile for Ken, a 15-year-old ninth grade student with language-learning disabilities, constructed using procedures recommended by Miller (1990).

* strong * stronger * strongest	relative degrees of willingness to engage in learning because it is reinforcing
** beginner	willing to engage in new learning, willing to not know something willing to make mistakes, willing to not be able to generalize easily. willing to take a long time getting better
*** prebeginner	unwilling to engage in new learning, unwilling to not know something unwilling to make mistakes, unwilling to not be able to generalize easily. unwilling to take a long time getting better

Note: From: Miller, L. (1990). *The Smart Profile: A qualitative approach for describing learners and designing instruction* (p. 4). Austin, TX: Smart Alternatives. Used by permission.

Self-advocacy involves the ability to explain one's strengths and specialized learning needs in new situations (academic, vocational, social) with each transition. Cronin and Patton (1993) recommended thinking of adult life skills in six domains: (1) employment/education, (2) home and family, (3) leisure pursuits, (4) personal responsibility and relationships, (5) physical/emotional health, and (6) community involvement. Each of these can be further specified as subdomains with major life demands and specific skills that can be targeted with instruction. In cases in which impairments result in continued functional limitations, individuals should be taught to advocate appropriately for selective accommodations that will help them overcome those limitations.

In a discussion with the Transition Coordinator at his high school, Ken established that he needed a few accommodations in his general education classes. These included: (1) unlimited time for testing, (2) the opportunity to use the Franklin Spelling Ace, and (3) the ability to use a word processor for written work. The transition plan included the annual goal:

> *Ken will identify needed accommodations/adaptations/ modifications in content area classes with his Transition Planning Team, and give this information in written form to his teachers at the beginning of each semester.*

His Transition Plan also included specification of desired long-term outcomes:

> *Employment:* I want to be employed full-time in a competitive employment setting.
> *Education/Training:* After high school I want to attend and graduate from college.
> *Adult Living:* I want to live independently in my own apartment or home.
> *Community Participation:* I want to be involved and independent in my community.

Independence

Objective 2. The student will demonstrate skills, strategies, and self-advocacy in life situations independent of special support.

A major goal of transition planning is to assist individuals to maintain skills and continue to grow independent of special supports. It is based on the philosophy that helping to establish one's own goals contributes to the individual's sense of ownership of them. Throughout the later stages of language acquisition, students with language disorders can provide input to define their own zones of significance and can practice restating their goals to demonstrate understanding.

A theme of this book has been to use questions to foster higher order problem solving and independence. Expecting independence is one of the keys to achieving it, but independence also needs active fostering. As students enter new situations and function well, they gain added confidence for risking new activities. An essential component of the scaffolding process is confirming independent demonstration of the scaffolded knowl-

edge, skill, or strategies in subsequent events. This is particularly characteristic of language intervention in the later stages of childhood and adolescence.

SUMMARY

This chapter presented consideration of the communicative contexts, abilities, and needs of children at later stages of language development. During this period, children consolidate their earlier language learning and gain confidence in using oral and written language for new and varied purposes. They expand their contacts with their peer group, and they work toward independence from their families. Techniques of curriculum-based language assessment and intervention were emphasized for working with language-learning needs within the context of real academic experiences, both written and oral.

Examples of later-stage intervention targets and strategies include the following: modify language-learning contexts with mediational and scaffolding techniques; foster metaskills and other executive strategies for school survival and higher order thinking, and focus on process rather than product; develop competence in varied discourse genres and events (conversational, narrative, and expository); encourage syntactic sophistication; develop abstract and nonliteral meanings; and facilitate transitions into adulthood.

As in previous chapters, no one intervention approach was advocated as best for all abilities and all children and adolescents. At the secondary level, however, strategy-based intervention approaches are particularly appropriate. The role of adults in the process as mediator or facilitator helps students gain access to more communicative events. The underlying message in this chapter is consistent with the message conveyed throughout the book. *Problems are not just within children–and neither are solutions.*

REVIEW TOPICS

- The language-learning contexts of later-stage language learning, including sociocultural factors, mediational discourse, classroom contexts, curriculum-based language intervention, and varied service delivery models (in-classroom direct, indirect consultation models, after-school computer writing labs and homework labs, alternate language classrooms, special workshops).

- Metaskills and intervention approaches, including learning strategy models, metapragmatic strategies and school survival skills, metacognitive strategies focused on memory (e.g., mnemonics) and higher order thinking, writing process approaches, SQ3R and other meta-approaches to develop reading comprehension.
- Intervention targets and strategies related to three discourse genres: conversational, narrative, and expository.
- Later-stage syntactic–semantic targets and intervention strategies, including morphological developments (particularly derivational), more complex sentences representing more abstract meanings, and cohesive relationships across sentences. Also, sentence combining and paraphrasing compared to discourse-based (whole language) approaches to intervention, crossing oral and written modalities.
- Later-stage lexical targets, including a "literate" lexicon, varieties of figurative language (idioms, similes, metaphors, and proverbs), and word retrieval strategies (focused on storage and retrieval processes).
- Transition plans and their roles in fostering independence.

REVIEW QUESTIONS

1. What are some of the executive demand differences of secondary school settings over the lower grades?
2. What are the six cognitive processes addressed in Bloom's taxonomy? What other techniques could you use to help students categorize their knowledge and what they need to know to solve particular academic problems?
3. How do conversational, narrative, and expository discourse structures differ? What variants can you identify within each type? What is the evidence that intervention can make a difference?
4. How should later-stage syntactic–semantic skills be encouraged? What does the literature say about targeting complex sentences within whole discourse, such as reading or telling stories, or as discrete language skills? How could you design a hybrid approach that would include elements of both?
5. Why is Tattershall's sequence "just me," "you and me," and "just you," a good reminder about setting up scaffolding for mediational teaching? The example related to the language of cohesion, but how

could you apply this sequence to other kinds of scaffolding discourse (e.g., related to teaching the language of mathematics)?
6. What criteria would you use to evaluate a computer software program designed to teach figurative language?
7. What would you want to know about an individual student before designing an intervention to target word finding difficulty?
8. What should a transition plan contain? How could you use it and other aspects of goal setting to help an adolescent be more independent and in control of his or her own future?

ACTIVITIES FOR EXTENDED THINKING

1. If you can obtain appropriate access, interview a group of adolescents with language-learning disabilities about what they like and don't like about the special interventions they have received over the years. What is their opinion of an ideal service delivery model for high school students?

2. Pull out a middle school or high school textbook. Analyze the discourse structure of selected passages. Look for evidence of cohesive devices (lexical, pronominal, conjunctive) and think about how you could frame them in scaffolding discourse so that a student with a language disorder could detect the logical and referential relationships. In a math book, look for evidence of direct versus indirect wording, extraneous information, and multistep operations. Try, yourself, to "first draw the problem, then do the math." In a literature selection, look for varieties of figurative language and literate vocabulary. Is there enough support in the surrounding context to infer meaning, or would one have to rely on prior world knowledge and experience with the specific forms?

3. Arrange to work with a student having difficulty in school. What evidence can you find that language weakness may be playing a role in the difficulty? Work with the student to scaffold the components of the pinball wizardry model that seem not to be lighting up for this particular student. Can you mediate the student to make connections and use language skills that were heretofore ignored or impossible? What functional outcomes can the two of you identify that demonstrate that change has made a real-life difference for the student?

13

Severe Communication Impairment: Assessment and Intervention

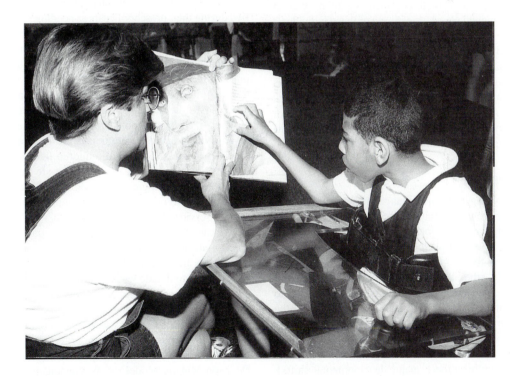

IDENTIFYING COMMUNICATION NEEDS
OF INDIVIDUALS WITH SEVERE
DISABILITIES

ASSESSMENT AND PLANNING MODELS

CONTEXTS FOR ASSESSMENT AND
INTERVENTION

COMMUNICATIVE INTENTIONS AND
INTERACTIONS

CONTENT–FORM DEVELOPMENTS

NARRATIVE AND LITERACY
DEVELOPMENTS

TRANSITIONS TO WORK AND ADULTHOOD

IDENTIFYING COMMUNICATION NEEDS OF INDIVIDUALS WITH SEVERE DISABILITIES

Children with such severe disabilities as moderate-to-severe cognitive impairment or autism are at risk to remain at earlier stages of language acquisition after their same-age peers have moved on. Severe sensory and motor deficits, particularly in combination with other problems, increase the risk for significant delay. For children with severe or mixed impairments, it is important to identify the extent of central cognitive and linguistic deficits and to separate those deficits as much as possible from more peripheral sensory and motor deficits. Intervention may involve provision of compensatory methods and technology, such as acoustic amplification and augmentative communication, along with environmental modifications and adaptations. This chapter considers the needs of individuals with severe communication impairments related to conditions such as autism, cerebral palsy, and mental retardation. Some of these individuals stay in the early stages of language acquisition. Others enter middle and later stages. In particular, a diagnosis of cerebral palsy predicts nothing about the state of a child's language system. Language intervention services needed by nonspeaking individuals should be matched to their language function levels with consideration of their chronological ages. They should also address written language as well as oral language.

Early-Stage Needs

In the early stages of normal language acquisition, children move from prelinguistic interactions, with others interpreting their behavior (including vocal behavior) as communicative (the **perlocutionary stage**), through a phase when they communicate intentionally but only nonverbally (the **illocutionary stage**), into a phase when they use verbal symbols to communicate and to express increasingly wide ranges of meanings (the **locutionary stage**). These gross landmarks in early communicative development can provide part of the map needed to establish early-stage intervention plans (Table 8.2 outlines these major developmental shifts). Children whose development is impeded by severe sensory, motor, and/or cognitive deficits may find some aspects of this process more accessible than others.

A premise underlying the treatment of all severely communicatively impaired children is that, just as no child is untestable, no child is incapable of achieving some level of communication. As some researchers have noted (Watzlawick, Beavin, & Jackson, 1967), it is impossible *not* to communicate:

> No matter how one may try, one cannot not *communicate. Activity or inactivity, words or silence all have message value: they influence others and these others, in turn, cannot not respond to these communications and are thus themselves communicating. It should be clearly understood that the mere absence of talking or of taking notice of each other is no exception to what had just been asserted. (p. 49)*

Middle-Stage Needs

Most children with multiple impairments, involving combinations of conditions such as hearing loss, mental retardation, autism, and physical impairment, are identified during their preschool years as needing special help, and they often continue to receive help over the years as they mature. Other children with multiple impairments may receive language intervention services during their preschool years but fail to meet eligibility criteria for specialized speech–language services as they advance in age. What criteria should be used for deciding which children need speech and language intervention services when speech and language delays are integral parts of other disabilities? Should all children like this qualify because their communicative abilities are inconsistent with their chronological ages? Should none of them qualify because other conditions are primary? In some school service–delivery systems, either of these extremes may be evident. Either approach may lead to inappropriate decisions about children when their needs as individuals are not considered.

One way to decide when to refer children with other disabilities for speech–language services is to look for mismatches between communicative skills and other developmental abilities, particularly cognitive ones. This is the cognitive-referencing criterion discussed in Chapters 3 and 6. It is a component of the Michigan Decision-Making Model (N. W. Nelson, 1989a; N. W. Nelson, Silbar, & Lockwood, 1981) discussed later in this chapter. But that model relates to what kind of communicative intervention should be provided, not *whether* it should be provided. Such a procedure, however, can have all of the pitfalls discussed previously.

As suggested throughout this book, professionals should remember to ask questions not only about what is wrong with children's communicative skills but also about what children need to be able to do in certain contexts (see Box 13.1). They should also ask about opportunities individuals have to participate in contexts that parents, teachers, and children identify as important. Regional rules should be written so that all children who need special education services are eligible to receive them in a way that does not limit their participation with same-age peers (see Personal Reflection 13.1).

Box 13.1 _____

Suggestions for Recognizing the Need for Consultation with a Communicative Specialist for Older Children and Adolescents with Moderate-to-Severe Multiple Disabilities

- **Failure to understand instructions.** When a person has difficulty performing essential job or daily living tasks, consider the possibility that the person may not understand the language of instructions and may not have sufficient communicative skill to ask for repetition or clarification.
- **Inability to use language to meet daily living needs.** When individuals can produce enough words to formulate a variety of utterances, including questions, then they can travel independently, shop independently, use the telephone when they need to, and ask for assistance in getting out of problem situations when they arise. If persons cannot function in a variety of working, shopping, and social contexts, consider that communicative impairments may be limiting their independence.
- **Violation of rules of politeness and other rules of social transaction.** The ability to function well in a variety of contexts with friends, acquaintances, and one-time contacts depends on sensitivity to the unspoken rules of social interaction. One of the most frequently cited reasons for failure of workers with disabilities to 'fit in' with fellow workers is their inability to engage in small-talk during work breaks. Examples that might cause difficulty are failure to take communicative turns when offered, or conversely, interrupting the turns of others; saying things that are irrelevant to the topic, not using politeness markers or showing interest in what the other person says; making blunt requests owing to lack of linguistic skill for softening them; failing to shift style of communication for different audiences (e.g., talking the same way to the boss as to co-workers); and any other communicative behavior that is perceived as odd or bizarre. If people seem to avoid interacting with the target person, referral may be justified.
- **Lack of functional ability to read signs and other symbols and to perform functional writing tasks.** The ability to recognize the communicative symbols of the culture enables people to know how to use public transportation, to find their way around buildings, to comply with legal and safety expectations, and to fill out forms or use bank accounts. Communicative specialists may be able to assist in identifying the best strategies for teaching functional reading and writing skills and encouraging the development of other symbol-recognition and use skills.
- **Problems articulating speech clearly enough to be understood, stuttering, or using an inaudible or inappropriate voice.** Other speech and voice disorders may interfere with the person's ability to communicate. When such problems are noted, the individual should be referred to a speech–language pathologist.

"We wanted more for Ted, but as we fought for his ed-ucation, we learned that we had to overcome prejudice and ignorance. Like the civil rights leaders who chal-lenged the cultural bias against minority children, we were pioneers, arguing that our child needed teachers and specialists who understood his differences, who wouldn't use standardized tests to deny him opportu-nities."

Charles Hart (1989, p. 116), writing about his son with autism in a book called *Without Reason,* in which Hart also writes about growing up with his own older brother who had autism as well. (Hart is also a member of the Board of Directors of the Autism Society of America.)

The challenge to professionals when working with older individuals with middle-stage communicative abilities is to offer services appropriate to individuals' developmental levels without relying on activities and materials that are either irrelevant or inappropriate to their age levels. A particular danger with older students who have not yet acquired skills that are common tar-gets of preschool curricula (e.g., independent dressing, shape recognition, color naming, or number identifica-tion) is that their programs will become mired in a focus on preschool level concerns. The danger is that the at-tention on developmental academic and self-help ob-jectives will cause other functional needs (e.g., for social interaction and even emergent literacy) to be ig-nored. It is not the case that self-dressing, color identi-fication, and shape naming are prerequisites for learning to read (Vellutino & Shub, 1982).

Students who have cognitive impairments, in partic-ular, need periodic program review to ensure that they are given opportunities to acquire skills that will enable them to function as independently as possible while in school and as they mature into adults. Their commu-nicative needs should be reassessed periodically in con-texts appropriate to their chronological age needs, because changing contexts may signal changes in their abilities to meet communicative demands of the new contexts.

Special education and language intervention pro-grams often focus on helping these individuals de-velop functional abilities for participating with as much

independence as possible in school, community, and job settings, and in **activities of daily living (ADL).** This focus on functionality is appropriate, but the professional should not overlook the possibility that functional literacy skills and other middle-stage lan-guage developments might be needed to support such activities. As functional goals are pursued, speech–language pathologists can collaborate with others to foster a better match, both by stretching individuals' comunicative abilities beyond their current limits and by increasing these youngsters' opportunities to partici-pate in activities from which they might acquire addi-tional middle-stage communicative skills. For example, some older children and adolescents with moderate-to-severe cognitive disabilities may acquire some literacy skills.

Later-Stage Needs

When individuals have severe or multiple disabilities, the challenge to offer services that are appropriate both for their developmental stage and chronological age levels is marked in the later-stage years. For each indi-vidual, communicative needs should be reassessed pe-riodically in age-appropriate contexts of home, school, community, and work, with a focus on activities of daily living and meaningful work.

Referral may be the best method for identifying these individuals, but referral criteria must be tailored to the purpose. Referral criteria based on discrete lan-guage abilities probably will not work, because most individuals with cognitive limitations have communi-cative skills considerably below those expected for their chronological ages. Shifting experiences in ado-lescence and adulthood may also bring new contextu-ally based communicative demands for which they are inadequately prepared. Box 13.1 offers a set of referral criteria to assist professionals such as employment counselors and special educators to know when a com-municative specialist might help to solve functional communication problems for older individuals with middle-stage (or even earlier) language abilities.

Some students with severe communicative impair-ments are nonspeaking but are functioning at the later stages of language development. These are individ-uals who may be in late elementary, middle school, high school, or post-secondary settings. They use augmentive and alternative communication (AAC) devices, techniques, and strategies to express their language, but they comprehend oral and written language at levels commensurate with their same-age peers, and they can meet the same academic standards. Beukelman and Mirenda (1992) called such students "academically competitive" (p. 207). They noted that meeting the same academic standards does not necessarily mean that students will complete all the same activities to the same degree:

> *For example, students with AAC systems often cannot write as rapidly as their peers and, therefore, the seat work they are expected to complete may be reduced, as long as the same academic standards are met. Some students may choose to reduce their total academic workloads in order to fulfill the requirements of classes in which they are competitive. For example, it is not uncommon for students with severe disabilities at the post-secondary level to enroll in only one or two classes each semester so that they can be academically successful and still have time to participate in the social opportunities available on a college campus. (p. 208)*

Students with multiple impairments that involve mental retardation as well as physical disability or autism, for example, may also have later-stage needs even though they cannot be academically competitive in any or all of their classes. Such individuals need an intervention team to consider ways to keep them "active" or "involved" (Beukelman & Mirenda, 1992, p. 208) with their same-age peers who are at the later stages of language acquisition. Jorgensen (1994b) described Matt, who had no traditional academic goals on his IEP, but was included in the eighth-grade science class. Jorgensen showed how objectives could be written that are appropriate both to a student's developmental needs and chronological age by contrasting "old" and "new" short-term objectives:

> ***Old Short-Term Objective:*** *Matt will sequence 5–6 pictures depicting a familiar activity correctly 9 times out of 10.*

> ***New Short-Term Objective:*** *During classroom activities, such as science lab, Matt will improve his skills in sequencing by assembling dissection trays or by documenting the steps of the experiment by taking instant*

photos and pasting them in order along the corresponding steps of the written report. (p. 92)

Augmentive and Alternative Communication Needs

When considering the needs of children whose motor development is severely impeded, it is important to recognize two things about relationships between speech and language: (1) Some individuals with severe physical disabilities will never speak intelligibly, and (2) being nonspeaking does not equate with being severely language impaired. As discussed in the previous section and originally in Chapter 2, differentiating factors related to language, speech, and communication can assist in planning appropriate intervention strategies. Nonspeaking children may have varying degrees of communicative and linguistic abilities. Some nonvocal individuals are quite verbal; they can use linguistic symbols in meaningful, productive, and conventional ways. Other communicative individuals who vocalize their needs and frustrations may be nonverbal.

Because the terminology associated with these conditions may be confusing, professionals in AAC have attempted to clarify it (Fried-Oken, 1987; Vanderheiden & Yoder, 1986). Those efforts are summarized in Box 13.2. A particularly important contrast, which is often misunderstood, is between **nonverbal communication** and **nonvocal verbal behavior.** Remember that "verbal," in the context of AAC discussions, refers to the presence of linguistic symbols, not speech. Therefore, **nonverbal communication** refers to actions that are received as communicative even though they involve no words. On the other hand, **nonvocal verbal behavior** is symbolic communication that involves unspoken linguistic transmission using a system like writing, sign language, or Blissymbols. A communication aid that uses synthetic speech is often referred to as a **voice output communication aid** (VOCA). Decisions about AAC for an individual depend on comprehensive assessments using all three models that have been discussed throughout this book (and later in this chapter), based on the work of Beukelman and Mirenda (1992): communication processes, communication needs, and participation.

In this chapter, AAC needs are not considered separately, but as an integral part of supporting communica-

Box 13.2 _____

Terminology Associated with Augmentative and Alternative Communication

Aided communication technique. Any augmentative and alternative communication (AAC) technique using some type of physical device or object (e.g., communication board, chart, mechanical or electronic aid).

Augmentative and alternative communication system. The total integrated network of techniques, aids, strategies, and skills an individual uses either to supplement (augmentative) or to replace (alternate) inadequate natural speaking capability. It includes (1) one or more communicative techniques, (2) a symbol set or system, and (3) a variety of communicative–interactive behaviors.

Communication. Process by which information is exchanged between individuals using both verbal and nonverbal behaviors.

Communication aid. A physical object or device that helps a person communicate (e.g., communication board, electronic aid, voice output communication aid).

Communicative mode. One of the several different major channels or forms of communication (e.g., speaking, listening, reading, writing, gesturing).

Nonspeaking person. Anyone whose speech is temporarily or permanently inadequate to meet all of his or her communication needs and whose inability to speak is not primarily due to a hearing impairment.

Nonverbal communication. Communication that does not involve the use of words (spoken, written, or signed); it does use nonverbal communicative behaviors such as kinesics (communicative posturing and bodily movements); paralinguistics (pitch height and range, stress, intonation, vocal intensity, articulatory control); proxemics (interpersonal distance); and chronemics (timing factors).

Nonvocal verbal behavior. The communication of information through some physical structure other than the vocal tract and oral musculature (e.g., written language, sign systems, and rule-governed graphic symbol systems, e.g., Blissymbols).

Skill. An ability developed over time and with practice (both strategies and skills, e.g., pointing or spelling, contribute to the relative competence a person exhibits when using AAC system components).

Strategy. A specific way of using aids or techniques more effectively for specific purposes (e.g., when communicating under time pressure, a more telegraphic style may be used; different strategies may be used for group communication).

Symbol. An abstract but recognized object, mark, or graphic design that stands for or represents something else (e.g., rebus, picture, Blissymbol, word, American Sign Language sign, gesture, or speech morpheme).

Technique. A method for transmitting ideas (e.g., linear scanning, row–column scanning, signing, common gestures, natural vocalizations, facial expressions, eye pointing).

Unaided communication technique. Any AAC technique that does not require a physical aid (e.g., manual, gestural, manual–visual sign, facial communication).

User interface. The physical means a person uses to control a communication aid (involves matching the most functional anatomical sites and positions for the person with a communication aid through, e.g., pointing, adaptive switches, touch panels, joysticks, or lightbeams and sensors).

Verbal communication. The use of words in written, spoken, and/or signed modes (synonymous with *linguistic*).

Vocal verbal behavior. The communication of information expressed with functional oral speech (synonymous with *speech*).

Based on Fried-Oken, 1987; Vanderheiden & Yoder, 1986.

_____

tion and encouraging language development. Although the details of service provision involving AAC are beyond the scope of this book (see, e.g., Beukelman & Mirenda, 1992; Reichle, York, & Sigafoos, 1991), the general principles are thoroughly interwoven with the discussions here. Most critically, AAC is not a matter of providing a single device, technique, or strategy, and it is certainly not intended to *replace* natural communicative gestures, facial expressions, and vocalizations, but to augment them. There is currently no evidence that AAC supports impede children's development of language. On the other hand, AAC can support children's inclusion in activities with their peers. To understand this distinction, consider the contrast offered by Calculator and Jorgensen (1991) between old short-term objectives designed to "train" a child to use an AAC device in the context of nonauthentic interactions, and a newer view, in which the AAC methods are designed to support authentic communication attempts and are learned in the context of real interactions:

> ***Old Short-term Objective.*** *John will accurately indicate yes and no 80% or more of the time, on 2 out of 3 consecutive days, in response to his mother's asking him a series of questions soliciting personal information (e.g., Is your name John?; Are you at school?; Are you a girl?). (p. 207)*

> ***New Short-term Objective.*** *In response to classmates' indicating that they do not understand John's speech during show and tell, John will attempt to clarify his message by supplementing his speech with other modes of communication (e.g., a gesture and/or his communication book), at least 80% of the time. (p. 207)*

ASSESSMENT AND PLANNING MODELS

When older children and adolescents have severe communicative impairments making it difficult for them to advance past early or middle stages of language acquisition, they probably also have multiple disabilities that justify intensive special education services. Most have been part of a special education services network for some time. Thus, these children do not need to be "found" in the same sense that infants and toddlers at risk do. However, they may need to be viewed from a fresh perspective (see Personal Reflection 13.2).

Periodically, difficult decisions must be made about the extent to which these children should be included in regular education buildings, classrooms, and activities. Inclusionary models of service delivery were discussed in Chapters 1 and 5. They present many challenges, but also opportunities for the development of true friendships and respect for diversity that benefit all students. With questions about placement and broad issues of service delivery, questions arise about the frequency

PERSONAL REFLECTION 13.2 _____

"At 7 months of age, we were thrown into a very strange and unfamiliar world of disbelief, of feeling incompetent and powerless. Andrew had been 'diagnosed' and our voyage took its first detour. He started in early intervention, and was 'provided' therapies (PT, OT, speech) four times a week. We waited and hoped that he would somehow be 'fixed' and returned to us as the child we had expected but somehow lost.

"Over the next 2 years, I realized that we hadn't lost anything. He was the same beautiful child I had brought home from the hospital. He had the same needs that all children have—to be fed, taken for walks, played with, read to, and loved and cared for by his family and close friends. It no longer mattered that early intervention hadn't 'fixed' him. We accepted Andrew for who he was." (p. xvii–xviii)

Beth Dixon, parent of Andrew and Educational Consultant, Institute on Disability/UAP—University of New Hampshire in the Prologue to Calculator and Jorgensen (1994).

and type of service to be provided by communicative disorders specialists. For example, "Should services be consultative or direct? Should they be daily or intermittent?" Calculator and Jorgensen (1994) sought to help varied individuals (teachers, speech-language pathologists, parents, school psychologists, and others) develop a:

> *vision of how communication and other skills can be taught to students with severe disabilities in regular classrooms and related settings. Communication is not conceptualized as an independent curriculum area nor as a goal in and of itself. Instead, it is presented as a means of enhancing students' active participation in meaningful activities in and out of school, and, as importantly, as a means for developing and maintaining relationships with family and friends. (p. ix)*

Other students may need assessment from a fresh perspective at multiple points across the preschool and school-age years and transition into adulthood. In particular, this group includes children who may have been underserved because no one had considered that they might need an AAC system.

Participation Model

As noted previously, the questions about whether older children with severe disabilities should be integrated into regular school buildings and classrooms are best answered by teams of professionals and parents on an individual basis. The specialist may find it helpful, however, to have a decision-making system based on more than one level of participation. The major steps in Beukelman and Mirenda's (1992) participation model of assessment are diagrammed in Figure 13.1. Notice that two kinds of barriers may be identified: opportunity and access. A focus on removing barriers related to policy and traditional practice and on assisting participants to acquire new knowledge and skills for working with children with severe disabilities may increase **opportunity.** A focus on increasing natural ability, environmental adaptation, and the use of assistive technology may increase **access.**

The outcome of all of the efforts illustrated in the flowchart of Figure 13.1 is increased participation. The standards for deciding who can participate in various settings may vary with the levels of participation expected. As noted in Chapter 5, Beukelman and Mirenda (1992) distinguished three patterns of academic and social participation. They suggested that, in either domain, children can be (1) competitive, (2) active, or (3) involved. Children who remain at early stages of language development would not be expected to be competitive, or even active, in regular classroom academic or social contexts, but they might be involved in at least some regular education or extracurricular activities during a school day. If the child is included, the specialist should conduct a contextually based assessment of how to best match the environment and the child.

The participation model is part of a three-phase assessment approach to meeting AAC needs (Beukelman & Mirenda, 1992). Phase I is **initial assessment for today.** Its goal is to gather information to design an initial intervention to match the individual's current needs and capabilities to support immediate communication interaction. Phase II is **detailed assessment for tomorrow.** Its goal is to develop a communication system that will "support the AAC user in a variety of specialized settings, beyond the familiar ones" (p. 101). Phase III is **follow-up assessment.** Its goal is to maintain a comprehensive AAC system that "meets the changing capabilities and life-style of the individual" (p. 103).

Michigan Decision-Making Model

Within a participation framework, questions about relative ability levels across developmental domains are appropriate. That was the purpose of the Michigan Decision-Making Model, originally developed by N. W. Nelson, Silbar, and Lockwood (1981) and described by N. W. Nelson (1989a). This approach focuses more on communicative processes than on communicative needs or opportunities. It includes four components: Two of them, a reference chart (see Chapter Appendix A) and a summary chart (Chapter Appendix B and Figure 13.2) are used to integrate information from other formal and informal assessment activities. Two additional components are a service-delivery decision-making chart (Figure 13.3) and an AAC decision-making chart (Figure 13.4).

The summary chart is used to estimate and compare a child's current levels of functioning across the four domains—cognitive bases, receptive language, expressive language, and social interaction and play. No single assessment tool is recommended for making the background judgments for shading in this chart, but the methods developed by Linder (1993), Norris and Hoffman (1990a), and A. M. Wetherby and Prizant (1993) (described in Chapter 7) are particularly suited for observational assessments that include compensation for sensory and motor deficits. For example, Linder (1993) described how a motorically involved child demonstrated age-level conceptualization of dramatic play even though her results on a standardized intelligence test indicated that she was mentally retarded. The more positive results were obtained because, in the play context, the girl was able to direct a facilitator's actions through a sequence of dramatic play events using her eyes and vocalizations to demonstrate a higher level of maturity.

The summary chart accompanying the Michigan Decision-Making Model (Figure 13.2 and Chapter Appendix B) is a condensation of the reference chart that appears in Chapter Appendix A. The reference chart may be used to fill in the summary chart by conducting interviews with parents and other participants to gain a picture of a child's best levels of functioning in real-life settings. For example, when parents are given clues as to what kinds of behavior represent development in a specific area and contexts that might elicit it, they may provide specific examples of their child's demonstration

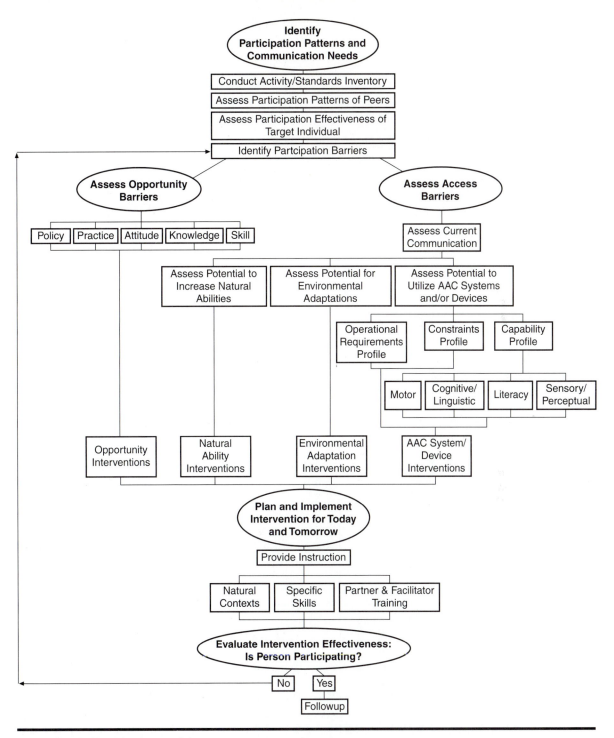

FIGURE 13.1   Participation model.

Note: From *Augmentative and Alternative Communication: Management of Severe Communication Disorders in Children and Adults* (p. 102) by D. R. Beukelman and P. Mirenda, 1992, Baltimore, MD: Paul H. Brookes Publishing Co. Copyright 1992 by Paul H. Brookes Publishing Co. Reprinted by permission.

FIGURE 13.2 Summary chart shaded to illustrate Andrea's profile.

Name: _____   BD: _____   Speech-Language Clinician: _____

Date: _____   Classroom Teacher: _____

COGNITIVE BASES	RECEPTIVE LANGUAGE	EXPRESSIVE LANGUAGE	SOCIAL INTERACTION AND PLAY
Preintentional (Birth to 8 months) *Sensorimotor I, II, III* ___ Infant moves from being purely reflexive to showing the initial beginnings of goal-oriented behavior ___ Developing object permanence	___ Startles to sound ___ Turns to sound ___ Reacts to human voice ___ Responds to tone of voice	___ Cry ___ Reflexive vocalizations	___ Engages in interaction ___ Manipulates interaction ___ Initiates interaction ___ Indicates preference for familiar people and objects
Early Intentional (8 to 12 months) *Sensorimotor IV* ___ Uses familiar means to achieve novel ends	___ No word comprehension yet ___ Imitates ongoing action ___ Looks where parent looks	___ Differentiated cries ___ Syllabic babbling	___ Plays nursery games ___ Plays with toys
Late Intentional (12 to 18 months) *Sensorimotor V* ___ Invents new means to achieve familiar ends	___ Responds appropriately to single words in context	___ Hi/bye routines ___ First words ___ Words used as "performatives" (to manipulate environment)	___ Solitary or onlooker play ___ Hugs doll, pulls toy
Representational Thought (18 to 24 months) *Sensorimotor VI* ___ Begins symbolic thinking	___ Understands words without context (points to pictures) ___ Follows two-word commands	___ Novel one-word utterances ___ Asks "What's that?" ___ Onset of two-word utterances	___ Parallel play
Early Preoperations (2 to 3½ yrs.) ___ Thought is preconceptual ___ Inference is sometimes but not always correct	___ Begins to understand Wh-questions ___ Answers yes/no questions	___ Two-word utterances ___ Basic sentences develop ___ Morphological markers develop	___ Symbolic play
Late Preoperations (3½ to 7 yrs.) ___ Begins to show intuitive thought ___ Problem solves by trial and error (not always correct)	___ Points to pictures representing sentences ___ Uses word order to understand agent-object relationships	___ Uses compound and complex sentences ___ Uses language to relate experiences ___ Talks about remote experiences ___ Adequate voice, articulation, fluency	___ Plays in small groups
Concrete Operations (7 to 12 yrs.) ___ Classifies on 2 characteristics	___ Understands conditional causal sentences	___ More clauses per sentence ___ Uses language to converse, persuade, tease	___ Genuine cooperative play

Recommendations:

Instructions:
1. Place a check mark beside characteristics demonstrated (reference chart in Chapter Appendix A or other evaluation tools may be used as necessary)
2. Shade in areas that describe functioning (areas may be partially shaded)
3. Refer to program decision chart

Note: From *The Michigan Decision-Making Strategy for Determining Appropriate Communicative Services for Physically and/or Mentally Handicapped Children* by N. W. Nelson, J. C. Silbar, and E. L. Lockwood, November 1981, presented at the annual conference of the American Speech-Language-Hearing Association. Los Angeles. Copyright 1981 by N. W. Nelson, J. C. Silbar, and E. L. Lockwood. Reprinted by permission.

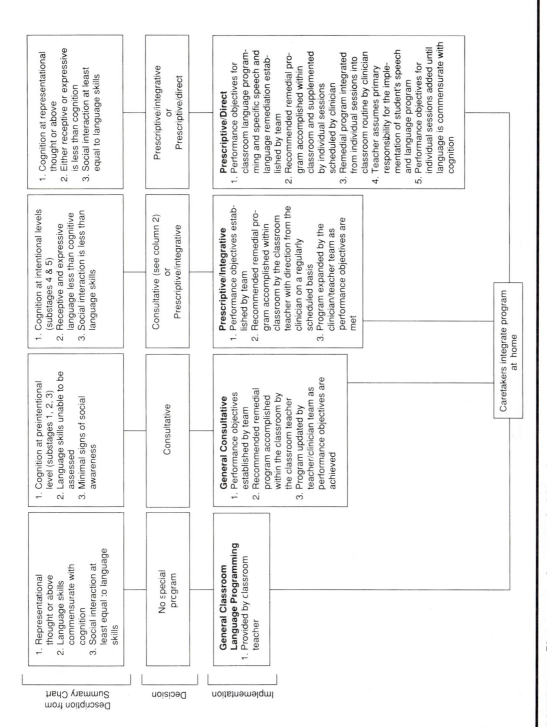

FIGURE 13.3 Placement and program decision chart.

Note: From *The Michigan Decision-Making Strategy for Determining Appropriate Communicative Services for Physically and/or Mentally Handicapped Children* by N. W. Nelson, J. C. Silbar, and E. L. Lockwood, November 1981, presented at the annual conference of the American Speech-Language-Hearing Association. Los Angeles. Copyright 1981 by N. W. Nelson, J. C. Silbar, and E. L. Lockwood. Reprinted by permission.

DOES CHILD NEED AUGMENTATIVE COMMUNICATION SYSTEM?

1. Cognition at intentional level (substage 4 or 5 or above), which may be impossible to demonstrate *until* an individual has an appropriate AAC system.
2. Receptive language at least equal to cognition and expressive language significantly less than receptive.
3. Expressive language unintelligible or extremely limited.
4. Social interaction significantly greater than expressive language.

Continue aural/oral training using placement and programming decision.

AND/OR

Select an augmentative system

AIDED

UNAIDED

If sufficient physical support for:

_____ Gesture

_____ Hand/face/body movements

_____ Other

Consider possible hardware:

_____ Communication board

_____ Lighted picture/ symbol board

_____ Synthetic speech device

_____ Computerized device

_____ Other

Consider possible accessing technologies:

_____ Eye/head pointing

_____ Direct select

_____ Coded select

_____ Scanning

_____ Combinations

_____ Other

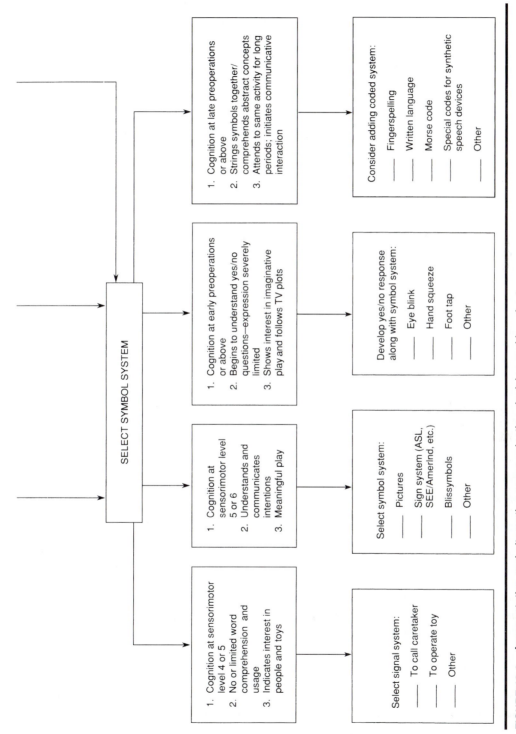

FIGURE 13.4 Augmentative and alternative communication decision-making chart.

Acknowledgement: The development of this chart was influenced by the work of David Yoder.

Note: From *The Michigan Decision-Making Strategy for Determining Appropriate Communicative Services for Physically and/or Mentally Handicapped Children* by N. W. Nelson, J. C. Silbar, and E. L. Lockwood, November 1981, presented at the annual conference of the American Speech-Language-Hearing Association. Los Angeles. Copyright 1981 by N. W. Nelson, J. C. Silbar, and E. L. Lockwood. Reprinted by permission.

of that behavior. Check-off boxes on the reference chart may be filled when this evidence is available. Remember that no matter how the information is gathered, allowances must be made for sensory and motor deficits that may interfere with demonstration of a particular level of functioning, and tasks should be modified as appropriate. The previously discussed (see Chapter 3) limitations of the Piagetian model for explaining contextually based cognitive development variations should also be kept in mind when using this system, because the system is tied most closely to that model (see Personal Reflection 13.3).

Following is a case example demonstrating use of the Michigan Decision-Making Model in developing services for Andrea, a 4-year-old student with suspected cognitive and related impairments functioning at a presymbolic level expressively. The summary chart shown in Figure 13.2 is shaded to illustrate Andrea's function profile. It is helpful, while sitting with parents and others in the planning group, to shade sections of the form while talking about the accomplishments they represent and gaining validation from parents and others that the profile accurately reflects the child's abilities. Later, the specialist may use this chart to mark progress by shading in new achievements with a different color or marking pattern.

Andrea shows evidence of being almost up to expectations for her 4-year-old chronological age in three of the four developmental domains, but in the area of ex-

PERSONAL REFLECTION 13.3

"When people were excluded from AAC services because of 'inadequate' capabilities, they were also usually excluded from the experiences, instruction, and practice necessary to improve their capabilities. Persons so excluded worked on 'perpetual readiness' activities that were hypothetically designed to teach them 'prerequisite' skills that they lacked. Most of these activities, such as learning about object permanence by finding toys hidden under towels, or learning about visual tracking by following stuffed animals moved across the line of visual regard, were nonfunctional and often age-inappropriate." (p. 100)

David Beukelman and *Pat Mirenda* (1992) in their descriptions of principles of assessment.

pressive language, she lags considerably behind. In nonverbal communicative attempts, Andrea demonstrates "hi–bye" routines and other forms of gestural, nonverbal communication to make her intentions known, and she can imitate a few signs taught to her by her parents, but she does not yet clearly use symbols spontaneously for communication. Thus, only a portion of the expressive language box at the 12- to 18-month level is shaded. When this profile is then used as input to the service-delivery decision-making chart (Figure 13.3), Andrea fits the needs profile of the fourth column. That is, she has one area (expressive language) significantly lower than others in combination with evidence of early preoperational thought, basically intact language comprehension, and symbolic play and social interaction skills that are close to age level. Andrea therefore is judged to need some fairly direct language and speech intervention services. In particular, because Andrea's problem seems to involve severe developmental oral–motor and speech apraxia, she may benefit from intensive direct focus on speech production as well as language use.

In addition, the fact that Andrea is 4 years old and cannot yet speak intelligibly indicates that she needs an augmentative communication system. It is increasingly rare to find AAC specialists who recommend waiting for 2 or 3 years to see if speech will develop, and Andrea probably should have been served in this way earlier. Every individual needs a way to communicate now, and all normally developing individuals use many different techniques and strategies to communicate their messages. The AAC system is now viewed primarily as a set of tools, techniques, and strategies *added* to a child's communication network rather than as a replacement for speech or as a sign that professionals have given up on assisting the child to acquire speech. However, the danger that an alternative mode may result in reduced efforts to help a child learn to speak naturally is real and should not be ignored.

For Andrea, all four indicators are present, suggesting a need to consider AAC options (see Figure 13.4). She clearly communicates intentionally, her receptive language skills and cognitive abilities are considerably more advanced than her expressive language, her expressive speech and language attempts are limited and unintelligible, and yet her social interactions suggest a desire and underlying ability to communicate much more. Even if Andrea demonstrated only one or two of these indicators, the need for AAC still should be deliberately considered. Furthermore, the communicative needs of children even more limited than Andrea, who do not yet show signs of intentional behavior, should be considered similarly. Remember that *no* nonspeaking child is too impaired for attention to his or her communicative needs and a child may not demonstrate intentionality *until* an appropriate AAC system is in place.

The recommendations for intervention differ based on the child's abilities. In the earliest stages of communicative development, more of the burden is on the communicative partner. With children in the preintentional (perlocutionary) communication stage (review Table 8.2), the specialist focuses on nudging the child into intentional (illocutionary) communication. The specialist responds to current behavioral signs as communicative and explores options that encourage the child to be aware of goal-directed communication and to begin to express intentions. Then the specialist assists the child to express those intentions more clearly, with more conventional means. Andrea has already moved beyond the earliest parts of this sequence. She is ready to acquire more conventional means of expression.

The AAC decision-making chart (Figure 13.4) can assist in this process by contributing to the selection of a symbol system, a display method, and accessing techniques (see a later section on early-stage word–symbol acquisition for a further discussion of the symbol-assessment process). Andrea's levels of symbolic play suggest that picture symbols might be explored for use in her preschool classroom. Furthermore, if she had a device with voice output, she could participate in activities such as circle time and reporting the weather audibly to her classmates. Because she has the cognitive development necessary and good general motor control, she can probably indicate yes–no responses with a combination of natural gestures and natural speech attempts, and she can use direct selection with her augmentative device by pointing or pressing a fairly small switch with her fingers.

The primary disadvantage of a communication *device* for Andrea would be that she would have to carry it around, and it might not be the most practical mode of communication for physically active Andrea in less formal settings. Therefore, her parents might be encouraged, in addition, to continue their efforts to learn a more sophisticated sign language system along with

Andrea and to use it in conjunction with speech. Andrea's parents are aware of the limitation that sign language is not generally intelligible to the public, but their acceptance of it, their awareness of Andrea's need to be able to express herself linguistically now, and their previous independent attempts to use such a system with her make it a good option to consider in conjunction with others. Whatever expressive language modalities Andrea uses, her level of receptive language also suggests that she should be encouraged to combine symbols expressively into at least two-word utterances. The specialist also should reassess her needs continually, because they are likely to change. Finally, the specialist should continue to give direct attention to Andrea's need for intelligible natural speech.

McGill Action Planning System

The McGill Action Planning System (MAPS; Vandercook, York, & Forest, 1989) was pioneered by Marsha Forest and Judith Snow as a system for encouraging a new level of conversation among students, families, and friends as students prepared to enter new school situations. It is now known as Making Action Plans (Falvey, Forest, Pearpoint, & Rosenberg, 1994). The focus of MAPS is on the student's characteristics as an individual rather than as a person with a disability. The conversation focuses on answering a series of questions: (1) Who is this person? (described in "regular" words, not special education language) (2) What is this person's history? (3) What is his or her dream? (4) What is the nightmare? (5) What are the person's gifts? (6) What does the person need right now to have a good life? (7) What needs to be done by us (student, parents, teachers, peers, other support staff) to help the person realize those needs?

Circle of Friends

One of the issues that arises when attempting to include individuals with severe disabilities in general education is how to encourage the establishment of sincere friendships. The Circle of Friends (Falvey et al., 1994) procedure helps students of all ages develop perspective taking. First they diagram their own Circles of Friends by putting: (1) themselves in the center circle along with their most intimate friends, those they cannot imagine living without; (2) good friends in the concentric second circle, who almost made the first circle; (3) people, organizations, and networks in the third circle (club members, the softball team, etc.); and (4) people paid to provide services in their lives in the fourth circle (medical professionals, teachers, etc.). After completing this process, students look at a Circle of Friends diagram for an individual with severe disabilities and reflect on how they would feel if that described their lives. They are then asked to brainstorm ways to fill in the circles for this individual from the outside in. They are specifically not asked, "Who wants to be Jane's friend?", which is "a question searching for failure" (p. 352). Rather they are asked, "Who knows Jane and is willing to brainstorm ways with me ideas for getting Jane more involved? For example, if Jane likes films, maybe we can identify someone who would invite her to the film club" (p. 352).

COACH Model

The COACH model also uses a family-focused team process (Giangreco, Cloninger, & Iverson, 1993). The acronym originally stood for Cayuga-Onandaga Assessment for Children with Severe Handicaps, but now stands for Choosing Options and Accommodations for Children with Handicaps. Like the MAPS approach, it starts with a positive student/family interview, in which quality-of-life indicators are explored, including the student's current living situation, health status and well-being, and how and with whom the student spends free time. Based on this discussion, the team establishes priorities for improvement during the current school year. These guide the development of goals and objectives and plans for how the student will participate within the regular education curriculum.

Needs-Based Discrepancy Analysis and Matrixing

Both MAPS and COACH cross professional disciplines and are aimed at comprehensive planning. They are based on needs assessments and deliberately avoid references to particular models of disability. Focusing more specifically on communication needs, Calculator (1994a) emphasized that "Students may be identified as having communication needs and yet be determined low priorities for contact with the SLP. Communication should nonetheless pervade students' curricula, with or without direct involvement from SLPs" (p. 119).

Calculator (1994b) also advocated for a philosophy of "zero exclusion," stating strongly that "There are no prerequisites to communication" (p. 198). He commented:

We believe very strongly that all students can benefit from communication intervention that focuses on fostering and enhancing interaction and participation in different settings. There are no minimal criteria or prerequisites that must be in place to justify communication services. (1994a, p. 120)

As an alternative to discrepancy formula (also questioned in Chapters 3, 5, and 6), Calculator and Jorgensen (1994) recommended that decisions about service delivery be based on careful consideration of an individual student's contextually based needs at particular points in time, through team consensus.

A primary tool of this process is the discrepancy analysis model, in which students' communication skills are examined relative to skills required for participation in an identified activity or event. This is a contextually based model, consistent with the major theme for this book. The approach is flexible. It starts with "an inventory of communication opportunities and demands in different settings" (Calculator, 1994a, p. 135). Next the student's communicative behaviors are examined within these situations. Discrepancies are noted between the demands and the student's current abilities. These become the targets of intervention. As in the curriculum-based language assessment model discussed previously, the process is guided by questions about: (1) what the context requires, (2) what the student currently does, (3) what the student might learn to do differently, and (4) how the context might be modified to enhance participation.

The results of this analysis feed back into the general planning process in constructing a matrix of how a student's needs can be accomplished within the context of general educational experiences. For example, Jorgensen (1994a) provided an example matrix for a fifth-grade student, Josh, with goals down the left margin and school activities across the top. The matrix was filled in with objectives for specific behaviors that would represent progress on his goals. Among Josh's eight goals were "Make choices," and "Sustain interactions." The matrix row for "Make choices" included the following: (1) Arrival—Walk in with friends of own choosing; (2) Writing—Choose topic from communication book or photo album; (3) Gym—As captain, choose team members; (4) Snack—Choose who to sit next to for snack; (5) Language Arts—Choose book; (6) Recycling [school job]—not applicable; (7) Lunch—Choose entree for hot lunch; (8) Recess—Choose equipment to play on or kids to hang around with; (9) Science—Choose station and project to work on; (10) Exploratories—Choose colors for painting sets for play; (11) Dismissal—Choose who to sit next to on bus (p. 52).

CONTEXTS FOR ASSESSMENT AND INTERVENTION

Routines, Mealtime, and Play

Social Interaction Routines.   The social routines discussed in Chapter 8 also provide appropriate intervention contexts for older students in earlier stages of development (see Personal Reflection 13.4). For example, "I'm gonna get you" and "knee-riding" routines allowed one mother to communicate with her 7-year-old daughter, Cathy, who was deaf (or profoundly hearing impaired) and blind. Yet, Cathy clearly communicated anticipation of sequence in the context of these routines and eventually learned to give a primitive sign to request more tickling in the context of the "I'm gonna get you" game. Like Cathy, many deaf–blind children learn best through predictable routines involving movement. Box 13.3 is a summary (from N. W. Nelson, 1988b) of five intervention levels in a "movement resonance," or "coactive movement" program based on a communication program developed originally by J. van Dijk (1965) for deaf–blind children in Europe. This particular summary includes adaptations developed for children with other severe and profound handicaps (L. Sternberg, 1982; L. Sternberg, Battle, & Hill, 1980; L. Sternberg, McNerney, & Pegnatore, 1985; L. Sternberg & Owens, 1984; L. Sternberg, Pegnatore, & Hill, 1983).

Siegel-Causey and Guess (1989) presented a comprehensive approach for enhancing nonsymbolic communication with individuals who have severe disabilities. It was based on five instructional guidelines related to:

1. Developing *nurturant* relationships
2. Enhancing *sensitivity* to nonsymbolic communication
3. Increasing *opportunities* for communication

4. *Sequencing* experiences in predictable order
5. Utilizing *movement* within natural interactions (p. 3)

Persons with developmental disabilities are particularly at risk for being socially disvalued because of inadequate communication abilities (see Personal Reflection 13.5). Part of the communication disorders specialist's role is to minimize the negative effects of external evaluations of their capabilities. Duchan (1986) suggested that clinicians can do this, within social interaction routines by using principles of sense making and fine tuning. By **sensemaking,** Duchan referred to "what the participants in the interaction think is going on and what ideas structure that thinking" (p. 188). By **fine tuning,** she meant "the various ways partners adjust their part of the interactions to be in accord with their model of the person they are interacting with" (p. 188). To use sensemaking in intervention, Duchan suggested that clinicians learn to focus on how children or young people make sense of events as whole processes. Some of the sense of events is based on the scripts that characterize them, and some events and aspects of events have stronger scripts than others. For example, ordering a Big Mac at McDonald's has a standard script, but deciding what to do if the sandwich falls

Box 13.3 _____

A Summary of the Five Levels of Early Communicative Interaction in a "Movement Resonance" or Coactive Movement Program for Children with Severe and Profound Handicaps

1. Preresonance
   a. Receptive indices
      (1) Moves, but not in response to stimulation
      (2) Changes behavior when stimulated (movement is encouraged in a same-plane, body-to-body motion of caretaker and child)
      (3) Repeats movement; focuses on own body
   b. Expressive indices
      (1) Produces undifferentiated cry
      (2) Produces different movements/vocalizations for specific discomforts
2. Resonance
   a. Receptive indices
      (1) Responds to another's cues by participating in movement modification (moving in an opposition plane; facing the caretaker)
      (2) Produces repetitive behavior on objects; focuses on what happens to object
   b. Expressive indices
      (1) Gives indication of recognition of familiar person/object
      (2) Participates in familiar motion after caretaker initiation; physical contact necessary
      (3) Signals caretaker to continue activity (such as pushing or pulling against a caretaker)
3. Coactive movement ("Movement Dialogue")
   a. Receptive indices
      (1) Responds to tactile signals for movement (when caretaker and child are separated in space but remain in close proximity)
      (2) Anticipates next movement in sequence

   b. Expressive indices
      (1) Imitates movements after caretaker stops movement as long as cues are provided by caretaker's position
      (2) Uses multiple signals to continue activities
      (3) Duplicates different movements while caretaker is moving; no physical contact necessary
4. Deferred imitation
   a. Receptive indices
      (1) Responds to simple gestural commands; no physical cues necessary
      (2) Anticipates routine event from cues
      (3) Responds to gesture for object provided gesture focuses on use of object and object is present
   b. Expressive indices
      (1) Imitates movements after caretaker finishes movement; no cues necessary
      (2) Uses gestures that are specific to certain situations; no generalization
      (3) Imitates new movements after caretaker finishes modeling movements
5. Natural gestures
   a. Receptive indices
      (1) Responds to gestures for objects provided gesture focuses on use; object need not be present
   b. Expressive indices
      (1) Uses gestures for objects/activities across various situations; generalization
      (2) Uses gestures instead of whole-hand pointing

Sources: L. Sternberg, 1982; L. Sternberg et al., 1980, 1983, 1985; L. Sternberg & Owens, 1984; L. Sternberg, Ritchey, Pegnatore, Wills, & Hill, 1986; J. van Dijk, 1965.

Note: From *Planning Individualized Speech and Language Intervention Programs*—Revised and Expanded, by Nickola Wolf Nelson, copyright 1988 by Communication Skill Builders, Inc., The Psychological Corporation, San Antonio, TX. Reprinted with permission.

_____

on the floor is an unforeseen part of the script. Both may be legitimate intervention targets.

The structure of some events may also influence clients' agendas regarding their participation. The agenda may be getting the sandwich or getting some tokens and pleasing the clinician. In the first case, the agenda is

more clearly the client's, and the clinician can fine tune the interaction to be consistent with that agenda. In the second, the locus of communicative control has shifted to the clinician, and opportunities for client-based fine tuning are diminished. Duchan now calls this philosophy of intervention "situated pragmatics" (Duchan,

1995a, 1997; Duchan, Hewitt, & Sonnenmeier, 1994). In 1986, she previewed its existence by summarizing the advantages of sensemaking and fine tuning over either traditional "pragmatics intervention" or "behavioral intervention" approaches:

> Clinicians can do more than model and expand on what they take the child to mean; they can be responsive to the child's intent, agenda, and overall sense of the event. They can do more than positively reinforce the child; they can also match the reinforcement to each act and to what the child wants to accomplish with it. (1986, p. 209)

Mealtimes and Feeding. Helping children organize their behavior into routines that involve increasingly conventional communicative exchanges involves focus on daily living scripts.

The following example from snacktime shows how predictable sequencing can help children function as communicative members of a social group:

> The service provider places a cup on the learner's tray to communicate that it is snack time. The learner, as a result of similar previous experiences, recognizes that the cup means snack and pushes the cup to the service provider to communicate "wanting juice." The service provider pours the juice and holds the filled cup out to the learner to determine if the learner's communication (i.e., pushing the cup) actually meant, "want juice." The learner smiles and reaches for the cup. The service provider responds by assisting the learner to bring the cup to his or her mouth. (Siegel-Causey & Guess, 1989, p. 8)

Another mealtime example comes from older children in school programs who stay at earlier stages of eating skill (e.g., children with cerebral palsy). For these students, Morris (1981) suggested a "Lunch Club." In a Lunch Club, all children in the child's regular education classroom take turns eating with one or more children with disabilities in a positive but quiet and controlled environment. Romski, Sevcik, and Pate (1988) also used mealtimes to facilitate symbolic communication in adolescents with severe retardation. Mealtime was one of the contexts that Lucariello (1990) identified as providing a familiar routine communicative event that can help children with higher cognitive abilities talk about more than the here-and-now.

When a child with severe impairments has feeding difficulties and needs to be fed by a variety of persons, problems may arise as each attempts to read the child's confusing communicative signals regarding the timing of bites, food choices, and facilitative techniques. The construction of a mealtime book, with personalized instructions and photographic illustrations, was suggested by S. E. Morris (1981). The following are entries drawn from the mealtime book of a 9-year-old boy with cerebral palsy:

> I enjoy my meals and like to enjoy being with the person who feeds me. My mealtime book will help you know me better. It will help you know the best ways for us to be real partners when you feed me. That makes it easier for me and for you too. . . .
>
> When I am ready for a bite of food, I will look at the food and open my mouth. I may also say "yeah" or "more" first. Please wait until I tell you with my open mouth and with my eyes that I am ready. . . .
>
> When the spoon is in my mouth, please keep it there until I have gently bitten on the spoon. This keeps my jaw steady and lets me begin to use my lips. Then you can pull the spoon out. (p. 231)

Age-Appropriate Play, Storytelling, and Story Enacting. When older children stay at early stages or have severe physical disabilities, how might play be used in intervention? Success may depend on staying within the limits of individuals' cognitive and physical abilities while not violating their needs for age-appropriate materials and experiences. Carlson (1982) provided a resource book for adapting toys for children with motoric handicaps. Musselwhite (1986) discussed broader aspects of encouraging children with cognitive and physical disabilities to play.

One approach my students and I used with a group of nonspeaking teenage boys with profound motor impairments and limited language and cognitive abilities was to collude with them in playing practical jokes on each other and the staff members in their school. For example, eye pointing and joint referencing were never so motivated as when these adolescents directed the teacher to put a plastic spider in her hair (or on the shirt of one of the boys) until other unsuspecting staff members arrived on the scene and were directed to notice it. Their eyes danced (and their minds were active) at those times.

When play is used to encourage language and cognitive development, it is essential to remember that *play is supposed to be fun.* Play is "what children do when they are *not* involved in activities that meet biological needs or that are required by adults" (Singer, quoted by Chance,

1979, p. 1). Therefore, to make play into a work session would be counterproductive. When adults do take part in play with children, it is important that they engage as "partners" (MacDonald, 1989), not just talk about playing (Chance, 1979). Although some evidence suggests that modeling of pretend play by adults may be an effective intervention strategy (S. Singer & Singer, 1977), it is probably most effective for adults to respond to child-initiated actions so as not to dominate the play with adults' ideas (this is the scaffolding strategy discussed previously). For children whose symbolic representational skills are just emerging, it may also be helpful to use real objects to set a meaningful context in which substitute objects can then be introduced for pretending (G. Fein, 1975). The most important thing is to keep play fun.

Storytelling and dramatization constitute a play context with relatively untapped potential for assisting children with severe communication impairments to grow linguistically, socially, and cognitively. As in other parts of this book, Vivian Paley's (1994) kindergarten teacher's voice offers special wisdom:

> Storytelling is of play, from play, about play, and ultimately, the essence of play. It is play under control, a compromise between the solitary soul and the outside culture. (p. 16)

Paley (1994) described three students, Dylan, Mary Ellen, and Serena, who were significantly different from the other 22 children in her kindergarten and from each other. They did, however, share three characteristics: "a deep distrust of teacher-led activities, a degree of self-absorption beyond the norm, and a varying inability to speak in coherent and familiar ways under ordinary circumstances" (p. 11). Dylan has shown unusual difficulty mastering a language or appropriate social behavior. He produces agrammatical sentences, like " 'They didn't I haven't in the way because they don't' " (p. 18). "Mary Ellen has been sexually abused and now lives with her grandmother. Her grammar poses no particular problem but she cannot keep unwanted memories, in the form of disconnected words and phrases, out of her sentences for very long" (p. 12). Serena, although not labeled by Paley, might be what specialists call "hyperlexic." She "speaks perfectly but stores her memories in verbal rituals and compulsive behaviors" (p. 12). Commenting on the temptation to label, and comparing professional lists with those Serena uses to communicate, Paley notes, "none of the lists, hers or ours, has anything to say about

storytelling" (p. 12). Then Paley proceeds to describe how the children's stories help them to organize themselves and their language to connect with their peers and to bring positive attention to their ideas in ways that free play has not the power to do:

> The logic and language of social and linguistic development are found in dramatic episodes. Here is the proper stage for those cognitive questions that need ballast and substance not found in workbooks or diagnostic tests: What does this word mean (so we can act it out)? What does this sentence mean (so we can act it out)? What do these characters say to each other (so we can act them out)?
>
> If you want us to know your story you must slow down and speak the words so that I am able to write them down. If your desire is to have the group act out your story (and it is universally so), then you can't pounce, or keep erasing, or disguise your ideas inside a private code all the time. (p. 18)

Culatta (1994) also recommended representational play, using props and assumed roles to recreate thematic scripts, and story enactments (with methods described later in this chapter in the section on narratives and literacy). She saw story enactment in play as an organized, motivational, and interactional context for facilitating and learning language and showed how play contexts can be structured to provide "opportunities for learning narrative structuring, turn taking, decontextualized language use, language form and function, and literacy skills" (p. 117).

Jorgensen (1994b) described how children with severe physical disabilities using augmentative communication systems could be included in the dramatic play and performances of classrooms:

> Julian is a second grader with severe cerebral palsy. This year he played the part of a prince in his class play. A friend tape-recorded the prince's dialogue and Julian activated a switch to say his lines at the appropriate time.
>
> **Old Short-Term Objective:** During speech and language therapy, Julian will activate the on-off switch to play a music tape within 15 seconds of a cue on 3 out of 4 consecutive trials.
>
> **New Short-Term Objective:** In the context of a variety of class activities, including class performances and book reports, Julian will activate a tape loop using a switch within 10 seconds of a clue. (pp. 91–92)

Butterfield (1994), working in New South Wales, Australia, described how Westby's (1980) play scales (see Tables 8.7 and 10.1) could be used for assessment and intervention with children with developmental disabilities. One nine-year-old girl with severe intellectual disabilities had more advanced language skills (at least on the surface) than play skills. As Butterfield described it, "If left undirected, she prefers her own idiosyncratic behaviours (poking objects into holes) to any form or involvement with toys" (p. 36). Although language skills appeared more advanced, "a language sample taken over several situations indicates that her vocabulary consists of several well known phrases often used inappropriately. For example, when in the dolls' corner she asked, 'Go in bus?', 'Sing tape?' and 'Go home mummy?' " (p. 36). This child could exhibit higher level play skills if prompted to do so, but she became aggressive if maintained in that situation. Thus, Butterfield recommended that in this case it would be preferable to use social routines and age-appropriate leisure activities than representational play. The only toys the girl did select to play with spontaneously were infant-stimulation toys of a musical kind, suggesting that a tape player or computer game might provide an appropriate context for interactions as well.

Participation in School and Community

In the past, students with severe disabilities commonly were segregated from their normal-learning peers into separate classrooms and separate buildings. As discussed previously, educators and parents now recognize that separate is generally not equal, and educators are providing more opportunities for people with severe disabilities to interact in significant ways within educational and social situations (Calculator & Jorgensen, 1994; Downing, 1996; Lipsky & Gartner, 1989; Murray-Seegert, 1989; Stainback & Stainback, 1990; Thousand, Villa, & Nevin, 1994; Villa, Thousand, Stainback, & Stainback, 1992). However, as Asch (1989) pointed out in Personal Reflection 13.6, the United States has a history of providing inadequate services to individuals with disabilities.

Now most professionals agree that change is needed. Strong advocacy and a few success stories currently must serve in place of solid models backed by extensive research (Cirrin & Penner, 1995). Professionals who are pioneering these approaches use philosophy to guide practice and experiment collaboratively in their neighborhood school settings.

The complex nature of severe and multiple disabilities demands collaboration among persons with disabilities, their parents, their regular and special educators, and possibly others. The contributions of speech–language pathologists and other communication specialists to the collaborative process are based on expertise in analyzing the communicative aspects of diverse events, as well as the speech, language, and communicative abilities of people who participate in them. Some of the intervention efforts of these professionals may aim directly at changing behaviors, thereby reducing impairment. Others may aim to help individuals meet important communicative demands through acquisition of new abilities or compensatory techniques, thereby reducing functional limitations. Still others may aim to expand environmental opportunities for persons with disabilities to participate in educational and community activities, thereby reducing disability.

Perhaps one of the greatest challenges facing professionals as they attempt to implement multifaceted intervention programs is to balance the need to modify contexts, so that individuals can experience communicative success without creating new contexts that are so different they practically ensure continued isolation of people with handicaps. The challenges apply across academic, social, and vocational settings.

When older children remain at earlier stages of development, assessment and intervention may take place in special and general education classrooms. The focus should be on the communicative demands and supports of contexts as well as on the intrinsic abilities of the child and the potential interactions between them. Both intervention needs and progress can be determined best when children are assessed within contexts where they are expected to participate. When conducting ecological assessments, Carta, Sainato, and Greenwood (1988) suggested that specialists ask questions not only about the effects of static environmental features, but also about dynamic features, such as the effects of teacher behavior. They could also ask how the current environment helps children develop survival skills they might need in the "next environment" (p. 225).

Students with severe peripheral sensory or motor impairments without cognitive impairments may need a different set of questions to keep them optimally independent in the later stages of language acquisition. Otherwise, in academic settings, what may look like harmless accommodations may actually "deprive students of achieving their full potential" (Asch, 1989, p. 186). In secondary schools, for example, note taking is a critical skill. As much as possible, students with severe disabilities involving peripheral sensory and motor systems should take their own notes rather than rely on the note-taking skills of others. Students with visual impairments may be provided laptop computers. Students with physical impairments may be provided microcomputers with special accessing, abbreviation characteristics, and printers. Students with hearing impairments or deafness may be provided interpreters. As Asch (1989) commented:

> If students are to develop the ability to sift out the essential from the illustrative in a lecture, they must themselves have the full text of that lecture communicated to them. If they are to join in class discussions, they must know what other students have said. For the student who must get information from lip-reading or sign, the only efficient and equivalent substitute for hearing is the interpreted class lecture and discussion. (p. 186)

In social settings, opportunities also may be limited (see Personal Reflection 13.7), particularly when severe central nervous systems deficits are involved, such as mental retardation or autism. Lack of opportunity may be exacerbated by the inappropriate and sometimes frightening communicative behaviors that appear among young people with severe disabilities who use aberrant communication styles. Schuler and Goetz

PERSONAL REFLECTION 13.7 _____

"Communication skills are a means for personal social interaction, not just the desired outcome of an intervention or development. Communication in social interaction is the fabric of children's lives." (p. 3)

Ann P. Kaiser (1993), Professor of Special Education and Psychology and Human Development, Peabody College of Vanderbilt University, Nashville, TN, in the introductory chapter to the book she co-edited. In the dedication, she wrote:

"One day when I was 7 years old, I stood watching my 5-year-old brother who could not yet talk or walk. I was overwhelmed with the sadness of not being able to connect with him and to understand him. For years afterward, I had a recurring dream of him talking to me."

(1981) pointed out that a lack of appropriate social and communicative skills may cause individuals with severe disabilities to communicate by using behaviors that others find unpleasant or frightening (e.g., tantrums or inappropriate hugging to communicate "I'm tired of doing this," or "Pay attention to me"). These concerns are addressed in the next section.

COMMUNICATIVE INTENTIONS AND INTERACTIONS

GOAL: The individual will use appropriate communication signals and strategies with adults and same-age peers.

- Prelinguistic Communicative Interaction
- Replacing Aberrant Expressions of Communicative Intention
- Improving the Assertive–Responsive Balance
- Expanding Social Interactions

OUTCOME: The child will participate in social interactions in a variety of contexts.

Prelinguistic Communicative Interaction

> _Objective 1:_ The child will use nonsymbolic communication strategies in social interaction routines that are both effective and socially acceptable.

As noted in Chapters 7 and 8 (see Table 8.2), children communicate before they use language. Older individuals with severe disabilities may use unconventional (and hence, often unrecognized) communication strategies that are intermittently effective. Intervention involves sensitivity to the communicative signals of students, matching those signals, and scaffolding the student to higher levels of communicative interaction. The goal is to help individuals move from preintentional (**perlocutionary level**) to intentional (**illocutionary level**) nonsymbolic communication in preparation for symbolic (**locutionary level**) communication. Forms of nonsymbolic communication are shown in Figure 13.5. The goal

FIGURE 13.5   Forms of learner nonsymbolic communications.

Generalized movements and changes in muscle tone
- Excitement in response to stimulation or in anticipation of an event
- Squirms and resists physical contact
- Changes in muscle tone in response to soothing touch or voice, in reaction to sudden stimuli, or in preparation to act

Vocalizations
- Calls to attract or direct another's attention
- Laughs or coos in response to pleasurable stimulation
- Cries in reaction to discomfort

Facial expressions
- Smiles in response to familiar person, object, or event
- Grimaces in reaction to unpleasant or unexpected sensation

Orientation
- Looks toward or points to person or object to seek or direct attention
- Looks away from person or object to indicate disinterest or refusal
- Looks toward suddenly appearing familiar or novel person, object, or event

Pause
- Ceases moving in anticipation of coming event
- Pauses to await service provider's instruction or to allow service provider to take turn

Touching, manipulating, or moving with another
- Holds or grabs another for comfort
- Takes or directs another's hand to something
- Manipulates service provider into position to start an activity or interactive "game"
- Touches or pulls service provider to gain attention
- Pushes away or lets go to terminate an interaction
- Moves with the movements of another

Acting on objects and using objects to interact with others
- Reaches toward, leans toward, touches, gets, picks up, activates, drops, or pushes away object to indicate interest or disinterest
- Extends, touches, or places object to show to another or to request another's action
- Holds out hands to prepare to receive object

Assuming positions and going places
- Holds up arms to be picked up, holds out hands to initiate "game," leans back on swing to be pushed
- Stands by sink to request drink, goes to cabinet to request material stored there

Conventional gestures
- Waves to greet
- Nods to indicate assent or refusal

Depictive actions
- Pantomimes throwing to indicate "throw ball"
- Sniffs to indicate smelling flowers
- Makes sounds similar to those made by animals and objects to make reference to them
- Draws picture to describe or request activity

Withdrawal
- Pulls away or moves away to avoid interaction or activity
- Curls up, lies on floor to avoid interaction or activity

Aggressive and self-injurious behavior
- Hits, scratches, bites, or spits at service provider to protest action or in response to frustration
- Throws or destroys objects to protest action or in response to frustration
- Hits, bites, or otherwise harms self or threatens to harm self to protest action, in response to frustration, or in reaction to pain or discomfort

Note: From *Enhancing Nonsymbolic Communication Interactions Among Learners with Severe Disabilities* (p. 7) by E. Siegel-Causey and D. Guess, 1989, Baltimore, MD: Paul H. Brookes Publishing Co. Copyright 1989 by Paul H. Brookes Publishing Co. Reprinted by permission.

is to build more interactive social interactive routines using the five principles suggested by Siegel-Causey and Guess (1989): *nurturance, sensitivity, opportunities, sequencing,* and *movement.*

In this approach, matching may involve nonsymbolic communicative expressions by the service provider as well as by the student. Table 13.1 summarizes how service providers may use different modalities to communicate to their students, both symbolically and non-symbolically. Siegel-Causey and Guess (1989) used a series of case studies to show how these principles and strategies could be implemented (see Box 13.4).

The **milieu teaching method,** introduced in Chapter 3 and discussed in Chapter 8, uses a hybrid of behavioral and social interactionist techniques to facilitate intentional requesting. Yoder, Warren, Kim, and Gazdag (1994) taught four children with mental retardation to replace preintentional signals with intentional requesting behaviors. Milieu teaching involves setting the context with interactive play routines, following the children's attentional lead, and using direct prompting techniques to facilitate intentional requesting. Intentional requests are defined as having three essential components: (1) a look to the object, (2) a look toward the adult, and (3) a discrete action or vocalization. If a child uses two, but not all three of these, the action is defined as preintentional signaling (called the **perlocutionary level** here), and the intervention consists of

TABLE 13.1   Forms of service providers' communicative expressions

MODALITY	SYMBOLIC	NONSYMBOLIC
Auditory	Service provider speaks to learner	Service provider turns on music to indicate the start of physical therapy Service provider uses a nonspeech vocalization to attract the learner's attention
Visual	Service provider signs to learner	Service provider makes pointing movement to draw learner's attention to an object Service provider holds out spoon to see if learner is ready for a bit of food Service provider draws a picture with learner to indicate the next activity Service provider makes a twisting motion over the lid of a container to demonstrate to the learner how to open it Service provider makes an exaggerated movement to elicit learner's attention
Tactile	Service provider fingerspells in learner's hand	Service provider taps learner's hand to prompt the learner to pick up an object Service provider puts hands under the under the learner's legs in a downward direction to request learner's assistance in pulling pants off Service provider ties bib on learner to indicate lunch
Kinesthetic	Service provider manipulates learner's hands through the "finish" sign to indicate that the activity is over	Service provider pauses while rocking with the learner to elicit a signal to continue Service provider manipulates the learner's hands through the start of pouring from a container to elicit the learner's participation
Olfactory		Service provider holds spoon near learner's nose to see if learner wants the particular food item

Note: From *Enhancing Nonsymbolic Communication Interactions Among Learners With Severe Disabilities* (p. 6) by E. Siegel-Causey and D. Guess, 1989. Baltimore, MD: Paul H. Brookes Publishing Co. Copyright 1989 by Paul H. Brookes Publishing Co. Reprinted by permission.

Box 13.4 _____

Case Study Example in Which Siegel-Causey and Guess (1989) Described How a New Teacher, Wendy, Developed a Nonsymbolic Communicative Relationship with Jennifer, Who Seemed Defensive at First

JENNIFER: Walks around the room stopping to look closely and intently at things with patterns. Sometimes she stops for long periods and rocks, shakes her head, and giggles. She smiles the entire time. Finally, she sits down at the table.

WENDY [using nurturance]: Goes over to the table and sits down. In order to avoid threatening Jennifer, she does not look at her or say anything.

JENNIFER: Immediately stops rocking and smiling. She seems to be waiting for something. After a few minutes, when Wendy does not do anything, Jennifer goes back to rocking and smiling, though she keeps her eye on Wendy.

WENDY [using movement]: Begins to imitate Jennifer's movements, because she knows this is an effective way of getting the student's attention as well as a good way to break the ice. She rocks, drums her fingers, picks up a book, examines it closely, stands up, and rocks while standing as Jennifer performs these actions. Of course, Wendy does not imitate any socially unacceptable behaviors such as eye poking, face slapping, light gazing, or light playing (e.g., moving arms/hands to play with shadows and brightness or light sources) because she does not want to encourage Jennifer's use of stereotypical behaviors.

[a little later in the interaction]

WENDY [using movement and nurturance]: Begins drawing and talking, but without addressing Jennifer. "I'm drawing Wendy," and points to herself. Wendy didn't really expect Jennifer to understand her words, but she continues to talk because she thinks it might be soothing to Jennifer. "I'm drawing Wendy's hair," and runs her hands through her hair. "I'm drawing Wendy's face," and points to her face. Wendy draws the nose and the mouth, but no eyes.

[providing opportunity] She puts the pen down and waits to give Jennifer a chance to participate without intruding on her.

JENNIFER: Who has been watching the drawing very closely, picks up the pen and draws the eyes.

Note: From *Enhancing Nonsymbolic Communication Interactions among Learners with Severe Disabilities* (pp. 145–147) by E. Siegel-Causey and D. Guess, 1989, Baltimore, MD: Paul H. Brookes Publishing Co. Copyright 1989 by Paul H. Brookes Publishing Co. Reprinted by permission.

_____

prompting the missing element. For example, the intervention might start with the adult imitating the child in a turn-taking routine, such as pushing a toy truck back and forth. Then, the adult stops the activity by holding onto the truck. If the child just looks at the truck, reaches, and vocalizes, without looking at the adult, the adult moves the desired object toward his or her face and directly prompts, "Look at me," before continuing the routine. If the child's response is incomplete due to lack of a discrete action or vocalization, the adult might say "What?" to indicate need for more information and use modeling or physical assistance to facilitate completion of the communication act. In the early stages, the adult might also directly prompt the child to request continuation of the routine, by asking "What do you want?" but as the requesting behaviors are learned, intentional requests are "elicited simply by stopping the routine" (p. 844). One of the positive outcomes of the work by Yoder and his colleagues was that when children began to replace their preintentional signals with intentional communication, parents began to map their children's actions linguistically, even though they were not instructed directly to do so. For example, parents began to say "Bye bye" as their children waved or to say "truck" as the child looked toward it and then them while pointing.

Some children need intensive scaffolding to move from preintentional to intentional communicative interactions. Klinger and Dawson (1992) described a social interaction approach for facilitating early social and communicative interactions for children with autism. They based the approach on four principles of normal development that have been promoted throughout this book:

(1) "social skills are facilitated naturally though play rather than taught explicitly"; (2) "strategies are based on knowledge of normal developmental sequences, progressing from very simple interactions to increasingly complex social interactive skills"; (3) "strategies seek to build an 'augmented scaffold' in which social experiences are not only geared toward the child's developmental level, but are also exaggerated and simplified so that the relevant aspects of social interaction are distilled and become highly salient and more easily assimilable"; and (4) "interventions seek to place the child in the role of initiator while maintaining a predictable environment" (p. 168).

The intervention described by Klinger and Dawson (1992) has two levels, each with multiple phases. **Level One** involves "facilitating attention to people, social contingency, and turn-taking" (p. 181). In *Phase One* of this level, adults imitate the child's actions with toys, body movements, and vocalizations, as simultaneously as possible, to establish a sense of contingency between the child's actions and an adult's actions. The goals are for the child to begin to: (1) attend to the adult's actions and (2) realize that the adult is following his or her actions. In *Phase Two* of Level One, adults encourage eye contact by holding toys directly in front of them as they imitate the child and show enjoyment when the child looks at them. The goals are for the child to: (1) begin to look at the adult's face and (2) continue to realize that the adult is following his or her actions. In *Phase Three* of this level, adults encourage turn taking in game routines, like bubble blowing, waiting for the child to signal a wish to continue turns. In this phase, the child should begin to show signs of participation, such as waiting to see if the adult will imitate him or her. In other words, the action becomes reciprocal. The goals are for the child to: (1) wait for the adult to imitate, (2) begin to change his or her behavior and watch to see what the adult does, and (3) show signs of participating in a game. In *Phase Four,* adults teach contingency through mimicry. "The purpose of this phase is to help the child learn that back-and-forth interaction can occur even when the adult is not exactly imitating his or her behavior" (p. 182). In this phase, the adult makes slight modifications in the behavior along with the imitations, for example, by moving faster or slower, using a different toy, or adding a phoneme to the child's syllable productions to

make a word, such as changing *ma-ma-ma* to *mom, mom, mom.* The goals are for the child to continue to: (1) anticipate the adult's imitations even though they are not exact and (2) enjoy the turn-taking interactions.

Level Two (Klinger & Dawson, 1992) has two sublevels: **imitation** (with two phases) and **early communication joint attention** skills (with four phases). In *Imitation Phase One,* the adult attempts to shift circumstances so the child begins to imitate the adult in the midst of familiar routines. Only this time, the adult switches the action slightly (perhaps to one recently shown by the child) and waits to see if the child imitates. The child's imitation may be delayed and may require several attempts by the adult, who should return to imitating the child after several attempts. The goals are for the child to imitate spontaneously: (1) familiar simple schemes with toys, (2) familiar vocalizations, and (3) complex schemes with toys and/or vocalizations. In *Imitation Phase Two,* novel schemes are introduced gradually by increasingly modifying familiar schemes. The goals are for the child to imitate spontaneously: (1) slight modifications of familiar schemes with toys and/or vocalizations, and (2) novel schemes with toys and/or vocalizations.

In *Early Communication and Joint Attention Phase One* (Klinger & Dawson, 1992), the purpose is "to motivate the child to communicate spontaneously with the adult in order to achieve a desired goal" (p. 183). The method is to use techniques called "communicative temptations" elsewhere in this book, so that the child needs the adult's assistance to reach an object or open a jar. Criteria for complying are either gesture, gaze, or language (not all three at this point). The goal is for the child to engage in spontaneous communication (gesture, gaze, or language) to request a desired object. In *Phase Two,* the purpose is to continue to build shared routines, in which the child "requests" the adult's assistance to blow bubbles, wind a toy, or make a train move. Phase Two is still at the **perlocutionary level** because adults respond "by interpreting a child's actions as if they were requests for a shared activity" (p. 184). The goals are for the child to: (1) engage in spontaneous communication to request help, (2) to request adult participation in a shared activity, and (3) to request adult engagement in shared social routines. *Phase Three* of Level Two is designed to move the child into the **illo-**

cutionary level because now the child must signal intentionality by making eye contact along with the reach and the vocalization. Klinger and Dawson noted that pausing before complying may facilitate face looking by lower functioning children. Acting confused about the nature of the request (e.g., to draw a "B" or "G"?) may facilitate face looking by higher functioning children. The goal is for the child to begin to request activities while looking at the adult's face, combining eye contact with requests. *Phase Four* is designed to assist the child to tune in to more complex nonverbal cues from the adult. The adult may feign inattention to the request or hesitance to comply, seeking to encourage more deliberate communicative attempts from the child. The goals are for the child to: (1) attend to nonverbal cues provided by the adult, and (2) direct the adult's attention to an object or activity.

Replacing Aberrant Expressions of Communicative Intention

Objective 2: The individual will replace aberrant expressions of communicative intention with alternative, communicatively acceptable forms.

Some individuals with profound developmental limitations communicate in highly unconventional ways. A general rule is that the more limited a person's abilities and the more unconventional the communicative signals, the greater is the burden for interpretation on interaction partners.

For some individuals in this category, "challenging" aberrant behaviors seem to be far more prevalent than behaviors that resemble positive communicative attempts. In spite of severe limitations in their ability to learn, these individuals may have learned well how to manipulate their environments and the adults in them. They do this through aberrant and aggressive behaviors such as screaming, biting, and self-abuse. Unfortunately, such behaviors tend to be reinforced and maintained when other more positive behaviors are not. Perhaps this is because these behaviors remove individuals from situations in which they do not want to participate (this is the negative reinforcement process of escaping an undesirable situation), or perhaps this is because such behaviors bring social attention (even if it is negative).

Reichle and Wacker (1993a) introduced their book on *Communicative Alternatives to Challenging Behavior* by noting that functional analysis is a recurring theme across the divergent chapters. "The extent to which we can identify the function of behavior is the single most important variable in establishing an effective intervention program" (p. 2). Reichle and Wacker characterized the interventions as reinforcement-based, starting with behavioral analysis of operant mechanisms. They noted the divergence among the strategies suggested by the authors of the book chapters and that the process must be highly individualized. Uniformly, however, the operant approach involves two essential steps. "First, the function of challenging behavior must be identified; we must identify the reinforcers maintaining behavior. Second, the identified reinforcers must be available only for one or more acceptable communicative responses and withheld for challenging behavior" (pp. 2–3).

Rather than using a purely behaviorist approach, Donnellan and colleagues (1984) recommended analyzing the communicative functions of aberrant behaviors and developing intervention tactics based on that analysis. These authors suggested that rather than trying to extinguish aberrant behaviors (through nonreinforcement) or to punish them, greater success might come from "teaching new functional behaviors that result in reinforcing consequences similar to those available following the aberrant behaviors" (p. 201). They likened this process to a pragmatic approach in which all behavior, regardless of its topography, is responded to for its functional message value (Schuler & Goetz, 1981). Thus, communicative intent can be determined only by examining the relationship between behavior and context, not by examining the topography (surface form) of behavior in isolation.

Contextually based analyses may show that some individuals with severe impairments produce communicative means that are function-specific—used to communicate only one message—whereas others may be observed to serve a variety of functions (Schuler & Goetz, 1981). For example, some individuals seem to use self-injurious behavior in different contexts to serve the varied functions of sensory stimulation, eliciting attention from others, and terminating undesirable situations. Donnellan and her colleagues (1984) analyzed these functions as having the respective pragmatic message values of: "I'm bored," "Pay attention to me," and "I don't want to do this anymore" (p. 202).

Intervention in aberrant behavior involves establishing goals to expand the individuals' limited response repertoires rather than eliminating their inappropriate behaviors. Donnellan and colleagues (1984) described three approach alternatives and gave clinical examples for each: (1) teach alternative communicative behaviors to replace aberrant responses, (2) teach other functionally related behaviors to replace aberrant responses, and (3) manipulate antecedent contexts.

Teaching Alternative Communicative Behaviors to Replace Aberrant Responses. The specialist may teach communicative behaviors explicitly to reduce aberrant behaviors. An example is Don, an 18-year-old with severe mental retardation whose formal communicative abilities were limited to about 15 signs, which he rarely used spontaneously. Don also engaged in self-injurious behaviors of head-banging, head-punching, and face-slapping, which his teacher inadvertently reinforced by paying social attention to him whenever the behavior occurred. Thus, this behavior seemed to carry the message value, "Pay attention to me, I need help" (Donnellan et al., 1984, p. 203).

Don's intervention consisted of prompting–fading and modeling techniques to teach him more conventional means to ask for assistance in the three-part sequence: (1) Elicit the teacher's attention by visually scanning the room for him, going over, and tapping him on the shoulder. (2) Make the manual sign for "help" to request assistance. (3) Specify the kind of help needed by walking back to the work area and pointing to the task at hand. The authors reported that "within six weeks, Don regularly performed the request-for-assistance sequence whenever he encountered task difficulty, and the self-injurious behavior was virtually eliminated" (Donnellan et al., 1984, p. 203).

Robinson and Owens (1995) reported on similar intervention with a 27-year-old woman with moderate–severe retardation. They used the scale designed by Donnellan and colleagues (1984) to perform an ecological analysis of the communicative value of this woman's intense disruptive and self-injurious behaviors, including stomping, head-banging, biting, and assaultiveness. Analysis suggested that:

These behaviors most likely served primarily as a request for medication for D's headaches, allergies, and consti-

pation. In addition, they also appeared to serve as requests for desired objects (i.e., oversized sunglasses or a colorful water wand) and declarations about events, actions, and feelings, particularly confusion and possibly fear, surrounding a change in her routine. (p. 209)

Although the woman had learned a few signs previously, they were not used functionally. Intervention involved construction of a temporal pictures board with photographs of D's daily activities and want and needs. On the first day, an intervention team detached a photograph from the board when it was time for an activity and laid it beside D while simultaneously signing and saying, "Time for ____." In response, D would pick up the photograph and reattach it to the board. By the second day, "D initiated detaching the photographs and replaced them with some prompting from the intervention team" (p. 209). It was evident that she understood the function of the board. Gradually, the temporal sequence pictures were used less and the wants and needs photographs more, but not excessively. Although the stomping did not disappear entirely, it rarely escalated to the other behaviors.

Teaching Other Functionally Related Behaviors to Replace Aberrant Responses. The second approach differs from the first in that the alternative responses taught are not designed to be specifically communicative. Sam, a 12-year-old boy with autism and moderate retardation, had a fairly extensive sign repertoire, which he used spontaneously. When he was in crowded, noisy, or novel situations (e.g., shopping malls, stores, and recreational facilities), however, he engaged in several auditory self-stimulatory behaviors, such as finger snapping and loud repetitive vocalizations. These behaviors seemed to communicate the message, "I'm anxious/tense/excited/overwhelmed by the input available" (Donnellan et al., 1984, p. 204).

Sam's treatment consisted of teaching an alternative, appropriate behavior that could serve the same function: Screen out high levels of sensory input from the environment. Donnellan and colleagues (1984) provided Sam with a portable cassette recorder with headphones and taught him in two phases: first, to operate the tape system and to listen to soothing music whenever overstimulated (this procedure took a few weeks and led to his being able to participate in community activities), and second, to remain for increasingly long periods of time in stimulating environments before using the tape system. Following the second phase, which took 3 months, "Sam was able to tolerate exposure to novel environments for up to one hour at a time before using the tape set for a 10-minute period" (p. 204).

Manipulating Antecedent Contexts.   In the third approach, the specialist manipulates antecedent conditions to reduce aberrant behavior. This approach is most useful when the aberrant behavior's message seems to be, "I don't want to do this anymore" (Donnellan et al., 1984, p. 204). Donnellan and her colleagues noted that treatment of this behavior starts with acceptance of the message as valid, followed by questioning why someone would want to escape from the particular situation. For example, the aberrant behavior of Sarah, a 7-year-old girl with autism and severe retardation, consisted primarily of aggression to staff members and throwing objects in the classroom.

For Sarah, Donnellan and colleagues (1984) devised a plan to assess her more carefully to determine her learning strengths, weaknesses, and modality preferences to more closely match learning tasks to her learning abilities. This meant reducing linguistic complexity and augmenting explanations with much nonverbal support and physical prompting while redesigning tasks to be more motivational and functional. The outcome was a program "designed to acknowledge the legitimacy of the communicative message of Sarah's behavior ('I don't understand'), and her aggression and tantrum behaviors decreased as they became unnecessary for terminating the activity" (p. 205).

Improving the Assertive–Responsive Balance

Objective 3: The child will adjust the frequency of assertive or responsive communicative acts to achieve an improved balance over baseline conversations.

Not all individuals with severe impairments exhibit aberrant behaviors; many are basically cooperative but highly passive communicators. As these individuals are taught linguistic symbols and structures, they have difficulty learning how to use them to communicate. The unintended outcome may be that language seems to function for them more as an academic task than as a means of communicating with others. The only communicative function they have mastered is to respond when prompted.

Mirenda and Santogrossi (1985) described one such individual. Amy was an 8½-year-old-girl who was non-speaking and who demonstrated severe retardation with autistic-like tendencies. Although Amy had learned to identify a fairly large number of symbols on her communication board in formal teaching contexts, she used them only when she was specifically prompted to do so (e.g., "Show me what you want"). For Amy, a revised primary treatment target was needed—**spontaneous functional communication.** It was defined as any communicative act that was not "performed in response to an instructional cue or prompt, such as 'What do you want?' or 'Show me what you want' " (pp. 143–144).

Teaching Amy the communicative value of her augmentative system involved returning to a level in which she had only one symbol available (a can of soda pop). Mirenda and Santogrossi used a prompt-free approach. Amy was first rewarded with a drink of the beverage whenever she accidentally touched the picture in the context of other learning activities. When she did so, the adult interactant poured Amy a drink and said something like, "Oh, you'd like a drink; Here." As Amy's touches became more frequent, and apparently intentional, the adult shaped them into even more deliberate communicative acts by honoring her "request" only when she searched for the symbol, located it, and looked at the teacher expectantly. This process included several stages in which the teacher replaced the original picture with a smaller, more symbolic drawing, which was gradually removed from her immediate range, covered with a translucent cover, and later placed in a notebook (see N. W. Nelson, 1988b, for a sequence of objectives related to this approach).

Eventually, the teacher introduced more pictures, and Amy began to communicate intentions with novel pictures in novel environments. Her communication book was built back up until she had 120 symbols in the categories of food, drink, activity, and self-care–clothing. Perhaps the most exciting outcome was a generalization of her original request behavior to varied communicative intentions. For example, at one point in school, after using her symbol book to request paper, crayons, and scissors, she drew a picture and cut it out. What was particularly remarkable about this event was that, after requesting and being given the crayons, Amy pointed back to the crayon symbol, communicating an intentional comment to her communicative partner. It was particularly remarkable because A. M. Wetherby,

Yonclas, and Bryan (1989) found that the production of comments by children with autism was extremely rare.

Not all individuals who demonstrate severe restrictions of communicative intentions are passive communicators. Gallagher and Craig (1984) described a 4-year-old boy named Clark who met criteria as a child with a severe specific language impairment. Initially, Clark produced the phrase "It's gone" 60 times within a 2-hour 10-minute videotaped sample. The phrase accounted for 17% of the utterances and seemed to serve varied communicative functions. Far from being passive, this child used the phrase, "It's gone," frequently during activity transitions to reestablish interaction with his partners in a game-like event similar to the nonexistence–disappearance ("all-gone") game played by infants and toddlers with their mothers. Gallagher and Craig noted that although Clark's repetitive phrase met criteria for syntactic productivity as a spontaneously rule-generated phrase, for him, it was best characterized as a memorized stereotypic phrase. They also noted that Clark's behavior illustrated the advisability of not discarding information about stereotypic, highly repetitive phrases from language samples, as is often done, but of analyzing them carefully for their communicative intent. Gallagher and Craig recommended establishing an intervention target to assist Clark to acquire an expanded repertoire of socially acceptable and recognizable access behaviors for gaining social attention. (Clark also may have been demonstrating a need to acquire more elaborated play routines, discussed in Chapter 10).

One of my students, Kim Schairer (Schairer & Nelson, 1996), investigated the possibility that participation in conversations might vary, particularly for students with autism, in the written modality. Schairer alternated holding 15 to 20 minute oral and written conversations with three adolescents with autism (to whom we gave the pseudonyms, Larry, Mark, and Becky) over a period of several weeks. In both modalities, she attempted to engage the students in meaningful conversation by showing interest in their interests (e.g., fishing books for Larry and dogs for Mark and Becky) and making comments contingent on their remarks. The written conversations were held by passing paper and pen back and forth. Larry, in particular, was more assertive in the written modality and produced more informative, non-obligatory utterances, with topics that matched prior comments. In oral conversations, he was often elliptical, sometimes failed to take obligatory turns (i.e., respond

to direct requests for information) and produced mismatching topics. For example, an oral exchange about videogames went like this (R = Researcher; L = Larry):

> **R:** *I'm an ace detective.*
>
> *pause*
>
> **L:** *On the bonus round, eight different countries.*
> **R:** *What's the bonus round?*
> **L:** *Eight markers.*
> **R:** *How do you get to that?*
> **L:** *Forty-five seconds. (p. 174)*

An excerpt from a written conversation, in which Larry and the Researcher were talking about videogames again, went like this:

> **R:** *It sounds like fun.*
> **L:** *Cody and Haggar are punching and jump-kicking.*
> **R:** *Cool! I bet you're really good at it.*
> **L:** *I have the new high score. (p. 175)*

Mark also used a style that was significantly less passive in writing than orally, and Becky was more informative in her written conversations. For Becky, a typical oral exchange was:

> **R:** *Why don't you tell me about some of the things you like to cook?*
> **B:** *Brownies.*
> **R:** *What else do you like to cook? Your mom says you really like recipes.*
> **B:** *Cake. (p. 176)*

In writing, Becky used more informative and complex language:

> **R:** *What do you do in music class?*
> **B:** *I do singing.*
> **R:** *That sounds like fun! I love to sing.*
> **B:** *I love music because it's fun. (p. 176)*

Expanding Social Interactions

Objective 4: The individual will increase the variety of communicative functions over baseline observations and will interact communicatively with more partners than previously.

Interpreting Functional Echolalia.   Expanding an individual's communicative repertoire beyond simple responsiveness may require changes in communicative contexts and partners as well as in modalities. It may also require looking below the surface of unconventional behaviors, such as echolalia, to mine them for their richer communicative potential. This can be done by mapping conventional communicative functions onto unconventional communicative forms to foster an expanded communicative repertoire.

Echolalia was regarded in early reports primarily as noncommunicative behavior representing signs of children's comprehension difficulties. Prizant (1987), however, pointed out that echolalic behaviors are best described along three continua regarding (1) exactness of the repetition, (2) degree of comprehension, and (3) underlying communicative intent. Prizant defined **immediate echolalia** as "utterances that are produced either following immediately or a brief time after the production of the model utterance" (p. 66) and **delayed echolalia** as "utterances repeated at a significantly later time" (p. 67). Others have suggested that the two kinds of echolalia might involve differential activation of echoic short-term and long-term memory (Hermelin & O'Connor, 1970). By providing a rich, contextually based analysis of the communicative intent underlying both immediate and delayed echolalia, Prizant and his colleagues (Prizant & Duchan, 1981; Prizant & Rydell, 1984) led clinicians beyond traditional views of echolalia as aberrant behavior to be ignored or extinguished. Varied functions that may be served by either immediate or delayed echolalia appear in Tables 13.2 and 13.3. The clinical implications are that this kind of analysis should be used to identify functional distinctions for echolalia produced by individual children in different contexts rather than lumping all occurrences into one category and targeting it for extinction.

Prizant (1987) provided intervention guidelines for incorporating echolalia into individualized intervention programs. He recommended using strategies that would (1) simplify language input, (2) respond to the child's apparent communicative intent when echolalia is used, (3) relate echolalic utterances to actions and objects in the child's environment, (4) follow Fay's (1979) suggestions to deemphasize correct pronominal usage in early stages, and (5) never punish or ignore a child for echolalia if it is intentful or interactive or the only means of communication available.

More generally, Prizant and Rydell (1993) noted the importance of understanding unconventional verbal behavior (UVB), which includes echolalia, in contexts of the person's communication system, emotional arousal, and the functions it serves—socioemotional, cognitive, and communicative. They reiterated that "many forms of UVB (e.g., echolalia) may be important compensatory strategies, and they may be part of an individual's natural transition to more conventional communication"

TABLE 13.2   Functional categories of immediate echolalia

CATEGORY	DESCRIPTION
Interactive	
1. Turn taking	1. Utterances used as turn fillers in an alternating verbal exchange.
2. Declaration	2. Utterances labeling objects, actions, or location (accompanied by demonstrative gestures).
3. "Yes" Answer	3. Utterances used to indicate affirmation of prior utterances.
4. Request	4. Utterances used to request objects or others' actions. Usually involves mitigated echolalia.
Noninteractive	
5. Nonfocused	5. Utterances produced with no apparent intent, and often in states of high arousal (e.g., fear, pain).
6. Rehearsal	6. Utterances used as a processing aid, followed by utterance or action indicating comprehension of echoed utterance.
7. Self-regulatory	7. Utterances that serve to regulate one's own actions. Produced in synchrony with motor activity.

Note: From "Theoretical and Clinical Implications of Echolalic Behavior in Autism" by B. M. Prizant in *Language and Treatment of Autistic and Developmentally Disordered Children* (p. 72) edited by T. Layton, 1987, Springfield, IL: Charles C. Thomas. Courtesy of Charles C. Thomas, Publisher, Springfield, Illinois.

TABLE 13.3   Functional categories of delayed echolalia

CATEGORY	DESCRIPTION
Prizant and Rydell (1984)	
Interactive	
1. Turn taking	1. Utterances used as turn fillers in alternating verbal exchange.
2. Verbal completion	2. Utterances that complete familiar verbal routines initiated by others.
3. Providing information	3. Utterances offering new information not apparent from situational context (may be initiated or respondent).
4. Labeling (interactive)	4. Utterances labeling objects or actions in environment.
5. Protest	5. Utterances protesting actions of others. May be used to prohibit others' actions.
6. Request	6. Utterances used to request objects.
7. Calling	7. Utterances used to call attention to oneself or to establish/maintain interaction.
8. Affirmation	8. Utterances used to indicate affirmation of previous utterances.
9. Directive	9. Utterances (often imperatives) used to direct others' actions.
Noninteractive	
10. Nonfocused	10. Utterances with no apparent communicative intent or relevance to the situational context. May be self-stimulatory.
11. Situation association	11. Utterances with no apparent communicative intent that appear to be triggered by an object, person, situation, or activity.
12. Self-directive	12. Utterances that serve to regulate one's own actions. Produced in synchrony with motor activity.
13. Rehearsal	13. Utterances produced with low volume followed by louder interactive production. Appears to be practice for subsequent production.
14. Label (noninteractive)	14. Utterances labeling objects or actions in environment with no apparent communicative intent. May be a form of practice for learning language.

Note: From "Theoretical and Clinical Implications of Echolalic Behavior in Autism" by B. M. Prizant in *Language and Treatment of Autistic and Developmentally Disordered Children* (p. 73) edited by T. Layton, 1987, Springfield, IL: Charles C. Thomas. Courtesy of Charles C. Thomas, Publisher, Springfield, Illinois.

(p. 293). Techniques for addressing problems of UVB include "indirect" strategies, such as modifying partners' communicative styles and situational determinants of UVB. These are appropriate when UVB becomes challenging or seems to be a function of limited comprehension. "Direct" strategies include helping the person acquire conventional language forms and augmentative communication options.

Alternative Methods and Partners.   Other clinical researchers have assisted adolescents with severe communicative impairments to expand their communicative functions and interactions by changing communicative contexts and partners. For example, Dalton and Bedro-

sian (1989) studied the effect of context on communication board use by adolescents functioning at preoperational cognitive levels. Prior studies consistently showed that such youngsters occupy the respondent role far more frequently than the initiator role in transactions with adults (e.g., Calculator & Dollaghan, 1982; D. Harris, 1982; Light, Collier, & Parnes, 1985a, 1985b, 1985c). Dalton and Bedrosian found that partner roles influenced outcomes, with adolescents assuming the respondent role primarily with their teachers. With nonspeaking peers, however, requests predominated, and with speaking peers, a variety of communicative functions appeared.

Wilkinson and Romski (1995) also explored the influence of encouraging conversational interactions with seven male adolescents with moderate to severe mental retardation. The youths, ages 13 to 20 years, were observed in conversations with other students without disabilities in the junior or senior high schools where their special education classrooms were housed. All of the youths with mental retardation had used augmented methods (including a portable voice output communication device called the WOLF) for at least 5 years. The results of analysis of the dyadic conversational samples showed that verbal questions and comments from peers were more likely to elicit conversational responses than directive prompts and that the male participants were more likely to respond to input from male peers than from females.

In a prior study with some of the same students, Romski, Sevcik, Robinson, and Bakeman (1994) had learned that parents and teachers had responded differently to natural (gestural and vocal) communication attempts and synthesized speech productions. The gestural and vocal attempts were more "**successful**" in that they opened communicative exchanges more frequently, particularly at home, but the augmented communicative attempts were more "**effective,**" particularly at school, because they conveyed information more clearly.

Goldstein and Kaczmarek (1992) reviewed the literature on promoting communicative interaction among children with severe disabilities at preschool age in integrated intervention settings and noted that "Surprisingly, remediating deficits in social skills and remediating deficits in communicative behavior have been studied separately" (p. 82). A more contemporary view might be to look at intervention as a means of fostering greater peer interaction than "remediating deficits," but in any event, "Researchers have repeatedly shown that simply placing preschool children with disabilities in the same educational environment as preschool children without disabilities does not automatically facilitate high quality social interactions" (p. 82). On a more promising note, children with disabilities do "become involved in more social interactions and verbal interactions" (p. 88) in integrated settings than in segregated settings. Variables that influence the interactions include types of toys and adult interventions. Social toys like blocks and toys relating to familiar daily routines promote the most interactions. Adult intervention might include prompting the child with disabilities to interact. An alternative focus has

been on fostering strategies among peer mediators: (1) to initiate frequent communicative initiations, for example, by asking peers with disabilities to play, offering assistance, and sharing toys, and (2) to respond with reinforcing interactions, for example, by handing out requested materials, providing social attention and offering hugs. Goldstein and Kaczmarek found three general strategies to hold particular promise:

1. Peers without disabilities can be taught to adopt the interest of a child with disabilities or to redirect the attention of the child with disabilities so that a shared focus of attention is established.
2. Peers without disabilities can be encouraged to be observant of ongoing activities and to talk about them to children with disabilities.
3. Peers without disabilities need to be taught how to detect both obvious and subtle verbal and nonverbal communicative attempts by children with disabilities and to respond to those attempts to set the stage for sustained interaction. (p. 104)

Peer Tutoring Approaches. The social interaction problems of individuals with severe disabilities have been summarized as failure to initiate, maintain, and terminate social interactions in socially acceptable ways (Murray-Seegert, 1989). Recognizing this, a first step in intervention might be to teach socially acceptable behaviors. Although social skills tend to be learned best in the context of natural social interactions, their absence may limit those interactions. Thus, by the adolescent years, a vicious cycle may be well established.

Murray-Seegert (1989) wrote about one attempt to break this cycle. By acting as a classroom aide in a San Francisco Bay area high school, Murray-Seegert used participant observation techniques to conduct an ethnographic study of social interactions in a program designed to integrate students with severe disabilities with regular education students. Adolescents with disabilities participated actively with regular education students, many of whom could themselves be considered at risk for school failure. The "regulars" volunteered to work with the students with disabilities, receiving course credit for their enrollment in the Internal Work Experience (IWE).

One part of the program involved peer tutoring. Murray-Seegert (1989) reported that it "proved to be an

important variable influencing the development of social relations between disabled and nondisabled students" (p. 114). A variation on peer tutoring involved
what Murray-Seegert called "mediated interactions,"
which were identified when nondisabled "helpers" promoted positive proximal or reciprocal contact between
another nondisabled student and a student with a severe
disability. One day Anita (a member of the group the
students dubbed the "Popular People") asked to bring
her "Thug" boyfriend, Denard (who had dropped out of
school), to class. After a card game with several special
education students, including Phuc Sanh and Dwayne,
Murray-Seegert described what happened when Denard
wanted to try out the computer:

*Anita says, "Phuc Sanh knows how to do it," and so the
two boys go to work. Phuc Sanh uses a single word utterance to help Denard: "Load . . . run . . . 5." Anita
comes to sit with them. Dwayne comes over to watch and
puts his hand on Anita's shoulder. Denard says, "Hey!
Don't you touch my woman!" Dwayne removes his hand.
Denard says, "I was just kiddin'." (p. 90)*

The program was not always successful in meeting
its primary objective of developing intergroup social relations. Ten of the 42 IWE students dropped out after a
few weeks, but many students in both groups benefited
from the interaction. Personal Reflection 13.8 describes
how one of the IWE students in the program described
his disabled peer. As Murray-Seegert noted, "remarks

PERSONAL REFLECTION 13.8 _____

"Dear Darryl,

How you been I been fine. I'm just out here in frisco going to school and waiting to
graduate out of High School.

   I go to my first period to sixth and I'm out at 2:00 pm. But in my third period class
I have a Special Ed class. It's students with a disability. Like one student Juan he's a
student that's a little slow in the mind and can't all the way speak yet. He's about 59
inches and black hair he's Spanish and he dress average. Sometimes he likes to play
games or go out side for a walk, but sometimes he just likes to Kick back. When he
wants something he yells and gives you sign language. He can go to the restroom by
his self he know his way around the school and sometimes he goes to lunch with a
peer tutor or to the wash house or to the store. He's kind of slow learning but he
catches on sooner or later. He needs a little help with yelling out loud or whistling, and
he needs help with his way of approaching people. Sometimes I will go to the church
and he likes to come along with me. He likes too go just about everywhere with any
of the peer tutors. I like to take him places with me because even though he's disabled we still are good friends and I wouldn't mind taking him anywhere with me. I
like to play games and baseball or running after each other. I can tell he's happy because everyday he comes in smiling about anything. And he always wants to go somewhere with me or play a game of battleship with me.

P.S. Write back soon. Sincerely yours, Preston."

Preston was a "Peer Tutor" writing to a hypothetical friend about his disabled classmate in an
assignment that he and fellow peer tutors were given. (Quoted by Murray-Seegert, 1989,
pp. 112–113.) Murray-Seegert noted the matter-of-fact way the regular students accepted behaviors that are often cited as evidence of lack of readiness for inclusion in integrated settings.
The letters written by peer tutors also showed that "dressing okay" was at least as important to
teenage peers as "acquisition of social skills" was to adult supervisors.

Note: From *Nasty Girls, Thugs, and Humans Like Us: Social Relations Between Severely Disabled and Nondisabled Students in High School* (pp. 112–113) by C. Murray-Seegert, 1989, Baltimore, MD: Paul H. Brookes. Copyright 1989 by Paul H. Brookes. Reprinted by permission.

like 'sometimes they get on my nerves' or 'sometimes I get bored' by the Regulars showed that they were relating to disabled students as fallible, multidimensional 'humans like us' rather than as idealized, infantilized Poster Children" (p. 105).

In some inclusion programs, techniques for promoting positive peer tutoring may be relatively more structured than those in Murray-Seegert's (1989) study. Some have used refinements of behavioral technology to structure interactions between adolescents with and without disabilities. In one two-study series, a group of researchers taught peer tutors to work with three young men with autism, first in their integrated high school and then in their off-campus jobs. In the first study (Gaylord-Ross, Haring, Breen, & Pitts-Conway, 1984), the peer tutors taught the young men to initiate, maintain, and terminate social interactions that were object-centered in that they revolved around things like offering chewing gum or listening to a personal stereo. After training, the students with autism had generalized the social skills across persons and were more often being approached themselves for social interaction. In the second study (Breen, Haring, Pitts-Conway, & Gaylord-Ross, 1985), nondisabled schoolmates taught the disabled individuals to participate in social interactions with co-workers during coffee breaks at their job sites. In this intervention program, the peer tutors learned to mediate a social skill chain that involved greeting a familiar co-worker, offering a cup of coffee, and elaborating the social exchange when the coworker showed a willingness to continue the interaction. The results again supported improvement in the students' abilities to make effective social bids. Few avoidance reactions occurred, and the bids "did lead to meaningful social responses of different types by the co-workers" (p. 14).

CONTENT–FORM DEVELOPMENTS

GOAL: The individual will use symbols and symbol combinations for expressing and understanding ideas.

- Selecting Symbol Systems
- Symbol Learning by Individuals with Severe Disabilities
- Using Multiword Constructions

OUTCOME: The individual will express and comprehend ideas that meet daily living needs and lead to greater social participation.

Selecting Symbol Systems

Early semantic intervention requires an appreciation of the relationships among words, referents, and meanings. **Meaning** is inherent in people, not things or words.

The word is a sign that signifies a referent, but the referent is not the meaning of the word. If, for example, you say to a child, "Look at the kitty," the actual cat is the referent but is not the meaning of kitty. *If the cat ran away or were run over by a truck, the word would still have the same meaning because meaning is an act of cognition. (Pease et al., 1989, p. 102)*

Words have arbitrary relationships to the things they represent, but some words are more arbitrary than others. This arbitrary relationship between signs (e.g., the word *kitty*) and their referents (e.g., the cat) is **symbolic.** Symbolic relationships may be represented by nonverbal signs (e.g., stop lights) as well as verbal signs, but not all signs are symbolic. Some do not have arbitrary relationships to the things they represent. A nonsymbolic sign that can be interpreted as having meaning is called an **index.** Examples are rain on the roof, footprints of animals, and cries of babies. They are less arbitrary and are also not symbolic. When a sign has a strong physical relationship to the thing it represents and can be recognized on the basis of physical similarity alone, the sign is said to be **iconic** or **transparent.**

It is not too surprising that, even in normal development, many of the early words or protowords learned by children are less arbitrary. For example, bumps on the knees may be called "owies," and clocks may be called "tick-tock." Parents provide some of these words, but others are children's own creations (Pease et al., 1989).

Older children who remain at early stages of language development may have particular difficulty learning arbitrary symbols. Some may never be able to say words and make them intelligible to others. What symbols, signs, and indexes should be used in trying to help such children acquire word knowledge? Mirenda and Locke (1989) considered this issue systematically by studying 11 different symbol sets and nonsymbolic means of representing objects with 40 nonspeaking individuals who experienced varying degrees of intellectual disabilities. Their review of the literature in this area showed that "persons with intellectual handicaps can learn symbol–referent associations and that some types of symbols are more difficult to learn than are others" (p. 131). Mirenda and Locke differentiated issues of **symbol transparency** (i.e., the degree to which a symbol looks like the thing it represents—its iconicity) from **symbol learnability** (i.e., how easy a symbol is to learn), although they recognized that the two are probably related. Mirenda and Locke did not attempt to teach the meaning of the symbols and thus measured only transparency and not learnability. Because of differences among the capabilities of the individuals taking part in the study, the authors assessed 29 with a standard receptive language protocol (3 used eye gaze to select objects), 1 with a yes–no protocol, and 10 with a matching protocol. As expected, all of the symbols assessed were found to be less transparent than were objects or pictures of objects. One of the most unexpected findings (although it had previously been hypothesized by Vanderheiden and Lloyd, 1986) was the low transparency of miniature objects. Apparently, some individuals with cognitive limitations have trouble seeing miniature objects as representative of real objects. In fact, color photographs are more transparent than miniature objects. Mirenda and Locke also noted that Blissymbols and written words were about equally transparent (although they may not necessarily be equally learnable).

Symbol Learning by Individuals with Severe Disabilities

Objective 1: The individual will demonstrate an understanding of a set of signs and symbols larger than at baseline.

Because of their cognitive limitations, some individuals may never learn to communicate with symbols; however, this does not mean that they will never learn to communicate (Siegel-Causey & Guess, 1989). The most appropriate service-delivery model for these individuals may be collaborative consultation in which the specialist assists caregivers to read communicative signs produced by the individuals and to teach them to make those signs in increasingly conventional ways so that they can be interpreted accurately by a wider range of partners. The long-term intervention process for receptive communication with these individuals may involve guiding them through stages in which they (1) recognize indexes provided by their caregivers (see Table 13.1 for a list of possibilities provided by Siegel-Causey & Guess); (2) associate real objects with the sequence of

the daily routine (e.g., a segmented wooden trough might be designed to hold objects that represent the major activities of the day in sequence); and (3) recognize photographs of objects to indicate where they are supposed to be and what they are supposed to be doing, and to represent available choices where appropriate.

Stephenson and Linfoot (1996) reviewed the literature on the use of pictures as communication symbols. They pointed out that picture recognition is essential to use of pictures for expressive and receptive communication, but "even in normal development, naming, comprehension, and matching skills do not emerge together, and they are likely to be displayed separately by persons with severe intellectual disability" (p. 253). Their review also showed that persons with profound disabilities can learn to use both arbitrary and pictographic symbols for communication even when they appear to have no receptive or expressive oral language skills.

For example, Romski, Sevcik, and Pate (1988) described how three out of four adolescent and young adult women with severe retardation acquired a vocabulary of 20 lexigrams (arbitrary printed symbols composed of geometric forms) in this way and used them in meaningful ways. Romski and her colleagues initially taught the women to use symbols to request their favorite foods, and later objects. The women's requesting skills did not initially generalize to labeling and to comprehension tasks. Additional request experiences, however, resulted in improvements in the other functional areas. Romski and co-workers also observed that the participants later began to initiate lexigram communications spontaneously and that spoken language comprehension and production attempts were facilitated.

Using Multiword Constructions

Objective 2: The individual will combine symbols to represent novel ideas and will demonstrate comprehension when others communicate with symbol combinations to him or her.

When individuals with severe disabilities reach the stage of language development that involves transition from early single symbols to forming two- and three-word utterances, intervention can follow the general strategies suggested in Chapter 8, but with age-appropriate topics and materials, and if necessary, AAC supports. Early attempts, as in normal development, may appear as stringing separate single symbols together. Early semantic–grammatic constructions can then be encouraged by arranging opportunities for the individual to participate in communicative interactions in which novel agents, actions, objects, locations, and attributes appear as real communicative choices. For example, an individual who uses a wheelchair might have options programmed into a communicative device to specify, "Jason push," or "Eduardo push" (agent + action) when it is time to change classrooms. If the IEP indicates the student can choose between attending gym class with peers or going to see the physical therapist, the device might be programmed with the options, "Go to gym" and "Go to PT" (action + locative).

In the early stages, such choices might be programmed as phrases so that they can be activated with one selection. As the student develops speed of activation and linguistic knowledge, however, it may be best to separate semantic roles into single words that have to be selected separately, especially in some contexts where speed is not the main issue. The question of whether to program phrases or single words into communicative devices is a difficult one, with linguistic implications. Clinicians should keep in mind that developing generative language skills, concepts of word boundaries, and syntactic knowledge may require a system that supports individuals in selecting novel word choices and sequencing them into sentences (Nelson, 1992a).

Intervention strategies for individuals with mental retardation aimed at developing multiword combinations are often grounded in a behaviorist paradigm (see Chapter 3). One of the most strictly behaviorist approaches, with a prescribed teaching sequence, was designed by Lovaas (1981) for children with developmental disabilities, particularly autism. The Lovaas approach first builds receptive and expressive object labeling and receptive and expressive action labeling, working from individual sounds as necessary, before working on word combinations. More advanced language is then built from the parts using similar techniques. For example, children may be directed to "Pick up the hammer before the ball" and be reinforced for correct sequencing or be punished if the sequence is incorrect, then directed to say again what they just did, again with reinforcement or punishment. Trials are discrete and reinforcers are delivered on planned schedules. After the child learns the responses in drill activities with small objects, responses are transferred to questions about pictures in books.

Milieu teaching (also called "incidental" teaching; Kaiser et al., 1987; Warren & Bambura, 1989; Warren & Kaiser, 1986), mand-model approaches (Warren et al., 1984), and matrix-training methods (Goldstein, 1985) share behaviorist foundations also. That is, they include particular focus on arranging the context to offer stimuli, to prompt imitation of responses, and to provide reinforcers contingent on the responses. Hamilton and Snell (1993) used the milieu approach to increase spontaneous communication book use across environments by an adolescent with autism and severe mental retardation. Ezell and Goldstein (1989) used a matrix training procedure to teach two moderately retarded children (a 6:1-year-old girl and a 9:11-year-old boy) to combine known and unknown words. When Ezell and Goldstein added imitation training to comprehension training, it not only facilitated comprehension learning but also helped the two students transfer the new constructions to expressive language.

More recent versions of approaches that have grown out of the behaviorist tradition have involved greater attention to social interactionist concerns (Bricker, 1992, 1993b; Warren & Yoder, 1994), but not always enough to satisfy those coming from a purely social interactionist perspective (Duchan, 1995a; Kirchner, 1991). Pure social interactionists emphasize that communicative interactions should be authentic and not contrived, that modeling is not the same as rote imitation, that successful communication does not equate with the delivery of a reinforcer, and that scaffolding is not the same as prompting. The distinctions may be primarily semantic, but my own belief is that language learning is most likely to be successful if adults seek to keep meaning making at the core of all communicative interactions and to be sincerely interested in how the infant, child, or adolescent is currently conceptualizing the world so he or she can be assisted to reach the next step in a way that fits with his or her own ways of knowing. Contextualizing the events in a social interactionist framework is critical, but so are understandings of behaviorist principles of learning, how experience might influence brain maturation, how information processes can be guided from executive levels, the signs that an individual is using linguistic communicative strategies, and how cognitive schemas can be modified in interactions with intentioned, goal-setting adults (using all six theoretical perspectives introduced in Chapter 3). It is the primary role of the language interventionist to frame cues and focus individuals to notice the connections between language and the natural features of the world and social interactions. Ultimately, success comes when the individual begins to construct new models of language and communication and to participate with individuals who do not have disabilities and who are not their caregivers or teachers.

NARRATIVE AND LITERACY DEVELOPMENTS

GOAL: The individual will demonstrate functional literacy skills for reading signs, interpreting a variety of print symbols, listening to material read aloud, participating in constructing stories, and producing written text.

- Ignoring Traditional Concepts of Readiness
- Building Narrative Understandings

OUTCOME: The individual will use emergent and functional literacy skills to participate more fully in the community.

Ignoring Traditional Concepts of Readiness

Objective 1. The individual will show understanding of print and other graphic symbols that communicate information about safety, where to find things (e.g., the men's and women's room, favorite cereals, soft drinks, and fast food restaurants), and personal meanings (e.g., names, labels, "I love you," creative stories), and will participate in opportunities to learn more.

Historically, educators assumed that individuals with severe disabilities were not "ready" to learn to read and write during their preschool and early elementary school years. Often, they have never been considered "ready" (see Personal Reflection 13.9). Parents have urged professionals to move beyond a strictly developmental model to write literacy goals in their children's IEPs even when they still could not tie their shoes or zip their pants. (Recall the personal reflections of parents reported in Chapter 1—"We'll buy him Velcro!," Personal Reflection 1.6—and Chapter 5—"You listen to

PERSONAL REFLECTION 13.9 _____

"He can read his story, and he doesn't even know his letters!"

Teacher quoted by *Kara McAlister* (1997) when relating the successful writing and reading experiences of a group of third- to fourth-grade students in a self-contained special education classroom. The students, who had severe language and learning disabilities, had not yet learned to name all the letters of the alphabet, but each constructed an original story for the class book of "Best Stories" using a Writer's Workshop approach. The students were scaffolded to organize their ideas using semantic webs in the prewriting stage. In the drafting stage, they constructed their own sentences, which they either spelled creatively or dictated to an adult. They reread and revised their stories, which were then typed into a computer for editing and publishing. None of these processes depends on knowing the alphabet.

_____

me politely, but you never write it down!"—Personal Reflection 5.9.)

Current trends are to include children with severe disabilities in activities where they will have opportunities to become literate and, if necessary, to provide them with microcomputer word processing systems with special switch access to help them learn to write. It is difficult, at this point, to establish a prognosis for learning to read and write because so many individuals with developmental disabilities did not have access to writing systems, or the same experiences to encourage emergent literacy as their peers (Koppenhaver et al., 1991; Koppenhaver & Yoder, 1993; Light, Binger, & Kelford Smith, 1994; Light & Kelford Smith, 1993; Light & McNaughton, 1993).

Phonological awareness seems to play an important role in literacy development among people who are nonspeaking, as it does for children who are normally developing (Blischak, 1994), but it is less predictive of reading success (Dahlgren Sandberg & Hjelmquist, 1996). Graphic symbol use may also contribute to children's metalinguistic concepts of print representations of words (McNaughton & Lindsay, 1995). The most critical step toward understanding concepts of literacy, however, may come from the use of graphic symbols for conveying meaningful messages (Rankin, Harwood, & Mirenda, 1994).

Following tradition, older individuals with severe cognitive and linguistic impairments should be taught to recognize written symbols and the international symbols needed for personal safety and daily living. Deliberate and early attempts should also be made to surround children who have severe disabilities with literate language and print, as discussed in Chapters 8 and 10. As programs are developed to incorporate literacy goals and related activities for students with severe disabilities, new discoveries may be made about their capacity to learn. It is certainly not a homogenous group, and decisions must be individualized.

Technological Assists to Emergent Literacy. Erickson and Koppenhaver (1995) described a transdisciplinary program for a class of eight children from ages 5 to 11 years whose intelligence was difficult to test due to their physical disabilities. The one child for whom a full scale IQ score had been obtained, scored "well below average" (p. 677). Seven of the eight children used wheelchairs. Six had cerebral palsy, one spina bifida, and one a degenerative disease. Literacy goals were built into language-rich classroom experiences all day long and integrated with physical therapy positioning objectives. The transdisciplinary team included a special education teacher, speech–language pathologist, two teacher assistants, and an aide. Erickson and Koppenhaver wrote that "This transdisciplinary approach did not occur naturally. The professionals struggled through 'turf' issues, conflicting pedagogies, and divergent theoretical bases, while holding onto a common commitment to the children" (p. 678). The intervention was supported with an array of high technology and light technology devices and techniques. It had four basic literacy components: "(a) writing during calendar time each morning; (b) directed reading in small groups or individually with the teacher; (c) use of computer software; and (d) group activities" (p. 680). Off-the-shelf software programs, with special accessing techniques and devices as needed, were used in the morning to work on language arts and math. In the afternoon, group activities included acting out favorite books. The authors wrote:

> Skits could be time consuming. Choreographing the movement of seven wheelchairs in a small classroom could be a feat in itself. In addition, several children had to use speech synthesis and loop tapes to say their lines, and the movements in general were slower. However, each child was provided with an opportunity to participate independently. (p. 679)

Attempts were made to keep the reading and writing activities "child directed and constructive rather than teacher directed and reactive" (p. 680). At the end of two years, four of the eight children returned to their neighborhood elementary schools, but they continued to have difficulty with a tendency for schools to "water down curriculum instead of providing alternative ways to participate in the standard curriculum" (pp. 682–683).

Facilitated Communication. Facilitated communication is a highly controversial approach that has been used with individuals who have autism and other severe developmental disabilities based on an assumption of hidden literacy abilities. Biklen (1988, 1990, 1993) has been the primary proponent of the approach in the United States, adapting the method from a program developed by Rosemary Crossley (1992a; 1992b) in Melbourne, Australia. Crossley first used the program with a young woman with cerebral palsy who had been institutionalized all her life but left the institution successfully when Crossley worked with her as she learned to read and write using facilitated communication (Crossley & MacDonald, 1984).

Using facilitated communication (FC), as developed further by Biklen (1988, 1990, 1992, 1993), the adult facilitator provides a keyboard writing system with print output (the Cannon communicator, an augmentative communication device, was used in the early studies). The adult supports the child's forearm, wrist, and index finger (if necessary). The adult then uses systematic steps to introduce the child to sound–letter correspondences, to teach simple words, to request simple words in response to fill-in tasks, and ultimately, to converse with the child in writing. In a significant proportion of cases, children have typed written messages that far exceeded expectations based on the child's ability to communicate orally.

The tempest surrounding questions of the authenticity of messages authored by individuals using FC has been strong. Duchan's (1993) tutorial about the approach stimulated letters to the editor of the *Journal of Speech and Hearing Research* that suggested that further research and clinical activity were a waste of time at best and unethical at worst (Fried-Oken, Paul, & Fay, 1995), an unproductive line of research (Yoder, 1995), or a situation that calls for dialogue rather than dogma (Duchan, 1995b; Silliman, 1995). Controlled studies (Wheeler, Jacobson, Paglieri, & Schwartz, 1993) and almost any review of them (Fried-Oken et al., 1995; Calculator & Hatch, 1995; Shane, 1994) provide basically uniform evidence that FC users are not authoring their own messages independently.

Questions have been promoted throughout this book as the guiding forces behind new insights and solid decision making. A primary question of research and discussions has been "Who is authoring the messages produced by FC users?" This is more than an academic question. Allegations of molestation by parents and others have been made in a number of cases. Although FC does not appear to be a generally valid form of testimony, validation should be accomplished on a case-by-case basis (Calculator & Hatch, 1995; Prizant, Wetherby, & Rydell, 1994).

My personal experiences with FC have been largely positive, enough to retain it as an option for seeking access to communication with individuals who seem largely noncommunicative but with sparks suggesting otherwise, such as sidewise glances and an apparent interest in literacy. I still think it is unwise to hold either an all or none position with regard to the efficacy of FC. When I asked Carole Cupps, inclusion consultant for Kalamazoo Public Schools, to validate the case description of the student described in Box 3.7, she responded (personal communication, September 3, 1996):

Your book page seems accurate and informative. It is so difficult to keep things short. For your information, we did reach the agreement or understanding that [the student's] screaming seemed to lessen over time as her interest and involvement through facilitated communication and choices in participation in academic tasks increased. She was extremely quiet when Mary read aloud to her. She especially enjoyed literature and science. [The student] ended the year by "writing" a research report on Autism.

AAC, FC, and the ABCs.   The heading for this subsection is the title of an article by Koppenhaver, Pierce, and Yoder (1995). They took the discussion about FC to a new level when they asked whether FC might be viewed as "a type of alternative access referred to as a selection technique" in AAC (p. 7). This moves the discussion beyond the question of authorship because it views facilitation as the first step toward traditional AAC values of independent message transmission. It

recognizes that individuals who seem to be candidates for FC are also candidates for AAC systems (both low- and high-technology approaches) that will allow them to become "more independent and competent communicators" (p. 8).

Koppenhaver, Pierce, and Yoder (1995) questioned all (especially) or none approaches to FC decision making. They described the experiences of Karen Erickson (see Erickson & Koppenhaver, 1995, described previously) when she acted as substitute teacher in a class of children during a 6-week summer session. Without using FC, Erickson was able to achieve "unexpected literacy" with six of seven students with severe disabilities "and unexpected amounts of functional spoken language in three of four students considered by previous teachers to be 'essentially nonverbal' " (p. 10). For example:

Johnny, a 7-year-old, was considered nonverbal, but was known to recognize a large number of words in isolation (tested in multiple-choice format) and to enjoy browsing through books. The regular staff assumed that he was not actually reading the books, because he was considered to be a beginning-level reader in his text comprehension. However, his reading comprehension had never been formally or informally assessed. One day during the summer program, the teacher presented a wordless picture book, Will's Mammoth, *to the class. The first day, she "read" the story to them. The second day, she modeled oral text generation, keeping her models to approximately three words per page. The next day, she went around the room, presenting one picture to each child, saying, "Your turn." When she got to Johnny, he said, "It looks like the elephants are eating snow." The next day, when she repeated the activity and came to him, he said, "Elephants don't eat snow." That is, this child, presumed to be nonverbal and possessing little language comprehension, generated orally a novel and related pair of statements about the pictures. After the teacher wrote on a chart all of the sentences about the pictures that the group had generated, Johnny then read it aloud verbatim. (p. 11)*

Building Narrative Understandings

Objective 2. The individual will participate in constructing stories, orally, in writing, and in dramatic representation, including characters' motives, goals, and feelings.

The previous discussions have added to the case for meaningful narratives of human interactions as the basic stuff of which all language and communication are made. Children with severe disabilities who reach higher than unexpected levels do so, almost uniformly, when someone, a parent (Butler, 1980) or a teacher (Erickson & Koppenhaver, 1995; Koppenhaver et al., 1995; Paley, 1990, 1994) encourages their sense of the narrative by fostering their opportunities to listen to and construct stories of their own lives and interests, no matter how rudimentary—often supported by written as well as oral communication (Schairer & Nelson, 1996). Another child described by Koppenhaver, Pierce, and Yoder (1995) was Allan, an 11-year-old, who wrote text willingly at times, but at other times became violent in his refusals:

> After seeing the moon low on the horizon one evening, he wrote in class, "I play ball summer. I play ball in the summer and in the winter. I saw the moon last night go to the earth." (p. 12)

It may have been opportunity and expectation that brought forth this moment of exquisite access to Allan's thoughts. The piece was written independently, but it appeared because his teacher had set up journal writing activities as a daily event.

Narratives as a Route to Subjectivity.   Play, story writing, and dramatization of stories from books and the children's own ideas have been described previously in this chapter and Chapters 8 and 10 as fruitful language intervention contexts. Hewitt (1994) described an intervention approach for an adolescent with autism based in appreciation of the importance of subjectivity to narrative comprehension. That is, Hewitt emphasized the representation of individual experience as the organizing motivation behind plot elements, cohesive devices, and other elements of story structure. She related this view to a cognitivist explanation of autism as a deficit in the theory of mind that makes it difficult to understand the perspectives of others (see Chapters 3 and 4) and to achieve subjectivity (Baron-Cohen, 1995; Hobson, l993). Her approach was not designed to teach uniform understandings of narrative structure. In fact, she noted that "looking at the child's system on its own terms allows for the possibility of discovering systematicity and structure that is unique to the individual" (p. 91). Hewitt

also recommended focusing on fictional narratives. She cited descriptions of fiction as "the only medium that offers us the illusion of directly experiencing the consciousness of another person" (p. 90).

The intervention approach Hewitt (1994) described for Barry, the adolescent with autism, had both cognitivist and social interactionist underpinnings. That is, Hewitt used a discourse-style lesson format (social interactionist in nature) while viewing her task primarily as a cognitive one of a "teacher presenting new information" (p. 98). Her intervention techniques have been described as scaffolding in this book, in that they involved framing, focusing, guiding, and feeding back data in the context of holistic experiences to make Barry aware of monitoring characters' psychological states in the texts they read together. Hewitt (coded as "L" for Lynne) provided a transcript of a typical session that illustrates these principles. I have added annotations in square brackets to highlight the elements of scaffolding:

> **L:** *Do you have any idea why she might have cried when her son said those bad things about himself? [framing]*
> **B:** *Uh uh.*
> **L:** *Why would that make a mother feel sad? [focusing]*
> **B:** *Itsa* It makes them afraid.*
> **L:** *It makes him afraid? Umm, what about her feelings, what is she feeling? [guiding]*
> **B:** *Her feelings were hurt.*
> **L:** *Um hm, I agree. How could her feelings have been hurt by him saying those things about himself? [focusing]*
> **B:** *I don't know. (almost inaudible)*
> **L:** *OK, let's think about mothers. Today's Mother's Day, right? That's one reason I picked this story. How do mothers usually feel about their kids? [framing]*
> **B:** *Sad.*
> **L:** *All the time? [feeding back]*
> **B:** *They feel happy.*
> **L:** *Do they love them or hate them or don't they care? [guiding]*
> **B:** *They love them. (pp. 98–99)*
>
> (* represents an abandoned start)

Over time, Barry learned to talk about characters' belief systems and to describe why they did things (e.g., in novels written for teenagers and in Charles Dickens' *Great Expectations,* read at school). He continued, however, to have difficulty understanding deception and dual identity, involving both the wolf in Little Red Riding Hood and Magwitch in *Great Expectations.*

Story Enactment.   Paley's (1990, 1994) uses of story dictation and dramatization in a general education kindergarten, sometimes with atypical children, have been described previously in this chapter and elsewhere in the book. Culatta (1994) also described play and story enactment as a language intervention context in which "the clinician guides the enactment of themes while implementing strategies to enhance a variety of linguistic goals" (p. 105).

For younger children, Culatta (1994) described how narratives can be facilitated in the context of representational play with four different strategies. First, the clinician can model selected narrative elements, to move the child a step beyond his or her current level of narrative understanding (see descriptions in Chapters 8 and 10), for example, by exemplifying temporally related events, causally related events, goal-directed behavior, or plans. Second, the clinician might engage the child in direct planning at the outset of play. Third, the clinician might impose an organized narrative framework on play by adopting different voices (stage manager, character, narrator) and suggest modifications during play. Fourth, the clinician could support the child's contributions to on-line planning, genuinely questioning the child's rationale if plot elements seem out of place and accepting the child's decisions as author and director, while encouraging the child to higher levels of narrative understanding. Culatta noted how such interactions could add to decontextualized language use and literacy by using abstract props and referring to remote events.

TRANSITIONS TO WORK AND ADULTHOOD

GOAL: The individual will use appropriate communicative skills for community-based and work interactions.

- Facilitating Transitions
- Functional Communication Life Skills
- Fostering Independence

OUTCOME: The individual will live in situations of increased independence.

Facilitating Transitions

One of the primary rites of passage in Western societies from childhood to adulthood involves making the transi-

tion from school to work. The data on employment of students with any disabilities, let along severe ones, after leaving school are generally discouraging. For many, the transition from school to work is far from complete.

> *Few handicapped students move from school to independent living in communities. Secondary special education programs appear to have little impact on students' adjustment to community life. More than 30% of the students enrolled in secondary special education programs drop out. (Edgar, 1987, p. 40)*

Comprehensive vocational transition programs for persons with severe handicaps have several characteristics. As summarized by Moon, Diambra, and Hill (1990), these include (1) a written, formal plan with goals and objectives, time lines, and responsible agencies and persons; (2) a functional school curriculum that uses community-based vocational instruction; and (3) concrete outcomes that include job placements. The development of Individualized Transition Plans (ITPs) requires a collaborative effort by a team of professionals. Sometimes missing from those plans is the consideration of the communicative demands of job settings and the students' related abilities. Contextually based assessments may increase the likelihood that students will succeed in their job placements.

Some students with severe disabilities may make transitions to higher education settings rather than jobs. Some make transitions to both (see Personal Reflection 13.10). When students with severe disabilities attend postsecondary educational programs, they often need additional support from student-service programs in their vocational training programs, community colleges, or universities. Language specialists may provide some of those services.

Functional Communication Life Skills

> *Objective 1.* The individual will demonstrate the functional communication skills to participate in important life contexts (changes documented from baseline descriptions in targeted context).

Adolescents or young adults in transition from school to work settings need functional communication skills. The National Joint Committee for the Communicative Needs of Persons with Severe Disabilities

PERSONAL REFLECTION 13.10 _____

"When J-P began college, he needed to find work to help support himself. He had never worked outside our home before, and again, we wondered if he ever could or would. I convinced a woman in the Microfiche Dept. of the college library to give J-P a chance. When he began to work, it took a lot of her time and patience to train him. He memorized the Microfiche system in several days, but he had to be painstakingly taught to do visual/motor tasks like using keys to unlock doors. J-P managed to create a niche for himself in the library over his four years there. He was always prompt and dependable. He worked hard and was willing to take on extra work when demand was high. He talked to and became friends with his co-workers."

Julia Donnelly (1991, p. 14), parent of Jean-Paul, a young man with autism, in an excerpt from a biographical series Donnelly wrote for *The Advocate,* the newsletter of the Autism Society of America.

(1992) identified functional communication as the intervention goal for persons with severe disabilities and noted that it includes abilities to:

1. Communicate for a variety of purposes relevant to the person's life experiences.
2. Use a variety of communication modes to accomplish these purposes effectively.
3. Initiate, maintain, and terminate social interactions as a critical dimension of communication. (p. 6)

The intervention team's job is to juggle concerns related to the young person's pattern of developmental levels with needs related to chronological age and stage of life expectations. Recall the general purpose of language intervention introduced earlier in this book: to make changes relevant to persons' needs in the domains of (1) social appropriateness, acceptance, and closeness; (2) formal and informal learning; and (3) gainful occupation (paid or unpaid). Keeping these broader purposes in mind will help professionals avoid missing the forest for the trees, which sometimes happens when people work for years on the same discrete skills.

What role should the communicative specialist play when it appears that young people will never master the

fine points of linguistic use usually acquired during the middle stages of language acquisition? In many U.S. school districts and community service plans, far too many of these individuals receive no services aimed specifically at their communicative needs because they do not show discrepancy between their cognitive and language levels using formal standardized tests. Yet, as noted in Personal Reflection 13.11, when their contextually based needs are considered, many appropriate goals emerge.

Most goals appropriate for older individuals with middle-stage developmental needs are related to functional outcome, and they are often expressed in situation-specific terms. For example, Mire and Chisholm (1990) listed seven goal areas, each of which related to a specific functional context: The client will independently (1) place an order in a fast-food restaurant, (2) use a telephone, (3) shop, (4) communicate needs and comments during leisure time, (5) communicate needs while traveling, (6) communicate while banking, and (7) communicate at the post office. Professionals then plan sequences of subobjectives based on task analysis. For example, in the goal area targeting communicating needs independently while traveling, subobjectives might include (1) requesting amount of bus fare and where to deposit it, (2) phoning for a taxi, (3) responding to questions about destination, and (4) requesting directions. Mire and Chisolm reported an increase in motivation among staff and clients as they worked toward skills that clients were eager to learn and that were clearly relevant.

The strategies of contextually based assessment and intervention discussed throughout this book mainly involve assessment of the abilities of persons with disabil-

PERSONAL REFLECTION 13.11 _____

"Individuals who are severely and moderately mentally handicapped may not be able to learn to use contractible copulas or past tense modals but they may be able to learn to order their own food, shop for themselves, use the phone, do their own banking, and communicate while having fun."

Stephen Mire and *Rebecca Chisholm* (1990, p. 57), writing about the need for functional communication goals for adolescents and adults with mental retardation.

ities within specific ecological contexts. L. Brown and colleagues (1979) called similar analyses, "Ecological and Student Repertoire Inventories." These inventories are charts that include three columns of information: (1) a contextually based ecological inventory of the demands of a key task, (2) an inventory of the student's current repertoire within that environment, and (3) recommendations for fostering a better match between the two.

One student's vocational plan included the need to interact with customers in the grocery store where he worked. Brown and colleagues (1979) analyzed the task demands to include three skills: (1) Look in the direction of a customer requesting assistance. (2) Answer the customer's question if possible. (3) If not possible, direct the customer to the manager's desk at the front of the store. The student's current repertoire for dealing with each of these situations was often hampered by problems that included looking at the floor when someone approached, insufficient verbal skills, and failure to direct customers when they needed it. Intervention involved extensive experiences interacting with others, the development of augmentative communicative aids, techniques, and strategies, and instruction for using them in actual communicative interactions.

Fostering Independence

Objective 2. The individual will function with increasing independence across a variety of natural contexts.

Learned helplessness is a hazard of growing up with a developmental disability. It occurs when a learner is habitually reinforced for minimal participation and becomes increasingly dependent on others to control interactions and make decisions (Guess, Benson, & Siegel-Causey, 1985; Seligman, 1975). Dependence has a way of obscuring individuality (see Personal Reflection 13.12), but it can be combated with a balance between personal acceptance and setting expectations a notch higher while scaffolding the person toward independence (see Personal Reflection 13.13).

Augmentative communication systems also support independence. A good place to start may be a system for making requests to fulfill personal needs and desires (Reichle, Mirenda, Locke, Piché, & Johnston, 1992). Organization aids also may be designed to promote in-

PERSONAL REFLECTION 13.12 _____

"Wouldn't you hate it if people were always helping you? Wouldn't it be awful if everybody pretended to accept everything you did, even when you were boring or obnoxious, just because you were 'special'? How would you like it if other people always initiated and terminated the interactions that involved you? Worst of all, how would it feel to experience that omnipresent strained politeness, lingering like a damp fog that obscured your individuality from every new person you met?"

Carola Murray-Seegert (1989, p. 91), encouraging perspective taking in her ethnographic study of an inner-city high school integration project that benefited students with obvious disabilities and the regular education students who volunteered to work with them.

Note: From *Nasty Girls, Thugs, and Humans Like Us: Social Relations Between Severely Disabled and Nondisabled Students in High School* (p. 91) by C. Murray-Seegert, 1989, Baltimore, MD: Paul H. Brookes. Copyright 1989 by Paul H. Brookes. Reprinted by permission.

_____

dependent functioning. For example, Doss and Reichle (1991) described a system that would support the independent development of shopping lists:

> To use a shopping list, a learner typically moves to the file box (or other storage location) containing logos and selects the logo that corresponds to the empty product container. The logo is then affixed to a magnetized board (or other display device) that is housed in a convenient location (e.g., on the refrigerator door). When it is time to go shopping, the symbols are transferred from the reminder list to the wallet (or other device for transporting symbols from the list to the store). When the learner finds an empty container, he or she is supposed to move to the storage location, gain access to the storage location, match the empty container to the appropriate symbol, and transfer the symbol to the reminder list. (p. 284)

Powers and Sowers (1994) described how a speech–language pathologist assisted a young adult, Devin, who was unable to speak, develop the communicative supports to live in his own apartment and to enjoy the community independently. The SLP consulted with Devin to tailor his communication to the varied situations in which he wanted to participate but where

PERSONAL REFLECTION 13.13 _____

IN ELEMENTARY SCHOOL:

"One day she sat, dejectedly, on a kitchen chair, her lunch box at her feet. She'd gotten dressed in time for the bus . . . almost.

" 'Good for you. Tie your shoes, and you'll be all done,' I said, as I sponged oatmeal out of Jill's hair and gave Matt a quick kiss before he started out the door.

" 'I can't tie them,' Nicole said.

" 'Why not?' I asked, reaching to grab Jill's milk cup before it tipped over.

" 'Cause I'm just a poor little retarded girl,' Nicole snuffled. She began to pick at a scab.

"What was this? Self-pity?"

" 'Get those shoes tied. Retarded doesn't mean helpless,' " I barked, as I began sopping up the spilt milk.

"She tied the shoes. And she never used her handicap to play on my sympathy again." (p. 36)

AT AGE 22, IN THE APARTMENT HER DAUGHTER INSISTED ON GETTING ON HER OWN:

"It was time to go. I lingered a moment while I arranged in a jelly glass a few flowers I'd brought from our garden. As I placed them on the kitchen counter, I thought of the pediatrician in the Panama Canal Zone. His words were as clear to me then as they'd been the day he'd said them twenty years before.

" 'She may never advance beyond the mental state of five years.' His prognosis had been accurate. Nicole's latest California Achievement test placed her at the first grade level. Yet here she was trying to live on her own. I wondered if psychologists had a way to measure *chutzpah*." (p. 72–73)

Sandra Z. Kaufman (1988), describing her relationship with her daughter who had mental retardation and her daughter's growing independence from childhood into adulthood in the book, *Retarded Isn't Stupid Mom!*

---

there was insufficient time for him to type out messages on his portable electronic communication device:

> For example, in the movie theatre, they decided Devin would type out the name of the movie on a typewriter at home and present the paper to the ticket taker. To enable Devin to order food at his favorite fast food Mexican restaurant, the SLP typed up the menu on a small card that Devin carried in his back pack. When he went to the restaurant, Devin pointed to the appropriate words on his card to communicate which food items he wanted. (p. 243)

Strategies for encouraging adult independence among people with severe disabilities, including mental retardation, are often based on principles articulated by Lou Brown and his colleagues (L. Brown, Nietupski, & Hamre-Nietupski, 1976). As summarized by Falvey,

Bishop, Grenot-Scheyer, and Coots (1988), those, include (1) preparation to function as independently as possible across as many integrated, heterogeneous environments as possible; (2) planning for generalization by teaching activities in environments that require them, using natural cues, corrections, and reinforcers specific to each environment; and (3) designing instructional strategies to be sufficiently flexible and individualized to meet the diverse needs of students with mental retardation.

When a person with a severe disability acquires sufficient communicative ability to live independently, it is a challenge to the parents and professionals who have guided the person's development along the way to let go. Eventually, and to varying degrees, letting go, however, may be the best form of intervention (see Personal Reflection 13.14).

"He does have talent, interest, and desire to pursue being a history professor. All his life I have taught, guided, and supported him. I have smoothed his path in what I thought were the best directions. Now he is 21 and I can no longer make his decisions. We have talked very honestly about his future. Jean-Paul is aware of his disabilities and the limited job market. He still chooses to work in the field that he loves and has ability in. What more can I say to him? His life has been a series of challenges, none of them easy, but he has always been willing to try. He has surprised us all with what he has achieved. All I can tell him now is, 'Yes, Jean-Paul, Go for it.' "

Julia Donnelly (1991, p. 15), parent of Jean-Paul, a young man with autism, in the closing comments of her biographical series about her son.

_____

SUMMARY _____

This chapter has addressed assessment and intervention concerns for individuals with severe communication impairments. It harks back to Chapter 2, in which the need to consider speech, language, and communication as highly integrated but separable systems was discussed. In this chapter, examples were provided of individuals who are nonspeaking but have later-stage language acquisition needs, as well as of individuals with severe cognitive and language impairments who can communicate nevertheless. An important point is that there are no prerequisites for communication. I would also remind readers that any of the procedures for fostering language acquisition that have been suggested in prior chapters might be adopted for individuals with severe communicative impairments to address their early-, middle-, and later-stage needs. A critical concern is that intervention contexts and materials be appropriate to an individual's chronological age, and not just the indiviual's cognitive development stage. The need to consider whether appropriate augmentative and alternative communication (AAC) options are available has also been a theme of this chapter.

Several assessment and planning models were described. The participation model (Beukelman & Mirenda, 1992) emphasizes opportunity and access. The Michigan Decision-Making Model (Nelson et al.,

1981) facilitates organization of assessment information from the four domains—cognition, receptive language, expressive language, social interaction and play—for use in collaborative decision making with parents and other professionals about communicative interventions for individual children. The MAPS model (Vandercook et al., 1989) involves parents and others in a process that considers a person's history, dreams, nightmares, gifts, and needs to plan for the future and to take immediate steps toward supporting a good life. The Circle of Friends approach (Falvey et al., 1994) offers a strategy for helping youths without disabilities look at peers with disabilities in a new way. The COACH model (Giangreco et al., 1993) starts with a student and family interview and moves to establish goals that can support a student within the regular education curriculum. Needs-based discrepancy analysis and matrixing (Calculator & Jorgensen, 1994) are used to inventory communicative demands and opportunities and to establish goals for addressing an individual's communicative needs within inclusive settings.

The contexts for assessment and intervention for individuals with severe communicative impairments are the same as those for other individuals. Social interaction and play routines were described as being important across the age span. The importance of mealtimes was also discussed. Fitting with the general theme of the book, an emphasis was placed on fostering participation in school and community.

Intervention goals and methods targeting communicative intentions and interactions were described. Prelinguistic interactions are designed to help individuals move from preintentional (perlocutionary level) to intentional (illocutionary level) communication, in preparation for movement to symbolic (locutionary level) communication. Nonsymbolic communication was viewed, however, as important in itself. Direct intervention for aberrant expressions of communicative intentions includes analysis of their message value or other functions and replacing them with alternative communicative behaviors or other functionally related behaviors. Indirect strategies include modifying contextual factors that seem to trigger aberrant responses. Improving the assertive–responsive balance is an important goal for individuals who are passive or inactive communicators. Expanding social interactions also can be targeted by seeking to understand the functions of unconventional communicative behaviors, such as echolalia. Bringing peers in as interacting partners or as peer tutors are particular advantages of working with individuals with severe disabilities in inclusive settings.

More advanced language content and forms are appropriate targets for many individuals with severe communicative impairments. Choices regarding symbol systems were discussed relative to their transparency (iconicity) and learnability. Advantages of real objects and color photographs were noted over miniature objects. Strategies for helping individuals develop multi-word constructions include: (1) linguistic and social interactionist approaches that set up a contextual need for linguistic semantic–grammatic (agent + action; action + locative) constructions; (2) strict behaviorist approaches (e.g., Lovaas, 1981); and (c) hybrid milieu teaching approaches. As noted in Chapter 3, no one approach has been shown to be superior over others.

Individuals with severe communicative impairments need opportunities to experience narrative discourse and exposure to a literacy-rich environment with technological supports to give them access to reading and writing ignoring traditional concepts of readiness. The controversy over facilitated communication was noted, and I indicated that I have not yet drawn any final conclusions of my own. With Koppenhaver and colleagues (1995), I did, however, recommend exploring independent literate uses of language that may have gone previously unrecognized, unexpected, and unsupported. I also think that we will learn even more about the power of narratives in human development and understandings over the next decade that will continue to support the importance of narratives for individuals with severe disabilities (e.g., Hewitt, 1994), as for all of us.

Transitions to work and adulthood need deliberate attention in plans for among individuals with severe communicative impairments. Communicative specialists can foster transitions by performing contextually based assessments and interventions. Goals may be set for functional communication life skills, but also to support some individuals in their goals to seek higher education. AAC options and other methods should be enlisted to help individuals with severe disabilities become as independent as possible, challenging all to reach higher than may seem "realistic" at first. This book ends as it started—with the reminder that *problems are not just within persons with communicative disorders, and neither are solutions.*

REVIEW TOPICS

- Speech, language, and communication as highly integrated but separable systems.
- Early-, middle-, later-stage, and AAC needs of individuals with severe communication impairments.
- Assessment and planning models including: the participation model, the Michigan Decision-Making Model, the MAPS model, the Circle of Friends model, the COACH model, and needs-based discrepancy analysis and matrixing models.
- Social interaction, mealtimes, play routines, school, and community as assessment and intervention contexts.
- Prelinguistic interactions: preintentional (perlocutionary level) to intentional (illocutionary level) to symbolic (locutionary level) communication.
- Nonsymbolic communication; three approaches to providing intervention for aberrant expressions of communicative intentions.
- Strategies for improving the assertive–responsive balance for individuals who are passive or inactive communicators (oral, written, and nonverbal).
- Expanding social interactions; analysis of functions of unconventional verbal behaviors, such as echolalia; soliciting peers as interactants; peer tutoring.
- Symbol systems and features of transparency and learnability; symbol combinations; strategies for encouraging more advanced content–form constructions.
- Relationships among narrative discourse, subjectivity, and literacy development; roles of phonological awareness for individuals who are nonspeaking; readiness issues for working on literacy with individuals with severe communicative impairments; facilitated communication.
- Strategies for fostering transitions to work and the multiple other contexts of adulthood.

REVIEW QUESTIONS

1. Are there any prerequisites for communication? If so, what? Why do most professionals who advocate for individuals with severe communicative impairments insist that there are no prerequisites? What implications does this view have for policy makers and service providers?

2. Describe circumstances that would lead you to select each of the following models for assessment and planning purposes: the participation model, the Michigan Decision-Making Model, the MAPS model, the Circle of Friends model, the COACH model, and needs-based discrepancy analysis and matrixing models.

3. What defines the transparency of a symbol system? What defines its learnability? What is the hierarchy of difficulty (for most individuals) of color photographs, miniature objects, and real objects?

4. Describe differences in the intervention approaches for teaching multiword constructions that would be taken by professionals guided by linguistic and social interactionist theories, behaviorist theories, and hybrid theories. Has the efficacy of one of these approaches been proved over the others? If so, which? Which approach would you most likely adopt and why?

5. What is the essence of the controversy over facilitated communication? [Hint: Think about authorship.] What does the preponderance of research show? How do questions about unexpected literacy abilities influence intervention choices besides whether or not to try facilitated communication?

6. What is meant by the concept of subjectivity? How does it relate to Theory of Mind discussions? What diagnostic group is thought to have greatest difficulty with this concept? What intervention methods might be used to help develop the concept of subjectivity and a theory of mind? Is deception or duality of identity an easier or more difficult concept to grasp than subjectivity, based on Hewitt's (1994) research?

7. What strategies can be used to foster transitions to adulthood and independence for individuals with severe disabilities?

ACTIVITIES FOR EXTENDED THINKING

1. Contact an inclusion specialist for a local school district. Ask if you can observe a MAPS, Circle of Friends, or COACH planning session, given the family's permission, of course. Pay close attention to the collaborative process. Did you observe any barriers that turned the activity into a more competitive or individualistic goal setting event? What elements did you observe in the discourse, turn-taking, and proxemic behaviors of the participants that supported the sense of collaborative problem solving? (e.g., How was space used? How were the participants positioned?)

2. Perform an ecological assessment of the communicative behaviors of a person who is nonspeaking, prelinguistic, and possibly preintentional. Can you assign message-value to any of the person's actions (or inactions)? Can you see opportunities for introducing other nonsymbolic communication options?

3. If you were given the opportunity to set up a self-contained summer school classroom for children with mixed physical and cognitive disabilities, told that you could spend up to $25,000 for hardware and software, and that your goal was to help them develop literacy and communication skills to help them be more academically competitive in their home schools in the following year, what would you ask for? How would you spend your instructional days?

Michigan Decision-Making Model Reference Chart

COGNITIVE BASES	RECEPTIVE LANGUAGE	EXPRESSIVE LANGUAGE	SOCIAL INTERACTION AND PLAY
Preintentional (Birth to 8 months) *Sensorimotor Stages I, II, III* ___ Little evidence of goal oriented actions at beginning of period ___ Assimilates new objects into reflex exercises ___ Explores objects by mouthing or banging ___ By end of period infant moves from being purely reflexive to showing the initial beginnings of goal oriented behavior ___ Gradually develops object permanence ___ Early: eyes focus on empty space where object was when it is dropped, fails to look under scarf for object ___ Later: eyes follow object as it is moved, looks under scarf for hidden object	*Precursors* (Birth to 8 months) ___ Startles to noise ___ Orients to sound source ___ Looks at person who calls name	*Precursors* (Birth to 8 months) ___ Undifferentiated cry ___ Reflexive vocalizations and comfort sounds	(Birth to 8 months) ___ Stares at large masses ___ Grasps object placed in hand ___ Makes eye contact briefly ___ Quiets when picked up ___ Actively seeks sound source ___ Looks intently and shakes toy in hand ___ Smiles at mirror image, familiar faces ___ Sobers at sight of strangers ___ Increases activity at sight of toy, familiar caretaker ___ Works for toy out of reach ___ Returns to activity after interruption
Early Intentional (8 to 12 months) *Sensorimotor IV* ___ Uses familiar means to achieve novel ends (tries to repeat or prolong an effect he/she has discovered) ___ Imitates ongoing actions already in repertoire (e.g., patty-cake, kiss mommy, peekaboo) ___ Object permanence now established (looks for object previously seen) ___ Looks at pictures in a book with adult ___ Stares to gain information ___ Reacts in anticipation prior to familiar event	*Precursors* (Strategies used prior to actual linguistic comprehension) (8 to 12 months) ___ Looks at objects that mother looks at ___ Acts on objects noticed ___ Imitates ongoing action or sound if it is already within repertoire ___ Laughs at familiar interaction sequences ___ Inhibits action in response to "no" ___ Responds to "bye-bye" ___ Follows caretaker's gaze to common objects when labeled	*Precursors* (8 to 12 months) ___ Differentiated cries ___ Syllabic babbling ___ Communication games ___ Intentional action	(8 to 12 months) ___ Responds to facial expressions ___ Frequently cries when parent leaves room ___ Drinks from cup, feeds self crackers ___ Imitates arm movements for games like peekaboo, pattycake ___ Squeezes toy to make it squeak ___ Drops toys and watches them fall ___ Puts small objects in and out of container ___ Stacks rings on peg ___ Holds crayon, imitates scribbling ___ Cooperates in dressing ___ Kisses, waves, holds out hands
Late Intentional (12 to 18 months) *Sensorimotor V* ___ Uses novel means to achieve familiar ends (e.g., communicative gestures and stereotyped vocalization used to achieve adult attention, particular object, object's removal) ___ Figures out ways to overcome some obstacles (opens door, reaches high objects)	*Lexical comprehension* (12 to 18 months) ___ Understands one word in some sentences when referents are present ___ Points to objects in response to "Show me ___" (e.g., body parts) *Nonverbal comprehension strategies* used to respond to commands: ___ Attend to object mentioned ___ Give evidence of notice ___ Do what is usually done in a situation	*First words* (12 to 18 months) ___ Performatives (gesture accompanies vocalization or word) ___ Hi/bye routines ___ Comment ___ Request object or attention ___ Reject ___ Communicates immediate needs by pulling or pointing	(12 to 18 months) ___ Reacts to emotions of others ___ Solitary or onlooker play, self-play ___ Scribbles spontaneously with crayon ___ Points to objects he/she wants and claims certain objects as own ___ Imitates sweeping, hair combing, etc. ___ Hugs doll, pulls toy

(continued)

COGNITIVE BASES	RECEPTIVE LANGUAGE	EXPRESSIVE LANGUAGE	SOCIAL INTERACTION AND PLAY
Representational Thought (18 to 24 months) *Sensorimotor VI* ___ Begins to replace sensorimotor activity of previous stages with internalized problem solving using images, memories, and symbols to represent actions and objects	*Lexical comprehension* (18 to 24 months) ___ Understanding of words when referent is not present ___ Understanding of action verbs out of routine context; carries out two-word commands, but often fails to understand three lexical elements ___ Understanding of routine forms of questions for agent, object, locative, and action *Nonverbal comprehension strategies* used to respond to commands: ___ Locate the objects mentioned ___ Give evidence of notice ___ Do what you usually do: objects into containers, conventional use ___ Act on the objects in the way mentioned ___ Child as agent	*Transition to two word combination* (18 to 24 months) ___ New semantic roles ___ Early: action–object relations; agent, action, object, recurrence, disappearance ___ Later: object–object relations, location, possession, nonexistence ___ Asks a "What's that" question ___ Answers some routine questions ___ Rapid acquisition of vocabulary ___ Successive one-word utterances ___ Increased frequency of talking ___ Onset of two-word utterances (MLU 1.5)	(18 to 24 months) ___ Parallel play (near others but not with them) ___ Talks to self while playing ___ Little social give and take—hugs, pushes, pulls, snatches, grabs, but pays little attention to what others say or do ___ Relates action to object or another person—washes, feeds doll in addition to self ___ Listens to short story ___ Demonstrates pleasure in make believe games (e.g., 2 sticks to represent "airplane")

COGNITIVE BASES	RECEPTIVE LANGUAGE	EXPRESSIVE LANGUAGE				SOCIAL INTERACTION AND PLAY
Early Preoperations (2 to 3½ yrs) ___ Arranges objects in patterns but not in categories ___ Initiates drawing of vertical line (by 30 mos) ___ Imitates drawing of horizontal line and circle (by 36 mos) ___ Matches identical objects ___ Draws 2 or more lines imitating a cross (by 3½ yrs) ___ Copies short line of beads by matching individual items but fails to put them in correct order, getting only adjacent pairs correct ___ Matches similar objects ___ Ability to represent one thing by another increases speed and range of thinking, particularly as language develops, but thinking remains tied closely to actions ___ Thought is preconceptual; inferences sometimes but not always correct	*Lexical comprehension* (2 to 3½ yrs) ___ Accepts or rejects, confirms or denies in response to yes/no questions ___ 2½ ___ What for object yrs. ___ What-do for action ___ Where for location (place) ___ 3 ___ Whose for possessor yrs. ___ Who for person ___ Why for cause or reason ___ How many for number ___ Understanding of gender contrasts in third person pronouns ___ 2–3 *Comprehension* yrs. *strategies* ___ Does what is usually done ___ Probable location strategy for in, on, under, beside ___ Probable event strategy for simple active reversible sentences ___ Supplies missing information (2 years) ___ Supply explanation (3 years) ___ Infers most probable speech act in context ___ Sequence for understanding Wh-questions	*Typ Brown's* (2 to 3½ yrs) *MLU Age Stage New (morph) Development*				(2 to 3½ yrs) ___ Parallel play predominates (24 mos) ___ Dramatization, imagination, and symbolic play (make believe and pretend) ___ Takes turns ___ Watches cartoons on TV ___ Associative group play begins (3½ yrs) ___ Organizes doll furniture accurately and plays imaginatively ___ Builds bridge from model
		2	___ I	Basic semantic relations ___ Agent–action ___ Action–object ___ Agent–object ___ Possessive ___ Entity–locative ___ Action–locative ___ Existence ___ Recurrence ___ Nonexistence ___ Rejection ___ Denial ___ Attributive	1.75	
			___ II	Grammatical inflections ___ Some articles, plurals, possessives ___ -ing on verbs ___ What doing? questions	2.25	
		2½	___ III	Differention of sentence Modalities ___ Possession ___ Number (noun plural) ___ Locative containment and support (in, on) ___ Temporary duration (ing)	2.75	
		3	___ IV	Sentence embedding ___ Immediate future gonna) ___ Regular past -ed ___ Inflects verb *be* (am, was, are)	3.50	

COGNITIVE BASES	RECEPTIVE LANGUAGE	EXPRESSIVE LANGUAGE	SOCIAL INTERACTION AND PLAY
Late preoperations (3½ to 7 yrs) ___ Applies systematic trial and error problem solving strategies to classification and seriation tasks ___ Sorts set of blocks varying in size, shape, and color into two piles on basis of single attribute (50% can do by age 3½) ___ Places seven blocks varying in height in order and places 3 missing blocks in sequences (50% can do by age 4½) ___ Begins differentiating open and closed shapes in drawings, and squares may have corners (by age 4½) ___ Develop concepts of time and space ___ Identifies one of the three pictures not in the same category ___ Matches pictures that "go together" ___ Draws person with 2 parts ___ Copies square (by age 4½) ___ Cuts and pastes—may finish project next day ___ Copies triangle (by age 5) ___ Draws person with body, arms, legs, feet, nose, and eyes	*Lexical comprehension* (3½ to 7 yrs) ___ Understands contrasts for topological locatives (in, on, under, beside) ___ Answers how questions with manner or instrument responses ("What do we eat with") ___ Comprehension of word order as cues to understand agent–object in active sentences (word order strategy) ___ Responds to two-stage action commands	Typ Age — Brown's Stage — New Development (3½ to 7 yrs) — MLU (morph) 3½ ___ V 3.75 ___ Sentence conjoining ___ Regular past -ed ___ Third pers. singular *Event relations* (sequence of emergence from 3½ to 7 years) ___ And (coordinate and temporal) ___ Because, so (causal) ___ But (contrastive) ___ When (conditional) ___ While (simultaneity) ___ After ___ Before ___ Past time (-ed) ___ Possibility (might) *Syntactic rule emergence from 4 to 6 years* ___ N + cont + cop + PN/PA/loc (He's sick) ___ There's expleture (There is a table) ___ Poss + N + V (Jim's dog bites) ___ Adj + N + V (the big truck rolled) ___ N + N + V (Joe and Jim race cars) ___ Reflexive (He sees himself) ___ S because S (He went because he wanted to) ___ S + V + indirect + N (He gave her a book) ___ When S + S (When I go to town, I will buy an ice cream cone) ___ Obligatory & emphatic do (He does not feel good. He does feel good) ___ Noninversion of aux/modal (Where daddy is?) ___ Aux/modal + aux modal (How can he can look? Is that's a rocket?) ___ Continued use of double negation. Some problems in the truth value of negatives. ___ Continued regularization of irregular forms. *Syntactic rule emergence from 6 to 7 years* ___ Passive transform (The boy was hit by the girl) ___ If transformation (If it rains, we won't go) ___ N + V + particle (He jumped up) ___ S/V concord (He likes candy) ___ Pronominalization (John knew he would win the race. He knew John would win the race) ___ Inversion of aux/modal + main V (When's going to be the party?) ___ Noninversion of aux/modal (Where she's going?)	(3½ to 7 yrs) ___ Increased dramatization in play ___ Suggests turns, but often bossy ___ Plays in group of 2 to 3 children ___ Shows off ___ Friendships stronger ___ Plays in groups of 2 to 5 ___ Able to play games by rules (by age 6) ___ Spends hours at one activity ___ Demands more realism in play (age 7)

(continued)

Michigan Decision-Making Model Reference Chart   continued

COGNITIVE BASES	RECEPTIVE LANGUAGE	EXPRESSIVE LANGUAGE	SOCIAL INTERACTION AND PLAY
Concrete Operations (7 to 12 yrs) ___ Formation of series and classes takes place mentally; physical actions are internalized as mental actions or 'operations' ___ Classifies in two ways at once (e.g., can sort by both color and shape in matrix) ___ Still solves problems primarily through trial and error rather than establishing general rules and testing hypotheses ___ Able to correct misconceptions through discussion	(7 to 12 yrs) ___ Understanding of conditional conjunctions *if* and *when* (usual rather than logical sense) ___ Probable relation of events strategy for causal conductions ___ Understanding of causal conjunctions *because* and *so* (8 years) ___ Understanding of contrastive conjunctions *but* and *although* as though they mean *and* (8 years) ___ Contrastive conjunctions *but* and *although* 10 years)	(7 to 12 years) *Marks of maturity in language* ___ Longer sentences ___ More clauses per sentence—8th graders use 150% more than 4th graders ___ Use of adverbial clauses (He was sleeping when I walked in the door) ___ Use of adjective clauses (The man with the broken foot limped along the highway) ___ Nominals (Flying airplanes is fun) ___ Sentence complements (They elected Jim president) ___ Infinitive complements (He told Jim to feed the dog) ___ Reduction of mazes and tangles (characteristic of younger children who begin a sentence that does not fulfill a communication unit and eventually drop it as if it is beyond them.) ___ Uses language to converse, persuade, tease	(7 to 12 years) ___ Genuine cooperation with others replaces isolated play or play in the company of others ___ Reduction in imaginary play but development of theatrical entertainment ___ Makes accurate replicas and working models ___ Enjoys categorizing collections of various sorts

Note: From *The Michigan Decision-Making Strategy for Determining Appropriate Communicative Services for Physically and/or Mentally Handicapped Children* by N. W. Nelson, J. C. Silbar, and E. L. Lockwood, 1981, November, presented at the annual conference of the American-Speech-Language-Hearing Association, Los Angeles. Copyright 1981 by N. W. Nelson, J. C. Silbar, and E. L. Lockwood. Reprinted by permission.

Michigan Decision-Making Model

SUMMARY CHART

Name: _____ BD: _____ Speech–Language Clinician: _____

Date: _____ Classroom Teacher: _____

COGNITIVE BASES	RECEPTIVE LANGUAGE	EXPRESSIVE LANGUAGE	SOCIAL INTERACTION & PLAY
Preintentional (Birth to 8 months) *Sensorimotor I, II, III* ___ Infant moves from being purely reflexive to showing the initial beginnings of goal-oriented behavior ___ Developing object permanence	___ Startles to sound ___ Turns to sound ___ Reacts to human voice ___ Responds to tone of voice	___ Cry ___ Reflexive vocalizations	___ Engages in interaction ___ Maintains interaction ___ Initiates interaction ___ Indicates preference for familiar people and objects
Early Intentional (8 to 12 months) *Sensorimotor IV* ___ Uses familiar means to achieve novel ends	___ No word comprehension yet ___ Imitates on-going action ___ Looks where parent looks	___ Differentiated cries ___ Syllabic babbling	___ Plays nursery games ___ Plays with toys
Late Intentional (12 to 18 months) *Sensorimotor V* ___ Invention of new means to achieve familiar ends	___ Responds appropriately to single words in context	___ Hi/bye routines ___ First words ___ Words used as 'performatives' (to manipulate environment	___ Solitary or onlooker play ___ Hugs doll, pulls toy
Representational Thought (18 to 24 months) *Sensorimotor VI* ___ Begins symbolic thinking	___ Understands words without context (points to pictures) ___ Follows two-word commands	___ Novel one-word utterances ___ Asks "What's that?" ___ Onset of two-word utterances	___ Parallel play
Early Preoperations (2 to 3½ years) ___ Thought is preconceptual ___ Inference is sometimes but not always correct	___ Begins to understand Wh- questions ___ Answers yes/no questions	___ Two-word utterances ___ Basic sentences develop ___ Morphological markers develop	___ Symbolic play
Late Preoperations (3½ to 7 years) ___ Beginning of intuitive thought ___ Problem solves by trial and error (not always correct)	___ Points to pictures representing sentences ___ Uses word order to understand agent–object relationships	___ Uses compound and complex sentences ___ Uses language to relate experiences ___ Talks about remote experiences ___ Adequate voice, articulation, fluency	___ Plays in small groups
Concrete Operations (7 to 12 years) ___ Classifies on 2 characteristics	___ Understands conditional causal sentences	___ More clauses per sentence ___ Uses language to converse, persuade, tease	___ Genuine cooperative play

Instructions:
1. Place a check mark beside characteristics demonstrated (reference chart or other evaluation tools may be used as necessary)
2. Shade in areas that describe functioning (areas may be partially shaded)
3. Refer to program decision chart.

Recommendations:

REFERENCES

Abikoff, H., & Gittelman, R. (1985). The normalizing effects of methylphenidate on the classroom behavior of ADHD children. *Journal of Abnormal Child Psychology, 13,* 33–44.

Abraham, W. (1984). *Figurative language* [Computer program]. Dimondale, MI: Hartley Courseware.

Ackerman, B. P. (1982). On comprehending idioms: Do children get the picture? *Journal of Experimental Child Psychology, 33,* 439–454.

Adler, S. (1991). Assessment of language proficiency of limited English proficient speakers: Implications for the speech-language specialist. *Language, Speech, and Hearing Services in Schools, 22,* 12–18.

Aitchison, J. (1976). *The articulate mammal: An introduction to psycholinguistics.* New York: Universe Books.

Algozzine, B., Morsink, C. V., & Algozzine, K. M. (1989). What's happening in self-contained special education classrooms? *Exceptional Children, 55,* 259–265.

Allen, J. P. B., & Van Buren, P. (1971). *Chomsky: Selected readings.* London: Oxford University Press.

Allen, R. E., & Oliver, J. M. (1982). The effects of child maltreatment on language development. *Child Abuse and Neglect, 6,* 299–305.

Allen, R. E., & Wasserman, G. A. (1985). Origins of language delay in abused infants. *Child Abuse and Neglect, 9,* 335–340.

Alley, G., & Deshler, D. (1979). *Teaching the learning disabled adolescent: Strategies and methods.* Denver: Love Publishing.

Als, H., Lester, B. M., Tronick, E., & Brazelton, T. B. (1982). Toward a research instrument for the assessment of preterm infants' behavior (APIB). In H. E. Fitzgerald, B. M. Lester, & M. W. Yogman (Eds.), *Theory and research in behavioral pediatrics, Vol. 1* (pp. 35–132). New York: Plenum Press.

American Educational Research Association, American Psychological Association, and National Council on Measurement in Education. (1985). Standards for educational and psychological testing. Washington, DC: American Psychological Association.

American Psychiatric Association. (1980). *Diagnostic and statistical manual of mental disorders, third edition (DSM III).* Washington, DC: Author.

American Psychiatric Association. (1987). *Diagnostic and statistical manual of mental disorders, third edition—revised (DSM III–R).* Washington, DC: Author.

American Psychiatric Association. (1994). *Diagnostic and statistical manual of mental disorders, fourth edition, revised (DSM IV).* Washington, DC: Author.

American Psychological Association. (1985). *Standards for educational and psychological testing.* Washington, DC: Author.

American Speech-Language-Hearing Association. (1982). Definitions: Communicative disorders and variations. *Asha, 24,* 949–950.

American Speech-Language-Hearing Association. (1990). Audiological assessment of central auditory processing: An annotated bibliography. *Asha, 32*(Suppl. 1), 13–30.

American Speech-Language-Hearing Association. (1991). Amplification as a remediation technique for children with normal peripheral hearing. *Asha, 33*(Suppl. 3), 22–24.

American Speech-Language-Hearing Association Joint Committee on Infant Hearing. (1991). 1990 position statement. *Asha, 33* (Suppl. 5) 3–6.

American Speech-Language-Hearing Association. (1993). Guidelines for caseload size and speech-language service delivery in the schools. *Asha, 35* (Suppl. 10), pp. 33–39.

American Speech-Language-Hearing Association. (1994). Guidelines for fitting and monitoring FM systems. *Asha, 36* (Suppl. 12), 1–9.

American Speech-Language-Hearing Association. (1996). Central auditory processing: Current status of research and implications for clinical practice. *American Journal of Audiology, 5*(2), 41–54.

American Speech-Language-Hearing Association. (1996, Spring). Inclusive practices for children and youths with communication disorders: Position statement and technical report. *Asha, 38* (Suppl. 16), pp. 33–44.

Amochaev, A. (1987). The infant hearing foundation—A unique approach to hearing screening of newborns. *Seminars in Hearing, 8*(2), 165–168.

Anderson, G. M., & Nelson, N. W. (1988). Integrating language intervention and education in an Alternate Adolescent Language Classroom. *Seminars in Speech and Language, 9*(4), 341–353.

Anderson, R. C. (1985). Role of the reader's schema in comprehension, learning, and memory. In H. Singer & R. B. Ruddell (Eds.), *Theoretical models and processes of reading* (3rd ed.) (pp. 372–384). Newark, DE: International Reading Association.

Anderson-Yockel, J., & Haynes, W. O. (1994). Joint book-reading strategies in working class African American and white mother-toddler dyads. *Journal of Speech and Hearing Research, 37,* 583–593.

Andreasen, N. C. (1984). *The broken brain: The biological revolution in psychiatry.* New York: Harper & Row.

Andrews, J. F., & Mason, J. M. (1991). Strategy usage among deaf and hearing readers. *Exceptional Children, 57,* 536–545.

Applebee, A. N. (1978). *The child's concept of story.* Chicago, IL: The University of Chicago Press.

Applebee, A. N., & Langer, J. A. (1983). Instructional scaffolding: Reading and writing as natural language activities. *Language Arts, 60,* 168–175.

Aram, D. M. (1984). *Seminars in speech and language: Vol 5. Assessment and treatment of developmental apraxia.* New York: Thieme-Stratton.

Aram, D. M. (1988). Language sequelae of unilateral brain lesions in children. In F. Plum (Ed.), *Language, communication, and the brain* (pp. 171–197). New York: Raven Press.

Aram, D. M. (1990, June). *Definition of child language disorders.* Paper presented at the 11th Symposium for Research on Child Language Disorders, The University of Wisconsin, June 1, 1990, Madison, WI.

Aram, D. M., & Ekelman, B. L. (1987). Unilateral brain lesions in children: Performance on the Revised Token Test. *Brain and Language, 32,* 137–158.

Aram, D. M., & Ekelman, B. L. (1988). Scholastic aptitude and achievement among children with unilateral brain lesions. *Neuropsychologia, 26,* 903–916.

Aram, D. M., Ekelman, B. L., & Gillespie, L. L. (1989). Reading and lateralized brain lesions in children. In K. von Euler, I. Lundberg, & G. Lennerstrand (Eds.), *Brain and reading* (pp. 61–75). Hampshire, England: MacMillan Press Ltd.

Aram, D. M., Ekelman, B. L., & Nation, J. E. (1984). Preschoolers with language disorders: 10 years later. *Journal of Speech and Hearing Research, 27,* 232–244.

Aram, D. M., Ekelman, B. L., & Whitaker, H. A. (1986). Spoken syntax in children with acquired unilateral hemisphere lesions. *Brain and Language, 27,* 75–100.

Aram, D. M., Ekelman, B. L., & Whitaker, H. A. (1987). Lexical retrieval in left and right brain lesioned children. *Brain and Language, 31,* 61–87.

Aram, D. M., Hack, M., Hawkins, S., Weissman, B. M., & Borawski-Clark, E. (1991). Very-low-birthweight children and speech and language development. *Journal of Speech and Hearing Research, 34,* 1169–1179.

Aram, D. M., Morris, R., & Hall, N. E. (1992). *Validity of discrepancy criteria for identifying children with developmental language disorders.* Cleveland, OH: Case Western Reserve University.

Aram, D. M., Morris, R., & Hall, N. E. (1993). Clinical and research congruence in identifying children with specific language impairment. *Journal of Speech and Hearing Research, 36,* 580–591.

Aram, D. M., & Nation, J. E. (1975). Patterns of language behavior in children with developmental language disorders. *Journal of Speech and Hearing Research, 18,* 229–241.

Aram, D. M., & Nation, J. E. (1980). Preschool language disorders and subsequent language and academic difficulties. *Journal of Communication Disorders, 13,* 159–170.

Aram, D., & Nation, J. (1982). *Child language disorders.* St. Louis, MO: C. V. Mosby.

Armbruster, B. B. (1984). The problem of 'inconsiderate' text. In G. G. Duffy, L. R. Roehler, & J. M. Mason (Eds.), *Comprehension instruction: Perspectives and suggestions* (pp. 202–217). New York: Longman.

Aronson, E., Blaney, N., Stephan, C., Sikes, J., & Snapp, M. (1978). *The jigsaw classroom.* Beverly Hill, CA: Sage Publications.

Arwood, E. (1983). *Pragmaticism: Theory and application.* Rockville, MD: Aspen.

Asch, A. (1989). Has the law made a difference? What some disabled students have to say. In D. K. Lipsky & A. Gartner (Eds.), *Beyond separate education: Quality education for all* (pp. 181–205). Baltimore: Paul H. Brookes.

ASHA Committee on Language, Speech, and Hearing Services in Schools. (1984). Guidelines for caseload size for speech-language services in the schools. *Asha, 26* (4), 53–58.

ASHA Committee on Language Learning Disabilities. (1989, March). Issues in determining eligibility for language intervention. *Asha, 31,* 113–118.

Astington, J. W. (1994). Children's developing notions of others' minds. In In J. F. Duchan, L. E. Hewitt, & R. M. Sonnenmeier (Eds.), *Pragmatics: From theory to practice* (pp. 72–87). Englewood Cliffs, NJ: Prentice Hall.

Atwell, N. (1987). *In the middle: Writing, reading, and learning with adolescents.* Portsmouth, NH: Heinemann.

Augustine, D. K., Gruber, K. D., & Hanson, L. R. (1990). Cooperation works! *Educational Leadership, 47*(4):4–7.

Augustinos, M. (1987). Developmental effects of child abuse: Recent findings. *Child Abuse and Neglect, 11,* 15–27.

Austin, J. (1962). *How to do things with words.* London: Oxford University Press.

Autism Society of America Board of Directors. (1988). Autism Society of America Resolution on abusive treatment and neglect. *Advocate* (journal of the ASA), *20*(3), 17.

Aylward, E. H. (1987). Psychological evaluation. In F. R. Brown III & E. H. Aylward (Eds.), *Diagnosis and management of learning disabilities* (pp. 33–57). Boston: College-Hill.

Aylward, E. H., & Brown, F. R. III. (1987). Interdisciplinary diagnosis. In F. R. Brown III & E. H. Aylward (Eds.), *Diagnosis and management of learning disabilities* (pp. 109–125). Boston: College-Hill.

Baddeley, A. (1986). *Working memory.* Oxford, England: Clarendon Press.

Bahr, C. M., Nelson, N. W., & Van Meter, A. (1996). The effects of text-base and graphics-based software tools on planning and organizing of stories. *Journal of Learning Disabilities, 2,* 355–370. This article also appears in a monograph, *Technology for students with learning disabilities: Educational applications,* with a print version and additional annotative text in a digital version. Austin, TX: Pro-Ed.

Bahr, C. M., Nelson, N. W., Van Meter, A., & Yanna, J. V. (1996). Children's use of desktop publishing features: Process and product. *Computing in Childhood Education, 7*(3/4), 149–177.

Bailey, D. B., Jr., & Brochin, H. A. (1989). Tests and test development. In D. B. Bailey & M. Wolery (Eds.), *Assessing infants and preschoolers with handicaps* (pp. 22–46). Columbus, OH: Merrill/Macmillan.

Bailey, D. B., Jr., & Simeonsson, R. J. (1988). Home-based early intervention. In S. L. Odom & M. B. Karnes (Eds). *Early intervention for infants and children with handicaps* (pp. 199–215). Baltimore: Paul. H. Brookes.

Bailey, D. B., Jr., Simeonsson, R. J., Yoder, D. E., & Huntington, G. S. (1990). Preparing professionals to serve infants and toddlers with handicaps and their families: An integrative analysis across eight disciplines. *Exceptional Children, 57,* 26–35.

Bailey, D. B., Jr., & Wolery, M. (1989). *Assessing infants and preschoolers with handicaps.* Columbus, OH: Macmillan.

Bain, B. A., & Olswang, L. B. (1995). Examining readiness for learning two-word utterances by children with specific expressive language impairment: Dynamic assessment validation. *American Journal of Speech-Language Pathology, 4*(1), 81–91.

Baker, L., & Brown, A. L. (1984). Metacognitive skills and reading. In P. D. Pearson (Ed.), *Handbook of reading research* (pp. 353–394). New York: Longman.

Baker, L., & Cantwell, D. P. (1982). Psychiatric disorder in children with different types of communication disorders. *Journal of Communication Disorders, 15,* 113–126.

Baker, L., & Cantwell, D. P. (1987a). Comparison of well, emotionally disordered and behaviorally disordered children with linguistic problems. *Journal of the American Academy of Child and Adolescent Psychiatry, 26,* 193–196.

Baker, L., & Cantwell, D. P. (1987b). A prospective psychiatric follow-up of children with speech/language disorders. *Journal of the American Academy of Child and Adolescent Psychiatry, 26,* 546–553.

Baldwin, D. A., & Markman, E. M. (1989). Establishing word-object relations: A first step. *Child Development, 60,* 381–398.

Baltaxe, C. A. M., & Simmons, J. Q. III. (1985). Prosodic development in normal and autistic children. In E. Schopler & G. B. Mesibov (Eds.), *Communication problems in autism* (pp. 95–125). New York: Plenum Press.

Baltaxe, C. A. M., & Simmons, J. Q. (1988). Communication deficits in preschool children with psychiatric disorders. *Seminars in Speech and Language, 8,* 81–90.

Baratz, J. C. (1969). Language and cognitive assessment of Negro children: Assumptions and research needs. *Asha, 10,* 87–91.

Barber, P. A., Turnbull, A. P., Behr, S. K., & Kerns, G. M. (1988). A family systems perspective on early childhood special education. In S. L. Odom & M. B. Karnes (Eds)., *Early intervention for infants and children with handicaps* (pp. 179–198). Baltimore: Paul. H. Brookes.

Barbero, G. (1982). Failure-to-thrive. In M. H. Klaus, T. Leger, & M. A. Trause (Eds.), *Maternal attachment and mothering disorders (Pediatric Round Table: 1)* (pp. 3–6). Skillman, NJ: Johnson & Johnson Baby Products Company.

Barkley, R. A. (1988). Poor self-control in preschool hyperactive children. *Medical Aspects of Human Sexuality, 21*(6), 176–180.

Barkley, R. A. (1995). *Taking charge of ADHD.* New York: The Guildford Press.

Baroff, G. S. (1986). *Mental retardation: Nature, cause, and management* (2nd ed.). New York: Hemisphere Publishing Corporation.

Baron-Cohen, S. (1995). Mindblindness: An essay on autism and theory of mind. Cambridge, MA: The MIT Press.

Baron-Cohen, S., Leslie, A., & Frith, U. (1985). Does the autistic child have a 'theory of mind'? *Cognition, 21,* 37–46.

Barrie-Blackley, S., Musselwhite, C. R., & Rogister, S. H. (1978). *Clinical oral language sampling.* Danville, IL: The Interstate Printers and Publishers, Inc.

Bashir, A. S. (1989). Language intervention and the curriculum. *Seminars in Speech and Language, 10*(3), 181–191.

Bashir, A. S., Wiig, E. H., & Abrams, J. C. (1987). Language disorders in childhood and adolescence: Implications for learning and socialization. *Pediatric Annals, 16,* 145–156.

Bass, P. M. (1988, November). *Attention deficit disorder/Management in preschool, adolescent, and adult populations.* Miniseminar presented at the Annual Conference of the American Speech-Language-Hearing Association, Boston, MA.

Bates, E. (1976). *Language and context: Studies in the acquisition of pragmatics.* New York: Academic Press.

Bates, E. (1979). *The emergence of symbols: Cognition and communication in infancy.* New York: Academic Press.

Bates, E., Benigni, L., Bretherton, I., Camaioni, L., & Volterra, V. (1979). *The emergence of symbols: Cognition and communication in infancy.* New York: Academic Press.

Bates, E., Bretherton, I., & Snyder, L. (1988). *From first words to grammar: Individual differences and dissociable mechanisms.* New York: Cambridge University Press.

Bates, E., Camaioni, L., & Volterra, V. (1975). The acquisition of performatives prior to speech. *Merrill-Palmer Quarterly, 21,* 205–226.

Bates, E., & MacWhinney, B. (1979). A functionalist approach to the acquisition of grammar. In E. Ochs & B. Schieffelin (Eds.), *Developmental pragmatics.* New York: Academic Press.

Bates, E., & MacWhinney, B. (1982). Functionalist approaches to grammar. In E. Wanner & L. Gleitman (Eds.), *Language acquisition: The state of the art.* New York: Cambridge University Press.

Bates, E., & MacWhinney, B. (1987). Competition, variation, and language learning. In B. MacWhinney (Ed.), *Mechanisms of language acquisition* (pp. 157–194). Hillsdale, NJ: Erlbaum.

Bates, E., & Snyder, L. (1985). The cognitive hypothesis in language development. In I. Uzigiris & J. M. Hunt (Eds.), *Research with scales of psychological development in infancy.* Champaign-Urbana: University of Illinois Press.

Bateson, M. (1971). The interpersonal context of infant vocalizations. *Quarterly progress report, Research laboratory of electronics, MIT, 100,* 170–176.

Bateson, M. (1975). Mother-infant exchanges: The epigenesis of conversational interaction. In D. Aronson & R. Rieber (Eds.), *Developmental psycholinguistics and communication disorders.* New York: New York Academy of Sciences.

Battle, D. E. (Ed.). (1993). *Communication disorders in multicultural populations.* Boston: Andover Medical Publishers.

Bayley, N. (1969). *Bayley Scales of Infant Development.* San Antonio, TX: Psychological Corporation.

Bean, C., Folkins, J. W., & Cooper, W. E. (1989). The effects of emphasis on passage comprehension. *Journal of Speech and Hearing Research, 32,* 707–712.

Bedore, L. M., & Leonard, L. B. (1995). Prosodic and syntactic bootstrapping and their clinical applications: A tutorial. *American Journal of Speech-Language Pathology, 4*(1), 66–72.

Beitchman, J. H., Nair, R., Clegg, M., & Patel, P. G. (1986). Prevalence of speech and language disorders in 5-year-old kindergarten children in the Ottawa-Carlton Region. *Journal of Speech and Hearing Disorders, 51,* 98–110.

Bellack, A. A., Kliebard, H. M., Hyman, R. T., & Smith, F. L., Jr. (1966). *The language of the classroom.* New York: Columbia University Teachers College Press.

Bellugi, U., Bihrle, A., Jernigan, T., Trauner, D., & Doherty, S. (1991). Neuropsychological, neurological, and neuroanatomical profile of Williams Syndrome. *American Journal of Medical Genetics Supplement, 6,* 115–125.

Bellugi, U., & Klima, E. (1982). The acquisition of three morphological systems in American Sign Language. *Papers and Reports on Child Language Development, 21,* 135.

Benedict, H. (1979). Early lexical development: Comprehension and production. *Journal of Child Language, 6,* 183–200.

Bennett, C. W. (1989). *Referential semantic analysis* [Computer program]. Woodstock, VA: Teaching Texts.

Bennett, C. W., & Alter, K. S. (1985). *Word class inventory for schoolage children* [Computer program]. San Diego, CA: College-Hill Press.

Bennett, C. W., & James, C. (1990, November). *TTR revisited: Selecting remedial targets.* Paper presented at the meeting of the American Speech-Language-Hearing Association, Seattle, WA.

Benson, D. F. (1967). Fluency in aphasia: Correlations with radioactive scan localization. *Cortex, 3,* 373–394.

Benson, D. F., & Geschwind, N. (1976). Aphasia and related disturbances. In A. B. Baker (Ed.), *Clinical neurology* (Vol. 1, pp. 1–28). New York: Harper & Row.

Berko, J. (1958). The child's learning of English morphology. *Word, 14,* 150–177.

Bernstein, B. B. (1972). A critique of the concept of compensatory education. In C. B. Cazden, V. P. John, & D. Hymes (Eds.), *Functions of language in the classroom* (pp. 135–154). New York: Columbia University Teachers College Press.

Bernstein, D. K. (1986). The development of humor: Implications for assessment and intervention. *Topics in Language Disorders, 6*(4), 65–72.

Bertalanffy, L. von. (1968). *General system theory: Foundations, development, applications.* New York: George Braziller.

Bess, F. H. (1982). Children with unilateral hearing loss. *Journal of Academy of Rehabilitation Audiology, 15,* 131–144.

Bess, F. H., Freeman, B., & Sinclair, J. S. (Eds.). (1981). *Amplification in education.* Washington, DC: A. G. Bell.

Bess, F. H., & McConnell, F. (1981). *Audiology, education, and the hearing impaired child.* St. Louis: C. V. Mosby.

Bettelheim, B. (1967). *The empty fortress.* New York: Free Press.

Beukelman, D. R. (1987). When you have a hammer, everything looks like a nail. *Augmentative and Alternative Communication, 3,* 94–96.

Beukelman, D. R., & Mirenda, P. (1988). Communication options for persons who cannot speak: Assessment and evaluation. In C. A. Coston (Ed.), *Proceedings of the national planners conference on assistive device service delivery: Planning and implementing augmentative communication service delivery* (pp. 151–165). Washington, DC: Rehabilitation Engineering Society of North America (RESNA), Association for the Advancement of Rehabilitation Technology.

Beukelman, D. R., & Mirenda, P. (1992). *Augmentative communication: Management of children and adults with severe communication disorders.* Baltimore: Paul H. Brookes.

Beukelman, D. R., & Tice, R. (programmer). (1990). *The vocabulary toolbox* [computer program]. Field test version under development at the University of Nebraska-Lincoln.

Beukelman, D. R., Tice, R., Garrett, K., & Lange, U. (1988). *Cue-write: Word processing with spelling assistance and practice* [computer software]. Tucson, AZ: Communication Skill Builders.

Beukelman, D. R., & Yorkston, K. M. (1991). Traumative brain injury changes the way we live. In D. R. Beukelman & K. M. Yorkston (Eds.), *Communication disorders following traumatic brain injury: Management of cognitive, language, and motor impairments* (pp. 1–13). Austin, TX: Pro-Ed.

Bickerton, D. (1983). Creole languages. *Scientific American, 249* (July), 116–122.

Biklen, D. (Producer). (1988). *Regular lives* [videotape]. Washington, DC: State of the Art.

Biklen, D. (1990). Communication unbound: Autism and praxis. *Harvard Educational Review, 60,* 291–314.

Biklen, D. (1992). Typing to talk: Facilitated communications. *American Journal of Speech-Language Pathology, 1* (2), 15–17.

Biklen, D. (1993). *Communication unbound.* New York: Teachers College Press.

Bird, J., Bishop, D. V. M., & Freeman, N. H. (1995). Phonological awareness and literacy development in children with expressive phonological impairments. *Journal of Speech and Hearing Research, 38,* 446–462.

Bishop, D. V. M., & Edmundson, A. (1987). Language-impaired 4-year-olds: Distinguishing transient from persistent impairment. *Journal of Speech and Hearing Disorders, 52,* 156–173.

Bivens, J. A., & Berk, L. E. (1990). A longitudinal study of the development of elementary school children's private speech. *Merrill-Palmer Quarterly, 36,* 443–463.

Bjorkland, D., & Bjorkland, B. (1988, January). Cultural literacy. *Parents,* 144.

Blachman, B. A. (1994). Early literacy acquisition: The role of phonological awareness. In G. P. Wallach & K. G. Butler (Eds.), *Language learning disabilities in school-age children and adolescents* (pp. 253–274). Boston: Allyn and Bacon.

Blackstone, S. (1989) Life is not a dress rehearsal. *Augmentative Communication News, 2*(5), 1–2.

Blager, F. B. (1979). The effect of intervention on the speech and language of abused children. *Child Abuse and Neglect, 5,* 991–996.

Blager, F. B., & Martin, H. P. (1976). Speech and language of abused children. In H. P. Martin (Ed.), *The abused child: A multidisciplinary approach to developmental issues and treatment* (pp. 83–92). Cambridge, MA: Ballinger Publishing Co.

Blank, M. (1973). *Teaching learning in the preschool: A dialogue approach.* Columbus, OH: Merrill.

Blank, M. (1975) Verbalization from young children in experimental tasks. *Child Development, 46,* 254–257.

Blank, M. (1982). Language and school failure: Some speculations on the relationship between oral and written language. In L. Feagans & D. Farran (Eds.), *The language of children reared in poverty* (pp. 75–93). New York: Academic Press.

Blank, M., McKirdy, L. S., & Payne, P. C. (1996a). Links to language I: Linguistic foundations of discourse. Boonton, NJ: Pathways to language, L. L. C.

Blank, M., McKirdy, L. S., & Payne, P. C. (1996b). Links to language II: Linguistic foundations of discourse. Boonton, NJ: Pathways to language, L. L. C.

Blank, M., McKirdy, L. S., & Payne, P. C. (1996c). Teaching tales: Foundations for narratives. Boonton, NJ: Pathways to language, L. L. C.

Blank, M., Rose, S. A., & Berlin, L. (1978). *The language of learning: The preschool years.* New York: Grune & Stratton.

Blank, M., & White, S. J. (1986). Questions: A powerful but misused form of classroom exchange. *Topics in Language Disorders, 6*(2), 1–12.

Blischak, D. M. (1994). Phonologic awareness: Implications for individuals with little or no functional speech. *Augmentative and Alternative Communication, 10*, 245–254.

Bliss, L. S. (1987). "I can't talk anymore; My mouth doesn't want to." The development and clinical applications of modal auxiliaries. *Language, Speech, and Hearing Services in Schools, 18*, 72–79.

Bloom, B. S. (Ed.). (1956). *Taxonomy of educational objectives. Handbook I. Cognitive domain.* New York: David McKay.

Bloom, L. (1967). A comment on Lee's "Developmental sentence types: A method for comparing normal and deviant syntactic development," *Journal of Speech and Hearing Disorders, 32*, 294–296.

Bloom, L. (1970). *Language development: Form and function in emerging grammars.* Cambridge, MA: MIT Press.

Bloom, L. (1973). *One word at a time: The use of single word utterances before syntax.* The Hague, Netherlands: Mouton.

Bloom, L. (1975). Communication skills of abused children (Doctoral dissertation, University of Pittsburgh, 1975) *Dissertation Abstracts Internationale, 36*, 7728A.

Bloom, L. (1988). What is language? In M. Lahey (Ed.). *Language disorders and language development* (pp. 1–19). New York: Macmillan.

Bloom, L., Hood, L., & Lightbown, P. (1974). Imitation in language development: If, when, and why. *Cognitive Psychology, 6*, 380–420.

Bloom, L., & Lahey, M. (1978). *Language development and language disorders.* New York: John Wiley & Sons.

Bloom, L., Lahey, M., Hood, L., Lifter, K., & Fiess, K. (1980). Complex sentences: Acquisition of syntactic connectives and the semantic relations they encode. *Journal of Child Language, 7*, 235–261.

Bloome, D., & Knott, G. (1985). Teacher-student discourse. In D. N. Ripich & F. M. Spinelli (Eds.), *School discourse problems* (pp. 53–76). San Diego: College-Hill.

Blosser, J. L., & DePompei, R. (1994). *Pediatric traumatic brain injury.* San Diego: Singular Publishing Group.

Boder, E., & Jarrico, S. (1982). *Boder Test of Reading-Spelling Patterns.* San Antonio, TX: The Psychological Corporation.

Bodner-Johnson, B. (1991). Family conversation style: Its effect on the deaf child's participation. *Exceptional Children, 57*, 502–509.

Boehm, A. E. (1971). *Boehm Test of Basic Concepts.* San Antonio, TX: Psychological Corporation.

Boehm, A. E. (1986). *Boehm Test of Basic Concepts-Revised.* San Antonio, TX: Psychological Corporation.

Bohannon, J. N., III, & Warren-Leubecker, A. (1989). Theoretical approaches to language acquisition. In J. B. Gleason (Ed.), *The development of language* (2nd ed.) (pp. 167–223). Columbus, OH: Merrill Publishing Co.

Bond, D. J., & Chandley, A. C. (1983). The origin and causes of aneuploidy in man. *Aneuploidy: Oxford monographs on medical genetics.* Oxford: Oxford University Press.

Boothroyd, A. (1982). *Hearing impairments in young children.* Englewood Cliffs, NJ: Prentice-Hall.

Bos, C. (1988). Process-oriented writing: Instructional implications for mildly handicapped students. *Exceptional Children, 54*, 521–527.

Bos, C. S., & Anders, P. L. (1990). Interactive practices for teaching content and strategic knowledge. In T. E. Scruggs & B. Y. L. Wong (Eds.), *Intervention research in learning disabilities* (pp. 116–185). New York: Springer-Verlag.

Botvin, G. J., & Sutton-Smith, B. (1977). The development of structural complexity in children's fantasy narratives. *Developmental Psychology, 13*, 377–388.

Bouvier, L. F., & Gardner, R. W. (1986). *Immigration to the U.S.: The unfinished story.* Washington, DC: Population Reference Bureau.

Bowerman, M. (1982). Reorganization processes in lexical and syntactic development. In E. Wanner & L. Gleitman (Eds.), *Language acquisition: The state of the art.* Cambridge: Cambridge University Press.

Boyce, N. L., & Larson, V. L. (1983). *Adolescents' communication: Development and disorders.* Eau Claire, WI: Thinking Publications.

Bracken, B. A. (1984). *Bracken Basic Concept Scale.* San Antonio, TX: Psychological Corporation.

Braddock, J. H. II, & McPartland, J. M. (1990). Alternatives to tracking. *Educational Leadership, 47*(7), 76–79.

Brannon, L. (1985). Toward a theory of composition. In B. W. McClelland & T. R. Donovan (Eds.), *Perspectives on research and scholarship in composition* (pp. 6–25). New York: The Modern Language Corporation of America.

Bransford, J. C., & Johnson, M. K. (1972). Contextual prerequisites for understanding: Some investigations of comprehension and recall. *Journal of Verbal Learning and Verbal Behavior, 11*, 717–726.

Bransford, J. C., & Nitsch, K. E. (1985). Coming to understand things we could not previously understand. In H. Singer & R. B. Ruddell (Eds.), *Theoretical models and processes of reading* (3rd ed., pp. 81–122). Newark, DE: International Reading Association.

Brazelton, T. B. (1973). *Neonatal behavioral assessment scale* (NBAS). Clinics in developmental medicine, No. 50. Philadelphia: J. P. Lippincott.

Brazelton, T. B. (1982). Mother-infant reciprocity. In M. H. Klaus, T. Leger, & M. A. Trause (Eds.), *Maternal attachment and mothering disorders (Pediatric Round Table: 1)* (pp. 49–54). Skillman, NJ: Johnson & Johnson Baby Products Company.

Brazelton, T. B. (1984). *Neonatal behavioral assessment scale* (NBAS, 2nd ed.). Clinics in developmental medicine, No. 50. Philadelphia: J. P. Lippincott.

Brazelton, T. B., Koslowski, B., & Main, M. (1974). The origins of reciprocity: The early mother-infant interaction. In M. Lewis & L. A. Rosenblum (Eds.), *The effect of the infant on its caretaker.* New York: John Wiley & Sons.

Breen, C., Haring, T., Pitts-Conway, V., & Gaylord-Ross, R. (1985). The training and generalization of social interaction during breaktime at two job sites in the natural environment. *The Journal of the Association for Persons with Severe Handicaps, 10,* 41–50.

Brenneis, D., & Lein, L. (1977). "You fruithead": A sociolinguistic approach to children's dispute settlement. In S. Ervin-Tripp & C. Mitchell-Kernan (Eds.), *Child discourse* (pp. 49–65). New York: Academic Press, Inc.

Bricker, D. (1992). The changing nature of communication and language intervention. In S. F. Warren & J. Reichle (Eds.), *Causes and effects in communication and language intervention* (pp. 361–375). Baltimore: Paul H. Brookes.

Bricker, D. (1993a). *Assessment, Evaluation, and Programming System (AEPS): Measurement for birth to three years* (Vol. 1; includes *Family Interest Survey*). Baltimore: Paul H. Brookes.

Bricker, D. (1993b). Then, now, and the path between: A brief history of language intervention. In A. P. Kaiser & D. B. Gray (Eds.), *Enhancing children's communication: Research foundations for intervention* (pp. 11–31). Baltimore: Paul H. Brookes.

Bricker, D., Squires, J., & Mounts, L. (1995). *Ages and Stages Questionnaires: A parent-completed, child-monitoring system.* Baltimore: Paul H. Brookes.

Brinton, B., & Fujiki, M. (1982). A comparison of request-response sequences in the discourse of normal and language-disordered children. *Journal of Speech and Hearing Disorders, 47,* 57–62.

Brinton, B., & Fujiki, M. (1984). Development of topic manipulation skills in discourse. *Journal of Speech and Hearing Research, 27,* 350–358.

Brinton, B., & Fujiki, M. (1989). *Conversational management with language-impaired children: Pragmatic assessment and intervention.* Rockville, MD: Aspen.

Brinton, B., & Fujiki, M. (1995). Conversational intervention with children with specific language impairment. In M. E. Fey, J. Windsor, & S. F. Warren (Eds.), *Language intervention: Preschool through the elementary years* (pp. 183–212). Baltimore: Paul H. Brookes.

Brinton, B., Fujiki, M., Winkler, E., & Loeb, D. F. (1986). Responses to requests for clarification in linguistically normal and language-impaired children. *Journal of Speech and Hearing Disorders, 51,* 370–378.

Britton, B., Glynn, S., & Smith, J. (1985). Cognitive demands of processing expository text: A cognitive workbench model. In B. Britton & J. Black (Eds.), *Understanding expository text.* Hillsdale, NJ: Erlbaum.

Britton, J. N. (1970). *Language and learning.* London: Penguin Press.

Britton, J. N. (1979). Learning to use language in two modes. In N. R. Smith & M. B. Franklin (Eds.), *Symbolic functioning in childhood.* Hillsdale, NJ: Erlbaum.

Bronfenbrenner, U. (1979). Foreword. In P. Chance (Ed.), *Learning through play* (pp. xv–xx) (Johnson & Johnson Pediatric Round Table Series No. 3). New York: Gardner Press.

Brooks, D. (1986). Otitis media with effusion and academic attainment. *International Journal of Pediatric Otorhinolaryngology, 12,* 39–47.

Brown, A. L., & Day, J. D. (1983). Macrorules for summarizing texts: The development of expertise. *Journal of Verbal Learning and Verbal Behavior, 22,* 1–14.

Brown, A. L., & Palincsar, A. (1982). Inducing strategic learning from texts by means of informed, self-control training. *Topics in Learning and Learning Disabilities, 2,* 1–17.

Brown, H., Sherbenou, R. J., & Johnsen, S. K. (1985). *Test of nonverbal intelligence: A language-free measure of cognitive ability* (TONI). Austin, TX: Pro-Ed.

Brown, J. (1977). *Mind, brain, and consciousness: The neuropsychology of cognition.* New York: Academic Press.

Brown, J. B., & Lloyd, H. (1975). A controlled study of children not speaking at school. *Journal of the Association of Workers for the Maladjusted Child,* 49–63.

Brown, L., Branston, M. B., & Hamre-Nietupski, S., Pumpian, I., Certo, N., & Gruenewald, L. (1979). A strategy for developing chronological age appropriate and functional curricular content for severely handicapped adolescents and young adults. *Journal of Special Education, 13*(1), 81–90.

Brown, L., Nietupski, J., & Hamre-Nietupski, S. (1976). The criterion of ultimate functioning and public school services for severely handicapped students. In M. A. Thomas (Ed.), *Hey, don't forget about me! Education's investment in the severely, profoundly, and multiply handicapped* (pp. 2–15). Reston, VA: Council for Exceptional Children.

Brown, L., Sherbenou, R. J., & Johnsen, S. K. (1985). *Test of nonverbal intelligence: A language-free measure of cognitive ability.* Austin, TX: Pro-Ed.

Brown, P. M., & Gustafson, M. S. (1995). Showing sensitivity to Deaf culture. *Asha, 37*(5), 46–47.

Brown, R. A.(1958). *Words and things.* New York: Free Press.

Brown, R. A. (1973). *A first language: The early stages.* Cambridge: Harvard University Press.

Brown, R. A. (1977). Introduction. In C. Snow & C. Ferguson (Eds.), *Talking to children.* New York: Cambridge University Press.

Brown, S. F. (Ed.). (1959). *The concept of congenital aphasia from the standpoint of dynamic differential diagnosis.* Washington, DC: American Speech and Hearing Association.

Brown, T. (1985). Foreword. In J. Piaget, *The equilibration of cognitive structures: The central problem of intellectual development* (translated by T. Brown and K. J. Thampy). Chicago, IL: University of Chicago Press.

Bruininks, V. L. (1978). Actual and perceived peer status of learning disabled students in mainstream programs. *Journal of Special Education, 12,* 51–58.

Bruner, J. (1968). *Processes of cognitive growth: Infancy (Vol. III, Heinz Werner Lecture Series).* Worcester, MA: Clark University Press.

Bruner, J. (1974/1975). From communication to language—A psychological perspective. *Cognition, 3,* 255–287.

Bruner, J. (1975). The ontogenesis of speech acts. *Journal of Child Language, 2,* 1–19.

Bruner, J. (1977). Early social interaction and language acquisition. In R. Schaffer (Ed.), *Studies in mother-infant interaction.* (pp. 271–289) New York: Academic Press.

Bruner, J. (1978). *The role of dialogue in language acquisition.* In A. Sinclair, R. J. Jarvella, & W. J. M. Levelt (Eds.), *The child's conception of language: Springer series in language and communication* (pp. 242–256). New York: Springer-Verlag.

Bruner, J. (1983). *Child's talk: Learning to use language.* New York: W. W. Norton.

Bruner, J. (1990). *Acts of meaning.* Cambridge: Harvard University Press.

Bruner, J., Oliver, R., & Greenfield, P. (1966). *Studies in cognitive growth.* New York: John Wiley & Sons.

Bryan, J. H., & Sherman, A. (1980). An observational analysis of classroom behaviors of children with learning disabilities. *Journal of Learning Disabilities, 1,* 23–34.

Bryan, T. (1986). A review of studies on learning disabled children's communicative competence. In R. L. Schiefel-busch (Ed.), *Language competence: Assessment and intervention* (pp. 227–259). Austin, TX: Pro-Ed.

Bullowa, M. (Ed.). (1979). *Before speech: The beginnings of interpersonal communication.* Cambridge: Cambridge University Press.

Bunce, B. H., Ruder, K. F., & Ruder, C. C. (1985). Using the miniature linguistic system in teaching syntax: Two case studies. *Journal of Speech and Hearing Disorders, 50,* 247–253.

Burke, C. L. (1980). Reading interview. In B. P. Farr & D. J. Stickler (Eds.), *Reading comprehension: An instructional videotape series recourse guide.* Bloomington, IN: Indiana University Press.

Butler, D. (1980). *Cushla and her books.* Boston: Horn Book.

Butler, K. G. (1981). Language processing disorder: Factors in diagnosis and remediation. In R. W. Keith (Ed.), *Central auditory and language disorders in children* (pp. 160–174). San Diego: College-Hill Press.

Butler, K. G. (1984a). Language processing: Halfway up the down staircase. In G. P. Wallach & K. G. Butler (Eds.), *Language learning disabilities in school-age children* (pp. 60–81). Baltimore: Williams & Wilkins.

Butler, K. G. (1984b). From the editor. *Topics in Language Disorders, 4*(2), iv.

Butler, K. G. (Ed.). (1985). From the editor (Introduction to issue entitled, "Language 1 and language 2: Implications for language disorders"). *Topics in Language Disorders, 5*(4), iv-vi.

Butterfield, N. (1994). Play as an assessment and intervention strategy for children with language and intellectual disabilities. In K. Linfoot (Ed.), *Communication strategies for people with developmental disabilities* (pp. 12–44). Baltimore, MD: Paul H. Brookes.

Buttrill, J., Niizawa, J., Biemer, C., Takakashi, C., & Hearn, S. (1989). Serving the language learning disabled adolescent: A strategies-based model. *Language, Speech, and Hearing Services in Schools, 20,* 185–204.

Byrnes, M. (1990). The Regular Education Initiative debate: A view from the field. *Exceptional Children, 56,* 345–349.

Cairns, H. S. (1996). *The acquisition of language* (2nd ed.). San Antonio, TX: Pro-Ed.

Calculator, S. N. (1988). Promoting the acquisition and generalization of conversational skills by individuals with severe handicaps. *Augmentative and Alternative Communication, 4,* 94–103.

Calculator, S. N. (1994a). Designing and implementing communicative assessments in inclusive settings. In S. N. Calculator & C. M. Jorgensen (Eds.), *Including students with* severe disabilities in schools: Fostering communication, interaction, and participation (pp. 113–181). San Diego, CA: Singular Publishing Group.

Calculator S. N. (1994b). Communicative intervention as a means to successful inclusion. In S. N. Calculator & C. M. Jorgensen (Eds.), Including students with severe disabilities in schools: Fostering communication, interaction, and participation (pp. 183–214). San Diego, CA: Singular Publishing Group.

Calculator, S., & Dollaghan, C. (1982). The use of communicative boards in a residential setting: An evaluation. Journal of Speech and Hearing Disorders, 47, 281–287.

Calculator, S. N. & Hatch, E. R. (1995). Validation of facilitated communication: A case study and beyond. American Journal of Speech-Language Pathology, 4(1), 49–58.

Calculator, S. N. & Jorgensen, C. M. (1991). Integrating AAC instruction into regular education settings: Expounding on best practices. Augmentative and Alternative Communication, 7, 204–214.

Calculator, S. N. & Jorgensen, C. M. (Eds.). (1994). Including students with severe disabilities in schools: Fostering communication, interaction, and participation. San Diego, CA: Singular Publishing Group.

Calfee, R., & Chambliss, M. (1988). Beyond decoding: Pictures of expository prose. Annals of Dyslexia, 38, 243–257.

Calfee, R., & Curley, R. (1984). Structure of prose in the content areas. In J. Flood (Ed.), Understanding reading comprehension (pp. 161–180). Newark, DE: International Reading Association.

Calkins, L. M. (1983). Lessons from a child: On the teaching and learning of writing. Portsmouth, NH: Heinemann.

Camarata, S. M., Nelson, K. E., & Camarata, M. N. (1994). Comparison of conversational-recasting and imitating procedures for training grammatical structures in children with specific language impairment. Journal of Speech and Hearing Research, 37, 1414–1423.

Campbell, S. B. (1985). Hyperactivity in preschoolers: Correlates and prognostic implications. Clinical Psychology Review, 5, 405–428.

Campbell, T. F., & Dollaghan, C. A. (1990). Expressive language recovery in severely brain-injured children and adolescents. Journal of Speech and Hearing Disorders, 55, 567–581.

Campione, J. C., & Brown, A. L. (1987). Linking dynamic assessment with school achievement. In C. S. Lidz (Ed.), Dynamic assessment: An interactional approach to evaluating learning potential (pp. 82–115). New York: Guilford Press.

Cantwell, D. P., & Baker, L. (1985). Interrelationship of communication, learning, and psychiatric disorders in children. In C. S. Simon (Ed.), Communication skills and classroom success: Assessment of language-learning disabled students (pp. 43–61). Austin, TX: Pro-Ed.

Cantwell, D. P., Baker, L., & Mattison, R. E. (1979). The prevalence of psychiatric disorder in children with speech and language disorder: An epidemiologic study. Journal of the American Academy of Child Psychiatry, 18, 450–461.

Capper, C. A. (1990). Students with low-incidence disabilities in disadvantaged rural settings. Exceptional Children, 56, 338–344.

Capra, F. (1982). The turning point: Science, society, and the rising culture. New York: Simon & Schuster.

Carey, S. (1978). The child as word learner. In M. Halle, J. Bresnan, & G. Miller (Eds.), Linguistic theory and psychological reality. Cambridge: MIT Press.

Carey, S., & Bartlett, E. (1978). Acquiring a single new word. Papers and Reports in Child Language Development, 15, 17–29.

Carignan-Belleville, L. (1989). Jason's story: Motivating the reluctant student to write. English Journal, 78, 57–60.

Carlson, C. C., & Nelson, N. W. (1994, November). Classroom amplification, middle ear pathology, and academic success. Poster presentation at the annual convention of the American Speech-Language-Hearing Association, New Orleans, LA.

Carlson, F. (1982). Prattle and play: Equipment recipes for nonspeech communication. Omaha, NB: Meyer Children's Rehabilitation Institute, University of Nebraska Medical Center.

Carnine, D., & Kinder, D. (1985). Teaching low-performing students to apply generative and schema strategies to narrative and expository material. Remedial and Special Education, 6, 20–30.

Carpenter, R., Mastergeorge, A., & Coggins, T. (1983). The acquisition of communicative intentions in infants eight to fifteen months of age. Language and Speech, 26, 101–116.

Carr, E., Newsom, C. D., & Binkhoff, J. A. (1980). Escape as a factor in the aggressive behavior of two retarded children. Journal of Applied Behavior Analysis, 13, 101–117.

Carrow, E. (1973a). Screening Test of Auditory Comprehension of Language. Austin, TX: Learning Concepts.

Carrow, E. (1973b). Test for Auditory Comprehension of Language. Austin, TX: Teaching Resources.

Carrow-Woolfolk, E. (1985). Test for auditory comprehension of language-revised (TACL-R). Austin, TX: Pro-Ed.

Carrow-Woolfolk, E. (1988). *Theory, assessment and intervention in language disorders: An integrative approach.* Philadelphia: Grune & Stratton (Harcourt Brace Jovanovich, Inc.).

Carta, J. J., Sainato, D. M., & Greenwood, C. R. (1988). Advances in the ecological assessment of classroom instruction for young children with handicaps. In S. L. Odom & M. B. Karnes (Eds.), *Early intervention for infants and children with handicaps* (pp. 217–239). Baltimore: Paul. H. Brookes.

Cartledge, G., Stupay, D., & Kaczala, C. (1988). Testing language in learning disabled and non-learning disabled Black children: What makes the difference? *Learning Disabilities Research, 3*(2), 101–106.

Casby, M. W. (1988). Speech-language pathologists' attitudes and involvement regarding language and reading. *Language, Speech, and Hearing Services in Schools, 19,* 352–358.

Casby, M. W. (1992a). An intervention approach for naming problems in children. *American Journal of Speech-Language Pathology, 1*(2), 35–42.

Casby, M. W. (1992b). The cognitive hypothesis and its influence on speech-language services in schools. *Language, Speech, and Hearing Services in Schools, 23,* 198–202.

Casby, M. W., & Ruder, K. F. (1983). Symbolic play and early language development in normal and mentally retarded children. *Journal of Speech and Hearing Research, 26,* 404–411.

Case, R. (1985). *Intellectual development: Birth to adulthood.* Orlando, FL: Academic Press.

Cattell, R. B. (1971). *Abilities: Their structure, growth, and action.* Boston: Houghton Mifflin.

Catts, H. W. (1989). Speech production deficits in developmental dyslexia. *Journal of Speech and Hearing Disorders, 54,* 422–428.

Catts, H. W. (1991). Facilitating phonological awareness: Role of speech-language pathologists. *Language, Speech, and Hearing Services in Schools, 22,* 196–203.

Catts, H. W., Hu, C. F., Larrivee, L., & Swank, L. (1994). Early identification of reading disabilities in children with speech-language impairments. In R. V. Watkins & M. L. Rice (Eds.), *Specific language impairments in children* (pp. 145–160). Baltimore, MD: Paul H. Brooks.

Cazden, C. B. (1972). Preface. In C. Cazden, V. John, & D. Hymes (Eds.), *Functions of language in the classroom.* New York: Teachers College, Columbia University.

Cazden, C. B. (1983). Adult assistance to language development: Scaffolds, models, and direct instruction. In R. Parker & F. Davis (Eds.), *Developing literacy: Young children's use of language* (pp. 3–18). Newark, DE: International Reading Association.

Cazden, C. B. (1988). *Classroom discourse: The language of teaching and learning.* Portsmouth, NH: Heinemann.

Cazden, C. B., John, V., & Hymes, D. (Eds.). (1972). *Functions of language in the classroom.* New York: Teachers College, Columbia University.

Chabon, S. S., & Prelock, P. A. (1989). Strategies of a different stripe: Our response to a zebra question about language and its relevance to the school curriculum. *Seminars in Speech and Language, 10*(3), 241–251.

Chadwick, O., Rutter, M., Brown, G., Shaffer, D., & Traub, M. (1981). A prospective study of children with head injuries: II. Cognitive sequelae. *Psychological Medicine, 11,* 49–61.

Chall, J. S. (1983). *Stages of reading development.* New York: McGraw-Hill.

Chance, P. (1979). *Learning through play* (Johnson & Johnson Pediatric Round Table Series No. 3). New York: Gardner Press.

Chapman, R. S. (1978). Comprehension strategies in children. In J. Kavanagh & P. Strange (Eds.), *Language and speech in the laboratory, school, and clinic.* Cambridge: MIT Press.

Chapman, R. S., & Miller, J. F. (1980). Analyzing language and communication in the child. In R. L. Schiefelbusch (Ed.), *Nonspeech language and communication* (pp. 159–196). Austin, TX: Pro-Ed.

Chappell, G. E. (1973). Childhood verbal apraxia and its treatment. *Journal of Speech and Hearing Disorders, 38,* 362–368.

Charney, R. (1980). Speech roles and the development of personal pronouns. *Journal of Child Language, 7,* 509–528.

Cheng, L. L. (1989). Service delivery to Asian/Pacific LEP children: A cross-cultural framework. *Topics in Language Disorders, 9*(3), 1–14.

Cherry, R. (1980). *The selective auditory attention test* (SAAT; manual and tape). St. Louis: Auditec.

Cherry, R., & Kruger, G. (1983). Delective auditory attention abilities of learning disabled and normal achieving children. *Journal of Learning Disabilities, 16,* 202–205.

Chi, J. G., Dooling, E. C., & Gilles, F. H. (1977). Left-right symmetries of the temporal speech areas of the human fetus. *Archives of Neurology, 34,* 346–346.

Chinn, P., Drew, E., & Logan, D. (1975). *Mental retardation: A life cycle approach.* St. Louis: C. V. Mosby Co.

Chipman, S., Segal, J., & Glaser, R. E. (Eds.). (1984). *Thinking and learning skills (Volume II): Current research and open questions.* Hillsdale, NJ: Erlbaum.

Chomsky, C. (1969). *The acquisition of syntax in children from 5 to 10.* Cambridge: MIT Press.

Chomsky, N. (1957). *Syntactic structures.* The Hague: Mouton.

Chomsky, N. (1965). *Aspects of the theory of syntax.* Cambridge: M. I. T. Press.

Chomsky, N. (1968). *Language and mind.* New York: Harcourt, Brace & World.

Chomsky, N. (1976). On the biological basis of language capacities. In R. W. Rieber (Ed.), *The neuropsychology of language.* New York: Plenum Press.

Chomsky, N. (1980). *Rules and representations.* New York: Columbia University Press.

Chomsky, N. (1981). *Lectures on government and binding.* Dordrecht, Holland: Foris.

Chua-Eoan, H. (1997, January 27). 'He was my hero.' *Time,* 23–27.

Churchill, D. W. (1972). The relation of infantile autism and early childhood schizophrenia to developmental language disorders of childhood. *Journal of Autism and Childhood Schizophrenia, 2,* 182–197.

Cirrin, F. M., & Penner, S. G. (1995). Classroom-based and consultative service delivery models for language intervention. In M. E. Fey, J. Windsor, & S. F. Warren (Eds.), *Language intervention: Preschool through the elementary years* (pp. 333–362). Baltimore: Paul H. Brookes.

Cirrin, R., & Rowland, C. (1985). Communicative assessment of nonverbal youths with severe/profound mental retardation. *Mental Retardation, 23,* 52–62.

Clark, D. A. (1989). Neonates and infants at risk for hearing and speech-language disorders. *Topics in Language Disorders, 10*(1), 1–12.

Clark, G. N., & Seifer, R. (1985). Assessment of parents' interactions with their developmentally delayed infants. *Infant Mental Health Journal, 6*(4), 214–225.

Clark, J. B., & Madison, C. L. (1986). *Clark-Madison test of oral language* (CMTOL). Austin, TX: Pro-Ed.

Clark, T., Morgan, E. C., & Wilson-Vlotman, A. L. (1984). *The INSITE model: A parent-centered, in-home, sensory intervention, training and educational program.* Logan, UT: Utah State University.

Clark, T., & Watkins, S. (1985). *SKI*HI curriculum manual: Programming for hearing impaired infants through home intervention.* Logan, UT: Utah State University.

Clarke-Klein, S. M. (1994). Expressive phonological deficiencies: Impact on spelling development. *Topics in Language Disorders, 14*(2), 40–55.

Clarke-Klein, S., & Hodson, B. W. (1995). A phonologically based analysis of misspellings by third graders with disordered phonology histories. *Journal of Speech and Hearing Research, 38,* 839–849.

Clarke, C. M., Edwards, J. H., & Smallpiece, V. (1961). 21 trisomy/normal mosaicism in an intelligent child with mongoloid characters. *Lancet, 1,* 1028.

Clay, M. M. (1979). *The early detection of reading difficulties* (3rd ed.). Auckland, New Zealand: Heinemann.

Cleary, L. M. (1988). A profile of Carlos: Strengths of a nonstandard dialect writer. *English Journal, 77*(5), 59–64.

Coggins, T. E., & Carpenter, R. L. (1981). The communicative intention inventory: A system for coding children's early intentional communication. *Applied Psycholinguistics, 2,* 235–252.

Coggins, T. E., Olswang, L. B., & Guthrie, J. (1987). Assessing communicative intents in young children: Low structured or observation tasks? *Journal of Speech and Hearing Disorders, 52,* 44–49.

Cohen, A. L. Torgesen, J. K., & Torgesen, J. L. (1988). Improving speed and accuracy of word recognition in reading disabled children: An evaluation of two computer program variations. *Learning Disability Quarterly, II,* 333–341.

Cole, A. J., Andermann, F., Taylor, L., Olivier, A., Rasmussen, T., Robitaille, Y., & Spire, J-P.(1988). The Landau-Kleffner syndrome of acquired epileptic aphasia: Unusual clinical outcome, surgical experience, and absence of encephalitis. *Neurology, 38,* 31–38.

Cole, K. N., & Dale, P. S. (1986). Direct language instruction and interactive language instruction with language delayed preschool children: A comparison study. *Journal of Speech and Hearing Research, 29,* 206–217.

Cole, K. N., Dale, P. S., & Mills, D. E. (1990). Defining language delay in young children by cognitive referencing: Are we saying more than we know? *Applied Psycholinguistics, 11,* 291–302.

Cole, K. N., Dale, P. S., & Mills, P. E. (1992). Stability of the intelligence quotient-language quotient relation: Is discrepancy modeling based on a myth? *American Journal on Mental Retardation, 97,* 131–143.

Cole, K. N., & Harris, S. R. (1992). Instability of the intelligence quotient–motor quotient relationship. *Developmental Medicine and Child Neurology, 34,* 633–641.

Cole, K. N., Mills, P. E., & Dale, P. S. (1989). Examination of test-retest and split-half reliability for measures derived from language samples of young handicapped children. *Language, Speech, and Hearing Services in Schools, 20,* 245–258.

Cole, K. N., Mills, P. E., & Kelley, D. (1994). Agreement of assessment profiles used in cognitive referencing.

Language, Speech, and Hearing Services in Schools, 25, 25–31.

Cole, L. (1989). E Pluribus Pluribus: Multicultural imperatives for the 1990s and beyond. *Asha, 31*(9), 65–70.

Cole, L. & Deal, V. R. (Eds.). (unpublished ms.). *Communication disorders in multicultural populations.* Rockville, MD: American Speech-Language-Hearing Association.

Coleman, M. (Ed.). (1976). *The autistic syndromes.* New York: American Elsevier.

Collins, W. A., Wellman, H., Keniston, A. H., & Westby, S. (1978). Age-related aspects of comprehension and inference from a televised dramatic narrative. *Child Development, 49,* 389–399.

Collins-Ahlgren, M. (1975). Language development of two deaf children. *American Annals of the Deaf, 120,* 524–539.

Committee on Amplification for the Hearing Impaired, American Speech-Language-Hearing Association. (1991). Amplification as a remediation technique for children with normal peripheral hearing. Supplement to the January 1991 *Asha, 33*(1), 22–24.

Committee on Language, American Speech-Language-Hearing Association. (1983, June). A definition of language. *Asha, 25*(6), 44.

Committee on Language, Speech, and Hearing Services in Schools, American Speech-Language-Hearing Association. (1982). Definitions: Communicative disorders and variations. *Asha, 24,* 949–950.

Connell, P. J. (1986a). Acquisition of semantic role by language-disordered children: Differences between production and comprehension. *Journal of Speech and Hearing Research, 29,* 366–374.

Connell, P. J. (1986b). Teaching subjecthood to language-disordered children. *Journal of Speech and Hearing Research, 29,* 481–492.

Connell, P. J. (1987). An effect of modelling and imitation teaching procedures on children with and without specific language impairment. *Journal of Speech and Hearing Research, 30,* 105–113.

Connell, P J.., & Myles-Zitzer, C. (1982). An analysis of elicited imitation as a language evaluation procedure. *Journal of Speech and Hearing Disorders, 47,* 390–396.

Conners, C. K. (1969). A teacher rating scale for use in drug studies with children. *American Journal of Psychiatry, 126,* 884–888.

Constable, C. M. (1987). Talking with teachers: Increasing our relevance as language interventionists in the schools. *Seminars in Speech and Language, 8*(4), 345–356.

Conti-Ramsden, G. (1990). Maternal recasts and other contingent replies to language-impaired children. *Journal of Speech and Hearing Disorders, 55,* 262–274.

Conti-Ramsden, G., & Friel-Patti, S. (1983). Mothers' discourse adjustments to language-impaired and non-language impaired children. *Journal of Speech and Hearing Disorders, 48,* 360–367.

Conti-Ramsden, G., Hutcheson, G. D., & Grove, J. (1995). Contingency and breakdown: Children with SLI and their conversations with mothers and fathers. *Journal of Speech and Hearing Research, 38,* 1290–1302.

Conti-Ramsden, G., North, T., & Ward, V. (1995). The number skills of children with specific language difficulties. *British Journal of Special Education, 22,* 81–88.

Cook-Gumperz, J. (1977). Situated instructions. In S. Ervin-Tripp & C. Mitchell-Kernan (Eds.), *Child discourse* (pp. 103–124). New York: Academic Press.

Cooper, C. R. (1976). Tonowanda Middle School's new writing program. *English Journal, 65,* 56–61.

Cooper, C. R. (1977). Holistic evaluation of writing. In C. R. Cooper & L. Odell (Eds.), *Evaluating writing: Describing, measuring, judging* (pp. 3–31). Urbana, IL: National Council of Teachers of English.

Cooper, C. R. & Odell, L. (Eds.). (1977). *Evaluating writing: Describing, measuring, judging.* Urbana, IL: National council of Teachers of English.

Cooper, D. C., & Anderson-Inman, L. (1988). Language and socialization. In M. A. Nippold (Ed.), *Later language development: Ages nine through nineteen* (pp. 225–245). Austin, TX: Pro-Ed.

Cooper, J. A., & Ferry, P. C. (1978). Acquired auditory verbal agnosia and seizures in childhood. *Journal of Speech and Hearing Disorders, 43,* 176–184.

Cooper, L. J., & Harding, J. (1993). Extending functional analysis procedures to outpatient and classroom settings for children with mild disabilities. In J. Reichle & D. P. Wacker (Eds.), *Communicative alternatives to challenging behavior: Integrating functional assessment and intervention strategies* (pp. 41–62). Baltimore: Paul H. Brookes.

Cooper, M. M. (1982). Context as vehicle: Implicature in writing. In M. Nystrand (Ed.), *What writers know: The language, process, and structure of written discourse* (pp. 106–129). New York: Academic Press.

Copeland, D. R., Fletcher, J. M., Pfefferbaum-Levine, B., Jaffe, N., Ried, H., & Maor, M. (1985). Neuropsychological sequelae of childhood cancer on long-term survivors. *Pediatrics, 75,* 745–753.

Cornett, R. (1967). Cued speech. *American Annals of the Deaf, 112,* 3–13.

Cornett, R. O. (1972). *Cued speech parent training and follow-up program.* Washington, DC: Bureau of Education for the Handicapped, DHEW.

Corrigan, R. (1978). Language development as related to stage six object permanence development. *Journal of Child Language, 5,* 173–190.

Costello, J. (1977). Programmed instruction. *Journal of Speech and Hearing Disorders, 42,* 3–28.

Courchesne, E. (1988). Hypoplasia of cerebellar vermal lobules VI and VII in autism. *New England Journal of Medicine, 318,* 1349–1354.

Cowley, J. (1988). *Dragon with a cold* (in the Sunshine Series). Bothell, WA: The Wright Group Publishers.

Cowley, H. (1990). *The jigaree* (in the Storybox Series). Bothell, WA: The Wright Group Publishers.

Crago, M. B. (1990). Development of communicative competence in Inuit children: Implications for speech-language pathology. *Journal of Childhood Communication Disorders, 13,* 73–83.

Crago, M. B., & Cole, E. (1991). Using ethnography to bring children's communicative and cultural worlds into focus. In T. M. Gallagher (Ed.), *Pragmatics of language: Clinical practice issues* (pp. 99–131). San Diego: Singular Publishing Group.

Craig, H. K. (1983). Application of pragmatic language models for intervention. In T. M. Gallagher & C. Prutting (Eds.), *Pragmatic assessment and intervention issues in language* (pp. 101–127). San Diego: College-Hill Press.

Craig, H. K. & Washington, J. A. (1995). African American English and linguistic complexity in reschool discourse: A second look. *Language, Speech, and Hearing Services in the Schools, 25,* 87–93.

Craik, F. I., & Lockhart, R. S. (1972). Levels of processing: A framework for memory research. *Journal of Verbal Learning and Verbal Behavior, 11,* 671–684.

Craik, K. (1943). *The nature of explanation.* Cambridge: Cambridge University Press.

Crain, S. (1994). Language acquisition in the absence of experience. In P. Bloom (Ed.), *Language acquisition* (pp. 364–409). Cambridge: The MIT Press. (Reprinted from *Behavioral and Brain Sciences, 14,* 1991).

Crais, E. R. (1990). World knowledge to word knowledge. World knowledge and language: Development and disorders. *Topics in Language Disorders, 10*(3), 45–62.

Crais, E. R. (1991). Moving from "parent involvement" to family-centered services. *American Journal of Speech-Language Pathology, 1* (1), 5–8.

Crais, E. R. (1995). Expanding the repertoire of tools and techniques for assessing the communication skills of infants and toddlers. *American Journal of Speech-Language Pathology, 4* (3), 47–59.

Crandell, C. C., Smaldino, J. J., & Flexer, C. (1995). *Soundfield FM amplification: Theory and practical applications.* San Diego: Singular Publishing Group.

Crary, M. A. (1984). A neurolinguistic perspective on developmental verbal dyspraxia. *Communicative Disorders, 9,* 33–48.

Crary, M. A. (1993). *Developmental motor speech disorders.* San Diego, CA: Singular Publishing Group.

Creaghead, N. A., & Tattershall, S. S. (1985). Observation and assessment of classroom pragmatic skills. In C. S. Simon (Ed.), *Communication skills and classroom success: Assessment of language-learning disabled students* (pp. 105–131). San Diego: College-Hill Press.

Cromer, R. F. (1981). Reconceptualizing language acquisition and cognitive development. In R. L. Schiefelbusch & D. Bricker (Eds.), *Early language: Acquisition and intervention* (pp. 51–138). Baltimore: University Park Press.

Cromer, R. F. (1991). The development of language and cognition: The cognition hypothesis. In R. F. Cromer, *Language and thought in normal and language handicapped children.* Cambridge, MA: Basil Blackwell. (Reprinted from B. Foss (Ed.) (1974). *New perspectives in child development* (pp. 184–252). Harmondsworth, Middx: Penguin.)

Cronin, M. E., & Patton, J. R. (1993). *Life skills instruction for all students with special needs.* Austin, TX: Pro-Ed.

Cross, T. G. (1984). Habilitating the language-impaired child: Ideas from studies of parent-child interaction. *Topics in Language Disorders, 4*(4), 1–14.

Crossley, R. (1992a). Getting the words out: Case studies in facilitated communication training. *Topics in Language Disorders, 12*(4), 46–49.

Crossley, R. (1992b). Lending a hand: A personal account of the development of facilitated communication training. *American Journal of Speech-Language Pathology, 1* (3), 15–18.

Crossley, R., & McDonald, A. (1984). *Annie's coming out.* New York: Viking Penguin.

Crouse, J. S. (1996). *Differences in the self-talk of students with language impairments when completing math computation and story problems.* Unpublished master's thesis, Western Michigan University, Kalamazoo, MI.

Crouse, J. S. & Nelson, N. W. (1996, November). *Self talk of students with language problems when completing math problems.* Poster session presented at the annual convention of the American Speech-Language Hearing Association, Seattle, WA.

Crowhurst, M. (1980). Syntactic complexity and teachers' quality ratings of narrations and arguments. *Research in the Teaching of English, 14,* 223–232.

Crystal, D. (1975). *The English tone of voice.* London: Edward Arnold.

Crystal, D. (1979). Prosodic development. In P. Fletcher & M. Garman (Eds.), *Language acquisition* (pp. 33–48). Cambridge: Cambridge University Press.

Crystal, D., Fletcher, P., & Garman, M. (1976). *The grammatical analysis of language disability.* London: Edward Arnold.

Cuda, R. A. (1976). *Analysis of speaking rate, syntactic complexity and speaking style of public school teachers.* Unpublished master's thesis, The Wichita State University, Wichita, KS.

Cuda, R., & Nelson, N. W. (1976, Nov.). *Analysis of teacher speaking rate, syntactic complexity, and hesitation phenomena as a function of grade level.* Paper presented at the Annual Conference of the American Speech-Language-Hearing Association, Houston, TX.

Culatta, B. (1994). Representational play and story enactments: Formats for language intervention. In J. F. Duchan, L. E. Hewitt, & R. M. Sonnenmeier (Eds.), *Pragmatics: From theory to practice* (pp. 105–119). Englewood Cliffs, NJ: Prentice Hall.

Culatta, B., Page, J. L., & Ellis, J. (1983). Story retelling as a communicative performance screening tool. *Language, Speech, and Hearing Services in Schools, 14,* 66–74.

Cullinan, B. E. (1989). Literature for young children. In D. S. Strickland & L. M. Morrow (Eds.), *Emerging literacy: Young children learn to read and write* (pp. 35–51). Newark, DE: International Reading Association.

Curtiss, S. (1977). *Genie: A linguistic study of a modern-day "wild child."* New York: Academic Press.

Curtiss, S. (1989). The independence and task-specificity of language. In A. Bornstein & J. Bruner (Eds.), *Interaction in human development.* Hillsdale, NJ: Erlbaum.

Curtiss, S., Fromkin, V., Krashen, S., Rigler, D., & Rigler, M. (1974). The linguistic development of Genie. *Language, 50,* 528–554.

Curtiss, S., Prutting, C. A., & Lowell, E. L. (1979). Pragmatic and semantic development in young children with impaired hearing. *Journal of Speech and Hearing Research, 22,* 534–552.

Dahlgren Sandberg, A., & Hjelmquist, E. (1996). Phonologic awareness and literacy abilities in nonspeaking preschool children with cerebral palsy. *Augmentative and Alternative communication, 12,* 138–153.

Dale, P. S. (1980). Is early pragmatic development measurable? *Journal of Child Language, 8,* 1–12.

Dalebout, S. D., Nelson, N. W., Hletko, P. J., & Frentheway, B. (1991). Selective auditory attention and children with attention-deficit hyperactivity disorder: Effects of repeated measurement with and without methylphenidate. *Language, Speech, and Hearing Services in Schools, 22,* 219–227.

Dalton, B. M., & Bedrosian, J. L. (1989). Communicative performance of adolescents with severe speech impairment: Influence of context. *Journal of Speech and Hearing Disorders, 54,* 403–421.

Damico, J. S. (1985/1991). Clinical discourse analysis: A functional approach to language assessment. In C. S. Simon (Ed.), *Communication skills and classroom success: Assessment of language-learning disabled students* (pp. 165–203). San Diego, CA: College-Hill. Reprinted in C. S. Simon (Ed.). (1991), *Communication skills and classroom success: Assessment and therapy methodologies for language and learning disabled students* (pp. 125–148). Eau Claire, WI: Thinking Publications.

Damico, J. S. (1987). Addressing language concerns in the schools: The SLP as consultant. *Journal of Childhood Communication Disorders, 11,* 17–40.

Damico, J. S. (1988). The lack of efficacy in language therapy: A case study. *Language, Speech, and Hearing Services in Schools, 19,* 51–66.

Damico, J., & Oller, J. W., Jr. (1980). Pragmatic versus morphological/syntactic criteria for language referrals. *Language, Speech, and Hearing Services in Schools, 11,* 85–94.

Damico, J. S., Oller, J. W., Jr., & Storey, M. E. (1983). The diagnosis of language disorders in bilingual children: Surface-oriented and pragmatic criteria. *Journal of Speech and Hearing Disorders, 48,* 385–394.

Davey, B. (1983). Think aloud: Modeling the cognitive process of reading comprehension. *Journal of Reading, 37,* 104–112.

Davis, G. Z. (1990). Skiing beyond the edge. *Perspectives on Dyslexia, 16*(1), 4.

Davis, J. M., Elfenbein, J., Schum, R., & Bentler, R. A. (1986). Effects of mild and moderate hearing impairments on language, educational, and psychosocial behavior of children. *Journal of Speech and Hearing Disorders, 51,* 53–62.

Davis, K. (1947). Final note on a case of extreme isolation. *American Journal of Sociology, 52,* 432–437.

Davis, W. E. (1989). The Regular Education Initiative debate: Its promises and problems. *Exceptional Children, 55,* 440–446.

Davis, W. E. (1990). Broad perspectives on the Regular Education Initiative: Response to Byrnes. *Exceptional Children, 56,* 349–356.

Deal, V. R., & Rodriguez, V. L. (1987). *Resource guide to multicultural tests and materials in communicative disorders.* Rockville, MD: American Speech-Language-Hearing Association.

DeMyer, M. K. (1975). Research in infantile autism: A strategy and its results. *Biological Psychiatry, 10,* 433–450.

DeMyer, M. K., Barton, S., DeMyer, W. E., Norton, J. A., Allen, J., & Steele, R. (1973). Prognosis in autism: A follow-up study. *Journal of Autism and Childhood Schizophrenia, 3,* 199–246.

DeMyer, M. K., Hingtgen, J. N., & Jackson, R. K. (1981). Infantile autism reviewed: A decade of research. *Schizophrenia Bulletin, 7,* 388–451.

Denckla, M. B. (1972). Clinical syndromes in learning disabilities: The case for "splitting" vs. "lumping." *Journal of Learning Disabilities, 5,* 401–406.

Denckla, M. B., & Rudel, R. G. (1976a). Naming of object drawings by dyslexic and other learning disabled children. *Brain and Language, 3,* 1–15.

Denckla, M. B., & Rudel, R. (1976b). Rapid "automatized" naming (RAN): Dyslexia differentiated from other learning disabilities. *Neuropsychologia, 14,* 471–478.

Denckla, M., Rudel, R., & Broman, M. (1981). Test that discriminate between dyslexic and other learning-disabled boys. *Brain and Language, 13,* 118–129.

Denham, C., & Lieberman, A. (Eds.). (1980). *Time to learn.* Washington, DC: National Institute of Education.

Deno, S. L. (1989). Curriculum-based measurement and special education services: A fundamental and direct relationship. In M. R. Shinn (Ed.), *Curriculum-based measurement: Assessing special children* (pp. 1–17). New York: Guilford Press.

Deshler, D. D., Alley, G. R., & Carlson, S. C. (1980). Learning strategies: An approach to mainstreaming secondary students with learning disabilities. *Education Unlimited, 2,* 6–11.

Deshler, D. D., Lowrey, N., & Alley, G. R. (1979). Programming alternatives for LD adolescents. *Academic Therapy, 14,* 389–397.

Despain, A. D., & Simon, C. S. (1987). Alternative to failure: A junior high school language development-based curriculum. *Journal of Childhood Communication Disorders, 11,* 139–179.

Deutch, M. (1949). An experimental study of the effects of cooperation and competition upon group process. *Human Relations, 2,* 199–232.

Deutsch, F. (1983). *Child services: On behalf of children.* Monterey, CA: Brooks/Cole.

De Villiers, J., & De Villiers, P. (1973). A cross-sectional study of the development of grammatical morphemes in child speech. *Journal of Psycholinguistic Research, 2,* 267–268.

Dietrich, K. N., Starr, R. H., & Kaplan, M. G. (1980). Maternal stimulation and care of abused infants. In T. M. Field, S. Goldberg, D. Stern, & A. M. Sostek (Eds.), *High-risk infants and children.* New York: Academic Press.

Dillard, J. L. (1972). *Black English: Its history and usage in the United States.* New York: Random House.

Dobie, R. A., & Berlin, C. I. (1979). Influence of otitis media on hearing and development. *Annals of Otology, Rhinology, and Laryngology, 88*(Suppl. 60), 48–53.

Dodd, B. (1976). The phonological systems of deaf children. *Journal of Speech and Hearing Disorders, 41,* 185–198.

Dollaghan, C. A. (1985). Child meets words: "Fast mapping" in preschool children. *Journal of Speech and Hearing Research, 28,* 449–454.

Dollaghan, C. A. (1987a). Fast mapping in normal and language impaired children. *Journal of Speech and Hearing Disorders, 52,* 218–222.

Dollaghan, C. A. (1987b). Comprehension monitoring in normal and language-impaired children. *Topics in Language Disorders, 7*(2), 45–60.

Dollaghan, C. A., Campbell, T. F., & Tomlin, R. (1990). Video narration as a language sampling context. *Journal of Speech and Hearing Disorders, 55,* 582–590.

Dollaghan, C., & Kaston, N. (1986). A comprehension monitoring program for language-impaired children. *Journal of Speech and Hearing Disorders, 51,* 264–271.

Dollaghan, C., & Miller, J. (1986). Observational methods in the study of communicative competence. In R. L. Schiefelbusch (Ed.), *Language competence: Assessment and intervention* (pp. 99–129). Austin, TX: Pro-Ed.

Donahue, M., & Bryan, T. (1984). Communicative skills and peer relations of learning disabled adolescents. *Topics in Language Disorders, 4*(2), 10–21.

Donahue, M. L., & Pearl, R. (1995). Conversational interactions of mothers and their preschool children who had been born preterm. *Journal of Speech and Hearing Research, 38,* 1117–1125.

Donahue, M., Pearl, R., Bryan, T. (1983). Communicative competence in learning disabled children. In K. D. Gadow & I. Bialer (Eds.), *Advances in learning and behavior disabilities* (Vol. 2, pp. 49–84). Greenwich, CT: JAI Press.

Donnellan, A. M., Mirenda, P. L., Mesaros, R. A., & Fassbender, L. L. (1984). Analyzing the communicative functions of aberrant behavior. *JASH* (Journal of the Association for Persons with Severe Handicaps), *9,* 202–212.

Donnelly, J. (1991, Summer). Jean Paul keeps on going. *The Advocate, Newsletter of the Autism Society of America, 23*(2), 14–15.

Dore, J. (1974). A pragmatic description of early language development. *Journal of Psycholinguistic Research, 4,* 343–350.

Dore, J. (1975). Holophrases, speech acts, and language universals. *Journal of Child Language, 2,* 21–40.

Dore, J. (1986). The development of conversational competence. In R. L. Schiefelbusch (Ed.), Language competence: Assessment and intervention (pp. 3–60). San Diego, CA: College-Hill (now Austin, TX: Pro-Ed).

Dorman, C. (1987). Reading disability subtypes in neurologically impaired students. *Annals of Dyslexia, 37,* 166–188.

Doss, L. S., & Reichle, J. (1991). Using graphic organization aids to promote independent functioning. In J. Reichle, J. York, & J. Sigafoos (Eds.), *Implementing augmentative and alternative communication* (pp. 275–288). Baltimore, MD: Paul H. Brookes.

Downing, J. E. (1996). *Including students with severe and multiple disabilities in typical classrooms.* Baltimore: Paul H. Brookes.

Drew, N. (1987). *Learning the skills of peacemaking.* Rolling Hills Estates, CA: Jalmar Press.

Dublinske, S. (1974). Planning for child change in language development/remediation programs carried out by teachers and parents. *Language, Speech, and Hearing Services in Schools, 5,* 225–237.

DuBose, R., Langley, M., & Stass, V. (1977). Assessing severely handicapped children. *Focus on Exceptional Children, 9,* 1–13.

Duchan, J. F. (1983). Language processing and geodesic domes. In T. M. Gallagher & C. Prutting (Eds.), *Pragmatic assessment and intervention issues in language* (pp. 83–99). San Diego: College-Hill.

Duchan, J. F. (1984). Clinical interactions with autistic children: The role of theory. *Topics in Language Disorders, 4*(4), 62–71.

Duchan, J. F. (1986). Language intervention through sense-making and fine tuning. In R. L. Schiefelbusch (Ed.), *Language competence: Assessment and intervention* (pp. 187–212). Austin, TX: Pro-Ed.

Duchan, J. F. (1993). Issues raised by facilitated communication for theorizing and research on autism. *Journal of Speech and Hearing Research, 36,* 1108–1119.

Duchan, J. F. (1995a). *Supporting language learning in everyday life.* San Diego, CA: Singular Publishing Group.

Duchan, J. F. (1995b). The role of experimental research in validating facilitated communication: A reply. *Journal of Speech and Hearing Research, 36,* 206–210.

Duchan, J. F. (1997). A situated pragmatics approach for supporting children with severe communication disorders. *Topics in Language Disorders, 17*(2), 1–18.

Duchan, J. F., Hewitt, L. E., & Sonnenmeier, R. M. (1994). Three themes: Stage two pragmatics, combating marginalization, and the relation of theory and practice. In J. F. Duchan, L. E. Hewitt, & R. M. Sonnenmeier (Eds.), *Pragmatics: From theory to practice* (pp. 1–9). Englewood Cliffs, NJ: Prentice Hall.

Duchan, J. F., & Katz, J. (1983). Language and auditory processing: Top down plus bottom up. In E. Z. Lasky & J. Katz (Eds.), *Central auditory processing disorders: Problems of speech, language, and learning* (pp. 31–45). Baltimore: University Park Press.

Duffy, F., & Geschwind, N. (1985). *Dyslexia: A neuroscientific approach to clinical evaluation.* Boston Little, Brown.

Dunlea, A. (1989). *Vision and the emergence of meaning: Blind and sighted children's early language.* New York: Cambridge University Press.

Dunn, C., & Newton, L. (1986). A comprehensive model for speech development in hearing-impaired children. *Topics in Language Disorders, 6*(3), 25–46.

Dunn, L. M., & Dunn, L. M. (1981). *Peabody Picture Vocabulary Test-Revised.* Circle Pines, MN: American Guidance Services.

Dunn, S. L., van Kleeck, A., & Rosetti, L. M. (1993). Current roles and continuing needs of speech-language pathologists working in neonatal intensive care units. *American Journal of Speech-Language Pathology, 2*(2), 52–64.

Dunst, C., & Lowe, L. (1986). From reflex to symbol: Describing, explaining, and fostering communicative competence. *Augmentative and Alternative Communication, 2,* 11–18.

Dunst, C., Lowe, L., & Bartholomew, P. (1990). Contingent social responsiveness, family ecology and infant communicative competence. *National Student Speech, Language, and Hearing Association Journal, 17,* 39–49.

Durgy, S. (1986). *Figuring out figurative language* [Computer program]. Fairfield, CT: Intellectual Software.

Edgar, E. (1987). Secondary programs in special education: Are many of them justifiable? *Exceptional Children, 53,* 555–561.

Edmonston, N. K., & Thane, N. L. (1992). Children's use of comprehension strategies in response to relational words: Implications for assessment. *American Journal of Speech-Language Pathology, 1*(2), 30–35.

Edwards, D. (1974). Sensory-motor intelligence and semantic relations in early child grammar. *Cognition, 2,* 395–434.

Egeland, B., & Sroufe, A. (1981). Developmental sequelae of maltreatment in infancy. *New Directions for Child Development, 11,* 77–92.

Ehren, B. J. (1994). New directions for meeting the academic needs of adolescents with language learning disabilities. In G. P. Wallach & K. G. Butler (Eds.), *Language learning disabilities in school-age children and adolescents* (pp. 393–417). Boston: Allyn and Bacon.

Ehren, B. J., & Lenz, B. K. (1989). Adolescents with language disorders: Special considerations in providing academically relevant language intervention. *Seminars in Speech and Language, 3,* 193–204.

Ehri, L. (1975). Word consciousness in readers and pre-readers. *Journal of Educational Psychology, 67,* 2–4, 212.

Ehri, L. C. (1989). The development of spelling knowledge and its role in reading acquisition and reading disability. *Journal of Learning Disabilities, 22,* 356–364.

Eichenger, J. (1990). Goal structure effects on social interaction: Nondisabled and disabled elementary students. *Exceptional Children, 56,* 408–416.

Eimas, P. D. (1975). Developmental studies in speech perception. In L. B. Cohen & P. Salapatek (Eds.), *Infant perception: From sensation to cognition* (Vol. 2, pp. 193–231). New York: Academic Press.

Eisenson, J. (1968). Developmental aphasia: A speculative view with therapeutic implications. *Journal of Speech and Hearing Disorders, 33,* 3–13.

Eisenson, J. (1972). *Aphasia in children.* New York: Harper & Row.

Elder, J. L., & Pederson, D. R. (1978). Preschool children's use of objects in symbolic play. *Child Development, 49,* 500–504.

Elksnin, L. K., & Capilouto, G. J. (1994). Speech-language pathologists' perceptions of integrated service delivery in school settings. *Language, Speech, and Hearing Services in the Schools, 25,* 258–267.

Elliott, L. L., Hammer, M. A., & Scholl, M. E. (1989). Fine-grained auditory discrimination in normal children and children with language-learning problems. *Journal of Speech and Hearing Research, 32,* 112–119.

Emig, J. (1971). *The composing processes of twelfth graders* (Research Report No. 13). Urbana, IL: National Council of Teachers of English.

Emig, J. (1977). Writing as a mode of learning. *College composition and communication, 28,* 122–127.

Englemann, S., & Osborn, J. (1976). *DISTAR language 1: An instructional system.* Chicago, IL: Science Research Associates.

Englert, C. S., & Mariage, T. V. (1991). Making students partners in the comprehension process: Organizing the reading "POSSE." *Learning Disability Quarterly, 14,* 123–138.

Englert, C. S., & Raphael, T. E. (1988). Constructing well-formed prose: Process, structure, and metacognitive knowledge. *Exceptional Children, 54,* 513–527.

Ensher, G. L. (1989). The first three years: Special education perspectives on assessment and intervention. *Topics in Language Disorders, 10*(1), 80–90.

Entus, A. K. (1977). Hemispheric asymmetry in processing of dichotically presented speech and nonspeech stimuli by infants. In S. Segalowitz & F. Gruber (Eds.), *Language development and neurological theory.* New York: Academic Press.

Entwisle, D. R., Forsyth, D. F., & Muuss, R. (1964). The syntagmatic-paradigmatic shift in children's word associations. *Journal of Verbal Learning and Verbal Behavior, 3,* 19–29.

Epstein, H. T. (1974). Phrenoblysis: Special brain and mind growth. II. Human mental development. *Developmental Psychobiology, 7,* 217–224.

Epstein, H. T. (1978). Growth spurts during brain development: Implications for educational policy and practice. In J. S. Chall & A. F. Mirsky (Eds.), *Education and brain yearbook of the N. S. S. E.* Chicago, IL: University of Chicago Press.

Erickson, F. (1977). Some approaches to inquiry in school-community ethnography. *Anthropology and Education Quarterly, 8*(2), 58–69.

Erickson, F., & Schultz, J. (1981). When is a context? Some issues and methods in the analysis of social competence. In J. Green & C. Wallat (Eds.), *Ethnography and language in educational settings* (pp. 147–160). Norwood, NJ: Ablex.

Erickson, J. G. (1981). Communication assessment of the bilingual bicultural child: An overview. In J. G. Erickson & D. R. Omark (Eds.), *Communication assessment of the bilingual bicultural child* (pp. 1–24). Austin, TX: Pro-Ed.

Erickson, J. G., & Omark, D. R. (Eds.). (1981). *Communication assessment of the bilingual bicultural child.* Austin, TX: Pro-Ed.

Erickson, K. A. & Koppenhaver, D. A. (1995). Developing a literacy program for children with severe disabilities. *The Reading Teacher, 48,* 676–684.

Erin, J. N. (1990). Language samples from visually impaired four- and five-year olds. *Journal of Childhood Communication Disorders, 13,* 181–191.

Ervin-Tripp, S., & Gordon, D. (1986). The development of requests. In R. L. Schiefelbusch (Ed.), *Language competence: Assessment and intervention* (pp. 61–95). Austin, TX: Pro-Ed.

Ervin-Tripp, S., & Mitchell-Kernan, C. (1977). Introduction. In S. Ervin Tripp & C. Mitchell-Kernan (Eds.), *Child discourse* (pp. 1–23). New York: Academic Press.

Esterreicher, C. (1986). *Figuring out figurative language* [Computer program]. San Antonio, TX: Communication Skill Builders.

Ewing-Cobbs, L., Fletcher, J. M., & Levin, H. S. (1985). In M. Ylvisaker (Ed.), *Head injury rehabilitation: Children and adolescents* (pp. 71–89). Austin, TX: Pro-Ed.

Ezell, H. K., & Goldstein, H. (1989). Effects of imitation on language comprehension and transfer to production in children with mental retardation. *Journal of Speech and Hearing Disorders, 54,* 49–56.

Ezell, H. K., & Goldstein, H. (1991). Comparison of idiom comprehension of normal children and children with mental retardation. *Journal of Speech and Hearing Research, 34,* 812–819.

Falvey, M. A., Bishop, K. B., Grenot-Scheyer, M., & Coots, J. (1988). Issues and trends in mental retardation. In S. N. Calculator & J. L. Bedrosian (Eds.), *Communication assessment and intervention for adults with mental retardation* (pp. 265–307). Austin, TX: Pro-Ed.

Falvey, M. A., Forest, M., Pearpoint, J., & Rosenberg, R. L. (1994). Building connections. In J. S. Thousand, R. A. Villan, & A. I. Nevin (Eds.), *Creativity and collaborative learning: A practical guide for empowering students and teachers* (pp. 347–368). Baltimore, MD: Paul H. Brookes.

Fasold, R. W., & Wolfram, W. (1970). Some linguistic features of Negro dialect. In R. W. Fasold & R. W. Shuy (Eds.), *Teaching standard English in the inner city* (pp. 41–86). Washington, DC: Center for Applied Linguistics.

Fawcett, R. P., & Perkins, M. R. (1980). *Child language transcripts 6–12* (Vols. 1–4). Pontypridd, Mid Galmorgan, Wales: Department of Behavioural and Communicative Studies, Polytechnic of Wales.

Fay, W. H. (1973). On the echolalia of the blind and the autistic child. *Journal of Speech and Hearing Disorders, 38,* 478–489.

Fay, W. (1979). Personal pronouns and the autistic child. *Journal of Autism and Developmental Disorders, 9,* 247–260.

Fay, W. H., & Schuler, A. L. (1980). *Emerging language in autistic children.* Baltimore, MD: University Park Press.

Fazio, B. B. (1994). The counting abilities of children with specific language impairment: A comparison of oral and gestural tasks. *Journal of Speech and Hearing Research, 37,* 358–368.

Fazio, B. B. (1996). Mathematical abilities of children with specific language impairment: A 2-year follow-up. *Journal of Speech and Hearing Research, 39,* 839–849.

Fein, D. (1983). The prevalence of speech and language impairments. *Asha, 25*(2), 37.

Fein, G. (1975). A transformational analysis of pretending. *Developmental Psychology, 11,* 291–296.

Fenson, L., Dale, P., Reznick, S., Thal, D., Bates, E., Hartung, J., Pethick, S., & Reilly, J. (1993). *MacArthur Communicative Development Inventories.* San Diego: Singular Publishing Group.

Fernald, A. (1989). Intonation and communicative intent in mothers' speech to infants: Is the melody the message? *Child Development, 60,* 1497–1510.

Ferry, P. C. (1981). In R. W. Keith (Ed.), *Central auditory and language disorders in children* (pp. 1–10). San Diego: College-Hill.

Feuerstein, R. (1979). *The dynamic assessment of retarded performers.* Austin, TX: Pro-Ed.

Feuerstein, R., Rand, Y., & Rynders, J. E. (1988). *Don't accept me as I am: Helping "retarded" people to excel.* New York: Plenum Press.

Fey, M. E. (1986). *Language intervention with young children.* San Diego: College-Hill (now available from Pro-Ed, Austin, TX).

Fey, M. E., Cleave, P. L., Long, S. H., & Hughes, D. L. (1993). Two approaches to the facilitation of grammar in children with language impairment: An experimental evaluation. *Journal of Speech and Hearing Research, 36,* 141–157.

Fey, M. E., Cleave, P. L., Ravida, A. I., Long, S. H., Dejmal, A. E., & Easton, D. L. (1994). Effects of grammar facilitation on the phonological performance of children with speech and language impairments. *Journal of Speech and Hearing Research, 37,* 594–607.

Fey, M. E., & Leonard, L. B. (1984). Partner age as a variable in the conversational performance of specifically language-impaired and normal-language children. *Journal of Speech and Hearing Research, 27,* 413–423.

Fey, M. E., Long, S. H., & Cleave, P. L. (1994). Reconsideration of IQ criteria in the definition of specific language impairment. In R. V. Watkins & M. L. Rice (Eds.), *Specific language impairments in children.* Baltimore: Paul H. Brookes.

Field, T. (1979). Interaction patterns of preterm and term infants. In T. Field, A. M. Sostek, S. Goldberg, & H. Shuman (Eds.), *Infants born at risk: Behavior and development.* New York: Spectrum Publications.

Fillmore, C. (1968). The case for case. In E. Bach & R. Harmas (Eds.), *Universals in linguistic theory.* New York: Holt, Rinehart, & Winston.

Fischler, R., Todd, N., & Feldman, C. (1985). Otitis media and language performance in a cohort of Apache Indian children. *American Journal of Diseases of Children, 139,* 355–360.

Fitzgerald, J. (1989). Research on stories: Implications for teachers. In K. D. Muth (Ed.), *Children's comprehension of text* (pp. 2–36). Newark, DE: International Reading Association.

Fletcher, P. (1979). The development of the verb phrase. In P. Fletcher & M. Garman (Eds.), *Language acquisition* (pp. 261–284). New York: Cambridge University Press.

Flexer, C. (1989). Turn on sound: An odyssey of sound field amplification. *Educational Audiology Association Newsletter, 5,* 6.

Flexer, C. (1994). *Facilitating hearing and listening in young children.* San Diego: Singular Publishing Group.

Flexer, C., Millin, J. P., & Brown, L. (1990). Children with developmental disabilities: The effect of sound field amplification on word identification. *Language, Speech, and Hearing Services in Schools, 21,* 177–182.

Flexer, C., Wray, D., & Ireland, J. (1989). Preferential seating is NOT enough: Issues in classroom management of hearing-impaired students. *Language, Speech, and Hearing Services in Schools, 20,* 11–21.

Flood, J., & Salus, M. W. (1982). Metalinguistic awareness: Its role in language development and its assessment. *Topics in Language Disorders, 2*(4), 56–64.

Flower, L., & Hayes, J. (1980). The dynamics of composing, making plans, and juggling constraints. In L. W. Gregg & E. R. Steinberg (Eds.), *Cognitive processes in writing: An interdisciplinary approach.* Hillsdale, NJ: Erlbaum.

Flynn, G. J. (1990, February/March). Quality education: Community or custody. *Newsletter of the Michigan Society for Autistic Citizens,* pp. 1, 5–6.

Fodor, J. (1983). *The modularity of mind.* Cambridge, MA: MIT Press.

Ford, J., & Fredericks, B. (1995). Perceptions of inclusion by parents of children who are deaf-blind. In N. G. Haring & L. T. Romer (Eds.), *Welcoming students who are deaf-blind into typical classrooms* (pp. 37–53). Baltimore, MD: Paul H. Brookes.

Forrest-Pressley, D. L., & Waller, T. G. (1984). *Cognition, metacognition, and reading.* Cambridge, MA: MIT Press.

Foss, D. J., & Hakes, D. T. (1978). *Psycholinguistics: An introduction to the psychology of language.* Englewood Cliffs, NJ: Prentice-Hall.

Foster, R., Giddan, J., & Stark, J. (1973). *Assessment of children's language comprehension* (2nd ed.). Austin, TX: Learning Concepts.

Fox, C. L. (1980). *Communicating to make friends.* Rolling Hills Estates, CA: B. L. Winch & Associates.

Fox, C. L. (1989). Peer acceptance of learning disabled children in the regular classroom. *Exceptional Children, 56,* 50–59.

Fox, L., Long, S. H., & Langlois, A. (1988). Patterns of language comprehension deficit in abused and neglected children. *Journal of Speech and Hearing Disorders, 53,* 239–244.

Fraiberg, S. (1977). *Insights from the blind: Comparative studies of blind and sighted infants.* New York: Basic Books.

Fraiberg, S. (1979). Blind infants and their mothers: An examination of the sign system. *Before speech: The beginning of interpersonal communication* (pp. 149–169). New York: Cambridge University Press.

Fraiberg, S. (1982). Billy: Psychological intervention for a failure-to-thrive infant. In M. H. Klaus, T. Leger, & M. A. Trause (Eds.), *Maternal attachment and mothering disorders* (pp. 6–14). Skillman, NJ: Johnson & Johnson Baby Products Co.

Francis, D. J., Fletcher, J. M., Shaywitz, B. A., Shaywitz, S. E., & Rourke, B. P. (1996). Defining learning and language disabilities: Conceptual and psychometric issues with the use of IQ tests. *Language, Speech, and Hearing Services in Schools, 27,* 132–143.

Frankenburg, W. K., Dodds, J. B., & Fandal, A. W. (1969). *Denver Developmental Screening Test* (Manual revised, 1970). Denver: University of Colorado Medical Center.

Frankenberger, W., & Fronzaglio, K. (1991). A review of states' criteria for identifying children with learning disabilities. *Journal of Learning Disabilities, 24,* 495–500.

Frassinelli, L., Superior, K., & Meyers, J. (1983). A consultation model for speech and language intervention. *Asha, 25*(11), 25–30.

Frattali, C., & Lynch, C. (1989). Functional assessment: Current issues and future challenges. *Asha, 25* (11), 25–30.

Frey, W. (1984). Functional assessment in the '80s. In A. Halpern & M. Fuhrer (Eds.), *Functional assessment in rehabilitation* (pp. 11–43). Baltimore: Paul H. Brookes.

Fried-Oken, M. (1987). Terminology in augmentative communication. *Language, Speech, and Hearing Services in Schools, 18,* 188–190.

Fried-Oken, M., Paul, R., Fay, W. (1995). Questions concerning facilitated communication: Response to Duchan. *Journal of Speech and Hearing Research, 38,* 200–202.

Friedman, R. J. (1980). The young child who does not talk: Observations on causes and management. *Clinical Pediatrics, 3,* 403–406.

Friel-Patti, S. (1994). Auditory linguistic processing and language learning. In G. P. Wallach & K. G. Butler (Eds.), *Language learning disabilities in school-age children and adolescents* (pp. 373–392). Boston: Allyn and Bacon.

Frith, U. (1980). *Cognitive processes in spelling.* Orlando, FL: Academic Press.

Fry, E. B. (1968). A readability formula that saves time. *Journal of Reading, 11,* 513–516, 575–578.

Frymier, B., & Gansneder, B. (1989). The Phi Delta Kappa study of students at risk. *The Phi Delta Kappan, 71,* 142–147.

Fuchs, D., & Fuchs, L. S. (1994). Inclusive schools movement and the radicalization of special education reform. *Exceptional Children, 60,* 294–309.

Fujiki, M., & Brinton, B. (1984). Supplementing language therapy: Working with the classroom teacher. *Language, Speech, and Hearing Services in Schools, 15,* 98–109.

Fujiki, M., & Brinton, B. (1994). Social competence and language impairment in children. In R. V. Watkins & M. L. Rice (Eds.), *Specific language impairments in children* (pp. 123–143). Baltimore, MD: Paul H. Brookes.

Fundudis, T., Kolvin, I., & Garside, R. F. (1979). *Speech retarded and deaf children: Their psychological development.* London: Academic Press.

Furth, H. (1966). *Thinking without language: Psychological implications of deafness.* New York: Free Press.

Furuno, S., O'Reilly, A., Hosaka, C. M., Inatsuka, T. T., Allman, T. L., & Zeisloft, B. (1979). *The Hawaii early learning profile (HELP).* Palo Alto, CA: VORT.

Gagné, J-P., Stelmacovich, P., & Yovetich, W. (1991). Reactions to requests for clarification used by hearing-impaired individuals. *The Volta Review, 93,* 129–143.

Galaburda, A. M. (1989). Ordinary and extraordinary brain development: Anatomical variation in developmental dyslexia. *Annals of Dyslexia, 39,* 67–80.

Galaburda, A. M., Corsiglia, J., Rosen, G. D., & Sherman, G. F. (1987). Planum temporale asymmetry: Reappraisal since Geschwind and Levitsky. *Neuropsychologia, 25,* 853–868.

Galaburda, A. M., & Kemper, T. L. (1979). Cytoarchitectonic abnormalities in developmental dyslexia: A case study. *Annals of Neurology, 6,* 94–100.

Gallagher, T. M. (1991). Language and social skills: Implications for assessment and intervention with school-age children. In T. M. Gallagher (Ed.), *Pragmatics of language: Clinical practice issues* (pp. 11–41). San Diego: Singular Publishing Group.

Gallagher, T. M., & Craig, H. K. (1984). Pragmatic assessment: Analysis of a highly frequent repeated utterance. *Journal of Speech and Hearing Disorders, 49,* 368–377.

Gallagher, T. M., & Prutting, C. (Eds.). (1983). *Pragmatic assessment and intervention issues in language.* San Diego: College-Hill.

Garbarino, J., & Crouter, A. (1978). Defining the community context of parent-child relations: The correlates of child maltreatment. *Child Development, 49,* 604–606.

Garcia, S. B., & Ortiz, A. A. (1988, June). Preventing inappropriate referrals of language minority students to special education. *New Focus (No. 5), Occasional Papers in Bilingual Education.* Wheaton, MD: The National Clearinghouse for Bilingual Education.

Gardner, H. (1983). *Frames of mind: The theory of multiple intelligences.* New York: Basic Books.

Garnett, K. (1986). Telling tales: Narratives and learning-disabled children. *Topics in Language Disorders, 6*(2), 44–56.

Gates, A. L., & McGinitie, W. E. (1972). *Gates McGinitie Reading Tests.* New York: Columbia University Teacher's College Press.

Gathercole, S. E., & Baddeley, A. D. (1990). Phonological memory deficits in language disordered children: Is there a connection? *Journal of Memory and Language, 29,* 336–360.

Gathercole, S. E., & Baddeley, A. D. (1995). Short-term memory may yet be deficient in children with language impairments: A comment on van der Lely & Howard (1993). *Journal of Speech and Hearing Research, 38,* 463–466.

Gaylord-Ross, R., Haring, T., Breen, C., & Pitts-Conway, V. (1984). The training and generalization of social interaction skills with autistic youth. *Journal of Applied Behavior Analysis, 17,* 229–247.

Gebers, J. L. (1990). *Books are for talking too!* San Antonio, TX: Communication Skill Builders.

Gee, K. (1995). Facilitating active and informed participation and learning in inclusive settings. In N. G. Haring & L. T. Romer (Eds.). *Welcoming students who are deaf-blind into typical classrooms* (pp. 369–404). Baltimore, MD: Paul H. Brookes.

Geers, A. E., & Moog, J. S. (1987). Predicting spoken language acquisition of profoundly hearing-impaired children. *Journal of Speech and Hearing Disorders, 52,* 84–94.

Geers, A., & Moog, J. (1989). Factors predictive of the development of literacy in profoundly hearing-impaired adolescents. *The Volta Review, 91,* 69–86.

Geers, A. E., & Schick, B. (1988). Acquisition of spoken and signed English by hearing-impaired children of hearing-impaired or hearing parents. *Journal of Speech and Hearing Disorders, 53,* 136–143.

Gerber, M. M., & Levine-Donnerstein, D. (1989). Educating all children: Ten years later. *Exceptional Children, 56,* 17–27.

Gerber, S. E. (1990). *Prevention: The etiology of communicative disorders in children.* Englewood Cliffs, NJ: Prentice Hall.

Gerhardt, J. (1989). Monologue as a speech genre. In K. Nelson (Ed.), *Narratives from the crib* (pp. 171–230). Cambridge, MA: Harvard University Press.

German, D. J. (1979). Word finding skills in children with learning disabilities. *Journal of Learning Disabilities, 12*(3), 43–48.

German, D. J. (1982). Word-finding substitutions in children with learning disabilities. *Language, Speech, and Hearing Services in Schools, 13,* 223–230.

German, D. J. (1983). I know it but I can't think of it: Word retrieval difficulties. *Academic Therapy, 18,* 539–545.

German, D. J. (1989). Revised manual for the *Test of Word Finding.* Allen, TX: DLM.

German, D. J. (1990). *Test of Adolescent/Adult Word Finding* (TAWF). Chicago, IL: Riverside.

German, D. J., (1991). *Test of Word Finding in Discourse.* Allen, TX: DLM.

German, D. J. (1992). Word-finding intervention for children and adolescents. *Topics in Language Disorders, 13*(1), 33–50.

German, D. J. (1993). *Word finding intervention program.* Austin, TX: Pro-Ed.

German, D. J. (1994). Word finding difficulties in children and adolescents. In G. P. Wallach & K. G. Butler (Eds.), *Language learning disabilities in school-age children and adolescents* (pp. 323–347). Boston: Allyn and Bacon.

Geschwind, N. (1984). The brain of a learning disabled individual. *Annals of Dyslexia, 34,* 319–327.

Geschwind, N., & Levitsky, W. (1968). Human brain: Left-right asymmetries in temporal speech region. *Science, 161,* 186–187.

Giangreco, M., Cloninger, C., & Iverson, V. (1993). *Choosing options and accommodations for children (COACH): A guide for planning inclusive education.* Baltimore: Paul H. Brookes.

Gibbs, R. W., Jr. (1991). Semantic analyzability in children's understanding of idioms. *Journal of Speech and Hearing Research, 34,* 613–620.

Gillam, R. B., Cowan, N., & Day, L. S. (1995). Sequential memory in children with and without language impairment. *Journal of Speech and Hearing Research, 38,* 393–402.

Gillam, R., McFadden, T. U., & van Kleeck, A. (1995). Improving narrative abilities: Whole language and language skills approaches. In M. E. Fey, J. Windsor, & S. F. Warren (Eds.), *Language intervention: Preschool through the elementary years* (pp. 145–182). Baltimore, MD: Paul H. Brookes.

Gillespie, S., & Cooper, E. (1973). Prevalence of speech problems in junior and senior high schools. *Journal of Speech and Hearing Research, 16*(4), 739–743.

Gillette, Y. (Ed.). (1992). *CATCH guide to planning services with families: Coordinated transitions from the hospital to the community and home.* San Antonio, TX: Communication Skill Builders.

Girolametto, L., & Tannock, R. (1994). Correlates of directiveness in the interactions of fathers and mothers of children with developmental delays. *Journal of Speech and Hearing Research, 37,* 1178–1192.

Gittelman-Klein, R., & Klein, D. (1976). Methylphenidate effects in learning disabilities. *Archives of General Psychiatry, 33,* 655–664.

Gittelman-Klein, R., Klein, D., Abikoff, H., Katz, S., Gloisten, A., & Kates, W. (1976). Relative efficacy of methylphenidate and behavior modification in hyperkinetic children: An interim report. *Journal of Abnormal Child Psychology, 4,* 361–379.

Glanville, B., Best, C., & Levenson, R. (1977). A cardiac measure of cerebral asymmetries in infant auditory perception. *Developmental Psychology, 13,* 54–59.

Gleitman, L. R., & Gleitman, H. (1981). Language. In H. Gleitman (Ed.), *Psychology* (pp. 353–411). New York: W. W. Norton.

Gleitman, L. R., Gleitman, H., Landau, B., & Wanner, E. (1988). Where learning begins: Initial representations for language learning. In F. Newmeyer (Ed.), *Linguistics: The Cambridge survey III. Language: Psychological and biological aspects* (pp. 150–193). Cambridge: Cambridge University Press.

Gleitman, L. R., Gleitman, H., & Shipley, E. F. (1972). The emergence of the child as grammarian. *Cognition, 1,* 137–164.

Gleitman, L. R., & Wanner, E. (1982). Language acquisition: The state of the art. In E. Wanner & L. Gleitman (Eds.), *Language acquisition: The state of the art.* Cambridge: Cambridge University Press.

Glover, M. E., Preminger, J. L., & Sanford, A. R. (1978). *The early learning accomplishment profile.* Winston-Salem, NC: Kaplan.

Golan, L. (1996). Dialogue of the Deaf: What Gallaudet won't teach. *Volta Voices* (news magazine of A. G. Bell Association for the Deaf), *3*(3), 3,5.

Goldgar, D., & Osberger, M. J. (1986). Factors related to academic achievement. In M. J. Osberger (Ed.), *Language and learning skills of hearing-impaired students* (pp. 87–91). *ASHA Monographs No. 23.* Rockville, MD: American Speech-Language-Hearing Association.

Goldin-Meadow, S., & Feldman, H. (1977). The development of language-like communication without a language model. *Science, 197,* 401–403.

Goldman-Rakic, P. S. (1981). Development and plasticity of primate frontal association cortex. In F. O. Schmidt, F. G. Worden, G. Adelman, & S. G. Dennis (Eds.), *The organization of the cerebral cortex. Proceedings of a neurosciences research program colloquium.* Cambridge, MA: MIT Press.

Goldstein, H. (1985). Enhancing language generalization using matrix and stimulus equivalence training. In S. Warren & A. Rogers-Warren (Eds.), *Teaching functional language* (pp. 225–249). Austin, TX: Pro-Ed.

Goldstein, H., & Kaczmarek, L. (1992). Promoting communicative interaction among children in integrated intervention settings. In S. F. Warren & J. Reichle (Eds.), *Causes and effects in communication and language intervention* (pp. 81–111). Baltimore, MD: Paul H. Brookes.

Goldstein, K. (1948). *Language and language disorders.* New York: Grune & Stratton.

Golin, A. K., & Ducanis, A. J. (1985). *The interdisciplinary team: A handbook for the education of exceptional children.* Rockville, MD: Aspen.

Golinkoff, R., Hirsh-Pasek, K., Cauley, K., & Gordon, L. (1987). The eyes have it: Lexical and syntactic comprehension in a new paradigm. *Journal of Child Language, 14,* 23–45.

Goodglass, H. (1981). The syndromes of aphasia: Similarities and differences in neurolinguistic features. *Topics in Language Disorders, 1*(4), 1–14.

Goodglass, H., & Kaplan, E. (1983). *The assessment of aphasia and related disorders* (2nd ed.) (Manual for *The Boston diagnostic aphasia examination* (BDAE)). Philadelphia: Lea & Febiger.

Goodman, K. S. (1969). Analysis of oral reading miscues: Applied psycholinguistics. *Reading Research Quarterly, 5*(1), 9–30.

Goodman, K. S. (1973a). Analysis of oral reading miscues: Applied psycholinguistics. In F. Smith (Ed.), *Psycholinguistics and reading* (pp. 158–176). New York: Holt, Rinehart, & Winston.

Goodman, K. S. (1973b). Psycholinguistic universals in the reading process. In F. Smith (Ed.), *Psycholinguistics and reading* (pp. 21–27). New York: Holt, Rinehart, & Winston.

Goodman, K. S. (1986). *What's whole in whole language?* Portsmouth, NH: Heinemann.

Goodman, Y. M., Watson, D. J., & Burke, C. L. (1987). *Reading miscue inventory: Alternative procedures.* New York: Richard C. Owen Publishers.

Gopnik, M. (1990). Feature blindness: A case study. *Language Acquisition: A Journal of Developmental Linguistics, 1,* 139–164.

Gopnik, M., & Crago, M. (1991). Familial aggregation of a developmental language disorder. *Cognition, 39,* 1–50.

Gordon, C. J., & Braun, C. (1983). Using story schema as an aid to reading and writing. *The Reading Teacher, 37,* 116–121.

Gough, P. B. (1972). One second of reading. In J. F. Kavanagh, & I. G. Mattingly (Eds.), *Language by ear and by eye: The relationships between speech and reading* (pp. 331–358). Cambridge: The MIT Press.

Gravel, J. S., & Wallace, I. (1995). Early otitis media, auditory abilities, and educational risk. *American Journal of Speech-Language Pathology, 4*(3), 89–94.

Graves, D. (1978). *Balance the basics: Let them write.* New York: Ford Foundation.

Graves, D. (1983). *Writing: Teachers and children at work.* Portsmouth, NH: Heinemann.

Gray, B., & Ryan, B. (1973). *A language program for the nonlanguage child.* Champaign, IL: Research Press.

Green, J. L., & Wallat, C. (1981). *Ethnography and language in educational settings.* Norwood, NJ: Ablex.

Greenfield, P. M., & Smith, J. H. (1976). *The structure of communication in early language development.* New York: Academic Press.

Greenspan, S. (1985). *First feelings: Milestones in the emotional development of your baby and child.* New York: Viking Penguin.

Greenspan, S. (1988). Fostering emotional and social development in infants with disabilities. *Zero to Three, 8,* 8–18.

Greenspan, S. I., Wieder, S., Nover, R. A., Lieberman, A. F., Lourie, R. S., & Robinson, M. E. (Eds.). (1987). *Infants in multirisk families.* Madison, WI: International Universities Press.

Gregory, M., & Carroll, S. (1978). *Language and situation: Language varieties and their social contexts.* London: Routledge and Kegan Paul.

Grice, H. P. (1975). Logic and conversation. In P. Cole & J. L. Morgan (Eds.), *Syntax and semantics 3: Speech acts* (pp. 41–58). New York: Academic Press.

Griffin, K., & Hannah, L. (1960). A study of the results of an extremely short instructional unit in listening. *Journal of Communication, 10,* 135–139.

Griffith, P. L., & Olson, M. W. (1992). Phonemic awareness helps beginning readers break the code. *The Reading Teacher, 45,* 516–523.

Grossman, H. (Ed.). (1983). *Classification in mental retardation.* Washington, DC: American Association on Mental Deficiency.

Gualtieri, C. T., Koriath, U., Van Bourgondien, M., & Saleeby, N. (1983). Language disorders in children referred for psychiatric services. *Journal of the American Academy of Child Psychiatry, 22,* 165–171.

Guess, D. (1989). Preface. In E. Siegel-Causey & D. Guess (Eds.), *Enhancing nonsymbolic communication interac-*

tions among learners with severe disabilities (pp. *xi-xii*). Baltimore: Paul H. Brookes.

Guess, D., & Baer, D. (1973). An analysis of individual differences in generalization between receptive and productive language in retarded children. *Journal of Applied Behavior Analysis, 6,* 311–329.

Guess, D., Benson, H., & Siegel-Causey, E. (1985). Concepts and issues related to choice making and autonomy among persons with severe disabilities. *Journal of the Association for Persons with Severe Handicaps, 10*(2), 79–86.

Guess, D., Sailor, W., & Baer, D. (1974). To teach language to retarded children. In R. Schiefelbusch & L. L. Lloyd (Eds.), *Language perspectives: Acquisition, retardation, and intervention.* Baltimore, MD: University Park Press.

Guess, D., Sailor, W., & Baer, D. (1978). Children with limited language. In R. Schiefelbusch (Ed.), *Language intervention strategies* (pp. 101–143). Baltimore, MD: University Park Press.

Guilford, J. P. (1967). *The nature of human intelligence.* New York: McGraw-Hill.

Guralnick, M. J., & Paul-Brown, D. (1977). The nature of verbal interactions among handicapped and nonhandicapped preschool children. *Child Development, 48,* 254–260.

Hack, M., Klein, N. K., & Taylor, H. G. (1995). Long-term developmental outcomes of low birth weight infants. In R. E. Bahrman (Ed.), *The future of children: Low birth-weight* (Vol. 5(1), pp. 176–196). Los Altos, CA: David and Lucile Packard Foundation.

Hagans, G. (1985). *Regions near and far.* Lexington, MA: D. C. Heath and Company.

Hagen, J. W., Barclay, C. R., & Schwethelm, B. (1982). In N. Ellis (Ed.), *International review of research in mental retardation* (pp. 1–4). New York: Academic Press.

Haley, K. L., Camarata, S. M., & Nelson, K. E. (1994). Social valence in children with specific language impairment during imitation-based and conversation-based language intervention. *Journal of Speech and Hearing Research, 37,* 378–388.

Hall, P. K., Jordan, L. S., & Robin, D. A. (1993). *Developmental apraxia of speech.* Austin, TX: Pro-Ed.

Hall, P. K., & Tomblin, J. B. (1978). A follow-up study of children with articulation and language disorders. *Journal of Speech and Hearing Disorders, 43,* 227–241.

Halliday, M. A. K. (1975). *Learning how to mean: Explorations in the development of language.* London: Edward Arnold.

Halliday, M. A. K., & Hasan, R. (1976). *Cohesion in English.* London: Longman.

Hamilton, B. L., & Snell, M. E. (1993). Using the milieu approach to increase spontaneous communication book use across environments by an adolescent with autism. *Augmentative and Alternative Communication, 9,* 259–272.

Hammill, D. D., & Larsen, S. C. (1974). The effectiveness of psycholinguistic training. *Exceptional Children, 40,* 5–14.

Hanline, M. F., & Halvorsen, A. (1989). Parent perceptions of the integration transition process: Overcoming artificial barriers. *Exceptional Children, 55,* 487–493.

Harber, J. (1980). Issues in the assessment of language and reading disorders in learning disabled children. *Learning Disability Quarterly, 3* (4), 20–28.

Haring, N. G., & Romer, L. T. (Eds.). (1995). *Welcoming students who are deaf-blind into typical classrooms.* Baltimore, MD: Paul H. Brookes.

Harris, A. J. (1983). How many kinds of reading disability are there? *Annual Review of Learning Disabilities, 1,* 50–56.

Harris, D. (1982). Communicative interaction processes involving nonvocal physically handicapped children. *Topics in Language Disorders, 2*(2), 21–37.

Harris, G. A. (1985). Considerations in assessing English language performance of Native American children. *Topics in Language Disorders, 5*(4), 42–52.

Harris, K. R., & Graham, S. (1996a). Constructivism and students with special needs: Issues in the classroom. *Learning Disabilities Research and Practice, 11,* 134–137.

Harris, K. R., & Graham, S. (1996b). *Making the writing process work: Strategies for composition and self-regulation.* Cambridge, MA: Brookline Books.

Harris, K. R., & Pressley, M. (1991). The nature of cognitive strategy instruction: Interactive strategy instruction. *Exceptional Children, 57,* 392–404.

Hart, B. (1985). Naturalistic language training techniques. In S. F. Warren & A. K. Rogers-Warren (Eds). *Teaching functional language* (pp. 63–88). Baltimore: University Park Press.

Hart, B., & Risley, T. R. (1968). Establishing the use of descriptive adjectives in the spontaneous speech of disadvantaged preschool children. *Journal of Applied Behavioral Analysis, 1,* 109–120.

Hart, B., & Risley, T. R. (1975). Incidental teaching of language in the preschool. *Journal of Applied Behavioral Analysis, 8,* 411–420.

Hart, B., & Risley, T. R. (1980). In vivo language training: Unanticipated and general effects. *Journal of Applied Behavioral Analysis, 12,* 407–432.

Hart, B., & Risley, T. R. (1986). Incidental strategies. In R. L. Schiefelbusch (Ed.), *Language competence: Assessment and intervention.* San Diego: College-Hill.

Hart, B., & Rogers-Warren, A. (1978). Milieu approach to teaching language. In R. L. Schiefelbusch (Ed.), *Language intervention strategies.* Baltimore, MD: University Park Press.

Hart, C. (1989). *Without reason: A family copes with two generations of autism.* New York: Harper & Row.

Hart, P. J. (1983). Classroom acoustical environments for children with central auditory processing disorders. In E. Z. Lasky & J. Katz (Eds.), *Central auditory processing disorders: Problems of speech, language, and learning* (pp. 343–352). Austin, TX: Pro-Ed.

Hart, V. (1977). The use of many disciplines with the severely and profoundly handicapped. In E. Sontag & N. Certo (Eds.), *Educational programming for the severely and profoundly handicapped.* Reston, VA: Division on Mental Retardation, Council for Exceptional Children.

Hartup, W. (1983). Peer interaction and the behavioral development of the individual child. In W. Damon (Ed.), *Social personality development: Essays on the growth of the child.* New York: W. W. Norton.

Hartwig, L. J. (1984). Living with dyslexia: One parent's experience. *Annals of Dyslexia, 34,* 313–318.

Hartzell, H. E. (1984). The challenge of adolescence. *Topics in Language Disorders, 4*(2), 1–9.

Hayden, T. L. (1980). The classification of elective mutism. *Journal of the American Academy of Child Psychology, 19,* 118–133.

Hayes, C. W., & Bahruth, R. (1985). Querer Es Poder. In J. T. Hansen, T. Newkirk, & D. Graves (Eds.), *Breaking ground: Teachers relate reading and writing in the elementary school.* Portsmouth, NH: Heinemann.

Hayes, J. R., & Flower, L. S. (1980). Identifying the organization of writing processes. In L. Gregg & E. Steinberg (Eds.), *Cognitive processes in writing* (pp. 3–30). Hillsdale, NJ: Erlbaum.

Hayes, J. R., & Flower, L. S. (1987). On the structure of the writing process. *Topics in Language Disorders, 7*(4), 19–30.

Haywood, H. C., Towery-Woolsey, J., Arbitman-Smith, R. & Aldridge, A. (1988). Cognitive education with deaf adolescents: Effects of instrumental enrichment. *Topics in Language Disorders, 8*(4), 23–40.

Hazel, J., Schumaker, J., Sherman, J., & Sheldon-Wildgen, J. (1981). *ASSET: A social skills program for adolescents.* Champaign, IL: Research Press.

Heath, S. B. (1982). What no bedtime story means: Narrative skills at home and school. *Language in Society, 11,* 49–76.

Heath, S. B. (1983). *Ways with words: Language, life and work in communities and classrooms.* New York: Cambridge University Press.

Heath, S. B. (1984, November). *Cross cultural acquisition of language.* Paper presented at the annual conference of the American Speech-Language-Hearing Association, San Francisco, CA.

Heath, S. B. (1986). Taking a cross-cultural look at narratives. *Topics in Language Disorders, 7*(1), 84–94.

Hecaen, H. (1976). Acquired aphasia in children and the ontogenesis of hemispheric functional specialization. *Brain and Language, 3,* 114–134.

Hecaen, H. (1983). Acquired aphasia in children: Revisited. *Neuropsychologia, 21,* 581–587.

Hedberg, N. L., & Westby, C. E. (1993). *Analyzing storytelling skills: Theory to practice.* Tucson, AZ: Communication Skill Builders.

Hedrick, D., Prather, E., & Tobin, A. (1984). *Sequenced inventory of communication development* (rev. ed.). Seattle, WA: University of Washington Press.

Heimlich, J. E., & Pittelman, S. D. (1986). *Semantic mapping: Classroom applications.* Newark, DE: International Reading Association.

Hermelin, B., & O'Connor, N. (1967). Remembering of words by psychotic and subnormal children. *British Journal of Psychology, 58,* 213–218.

Hermelin, B., & O'Connor, N. (1970). *Psychological experiments with autistic children.* Oxford: Pergamon.

Hess, L. J., & Fairchild, J. L. (1988). Model, analyse, practise (MAP): A language therapy model for learning-disabled adolescents. *Child Language Teaching and Therapy, 4,* 325–338.

Hewitt, L. E. (1994). Narrative comprehension: The importance of subjectivity. In J. F. Duchan, L. E. Hewitt, & R. M. Sonnenmeier (Eds.), *Pragmatics: From theory to practice* (pp. 88–104). Englewood Cliffs, NJ: Prentice Hall.

Hier, D., LeMay, M., Rosenberger, P., et al. (1978). Developmental dyslexia. *Archives of Neurology, 35,* 90–92.

Hier, D., & Rosenberger, P. (1980). Focal left temporal lobe lesions and delayed speech acquisition. *Developmental and behavioral pediatrics, 1,* 54–57.

Higginbotham, D. J., & Yoder, D. E. (1982). Communication within natural conversational interaction: Implications for severe communicatively impaired persons. *Topics in Language Disorders, 2*(2), 1–19.

Hill, B. P., & Singer, L. T. (1990). Speech and language development after infant tracheostomy. *Journal of Speech and Hearing Disorders, 55,* 15–20.

Hillocks, G., Jr. (1986). *Research on written composition.* Urbana, IL: ERIC Clearinghouse on Reading and Communication Skills.

Hobson, R. P. (1993). *Autism and the development of mind.* U. K.: Hove.

Hodson, B. W. (1994). Helping individuals become intelligible, literate, and articulate: The role of phonology. *Topics in Language Disorders, 14*(2), 1–16.

Hodson, B., & Paden, E. (1990). *Targeting intelligible speech: A phonological approach to remediation.* (2nd ed.). San Antonio, TX: Pro-Ed.

Hoffman, L. P. (1990). The development of literacy in a school-based program. *Topics in Language Disorders, 10* (2), 81–94.

Hoffman, P. R. (1990). Spelling, phonology, and the speech-language pathologist: A whole language perspective. *Language, Speech, and Hearing Services in Schools, 21,* 238–243.

Hohmann, M., Banet, B., & Weikert, D. P. (1979). *Young children in action: A manual for preschool educators.* Ypsilanti, MI: High/Scope Press.

Holden, M. H., & MacGinitie, W. H. (1972). Children's conceptions of word boundaries in speech and print. *Journal of Educational Psychology, 63,* 551–557.

Hood, L., & Bloom, L. (1979). What, when, and how about why: A longitudinal study of early expressions of causality. *Monographs of the Society for Research in Child Development, 44.*

Horgan, D. (1979). *Nouns: Love 'em or leave 'em.* Address to the New York Academy of Sciences, New York.

Horn, J. L. (1968). Organization of abilities and the development of intelligence. *Psychological Review, 75,* 242–259.

Hoskins, B. (1987). *Conversations: Language intervention for adolescents.* Allen, TX: DLM Teaching Resources.

Hoskins, B. (1990). Language and literacy: Participating in the conversation. *Topics in Language Disorders, 10*(2), 46–62.

Hoskins, B. (1997). What is classroom-based instruction? In N. W. Nelson & B. Hoskins (Eds.). *Strategies for supporting classroom success: Focus on communication* (30 minute segment of an audioworkshop). San Diego: Singular Publishing Group.

House, T. D., & House, L. I. (1989, November). *Pragmatic deficits in visually impaired children.* Paper presented at the annual conference of the American Speech-Language-Hearing Association, St. Louis, MO.

Howes, C. (1985). Sharing fantasy: Social pretend play in toddlers. *Child Development, 56,* 1253–1258.

Hresko, W. P., Reid, D. K., & Hammill, D. D. (1981). *The test of early language development* (TELD). Austin, TX: Pro-Ed.

Hresko, W. P., Reid, D. K., & Hammill, D. D. (1991). *Test of early language development,* 2nd ed. (TELD-2). Austin, TX: Pro-Ed.

Hubbell, R. (1981). Children's language disorders: An integrated approach. Englewood Cliffs, NJ: Prentice Hall.

Hubbell, R. D. (1988). *A handbook of English grammar and language sampling.* Englewood Cliffs, NJ: Prentice Hall.

Hughes, D. L. (1985). *Language treatment and generalization.* San Diego: College-Hill.

Hughes, D. L. (1989). *Seminars 1989, 10*(3), 218–230.

Hughes, D. L., & Carpenter, R. (1983, November). *Effects of two grammar treatment programs on target generalization to spontaneous language.* Paper presented at the Annual Conference of the American Speech-Language-Hearing Association, Cincinnati, OH.

Huisingh, R., Barrett, M., Zachman, L., Blagden, C., & Orman, J. (1990). *Word Test-R: Elementary.* Moline, IL: LinguiSystems.

Humphrey, N. (1984). *Consciousness regained.* Oxford, England: Oxford University Press.

Hunt, K. W. (1965). *Grammatical structures written at three grade levels.* Urbana, IL: National Council of Teachers of English.

Hunt, K. W. (1970). Syntactic maturity in school children and adults. *Monographs of the Society for Research in Child Development,* No. 134.

Hunt, K. W. (1977). Early blooming and late blooming syntactic structures. In C. R. Cooper & L. Odell (Eds.), *Evaluating writing: Describing, measuring, judging* (pp. 91–106). Urbana, IL: National Council of Teachers of English.

Hutchinson, D. (1974). *A model for transdisciplinary staff development* (technical report developed as part of the National Collaborative Infant Project). New York: United Cerebral Palsy Association of America.

Hutchinson, T. A. (1996). What to look for in the technical manual: Twenty questions for users. *Language, Speech, and Hearing Services in Schools, 27,* 109–121.

Huttenlocher, J. (1974). The origins of language comprehension. In R. Solso (Ed.), *Theories in cognitive psychology: The Loyola symposium* (pp. 331–368). New York: John Wiley & Sons.

Hutter, J. J. (1986). Late effects in children with cancer [letter to the editor]. *American Journal of Diseases of Children, 140,* 17–18.

Hyman, C. A., Parr, R., & Browne, K. (1979). An observational study of mother-infant interaction in abusing families. *Child Abuse and Neglect, 3,* 241–246.

Hymes, D. (1972). On communicative competence. In J. B. Pride & J. Holmes (Eds.), *Sociolinguistics.* Harmondsworth, England: Penguin.

Hynd, G. W., Marshall, R., & Gonzalez, J. (1991). Learning disabilities and presumed central nervous system dysfunction. *Learning Disability Quarterly, 14,* 283–296.

Hyter, Y. (1984). *Reliability and validity of the Black English Sentence Scoring system.* Unpublished master's thesis, Western Michigan University, Kalamazoo.

Idol, L., Nevin, A., & Paolucci-Whitcomb, P. (1986). *Models of curriculum-based assessment.* Rockville, MD: Aspen Publishers.

Idol, L., Paolucci-Whitcomb, P., & Nevin, A. (1986). *Collaborative consultation.* Rockville, MD: Aspen Publishers.

Iglesias, A. (1985). Communication in the home and classroom: Match or mismatch? *Topics in Language Disorders, 5*(4), 29–41.

Iglesias, A. (1989). My dream. *Asha, 31*(9), 75.

Ingram, D. (1974). The relationship between comprehension and production. In R. Schiefelbusch & L. Lloyd (Eds.), *Language perspectives—Acquisition, retardation, and intervention* (pp. 313–364). Baltimore, MD: University Park Press.

Ingram, D. (1976). *Phonological disability in children.* New York: American Elsevier.

Ingram, D. (1986). Foreword. In J. R. Muma, *Language Acquisition: A functionalist perspective* (pp. xi-xiii). Austin, TX: Pro-Ed.

Irwin, J. W. (1988). Linguistic cohesion and the developing reader/writer. *Topics in Language Disorders, 8*(3), 14–23.

Isaacson, S. (1985). Assessing written language skills. In C. S. Simon (Ed.), *Communication skills and classroom success: Assessment of language-learning disabled students* (pp. 403–425). San Diego: College-Hill. Reprinted in C. S. Simon (Ed.). (1991), *Communication skills and classroom success: Assessment and therapy methodologies for language and learning disabled students* (pp. 224–237). Eau Claire, WI: Thinking Publications.

Jakobson, R. (1968). *Child language, aphasia and phonological universals.* The Hague: Mouton.

Jakobson, R., & Halle, M. (1956). *Fundamentals of language.* The Hague: Mouton.

Jaffe, M. B. (1989). Feeding at-risk infants and toddlers. *Topics in Language Disorders, 10*(1), 13–25.

Jagiello, G. M., Fang, J-S., Ducayen, M. B., & Sung, W. K. (1987). Etiology of human trisomy 21. In S. M. Pueschel, C. Tingey, J. E. Rynders, A. C. Crocker, & D. M. Crutcher (Eds.), *New perspectives on Down syndrome* (pp. 23–38). Baltimore: Paul H. Brookes.

James, S. (1989). Assessing children with language disorders. In D. K. Bernstein & E. Tiegerman (Eds.), *Language and communication disorders in children* (pp. 157–207). Columbus, OH: Merrill.

Jenkins, J. R., & Heinen, A. (1989). Students' preferences for service delivery: Pull-out, in-class, or integrated models. *Exceptional Children, 55,* 516–523.

Jenkins, J. R., Odom, S. L., & Speltz, M. L. (1989). Effects of social integration of preschool children with handicaps. *Exceptional Children, 55,* 420–428.

Jenkins, J. R., Speltz, M. L., & Odom, S. L. (1985). Integrating normal and handicapped preschoolers: Effects on child development and social interaction. *Exceptional Children, 52,* 7–17.

Johnson, C. (1985). The emergence of present perfect verb forms: Semantic influences on selective imitation. *Journal of Child Language, 12,* 325–352.

Johnson, C. J. (1995). Expanding norms for narration. *Language, Speech, and Hearing Services in Schools, 26,* 326–341.

Johnson, D. J. (1985). Using reading and writing to improve oral language skills. *Topics in Language Disorders, 3*(3), 55–69.

Johnson, D. J., & Myklebust, H. (1967). *Learning disabilities: Educational principles and practices.* New York: Grune & Stratton.

Johnson, D. W. (1989, September). *Cooperative learning in postsecondary education.* Paper presented at a workshop, Western Michigan University, Kalamazoo.

Johnson, D. W., & Johnson, R. (1975). *Learning together and alone.* Englewood Cliffs, NJ: Prentice Hall.

Johnson, D. W., & Johnson, R. T. (1990). Social skills for successful group work. *Educational Leadership, 47*(4), 29–33.

Johnson, D. W., Johnson, R. T., & Holubec, E. (1988). *Cooperation in the classroom* (rev. ed.). Edina, MN: Interaction Book Company.

Johnson, N. S., & Mandler, J. M. (1980). A tale of two structures: Underlying and surface forms in stories. *Poetics, 9,* 51–86.

Johnson, W., Darley, F. L., & Spriesterbach, D. (1952). *Diagnostic methods in speech correction.* New York: Harper & Row.

Johnson-Laird, P. N. (1983). *Mental models: Towards a cognitive science of language, inference, and consciousness.* Cambridge, MA: Harvard University Press.

Johnson-Martin, N., Jens, K. G., & Attermeier, S. M. (1986). *The Carolina curriculum for handicapped infants and infants at risk.* Baltimore, MD: Paul H. Brookes.

Johnston, J. R. (1982a). Interpreting the Leiter IQ: Performance profiles of young normal and language-disordered children. *Journal of Speech and Hearing Research, 25,* 291–296.

Johnston, J. R. (1982b). Narratives: A new look at communication problems in older language-disordered children.

Language, Speech, and Hearing Services in Schools, 13, 144–155.

Johnston, J. R. (1985). The discourse symptoms of developmental disorders. In T. A. Van Dijk (Ed.), *Handbook of discourse analysis, Vol. 3: Discourse and dialogue* (pp. 79–93). Orlando, FL: Academic Press.

Johnston, J. R. (1991). Questions about cognition in children with specific language impairment. In J. Miller (Ed.), *Research on child language disorders* (pp. 299–307). Austin, TX: Pro-Ed.

Johnston, J. R. (1994). Cognitive abilities of children with language impairment. In R. V. Watkins & M. L. Rice (Eds.), *Specific language impairments in children* (pp. 107–121). Baltimore, MD: Paul H. Brookes.

Johnston, J., & Kamhi, A. (1984). Syntactic and semantic aspects of the utterances of language impaired children: Can same be less? *Merrill-Palmer Quarterly, 30,* 65–85.

Jordan, F. M., Murdoch, B. E., & Buttsworth, D. L. (1991). Closed-head-injured children's performance on narrative tasks. *Journal of Speech and Hearing Disorders, 34,* 572–582.

Jordan, L. S. (1980). Receptive and expressive language problems occurring in combination with a seizure disorder: A case report. *Journal of Communication Disorders, 13,* 295–303.

Jorgensen, C. M. (1994a). Developing individualized inclusive educational programs. In S. N. Calculator & C. M. Jorgensen (Eds.), *Including students with severe disabilities in schools: Fostering communication, interaction, and participation* (pp. 27–74). San Diego, CA: Singular Publishing Group.

Jorgensen, C. M. (1994b). Modifying the curriculum and short-term objectives to foster inclusion. In S. N. Calculator & C. M. Jorgensen (Eds.), *Including students with severe disabilities in schools: Fostering communication, interaction, and participation* (pp. 75–111). San Diego, CA: Singular Publishing Group.

Just, M. A., & Carpenter, P. A. (1987). *The psychology of reading and language comprehension.* Boston: Allyn and Bacon.

Kagan, J. (1989). The young child at risk. In B. A. Stewart (Ed.), *Partnerships in education: Toward a literate America* (pp. 8–17). *ASHA Reports 17.* Rockville, MD: American Speech-Language-Hearing Association.

Kagan, S. (1990). The structural approach to cooperative learning. *Educational Leadership, 47*(4), 12–15.

Kail, R., & Leonard, L. B. (1986). Word-finding abilities in language-impaired children. *ASHA Monographs Number 25.* Rockville, MD: American Speech-Language-Hearing Association.

Kaiser, A. P. (1993). Introduction: Enhancing children's social communication. In A. P. Kaiser & D. B. Gray (Eds.), *Enhancing children's communication: Research foundations for intervention* (pp. 1–9). Baltimore: Paul H. Brookes.

Kaiser, A. P., Alpert, C. L., & Warren, S. L. (1987). Teaching functional language: Strategies for intervention. In M. E. Snell (Ed.), *Systematic instruction for persons with severe handicaps* (pp. 247–272). Columbus, OH: Merrill.

Kaiser, A. P., & Hester, P. P. (1994). Generalized effects of enhanced milieu teaching. *Journal of Speech and Hearing Research, 37,* 1320–1340.

Kaiser, A. P., & Warren, S. F. (1988). Pragmatics and generalization. In R. L. Schiefelbusch & L. L. Lloyd (Eds.), *Language perspectives II.* Austin, TX: Pro-Ed.

Karlsen, B., & Gardner, E. F. (1984). *Stanford diagnostic reading test* (SDRT) (3rd ed.). San Antonio, TX: The Psychological Corporation.

Kamhi, A. G. (1981). Developmental vs. different theories of mental retardation: A new look. *American Journal of Mental Deficiency, 86,* 1–7.

Kamhi, A. G. (1982). The effect of self-initiated and other-initiated actions on linguistic performance. *Journal of Speech and Hearing Research, 25,* 177–183.

Kamhi, A. G. (1990, June). Unpublished discussion at the 11th Symposium for Research on Child Language Disorders, The University of Wisconsin, Madison.

Kamhi, A. G. (1993). Some problems with the marriage between theory and clinical practice. *Language, Speech, and Hearing Services in Schools, 24,* 57–60.

Kamhi, A. G. (1996). Linguistic and cognitive aspects of specific language impairment. In M. D. Smith & J. S. Damico (Eds.), *Childhood language disorders* (pp. 97–116). New York: Thieme Medical Publishers.

Kamhi, A. G., & Catts, H. (1986). Toward an understanding of developmental language and reading disorders. *Journal of Speech and Hearing Disorders, 51,* 337–347.

Kamhi, A. G., & Catts, H. W. (1989). *Reading disabilities: A developmental language perspective.* Austin, TX: Pro-Ed.

Kamhi, A. G., Catts, H., Mauer, D., Apel, K., & Gentry, B. F. (1988). Phonological and spatial processing abilities in language- and reading-impaired children. *Journal of Speech and Hearing Disorders, 53,* 316–327.

Kamhi, A. G., Gentry, B., Mauer, D., & Gholson, B. (1990). Analogical learning and transfer in language-impaired children. *Journal of Speech and Hearing Disorders, 55,* 140–148.

Kamhi, A. G., & Lee, R. F. (1988). Cognition. In M. A. Nippold (Ed.), *Later language development: Ages 9 through 19* (pp. 127–158). Austin, TX: Pro-Ed.

Kamhi, A. G., Minor, J. S., & Mauer, D. (1990). Content analysis and intratest performance profiles on the Columbia and the TONI. *Journal of Speech and Hearing Research, 33,* 375–379.

Kamhi, A. G., Pollock, K. E., & Harris, J. L. (Eds.). (1996). *Communication development and disorders in African American children.* Baltimore: Paul H. Brookes.

Kandel, E. R. (1977). Neuronal plasticity and the modification of behavior. In E. R. Kandel (Ed.), *Cellular biology of neurons, Vol. 1: The nervous system* (pp. 1137–1182). Amsterdam: Elsevier.

Kanner, L. (1943). Autistic disturbance of affective contact. *Nervous Child, 2,* 217–250.

Kanter, R. M. (1983). *The change masters: Innovation and entrepreneurship in the American corporation.* New York: Simon & Schuster.

Kaplan, G. K., Fleshman, J. K., Bender, T. R., et al. (1973). Long-term effects of otitis media: A 10-year cohort study of Alaska Eskimo children. *Pediatrics, 52,* 577–585.

Kaplan, E., & Goodglass, H. (1981). Aphasia-related disorders. In M. T. Sarno (Ed.), *Acquired aphasia* (pp. 303–325). New York: Academic Press.

Karmiloff-Smith, A. (1993). Innate constraints and developmental change. In P. Bloom (Ed.), *Language acquisition* (pp. 563–590). Cambridge: The MIT Press.

Kaufman, A. S., & Kaufman, N. L. (1983). *Kaufman Assessment Battery for Children* (K-ABC). Circle Pines, MN: American Guidance Service.

Kaufman, S. Z. (1988). *Retarded isn't stupid, Mom!* Baltimore: Paul H. Brookes.

Kawakami, A. J., & Au, K. H. (1986). Encouraging reading and language development in cultural minority children. *Topics in Language Disorders, 6*(2), 71–80.

Kayser, H. (1989). Speech and language assessment of Spanish-English speaking children. *Language, Speech, and Hearing Services in Schools, 20,* 226–244.

Keeler, W. R. (1958). Autistic patterns and defective communication in blind children with retrolental fibroplasia. In P. H. Hoch & J. Subin (Eds.), *Psychopathology of communication.* New York: Grune & Stratton.

Keith, R. W. (1977). (Ed.), *Central auditory dysfunction.* New York: Grune & Stratton.

Keith, R. W. (1981). (Ed.), *Central auditory and language disorders in children.* San Diego: College Hill.

Keith, R. W. (1986). Screening test for auditory processing disorders (SCAN). San Antonio, TX: The Psychological Corporation.

Kekelis, L. S., & Anderson, E. S. (1984). Family communication styles and language development. *Journal of Visual Impairment and Blindness, 78,* 54–65.

Kelford-Smith, A., Thurston, S., Light, J., Parnes, P., & O'Keefe, B. (1989). The form and use of written communication produced by physically disabled individuals using microcomputers. *Augmentative and Alternative Communication, 5,* 115–124.

Kelly, C. A., & Dale, P. S. (1989). Cognitive skills associated with the onset of multiword utterances. *Journal of Speech and Hearing Research, 32,* 645–656.

Kendall, P. C., & Braswell, L. (1985). *Cognitive-behavioral therapy for impulsive children.* New York: Guilford Press.

Kent, L. (1974). *Language acquisition program for the severely retarded.* Champaign, IL: Research Press.

Kent, R., Osberger, M., Netsell, R., & Hustedde, C. (1987). Phonetic development in identical twins differing in auditory function. *Journal of Speech and Hearing Disorders, 52,* 64–75.

Kernan, K. (1977). Semantic and expressive elaborations in children's narratives. In S. Ervin-Tripp & C. Mitchell-Kernan (Eds.), *Child discourse* (pp. 91–102). New York: Academic Press.

King, D. F., & Goodman, K. S. (1990). Whole language: Cherishing learners and their language. *Language, Speech, and Hearing Services in Schools, 21,* 221–227.

King, R. R., Jones, C., & Lasky, E. (1982). In retrospect: A fifteen-year follow-up report of speech-language-disordered children. *Language, Speech, and Hearing Services in Schools, 13,* 24–32.

Kinney, P., Ouellette, T., & Wolery, M. (1989). Screening and assessing sensory functioning. In D. B. Bailey, Jr. & M. Wolery (Eds.), *Assessing infants and preschoolers with handicaps* (pp. 144–165). Columbus, OH: Merrill.

Kinsbourne, M. (1981). The development of cerebral dominance. In S. D. Filskov & T. J. Boll (Eds.), *Handbook of clinical neuropsychology.* New York: John Wiley & Sons.

Kirchner, D. M. (1991). Using verbal scaffolding to facilitate conversational participation and language acquisition in children with pervasive developmental disorders. *Journal of Childhood Communication Disorders, 14,* 81–98.

Kirk, S. A., McCarthy, J. J., & Kirk, W. D. (1968). *The Illinois Test of Psycholinguistic Abilities* (rev. ed.). Urbana, IL: University of Illinois Press.

Kirk, U. (1983). Introduction: Toward an understanding of the neuropsychology of language, reading, and spelling. In U. Kirk (Ed.), *Neuropsychology of language, reading, and spelling* (pp. 3–31). Orlando, FL: Academic Press.

Klecan-Aker, J. S. (1985). Syntactic abilities in normal and language deficient middle school children. *Topics in Language Disorders, 5*(3), 46–54.

Klecan-Aker, J. S., & Hedrick, L. D. (1985). A study of the syntactic language skills of normal school-age children. *Language, Speech, and Hearing Services in Schools, 16,* 187–198.

Klee, T., Schaffer, M., May, S., Membrino, I., & Mougey, K. (1989). A comparison of the age-MLU relation in normal and specifically language-impaired preschool children. *Journal of Speech and Hearing Disorders, 54,* 226–233.

Klein, J., Chase, C., Teele, D., Menyuk, P., & Rosner, B. (1988). Otitis media and the development of speech, language, and cognitive abilities at seven years of age. In D. Lim, C. Bluestone, J. Klein, & J. Nelson (Eds.), *Recent advances in otitis media* (pp. 396–400). Toronto: B. C. Decker, Inc.

Klein, M. D., & Briggs, M. H. (1987). Facilitating mother-infant communicative interaction in mothers and high-risk infants. *Journal of Communication Disorders, 10,* 95–106.

Klinger, L. G., & Dawson, G. (1992). Facilitating early social and communicative development in children with autism. In S. F. Warren & J. Reichle (Eds.), *Causes and effects in communication and language intervention* (pp. 157–186). Baltimore: Paul H. Brookes.

Knapczyk, D. (1991). Effects of modeling in promoting generalization of student question asking and question answering. *Learning Disabilities Research and Practice, 6,* 75–82.

Knapp, M. S., Turnbull, B. J., & Shields, P. M. (1990). New directions for educating the children of poverty. *Educational Leadership, 48*(1), 4–8.

Knobloch, H., Stevens, F., & Malone, A. F. (1980). *Manual of developmental diagnosis.* New York: Harper & Row.

Knoll, J. A., & Meyer, L. (1987). Integrated schooling and educational quality: Principles and effective practices. In M. S. Berres & P. Knoblock (Eds.), *Program models for mainstreaming: Integrating students with moderate to severe disabilities* (pp. 41–59). Rockville, MD: Aspen Publishers.

Kochanek, T. T., Kabacoff, R. I., & Lipsitt, L. P. (1990). Early identification of developmentally disabled and at-risk preschool children. *Exceptional Children, 56,* 528–538.

Koegel, R. L., & Traphagen, J. (1982). Selection of initial words for speech training with nonverbal children. In R. L. Koegel, A. Rincover, & A. L. Egel (Eds.), *Educating and understanding autistic children* (pp. 65–77). San Diego, CA: College-Hill Press.

Kolvin, T., & Fundudis, T. (1981). Elective mute children: Psychological development and background factors. *Journal of Child Psychology and Psychiatry, 22,* 219–232.

Koppenhaver, D. A., Coleman, P. P., Kalman, S. L., & Yoder, D. E. (1991). The implications of emergent literacy research for children with developmental disabilities. *American Journal of Speech-Language Pathology, 1,* 38–44.

Koppenhaver, D. A., Pierce, P. L., & Yoder, D. E. (1995). AAC, FC, and the ABCs: Issues and relationships. *American Journal of Speech-Language Pathology, 4*(4), 5–14.

Koppenhaver, D. A., & Yoder, D. E. (1988, October). *Literacy and the augmentative and alternative communication user.* Paper presented at the conference of the International Society for Augmentative and Alternative Communication. Annaheim, CA.

Koppenhaver, D. A., & Yoder, D. E. (1993). Classroom literacy instruction for children with severe speech and physical impairments (SSPI): What is and what might be. *Topics in Language Disorders, 13*(2), 1–15.

Kotulak, R. (1996, January 5). Games kids play improve speech skills. *Chicago Tribune,* pp. 1, 14.

Kovarsky, D., & Crago, M. (1991). Toward the ethnography of communication disorders. *Journal of the National Student Speech-Language-Hearing Association.*

Kramer, C., James, S., & Saxman, J. (1979). A comparison of language samples elicited at home and in the clinic. *Journal of Speech and Hearing Disorders, 44,* 321–330.

Kramer, J. H., Norman, D., Grant-Zawadzki, M., Albin, A., & Moore, I. (1988). Absence of white matter changes on magnetic resonance imaging in children treated with CNS prophylaxis therapy for leukemia. *Cancer, 61,* 928–930.

Krauss, M. W. (1990). New precedent in family policy: Individualized Family Service Plan. *Exceptional Children, 56,* 388–395.

Kuczaj, S., & Maratsos, M. (1975). What children *can* say before they *will. Merrill-Palmer Quarterly, 21,* 89–111.

Kuhl, P. (1992). Psychoacoustics and speech perception: Internal standards, perceptual anchors, and prototypes. In L. A. Werner & E. Rubel (Eds.), *Developmental psychoacoustics.* Washington, DC: American Psychological Association.

LaBerge, D., & Samuels, S. J. (1987). Toward a theory of automatic information processing in reading. In H. Singer & R. B. Ruddell (Eds.), *Theoretical models and processes of reading* (3rd ed.) (pp. 689–718). Newark, DE: International Reading Association.

Labov, W. (1966). *The social stratification of English in New York City.* Washington, DC: Center for Applied Linguistics.

Labov, W. (1969). The logic of nonstandard English. In J. E. Alatis (Ed.), *Report of the twentieth annual round table meeting on linguistics and language studies.* Washington, DC: Georgetown University Press.

Ladas, H. (1980). Note-taking on lectures: An information-processing approach. *Educational Psychologist, 15,* 44–53.

LaGreca, A., & Mesibov, G. (1981). Facilitating interpersonal functioning with peers in learning disabled children. *Journal of Learning Disabilities, 14,* 197–199.

Lahey, M. (1988). *Language disorders and language development.* New York: Macmillan.

Lahey, M. (1990). Who shall be called language disordered? Some reflections and one perspective. *Journal of Speech and Hearing Disorders, 55,* 612–620.

Lahey, M. (1992). Linguistic and cultural diversity: Further problems for determining who shall be called language disordered. *Journal of Speech and Hearing Disorders, 56,* 638–639.

Lahey, M., & Bloom, L. (1977). Planning a first lexicon: Which words to teach first. *Journal of Speech and Hearing Disorders, 42,* 340–350.

Lahey, M., & Bloom, L. (1994). Variability and language learning disabilities. In G. P. Wallach & K. G. Butler (Eds.), *Language learning disabilities in school-age children and adolescents* (pp. 354–373). Boston: Allyn and Bacon.

Lakoff, G. (1987). *Women, fire, and dangerous things: What categories reveal about the mind.* Chicago: The University of Chicago Press.

Lamphear, V. S. (1985). The impact of maltreatment on children's psychosocial adjustment: A review of the research. *Child Abuse and Neglect, 9,* 251–263.

Landau, W. M., & Kleffner, F. R. (1957). Syndrome of acquired aphasia with convulsive disorder in children. *Neurology, 7,* 523–530.

Lane, H. (1992). *The mask of benevolence: Disabling the deaf community.* New York: Alfred A. Knopf.

Langer, J. (1982). Facilitating text processing: The elaboration of prior knowledge. In J. Langer & M. T. Smith-Burke (Eds.), *Reader meets author/Bridging the gap.* Newark, DE: International Reading Association.

Larson, V. L., & McKinley, N. L. (1987). *Communication assessment and intervention strategies for adolescents.* Eau Claire, WI: Thinking Publications.

Lasky, E. Z., & Cox, L. C. (1983). Auditory processing and language interaction: Evaluation and intervention strategies. In E. Z. Lasky & J. Katz (Eds.), *Central auditory processing disorders: Problems of speech, language, and learning* (pp. 243–268). Baltimore, MD: University Park Press.

Lasky, E. Z., & Katz, J. (Eds.). (1983). *Central auditory processing disorders: Problems of speech, language, and learning.* Austin, TX: Pro-Ed.

Lasky, E. Z., & Klopp, K. (1982). Parent-child interactions in normal and language-disordered children. *Journal of Speech and Hearing Disorders, 47,* 7–18.

Lasky, E., & Tobin, H. (1973). Linguistic and nonlinguistic competing message effects. *Journal of Learning Disabilities, 6,* 46–53.

Laughton, J., & Hasenstab, M. S. (1986). *The language learning process.* Rockville, MD: Aspen Publishers.

Launer, P. B., & Lahey, M. (1981). Passages: From the fifties to the eighties in language assessment. *Topics in Language Disorders, 1*(3), 11–29.

Lazar, R. T., Warr-Leeper, G. A., Nicholson, C. B., & Johnson, S. (1989). Elementary school teachers' use of multiple meaning expressions. *Language, Speech, and Hearing Services in Schools, 20,* 420–430.

Leadholm, B. J., & Miller, J. F. (1992). *Language sample analysis: The Wisconsin guide.* Madison, WI: Wisconsin Department of Public Instruction.

Lederberg, A. (1980). The language environment of children with language delays. *Journal of Pediatric Psychology, 5,* 141–159.

Lee, L. L. (1966). Developmental sentence types: A method for comparing normal and deviant syntactic development. *Journal of Speech and Hearing Disorders, 31,* 311–330.

Lee, L. L. (1974). *Developmental sentence analysis.* Evanston, IL: Northwestern University Press.

Lefebvre, M., & Pinard, A. (1972). Apprentisage de la conservation des qualités par une méthode de conflict cognitif. *Canadian Journal of the Behavioral Sciences, 4*(1), 1–12.

Leiter, R. G. (1959). Part I of the manual for the 1948 revision of the Leiter International Performance Scale. *Psychological Service Center Journal, 11,* 1–72.

Lenneberg, E. H. (1967). *Biological foundations of language.* New York: John Wiley & Sons.

Leonard, L. B. (1972). What is deviant language? *Journal of Speech and Hearing Disorders, 37,* 427–446.

Leonard, L. B. (1973). The role of intonation in recall of various linguistic stimuli. *Language and Speech, 16,* 327–335.

Leonard, L. B. (1980). The speech of language-disabled children. *Bulletin of the Orton Society* (now *Annals of Dyslexia*), *30,* 141–152.

Leonard, L. B. (1987). Is specific language impairment a useful construct? In S. Rosenberg (Ed.), *Advances in applied psycholinguistics, Vol. 1: Disorders of first language acquisition* (pp. 1–39). New York: Cambridge University Press.

Leonard, L. B. (1989). Language learnability and specific language impairment in children. *Applied Psycholinguistics, 10,* 179–202.

Leonard, L. B. (1991). Specific language impairment as a clinical category. *Language, Speech, and Hearing Services in Schools, 22,* 66–68.

Leonard, L. B. (1994). Some problems facing accounts of morphological deficits in children with specific language impairments. In R. V. Watkins & M. L. Rice (Eds.), *Specific language impairments in children.* (pp. 91–105). Baltimore, MD: Paul H. Brookes.

Leonard, L. B., Bortolini, U., Caselli, M. C., McGregor, K. K., & Sabbadini, L. (1992). Morphological deficits in children with specific language impairment: The status of features in the underlying grammar. *Language Acquisition: A Journal of Developmental Linguistics, 2,* 151–180.

Leonard, L. B., & Fey, M. E. (1991). Facilitating grammatical development: The contributions of pragmatics. In T. M. Gallagher (Ed.), *Pragmatics of language: Clinical practice issues* (pp. 333–355). San Diego: Singular Publishing Group.

Leonard, L. B., & Loeb, D. F. (1988). Government binding theory and some of its applications: A tutorial. *Journal of Speech and Hearing Research, 31,* 515–524.

Leonard, L., Schwartz, R., Chapman, K., Rowan, L., Prelock, P., Terrell, B., Weiss, A., & Messick, C. (1982). Early lexical acquisition in children with specific language disorder. *Journal of Speech and Hearing Research, 25,* 554–564.

Leonard, L., Schwartz, R., Folger, M., & Wilcox, M. (1978). Some aspects of child phonology in imitative and spontaneous speech. *Journal of Child Language, 5,* 403–415.

Leonard, L., Steckol, K. F., & Panther, K. M. (1983). Returning meaning to semantic relations: Some clinical applications. *Journal of Speech and Hearing Disorders, 48,* 25–36.

Leslie, A. M. (1994). ToMM, ToBy, and agency: Core architecture and domain specificity. In L. Hirschfeld & S. Gelman (Eds.), *Mapping the mind: Domain specificity in cognition and culture.* New York: Cambridge University Press.

Levi, G., Capozzi, F., Fabrizi, A., & Sechi, E. (1982). Language disorders and prognosis for reading disabilities in developmental age. *Perceptual and Motor Skills, 54,* 1119–1122.

Levin, H. S., & Eisenberg, H. M. (1979). Neuropsychological impairment after closed head injury in children and adolescents. *Journal of Pediatric Psychology, 4,* 389–402.

Levin, H. S., Ewing-Cobbs, L., & Benton, A. L. (1984). Age and recovery from brain damage: A review of clinical studies. In S. W. Scheff (Ed.), *Aging and recovery of function in the central nervous system* (pp. 169–205). New York: Plenum Press.

Levine, M. (1987). Developmental variation and learning disorders. Cambridge, MA: Educators Publishing Service.

Levinson, S. (1983). *Pragmatics.* Cambridge: Cambridge University Press.

Levitt, H., McGarr, N., & Geffner, D. (1988). Development of language and communication skills in hearing-impaired children. *ASHA Monographs,* Rockville, MD: American Speech-Language-Hearing Association. (No. 26).

Liberman, A. M., Cooper, F. S., Shankweiler, D. P., & Studdert-Kennedy, M. (1967). Perception of the speech code. *Psychological Review, 74,* 431–461.

Liberman, I. Y., & Liberman, A. M. (1990). Whole language vs. code emphasis: Underlying assumptions and their implications for reading instruction. *Annals of Dyslexia, 40,* 51–76.

Liberman, I. Y., Shankweiler, D., Liberman, A. M., Fowler, C., & Fischer, F. W. (1977). Phonetic segmentation and recording in the beginning reader. In S. S. Reber & D. Scarborough (Eds.), *Toward a psychology of reading.* Hillsdale, NJ: Erlbaum.

Lidz, C. S. (1991). *Practitioner's guide to dynamic assessment.* New York: Guilford Press.

Liebergott, J. W., Bashir, A. S., & Schultz, M. C. (1984). Dancing around and making strange noises: Children at risk. In A. Holland (Ed.), *Language disorders in children* (pp. 37–56). San Diego, CA: College-Hill Press.

Lieberman, I., & Shankweiler, D. (1985). Phonology and problems of learning to read and write. *Remedial and Special Education, 6,* 8–17.

Lieven, E. V. M. (1984). Interactional style and children's language learning. *Topics in Language Disorders, 4*(4), 15–23.

Light, J. (1988). Interaction involving individuals using augmentative and alternative communication systems: State of the art and future directions. *Augmentative and Alternative Communication, 4,* 66–82.

Light, J., Binger, C., & Kelford Smith, A. (1994). Story reading interactions between preschoolers who use AAC and their mothers. *Augmentative and Alternative Communication, 10,* 255–268.

Light, J., Collier, B., & Parnes, P. (1985a). Communicative interaction between young nonspeaking physically disabled children and their primary caregivers: Part I—Discourse patterns. *Augmentative and Alternative Communication, 1,* 74–83.

Light, J., Collier, B., & Parnes, P. (1985b). Communicative interaction between young nonspeaking physically disabled children and their primary caregivers: Part II—Communicative function. *Augmentative and Alternative Communication, 1,* 98–107.

Light, J., Collier, B., & Parnes, P. (1985c). Communicative interaction between young nonspeaking physically disabled children and their primary caregivers: Part III—Modes of communication. *Augmentative and Alternative Communication, 1,* 125–133.

Light, J., & Kelford Smith, A. (1993). The home literacy experiences of preschoolers who use augmentative communicative systems and of their nondisabled peers. *Augmentative and Alternative Communication, 9,* 10–25.

Light, J., Kelford-Smith, A., & McNaughton, D. (1990, August). *The literacy experiences of preschoolers who use augmentative and alternative communication systems.* Paper presented at the biennial meeting of the International Society for Augmentative and Alternative Communication, Stockholm, Sweden.

Light, J., & McNaughton, D. (1993). Literacy and augmentative and alternative communication: The experiences and priorities of parents and teachers. *Topics in Language Disorders, 13*(2), 33–46.

Liles, B. Z. (1985). Cohesion in the narratives of normal and language-disordered children. *Journal of Speech and Hearing Research, 28,* 123–133.

Liles, B. Z., Duffy, R. J., Merritt, D. D., Purcell, S. L. (1995). Measurement of narrative discourse ability in children with language disorders. *Journal of Speech and Hearing Research, 38,* 415–425.

Lindamood, C. H., & Lindamood, P. C. (1969). *Auditory discrimination in depth.* Austin, TX: DLM Teaching Resources.

Linder, T. W. (1990). *Transdisciplinary play-based assessment* (TPBA). Baltimore: Paul H. Brookes.

Linder, T. (1993). *Transdisciplinary play-based assessment: A functional approach to working with young children* (rev. ed.). Baltimore, MD: Paul H. Brookes.

Lindfors, J. W. (1987). *Children's language and learning* (2nd ed.). Englewood Cliffs, NJ: Prentice Hall.

Ling, D. (1976). *Speech and the hearing-impaired child: Theory and practice.* Washington, DC: A. G. Bell.

Ling, D. (Ed.). (1984a). *Early intervention for hearing impaired children: Oral options.* Austin, TX: Pro-Ed.

Ling, D. (Ed.). (1984b). *Early intervention for hearing impaired children: Total communication options.* Austin, TX: Pro-Ed.

Ling, D., & Clarke, B. R. (1975). Cued speech: An evaluative study. *American Annals of the Deaf, 120,* 480–488.

Ling, D., & Clarke, B. R. (1976). The effects of using cued speech: A follow-up study. *Volta Review, 78,* 23–34.

Ling, D., & Ling, A. H. (1978). *Aural habilitation: The foundations of verbal learning in hearing-impaired children.* Washington, DC: A. G. Bell Association for the Deaf.

Lingerfelt, B. V., Bennett, T., & Nelson, D. E. (1992). *Facilitating family-centered training in early intervention.* San Antonio, TX: Communication Skill Builders/The Psychological Corporation.

Lipsky, D. K. & Gartner, A. (Eds.). (1989). *Beyond separate education: Quality education for all.* Baltimore: Paul H. Brookes.

Lloyd, J. (1980). Academic instruction and cognitive behavior modification: The need for attack strategy training. *Exceptional Education Quarterly, 1,* 53–63.

Loban, W. D. (1963). *The language of elementary school children. NCTE Research Report No. 1.* Urbana, IL: National Council of Teachers of English.

Loban, W. D. (1976). *Language development: Kindergarten through grade twelve.* Urbana, IL: National Council of Teachers of English.

Longhurst, T. M. (Ed.). (1974). *Linguistic analysis of children's speech: Readings.* New York: MSS Information Corporation.

Lovaas, O. I. (1981). *Teaching developmentally disabled children: The me book.* Austin, TX: Pro-Ed.

Lovaas, O. I. (1987). Behavioral treatment and normal educational and intellectual functioning in young autistic children. *Journal of Consulting and Clinical Psychology, 55,* 3–9.

Lovaas, O. I., Schaeffer, B., & Simmons, J. Q. (1965). Experimental studies in childhood schizophrenia: Building social behavior in autistic children by use of electric shock. *Journal of Experimental Research in Personality, 1,* 99–109.

Love, R. J., & Webb, W. G. (1986). *Neurology for the speech-language pathologist.* Stoneham, MA: Butterworth Publishers.

Lowe, M., & Costello, A. (1976). *Manual for Symbolic Play Test.* London: National Foundation of Educational Research.

Lucariello, J. (1990). Freeing talk from the here-and-now: The role of event knowledge and maternal scaffolds. *Topics in Language Disorders, 10*(3), 14–29.

Lucas, E. V. (1980). *Semantic and pragmatic language disorders: Assessment and remediation.* Rockville, MD: Aspen Publishers.

Lund, N. J., & Duchan, J. F. (1993). *Assessing children's language in naturalistic contexts* (3rd ed.). Englewood Cliffs, NJ: Prentice-Hall.

Lundsteen, S. W. (1979). *Listening: Its impact at all levels on reading and the other language arts.* Urbana, IL: National Council of Teachers of English.

Luterman, D. (1979). *Counseling parents of hearing impaired children.* Boston: Little, Brown, & Company.

Lyman, H. (1986). *Test scores and what they mean* (4th ed.). Englewood Cliffs, NJ: Prentice-Hall.

Lynch, M. P., Eilers, R. E., Oller, D. K., & Cobo-Lewis, A. (1989). Multisensory speech perception by profoundly hearing-impaired children. *Journal of Speech and Hearing Disorders, 54,* 57–67.

Lynch-Fraser, D., & Tiegerman, E. (1987). *Baby signals.* New York: Walker and Company.

Lyon, S., & Lyon, G. (1980). Team functioning and staff development: A role release approach to providing integrated educational services for severely handicapped students. *JASH* (Journal of the Association for Persons with Severe Handicaps), *5*(3), 250–263.

Mabbett, B. (1990). The New Zealand story. *Educational Leadership, 47*(6), 59–61.

MacDonald, J. (1989). *Becoming partners with children: From play to conversation.* San Antonio, TX: Special Press.

MacKeith, R. C., & Rutter, M. (1972). A note on the prevalence of language disorders in young children. In M. Rutter & J. A. M. Martin (Eds.), *The child with delayed speech. Clinics in developmental medicine.* (No. 43, pp. 48–51). London: Heineman Medical Books, Ltd.

MacMurray, J. (1961). *Persons in relation.* London: Faber.

MacWhinney, B. (1987). The competition model. In B. MacWhinney (Ed.), *Mechanisms of language acquisition* (pp. 249–308). Hillsdale, NJ: Erlbaum.

MacWhinney, B. (1996). The CHILDES system. *American Journal of Speech-Language Pathology, 5*(1), 5–14.

Magnotta, O. H. (1991). Looking beyond tradition. *Language, Speech, and Hearing Services in Schools, 22,* 150–151.

Mahoney, T. M., & Eichwald, J. G. (1987). The ups and "Downs" of high-risk screening: The Utah statewide program. *Seminars in Hearing, 8*(2), 155–163.

Mandler, J., & Johnson, N. L. (1977). Remembrance of things parsed: Story structure and recall. *Cognitive Psychology, 9,* 111–191.

Manis, F. R., Szeszulski, P. A., Holt, L. K., & Graves, K. (1988). A developmental perspective on dyslexic subtypes. *Annals of Dyslexia, 38,* 139–153.

Manolson, A. (1992). *It takes two to talk: A parent's guide to helping children communicate.* Toronto, Ontario: The Hanen Centre.

Manolson, A. (1995). *You make the difference: In helping your child learn.* Toronto, Ontario: The Hanen Centre.

Mantovani, J. F., & Landau, W. M. (1980). Acquired aphasia with convulsive disorder: Course and prognosis. *Neurology, 30,* 524–529.

Mardell, C., & Goldenberg, D. (1975). *The Developmental Indicators for the Assessment of Learning (DIAL).* Chicago, IL: Childcraft Education.

Mardell-Czudnowski, C., & Goldenberg, D. (1984). Revision and restandardization of a preschool screening test: DIAL becomes DIAL-R. *Journal of the Division for Early Childhood, 11,* 238–246.

Mardell-Czudnowski, C., & Goldenberg, D. (1990). *Developmental Indicators for the Assessment of Learning-Revised (DIAL-R).* Circle Pines, MN: AGS.

Marin-Padilla, M. (1975). Neuron differences in mental retardation. In D. Bergsma (Ed.), *Morphogenesis and malformation of the face and brain.* New York: Allen R. Liss.

Markus, D. (1988, November). Out of the shadows. *Parenting,* 113–114.

Marshall, J. C. (1979). Language acquisition in a biological frame of reference. In P. Fletcher & M. Garman (Eds.), *Language acquisition* (pp. 437–453). Cambridge: Cambridge University Press.

Marston, D. B. (1989). A curriculum-based measurement approach to assessing academic performance: What it is and why do it. In M. R. Shinn (Ed.), *Curriculum-based measurement: Assessing special children* (pp. 18–78). New York: Guilford Press.

Martin Luther King Junior Elementary School Children et al. v. Ann Arbor School District Board, Civil Action No. 7–71861, 451 F. Supp. 1324 (1978), 463 F. Supp. 1027 (1978) and 473 F. Supp. 1371 (1979, E. D. Detroit, Michigan).

Martin, V. E. (1974). Consulting with teachers. *Language, Speech, and Hearing Services in Schools, 5,* 176–179.

Marvin, C. A. (1987). Consultation services: Changing roles for SLPs. *Journal of Childhood Communication Disorders, 11,* 1–15.

Marx, M. H., & Hillix, W. A. (1979). *Systems and theories in psychology.* New York: McGraw-Hill.

Marzano, R., Hagerty, P., Valencia, S., & DiStefano, P. (1987). *Reading diagnosis and instruction: Theory into practice.* Englewood Cliffs, NJ: Prentice-Hall.

Mason, J. (1980). When do children begin to read?: An exploration of four-year-old children's letter and word reading competencies. *Reading and Research Quarterly, 15,* 203–227.

Massaro, D. W. (1973). Perception of letters, words, and nonwords. *Journal of Experimental Psychology, 100,* 349–353.

Matarazzo, J. D. (1972). *Wechsler's measurement and appraisal of adult intelligence.* Baltimore, MD: Williams & Wilkins.

Mattis, S. (1978). Dyslexia syndromes: A working hypothesis that works. In A. L. Benton & D. Pearl (Eds.), *Dyslexia: An appraisal of current knowledge.* New York: Oxford University Press.

Mattis, S., French, J. H., & Rapin, I. (1975). Dyslexia in children and young adults: Three independent neuropsychological syndromes. *Developmental Medicine and Child Neurology, 17,* 150–163.

Matsuyama, U. K. (1983). Can story grammar speak Japanese? *The Reading Teacher, 36,* 666–669.

Maurice, C. (1996). *Behavioral intervention for young children with autism: A manual for parents and professionals.* Austin, TX: Pro-Ed.

Mautner, T. S. (1984). Dyslexia—My "invisible handicap." *Annals of Dyslexia, 34,* 299–311.

Maxon, A., & Brackett, D. (1987). The hearing-impaired child in regular schools. *Seminars in Speech and Language, 8*(4), 393–413.

Maxwell, D. L. (1984). The neurology of learning and language disabilities: Developmental considerations. In G. P. Wallach & K. G. Butler (Eds.), *Language learning disabilities in school-age children* (pp. 35–59). Baltimore, MD: Williams & Wilkins.

Maxwell, S. E., & Wallach, G. P. (1984). The language-learning disabilities connection: Symptoms of early language disability change over time. In G. P. Wallach & K. G. Butler (Eds.), *Language learning disabilities in school-age children* (pp. 15–34). Baltimore, MD: Williams & Wilkins.

McAlister, K. (1997, February). *A writer's workshop approach for students with severe language impairments.* Paper presented at Western Michigan University, Kalamazoo, MI.

McCabe, A., & Rollins, P. R. (1994). Assessment of preschool narrative skills. *American Journal of Speech-Language Pathology, 3*(1), 45–56.

McCalla, J. L. (1985). A multidisciplinary approach to identification and remedial intervention for adverse late effects of cancer therapy. *Nursing Clinics of North America, 20,* 117–129.

McCarthy, D. A. (1930). The language development of the pre-school child. *University of Minnesota Institute of Child Welfare Monograph Series IV.* Minneapolis, MN: University of Minnesota Press.

McCarthy, D. (1954). Language development in children. In L. Carmichael (Ed.), *Manual of child psychology.* New York: John Wiley & Sons.

McCarthy, D. (1972). *McCarthy scales of children's abilities.* San Antonio, TX: The Psychological Corporation.

McCauley, R. J. (1996). Familiar strangers: Criterion-referenced measures in communication disorders. *Language, Speech, and Hearing Services in Schools, 27,* 122–131.

McCauley, R. J., & Swisher, L. (1984). Psychometric review of language and articulation tests for preschool children. *Journal of Speech and Hearing Disorders, 49,* 34–42.

McCauley, R. J., & Swisher, L. (1987). Are maltreated children at risk for speech or language impairment?: An unanswered question. *Journal of Speech and Hearing Disorders, 52,* 301–303.

McClelland, J., Rumelhart, D., & PDP Research Group. (1986). *Parallel distributed processing: Explorations in the microstructure of cognition* (Vol. 2). Cambridge, MA: Bradford Books.

McClure, E., Mason, J., & Williams, J. (1983). Sociocultural variables in children's sequencing of stories. *Discourse Processes, 6,* 131–143.

McConkey, R. (1984). The assessment of representational play: A springboard for language remediation. In D. Mueller (Ed.), *Remediating children's language: Behavioral and naturalistic approaches* (pp. 1113–1134). Austin, TX: Pro-Ed.

McCormick, L. (1990a). Developing objectives. In L. McCormick & R. L. Schiefelbusch (Eds.), *Early language intervention: An introduction* (2nd ed.) (pp. 181–214). Columbus, OH: Merrill.

McCormick, L. (1990b). Intervention processes and procedures. In L. McCormick & R. L. Schiefelbusch (Eds.), *Early language intervention: An introduction* (2nd ed.) (pp. 216–260). Columbus, OH: Merrill.

McCormick, L. (1990c). Extracurricular roles and relationships. In L. McCormick & R. L. Schiefelbusch (Eds.), *Early language intervention: An introduction* (2nd ed.) (pp. 262–301). Columbus, OH: Merrill.

McCormick, L., & Goldman, R. (1979). The transdisciplinary model: Implications for service delivery and personnel preparation for the severely and profoundly handicapped. *AAESPH Review, 4*(2), 152–161.

McCormick, L. & Schiefelbusch, R. L. (Eds.). (1990). *Early language intervention: An introduction* (2nd ed.). Columbus, OH: Merrill.

McCormick, M. C. (1989). Long-term follow-up of infants discharged from neonatal intensive care units. *Journal of the American Medical Association, 261,* 1767–1772.

McCune-Nicolich, L. (1981). Toward symbolic functioning: Structure of early pretend games and potential parallels with language. *Child Development, 52,* 785–797.

McCune-Nicolich, L., & Fenson, L. (1984). Methodological issues in studying pretend play. In T. D. Yawkey & A. D. Pelligrini (Eds.), *Child's play: Developmental and applied.* (pp. 81–104). Hillsdale, NJ: Erlbaum.

McDermott, R. P. (1977). Social relations as contexts for learning in school. *Harvard Educational Review, 47,* 198–213.

McFadden, T. U., & Gillam, R. B. (1996). An examination of the quality of narratives produced by children with language disorders. *Language, Speech, and Hearing Services in Schools, 27,* 48–56.

McGee, L. M., & Richgels, D. J. (1990). *Literacy's beginnings: Supporting young readers and writers.* Boston: Allyn and Bacon.

McGregor, K. K. (1994). Use of phonological information in a word-finding treatment for children. *Journal of Speech and Hearing Research, 37,* 1381–1393.

McGregor, K. K., & Leonard, L. B. (1995). Intervention for word-finding deficits in children. In M. E. Fey, J. Windsor, & S. F. Warren (Eds.), *Language intervention: Preschool through the elementary years* (pp. 85–105). Baltimore: Paul H. Brookes.

McInnes, J. M., & Treffry, J. A. (1982). *Deaf-blind infants and children: A developmental guide.* Toronto, Canada: University of Toronto Press.

McKenzie, R. G. (1991). Content area instruction delivered by secondary learning disabilities teachers: A national survey. *Learning Disability Quarterly, 14,* 115–122.

McKinley, N. L., & Lord-Larson, V. (1985). Neglected language-disordered adolescents: A delivery model. *Language, Speech, and Hearing Services in Schools, 16,* 2–15.

McKirdy, L. S., & Blank, M. (1982). Dialogue in deaf and hearing preschoolers. *Journal of Speech and Hearing Research, 25,* 487–499.

McLean, J. E., & Snyder-McLean, L. K. (1978). *A transactional approach to early language training: Derivation of a model system.* Columbus, OH: Merrill.

McNaughton, S., & Lindsay, P. (1995). Approaching literacy with AAC graphics. *Augmentative and Alternative Communication, 11,* 212–228.

McNeill, D. (1966). Developmental psycholinguistics. In F. Smith & G. Miller (Eds.), *The genesis of language.* Cambridge, MA: MIT Press.

McNeill, D. (1970). *The acquisition of language: The study of developmental psycholinguistics.* New York: Harper & Row.

Mehan, H. (1979). *Learning lessons: Social organization in the classroom.* Cambridge, MA: Harvard University Press.

Meier, R. P. (1991). Language acquisition by deaf children. *American Scientist, 79*(1), 60–70.

Menyuk, P. (1964). Comparison of grammar of children with functionally deviant and normal speech. *Journal of Speech and Hearing Research, 7,* 109–121.

Menyuk, P. (1968). Children's learning and reproduction of grammatical and nongrammatical phonological sequences. *Child Development, 39,* 849–959.

Mercer, J. R. (1973). *Labeling the mentally retarded.* Berkeley: University of California Press.

Mercer, J. R., & Denti, L. (1989). Obstacles to integrating students in a "two-roof" elementary school. *Exceptional Children, 56,* 30–38.

Mercer, J. R., & Lewis, J. P. (1975). *System of multicultural pluralistic assessment. Technical manual.* Unpublished manuscript. University of California at Riverside.

Merzenich, M. M., Jenkins, W. M., Johnston, P., Schreiner, C., Miller, S. L., & Tallal, P. (1996, January 5). Temporal processing deficits of language-learning impaired children ameliorated by training. *Science, 271,* 77–81.

Meyer, B. J. F. (1975). *The organization of prose and its effects on memory.* Amsterdam: North Holland.

Miedzianik, D. (1990, Spring). I hope some lass will want me after reading all this. *The Advocate* (newsletter of the Autism Society of America), *22*(1), 7.

Miller, B. L. (1988). *Effects of intervention on the ability of students with hearing impairments to write personal narrative stories.* Unpublished master's thesis, Western Michigan University, Kalamazoo, MI.

Miller, G. A. (1956). The magical number seven, plus or minus two: Some limits on our capacity for processing information. *Psychological Review, 63,* 81–97.

Miller, G. A., & Gildea, P. M. (1987). How children learn words. *Scientific American, 257,* 94–99.

Miller, J. F. (1981). *Assessing language production in children: Experimental procedures.* Austin, TX: Pro-Ed.

Miller, J. F. (1987). Language and communication characteristics of children with Down syndrome. In S. M. Pueschel, C. Tingey, J. E. Rynders, A. C. Crocker, & D. M. Crutcher (Eds.), *New perspectives on Down syndrome* (pp. 233–262). Baltimore: Paul H. Brookes.

Miller, J. F., Campbell, T. F., Chapman, R. S., & Weismer, S. E. (1984). Language behavior in acquired childhood aphasia. In A. Holland (Ed.), *Language disorders in children* (pp. 57–99). San Diego: College Hill.

Miller, J. F., & Chapman, R. S. (1981). The relation between age and mean length of utterance in morphemes. *Journal of Speech and Hearing Research, 24,* 154–161.

Miller, J., & Chapman, R. (1991). *Systematic analysis of language transcripts (SALT)* [Computer program; A. Nockerts, Programmer]. Madison, WI: Language Analysis Laboratory, Waisman Center on Mental Retardation and Human Development.

Miller, J. F., Chapman, R., Branston, M. B., & Reichle, J. (1980). Language comprehension in sensorimotor Stages V and VI. *Journal of Speech and Hearing Research, 23,* 284–311.

Miller, J. F., & Paul, R. (1995). *The clinical assessment of language comprehension.* Baltimore: Paul H. Brookes.

Miller, J. F., Sedey, A. L., & Miolo, G. (1995). Validity of parent report measures of vocabulary development for children with Down syndrome. *Journal of Speech and Hearing Research, 38,* 1037–1044.

Miller, L. (1978). Pragmatics and early childhood language disorders: Communicative interactions in a half-hour sample. *Journal of Speech and Hearing Disorders, 43,* 419–436.

Miller, L. (1989). Classroom-based language intervention. *Language, Speech, and Hearing Services in Schools, 20,* 153–169.

Miller, L. (1990). *The smart profile: A qualitative approach for describing learners and designing instruction.* Austin, TX: Smart Alternatives.

Miller, L. (1993). *What we call smart: A new narrative for intelligence and learning.* San Diego: Singular Publishing Group.

Mills, A. E. (Ed.). (1983). *Language acquisition in the blind child: Normal and deficient.* San Diego: College Hill.

Milosky, L. M. (1987). Narratives in the classroom. *Seminars in Speech and Language, 8*(4), 329–343.

Milosky, L. M. (1990). The role of world knowledge in language comprehension and language intervention. *Topics in Language Disorders, 10*(3), 1–13.

Minskoff, E. (1982). Sharpening language skills in secondary LD students. *Academic Therapy, 18*(1), 53–60.

Minuchin, P. (1985). Families and individual development: Provocations from the field of family therapy. *Child Development, 56,* 289–302.

Mire, S. P., & Chisholm, R. W. (1990). Functional communication goals for adolescents and adults who are severely and moderately mentally handicapped. *Language, Speech, and Hearing Services in Schools, 21,* 57–58.

Mirenda, P., & Locke, P. A. (1989). A comparison of symbol transparency in nonspeaking persons with intellectual disabilities. *Journal of Speech and Hearing Disorders, 54,* 131–140.

Mirenda, P., & Santogrossi, J. (1985). A prompt-free strategy to teach pictorial communication system use. *Augmentative and Alternative Communication, 1,* 143–150.

Mishler, E. G. (1979). Meaning in context: Is there any other kind? *Harvard Educational Review, 49,* 1–19.

Moeller, M. P. (1989, November). *Strategies for enhancing hearing parent's sign communication with deaf children.* Paper presented at the Annual Convention of the American Speech-Language-Hearing Association, St. Louis, MO.

Moeller, M. P., Osberger, M. J., & Eccarius, M. (1986). Cognitively based strategies for use with hearing-impaired students with comprehension deficits. *Topics in Language Disorders, 6*(4), 37–50.

Molfese, D., Freeman, R., & Palermo, D. (1975). The ontogeny of brain lateralization for speech and nonspeech stimuli. *Brain and Language, 2,* 356–368.

Montague, M., Graves, A., & Leavell, A. (1991). Planning, procedural facilitation, and narrative composition of junior high students with learning disabilities. *Learning Disabilities Research and Practice, 6,* 219–224.

Montgomery, J. W. (1995). Sentence comprehension in children with specific language impairment: The role of phonological working memory. *Journal of Speech and Hearing Research, 38,* 187–199.

Moon, M. S., Diambra, T., & Hill, M. (1990). An outcome-oriented vocational process for students with severe handicaps. *Teaching Exceptional Children, 23*(1), 47–50.

Moores, D. (1969). Cued speech: Some practical and theoretical considerations. *American Annals of the Deaf, 114,* 23–27.

Moran, M. R. (1987). Individualized objectives for writing instruction. *Topics in Language Disorders, 7*(4), 42–54.

Moran, M. R. (1988). Rationale and procedures for increasing the productivity of inexperienced writers. *Exceptional Children, 54,* 552–558.

Morgan, D., & Guilford, A. (1984). *Adolescent Language Screening Test* (ALST). Tulsa, OK: Modern Educational Corp.

Morley, M. E. (1972). *The development and disorders of speech in childhood.* London: Churchill Livingstone.

Morris, C. (1946). *Foundation of the theory of signs. International encyclopedia of unified science.* Chicago: University of Chicago Press.

Morris, N. T., & Crump, W. D. (1982). Syntactic and vocabulary development in the written language of learning disabled and non-disabled students at four age levels. *Learning Disability Quarterly, 5,* 163–172.

Morris, S. E. (1981). Communication/interaction development at mealtimes for the multiply handicapped child: Implications for the use of augmentative communication systems. *Language, Speech, and Hearing Services in Schools, 12,* 216–232.

Morris, S. E. (1982). *Prespeech assessment scale.* Clifton, NJ: J. A. Preston.

Morris, S. E., & Klein, M. D. (1987). *Pre-feeding skills.* Tucson, AZ: Communication Skill Builders.

Moses, K. L. (1985). Infant deafness and parental grief: Psychosocial early intervention. In F. Powell, T. Finitzo-Hieber, S. Friel-Patti, & D. Henderson (Eds.), *Education of the hearing impaired child* (pp. 85–102). Austin, TX: Pro-Ed.

Mroczkowski, M. M. (1988). Self-contained language classes for kindergartners—Nine years of data. *Seminars in Speech and Language, 9,* 329–339.

Mulac, A., & Tomlinson, C. (1977). Generalization of an operant remediation program for syntax with language delayed children. *Journal of Communication Disorders, 10,* 231–243.

Mulligan, M., Guess, D., Holvoet, J., & Brown, F. (1980). The individualized curriculum sequencing model: Implications from research on massed, distributed, or spaced trial training. *JASH* (Journal for the Association for Persons with Severe Handicaps), *5,* 325–336.

Muma, J. (1978). *Language handbook: Concepts, assessment, intervention.* Englewood Cliffs, NJ: Prentice Hall.

Muma, J. (1983). Speech-language pathology: Emerging clinical expertise in language. In T. M. Gallagher & C. Prutting (Eds.), *Pragmatic assessment and intervention issues in language* (pp. 195–214). San Diego, CA: College-Hill Press.

Mundy, P., Kasari, C., Sigman, M., & Ruskin, E. (1995). Nonverbal communication and early language acquisition in children with Down syndrome and in normally developing children. *Journal of Speech and Hearing Research, 38,* 157–167.

Murray-Seegert, C. (1989). *Nasty girls, thugs, and humans like us: Social relations between severely disabled and nondisabled students in high school.* Baltimore: Paul H. Brookes.

Musselwhite, C. R. (1986). *Adaptive play for special needs children.* Austin, TX: Pro-Ed.

Muth, K. D. (1989). *Children's comprehension of text.* Newark, DE: International Reading Association.

Myklebust, H. R. (1954). *Auditory disorders in children.* New York: Grune & Stratton.

Myklebust, H. R. (1957). Aphasia in children—diagnosis and training. In L. E. Travis (Ed.), *Handbook of speech pathology and audiology.* Englewood Cliffs, NJ: Prentice-Hall.

Myklebust, H. R. (1964). *The psychology of deafness* (2nd ed.). New York: Grune & Stratton.

Nash, J. M. (1996, January 29). Zooming in on dyslexia. *Time,* pp. 62–64.

National Assessment of Educational Progress. (1980). Writing achievement, 1969–1979: Results from the Third National Writing Assessment. Denver, CO: Author. (ERIC Document Reproduction Service Nos. ED 196 043, ED 196 044).

National Association of State Boards of Education. (1992). *Winners all: A call for inclusive schools.* Washington, DC: Author.

National Joint Committee for the Communicative Needs of Persons with Severe Disabilities. (1992). Guidelines for meeting the communication needs of persons with severe disabilities. *Asha, 34* (March, Suppl. 7), 1–8.

National Joint Committee on Learning Disabilities. (1985). *Learning disabilities and the preschool child.* (A position paper of the National Joint Committee on Learning Disabilities, February 10, 1985). Baltimore, MD: The Orton Dyslexia Society.

National Joint Committee on Learning Disabilities. (1991). Learning disabilities: Issues on definition (A position paper of the National Joint Committee on Learning Disabilities). *Asha, 33* (Suppl. 5), 18–20.

Neisworth, J. T., & Bagnato, S. J. (1988). Assessment in early childhood special education: A typology of dependent measures. In S. L. Odom & M. B. Karnes (Eds.), *Early intervention for infants and children with handicaps* (pp. 23–50). Baltimore: Paul. H. Brookes.

Nelson, K. (1973). Structure and strategy in learning to talk. *Monographs of the Society for Research in Child Development,* Serial No. 38.

Nelson, K. (1985). *Making sense: The acquisition of shared meaning.* New York: Academic Press.

Nelson, K. (1986). *Event knowledge: Structure and function in development.* Hillsdale, NJ: Erlbaum.

Nelson, K. (Ed.). (1989). *Narratives from the crib.* Cambridge, MA: Harvard University Press.

Nelson, K., Benedict, H., Gruendel, J., & Rescorla, L. (1977). *Lessons from early lexicons.* Paper presented at the biennial meeting of the Society for Research in Child Development, New Orleans, LA.

Nelson, N. W. (1981a). An eclectic model of language intervention for disorders of listening, speaking, reading, and writing. *Topics in Language Disorders, 1*(2), 1–23.

Nelson, N. W. (1981b). Tests and materials in speech and language screening. *Seminars in Speech, Language, and Hearing, 2,* 11–36.

Nelson, N. W. (1984). Beyond information processing: The language of teachers and textbooks. In G. P. Wallach & K. G. Butler (Eds.), *Language learning disabilities in school-age children* (pp. 154–178). Baltimore, MD: Williams & Wilkins.

Nelson, N. W. (1985). Teacher talk and child listening—Fostering a better match. In C. S. Simon (Ed.), *Communication skills and classroom success: Assessment of language-learning disabled students* (pp. 65–102). San Diego, CA: College-Hill Press. Reprinted in C. S. Simon (Ed.). (1991), *Communication skills and classroom success: Assessment and therapy methodologies for language and learning disabled students* (pp. 78–103). Eau Claire, WI: Thinking Publications.

Nelson, N. W. (1986a). Individual processing in classroom settings. *Topics in Language Disorders, 6*(2), 13–27.

Nelson, N. W. (1986b). What is meant by meaning (and how can it be taught)? *Topics in Language Disorders, 6*(4), 1–14.

Nelson, N. W. (1988a). The nature of literacy. In M. A. Nippold (Ed.), *Later language development: Ages nine through nineteen* (pp. 11–28). Austin, TX: Pro-Ed.

Nelson, N. W. (1988b). *Planning individualized speech and language intervention programs* (2nd ed.). Tucson, AZ: Communication Skill Builders.

Nelson, N. W. (1988c). Reading and writing. In M. A. Nippold (Ed.), *Normal language development: Ages nine through nineteen* (pp. 97–126). Austin, TX: Pro-Ed.

Nelson, N. W. (1989a). Language intervention in school settings. In D. K. Bernstein & E. Tiegerman (Eds.), *Language and communication disorders in children* (2nd ed.), (pp. 417–468). Columbus, OH: Merrill.

Nelson, N. W. (1989b). Curriculum-based language assessment and intervention. *Language, Speech, and Hearing Services in Schools, 20,* 170–184.

Nelson, N. W. (1990). Only relevant practices can be best. *Best Practices in School Speech-Language Pathology* (a publication of The Psychological Corporation, Inc.), *1,* 15–27.

Nelson, N. W. (1992a). Performance is the prize: Language competence and performance among AAC users. *Augmentative and Alternative Communication, 8,* 3–18.

Nelson, N. W. (1992b). Targets of curriculum-based language assessment and intervention. J. Damico (Ed.), Volume two of series on *Best Practices in School Speech-Language Pathology* (pp. 73–85) San Antonio, TX: The Psychological Corporation, Harcourt, Brace, Jovanovich.

Nelson, N. W. (1994). Curriculum-based language assessment and intervention across the grades. In G. P. Wallach & K. G. Butler (Eds.), *Language learning disabilities in school-age children and adolescents* (pp. 104–131). Boston: Allyn and Bacon.

Nelson, N. W. (1995). Scaffolding in the secondary school. In D. Tibbits (H. Winnitz, Series Ed.), *Language intervention: Beyond the primary grades* (pp. 375–419). Austin, TX: Pro-Ed.

Nelson, N. W. (1997). Implementing a language-based homework lab: A plan for curriculum-based intervention. In N. W. Nelson & B. Hoskins (Eds.). *Strategies for supporting classroom success: Focus on communication* (30 minute segment of an audioworkshop). San Diego: Singular Publishing Group.

Nelson, N. W., Bahr, C. M., & Van Meter, A. M. (in press). *Writing process instruction and computers: Making connections and building language.* Baltimore: Paul H. Brookes.

Nelson, N. W., & Friedman, K. K. (1988). *Development of the concept of story in narratives written by older children.* Unpublished paper. Kalamazoo, MI: Western Michigan University.

Nelson, N. W., & Gillespie, L. (1991). *Analogies for thinking and talking.* Tucson, AZ: Communication Skill Builders.

Nelson, N. W., & Hyter, Y. D. (1990a). *Black English Sentence Scoring: Development and Use as a Tool for Non-Biased Assessment.* Unpublished manuscript. Western Michigan University.

Nelson, N. W., & Hyter, Y. D. (1990b, November). *How to use Black English Sentence Scoring.* Short course presented at the Annual Conference of the American Speech-Language-Hearing Association, Seattle, WA.

Nelson, N. W., & Schwentor, B. A. (1990). Reading and writing. In D. R. Beukelman & K. M. Yorkston (Eds.), *Management of the communication and swallowing disorders of persons with traumatic brain injury* (pp. 191–249). Austin, TX: Pro-Ed.

Nelson, N. W., Silbar, J. C., & Lockwood, E. L. (1981, November). *The Michigan decision-making strategy for determining appropriate communicative services for physically and/or mentally handicapped children.* Paper presented at the annual conference of the American Speech-Language-Hearing Association, Los Angeles, CA.

Nelson, N. W., & Snyder, T. [programmer]. (1990). *Planning individualized speech and language intervention programs: Software version* (rev. ed.) (computer program). Tucson, AZ: Communication Skill Builders.

Nelson, N. W., & Van Meter, A. (1996, November). *Language-based homework lab: A context for curriculum-based language intervention.* Miniseminar presented at the Annual Convention of the American Speech-Language Hearing Association, Seattle, WA.

Newborg, J., Stock, J. R., Wnek, L., Guidubaldi, J., & Svinicki, J. (1984). *The Battelle Developmental Inventory.* Allen, TX: DLM/Teaching Resources.

Newcomer, P. L., & Hammill, D. D. (1988). *Test of Language Development-2: Primary* (TOLD-2). Austin, TX: Pro-Ed.

Newhoff, M. (1986). Attentional deficit—What it is, what it is not. *The Clinical Connection, Fall,* 10–11.

Newhoff, M. (1990). Attention deficit hyperactivity disorder: Defining our role. *The Clinical Connection, 1st Quarter,* 10–12.

Newman, P., Creaghead, N. A., & Secord, W. (1985). *Assessment and remediation of articulatory and phonological disorders.* Columbus, OH: Merrill.

Newport, E. L., & Ashbrook, E. (1977). The emergence of semantic relations in American Sign Language. *Papers and Reports on Child Language Development, 13,* 16–21.

Newton, L. (1985). Linguistic environment of the deaf child: A focus on teachers' use of nonliteral language. *Journal of Speech and Hearing Research, 28,* 336–344.

Ninio, A. (1983). Joint book reading as a multiple vocabulary acquisition device. *Developmental Psychology, 19,* 445–451.

Ninio, A., & Bruner, J. S. (1978). The achievements and antecedents of labelling. *Journal of Child Language, 5,* 1–16.

Nippold, M. A. (1985). Comprehension of figurative language in youth. *Topics in Language Disorders, 5*(3), 1–20.

Nippold, M. A. (1986). Verbal analogical reasoning in children and adolescents. *Topics in Language Disorders, 6*(4), 51–63.

Nippold, M. A. (1988a). Figurative language. In M. A. Nippold (Ed.), *Later language development: Ages nine through nineteen* (pp. 179–210). Austin, TX: Pro-Ed.

Nippold, M. A. (1988b). Introduction. In M. A. Nippold (Ed.), *Later language development: Ages nine through nineteen* (pp. 1–10). Austin, TX: Pro-Ed.

Nippold, M. A. (1988c). The literate lexicon. In M. A. Nippold (Ed.), *Later language development: Ages nine through nineteen* (pp. 29–47). Austin, TX: Pro-Ed.

Nippold, M. A. (1988d). Verbal reasoning. In M. A. Nippold (Ed.), *Later language development: Ages nine through nineteen* (pp. 159–177). Austin, TX: Pro-Ed.

Nippold, M. A. (1988e). Figurative language. In M. A. Nippold (Ed.), *Later language development: Ages nine through nineteen* (pp. 179–210). Austin, TX: Pro-Ed.

Nippold, M. A. (1991). Evaluating and enhancing idiom comprehension in language-disordered students. *Language, Speech, and Hearing Services in Schools, 22,* 100–106.

Nippold, M. A. (1995). School-age children and adolescents: Norms for word definition. *Language, Speech, and Hearing Services in Schools, 26,* 320–325.

Nippold, M. A., Erskine, B. A., & Freed, D. B. (1988). Proportional and functional analogical reasoning in normal and language-impaired children. *Journal of Speech and Hearing Disorders, 53,* 440–448.

Nippold, M. A., & Fey, S. H. (1983). Metaphoric understanding in preadolescents having a history of language acquisition difficulties. *Language, Speech, and Hearing Services in Schools, 14,* 171–180.

Nippold, M. A., & Haq, F. S. (1996). Proverb comprehension in youths: The role of concreteness and familiarity. *Journal of Speech and Hearing Research, 39,* 166–176.

Nippold, M. A., Leonard, L. B., & Anastopoulos, A. (1982). Development in the use and understanding of polite forms in children. *Journal of Speech and Hearing Research, 25,* 193–202.

Nippold, M. A., & Martin, S. T. (1989). Idiom interpretation in isolation versus context: A developmental study with adolescents. *Journal of Speech and Hearing Research, 32,* 59–66.

Nippold, M. A., & Rudzinski, M. (1993). Familiarity and transparency in idiom explanation: A developmental study of children and adolescents. *Journal of Speech and Hearing Research, 36,* 728–737.

Nippold, M. A., Schwarz, I. E., & Lewis, M. (1992). Analyzing the potential benefit of microcomputer use for teaching figurative language. *American Journal of Speech-Language Pathology, 1*(2), 36–43.

Nippold, M. A., & Taylor, C. (1995). Idiom understanding in youth: Further examination of familiarity and transparency. *Journal of Speech and Hearing Research, 36,* 728–737.

Nisbett, R. E., & Wilson, T. D. (1977). The halo effect: Evidence for unconscious alteration of judgements. *Journal of Personality and Social Psychology, 35,* 250–256.

Nordenbrock, D. C. (1995). *Development in drawing and language of young children with hearing impairments.* Unpublished master's thesis, Western Michigan University, Kalamazoo, MI.

Norlin, P. F. (1986). Familiar faces, sudden strangers: Helping families cope with the crisis of aphasia. In R. Chapey (Ed.), *Language intervention strategies in adult aphasia* (pp. 174–186). Baltimore, MD: Williams & Wilkins.

Norman, J. B. (1983, November). *A holistic treatment approach to elective mutism.* Paper presented at the Annual Conference of the American Speech-Language-Hearing Association, Cincinnati, OH.

Norris, J. A. (1988). Using communication strategies to enhance reading acquisition. *The Reading Teacher, 47,* 668–673.

Norris, J. A. (1989). Providing language remediation in the classroom: An integrated language-to-reading intervention method. *Language, Speech, and Hearing Services in Schools, 20,* 205–218.

Norris, J. A. (1995). Expanding language norms for school-age children and adolescents: Is it pragmatic? *Language, Speech, and Hearing Services in Schools, 26,* 342–352.

Norris, J. A., & Bruning, R. H. (1988). Cohesion in the narratives of good and poor readers. *Journal of Speech and Hearing Research, 53,* 416–424.

Norris, J. A., & Damico, J. S. (1990). Whole language in theory and practice: Implications for language intervention. *Language, Speech, and Hearing Services in Schools, 21,* 212–220.

Norris, J. A., & Hoffman, P. R. (1990a). Comparison of adult-initiated vs. child-initiated interaction styles with handicapped pre-language children. *Language, Speech, and Hearing Services in Schools, 21,* 28–36.

Norris, J. A., & Hoffman, P. R. (1990b). Language intervention within naturalistic environments. *Language, Speech, and Hearing Services in Schools, 21,* 72–84.

Norris, J., & Hoffman, P. (1993). *Whole language intervention for school-age children.* San Diego: Singular Publishing Group.

Northcott, W. H. (Ed.). (1977). *Curriculum guide: Hearing impaired children—birth to three years—and their parents* (rev. ed.). Washington, DC: A. G. Bell Association for the Deaf.

Northern, J. L., & Downs, M. P. (1984). *Hearing in children* (3rd ed.). Baltimore, MD: Williams & Wilkins.

Northern, J. L., & Downs, M. P. (1991). *Hearing in children* (4th ed.). Baltimore, MD: Williams & Wilkins.

Nye, C., & Montgomery, J. K. (1989, Spring). Identification criteria for language disordered children: A national survey. *Hearsay* (Journal of the Ohio Speech and Hearing Association), *Spring,* 26–33.

Nystrand, M. (Ed.). (1982). *What writers know: The language, process, and structure of written discourse.* New York: Academic Press.

O'Brien, M. A., & O'Leary, T. S. (1988). Evolving to the classroom model: Speech-language service for the mentally retarded. *Seminars in Speech and Language, 9,* 355–366.

O'Connor, L., & Eldridge, P. (1981). *Communication disorders in adolescence: Program planning, diagnostics, and practical remediation techniques.* Springfield, IL: Charles C. Thomas.

Odell, L. (1981). Defining and assessing competence in writing. In C. R. Cooper (Ed.), *The nature and measurement of competency in English* (pp. 95–138). Urbana, IL: National Council of Teachers of English.

Odom, S. L., & Karnes, M. B. (Eds.). (1988). *Early intervention for infants and children with handicaps.* Baltimore: Paul H. Brookes.

Odom, S. L., & Warren, S. F. (1988). Early childhood education in the year 2000. *Journal of the Division for Early Childhood, 12,* 262–273.

O'Donnell, K. J., & Oehler, J. M. (1989). Neurobehavioral assessment of the newborn infant. In D. B. Bailey, Jr. & M. Wolery (Eds.), *Assessing infants and preschoolers with handicaps* (pp. 167–201). Columbus, OH: Merrill.

O'Donnell, R. C., Griffin, W. J., & Norris, R. D. (1967). *Syntax of kindergarten and elementary school children: A transformational analysis.* (Research Report No. 8). Champaign, IL: National Council of Teachers of English.

Oetting, J. B., Rice, M. L., & Swank, L. K. (1995). Quick incidental learning (QUIL) of words by school-age children with and without SLI. *Journal of Speech and Hearing Research, 38,* 434–445.

Office of Special Education and Rehabilitative Services, U. S. Department of Education. (1989, Summer). Community integration: The next step. *OSERS News in Print!,* p. 1.

Oller, D. K. (1978). Infant vocalization and the development of speech. *Allied Health and Behavioral Sciences, 1,* 523–549.

Oller, D. K. (1980). The emergence of sounds of speech in infancy. In G. Yeni-Komshian, J. F. Kavanagh, & C. A. Ferguson (Eds.), *Child phonology: Production* (Vol. 1, pp. 93–112). New York: Academic Press.

Oller, D. K., Eilers, R., Bull, D., & Carney, A. (1985). Prespeech vocalizations of a deaf infant: A comparison with normal metaphonological development. *Journal of Speech and Hearing Research, 28,* 47–63.

Oller, D. K., Jensen, H., & Lafayette, R. (1978). The relatedness of phonological processes of a hearing impaired child. *Journal of Communication Disorders, 11,* 97–105.

Olson, C., & Bennett, C. W. (1987a, March). *Regional differences in receptive and expressive vocabulary skills of normal children.* Paper presented at the meeting of the Speech and Hearing Association of Virginia, Roanoke, VA.

Olson, C., & Bennett, C. W. (1987b, March). *Referential semantic analysis: Test-retest reliability.* Paper presented at the meeting of the Speech and Hearing Association of Virginia, Roanoke, VA.

Olswang, L. B., & Bain, B. A. (1991). Treatment efficacy: When to recommend intervention. *Language, Speech, and Hearing Services in Schools, 22,* 255–263.

Olswang, L. B., & Bain, B. A. (1996). Assessment information for predicting upcoming change in language production. *Journal of Speech and Hearing Research, 39,* 414–423.

Olswang, L. B., Bain, B. A., & Johnson, G. A. (1992). Using dynamic assessment with children with language disorders. In S. Warren & J. Reichle (Eds.), *Causes and effects in communication and language intervention* (pp. 187–216). Baltimore, MD: Paul H. Brookes.

Olswang, L. B., Bain, B. A., Rosendahl, P. D., Oblak, S. B., & Smith, A. E. (1986). Language learning: Moving performance from a context-dependent to -independent state. *Child Language Teaching and Therapy, 2,* 180–210.

Olswang, L., & Carpenter, R. (1978). Elicitor effects on the language obtained from language-impaired children. *Journal of Speech and Hearing Disorders, 43,* 76–88.

Olswang, L. B., & Carpenter, L. B. (1982a). The ontognesis of agent: Cognitive notion. *Journal of Speech and Hearing Research, 25,* 297–306.

Olswang, L. B., & Carpenter, L. B. (1982b). The ontognesis of agent: Linguistic expression. *Journal of Speech and Hearing Research, 25,* 306–314.

Olswang, L., Stoel-Gammon, C., Coggins, T., & Carpenter, R. (1987). *Assessing linguistic behaviors: Assessing prelinguistic and early linguistic behaviors in developmentally young children.* Seattle, WA: University of Washington Press.

O'Neil, W. (1990). Dealing with bad ideas: Twice is less. *English Journal, 79*(4), 80–88.

O'Neill, T. J. (1987). Foreword: The person comes first. In S. M. Pueschel, C. Tingey, J. E. Rynders, A. C. Crocker, & D. M. Crutcher (Eds.), *New perspectives on Down syndrome* (pp. xviii-xix). Baltimore: Paul H. Brookes.

Ornitz, E., & Ritvo, E. (1976). The syndrome of autism: A critical review. *The American Journal of Psychiatry, 133,* 609–621.

Orr, E. W. (1987). *Twice as less: Black English and the performance of Black students in mathematics and science.* New York: Norton.

Orton, S. (1937). *Reading, writing, and speech problems in children.* New York: Norton.

Osberger, M. J. (1986). Introduction. In M. J. Osberger (Ed.), *Language and learning skills of hearing-impaired students* (pp. 3–5). *ASHA Monographs No. 23.* Rockville, MD: American Speech-Language-Hearing Association.

Osgood, C. E. (1967). The nature of meaning. In J. P. DeCecco (Ed.), *The psychology of language, thought, and instruction* (pp. 156–164). New York: Holt, Rinehart, & Winston.

Osgood, C. E. (1968). Toward a wedding of insufficiencies. In T. R. Dixon & D. L. Horton (Eds.), *Verbal behavior and general behavior theory* (pp. 495–519). Englewood Cliffs, NJ: Prentice-Hall.

Osgood, C. E., & Miron, M. S. (1963). *Approaches to the study of aphasia.* Urbana, IL: University of Illinois Press.

Osofsky, J. D. (1990). Risk and protective factors for teenage mothers and their infants. *Newsletter of the Society for Research in Child Development, Winter,* 1–2.

Owens, R. E., Jr. (1988). *Language development: An introduction* (2nd ed.). Columbus, OH: Merrill/Macmillan.

Owens, R. E., Jr. (1989). Mental retardation: Difference or delay? In D. K. Bernstein & E. Tiegerman (Eds.), *Language and communication disorders in children* (2nd ed.) (pp. 229–297). Columbus, OH: Merrill.

Owens, R. E., Jr. (1992). *Language development: An introduction* (3rd ed.). Columbus, OH: Merrill/Macmillan.

Owens, R. E., Jr. (1996). Language development: An introduction (4th ed.). Boston: Allyn and Bacon.

Padgett, S. Y. (1988). Speech- and language-impaired three and four year olds: A five year follow-up study. In R. L. Masland & M. W. Masland (Eds.), *Preschool prevention of reading failure* (pp. 52–77). Parkton, MD: York Press.

Page, J. L., & Stewart, S. R. (1985). Story grammar skills in school-age children. *Topics in Language Disorders, 5*(2), 16–30.

Paley, V. G. (1981). *Wally's stories: Conversations in the kindergarten.* Cambridge, MA: Harvard University Press.

Paley, V. G. (1990). *The boy who would be a helicopter.* Cambridge, MA: Harvard University Press.

Paley, V. G. (1992). *You can't say you can't play.* Cambridge, MA: Harvard University Press.

Paley, V. G. (1994). Every child a storyteller. In J. F. Duchan, L. E. Hewitt, and R. M. Sonnenmeier (Eds.), *Pragmatics: From theory to practice* (pp. 10–19). Englewood Cliffs, NJ: Prentice Hall.

Palincsar, A. S., & Brown, D. (1984). Reciprocal teaching of comprehension-fostering and comprehension-monitoring activities. *Cognition and Instruction, 1,* 117–175.

Palinscar, A. S., & Brown, D. (1987). Enhancing instructional time through attention to metacognition. *Journal of Learning Disabilities, 20,* 66–75.

Palincsar, A. S., Brown, A. L., & Campione, J. C. (1994). Models and practices of dynamic assessment. In G. P. Wallach & K. G. Butler (Eds.), *Language learning disabilities in school-age children and adolescents* (pp. 132–144). Boston: Allyn and Bacon.

Palincsar, A. S., & Ransom, K. (1988). From the mystery spot to the thoughtful spot: The instruction of metacognitive strategies. *The Reading Teacher, 41,* 784–789.

Panagos, J. M., & Prelock, P. A. (1982). Phonological constraints on the sentence productions of language-disordered children. *Journal of Speech and Hearing Research, 25,* 171–177.

Pang, D. (1985). In M. Ylvisaker (Ed.), *Head injury rehabilitation: Children and adolescents* (pp. 3–70). Austin, TX: Pro-Ed.

Papanicolaou, A. C., DiScenna, A., Gillespie, L., & Aram, D. M. (1990). Probe evoked potential findings following unilateral left hemisphere lesions in children. *Archives of Neurology, 47,* 562–566.

Parker, F. (1986). *Linguistics for non-linguists.* Boston: College-Hill, A division of Little, Brown, & Company.

Parmar, R. S., Cawley, J. F., & Frazita, R. R. (1996). Word problem-solving by students with and without mild disabilities. *Exceptional Children, 62,* 415–429.

Pascual-Leone, J. (1969). *Cognitive development and cognitive style.* Unpublished doctoral dissertation, University of Geneva.

Pascual-Leone, J. (1984). Attentional, dialectic, and mental effort. In M. L. Commons, F. A. Richards, & C. Armon (Eds.), *Beyond formal operations.* New York: Plenum.

Paul, L. (1985). Programming peer support for functional language. In S. F. Warren, & A. K. Rogers-Warren (Eds)., *Teaching functional language* (pp. 289–307). Baltimore, MD: University Park Press.

Paul, R. (1981). In J. Miller (Ed.)., *Assessing language production in children: Experimental procedures.* Baltimore, MD: University Park Press.

Paul, R. (1990). Comprehension strategies: Interactions between world knowledge and the development of sentence comprehension. *Topics in Language Disorders, 10*(3), 63–75.

Pearl, L. F. (1993). Providing family-centered early intervention. In W. Brown, S. K. Thurman, & L. F. Pearl (Eds.), *Family-centered early intervention with infants and toddlers: Innovative cross-disciplinary approaches* (pp. 81–101). Baltimore, MD: Paul H. Brookes.

Pease, D. M., Gleason, J. B., & Pan, B. A. (1989). Gaining meaning: Semantic development. In J. B. Gleason (Ed.), *The development of language* (2nd ed.) (pp. 101–134). Columbus, OH: Merrill.

Pehrsson, R. S., & Denner, P. R. (1988). Semantic organizers: Implications for reading and writing. *Topics in Language Disorders, 8*(3), 24–37.

Peña, E., Quinn, R., & Iglesias, A. (1992). The application of dynamic methods to language assessment: A non-biased procedure. *Journal of Special Education, 26*(3), 269–280.

Perera, K. (1984). *Children's writing and reading.* London: Blackwell.

Peters, A. (1977). Does the whole equal the sum of the parts? *Language, 53,* 560–573.

Peterson, C. & McCabe, A. (1983). *Developmental psycholinguistics: Three ways of looking at a child's narrative.* New York: Plenum Press.

Pettito, L. A. (1994). Modularity and constraints in early lexical acquisition: Evidence from children's early language and gesture. In P. Bloom (Ed.), *Language acquisition* (pp. 95–126). Cambridge, MA: The MIT Press. (Reprinted from *Minnesota Symposium in Child Psychology, 25,* 1992, Lawrence Erlbaum Associates).

Petitto, L. A., & Marentette, P. F. (1991). Babbling in the manual mode: Evidence for the ontogeny of language. *Science, 251,* 1493–1496.

Philips, S. U. (1983). *The invisible culture.* New York: Longman, Inc.

Piaget, J. (1926). *The language and thought of the child.* London: Routledge & Kegan Paul.

Piaget, J. (1952). *The origins of intelligence in children.* New York: International Universities Press.

Piaget, J. (1962). *Play, dreams, and imitation in childhood.* London: Routledge & Kegan Paul.

Piaget, J. (1964). Development and learning. In R. E. Ripple & V. N. Rockcastle (Eds.), *Piaget rediscovered* (pp. 7–20). Ithaca, NY: Cornell School of Education Press.

Piaget, J. (1969). *Psychology of intelligence.* Totowa, NJ: Littlefield, Adams.

Piaget, J. (1970). Piaget's theory. In P. H. Mussen (Ed.), *Carmichael's manual of child psychology* (3rd ed., Vol. 1) (pp. 703–732). New York: John Wiley & Sons.

Piaget, J. (1977). The mission of the idea. Trans. H. E. Gruber & J. J. Von`eche. In H. E. Gruber & J. J. Von`eche (Eds.), *The essential Piaget.* New York: Basic Books.

Piaget, J., & Inhelder, B. (1971). *Mental imagery in the child.* London: Routledge & Kegan Paul.

Piccolo, J. (1987). Expository text structure: Teaching and learning strategies. *The Reading Teacher, 40,* 838–847.

Pickering, M., & Kaelber, P. (1978). The speech-language pathologist and the classroom teacher: A team approach to language development. *Language, Speech, and Hearing Services in Schools, 9,* 43–49.

Pinker, S. (1984). *Language learnability and language development.* Cambridge, MA: Harvard University Press.

Pinker, S. (1987). The bootstrapping problem in language acquisition. In B. MacWhinney (Ed.), *Mechanisms of language acquisition.* Hillsdale, NJ: Erlbaum.

Pinker, S. (1990). *Learnability and cognition: The acquisition of argument structure.* Cambridge, MA: MIT Press.

Pinker, S. (1994). *The language instinct.* New York: William Morrow and Company.

Pitcher, E. G., & Prelinger, E. (1963). *Children tell stories: An analysis of fantasy.* New York: International Universities Press.

Plante, E., Swisher, L., & Vance, R. (submitted). MRI findings in four consecutive cases of specific language impairment. Unpublished manuscript, University of Arizona, at Tucson.

Plante, E., & Vance, R. (1994). Selection of preschool language tests: A data-based approach. *Language, Speech, and Hearing Services in Schools, 25,* 15–25.

Platt, J., & Coggins, T. (1990). Comprehension of social-action games in prelinguistic children: Levels of participation and effect of adult structure. *Journal of Speech and Hearing Disorders, 55,* 315–316.

Poirer, M., Jackson, V., & Boonyasopan, J. (1985). *Focusing on language arts: Figurative language* (Computer program). New York: Random House.

Polani, P. E., Briggs, J. H., Ford, C. E., Clarke, C. M., & Berg, J. M. (1960). A mongol girl with 46 chromosomes. *Lancet, 1,* 1028.

Pollack, D. (1984). An acoupedic program. In D. Ling (Ed.), *Early intervention for hearing impaired children: Oral options* (pp. 181–254). Austin, TX: Pro-Ed.

Pope, A. M., & Tarlov, A. R. (Eds.). (1991). *Disability in America: Toward a national agenda for prevention.* Washington, DC: National Academy Press.

Powers, L. E., & Sowers, J. A. (1994). Transitions to adult living: Promoting natural supports and self-determination. In S. N. Calculator & C. M. Jorgensen (Eds.), *Including students with severe disabilities in schools: Fostering communication, interaction, and participation* (pp. 215–247). San Diego, CA: Singular Publishing Group.

Poyadue, F. (1979). *Visiting parents: Peer counselling training manual.* San Jose, CA: Parents Helping Parents (535 Race St., Suite 20).

Prather, E., Beecher, S., Stafford, M., & Wallace, E. (1980). *Screening Test of Adolescent Language* (STAL). Seattle, WA: University of Washington Press.

Prather, E., Hedrick, D., & Kern, C. (1975). Articulation development in children aged two to four years. *Journal of Speech and Hearing Disorders, 40,* 179–191.

Prelock, P. A., Miller, B. E. L., & Reed, N. L. (1993). *Working with the classroom curriculum: A guide for analysis and use in speech therapy.* San Antonio, TX: Communication Skill Builders.

Premack, D., & Woodruff, G. (1978). Does the chimpanzee have a "theory of mind"? *Behavior and Brain Sciences, 4,* 515–526.

President's Committee on Mental Retardation. (1978). *Mental retardation: The leading edge.* Washington, DC: U.S. Government Printing Office, Pub. No. (OHDS) 79–21018.

Pressley, M., & Harris, K. R. (1990). What we really know about strategy instruction. *Education Leadership, 48*(1), 31–34.

Prizant, B. M. (1983). Language acquisition and communicative behavior in autism: Toward an understanding of the "whole" of it. *Journal of Speech and Hearing Disorders, 48,* 296–307.

Prizant, B. M. (1984). Assessment and intervention of communicative problems in children with autism. *Communication Disorders, 9,* 127–142.

Prizant, B. M. (1987). Theoretical and clinical implications of echolalic behavior in autism. In T. L. Layton (Ed.), *Language and treatment of autistic and developmentally disordered children* (pp. 65–88). Springfield, IL: Charles C. Thomas.

Prizant, B. M., Audet, L. R., Burke, G. M., Hummel, L. J., Maher, S. R., & Theadore, G. (1990). Communication disorders and emotional/behavioral disorders in children and adolescents. *Journal of Speech and Hearing Disorders, 55,* 179–192.

Prizant, B. M., & Duchan, J. F. (1981). The functions of immediate echolalia in autistic children. *Journal of Speech and Hearing Disorders, 46,* 241–249.

Prizant, B. M., & Rydell, P. J. (1984). Analysis of functions of delayed echolalia in autistic children. *Journal of Speech and Hearing Research, 27,* 183–192.

Prizant, B. M., & Rydell, P. J. (1993). Assessment and intervention considerations for unconventional verbal behavior. In J. Reichle & D. P. Wacker (Eds.), *Communicative alternatives to challenging behavior* (pp. 263–297). Baltimore: Paul H. Brookes.

Prizant, B. M., & Wetherby, A. M. (1990). Toward an integrated view of early language and communication development and socioemotional development. *Topics in Language Disorders, 10*(4), 1–16.

Prizant, B. M., Wetherby, A. M., & Rydell, P. J. (1994). Implications of facilitated communication for educational and communication enhancement practices for persons with autism. In H. C. Shane (Ed.), *Facilitated communication: The clinical and social phenomenon* (pp. 123–155). San Diego, CA: Singular Publishing Group.

Proctor, A. (1989). Stages of normal noncry vocal development: A protocol for assessment. *Topics in Language Disorders, 10*(1), 26–42.

Prutting, C., Gallagher, T., & Mulac, A. (1975). The expressive portion of the NSST compared to a spontaneous language sample. *Journal of Speech and Hearing Disorders, 40,* 40–68.

Prutting, C. A. (1982). Pragmatics as social competence. *Journal of Speech and Hearing Disorders, 47,* 123–134.

Prutting, C. A., & Kirchner, D. M. (1987). A clinical appraisal of the pragmatic aspects of language. *Journal of Speech and Hearing Disorders, 52,* 105–119.

Public Law 94–142. (1977, August). Implementation of Part B of the Education of the Handicapped Act. *Federal Register.*

Public Law 99–457. (1986, October). Education of Handicapped Amendments of 1986. *Federal Register.*

Public Law 101–476. (1990). Individuals with Disabilities Education Act (IDEA). *Federal Register.*

Pueschel, S. M. (1987). Health concerns in persons with Down syndrome. In S. M. Pueschel, C. Tingey, J. E. Rynders, A. C. Crocker, & D. M. Crutcher (Eds.), *New perspectives on Down syndrome* (pp. 113–148). Baltimore: Paul H. Brookes.

Purves, A. (1981). Competence in reading. In C. R. Cooper (Ed.), *The nature and measurement of competency in English* (pp. 65–94). Urbana, IL: National Council of Teachers of English.

Quigley, S. P., & Paul, P. V. (1984). *Language and deafness.* Austin, TX: Pro-Ed.

Quigley, S. P., Power, D. J., & Steinkamp, M. W. (1977). The language structure of deaf children. *The Volta Review, 79,* 73–84.

Quigley, S. P., Smith, N. L., & Wilbur, R. B. (1974). Comprehension of relativized sentences by deaf students. *Journal of Speech and Hearing Research, 17,* 325–341.

Ramey, C. T., Trohanis, P. L., & Hostler, S. L. (1982). An introduction. In C. T. Ramey & P. L. Trohanis (Eds.), *Finding and educating high-risk and handicapped infants.* San Antonio, TX: Pro-Ed.

Randall, D., Rynell, J., & Curwen, M. (1974). A study of language development in a sample of three-year-old children. *British Journal of Disorders of Communication, 9,* 3.

Rankin, J. L., Harwood, K., & Mirenda, P. (1994). Influence of graphic symbol use on reading comprehension. *Augmentative and Alternative Communication, 10,* 269–281.

Raphael, T. E. (1982). Question-answer strategies for children. *The Reading Teacher, 36,* 186–190.

Raphael, T. E. (1986). Teaching question-answer relationships, revisited. *The Reading Teacher, 39,* 516–522.

Raphael, T. E., & Pearson, P. D. (1982). *The effects of metacognitive strategy awareness training on students' question answering behavior* (Tech. Rep. No. 238). Urbana, IL: University of Illinois, Center for the Study of Reading.

Rapin, I., & Allen, D. A. (1983). Developmental language disorders: Nosologic consideration. In U. Kirk (Ed.), *Neuropsychology of language, reading, and spelling* (pp. 155–184). Orlando, FL: Academic Press, Inc.

Rapin, I., Mattis, S., Rowan, A. J., & Golden, G. G. (1977). Verbal auditory agnosia in children. *Developmental Medicine and Child Neurology, 19,* 192–207.

Rapport, M., Stoner, G., DuPaul, G., Birmingham, B., & Tucker, S. (1985). Methylphenidate in hyperactive children: Differential effects of dose on academic, learning and social behavior. *Journal of Abnormal Child Psychology, 13,* 227–244.

Ray, H., Sarff, L. S., & Glassford, J. E. (1984, Summer/Fall). Sound field amplification: An innovative educational intervention for mainstreamed learning disabled students. *The Directive Teacher,* 18–20.

Records, N. L., & Tomblin, J. B. (1994). Clinical decision making: Describing the decision rules of practicing speech-language pathologists. *Journal of Speech and Hearing Research, 37,* 144–156.

Records, N. L., Tomblin, J. B., & Freese, P. R. (1992). The quality of life of young adults with histories of specific language impairments. *American Journal of Speech-Language Pathology, 1*(2), 44–53.

Reed, V. A. (1986). Language disordered adolescents. In V. A. Reed (Ed.), *An introduction to children with language disorders* (pp. 228–249). New York: Macmillan Publishing Company.

Rees, N. (1973). Auditory processing factors in language disorders: The view from Procrustes' bed. *Journal of Speech and Hearing Disorders, 38,* 304–315.

Rees, N. (1981). Saying more than we know: Is auditory processing disorder a meaningful concept? In R. Keith (Ed.), *Central auditory and language disorders in children* (pp. 94–120). San Diego, CA: College-Hill Press.

Reichle, J., Mirenda, P., Locke, P., Piché, L., & Johnston, S. (1992). Beginning augmentative communication systems. In S. F. Warren & J. Reichle (Eds.), *Causes and effects in communication and language intervention* (pp. 131–156). Baltimore, MD: Paul H. Brookes.

Reichle, J., & Wacker, D. P. (Eds.). (1993a). *Communicative alternatives to challenging behavior: Integrating functional assessment and intervention strategies.* Baltimore: Paul H. Brookes.

Reichle, J., & Wacker, D. P. (1993b). Functional communication training as an intervention for problem behavior. In J. Reichle & D. P. Wacker (Eds.), *Communicative alternatives to challenging behavior* (pp. 1–8). Baltimore: Paul H. Brookes.

Reichle, J., York, J., & Sigafoos, J. (Eds.). (1991). *Implementing augmentative and alternative communication: Strate-*

gies for learners with severe disabilities. Baltimore, MD: Paul H. Brookes.

Reid, D. K., & Button, L. J. (1995). Anna's story: Narratives of personal experience about being labeled learning disabled. *Journal of Learning Disabilities, 28,* 602–614.

Renfrew, C. E. (1969). *The Bus Story: A test of continuous speech.* (Available from the author at North Place, Old Headington, Oxford, England)

Rescorla, L. (1989). The language development survey: A screening tool for delayed language in toddlers. *Journal of Speech and Hearing Disorders, 54,* 587–599.

Rescorla, L. & Fechnay, T. (1996). Mother-child synchrony and communicative reciprocity in late-talking toddlers. *Journal of Speech and Hearing Research, 39,* 200–208.

Rescorla, L., & Manzella, L. (1990, June). *Toddlers with specific expressive language delay (SELD): Language outcome at age 3.* Paper presented at the 11th annual Symposium for Research on Child Language Disorders, Madison, WI.

Rescorla, L. & Ratner, N. B. (1996). Phonetic profiles of toddlers with specific expressive language impairment (SLI-E). *Journal of Speech and Hearing Research, 39,* 153–165.

Restak, R. M. (1979). *The brain: The last frontier.* New York: Warner Books.

Reveron, W. W. (1984). Language assessment of Black children: The state of the art. *Papers in the Social Sciences, 4,* 79–94.

Reveron, W. W. (in press). Issues in nondiscriminatory assessment of minority populations. In L. T. Cole (Ed.), *Training manual on communication disorders in multicultural populations.* Rockville, MD: American Speech-Language-Hearing Association.

Reynolds, M. C., & Wang, M. C. (1983). Restructuring "special" school programs: A position paper. *Policy Studies Review, 2*(1), 189–212.

Rice, M. L. (1980). *Cognition to language: Categories, word meanings, and training.* Baltimore, MD: University Park Press.

Rice, M. L. (1983). Contemporary accounts of the cognition/language relationship: Implications for speech-language clinicians. *Journal of Speech and Hearing Disorders, 48,* 347–359.

Rice, M. L. (1994). Grammatical categories of children with specific language impairments. In R. V. Watkins & M. L. Rice (Eds.), *Specific language impairments in children* (pp. 69–89). Baltimore, MD: Paul H. Brookes.

Rice, M. L. (1997). Speaking out: Evaluating new training programs for language impairment. *Asha, 39*(3), 13.

Rice, M. L., Buhr, J. C., & Nemeth, M. (1990). Fast mapping word-learning abilities of language-delayed preschoolers. *Journal of Speech and Hearing Disorders, 55,* 33–42.

Rice, M. L. & Oetting, J. B. (1993). Morphological deficits of children with SLI: Evaluation of number marking and agreement. *Journal of Speech and Hearing Research, 36,* 1249–1257.

Rice, M. L., Oetting, J. B., Marquis, J., Bode, J., & Pae, S. (1994). Frequency of input effects on word comprehension of children with specific language impairment. *Journal of Speech and Hearing Research, 37,* 106–122.

Rice, M. L., Sell, M. A., & Hadley, P. A. (1990). The Social Interactive Coding System (SICS): An on-line, clinically relevant descriptive tool. *Language, Speech, and Hearing Services in Schools, 21,* 2–14.

Rice, M. L., & Wexler, K. (1996a). A phenotype of specific language impairment: Extended optional infinitives. In M. L. Rice (Ed.), *Toward a genetics of language* (pp. 215–237). Mahwah, NJ: Erlbaum.

Rice, M. L., & Wexler, K. (1996b). Tense over time: The persistence of optional infinitives in English in children with SLI. In A. Stringfellow, D., Cahana-Amitay, E. Hughes, & A. Zukowski (Eds.), *Proceedings of the 20th annual Boston University Conference on Language Development (Vol 2.),* (pp. 610–621). Boston: Boston University.

Rice, M. L., & Wexler, K. (1996c). Toward tense as a clinical marker of specific language impairment in English-speaking children. *Journal of Speech and Hearing Research, 39,* 1239–1257.

Rice, M. L., Wexler, K., & Cleave, P. L. (1995). Specific language impairment as a period of extended optional infinitive. *Journal of Speech and Hearing Research, 38,* 850–863.

Rich, H. L., & Ross, S. M. (1989). Students' time on learning tasks in special education. *Exceptional Children, 55,* 508–515.

Richardson, J. S., & Morgan, R. F. (1990). *Reading to learn in the content areas.* Belmont, CA: Wadsworth.

Richardson, K., Calnan, M. Essen, J., & Lambert, L. (1976). The linguistic maturity of 11-year-olds: Some analysis of the written composition of children in the National Development Study. *Journal of Child Language, 3,* 99–115.

Richgels, D., McGee, L. M., Lomax, R., & Sheard, C. (1987). Awareness of four text structures: Effects on recall of expository text. *Reading Research Quarterly, 22,* 177–196.

Rie, E., & Rie, H. (1977). Recall, retention and Ritalin. *Journal of Consulting and Clinical Psychology, 45,* 967–972.

Rie, H., Rie, E., & Stewart, S. (1976). Effects of methylphenidate on underachieving children. *Journal of Consulting and Clinical Psychology, 44,* 250–260.

Rief, L. (1990). Finding the value in evaluation: Self-assessment in a middle school classroom. *Educational Leadership, 47*(6), 24–29.

Rimland, B. (1964). *Infantile autism.* New York: Appleton-Century-Crofts.

Ripich, D. N., & Griffith, P. L. (1985, November). *Story structure, cohesion and propositions in learning disabled children.* Paper presented at the meeting of the American Speech-Language-Hearing Association, Washington, DC.

Ritvo, E. R., & Freeman, B. J. (1978). National Society for Autistic Children definition of the syndrome of autism. *Journal of Autism and Childhood Schizophrenia, 8,* 162–167.

Robbins, A. M. (1986). Facilitating language comprehension in young hearing-impaired children. *Topics in Language Disorders, 6*(3), 12–24.

Roberts, J. E., & Crais, E. R. (1989). Assessing communication skills. In D. B. Bailey, Jr. & M. Wolery (Eds.), *Assessing infants and preschoolers with handicaps* (pp. 339–389). Columbus, OH: Merrill.

Roberts, J. E., & Medley, L. P. (1995). Otitis media and speech-language sequelae in young children: Current issues in management. *American Journal of Speech-Language Pathology, 4*(1), 15–24.

Roberts, J., Sanyal, M., Burchinal, M., Collier, A. M., Ramey, C. T., & Henderson, F. W. (1986). Otitis media in early childhood and its relationship to later verbal and academic performance. *Pediatrics, 78,* 423–430.

Robinson, F. P. (1970). *Effective study.* New York: Harper & Row.

Robinson, L. A., & Owens, R. E., Jr. (1995). Clinical notes: Functional augmentative communication and positive behavior change. *Augmentative and Alternative Communication, 11,* 207–211.

Roeser, R. J. (1988). Cochlear implants and tactile aids for the profoundly deaf student. In R. J. Roeser & M. P. Downs (Eds.), *Auditory disorders in school children* (pp. 260–280). New York: Thieme Medical Publishers.

Roeser, R. J., & Downs, M. P. (Eds.). (1988). *Auditory disorders in school children.* New York: Thieme Medical Publishers.

Rogers, S. J., D'Eugenio, D. B., Brown, S. L., Donovan, C. M., & Lynch, E. W. (1981). *Early Intervention Developmental Profile.* Ann Arbor, MI: University of Michigan Press.

Rogers-Warren, A., & Warren, S. (1980). Mands for verbalization: Facilitating the display of newly-taught language. *Behavior Modification, 4,* 361–382.

Rohwer, W. D., Jr., & Dempster, F. N. (1977). Memory development and educational processes. In R. V. Kail & J. W. Hagen (Eds.), *Perspectives on the development of memory and cognition* (pp. 407–435). Hillsdale, NJ: Erlbaum.

Romski, M. A. (1989, May). Two decades of language research with great apes. *Asha, 31,* 81–82,83.

Romski, M. A., Sevcik, R. A., & Pate, J. L. (1988). Establishment of symbolic communication in persons with severe retardation. *Journal of Speech and Hearing Disorders, 53,* 94–107.

Romski, M. A., Sevcik, R. A., Robinson, B., & Bakeman, R. (1994). Adult-directed communications of youth with mental retardation using the system for augmenting language. *Journal of Speech and Hearing Research, 37,* 617–628.

Rosen, C. D., & Gerring, J. P. (1986). *Head trauma: Educational reintegration.* Austin, TX: Pro-Ed.

Rosenbek, J. C., & Wertz, R. T. (1972). A review of 50 cases of developmental apraxia of speech. *Language, Speech, and Hearing Services in Schools, 3,* 23–33.

Rosenberg, J. B., & Lindblad, M. B. (1978). Behavior therapy in a family context: Treating elective mutism. *Family Process, 17,* 77–82.

Rosenthal, R., & Jacobson, L. (1968). *Pygmalion in the classroom: Teacher expectation and pupils' intellectual development.* New York: Holt, Rinehart, & Winston.

Rosenzweig, M. R., & Bennett, E. L. (1976). Enriched environments: Facts, factors, and fantasies. In L. Petrinovitch & J. L. McGaugh (Eds.), *Knowing, thinking, and believing* (pp. 179–213). New York: Plenum Press.

Rosetti, L. (1990). *Infant-Toddler Language Scale.* East Moline, IL: LinguiSystems.

Ross, G. S. (1982). Language functioning and speech development of six children receiving tracheostomy in infancy. *Journal of Communication Disorders, 15,* 95–111.

Ross, M. (1977). Definitions and descriptions. In J. Davis (Ed.), *Our forgotten children: Hard-of-hearing pupils in the schools.* Minneapolis, MN: National Support Systems Project and Division of Personnel Preparation, Bureau of Education for the Handicapped, Department of Health Education, and Welfare.

Ross, M. (1978). Classroom acoustics and speech intelligibility. In J. Katz (Ed.), *Handbook of clinical audiology* (pp. 469–478). Baltimore, MD: Williams & Wilkins.

Ross, M. (1982). *Hard of hearing children in regular schools.* Englewood Cliffs, NJ: Prentice Hall.

Ross, M., & Calvert, D. R. (1973). The semantics of deafness. In W. H. Northcott (Ed.), *The hearing impaired child in a regular classroom.* Washington, DC: The A. G. Bell Association for the Deaf.

Roth, F. P., & Cassatt-James, E. L. (1989). The language assessment process: Clinical implications for individuals with severe speech impairments. *Augmentative and Alternative Communication, 5,* 165–172.

Roth, F. P., & Clark, D. M. (1987). Symbolic play and social participation abilities of language-impaired and normally developing children. *Journal of Speech and Hearing Disorders, 52,* 17–29.

Roth, F. P., & Perfetti, C. A. (1980). A framework for reading, language comprehension, and language disability. *Topics in Language Disorders, 1*(1), 15–27.

Roth, F. P., & Spekman, N. J. (1984). Assessing the pragmatic abilities of children: Part I. Organizational framework and assessment parameters. *Journal of Speech and Hearing Disorders, 49,* 2–11.

Roth, F. P., & Spekman, N. J. (1986). Narrative discourse: Spontaneously generated stories of learning-disabled and normally achieving students. *Journal of Speech and Hearing Disorders, 51,* 8–23.

Roth, F. P., & Spekman, N. J. (1989). Higher-order language processes and reading disabilities. In A. G. Kamhi & H. W. Catts (Eds.), *Reading disabilities: A developmental language perspective* (pp. 159–197). Austin, TX: Pro-Ed.

Ruben, D. (1988, November). Triumph of the heartland: How two mothers and their disabled sons made their Iowa town a beacon for the nation. *Parenting,* 120–126.

Rubin, D. L. (1982). Adapting syntax in writing to varying audiences as a function of age and social cognitive ability. *Journal of Child Language, 9,* 497–510.

Rubin, D. L. (1984). The influence of communicative context on stylistic variation in writing. In A. Pelligrini & T. Yawkey (Eds.), *The development of oral and written language in social contexts* (pp. 213–231). Norwood, NJ: Ablex.

Rubin, D. L. (1987). Divergence and convergence between oral and written communication. *Topics in Language Disorders, 7*(4), 1–18.

Ruder, K., Bunce, B., & Ruder, C. (1984). Language intervention in a preschool classroom setting. In L. McCormick & R. Schiefelbusch (Eds.), *Early language intervention: An introduction* (pp. 267–297). Columbus, OH: Merrill.

Rueda, R. (1989). Defining mild disabilities with language-minority students. *Exceptional Children, 56,* 121–128.

Rumelhart, D. E. (1975). Notes on a schema for stories. In D. G. Bobrow & A. Collins (Eds.), *Representation and understanding: Studies in cognitive science* (pp. 211–236). New York: Academic Press.

Rumelhart, D. E., & McClelland, J. L. (1981). Interactive processing through spreading activation. In A. M. Lesgold & C. A. Perfetti (Eds.), *Interactive processes in reading* (pp. 37–60). Hillsdale, NJ: Erlbaum.

Rumelhart, D. E., & McClelland, J. L. (1994). On learning the past tenses of English verbs. In P. Bloom (Ed.), *Language acquisition* (pp. 423–471). Cambridge, MA: The MIT Press. (Reprinted from *Parallel Distributed Processing,* Vol. 2, 1986, The MIT Press)

Russell, W. K., Quigley, S. P., & Power, D. J. (1976). *Linguistics and deaf children.* Washington, DC: The A. G. Bell Association for the Deaf.

Rutter, M. (1965). Speech disorders in a series of autistic children. In A. W. Franklin (Ed.), *Children with communication problems.* London: Plenum Press.

Rutter, M. (1983). Cognitive deficits in the pathogenesis of autism. *Journal of Child Psychology and Psychiatry, 24,* 513–531.

Rutter, M., Graham, P. J., & Yule, W. (1970). *A neuropsychiatric study in childhood. Clinics in developmental medicine* (No. 35/36). London: S. I. M. P. with Heinemann.

Rutter, M., Tizard, J., & Whitmore, K. (Eds.). (1970). *Education, health, and behavior.* London: Longmans Green.

Rynders, J. E. (1987). History of Down syndrome: The need for a new perspective. In S. M. Pueschel, C. Tingey, J. E. Rynders, A. C. Crocker, & D. M. Crutcher (Eds.), *New perspectives on Down syndrome* (pp. 1–17). Baltimore: Paul H. Brookes.

Sabers, D., & Hutchinson, T. A. (1990). *User norms software.* San Antonio, TX: Special Press, Inc.

Sameroff, A., & Chandler, M. (1975). Reproductive risk and the continuum of caretaking causality. In F. Horowitz (Ed.), *Review of child development research* (Vol. 4). Chicago: University of Chicago Press.

Sameroff, A., & Fiese, B. (1990). Transactional regulation and early intervention. In S. Meisels & P. Shonkoff (Eds.), *Early intervention: A handbook of theory, practice, and analysis.* New York: Cambridge University Press.

Samples, J. M., & Lane, V. W. (1985). Genetic possibilities in six siblings with specific language learning disorders. *Asha, 27*(12), 27–32.

Sandler, A., Coren, A., & Thurman, S. (1983). A training program for parents of handicapped preschool children: Effects upon mother, father, and child. *Exceptional Children, 49,* 355–357.

Sanford, A. R., & Zelman, J. G. (1981). *The Learning Accomplishment Profile.* Winston-Salem, NC: Kaplan.

Sapir, E. (1949). *Language.* New York: Harcourt, Brace, and World.

Sarachan-Deily, A. B., Hopkins, C., & DeVivo, S. (1983). Correlating the DIAL and the BTBC. *Language, Speech, and Hearing Services in Schools, 14,* 54–59.

Sarff, L., Ray, H., & Bagwell, C. (1981). Why not amplification in every classroom? *Hearing Aid Journal, 34*(10), 11, 47–52.

Sattler, J. M. (1988). *Assessment of children* (3rd ed.). San Diego:Author.

Satz, P., & Bullard-Bates, C. (1981). Acquired aphasia in children. In M. T. Sarno (Ed.), *Acquired aphasia* (pp. 399–426). New York: Academic Press.

Satz, P., & Morris, R. (1981). Learning disability subtypes: A review. In F. J. Pirozzolo & M. C. Wittrock (Eds.), *Neuropsychological and cognitive processes in reading* (pp. 109–141). New York: Academic Press.

Saville-Troike, M. (1993). Anthropological considerations in the study of communication. In O. L. Taylor (Ed.), *Nature of communication disorders in culturally and linguistically diverse populations* (pp. 47–72). San Diego, CA: College-Hill Press.

Sawyer, D. J., Dougherty, C., Shelly, M., & Spaanenburg, L. (1985). Auditory segmenting performance and reading acquisition. In C. S. Simon (Ed.), *Communication skills and classroom success: Assessment of language-learning disabled students* (pp. 375–400). San Diego, CA: College-Hill Press.

Scarborough, H. S., & Dobrich, W. (1985). Illusory recovery from language delay. *Proceedings of the Symposium on Research in Child Language Disorders, 6,* 90–99.

Scarborough, H. S., & Dobrich, W. (1990). Development of children with early language delay. *Journal of Speech and Hearing Disorders, 33,* 70–83.

Schaeffer, A. L., Zigmond, N., Kerr, M. M., & Farra, H. E. (1990). Helping teenagers develop school survival skills. *Teaching Exceptional Children, 23*(1), 6–9.

Schaffer, R. (Ed.). (1977). *Mothering.* Cambridge, MA: Harvard University Press.

Schairer, K. S., & Nelson, N. W. (1996). Communicative possibilities of written conversations with adolescents who have autism. *Child Language Teaching and Therapy, 12,* 164–180.

Schein, E. (1978). The role of the consultant: Content expert or process facilitator? *Personnel and Guidance Journal, 6,* 339–343.

Scherer, N. J., & Olswang, L. B. (1989). Using structured discourse as a language intervention technique with autistic children. *Journal of Speech and Hearing Disorders, 54,* 383–394.

Schery, T. K. (1985). Correlates of language development in language disordered children. *Journal of Speech and Hearing Disorders, 50,* 73–83.

Schickedanz, J. A. (1989). The place of specific skills in preschool and kindergarten. In D. S. Strickland & L. M. Morrow (Eds.), *Emerging literacy: Young children learn to read and write* (pp. 96–106). Newark, DE: International Reading Association.

Schiff-Myers, N. (1983). From pronoun reversals to correct pronoun usage: A case study of a normally developing child. *Journal of Speech and Hearing Disorders, 48,* 394–402.

Schildroth, A. N., & Karchmer, M. A. (Eds.). (1986). *Deaf children in America.* Austin, TX: Pro-Ed (formerly College-Hill).

Schirmer, B. R. (1989). Framework for using a language acquisition model in assessing semantic and syntactic development and planning instructional goals for hearing-impaired children. *The Volta Review, 91,* 87–94.

Schlesinger, H. S., & Meadow, K. P. (1972). *Sound and sign: Childhood deafness and mental health.* Berkeley: University of California Press.

Schlesinger, I. M. (1981). Semantic assimilation in the development of relational categories. In H. Whitaker & H. A. Whitaker (Eds.), *Studies in neurolinguistics* (pp. 1–58). New York: Academic Press.

Schneider, P. (1996). Effects of pictures versus orally presented stories on story retellings by children with language impairment. *American Journal of Speech-Language Pathology, 5*(1), 86–96.

Schneider, P., & Watkins, R. V. (1996). Applying Vygotskian developmental theory to language intervention. *Language, Speech, and Hearing Services in Schools, 27,* 157–170.

Schopler, E., & Mesibov, G. B. (Eds.). (1985). *Communication problems in autism.* New York: Plenum Press.

Schopler, E., & Mesibov, G. (Eds). (1986). *Social behavior in autism.* New York: Plenum Press.

Schory, M. E. (1990). Whole language and the speech-language pathologist. *Language, Speech, and Hearing Services in Schools, 21,* 206–211.

Schrag, J. (public letter, August, 1990) (Reprinted in *Governmental Affairs Review,* December, 1991, Rockville, MD: American Speech-Language-Hearing Association).

Schreibman, L. (1988). *Autism* (Vol. 15 in Developmental Clinical Psychology and Psychiatry series). Newbury Park, CA: Sage Publications, Inc.

Schuler, A. L., & Goetz, C. (1981). The assessment of severe language disabilities: Communicative and cognitive considerations. *Analysis and Intervention in Developmental Disabilities, 1,* 333–346.

Schumaker, J. B., & Deshler, D. D. (1984). Setting demand variables: A major factor in program planning for the LD adolescent. *Topics in Language Disorders, 4*(2), 22–40.

Schumaker, J., Deshler, D., Alley, G., & Warner, M. (1983). Toward the development of an intervention model for learning disabled adolescents: The University of Kansas Institute. *Exceptional Education Quarterly, 4,* 45–74.

Schumaker, J. B., Deshler, D. D., Alley, G. R, Warner, M. M., & Denton, P. H. (1982). Multipass: A learning strategy for improving reading comprehension. *Learning Disability Quarterly, 5,* 295–304.

Schumaker, J. B., Sheldon-Wildgen, J., & Sherman, J. A. (1980). *An observational study of the academic and social behaviors of learning disabled adolescents in the regular classroom.* (Research Report No. 22). Lawrence, KS: University of Kansas Institute for Research in Learning Disabilities.

Schwartz, R., & Leonard, L. (1982). Do children pick and choose? An examination of phonological selection and avoidance in early lexical acquisition. *Journal of Child Language, 9,* 319–336.

Schwartz, R., & Leonard, L. (1984). Words, objects, and actions in early lexical acquisition. *Journal of Speech and Hearing Research, 27,* 119–127.

Schwartz, L., & McKinley, N. K. (1984). *Daily communication: Strategies for the language disordered adolescent.* Eau Claire, WI: Thinking Publications.

Scinto, L. (1986). *Written language and psychological development.* Boston: Academic Press.

Scott, C. M. (1984). *What happened in that: Structural characteristics of school children's narratives.* Paper presented at the Annual Convention of the American Speech-Language-Hearing Association, San Francisco, CA.

Scott, C. M. (1988a). A perspective on the evaluation of school children's narratives. *Language, Speech, and Hearing, Services in Schools, 19,* 67–82.

Scott, C. M. (1988b). Spoken and written syntax. In M. A. Nippold (Ed.), *Later language development: Ages nine through nineteen* (pp. 49–95). Austin, TX: Pro-Ed.

Scott, C. M. (1988c). Producing complex sentences. *Topics in Language Disorders, 8*(2), 44–62.

Scott, C. M. (1989). Problem writers: Nature, assessment, and intervention. In A. G. Kamhi & H. W. Catts (Eds.), *Reading disabilities: A developmental language perspective* (pp. 303–344). Austin, TX: Pro-Ed.

Scott, C. M. (1994). A discourse continuum for school-age students: Impact of modality and genre. In G. P. Wallach & K. G. Butler (Eds.), *Language learning disabilities in school-age children and adolescents* (pp. 219–252). Boston: Allyn and Bacon.

Scott, C. M. (1995). Syntax for school-age children: A discourse perspective. In M. E. Fey, J. Windsor, & S. F. Warren (Eds.), *Language intervention: Preschool through the elementary years* (pp. 107–143). Baltimore, MD: Paul H. Brookes.

Scott, C. M., & Stokes, S. L. (1995). Measures of syntax in school-age children and adolescents. *Language, Speech, and Hearing Services in Schools, 26,* 309–319.

Scribner, S., & Cole, M. (1978). Literacy without schooling: Testing for intellectual effects. *Harvard Educational Review, 48,* 448–461.

Scribner, S., & Cole, M. (1980). Literacy without schooling: Testing for intellectual effects. In M. Wolf, M. K. McQuillan, & E. Radwin (Eds.), *Thought and language/Language and reading* (pp. 382–395). Reprint Series No. 14. Cambridge: Harvard Educational Review. (Reprinted from *Harvard Educational Review,* 1978, 48, 448–461.)

Scruggs, T. E., & Mastropieri, M. A. (1990). Mnemonic instruction for students with learning disabilities: What it is and what it does. *Learning Disability Quarterly, 13,* 271–280.

Searle, J. R. (1969). *Speech acts.* Cambridge, England: Cambridge University Press.

Searle, J. R. (1975). Indirect speech acts. In P. Cole & J. L. Morgan (Eds.), *Syntax and semantics 3: Speech acts* (pp. 59–82). New York: Academic Press.

Searle, J. R. (1976). The classification of illocutionary acts. *Language in Society, 5,* 1–24.

Seashore, H. G. (1955). Methods of expressing test scores. *Test Service Bulletin,* No. 48. (Reprinted in W. A. Mehrens (Ed.). (1976). *Readings in Measurement and evaluation in education and psychology* (pp. 65–72). New York: Holt, Rinehart, & Winston.)

Seidel, U. P., Chadwick, O., & Rutter, M. (1975). Psychological disorders in crippled children with and without brain damage. *Developmental Medicine and Child Neurology, 17,* 563–573.

Seidenberg, P. L. (1988). Cognitive and academic instructional intervention for learning disabled adolescents. *Topics in Language Disorders, 8*(3), 56–71.

Seidenberg, P. L., & Bernstein, D. K. (1986). The comprehension of similes and metaphors by learning-disabled and nonlearning-disabled children. *Language, Speech, and Hearing Services in Schools, 17,* 219–229.

Seligman, M. (1975). *Helplessness: On depression, development and death.* San Francisco, CA: W. H. Freeman.

Seliger, H. W., Krashen, S. D., & Ladefoged, P. (1975). Maturational constraints on acquisition of second language accents. *Language Sciences, 36,* 20–22.

Semel, E. (1976). *Semel auditory processing program.* Chicago: Follett Publishing Company.

Semel, E., & Wiig, E. (1980). *Clinical evaluation of language functions.* Columbus, OH: Merrill.

Semel, E., Wiig, E. H., & Secord, W. (1987). *Clinical evaluation of language fundamentals* (revised ed.). San Antonio, TX: The Psychological Corporation.

Semel, E., Wiig, E. H., & Secord, W. (1995). *Clinical evaluation of language fundamentals* (3rd ed.). San Antonio, TX: The Psychological Corporation.

Seymour, H. N. (1986). Clinical intervention for language disorders among nonstandard speakers of English. In O. L. Taylor (Ed.), *Treatment of communication disorders in culturally and linguistically diverse populations* (pp. 135–153). Austin, TX: Pro-Ed.

Seymour, H. N. (1992). The invisible children: A reply to Lahey's perspective. *Journal of Speech and Hearing Disorders, 56,* 640–641.

Shaffer, D. (1985). *Developmental psychology.* Monterey, CA: Brooks/Cole.

Shaffer, D., Bijur, P., Chadwick, O. F. D., & Rutter, M. (1980). Head injury and later reading disability. *Journal of the American Academy of Child Psychiatry, 19,* 592–610.

Shane, H. (Ed.). (1994). *Facilitated communication: The clinical and social phenomenon.* San Diego, CA: The Singular Publishing Group.

Shapiro, H. R. (1992). Debatable issues underlying whole-language philosophy: A speech-language pathologist's perspective. *Language, Speech, and Hearing Services in Schools, 23,* 308–311.

Shapiro, N. Z., & Anderson, R. (1985). Toward an ethics and etiquette for electronic mail. National Science Foundation Report. (Cited in "Stop reading my e-mail!" *Academic Technology,* Vol. 1, No. 3, Nov. 28, 1988.)

Shepard, N. T., Davis, J. M., Gorga, M. P., & Stelmachowicz, P. G. (1981). Characteristics of hearing-impaired children in the public schools: Part I—Demographic data. *Journal of Speech and Hearing Disorders, 46,* 123–129.

Shiff-Myers, N. B. (1983). From pronoun reversals to correct pronoun usage: A case study of a normally developing child. *Journal of Speech and Hearing Disorders, 48,* 394–402.

Shinn, M. R. (Ed.). (1989). *Curriculum-based measurement: Assessing special children.* New York: Guilford Press.

Shriberg, L. D., & Kwiatkowski, J. (1980). *Natural process analysis (NPA).* New York: John Wiley & Sons.

Shriberg, L. D., & Kwiatkowski, J. (1982a). Phonological disorders I: A diagnostic classification system. *Journal of Speech and Hearing Disorders, 47,* 226–241.

Shriberg, L. D., & Kwiatkowski, J. (1982b). Phonological disorders II: A conceptual framework for management. *Journal of Speech and Hearing Disorders, 47,* 242–256.

Shriberg, L. D., & Kwiatkowski, J. (1982c). Phonological disorders III: A procedure for assessing severity of involvement. *Journal of Speech and Hearing Disorders, 47,* 256–270.

Siegel, G. M., Cooper, M., Morgan, J. L., & Brenneise-Sarshad, R. (1990). Imitation of intonation by infants. *Journal of Speech and Hearing Research, 33,* 9–15.

Siegel, L. S. (1992). An evaluation of the discrepancy definition of dyslexia. *Journal of Learning Disabilities, 25,* 618–629.

Siegel-Causey, E., Ernst, B., & Guess, D. (1987). Elements of nonsymbolic communication and early interactional processes. In M. Bullis (Ed.), *Communication development in young children with deaf blindness: Literature review III.* Eugene, OR: Communication Skill Center for Young Children with Deaf-Blindness.

Siegel-Causey, E., & Guess, D. (1989). *Enhancing nonsymbolic communication interactions among learners with severe disabilities.* Baltimore, MD: Paul H. Brookes.

Silliman, E. R. (1987). Individual differences in the classroom performance of language-impaired students. *Seminars in Speech and Language, 8*(4), 357–375.

Silliman, E. R. (1995). Issues raised by facilitated communication for theorizing and research on autism: Comments on Duchan's (1993) tutorial. *Journal of Speech and Hearing Research, 38,* 204–206.

Silliman, E. R., & Lamanna, M. L. (1986). Interactional dynamics of turn disruption: Group and individual effects. *Topics in Language Disorders, 6*(2), 28–43.

Silliman, E. R., & Wilkinson, L. C. (1991). *Communicating for learning: Classroom observation and collaboration.* Gaithersburg, MD: Aspen Publishers.

Silliman, E. R., & Wilkinson, L. C. (1994a). Discourse scaffolds for classroom intervention. In G. P. Wallach & K. G. Butler (Eds.), *Language learning disabilities in school-age children and adolescents* (pp. 27–52). Boston: Allyn and Bacon.

Silliman, E. R., & Wilkinson, L. C. (1994b). Observation is more than looking. In G. P. Wallach & K. G. Butler (Eds.), *Language learning disabilities in school-age children and adolescents* (pp. 145–173). Boston: Allyn and Bacon.

Silva, P. A. (1980). The prevalence, stability and significance of language delay in preschool children. *Developmental Medicine and Child Neurology, 22,* 768–777.

Silva, P. A., Kirkland, C., Simpson, A., Stewart, I., & Williams, S. (1982). Some developmental and behavioral problems associated with bilateral otitis media with effusion. *Journal of Learning Disabilities, 15,* 417–421.

Simmons, A. A. (1962). A comparison of type-token ratios of spoken and written language of deaf and hearing children. *Volta Review, 64,* 417–421.

Simon, C., & Fourcin, A. J. (1978). Cross-language study of speech pattern learning. *Journal of the Acoustical Society of America, 63,* 925–935.

Simon, C. S. (1977). Cooperative programming: A partnership between the learning disabilities teacher and the speech-language pathologist. *Language, Speech, and Hearing Services in Schools, 8,* 188–200.

Simon, C. S. (1985). Teaching logical thinking and discussion skills. In C. Simon (Ed.), *Communication skills and classroom success: Therapy methodologies for language-learning disabled students* (pp. 219–237). San Diego: College Hill Press.

Simon, C. S. (1987). Out of the broom closet and into the classroom: The emerging SLP. *Journal of Childhood Communication Disorders, 11,* 41–66.

Simons, R. (1987). *After the tears: Parents talk about raising a child with a disability.* San Diego, CA: Harcourt, Brace, Jovanovich.

Singer, H., & Ruddell, R. B. (Eds.). (1985). *Theoretical models and processes of reading* (3rd ed.). Newark, DE: International Reading Association.

Singer, S., & Singer, J. (1977). *Partners in play.* New York: Harper & Row.

Sitnick, V. N., Rushmer, N., & Arpan, R. (1982). *Parent-infant communication: A program of clinical and home training for parents and hearing impaired infants* (rev. ed.). Portland, OR: IHR Publications, Good Samaritan Hospital and Medical Center.

Skarakis-Doyle, E., MacLellan, N., & Mullin, K. (1990). Nonverbal indicants of comprehension monitoring in language-disordered children. *Journal of Speech and Hearing Disorders, 55,* 461–467.

Skarakis-Doyle, E., & Mullin, K. (1990). Comprehension monitoring in language-disordered children: A preliminary investigation of cognitive and linguistic factors. *Journal of Speech and Hearing Disorders, 55,* 700–705.

Skinner, B. F. (1957). *Verbal behavior.* New York: Appleton-Century-Crofts.

Skinner, B. F. (1983). *A matter of consequences.* New York: Albert A. Knopf.

Skinner, M. W. (1978). The hearing of speech during language acquisition. *Otolaryngology Clinics of North America, 11,* 631–650.

Slater, W. H., & Graves, M. F. (1989). Research on expository text: Implications for teachers. In K. D. Muth (Ed.), *Children's comprehension of text* (pp. 140–166). Newark, DE: International Reading Association.

Slavin, R. E. (1983). *Cooperative learning.* New York: Longman.

Slingerland, B. H. (1981). Specific language disability: Some general characteristics. In *Slingerland multi-sensory approach to language arts for specific language disability children in the primary grades.* Cambridge, MA: Educators Publishing Service.

Sloan, C. (1986). *Treating auditory processing difficulties in children.* Austin, TX: Pro-Ed.

Sloane, H., & MacAulay, B. (Eds.). (1968). *Operant procedures in remedial speech and language training.* Boston: Houghton Mifflin.

Slobin, D. (1979). *Psycholinguistics* (2nd ed.). Glenview, IL: Scott, Foresman.

Smith v. Robinson, 104 S. Ct. 3457 (1984).

Smith, C. (1970). An experimental approach to children's linguistic competence. In J. Hayes (Ed.), *Cognition and the development of language.* New York: John Wiley & Sons.

Smith, F. (1973). *Psycholinguistics and reading.* New York: Holt, Rinehart, & Winston.

Smith, F. (1975). *Comprehension and learning: A conceptual framework for teachers.* New York: Holt, Rinehart, & Winston.

Smith, P. L., & Friend, M. (1986). Training learning disabled adolescents in a strategy for using text structure to aid recall of instructional prose. *Learning Disabilities Research, 2,* 38–44.

Smitherman, G. (1985). "What go round come round": King in perspective. In C. K. Brooks (Ed.), *Tapping potential: English and language arts for the Black learner.* Urbana, IL: National Council of Teachers of English.

Snow, C. E. (1977a). The development of conversation between mothers and babies. *Journal of Child Language, 4,* 1–22.

Snow, C. E. (1977b). Mothers' speech research: From input to interaction. In C. E. Snow & C. A. Ferguson (Eds.), *Talking to children: Language input and acquisition* (pp. 31–49). Cambridge: Cambridge University Press.

Snow, C. E. (1983). Literacy and language: Relationships during the preschool years. *Harvard Educational Review, 53*(2), 165–189.

Snow, C. E. (Ed.). (1984). *Language development and disorders in the social context.* An issue of *Topics in Language Disorders, 4*(4).

Snow, C. E. (1991). Diverse conversational contexts for the acquisition of various language skills. In J. Miller (Ed.), *Research on child language disorders* (p. 105–124). Austin, TX: Pro-Ed.

Snow, C. E., & Ferguson, C. (1977). *Talking to children.* New York: Cambridge University Press.

Snow, C. E., & Ninio, A. (1986). The contracts of literacy: What children learn from learning to read books. In W. Teale & E. Sulzby (Eds.), *Emergent literacy.* Norwood, NJ: Ablex.

Snyder, L. S., & Downey, D. M. (1983). Pragmatics and information processing. *Topics in Language Disorders, 4*(1), 75–86.

Snyder, L. S., & Downey, D. M. (1991). The language-reading relationship in normal and reading-disabled children. *Journal of Speech and Hearing Research, 34,* 129–140.

Snyder, L. S., & Downey, D. M. (1995). Serial rapid naming skills in children with reading disabilities. *Annals of Dyslexia, 45,* 31–49.

Sparks, S. N. (1984). *Birth defects and speech-language disorders.* Austin, TX: Pro-Ed.

Sparks, S. N. (1989a). Speech and language in maltreated children: Response to McCauley and Swisher (1987). *Journal of Speech and Hearing Disorders, 54,* 124–126.

Sparks, S. N. (1989b). Assessment and intervention with at-risk infants and toddlers: Guidelines for the speech-language pathologist. *Topics in Language Disorders, 10*(1), 43–56.

Sparks, S. N. (1993). *Children of prenatal substance abuse.* San Diego, CA: Singular Publishing Group.

Spearman, C. E. (1923). *The nature of intelligence and the principles of cognition.* London: Macmillan.

Spearman, C. E. (1927). *The abilities of man.* New York: Macmillan.

Springer, S. P., & Deutsch, G. (1985). *Left brain, right brain* (rev. ed.). New York: W. H. Freeman and Company.

Squire, J. R. (1964). *The responses of adolescents while reading four short stories.* NCTE Research Report No. 2. Urbana, IL: National Council of Teachers of English.

Staats, A. (1971). Linguistic-mentalistic theory versus an explanatory S-R learning theory of language development. In D. Slobin (Ed.), *The ontogenesis of grammar.* New York: Academic Press.

Stainback, S., & Stainback, W. (1988). *Understanding and conducting qualitative research.* Reston, VA: The Council for Exceptional Children.

Stainback, W., & Stainback, S. (1990). *Support networks for inclusive schooling: Interdependent integrated education.* Baltimore: Paul H. Brookes.

Stainback, W., Stainback, S., Courtnage, L., & Jaben, T. (1985). Facilitating mainstreaming by modifying the mainstream. *Exceptional Children, 52,* 144–152.

Stampe, D. (1969). The acquisition of phonetic representation. In R. I. Binnick, A. Davison, G. M. Greene, & J. L. Morgan (Eds.), *Papers from the fifth regional meeting, Chicago Linguistic Society.* Chicago: Chicago Linguistic Society.

Stanovich, K. E. (1985). Explaining the variance in reading ability in terms of psychological processes: What have we learned? *Annals of Dyslexia, 35,* 67–96.

Stanovich, K. E. (1988). The right and wrong places to look for the cognitive locus of reading disability. *Annals of Dyslexia, 38,* 154–177.

Stark, R. E., Bernstein, L. E., Condino, R., Bender, M., Tallal, P., & Catts, H. (1984). Four-year follow-up study of language impaired children. *Annals of Dyslexia, 34,* 49–68.

Stark, R., & Tallal, P. (1981). Selection of children with specific language deficits. *Journal of Speech and Hearing Disorders, 46,* 114–122.

Statewide Project for the Deaf. (1982). *Developmental language centered curriculum for hearing impaired children: Stage 0.* Austin, TX: Texas Education Agency, Resource Center and Publications.

Stauffer, R. G. (1975). *Directing the reading-thinking process.* New York: Harper & Row.

Steckol, K. F., & Leonard, L. B. (1981). Sensorimotor development and the use of prelinguistic performatives. *Journal of Speech and Hearing Research, 24,* 262–268.

Stein, N., & Glenn, C. (1979). An analysis of story comprehension in elementary school children. In R. Freedle (Ed.), *New directions in discourse processing* (Vol. 2). (pp. 53–120). Norwood, NJ: Ablex.

Stein, N. L., & Glenn, C. G. (1982). Children's concept of time: The development of a story schema. In W. Freeman (Ed.), *The developmental psychology of time* (pp. 255–282). New York: Academic Press.

Stephens, M. I., & Montgomery, A. A. (1985). A critique of recent relevant standardized tests. *Topics in Language Disorders, 5*(3), 21–45.

Stephenson, J., & Linfoot, K. (1996). Pictures as communication symbols for students with severe intellectual disability. *Augmentative and Alternative Communication, 12,* 244–255.

Stern, D. (1985). *The interpersonal world of the infant.* New York: Basic Books.

Sternberg, L. (1982). Communication instruction. In L. Sternberg & G. L. Adams (Eds.), *Educating severely and profoundly handicapped students* (pp. 209–241). Rockville, MD: Aspen Publishers.

Sternberg, L., Battle, C., & Hill, J. (1980). Prelanguage communication programming for the severely and profoundly handicapped. *JASH* (Journal of the Association for Persons with Severe Handicaps), *5,* 224–233.

Sternberg, L., McNerney, C. D., & Pegnatore, L. (1985). Developing co-active imitative behaviors with profoundly mentally handicapped students. *Education and Training of the Mentally Retarded, 20,* 260–267.

Sternberg, L., & Owens, A. (1984). Establishing pre-language signalling behaviour with profoundly mentally handicapped students: A preliminary investigation. *Journal of Mental Deficiency Research, 29,* 81–93.

Sternberg, L., Pegnatore, L., & Hill, C. (1983). Establishing interactive communication behaviors with profoundly mentally handicapped students. *JASH* (Journal of the Association for Persons with Severe Handicaps), *8,* 39–46.

Sternberg, L., Ritchey, H., Pegnatore, L., Wills, L., & Hill, C. (1986). *A curriculum for profoundly handicapped students.* Rockville, MD: Aspen Publishers.

Sternberg, R. J. (1979). The nature of mental abilities. *American Psychologist, 34,* 214–230.

Sternberg, R. J. (1981). The nature of intelligence. *New York University Education Quarterly, 12,* 10–17.

Sternberg, R. J. (1985). *Beyond IQ: A triarchic theory of human intelligence.* New York: Cambridge University Press.

Sternberg, R. J. (1988). *The triarchic mind.* New York: Viking.

Sternberg, R. J., Okagaki, L., & Jackson, A. S. (1990). Practical intelligence for success in school. *Educational Leadership, 48*(1), 35–39.

Stevens, L. J., & Bliss, L. S. (1995). Conflict resolution abilities of children with specific language impairment and children with normal language. *Journal of Speech and Hearing Research, 38,* 599–611.

Stewart, S. R. (1985). Development of written language proficiency: Methods for teaching text structure. In C. Simon (Ed.), *Communication skills and classroom success: Therapy methodologies for language-learning disabled students* (pp. 341–361). San Diego, CA: College-Hill. Reprinted in C. S. Simon (Ed.). (1991), *Communication skills and classroom success: Assessment and therapy methodologies for language and learning disabled students* (pp. 419–432). Eau Claire, WI: Thinking Publications.

Stockman, I. J. (1996). The promises and pitfalls of language sample analysis as an assessment tool for linguistic minority children. *Language, Speech, and Hearing Services in Schools, 27,* 355–366.

Stockman, I. J., & Vaughn-Cooke, F. B. (1986). Implications of semantic category research for the language assessment of nonstandard speakers. *Topics in Language Disorders, 6*(4), 15–25.

Stoel-Gammon, C. (1987). Phonological skills of 2-year-olds. *Language, Speech, and Hearing Services in Schools, 18,* 323–329.

Stoel-Gammon, C. (1988). Prelinguistic vocalizations of hearing-impaired and normally hearing subjects: A comparison of consonantal inventories. *Journal of Speech and Hearing Disorders, 53,* 302–315.

Stoel-Gammon, C., & Otomo, K. (1986). Babbling development of hearing-impaired and normally hearing subjects. *Journal of Speech and Hearing Disorders, 51,* 33–41.

Stokes, T. F., & Baer, D. M. (1977). An implicit technology of generalization. *Journal of Applied Behavioral Analysis, 10,* 349–367.

Stremel-Campbell, K., & Campbell, C. R. (1985). Training techniques that may facilitate generalization. In S. F. Warren & A. K. Rogers-Warren (Eds.), *Teaching functional language* (pp. 251–285). Austin, TX: Pro-Ed.

Strickland, D. S., & Taylor, D. (1989). Family storybook reading: Implications for children, families, and curriculum. In D. S. Strickland & L. M. Morrow (Eds.), *Emerging literacy: Young children learn to read and write* (pp. 27–34). Newark, DE: International Reading Association.

Strominger, A. Z., & Bashir, A. S. (1977, November). *Longitudinal study of language-delayed children.* Paper presented at the Annual Convention of the American Speech-Language-Hearing Association, Chicago, IL.

Strong, W. (1986). *Creative approaches to sentence combining.* Theory and Research into Practice (TRIP). Urbana, IL: ERIC Clearinghouse on Reading and Communication Skills.

Sturm, J. M. (1990). *Teacher and student discourse variables in academic communication.* Unpublished masters thesis, Western Michigan University, Kalamazoo, MI.

Sturm, J. M., & Nelson, N. W. (1989, November). *Mediated language and cognitive intervention for post-leukemia encephalopathy—Sarah's story.* Poster presentation at the Annual Conference of the American Speech-Language-Hearing Association, Nov. 19, St. Louis, Mo.

Sturm, J. M., & Nelson, N. W. (1997). Formal classroom lessons: New perspectives on a familiar discourse event, *Language Speech and Hearing Services in Schools, 28.* 255–273.

Sturner, R. A., Kunze, L., Funk, S. G., & Green, J. (1993). Elicited imitation: Its effectiveness for speech and language screening (SRST). *Developmental Medicine and Child Neurology, 35,* 715–726.

Sturner, R. A., Layton, T. A., Evans, A. W., Heller, J. H., Funk, S. G., & Machon, M. W. (1994). Preschool speech and language screening: A review of currently available tests. *American Journal of Speech-Language Pathology, 3*(1), 25–36.

Suritsky, S. K., & Hughes, C. A. (1991). Benefits of notetaking: Implications for secondary and postsecondary students with learning disabilities. *Learning Disability Quarterly, 14,* 7–18.

Sussman, H. M. (1989, May). A bird brain approach to language. *Asha, 31,* 83–86.

Sutter, J., & Johnson, C. J. (1988, November). *Production of later acquired verb forms: An issue of oral vs. literate language.* Paper presented at the American Speech-Language-Hearing Association Convention, New Orleans, LA.

Sutter, J. C., & Johnson, C. J. (1990). School-age children's metalinguistic awareness of grammaticality in verb form. *Journal of Speech and Hearing Research, 33,* 84–95.

Sutter, J. C. L., & Johnson, C. J. (1995). Advanced verb form production in story retelling. *Journal of Speech and Hearing Research, 38,* 1067–1080.

Sutton, A. C. (1989). The social-verbal competence of AAC users. *Augmentative and Alternative Communication, 5,* 150–164.

Sutton-Smith, B. (1986). The development of fictional narrative performances. *Topics in Language Disorders, 7*(1), 1–10.

Swisher, L., & Demetras, M. J. (1985). The expressive language characteristics of autistic children compared with mentally retarded or specific language-impaired children. In E. Schopler & G. B. Mesibov (Eds.), *Communication problems in autism* (pp. 147–162). New York: Plenum Press.

Swisher, L., Restrepo, M. A., Plante, E., & Lowell, S. (1995). Effect of implicit and explicit "rule" presentation on bound-morpheme generalization in specific language impairment. *Journal of Speech and Hearing Research, 38,* 168–173.

Swoger, P. A. (1989). Scott's gift. *English Journal, 78,* 61–65.

Szekeres, S. F., Ylvisaker, M., & Holland, A. L. (1985). Cognitive rehabilitation therapy: A framework for intervention. In M. Ylvisaker, M. (Ed.), *Head injury rehabilitation: Children and adolescents* (pp. 219–246). Austin, TX: Pro-Ed.

Taff, T. G. (1990). Success for the unsuccessful. *Educational Leadership, 48*(1), 71–72.

Tager-Flusberg, H. (1985). Putting words together: Morphology and syntax in the preschool years. In J. B. Gleason (Ed.), *The development of language* (pp. 135–171). Columbus, OH: Merrill.

Tallal, P. (1980). Auditory temporal processing, phonics, and reading disabilities in children. *Brain and Language, 9,* 182–198.

Tallal, P. (1988). Developmental language disorders. J. F. Kavanagh & T. J. Truss, Jr. (Eds.). *Learning disabilities: Proceedings of the National Conference* (pp. 181–272). Parkton, MD: York Press.

Tallal, P. (1996, August). Temporal processing deficits in children with LLI: Integrating research and remediation. *Newsletter of ASHA Special Interest Division 1: Language Learning and Education, 3*(2), 3–8.

Tallal, P. (1997). Speaking out: Evaluating new training programs for language impairment. *Asha, 39*(3), 12.

Tallal, P., Miller, S. L., Bedi, G., Byma, G., Wang, X., Nagarajan, S. S., Schreiner, C., Jenkins, W. M., & Merzenich, M. M. (1996, January 5). Language comprehension in language-learning impaired children improved with acoustically modified speech. *Science, 271,* 81–84.

Tallal, P., & Piercy, M. (1973). Developmental aphasia: Impaired rate of non-verbal processing as a function of sensory modality. *Neuropsychologia, 11,* 389–398.

Tallal, P., & Piercy, M. (1975). Developmental aphasia: The perception of brief vowels and extended stop consonants. *Neuropsychologia, 13,* 69–74.

Tallal, P., & Piercy, M. (1978). Defects of auditory perception in children with developmental dysphasia. In N. A. Wyke (Ed.), *Developmental dysphasia* (pp. 63–84). New York: Academic Press.

Tallal, P., Ross, R., & Curtiss, S. (1989). Familial aggregation in specific language impairment. *Journal of Speech and Hearing Disorders, 54,* 167–173.

Tallal, P., & Stark, R. (1976). Relation between speech perception and speech production impairment in children with developmental dysphasia. *Brain and Language, 3,* 305–317.

Tallal, P., Stark, R., Kallman, C., & Mellits, D. (1981). A reexamination of some nonverbal perceptual abilities of language-impaired and normal children as a function of age and sensory modality. *Journal of Speech and Hearing Research, 24,* 351–357.

Tamaroff, M., Miller, D. R., Murphy, M. L., Salwen, R., Ghavini, F., & Nir, Y. (1982). Immediate and long-term posttherapy neuropsychologic performance in children with acute lymphoblastic leukemia treated without central nervous system radiation. *Journal of Pediatrics, 101,* 524–529.

Tannen, D. (1982). *Spoken and written language: Exploring orality and literacy.* Norwood, NJ: Ablex.

Tateyama-Sniezek, K. M. (1990). Cooperative learning: Does it improve the academic achievement of students with handicaps? *Exceptional Children, 56,* 426–437.

Tattershall, S. (1987). Mission impossible: Learning how a classroom works before it's too late! *Journal of Childhood Communication Disorders, 11,* 181–184.

Tattershall, S. S. (1994). Upping the ante: Increasing demands for literacy and discourse skills in adolescence. In D. N. Ripich & N. A. Creaghead (Eds.), *School discourse problems* (2nd ed.) (pp. 63–89). San Diego, CA: Singular Publishing Group.

Tattershall, S. (in preparation). *Adolescents with language and learning needs: Solving their problems shoulder to shoulder.* To appear as a volume in the School-Age Children Series (N. W. Nelson, series editor). San Diego, CA: Singular Publishing Group.

Taylor, B. M., & Beach, R. W. (1984). The effects of text structures instruction on middle grade students' comprehension and production of expository text. *Reading Research Quarterly, 19,* 134–146.

Taylor, D. (1983). *Family literacy: Young children learning to read and write.* Portsmouth, NH: Heinemann.

Taylor, D., & Dorsey-Gaines, C. (1987). *Growing up literate: Learning from inner city families.* Portsmouth, NH: Heinemann.

Taylor, O. L. (1972). An introduction to the historical development of Black English. *Language, Speech, and Hearing Services in Schools, 3*(4), 5–15.

Taylor, O. L. (1985). *Nature of communication disorders in culturally and linguistically diverse populations.* Austin, TX: Pro-Ed.

Taylor, O. L. (Ed.). (1986). *Nature of communication disorders in culturally and linguistically diverse populations.* San Diego, CA: College-Hill Press.

Taylor, O. L. (unpublished manuscript). Clinical practice as a social occasion. In L. Cole & V. R. Deal (Eds.), *Communication disorders in multicultural populations.* Rockville, MD: American Speech-Language-Hearing Association.

Taylor, O. (1995). Foreword. In H. Kayser, *Bilingual speech-language pathology: An Hispanic focus* (pp. ix-xii). San Diego, CA: Singular Publishing Group.

Taylor, O. L., & Payne, K. T. (1983). Culturally valid testing: A proactive approach. *Topics in Language Disorders, 3* (3), 8–20.

Taylor, O., Stroud, V., Moore, E., Hurst, C., & Williams, R. (1969). Philosophies and goals of ASHA Black Caucus. *Asha, 11,* 216–218.

Templin, M. (1957). *Certain language skills in children.* Minneapolis, MN: University of Minnesota Press.

Templin, M., & Darley, F. (1960). *The Templin-Darley Test of Articulation.* Iowa City, IA: University of Iowa, Iowa City Bureau of Educational Research.

Terrell, B. Y., Schwartz, R. G., Prelock, P. A., & Messick, C. K. (1984). Symbolic play in normal and language-impaired children. *Journal of Speech and Hearing Research, 27,* 424–429.

Terrell, S. L., & Terrell, F. (1983). Distinguishing linguistic differences from disorders: The past, present, and future of nonbiased assessment. *Topics in Language Disorders, 3* (3), 1–7.

Thal, D., & Tobias, S. (1994). Relationships between language and gesture in normally developing and late-talking toddlers. *Journal of Speech and Hearing Research, 37,* 157–170.

Tharp, R. G., & Gallimore, R. (1988). *Rousing minds to life: Teaching, learning, and schooling in social context.* New York: Cambridge Press.

Thatcher, V. S. (Ed.). (1980). *The new Webster encyclopedic dictionary of the English language.* Chicago, IL: Consolidated Book Publishers.

Thomas, C., Englert, C. S., & Morsink, C. (1984). Modifying the classroom program in language. In C. V. Morsink (Ed.), *Teaching special needs students in regular classrooms* (pp. 239–276). Boston, MA: Little, Brown & Company.

Thorndike, E. L. (1917). Reading as reasoning: A study of mistakes in paragraph reading. *Journal of Educational Psychology, 8,* 323–332.

Thorndike, R. L., Hagen, E. P., & Sattler, J. M. (1986). *Stanford-Binet Intelligence Scale—Revised.* Chicago: The Riverside Publishing Company.

Thorndyke, P. W. (1977). Cognitive structures in comprehension and memory of narrative discourse. *Cognitive Psychology, 9,* 77–110.

Thousand, J. S., Villa, R. A., & Nevin, A. I. (Eds.). (1994). *Creativity and collaborative learning: A practical guide to empowering students and teachers.* Baltimore: Paul H. Brookes.

Tibbits, D. (1982). *Language disorders in adolescents.* Lincoln, NE: Cliff Notes.

Tiegerman, E. (1989). Autism: Learning to communicate. In D. Bernstein & E. Tiegerman (Eds.), *Language and communication disorders in children* (2nd ed.) (pp. 298–338). Columbus, OH: Merrill.

Tiegerman, E., & Siperstein, M. (1984). Individual patterns of interaction in the mother-child dyad: Implications for parent intervention. *Topics in Language Disorders, 4*(4), 50–61.

Tierney, R. J. (1990). Redefining reading comprehension. *Educational Leadership, 47*(6), 37–42.

Tierney, R. J., & Cunningham, J. W. (1984). Research on teaching reading comprehension. In P. D. Pearson (Ed.), *Handbook of reading research* (pp. 609–655). New York: Longman.

Timothy W. v. Rochester School District. 875 F.2d 954 (1st Cir. New Hampshire 1989).

Tindal, G., & Parker, R. (1991). Identifying measures for evaluating written expression. *Learning Disabilities Research and Practice, 6,* 211–218.

Tizard, B., Philips, J., & Plewis, J. (1976). Play in preschool centers: Play measures and their relation to age, sex and

IQ. *Journal of Child Psychology and Psychiatry, 17,* 251–264.

Tjossem, T. D. (1976). Early intervention: Issues and approaches. In T. D. Tjossem (Ed.), *Intervention strategies for high risk infants and young children.* San Antonio, TX: Pro-Ed.

Tomblin, J. B. (1983). An examination of the concept of disorder in the study of language variation. *Proceedings from the Symposium on Research in Child Language Disorders, 4,* 81–109.

Tomblin, J. B. (1989, November). *Comments on causation in specific language disorders.* Paper presented at the annual convention of the American Speech-Language-Hearing Association, St. Louis, MO.

Tomblin, J. B. (1994). Perspectives on diagnosis. In J. B. Tomblin, H. L. Morris, & R. D. C. Spriestersbach (Eds.), *Diagnosis in speech-language pathology* (pp. 1–28). San Diego, CA: Singular Publishing Group.

Tomblin, J. B., Abbas, P. J., Records, N. L., & Brenneman, L. M. (1995). Auditory evoked responses to frequency-modulated tones in children with specific language impairment. *Journal of Speech and Hearing Research, 38,* 387–392.

Tomblin, J. B., Freese, P., & Records, N. (1990, June). *Language, cognition, and social characteristics of young adults with histories of developmental language disorder.* Paper presented at the Symposium for Research on Child Language Disorders, Madison, WI.

Tonjes, M. J., & Zintz, M. V. (1987). *Teaching reading thinking study skills in content classrooms.* Dubuque, IA: Wm. C. Brown.

Torgesen, J. K. (1982). The learning disabled child as an interactive learner: Educational implications. *Topics in Learning and LD, 2,* 45–52.

Torgesen, J. K., & Licht, B. G. (1983). The learning disabled child as an inactive learner: Retrospect and prospects. In J. D. McKinney & L. Feagans (Eds.), *Current topics in learning disabilities* (pp. 3–31). Norwood, NJ: Ablex Publishing.

Torgesen, J. K., & Torgesen, J. L. (1995) *WORDS* [Computer program]. Tallahassee: Florida State University.

Trapani, C. (1990). *Transition goals for adolescents with learning disabilities.* Boston: Little, Brown, & Company.

Trevarthen, C. (1974). Prespeech in communication of infants with adults. *Journal of Child Language, 1,* 335–337.

Trevarthen, C. (1979). Communication and cooperation in early infancy: A description of primary intersubjectivity. In M. Bullows (Ed.), *Before speech* (pp. 321–347). Cambridge, England: Cambridge University Press.

Tronick, E. (1989). Emotions and emotional communication in infants. *American Psychologist, 44,* 112–119.

Tronick, E., Als, H., & Adamson, L. (1979). Structure of early face-to-face communicative interactions. In M. Bullowa (Ed.), *Before speech.* New York: Cambridge University Press.

Trout, M., & Foley, G. (1989). Working with families of handicapped infants and toddlers. *Topics in Language Disorders, 10*(1), 57–67.

Tucher, A. (Ed.). (1990). *Bill Moyers: A world of ideas (II): Public opinions from private citizens.* New York: Doubleday.

Tucker, J. A. (1985). Curriculum-based assessment: An introduction. *Exceptional Children, 52,* 199–204.

Turner, R. G. (1990, September). Recommended guidelines for infant hearing screening: Analysis. *Asha, 32,* 57–61, 66.

Tyack, D. L. (1981). Teaching complex sentences. *Language, Speech, and Hearing Services in Schools, 12,* 49–56.

Tyack, D. L., & Gottsleben, R. H. (1977). *Language sampling, analysis, and training: A handbook for teachers and clinicians.* Palo Alto, CA: Consulting Psychologists Press.

Tyack, D. L., & Gottsleben, R. H. (1986). Acquisition of complex sentences. *Language, Speech, and Hearing Services in Schools, 17,* 160–174.

U. S. Department of Health, Education, and Welfare. (1969). *Minimal brain dysfunction in children.* Public Health Service Publication No. 2015. Washington, DC: U.S. Government Printing Office.

U. S. Department of Health and Human Services. (1981). *Study findings of the National Study of the Incidence and Severity of Child Abuse and Neglect* (DHHS Publication No. [OHDS] 82–30325). Washington, DC: U. S. Government Printing Office.

U. S. Office of Education. (1997). Assistance to states for education for handicapped children: Procedure for evaluating specific learning disabilities. *Federal Register, 42,* G1082-G1085.

Vail, P. L. (1987). *Smart kids with school problems: Things to know and ways to help.* New York: E. P. Dutton.

Vandercook, T., York, J., & Forest, M. (1989). The McGill action planning system (MAPS): A strategy for building the vision. *Journal of the Association for Persons with Severe Handicaps, 14,* 205–215.

Vanderheiden, G. C., & Lloyd, L. L. (1986). Communication systems and their components. In S. W. Blackstone (Ed.), *Augmentative communication: An introduction* (pp. 49–161). Rockville, MD: American Speech-Language-Hearing Association.

Vanderheiden, G. C., & Yoder, D. E. (1986). Overview. In S. W. Blackstone (Ed.), *Augmentative communication: An introduction* (pp. 1–28). Rockville, MD: American Speech-Language-Hearing Association.

van der Lely, H. K. J., & Harris, M. (1990). Comprehension of reversible sentences in specifically language-impaired children. *Journal of Speech and Hearing Disorders, 55,* 101–117.

van Dijk, J. (1965). The first steps of the deaf/blind child toward language. *Proceedings of the conference on the deaf/blind, Refsnes, Denmark.* Boston: Perkins School for the Blind.

van Dijk, T., & Kintsch, W. (1978). Cognitive psychology and discourse: Recalling and summarizing stories. In W. U. Dressler (Eds.), *Current trends in textlinguistics.* New York: Walter de Druyter.

Van Dongen, R., & Westby, C. E. (1986). Building the narrative mode of thought through children's literature. *Topics in Language Disorders, 7*(1), 70–83.

Vane, J. (1975). Vane Evaluation of Language Scale. *Archives of Behavioral Sciences, 49,* 3–33.

van Kleeck, A. (1984). Metalinguistic skills: Cutting across spoken and written language and problem-solving abilities. In G. P. Wallach & K. G. Butler (Eds.), *Language learning disabilities in school-age children* (pp. 128–153). Baltimore, MD: Williams & Wilkins.

van Kleeck, A. (1990). Emergent literacy: Learning about print before learning to read. *Topics in Language Disorders, 10*(2), 25–45.

van Kleeck, A. (1994a). Metalinguistic development. In G. P. Wallach & K. G. Butler (Eds.), *Language learning disabilities in school-age children and adolescents* (pp. 53–98). Boston: Allyn and Bacon.

van Kleeck, A. (1994b). Potential cultural bias in training parents as conversational partners with their children who have delays in language development. *American Journal of Speech-Language Pathology, 3*(1), 67–78.

van Kleeck, A., & Richardson, A. (1986). What's in an error? Using children's wrong responses as language teaching opportunities. *Journal of the National Student Speech-Language-Hearing Association, 14,* 25–50.

Van Riper, C., & Erickson, R. L. (1996). *Speech correction: An introduction to speech pathology and audiology* (9th ed.). Boston: Allyn and Bacon.

Vaughn, S., McIntosh, R., & Spencer-Rowe, J. (1991). Peer rejection is a stubborn thing: Increasing peer acceptance of rejected students with learning disabilities. *Learning Disabilities Research and Practice, 6,* 83–88.

Vaughn-Cooke, F. B. (1983). Improving language assessment in minority children. *Asha, 25*(9), 29–34.

Vaughn-Cooke, F. B. (1989). Speech-language pathologists and educators: Time to strengthen the partnership. In B. A. Stewart (Ed.), *ASHA Reports No. 17, Partnerships in education: Toward a literate America* (pp. 67–72). Rockville, MD: American Speech-Language-Hearing Association.

Vavra, E. (1987). Grammar and syntax: The student's perspective. *English Journal, 76*(6), 42–48.

Vellutino, F. (1979). *Dyslexia: Theory and research.* Cambridge, MA: MIT Press.

Vellutino, F. R., & Schub, M. J. (1982). Assessment of disorders in formal school language: Disorders in reading. *Topics in Language Disorders, 2*(4), 20–33.

Venezky, R. L. (1970). *The structure of English orthography.* The Hague: Mouton.

Vernon, M. (1969). Sociological and psychological factors associated with hearing loss. *Journal of Speech and Hearing Research, 12,* 541–563.

Villa, R. A., Thousand, J. S., Stainback, W., & Stainback, S. (Eds.). (1992). *Restructuring for caring and effective education.* Baltimore: Paul H. Brookes.

Vygotsky, L. S. (1962). *Thought and language.* (Edited and translated by E. Hanfmann & G. Vakar from the original work, published posthumously in 1934). Cambridge: MIT Press.

Vygotsky, L. S. (1967). Play and its role in the mental development of the child. *Soviet Psychology, 5,* 6–18.

Vygotsky, L. S. (1978). *Mind in society: The development of higher psychological processes.* Cambridge, MA: Harvard University Press.

Wada, J. A. (1977). Prelanguage and functional asymmetry of the infant brain. *Annals of the New York Academy of Sciences, 299,* 370–379.

Wada, J. A., Clark, R., & Hamm, A. (1975). Cerebral hemispheric asymmetry in humans. *Archives of Neurology, 32,* 239–246.

Wallace, G., & Hammill, D. D. (1994).*Comprehensive Receptive and Expressive Vocabulary Test (CREVT).* Austin, TX: Pro-Ed.

Wallach, G. P. (1984). Later language learning: Syntactic structures and strategies. In G. P. Wallach & K. G. Butler (Eds.), *Language learning disabilities in school-age children* (pp. 82–102). Baltimore, MD: Williams & Wilkins.

Wallach, G. P. (1989). Current research as a map for language intervention in the school years. *Seminars in Speech and Language, 10*(3), 205–217.

Wallach, G. P. (1990). Magic Buries Celtics: Looking for broader interpretations of language learning and literacy. *Topics in Language Disorders, 10*(2), 63–80.

Wallach, G. P., & Butler, K. G. (1994). Creating communication, literacy, and academic success. In G. P. Wallach & K. G. Butler (Eds.), *Language learning disabilities in school-age children and adolescents* (pp. 2–26). Boston: Allyn and Bacon.

Wallach, G. P., & Miller, L. (1988). *Language intervention and academic success.* Austin, TX: Pro-Ed.

Wanat, P. (1983). Social skills: An awareness program with learning disabled adolescents. *Journal of Learning Disabilities, 16,* 35–38.

Wang, M. C., & Reynolds, M. C. (1985). Avoiding the "Catch 22" in special education reform. *Exceptional Children, 51,* 497–502.

Warren, D. H. (1984). *Blindness and early childhood development.* New York: Academic Foundation for the Blind.

Warren, S. F. (1988). A behavioral approach to language generalization. *Language, Speech, and Hearing Services in Schools, 19,* 292–303.

Warren, S. F., & Bambara, L. M. (1989). An experimental analysis of milieu language intervention: Teaching the action-object form. *Journal of Speech and Hearing Disorders, 54,* 448–461.

Warren, S. F., & Kaiser, A. P. (1986). Incidental language teaching: A critical review. *Journal of Speech and Hearing Disorders, 51,* 291–299.

Warren, S. F., McQuarter, R. J., & Rogers-Warren, A. K. (1984). The effects of mands and models on the speech of unresponsive language-delayed preschool children. *Journal of Speech and Hearing Disorders, 49,* 43–52.

Warren, S. F., & Rogers-Warren, A. K. (1983). A longitudinal analysis of language generalization among adolescents with severely handicapping conditions. *JASH* (Journal of the Association for Persons with Severe Handicaps), *8*(4), 18–31.

Warren, S. F., & Rogers-Warren, A. K. (Eds.). (1985). *Teaching functional language.* Baltimore, MD: University Park Press.

Warren, S. F., & Yoder, P. J. (1994). Communication and language intervention: Why a constructivist approach is insufficient. *The Journal of Special Education, 28,* 248–258.

Waryas, C., & Stremel-Campbell, K. (1983). *Communication Training Program.* New York: Teaching Resources.

Washington, J. A. (1996). Issues in assessing the language abilities of African American children. In A. G. Kamhi, K. E. Pollock, & J. L. Harris (Eds.), *Communication development and disorders in African American children* (pp. 35–54). Baltimore, MD: Paul H. Brookes.

Washington, J. A., & Craig, H. K. (1992). Performances of low-income, African American preschool and kindergarten children on the Peabody Picture Vocabulary Test-Revised. *Language, Speech, and Hearing Services in the Schools, 23,* 329–333.

Washington, J. A., & Craig, H. K. (1994). Dialectal forms during discourse of poor, urban, African American preschoolers. *Journal of Speech and Hearing Research, 37,* 816–823.

Wasserman, G. A., Green, A., & Allen, R. (1983). Going beyond abuse: Maladaptive patterns of interaction in abusing mother-infant pairs. *Journal of the American Academy of Child Psychiatry, 22,* 245–252.

Watkins, R. V. (1994). Specific language impairments in children: An introduction. In R. V. Watkins & M. L. Rice (Eds.), *Specific language impairments in children* (pp. 1–15). Baltimore, MD: Paul H. Brookes.

Watkins, R. V., Kelly, D. J., Harbers, H. M., & Hollis, W. (1995). Measuring children's lexical diversity: Differentiating typical and impaired learners. *Journal of Speech and Hearing Research, 38,* 1349–1355.

Watson, B. U., Sullivan, P. M., Moeller, M. P., & Jensen, J. K. (1982). Nonverbal intelligence and English language ability in deaf children. *Journal of Speech and Hearing Disorders, 47,* 199–204.

Watson, L., Lord, C., Schaffer, B., & Schopler, E. (1989). *Teaching spontaneous communication to autistic and developmentally handicapped children.* New York: Irvington Publishers.

Watzlawick, P., Beavin, J. H., & Jackson, D. D. (1967). *Pragmatics of human communication.* New York: W. W. Norton.

Weaver, C. (1982). Welcoming errors as signs of growth. *Language Arts, 59,* 438–444.

Weaver, C. (1993). Understanding and educating students with Attention Deficit Hyperactive Disorder: Toward a system theory and whole language perspective. *American Journal of Speech-Language Pathology, 2,* 79–89.

Weaver, C. (1994a). *Reading process and practice: From socio-psycholinguistics to whole language* (2nd ed.). Portsmouth, NH: Heinemann.

Weaver, C. (Ed.). (1994b). *Success at last! Helping students with ADHD achieve their potential.* Portsmouth, NH: Heinemann.

Weaver, J. (1994). What I've learned as an ADHDer about the problems and needs of students with ADHD. In C. Weaver (Ed.), *Success at last! Helping students with ADHD achieve their potential* (pp. 46–62). Portsmouth, NH: Heinemann.

Weber-Olsen, M., Putnam-Sims, P., & Gannon, J. D. (1983). Elicited imitation and the *Oral Language Sentence Imitation Screening Test* (OLSIST): Content or context? *Journal of Speech and Hearing Disorders, 48,* 368–378.

Wechsler, D. (1967). *Wechsler Preschool and Preprimary Scale of Intelligence* (WISC-R). San Antonio, TX: The Psychological Corporation.

Wechsler, D. (1974). *Wechsler Intelligence Scale for Children-Revised* (WISC-R). San Antonio, TX: The Psychological Corporation.

Wechsler, D. (1981). *Wechsler Adult Intelligence Scale-Revised.* San Antonio, TX: Psychological Corporation.

Weicker, L. (1989). Testimony on ADA. *Word from Washington.* UCPA. p. 17–18.

Weiner, B. (1979). A theory of motivation for some classroom experiences. *Journal of Educational Psychology, 71,* 3–25.

Weiner, B. (1980). The role of affect in rational (attributional) approaches to human motivation. *Educational Researcher, 9,* 4–11.

Weiner, P. S. (1985). The value of follow-up studies. *Topics in Language Disorders, 5*(3), 78–92.

Weir, R. (1962). *Language in the crib.* The Hague: Mouton.

Weismer, S. E., & Hesketh, L. J. (1996). Lexical learning by children with specific language impairment: Effects of linguistic input presented at varying speaking rates. *Journal of Speech and Hearing Research, 39,* 177–190.

Weitzman, E. (1992). *Learning language and loving it: A guide to promoting children's social and language development in early childhood settings.* Toronto, Ontario: The Hanen Centre.

Wells, G. (1986). *The meaning makers: Children learning language and using language to learn.* Portsmouth, NH: Heinemann.

Wepman, J. M., Jones, L. V., Bock, R. D., & van Pelt, D. (1960). Studies in aphasia: Background and theoretical formulations. *Journal of Speech and Hearing Disorders, 25,* 323–332.

Werker, J. F., & Lalonde, C. E. (1988). The development of speech perception: Initial capabilities and the emergence of phonemic categories. *Developmental Psychology, 24,* 672–683.

Werner, H., & Kaplan, E. (1950). The acquisition of word meanings: A developmental study. *Monographs of the Society of Research in Child Development, 15,* Serial No. 51.

Werner, E., & Kresheck, J. D. (1983). *Structured photographic expressive language test-II.* Sandwich, IL: Janelle Publications.

Wertsch, J. V. (1985). *Vygotsky and the social formation of mind.* Cambridge, MA: Harvard University Press.

Wertsch, J. V. (1991). *Voices of the mind: A sociocultural approach to mediated action.* Cambridge, MA: Harvard University Press.

West, J., & Weber, J. (1973). A phonological analysis of the spontaneous language of a four-year-old hard-of-hearing child. *Journal of Speech and Hearing Disorders, 38,* 25–35.

Westby, C. E. (1980). Assessment of cognitive and language abilities through play. *Language, Speech, and Hearing Services in Schools, 11,* 154–168.

Westby, C. E. (1982). *Cognitive and linguistic aspects of children's narrative development* [Audiotaped journal]. New York: Grune & Stratton, Vol. 7, no. 1.

Westby, C. E. (1984). Development of narrative language abilities. In G. P. Wallach & K. G. Butler (Eds.), *Language learning disabilities in school-age children* (pp. 103–127). Baltimore, MD: Williams & Wilkins.

Westby, C. E. (1985). Learning to talk—Talking to learn: Oral-literate language differences. In C. Simon (Ed.), *Communication skills and classroom success: Therapy methodologies for language-learning disabled students* (pp. 181–213). San Diego, CA: College-Hill. Reprinted in C. S. Simon (Ed.). (1991), *Communication skills and classroom success: Assessment and therapy methodologies for language and learning disabled students* (pp. 334–355). Eau Claire, WI: Thinking Publications.

Westby, C. E. (1988). Children's play: Reflections of social competence. *Seminars in Speech and Language, 9,* 1–14.

Westby, C. E. (1989). Assessing and remediating text comprehension problems. In A. G. Kamhi & H. W. Catts (Eds.), *Reading disabilities: A developmental language perspective* (pp. 199–259). Austin, TX: Pro-Ed.

Westby, C. E. (1990). Ethnographic interviewing: Asking the right questions to the right people in the right ways. *Journal of Childhood Communication Disorders, 13,* 101–111.

Westby, C. E. (1991). *Understanding classroom texts.* Presented as part of an audioteleconference on *Steps to Developing and Achieving Language Based Curriculum in the Classroom,* originating from the American Speech-Language-Hearing Association, Rockville, MD, October, 4, 1991.

Westby, C. E. (1994). The effects of culture on genre, structure, and type of oral and written texts. In G. P. Wallach & K. G. Butler (Eds.), *Language learning disabilities in school-age children and adolescents* (pp. 180–218). Boston: Allyn and Bacon.

Westby, C. E., StevensDominguez, M., & Oetter, P. (1996). A performance/competence model of observational assessment. *Language, Speech, and Hearing Services in Schools, 27,* 144–156.

Wetherby, A. M., Cain, D., Yonclas, D., & Walker, V. (1988). Analysis of intentional communication of normal children from the prelinguistic to the multi-word stage. *Journal of Speech and Hearing Research, 31,* 240–252.

Wetherby, A. M., & Prizant, B. M. (1990). *Communication and Symbolic Behavior Scales.* Chicago: Riverside.

Wetherby, A. M., & Prizant, B. M. (1993). *Communication and Symbolic Behavior Scales.* Chicago: Applied Symbolix.

Wetherby, A. M., & Prutting, B. M. (1984). Profiles of communicative and cognitive-social abilities in autistic children. *Journal of Speech and Hearing Research, 27,* 364–377.

Wetherby, A. M., Yonclas, D. G., & Bryan, A. A. (1989). Communication profiles of preschool children with handicaps: Implications for early identification. *Journal of Speech and Hearing Disorders, 54,* 148–158.

Wetherby, B., & Striefel, S. (1978). Application of a miniature linguistic system on matrix-training procedures. In R. L. Schiefelbusch (Ed.), *Language intervention strategies* (pp. 317–356). Austin, TX: Pro-Ed.

Wexler, K. (1982). A principle theory for language acquisition. In E. Wanner & L. Gleitman (Eds.), *Language acquisition: The state of the art.* Cambridge: Cambridge University Press.

Wheeler, D., Jacobson, J., Paglieri, R., & Schwartz, A. (1993). An experimental assessment of facilitated communication. *Mental Retardation, 31,* 49–60.

Whitaker, H. & Whitaker, H. A. (1979). *Studies in neurolinguistics. Vol. 4.* New York: Academic Press.

White, S. H. (1980). Cognitive competence and performance in everyday environments. *Bulletin of the Orton Society* (now called *Annals of Dyslexia*), *30,* 29–45.

White, S. J., & White, R. E. C. (1984). The deaf imperative: Characteristics of maternal input to hearing-impaired children. *Topics in Language Disorders, 4*(4), 38–49.

Whiteman, M. F. (Ed.). (1981). *Writing: The nature, development, and teaching of written communication: Volume 1, Variation in writing: Function and linguistic-cultural differences.* Hillsdale, NJ: Erlbaum.

Wieder, S., & Findikoglu, P. (1987). The infant center: A developmentally based environment to support difficult lives. In S. I. Greenspan, S. Wieder, R. A. Nover, A. F. Lieberman, R. S. Lourie, & M. E. Robinson (Eds.), *Infants in multirisk families: Case studies in preventive intervention* (pp. 23–37). Clinical Infant Reports Series of the National Center for Clinical Infant Programs. Madison, WI: International Universities Press.

Wieder, S., & Greenspan, S. I. (1987). Staffing, process, and structure of the clinical infant development program. In S. I. Greenspan, S. Wieder, R. A. Nover, A. F. Lieberman, R. S. Lourie, & M. E. Robinson (Eds.), *Infants in multirisk families: Case studies in preventive intervention* (pp. 9–21). Clinical Infant Reports Series of the National

Center for Clinical Infant Programs. Madison, WI: International Universities Press.

Wiener, F. D., Lewnau, L. E., & Erway, E. (1983). Measuring language competency in speakers of Black American English. *Journal of Speech and Hearing Disorders, 48,* 76–84.

Wiess, A. L. (1986). Classroom discourse and the hearing-impaired child. *Topics in Language Disorders, 6* (3), 60–70.

Wiig, E. H. (1982). *Let's talk: Developing prosocial communication skills.* Columbus, OH: Merrill.

Wiig, E. H. (1984). Language disabilities in adolescents: A question of cognitive strategies. *Topics in Language Disorders, 4*(2), 41–58.

Wiig, E. H. (1989, May). The interpretation of CELF-R results: A process. *CELF-R Update 2* (Newsletter published by The Psychological Corporation, San Antonio, TX), *2,* 8–10.

Wiig, E. H., & Secord, W. (1992). *Test of Word Knowledge* (TOWK). San Antonio, TX: The Psychological Corporation.

Wiig, E. H., & Semel, E. M. (1976). *Language disabilities in children and adolescents.* Columbus, OH: Merrill.

Wiig, E. H., & Semel, E. M. (1980). *Language assessment and intervention for the learning disabled.* Columbus, OH: Merrill.

Wilbur, R. (1976). The linguistics of manual languages and manual systems. In L. Lloyd (Ed.), *Communication assessment and intervention strategies* (pp. 423–500). Austin, TX: Pro-Ed.

Wilbur, R. B. (1977). An explanation of deaf children's difficulty with certain syntactic structures of English. *Volta Review, 79,* 85–91.

Wilcox, M. J. (1989). Delivering communication-based services to infants, toddlers, and families: Approaches and models. *Topics in Language Disorders, 10*(1), 68–79.

Wilkins, R. (1985). A comparison of elective mutism and emotional disorders in children. *British Journal of Psychiatry, 146,* 198–203.

Wilkinson, K. M., & Romski, M. A. (1995). Responsiveness of male adolescents with mental retardation to input from nondisabled peers: The summoning power of comments, questions, and directive prompts. *Journal of Speech and Hearing Research, 38,* 1045–1053.

Wilkinson, L. C., & Milosky, L. M. (1987). School-age children's metapragmatic knowledge of requests and responses in the classroom. *Topics in Language Disorders, 7*(2), 61–70.

Wilkinson, L. C., Milosky, L. M., & Genishi, C. (1986). Second language learners' use of requests and responses in elementary classrooms. *Topics in Language Disorders, 6*(2), 57–70.

Will, M. (1986). *Educating students with learning problems: A shared responsibility. A report to the Secretary.* Office of Special Education and Rehabilitative Services. Washington, DC: Dept. of Education.

Willeford, J. A., & Burleigh, J. M. (1985). *Handbook of central auditory processing disorders in children.* Orlando, FL: Grune & Stratton.

Williams, J. P. (1988). Identifying main ideas: A basic aspect of reading comprehension. *Topics in Language Disorders, 8*(3), 1–13.

Windsor, J. (1995). Language impairment and social competence. In M. E. Fey, J. Windsor, & S. F. Warren (Eds.), *Language intervention: Preschool through the elementary years* (pp. 213–238). Baltimore, MD: Paul H. Brookes.

Wing, L. (1983). Social and interpersonal needs. In E. Schopler & G. B. Mesibov (Eds.), *Autism in adolescents and adults* (pp. 337–354). New York: Plenum Press.

Winitz, H. (1973). Problem solving and the delay of speech as strategies in the teaching of language. *Asha, 15,* 583–586.

Winograd, P., & Niquette, G. (1988). Assessing learned helplessness in poor readers. *Topics in Language Disorders, 8* (3), 38–55.

Wixson, K., Boskey, A., Yochum, M., & Alverman, D. (1984). An interview for assessing students' perceptions of classroom reading tasks. *The Reading Teacher, 37,* 348.

Wolery, M. (1989). Child find issues and screening. In D. B. Bailey, Jr. & M. Wolery (Eds.), *Assessing infants and preschoolers with handicaps* (pp. 119–143). Columbus, OH: Merrill.

Wolf, M., & Segal, D. (1992). Word finding and reading in the developmental dyslexias. *Topics in Language Disorders, 13,* 51–65.

Wolff, P. H. (1963). Observations on the early development of smiling. In B. M. Foss (Ed.), *Determinants of infant behaviour* (Vol. 2). London: Metheun; New York: John Wiley & Sons.

Wolff, S., & Barlow, A. (1979). Schizoid personality in childhood. *Journal of Child Psychology and Psychiatry, 20,* 29–46.

Wolfram, W. (1979). *Speech pathology and dialect differences.* Arlington, VA: Center for Applied Linguistics.

Wolfram, W. (1983). Test interpretation and sociolinguistic differences. *Topics in Language Disorders, 3*(3), 21–34.

Wolfram, W., Williams, R., & Taylor, O. L. (1972). *Dialectal bias of language assessment instruments.* Short course presented at the annual meeting of the American Speech and Hearing Association, San Francisco, CA.

Wolfus, B., Moskovitch, M., & Kinsbourne, M. (1980). Subgroups of language development. *Brain and Language, 10,* 152–171.

Wong, B. Y., & Jones, W. (1982). Increasing metacomprehension in learning disabled and normally achieving students through self-questioning training. *Learning Disability Quarterly, 5,* 228–240.

Wong, B. Y. L., Wong, R., Darlington, D., & Jones, W. (1991). Interactive teaching: An effective way to teach revision skills to adolescents with learning disabilities. *Learning Disabilities Research & Practice, 6,* 117–127.

Wood, B. S. (1976). *Children and communication: Verbal and nonverbal language development.* Englewood Cliffs, NJ: Prentice Hall.

Wood, D. J., Bruner, J., & Ross, G. (1976). The role of tutoring in problem solving. *Journal of Child Psychiatry, 17,* 89–100.

Wood, D., Wood, H., & Middleton, D. (1978). An experimental evaluation of four face to face teaching strategies. *International Journal of Behavioral Development, 1,* 131–147.

Wood, P. (1980). Appreciating the consequences of disease: The classification of impairments, disabilities, and handicaps. *The World Health Organization Chronicle, 34,* 376–380.

Woodcock, R., & Johnson, M. B. (1989). *Woodcock-Johnson Psycho-Educational Test Battery—Revised.* Austin, TX: DLM Teaching Resources.

Woodruff, G., & McGonigel, M. J. (1988). Early intervention team approaches: The transdisciplinary model. In J. B. Jordan, J. J. Gallagher, P. L. Hutinger, & M. B. Karnes (Eds.), *Early childhood special education: Birth to three* (pp. 163–182). Reston, VA: Council for Exceptional Children and the Division for Early Childhood.

Worster-Drought, C. (1971). An unusual form of acquired aphasia in children. *Developmental Medicine and Child Neurology, 13,* 563–571.

Wurman, R. S. (1989). *Information anxiety.* New York: Doubleday.

Yell, M. L., & Espin, C. A. (1990). The Handicapped Children's Protection Act of 1986: Time to pay the piper? *Exceptional Children, 56,* 396–407.

Ylvisaker, M. (Ed.). (1985). *Head injury rehabilitation: Children and adolescents.* San Diego, CA: College-Hill Press. (Now available from Pro-Ed, Austin, TX.)

Ylvisaker, M., & Szekeres, S. F. (1986). Management of the patient with closed head injury. In R. Chapey (Ed.), *Language intervention strategies in adult aphasia* (pp. 474–490). Baltimore, MD: Williams & Wilkins.

Yoder, D. (1980). Communication systems for nonspeech children. *New Directions in the Exceptional Child, 2,* 63–78.

Yoder, P. J. (1989). Maternal question use predicts later language development in specific-language-disordered children. *Journal of Speech and Hearing Disorders, 54,* 347–355.

Yoder, P. J. (1995). Validity of facilitated communication intervention: Response to Duchan. *Journal of Speech and Hearing Research, 38,* 202–204.

Yoder, P. J., Davies, B., Bishop, K., & Munson, L. (1994). Effect of adult continuing Wh-Questions on conversational participation in children with developmental disabilities. *Journal of Speech and Hearing Research, 73,* 193–204.

Yoder, P. J., Kaiser, A. P., & Alpert, C. L. (1991). An exploratory study of the interaction between language teaching methods and child characteristics. *Journal of Speech and Hearing Research, 34,* 155–167.

Yoder, P. J., Warren, S. F., Kim, K., & Gazdag, G. E. (1994). Facilitating prelinguistic skills in young children with developmental delay II: Systematic replication and extension. *Journal of Speech and Hearing Research, 37,* 841–851.

Yoshida, R. K. (1983). Are multidisciplinary teams worth the investment? *School Psychology Review, 12,* 127–143.

Yoshinago-Itano, C., & Downey, D. M. (1986). A hearing-impaired child's acquisition of schemata: Something's missing. *Topics in Language Disorders, 7*(1), 45–57.

Yoss, K. A., & Darley, F. L. (1974). Developmental apraxia of speech in children with defective articulation. *Journal of Speech and Hearing Research, 17,* 399–416.

Ysseldyke, J. R., & Algozzine, B. (1982). *Critical issues in special and remedial education.* Boston: Houghton Mifflin.

Ysseldyke, J. E., Thurlow, M., Graden, J., Wesson, C., Algozzine, B., & Deno, S. (1983). Generalizations from five years of research on assessment and decision making: The University of Minnesota Institute. *Exceptional Education Quarterly, 4,* 75–93.

Zachman, L., Huisingh, R., Barrett, M., Orman, J., & Blagden, C. (1989). *The Word Test: Adolescent.* Moline, IL: LinguiSystems.

Zametkin, A. J., & Rapoport, J. L. (1987). Neurobiology of attention deficit disorder with hyperactivity: Where have we come in 50 years? *Journal of American Academy of Child and Adolescent Psychiatry, 26,* 676–686.

Zinkus, P., & Gottlieb, M. (1980). Patterns of perceptual and academic deficits related to early chronic otitis media. *Pediatrics, 66,* 246–253.

Zwitman, D., & Sonderman, J. (1979). A syntax program designed to present base linguistic structures to language-disordered children. *Journal of Communication Disorders, 2,* 323–335.